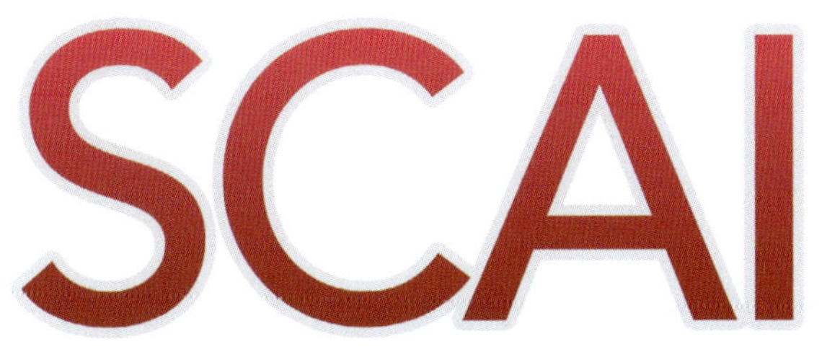

Interventional Cardiology Review

FOURTH EDITION

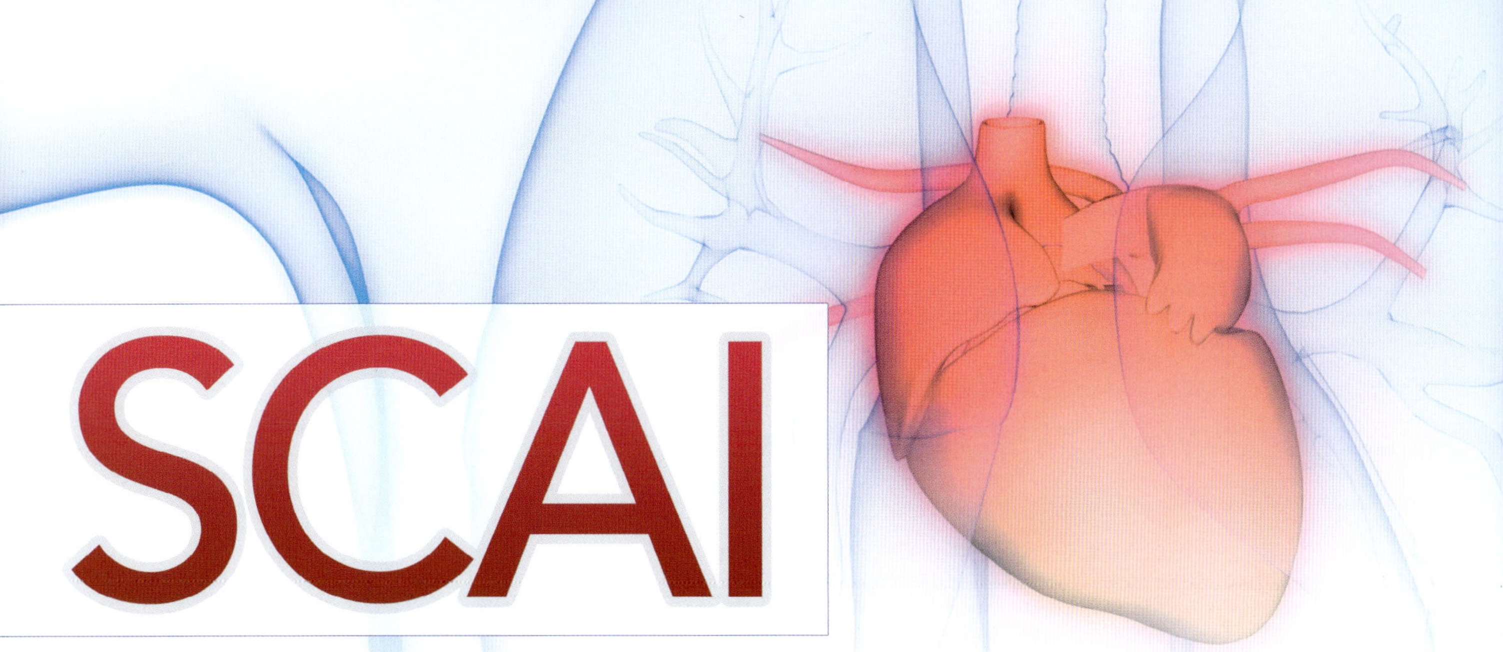

SCAI

Interventional Cardiology Review

FOURTH EDITION

Morton J. Kern, MD, MSCAI, FAHA, FACC
Professor of Medicine
University California, Irvine School of Medicine
Irvine, California
Long Beach Veterans Administration Health Care System
Long Beach, California

Arnold H. Seto, MD MPA FSCAI, FACC
Associate Professor of Medicine
University California, Irvine School of Medicine
Irvine, California
Long Beach Veterans Administration Health Care System
Long Beach, California

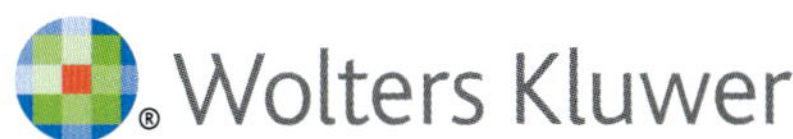

Philadelphia • Baltimore • New York • London
Buenos Aires • Hong Kong • Sydney • Tokyo

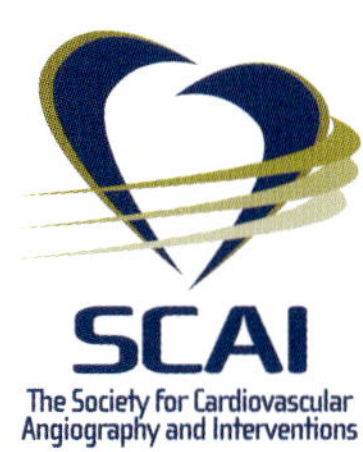

Acquisitions Editor: James Sherman
Senior Development Editor: Ashley Fischer
Editorial Coordinator: Vinoth Ezhumalai
Marketing Manager: Kirsten Watrud
Production Project Manager: Matthew West
Manager, Graphic Arts & Design: Stephen Druding, Leslie Caruso
Manufacturing Coordinator: Margie Orzech-Zeranko
Prepress Vendor: TNQ Tech

Fourth Edition

Copyright © 2025 Wolters Kluwer.

Copyright © 2018 Wolters Kluwer.

Copyright © 2014 by LIPPINCOTT WILLIAMS & WILKINS, a WOLTERS KLUWER business Two Commerce Square 2001 Market Street, Philadelphia, PA 19103 USA LWW.com

1st Edition © 2007 by LIPPINCOTT WILLIAMS & WILKINS, a WOLTERS KLUWER business.

All rights reserved. This book is protected by copyright. No part of this book may be reproduced or transmitted in any form or by any means, including as photocopies or scanned-in or other electronic copies, or utilized by any information storage and retrieval system without written permission from the copyright owner, except for brief quotations embodied in critical articles and reviews. Materials appearing in this book prepared by individuals as part of their official duties as U.S. government employees are not covered by the above-mentioned copyright. To request permission, please contact Wolters Kluwer at Two Commerce Square, 2001 Market Street, Philadelphia, PA 19103, via email at permissions@lww.com, or via our website at shop.lww.com (products and services).

9 8 7 6 5 4 3 2 1

Printed in Mexico

Library of Congress Cataloging-in-Publication Data

ISBN-13: 978-1-975212-61-2

Cataloging in Publication data available on request from publisher.

This work is provided "as is," and the publisher disclaims any and all warranties, express or implied, including any warranties as to accuracy, comprehensiveness, or currency of the content of this work.

This work is no substitute for individual patient assessment based upon healthcare professionals' examination of each patient and consideration of, among other things, age, weight, gender, current or prior medical conditions, medication history, laboratory data and other factors unique to the patient. The publisher does not provide medical advice or guidance and this work is merely a reference tool. Healthcare professionals, and not the publisher, are solely responsible for the use of this work including all medical judgments and for any resulting diagnosis and treatments.

Given continuous, rapid advances in medical science and health information, independent professional verification of medical diagnoses, indications, appropriate pharmaceutical selections and dosages, and treatment options should be made and healthcare professionals should consult a variety of sources. When prescribing medication, healthcare professionals are advised to consult the product information sheet (the manufacturer's package insert) accompanying each drug to verify, among other things, conditions of use, warnings and side effects and identify any changes in dosage schedule or contraindications, particularly if the medication to be administered is new, infrequently used or has a narrow therapeutic range. To the maximum extent permitted under applicable law, no responsibility is assumed by the publisher for any injury and/or damage to persons or property, as a matter of products liability, negligence law or otherwise, or from any reference to or use by any person of this work.

shop.lww.com

QUADM0824

To Margaret and Anna Rose, who provide unwavering support without measure.

—Morton J. Kern

To Lily for her inexhaustible understanding, and to Dr. Kern for opening so many doors for me.

—Arnold H. Seto

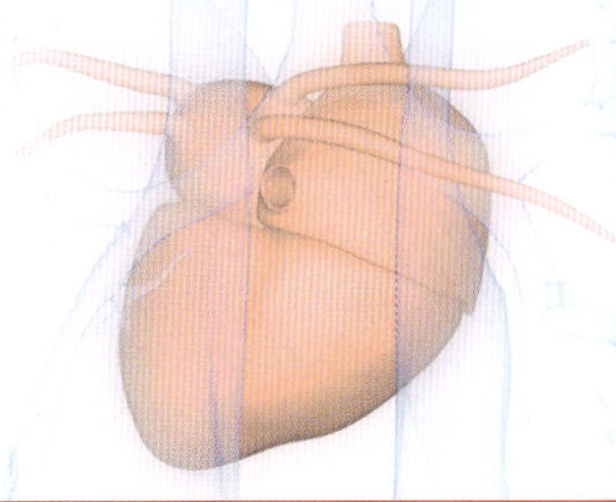

CONTRIBUTORS

Owais S. Abdul-Kafi, MD, MA
Fellow
Division of Cardiology
Department of Medicine
University of Illinois College of Medicine at Chicago
Chicago, Illinois

Mazen Abu-Fadel, MD, FACC, FSCAI
Associate Professor of Medicine
Vice Chief, Section of Cardiovascular Medicine
Director, Interventional Cardiology & Cardiac Cath Lab
Program Director, Interventional Cardiology Fellowship
University of Oklahoma Health Sciences Center
Oklahoma City, Oklahoma

Abdullah Al-Abcha, MD
Fellow
Department of Cardiovascular Medicine
Mayo Clinic
Rochester, Minnesota

Karim M. Al-Azizi, MD, FACC, FSCAI, FESC
Clinical Assistant Professor
Texas A&M University College of Medicine
Medical Director, Cardiac Catheterization Laboratories
Associate Program Director, Cardiology Fellowship
Baylor Scott & White The Heart Hospital - Plano
College Station, Texas

Ziad A. Ali, MD,MPhil
Director, DeMatteis Cardiovascular Institute
Department of Cardiology
St. Francis Hospital and Heart Center
Roslyn, New York

Salman S. Allana, MD, FACC, FSCAI
Fellow
Minneapolis Heart Institute Foundation
Minneapolis, Minnesota

Modar Alom, MD
Fellow
Department of Cardiovascular Disease
Baylor Scott & White The Heart Hospital – Plano
Plano, Texas

Jayant Bagai, MD, MMHC, FSCAI, FACC
Associate Professor of Medicine
Department of Medicine
Vanderbilt University School of Medicine
Vanderbilt University Medical Center
Nashville, Tennessee

Atul D. Bali, MD
Interventional Cardiologist
Department of Cardiology
Donald and Barbara Zucker School of Medicine at Hofstra/Northwell
Lenox Hill Hospital
New York, New York

Suzanne J. Baron, MD, MSc
Director of Interventional Cardiology Research
Department of Cardiology
Massachusetts General Hospital
Boston, Massachusetts

Mir Basir, DO
Physician
Department of Cardiology
Henry Ford Hospital
Detroit, Michigan

Emmanouil S. Brilakis, MD, PhD
Director
Center for Complex Coronary Interventions
Minneapolis Heart Institute Foundation
Minneapolis, Minnesota

Neel M. Butala, MD, MBA
Assistant Professor of Medicine
Department of Medicine
University of Colorado School of Medicine
Medical Director of Structural Heart Disease and Intervention
VA Eastern CO Healthcare System
Aurora, Colorado

Emily Cendrowski, MD
Fellow
Department of Interventional Cardiology
Mayo Clinic
Rochester, Minnesota

Yiannis Chatzizisis, MD, PhD
Professor and Chief
Division of Cardiovascular Medicine
University of Miami Miller School of Medicine
Miami, Florida

Adnan K. Chhatriwalla, MD, FACC, FSCAI
Assistant Professor
Section of Cardiology
Department of Internal Medicine
University of Missouri-Kansas City School of Medicine
Medical Director, Structural Intervention
Saint Luke's Mid America Heart Institute
Kansas City, Missouri

Christine J. Chung, MD
Assistant Professor
Division of Cardiology
University of Washington School of Medicine
Seattle, Washington

Fareed Moses S. Collado, MD, FACC, FSCAI
Assistant Professor of Medicine
Department of Cardiology (Interventional Cardiology and Structural Heart Disease)
Rush University Medical Center
Chicago, Illinois

Gregory J. Condos, MD
Interventional Cardiologist
Division of Cardiology
Department of Medicine
University of Washington School of Medicine
Seattle, Washington

Abdulla Damluji, MD, PhD
Director
Inova Center of Outcomes Research
Inova Heart and Vascular Institute
Inova Health
Fairfax, Virginia

Kaushik Darbha, MBBS, MD
Resident
Department of Internal Medicine
Charles R. Drew University of Medicine and Science
Los Angles, California

Rhian E. Davies, DO, MS
Director of Complex Coronary (Interventional Cardiology)
Department of Cardiology
WellSpan Health
York, Pennsylvania

Teodora Donisan, MD
Fellow
Department of Cardiovascular Disease
Mayo Clinic
Rochester, Minnesota

Douglas E. Drachman, MD, FACC, MSCAI
Assistant Professor
Department of Medicine
Harvard Medical School
Director of Education, Heart Center
Massachusetts General Hospital
Boston, Massachusetts

Marvin Eng, MD
Director, Structural Heart Disease Program
Department of Medicine
Banner University Medical Center
Phoenix, Arizona

Georges Ephrem, MD, MSc
Assistant Professor
Department of Medicine
University of Tennessee Health Science Center
Memphis, Tennessee

Dimitry Feldman, MD
Professor of Medicine
Department of Cardiology
Weill Cornell Graduate School of Medical Sciences
New York, New York

Francesco Franchi, MD
Associate Professor of Medicine
Division of Cardiology
University of Florida College of Medicine-Jacksonville
Medical Director, UF Health North Cardiovascular Center
Jacksonville, Florida

Keyvan Karimi Galougahim, MD, PhD
Interventional Cardiologist
DeMatties Center for Cardiac Research
New York, New York

Sareena George, MD
Assistant Professor
Department of Cardiology and Vascular Medicine
Lahey Hospital & Medical Center
Burlington, Massachusetts

Salvatore Giordano, MD
Fellow
Division of Cardiology
University of Florida College of Medicine
Jacksonville, Florida

Andrew Goldsweig, MD, MS
Director, Cardiac Catheterization Laboratory
Director Cardiovascular Clinical Research
Department of Cardiovascular Medicine
Baystate Medical Center
Springfield, Massachusetts

Mayra Elizabeth Guerrero, MD
Professor of Medicine
Department of Cardiovascular Medicine
Mayo Clinic
Rochester, Minnesota

Ada Ip, MD
Assistant Professor of Medicine
Division of Cardiology
University of California, San Francisco School of Medicine
San Francisco, California

Farouc A. Jaffer, MD, PhD
Cardiology Division
Department of Medicine
Associate Professor
Harvard Medical School
Massachusetts General Hospital
Boston, Massachusetts

Judit Karacsonyi, MD, PhD
Senior research fellow
Center for Coronary Artery Disease, Minneapolis Heart Institute Foundation
Minneapolis, Minnesota

Prashant Kaul, MD, FACC, FSCAI
Director, Cardiac Catheterization Laboratory
Piedmont Heart Institute
Atlanta, Georgia

Clifford J. Kavinsky, MD, PhD, FACC, MSCAI
Associate Professor of Medicine
Harvard Medical School
Beth Israel Deaconess Medical Center
Boston, Massachusetts

Ahmed E. Kazem, DO
Fellow
Department of Cardiovascular Medicine
Baylor Scott & White The Heart Hospital – Plano
Plano, Texas

Kathleen E. Kearney, MD
Assistant Professor, Interventional Cardiology
Division of Cardiology
Department of Medicine
University of Washington School of Medicine
Seattle, Washington

Morton J. Kern, MD, MSCAI, FAHA, FACC
Professor of Medicine
University California, Irvine School of Medicine
Irvine, California
Long Beach Veterans Administration Health Care System
Long Beach, California

Ajay J. Kirtane, MD, SM, FACC, FSCAI
Chief Academic Officer
Center for Interventional Vascular Therapy
Director, Interventional Cardiology
Fellowship Program
Assistant Professor of Clinical Medicine
Division of Cardiology
Department of Medicine
Columbia University Vagelos College of Physicians and Surgeons
Columbia University Medical Center
New York-Presbyterian Hospital
New York, New York

Andrew J.P. Klein, MD, FACC, FSVM, FSCAI
Interventional Cardiologist
Piedmont Heart Institute
Atlanta, Georgia

Dhaval Kolte, MD, PhD, MPH
Assistant Professor
Department of Medicine
Harvard Medical School
Cardiologist
Massachusetts General Hospital
Boston, Massachusetts

Katherine J. Kunkel, MD, MSEd, FSCAI
Interventional Cardiologist
Piedmont Heart Institute
Atlanta, Georgia

Rony Lahoud, MD, MPH, FSCAI, FACC
The Robert Larner, M.D. College of Medicine at The University of Vermont
Burlington, Vermont
Director, Structural Heat Disease Fellowship

Alexandra J. Lansky, MD
Associate Professor, Cardiovascular Medicine
Director, Interventional Cardiovascular Research
Co-Director, Valve Program
Yale School of Medicine
New Haven, Connecticut

Faisal Latif, MD, FACC, FSCAI
Clinical Associate Professor of Medicine
University Of Oklahoma College of Medicine
Oklahoma City, Oklahoma

Jun Li, MD, FSCAI, FACC
Co-Director, Vascular Center
Co-Director, Pulmonary Embolism Response Team
University Hospitals Harrington Heart & Vascular Institute
Cleveland, Ohio

David W. Louis, MD
Fellow
Cardiovascular Institute
Lifespan/Brown University
Providence, Rhode Island

Angela M. Lowenstern, MD, MHS
Assistant Professor of Medicine
Department of Medicine
Vanderbilt University School of Medicine
Vanderbilt University Medical Center
Nashville, Tennessee

Max W. Maffey, MBBS, FRACP
Fellow
Division of Cardiology
Department of Medicine
London Health Sciences Centre
Schulich School of Medicine & Dentistry, Western University
London, Ontario, Canada

Perwaiz M. Meraj, MD, FACC, FSCAI
Director, Cardiac Catheterization Laboratory
Director, CHIP/CTO Program
Sandra Atlas Bass Heart Hospital
Manhasset, New York

Jefferson T. Miley, MD
Assistant Professor of Neurology
Department of Neurology
Dell Medical School – The University of Texas at Austin
Austin, Texas

Ari J. Mintz, DO
Assistant Professor of Medicine
Department of Medicine
Columbia University Vagelos College of Physicians and Surgeon
Columbia University Medical Center
New York, New York

Peter P. Monteleone, MD, FACC, FSCAI
Assistant Professor
Department of Internal Medicine
Dell Medical School - The University of Texas at Austin
Director, Ascension Seton Cardiovascular Research
Director, Ascension Seton Cardiac Catheterization Laboratory
Austin, Texas

Mohamad B. Moumneh, MD
Fellow
Inova Center of Outcomes Research Inova Heart and Vascular Institute
Fairfax, Virginia

Srihari S. Naidu, MD, FACC, FAHA, FSCAI
Professor of Medicine
New York Medical College
President-Elect, SCAI / Trustee Emeritus, Brown University
System Director, Cardiac Catheterization Labs & Director, Hypertrophic Cardiomyopathy Center
Department of Cardiology
Westchester Medical Center
WMCHealth Network
Providence, Rhode Island

Michael G. Nanna, MD, MHS
Assistant Professor
Department of Internal Medicine
Yale School of Medicine
New Haven, Connecticut

Vivian G. Ng, MD
Assistant Professor of Medicine
Division of Cardiology
Department of Medicine
Columbia University Vagelos College of Physicians and Surgeons
Columbia University Medical Center
New York, New York

Eric A. Osborn, MD, PhD, FSCAI, FACC
Instructor
Harvard Medical School
Beth Israel Deaconess Medical Center
Boston, Massachusetts

Sahil A. Parikh, MD
Associate Professor of Medicine
Division of Cardiology
Department of Medicine
Columbia University Vagelos College of Physicians and Surgeons
Columbia University Irving Medical Center
New York, New York

Sridevi R. Pitta, MD, MBA
Interventional Cardiologist
Associate Clinical Professor of Medicine
Cardiology
Texas Health Physicians Group
Denton, Texas

Anshul Pranva, MBBS
Research Assistant
Division of Cardiology
Department of Medicine
University of Illinois College of Medicine at Chicago
Chicago, Illinois

Megha Prasad, MD, MS
Assistant Professor of Medicine
Director, Cardiorenal Medicine and Interventions
Division of Cardiology
Department of Medicine
Columbia University Vagelos College of Physicians and Surgeons
Columbia University Medical Center
New York, New York

Sonal Pruthi, MD
Assistant Professor
Division of Cardiology
Department of Medicine
Columbia University Vagelos College of Physicians and Surgeons
Columbia University Medical Center
New York, New York

Hussein Rahim, MD
Structural Interventional Cardiologist
Department of Cardiology
Valley Health System
Ridgewood, New Jersey

Leah M. Raj, MD
Assistant Professor
Department of Internal Medicine
Vanderbilt University School of Medicine
Vanderbilt University Medical Center
Nashville, Tennessee

Jeremy D. Rier, DO
Fellow
Penn State Hershey Medical Center
Hershey, Pennsylvania
Durham, North Carolina

Yader Sandoval, MD, FACC, FSCAI, FESC
Interventional Cardiologist
Center for Coronary Artery Disease
Minneapolis Heart Institute Foundation
Minneapolis, Minnesota

John T. Saxon, MD, FSCAI
Associate Professor
Division of Cardiovascular Medicine
Director, Advanced Cardiac Valve Center
University of Virginia School of Medicine
University of Virginia Health
Charlottesville, Virginia

Sanjum S. Sethi, MD, MPH
Assistant Professor of Medicine
Division of Cardiology
Department of Medicine
Columbia University Vagelos College of Physicians and Surgeons
Columbia University Medical Center
New York- Presbyterian
New York, New York

Arnold H. Seto, MD, MPA, FSCAI, FACC
Associate Professor of Medicine
University California, Irvine School of Medicine
Irvine, California
Long Beach Veterans Administration Health Care System
Long Beach, California

Marco Shaker, MD, MS
Fellow
Division of Cardiology
Department of Medicine
University of Illinois College of Medicine at Chicago
Chicago, Illinois

Prateek Sharma, MD
Assistant Professor of Medicine, Interventional Cardiology
Section of Cardiology
Department of Medicine
University of Chicago Pritzker School of Medicine
Chicago, Illinois

Doosup Shin, MD
Interventional Cardiologist
St Francis Hospital and Heart Center
Roslyn, New York

Daniel Shpilsky, MD
Cardiologist
Cardiology Maine Medical Center
Portland, Maine

Adhir Shroff, MD, MPH
Professor of Medicine
Chief, Clinical Cardiology Services
Director, Cardiovascular Catheterization Laboratories
Director, Interventional Cardiology Fellowship Program
Division of Cardiology
Department of Medicine
University of Illinois College of Medicine at Chicago
Chicago, Illinois

Trevor Simard, MD, PhD
Interventional Cardiologist
Department of Cardiovascular Medicine
Mayo Clinic
Rochester, Minnesota

Nathaniel Smilowitz, MD, MS, FACC, FSCAI
Assistant Professor of Medicine
The Leon H. Charney Division of Cardiology
NYU Grossman School of Medicine
NYU Langone Health
New York, New York

Daniel Snyder, MD
Physician
Division of Cardiology
Department of Medicine
Columbia University Irving Medical Center
New York, New York

Sumit Sohal, MD, MS
Physician
Division of Cardiology
Department of Internal Medicine
Newark Beth Israel Medical Center
Newark, New Jersey

Nadia R. Sutton, MD, MPH
Assistant Professor
Department of Internal Medicine
Department of Biomedical Engineering
Vanderbilt University School of Medicine
Vanderbilt University Medical Center
Nashville, Tennessee

Jacqueline Tamis-Holland, MD
Interventional Cardiologist
Mount Sinai Morningside
New York, New York

Raj Tayal, MD, MPH, FACC, FSCAI
Clinical Assistant Professor of Medicine
Icahn School of Medicine at Mount Sinai
Director, Cardiac Catheterization Lab
Director, Structural Heart Disease
Valley Health System
New York, New York

Carlos E. Uribe, MD, FSCAI
Interventional Cardiologist
Division of Cardiology
Medellin Clinic Universidad UPB
Medellin, Colombia

Raghava S. Velagaleti, MD, MPH
Interventional Cardiologist
Department of Cardiology
Boston VA Healthcare System
West Roxbury, Massachusetts

Mladen I. Vidovich, MD, FACC, FSCAI
Professor of Medicine
Division of Cardiology
Department of Medicine
University of Illinois College of Medicine at Chicago
Chicago, Illinois

Stephen W. Waldo, MD
Professor of Medicine
University of Colorado School of Medicine
Director, Interventional Cardiology
Rocky Mountain Regional VA Medical Center
Aurora, Colorado
Clinical Director, CART Program
VHA Office of Quality and Patient Safety
Washington DC

Dee Dee Wang MD, FACC, FASE, FSCCT, FSCAI
Director, Structural Heart Imaging
Henry Ford Health System
Detroit, Michigan

Luiz F. Ybarra, MD, PhD, MBA, FSCAI
Assistant Professor
Division of Cardiology
Department of Medicine
London Health Sciences Centre
Schulich School of Medicine & Dentistry, Western University
London, Ontario, Canada

David A. Zidar, MD, PhD
Associate Professor
Departments of Pathology and Medicine
Case Western Reserve School of Medicine
Cleveland, Ohio

Robert S. Zilinyi, MD
Fellow
Division of Cardiology
Department of Medicine
Columbia University Irving Medical Center
New York, New York

Olivia Zurawska
Research Assistant
Division of Cardiology
Department of Medicine
University of Illinois College of Medicine at Chicago
Chicago, Illinois

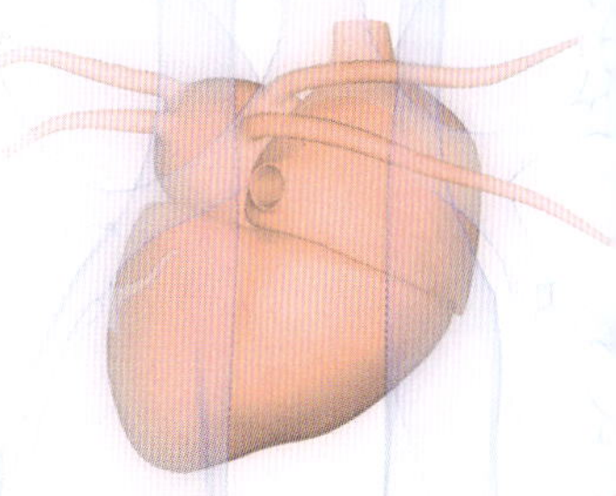

PREFACE

Interventional cardiology continues to demonstrate that it is among the most dynamic and rapidly changing specialties in the field of medicine. Since the inception of the ABIM Interventional Cardiology Specialty in 1999, new procedures and new data are generated yearly. Because certifying examinations test updated cognitive knowledge, a concise yet comprehensive review of the pertinent material is important. As continuing education in interventional cardiology is one of the major missions of the SCAI, we believe this SCAI Interventional Cardiology Board review book fulfills that mission in assisting fellows-in-training, students, residents, and those physicians wishing to review and renew their knowledge base and pass the test.

Coronary interventions still occupy a major part of testable material, but percutaneous structural heart disease interventions as well as some peripheral vascular interventions are now commonplace and will certainly be part of this testable knowledge base. As part of that knowledge base, a few of the most well-known studies are used to demonstrate an understanding of the underpinnings for use of modern pharmacologic therapies and pathophysiologic mechanisms directing selection of interventional modalities. Current practice guidelines are highly likely to be included by the examiners.

In this new fourth edition, the sections on structural heart interventions focusing on transcatheter aortic valve replacement, percutaneous mitral valve repair (MitraClip), closure of atrial septal defects, and left atrial appendage occluder indications have been expanded. While most of the sections on basic science, the fundamentals of atherosclerosis, including endothelial function and restenosis, the pharmacology of interventional practice has been updated. More attention has been paid to the principles of imaging, anatomy, and coronary physiology for application in PCI. Specific commonly encountered coronary interventional patient subsets, critical aspects of patient management, peripheral vascular disease, and finally, guidelines are reviewed.

As with any review textbook, it is impossible to include all aspects of every topic of a complex medical field. Each expert has revised the earlier versions of the chapters and provided several sample questions, which we believe the reader will find useful in their study for the examination. Study questions have been included in the online supplement.

I want to acknowledge the continued and highly supportive role that the Society of Cardiac Angiography and Intervention plays in the education of interventional cardiologists. The mission of SCAI is to be the leading society for interventional cardiologists in education, representation, and advocacy. It is our hope that the *SCAI Interventional Cardiology Review* will benefit all those interested in interventional cardiology, whether or not they are preparing for their Board Exam. We as the SCAI also believe that providing interventional cardiologists with high-quality education will lead to better patient care, our ultimate career goal.

On a personal note, I thank my co-editor, Dr. Arnold Seto and my colleagues, who contributed their knowledge and precious time. Many of the contributors are members of the SCAI Early Career Interventional Committee or Early Leadership Mentor Award recipients. Their contributions further reflect their competence and commitment.

The SCAI plays a unique role in the life of an interventional cardiologist. Now more than 4000 members strong, the SCAI fills a vital need in our professional community and the cardiologist's professional life. The SCAI is a stable home for interventional cardiologists, and a strong resource for communication, education, and professional support to the filed. I remain indebted to my friends and staff of the SCAI.

Morton J. Kern, MD, MSCAI, FAHA, FACC
Professor of Medicine
University California, Irvine School of Medicine
Irvine, California
Long Beach Veterans Administration Health Care System
Long Beach, California

How we share medical knowledge continues to evolve in the internet age, and now the age of artificial intelligence. The majority of journals themselves have become fully electronic and open-access, leading to a flood of information often of variable quality. You are more likely to consult the latest journal article from a smartphone than to pick up a book, and by the time any book is published, it may already seem out-of-date. Google and Chat-GPT can come up with some reasonable initial answers to questions you might have.

A review book may seem an antiquated way to learn, and yet, nowhere else can you find the expert summary, curation, and evaluation of a vast amount of accumulated knowledge. This is where you can learn what questions to ask and what expert reviewers really think, something that AI can't provide (yet).

I thank all of the contributors to this endeavor for their hard (and very human) work, and hope you make the most of the collective knowledge, judgment, and experience contained in this book.

Arnold H. Seto, MD, MPA, FSCAI, FACC
Associate Professor of Medicine
University California, Irvine School of Medicine
Irvine, California
Long Beach Veterans Administration Health Care System
Long Beach, California

ACKNOWLEDGMENT

We thank the SCAI leadership and membership for their support and the opportunity to further their educational mission through this book.

—Morton J. Kern and Arnold H. Seto

CONTENTS

SECTION VI. Vascular Access and Hemostasis

SECTION VII. Women, Prevention, and Guidelines

SECTION VIII. Peripheral Vascular Disease and Interventions

SECTION IX. Structural Heart Disease and Interventions

Arterial Disease—Atherosclerosis

Michael G. Nanna, Leah M. Raj, Angela M. Lowenstern, and Nadia R. Sutton

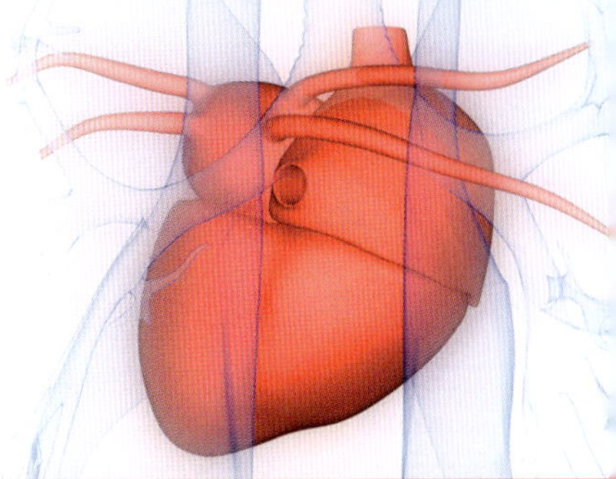

INTRODUCTION

Atherosclerosis refers to the buildup of plaque inside blood vessels and is closely related and often present alongside arteriosclerosis, which refers to hardening or stiffening of the vessel wall. Much has been learned about the pathophysiology of atherosclerosis in recent decades, and cardinal features of atherosclerosis include accumulation of lipids, infiltration with inflammatory cells, and a fibrous cap of variable thickness and stability. Knowledge of the underlying pathophysiology of atherosclerosis is necessary to understand the natural history of untreated atherosclerosis, as well as the potential utility of secondary prevention strategies and percutaneous coronary intervention. This chapter will review the pathophysiology of atherosclerosis and characteristics of stable versus unstable atherosclerotic plaques.

Atherosclerosis

Atherosclerosis is a pathologic process that is stimulated by a multitude of risk factors (**Table 1.1**) and ultimately translates into the leading cause of death worldwide, ischemic heart disease.[1,2] Risk factors can be broadly categorized as metabolic, environmental, genetic, or infectious, and from a prevention standpoint are often considered as modifiable or nonmodifiable. Intrinsic to the pathophysiology of atherosclerosis, and underlying many of these risk factors is the unifying theme of inflammation. The central role of inflammation in the pathogenesis of atherosclerosis is evidenced by numerous epidemiologic studies that demonstrate a correlation between circulating markers of inflammation (eg, fibrinogen, C-reactive protein [CRP], serum amyloid protein, myeloperoxidase) and subsequent risk of coronary events.[3,4] One of the strongest risk factors for the development of atherosclerosis is chronological aging. A hallmark of biological aging is inflammation, termed *inflammaging*.[5]

Atherosclerosis: Pathogenesis

There are several key biological events involved in atherogenesis: extracellular lipid accumulation, leukocyte recruitment, foam cell formation, neointimal growth (as a result of smooth muscle cell (SMC) migration and proliferation and extracellular matrix deposition), as well as vessel remodeling (**Fig. 1.1**).[6]

Extracellular and Intracellular Lipid Accumulation

The key event in the creation of the incipient atherosclerotic lesion is the accumulation of lipoproteins within the intima. These lipoproteins may be modified subsequently by processes such as oxidation and glycation, as may occur in the process of aging and in the setting of hyperglycemia. Lipoprotein modifications elicit a cascade of molecular and cellular events, including stimulation of cytokine production from endothelial and SMCs. These early events lead to recruitment of leukocytes and eventually to SMC proliferation and migration, all of which act to develop the atherosclerotic plaque.

Hyperlipidemia incites inflammation, as is made evident by the presence of foam cells, a hallmark of the fatty streak, which is the initial stage of atherosclerosis. Macrophages bind and internalize modified lipoprotein particles via a number of scavenger receptors, including scavenger receptor-A family members, CD36, and macrosialin. Macrophages that have ingested lipids develop a foamy appearance and are termed *foam cells*, which are able to further modify lipoproteins. Oxidized lipoproteins can lead to foam cell death, resulting in necrotic debris and free cholesterol clefts and ester within the lesion.[7] Foam cells undergo programmed cell death through diverse pathways including apoptosis and autophagy.

TABLE 1.1 Factors Associated with the Development of Atherosclerosis and Cardiac Events

Metabolic
Hyperlipidemia Hyperglycemia Hyperhomocysteinemia Obesity
Physical
Hypertension Shear forces (eg, bifurcations)
Environmental
Tobacco use Diet/Lifestyle Pollution
Genetic
Sex Monogenic (single gene) risk (eg, familial defective apolipoprotein B (apoB)) Polygenic risk (eg, familial hypercholesterolemia (FH)).
Age
Illicit Drug Use
Mental Health
Depression and anxiety Allostatic load: cumulative burden of chronic stress and life events
Peripartum Cardiovascular Factors
Gestational hypertension Pre-eclampsia Gestational diabetes
Infectious
Chlamydia pneumoniae *Porphyromonas gingivalis* *Helicobacter pylori* Influenza A virus Hepatitis C virus Cytomegalovirus (CMV) Human immunodeficiency virus (HIV) COVID-19

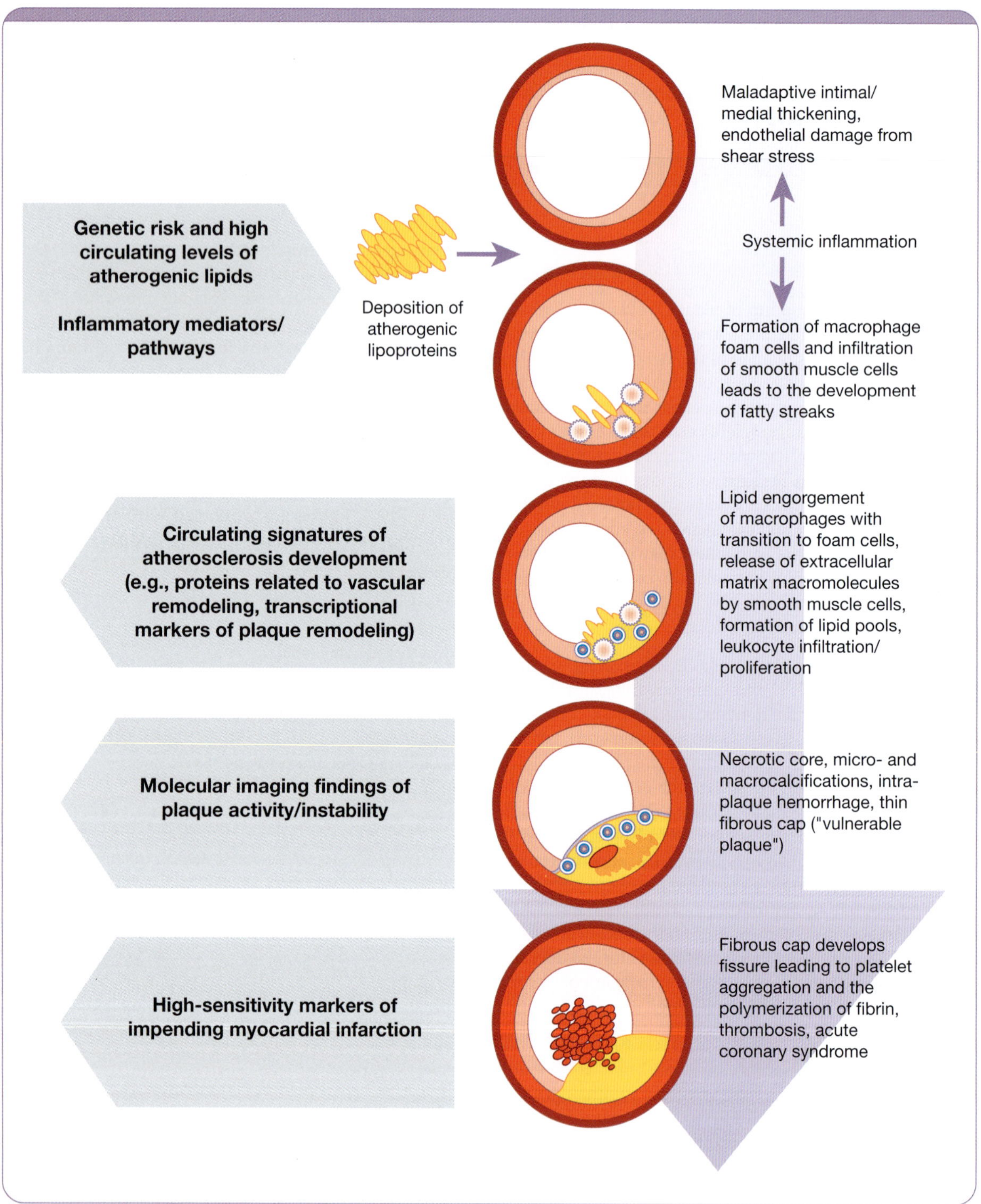

FIGURE 1.1 The molecular biology of atherosclerotic cardiovascular disease (ASCVD). Atherosclerosis begins with a proatherogenic, lipid-rich, inflammatory milieu leading to focal inflammation, maladaptive intimal and medial thickening, and endothelial damage. Blood lipids and inflammatory markers are elevated in the circulation. As atherosclerosis progresses, fatty streaks develop into atherosclerotic plaques through lipid accumulation and vascular smooth muscle cell migration. This process is influenced by macrophage and transition to foam cells and lymphocyte infiltration. Cell death leads to a necrotic core. Micro-calcifications and thin fibrous caps are characteristic of vulnerable plaques prone to rupture. Complications of ASCVD occur as a result of obstruction by plaque and plaque rupture events, leading to thrombosis and acute ischemia. (Adapted from Nayor M, Brown KJ, Vasan RS. The molecular basis of predicting atherosclerotic cardiovascular disease risk. *Circ Res.* 2021;128:287-303. doi:10.1161/CIRCRESAHA.120.315890.)

The necrotic debris within the plaque, along with the presence of prothrombotic tissue factor, results in a scenario whereby if exposure of the plaque contents to blood occurs due to cap erosion or rupture, the plaque contents quickly stimulate thrombus formation and, in some cases, obstruction of blood flow.

Leukocyte Recruitment

Leukocytes, especially macrophages, play an important role in atherosclerosis through the release of cytokines and growth factors that influence atherogenesis, plaque rupture, and thrombosis. The process of leukocyte recruitment, attachment, and migration into the plaque is under the influence of a variety of molecules. In response to injury, including lipoprotein accumulation, endothelial cells express adhesion molecules such as E-selectin, which interacts with ligands on the surface of circulating leukocytes to begin a process of leukocyte rolling along the surface of the vessel.[8] Subsequent tight binding mediated by the integrin class of adhesion molecules stops the leukocyte, prior to the process of diapedesis. Human studies have demonstrated that plasma levels of intracellular cell adhesion molecules (ICAM-1) and E-selectin correlate with clinical manifestations of coronary atherosclerosis.[9]

Chemokines are secreted cytokines that induce leukocyte cell migration to the plaque. For example, monocyte chemoattractant protein-1 (MCP-1) participates in the recruitment of monocytes.[10] Interleukin-8 (IL-8) recruits neutrophils to areas of vascular injury.[11]

Leukocytes tend to accumulate at the "shoulder" regions of plaques where the plaque merges with the more normal vessel architecture. This clustering is thought to account for the increased vulnerability of this plaque region to rupture.[12] It has long been observed that atherosclerosis develops preferentially at bifurcations and regions of turbulent or high-shear-stress regions within the coronary arteries. This has been attributed to upregulation of adhesion molecules and increased leukocyte recruitment in those regions.[13] In addition, monocytes may contribute to vascular calcification in response to monocyte colony–stimulating factor and receptor activator of nuclear factor kappa beta (NF-κB) (receptor activator of NF-κB [RANKL]), although vascular calcification occurs in both a reactive and orchestrated fashion by vascular SMCs.[14] Atherosclerotic plaque micro-calcifications are also associated with increased vulnerability to plaque rupture and cardiovascular events.[15]

Innate Versus Adaptive Immunity

There are two major branches of the immune system: the innate or nonspecific arm and the adaptive or specific arm.[16] There are several key distinguishing features between these two arms. The innate arm relies predominantly on phagocytic cells, such as neutrophils and monocyte/macrophages, the cells most classically associated with atherosclerosis. The innate arm is not antigen-dependent and is an immediate response to injury or infection. On the other hand, the adaptive arm is characterized by a specific antigen-dependent response that has the characteristic of conferring memory against the pathogen. Unlike the immediate response of the innate arm, the adaptive arm involves a lag time between exposure to the pathogen and response. The primary effector cells of this adaptive arm are lymphocytes. These two arms work with dendritic cells of the innate immune system, which link innate and adaptive immunity by presenting antigens to cells of the adaptive system.[17]

Innate Immune Response in Atherosclerosis

The monocyte is thought to be the first leukocyte recruited to the incipient atheroma after encountering complex signals that include soluble (circulating) and local factors and becomes a macrophage after migrating into the plaque. Monocytes are stimulated to become macrophages and may differentiate into specific macrophage phenotypes based on environmental signals. Although simplified and, in actuality, gradations of macrophage phenotypes exist, macrophages are sometimes categorized as type 1, induced by interferon (IFN)-γ or lipopolysaccharide (LPS) signaling and displaying a proinflammatory phenotype, and type 2, induced by IL-4 or IL-13, conferring an anti-inflammatory/reparative macrophage phenotype. Type 1 macrophages (M1) produce high amounts of reactive oxygen species and inflammatory cytokines such as tumor necrosis factor (TNF) or IL-1β. Type 2 macrophages show a high expression of scavenger receptors that produce extracellular matrix components and remodeling enzymes and secrete anti-inflammatory cytokines IL-1ra, chemokine ligand 18, and IL-10.[18,19] The phenotypes of plaque-associated macrophages (PAMs) are mixed because infiltrating monocytes/macrophages express markers of both M1- and M2-type macrophages.[20] Macrophages further amplify the inflammatory response through the secretion of cytokines such as TNF-α and IL-1β.[16] Other cells of the innate immune response that have been implicated in atherosclerosis include mast cells, natural killer cells, and neutrophils.[21]

Adaptive Immune Response in Atherosclerosis

In contrast to the monocyte, the $CD4^+$ T cell is the primary cell of the adaptive arm of the immune response present at atherosclerotic sites. It is believed that these T cells and their secreted cytokines influence progression and vulnerability of plaques.[21] For example, IFN-γ inhibits the growth of SMCs and promotes apoptosis (programmed cell death) of these cells, leading to plaque vulnerability. In addition, IFN-γ limits production of structural proteins (collagen and elastin) that SMCs secrete and may lead to the increased risk of plaque rupture.[22] $CD4^+$ T cells also express a CD40 ligand on their surface, which is subsequently released as a soluble factor. Among its effects, the soluble CD40 ligand influences a variety of cell types to produce a highly procoagulant tissue factor. There are subsets of $CD4^+$ T cells that have been identified by cellular receptors and the typical cytokines released from these cells. $CD4^+$ T_H1 T cells are the predominant types in atherosclerotic lesions and are believed to promote atherosclerosis.[23] $CD4^+$ T_H2 T cells, on the other hand, are likely antiatherogenic. In addition, regulatory T cells are present, which suppress activation of other T cells and may be either pro- or anti-atherogenic.

Lastly, B cells can also be identified within atherosclerosis. Antibodies to oxidized low-density lipoprotein (LDL) can be identified in human and animal models,[21] and it is thought that this humoral immune response acts as a protectant against atherosclerosis, possibly by intercepting and neutralizing antigens prior to reaching the sites of atherosclerosis. There is other evidence to suggest that infection with agents such as *Chlamydia pneumonia* or viruses can create antibodies with auto-immune features that promote atherogenesis.[24]

Smooth Muscle Migration, Proliferation, and Extracellular Matrix Deposition

SMCs and their products are responsible for providing structure to the mature atherosclerotic plaque, which is initially little more than a collection of lipids and foam cells. Under the influence of growth factors and chemoattractants, such as platelet-derived growth factors and thrombin, SMCs migrate out from the media into the neointima where they begin to proliferate. In addition, SMCs produce extracellular matrix constituents, including collagen, proteoglycans, elastin, fibrinogen, fibronectin, and vitronectin. These proteins often account for a substantial volume of the plaque and are important in determining the structural integrity of the fibrous cap. There is evidence that these cells express bone matrix proteins that have been subsequently corroborated by other investigators.[25-27] This highlights the role of SMC in vascular calcification.[15]

Plaque Angiogenesis and Hypoxia

New vasculature, under the influence of angiogenic growth factors, such as hypoxia inducible factor (HIF)/vascular endothelial growth factor (VEGF),[28] may grow from the vasa vasorum within the adventitia into the plaque. These vessels may be disrupted and cause plaque hemorrhage independent of plaque rupture.

In addition, analogous to tumor growth, these vessels may stimulate plaque growth. There is experimental evidence demonstrating inhibition of plaque growth by angiogenic inhibitors in a murine model of atherosclerosis.[29] Furthermore, neo vessel density is higher in nonstenotic segments and stenotic noncalcified plaques than in normal segments or calcified lesions.[30]

Hypoxemia not only promotes angiogenesis but also contributes to proteolysis through the promotion of matrix metalloproteinases (MMPs), a family of interstitial collagenases that weaken the fibrous cap, and gelatinases capable of catabolizing nonfibrillar collagen, to which endothelial cells adhere.[31-33] Proteolysis leads to dissolution of the plaque extracellular matrix and plaque vulnerability. Hypoxemia promotes the formation of proinflammatory cytokines and leukotrienes and activates the Akt and beta-catenin pathways with subsequent macrophage activation.[32,34] In addition, conditions resulting in lipid accumulation in macrophages are amplified with accumulation of triglyceride containing cytosolic lipid droplets and adipose differentiation protein (ADRP) expression, even in the absence of exogenous lipids. The lipid accumulation is a result of increased triglyceride biosynthesis, reduced [beta]-oxidation of fatty acids, and increased expression of stearoyl-coenzyme A desaturase (SCD-1), an enzyme involved in the synthesis of fatty acids.[34-36]

The Mature Atherosclerotic Plaque

The mature atherosclerotic plaque is composed of a fibrous cap consisting of SMCs and extracellular matrix proteins overlying a necrotic lipid core, which includes free cholesterol esters, foam cells, other leukocytes (such as T cells), and necrotic debris of dead foam cells (**Fig. 1.1**).[6] These plaques are commonly eccentric in nature with a variety of cap thicknesses and distribution of leukocytes. Both these features impact the likelihood of plaque rupture events that lead to acute coronary syndromes.

Vascular Remodeling

While angiography remains the gold standard to diagnose coronary artery disease, there are major limitations that include the inability to visualize the architecture of the vessel wall. The use of intravascular imaging during coronary angiography allows for characterization of plaque for specific flow-obstructing lesions and throughout the vessel. Obstructive lesions due to atherosclerosis are often the first to be recognized; however, atherosclerosis is almost always diffuse, although more difficult to detect without intravascular imaging. The amount of impingement of the plaque on the lumen is determined by the growth of the plaque volume and vascular remodeling.

Vascular remodeling involves restructuring of cellular or noncellular components of the wall and can occur in response to a variety of stimuli (commonly known as risk factors for coronary atherosclerosis).[37] For example, in the setting of hypertension, muscle mass of the vessel wall can increase to normalize wall stress. In atherosclerosis, remodeling often consists of compensatory enlargement of the vessel to preserve luminal area (**Fig. 1.2**).[38] Central to the process of vascular remodeling are the MMPs, a family of zinc-dependent proteases that have been demonstrated to be upregulated in areas of vessel wall remodeling and are thought to also play a role in plaque rupture.[39]

Clinical Sequelae of Atherosclerosis

Coronary artery disease manifests as a spectrum of syndromes from stable angina to ST-segment-elevation myocardial infarction (MI). The syndromes of unstable angina and non–ST-elevation MI (NSTEMI) exist between these two extremes. Unstable angina, NSTEMI, and ST-segment elevation MI are collectively termed as the acute coronary syndromes due to their similar pathophysiology and worse prognosis compared to stable angina. Complications from these events can result from two related but distinct mechanisms. Simple luminal narrowing can lead to an imbalance between supply and demand for blood, typically resulting in stable exertional angina or atheromatous plaque rupture, resulting in a thrombus with varying degrees of occlusion.[40] The propensity for thrombotic complications depends on the degree of stenosis and a variety of vascular biologic factors. The atherosclerotic process fundamentally alters the normal vasomotor functions of the endothelium necessary to autoregulate blood flow in accordance with the demands of hemodynamics, a condition termed *endothelial dysfunction*.

Progressive Lumen Encroachment and Stable Angina

As atherosclerotic lesions grow in size, depending on the amount of compensatory vascular remodeling that occurs, they gradually encroach upon the lumen of the vessel (**Fig. 1.2**).[38] As a response

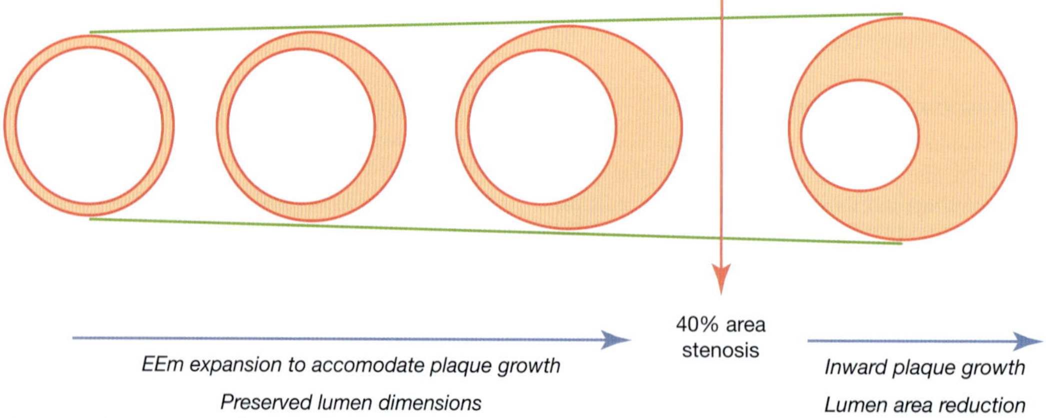

FIGURE 1.2 Schematic of positive vascular remodeling. Initially, the external elastic lamina (external red circle) enlarges to accommodate plaque growth. As the plaque size increases, the luminal area is compromised. EEM, external elastic membrane, also called external elastic lamina. (Adapted from Gonzalo N, Rodriguez V, Broyd CJ, Jimenez-Quevedo P, Escaned J. Remodeling of epicardial coronary vessels. In: Escaned J, Davies J, eds. *Physiological Assessment of Coronary Stenoses and the Microcirculation*. London: Springer; 2017:55-63.)

to reduction in flow, there is vasodilation of the distal microcirculation to increase flow. This reduces the ability of the coronary circulation to increase blood flow in response to demand, which typically leads to exertional angina. At what point luminal encroachment causes symptoms depends on many factors, including the severity of the lesion, the demand of the distal cardiac bed, and the oxygen-carrying capacity of the blood stream. In general, however, lesions begin to produce symptoms when they reach approximately 60% to 70% diameter stenosis. Modern techniques of interrogating intracoronary hemodynamics with flow and pressure wires have allowed interventional cardiologists to objectively identify lesions that result in hemodynamic consequences.[41]

Plaque Rupture, Thrombosis, and the Acute Coronary Syndromes

Insights into acute coronary syndromes come from studies with mandated angiography after randomization to either placebo or thrombolytic therapy. The angiograms demonstrated that the majority of lesions responsible for MI were <50% in diameter stenosis.[42,43] In addition, other angiographic studies have shown that mild and moderate stenoses may progress to produce MI in a matter of weeks to months. In the analysis of four serial angiographic studies, only 15% of acute MIs were found to arise from lesions with degrees of stenosis >60% on an antecedent angiogram (**Fig. 1.3**). This suggests that the vascular biologic state of the lesion is predominantly responsible for its propensity to cause an infarct, not the severity of stenosis. However, it should not be misinterpreted to suggest that lesion severity is correlated with the danger of infarction. Rather, noncritical lesions represent a larger population than critical lesions. As described earlier, compensatory enlargement of the vessel often accompanies atherosclerosis; therefore, even mildly stenotic lesions may represent large plaques by volume. In summary, thrombosis, often on a noncritical stenosis, caused by lesion disruption causes the majority of MIs.

The proximate event leading to thrombosis at a lesion is plaque rupture leading to exposure of blood to highly thrombotic subendothelial components of the plaque. Histologic studies have identified several features that appear to be associated with plaques more vulnerable to rupture. These include a thin fibrous cap, a large lipid core, and an abundance of inflammatory cells largely concentrated at the shoulder regions of the plaque (**Fig. 1.4**).[12]

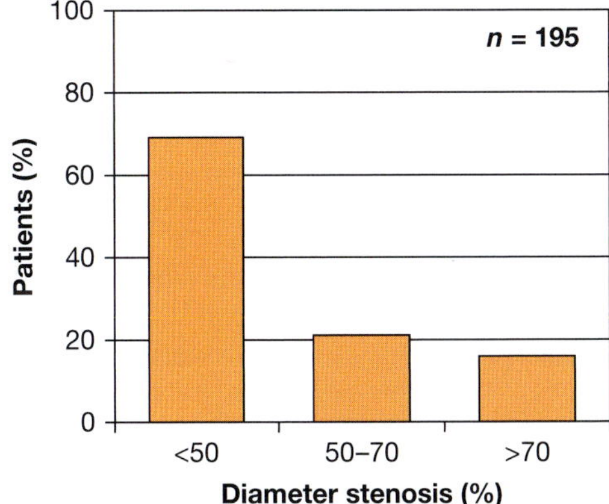

FIGURE 1.3 Compiled data from four thrombolytic trials showing that the majority of underlying lesions responsible for acute myocardial infarction are less than 50% diameter stenosis. (From Smith SC. Risk-reduction therapy: the challenge to change. Paper presented at the 68th scientific session of the American Heart Association, November 13, 1995, Anaheim, California. *Circulation.* 1996;93:2205-2211.)

Inflammation is a key regulator of the structural integrity of the plaque. One of the largest trials to date to examine the natural history of atherosclerosis is the Providing Regional Observations to Study Predictors of Events in the Coronary Tree (PROSPECT) study.[44] In this trial, 697 patients with acute coronary syndrome undergoing percutaneous intervention had all their major epicardial arteries checked with intravascular ultrasound. Patients were followed up for over 2 years. One hundred and six nonculprit lesions were subsequently associated with adverse cardiac events. Correlates that predicted a subsequent event were a plaque burden greater than 70%, the presence of a thin-capped fibroatheroma, and a minimal luminal area less than 4 mm^2.

The structural integrity of the plaque is dependent on a balance between two components: SMC mass and extracellular matrix content. SMC mass is a balance between cell accumulation (via migration from the media and proliferation) in the neointima and cell death. There is evidence to suggest that cytokines released from inflammatory cells control apoptosis, or programmed cell death.[45] Extracellular matrix content is a balance between production from SMCs and degradation by a variety of proteases (**Fig. 1.5**). Production of extracellular matrix content is dependent on the number of cells present and their activity. Activated T cells in the plaque secrete IFN-γ, an inhibitor of SMC collagen synthesis. Inflammatory cells in atherosclerotic plaques also produce enzymes, such as MMP and cathepsins, which are capable of degrading important constituents of the extracellular matrix (ie, collagens, elastin).[12] Therefore, inflammatory cells can contribute to plaque weakening by decreasing SMC mass, decreasing extracellular matrix content, and by increasing extracellular matrix degradation.

There are still several unanswered questions in this area: most importantly—how and why plaques rupture when they do. The variability of plaque rupture involves a number of postulated mechanisms, including circadian variation,[46] stress events,[47] the abrupt release of cortisol and adrenaline, and high-circumferential biomechanical forces acting at the shoulder regions of plaques.[48] Therefore, there is an interesting combination of both biochemical and biophysical characteristics that make plaques prone to rupture.

While frank plaque rupture is the major antecedent cause of thrombotic complications of the acute coronary syndromes, other processes may also be responsible. Local superficial denudation of endothelial cells may expose the internal elastic membrane, representing an important thrombotic substrate. This has implications for therapy; due to the lack of ruptured plaque and the unique nature of the adherent thrombus, plaque erosion pathophysiology is more based in platelet adhesion and aggregation (**Fig. 1.6**).

Irrespective of the inciting factor (plaque rupture or endothelial denudation), flow alterations result from vessel thrombosis. Exposure of blood to the lipid core is a potent stimulus for thrombus formation, largely due to exposure to the prothrombotic tissue factor associated with lipid-laden and necrotic macrophages. Variations in procoagulant–anticoagulant and fibrinolytic–antifibrinolytic factors in the blood stream between individuals likely determines the consequences of any given plaque disruption. In the presence of an intact and robust fibrinolytic milieu, a mural thrombus might undergo rapid lysis, limiting its clinical consequences to unstable angina or NSTEMI. In the presence of prothrombotic factors, such as elevated levels of fibrinogen or plasminogen activator inhibitor-1 (PAI-1), growth of a thrombus to occlusion may occur more frequently. A nonocclusive mural thrombus may be incorporated into the plaque during the process of healing, providing a mechanism for plaque growth.

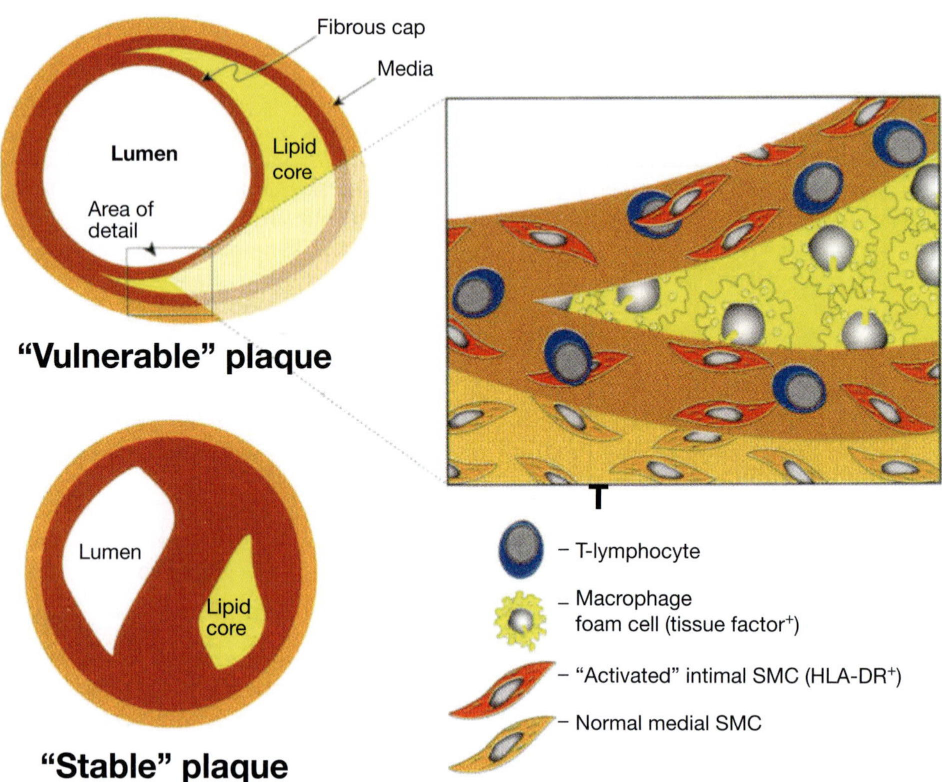

FIGURE 1.4 Characteristics of stable versus vulnerable plaques. Vulnerable plaques have thinner fibrous caps and larger, more inflammatory, cell-rich lipid cores. SMC, smooth muscular cell. (From Libby P. Molecular bases of the acute coronary syndromes. *Circulation*. 1995;91:2844-2850.)

There are numerous trials of antiplatelet therapy that corroborate the thrombotic paradigm of the acute coronary syndromes. Trials of lipid-lowering therapy have corroborated theories of plaque vulnerability, suggesting marked reductions in subsequent coronary events associated with lipid lowering, with essentially no change in lesion severity.[49] As stated earlier, lipids within the plaque provide the critical initiating and sustaining inflammatory stimulus for plaque growth and rupture, and the beneficial actions of "statin" lipid-lowering agents may derive in part from the reduction of inflammation leading to stabilization of the fibrous cap and reduced thrombogenicity of the inner core. There is increasing evidence to support lipid-lowering therapy as a vital therapy in both acute and chronic ischemic heart disease.

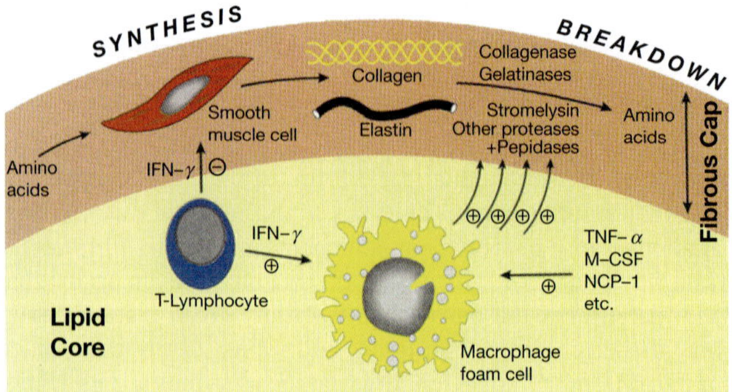

FIGURE 1.5 Thickness of the fibrous cap is a balance between synthesis of extracellular matrix proteins by smooth muscle cells and the breakdown of these products by degradative enzymes. These processes are largely under the influence of inflammatory cells. CSF, colony-stimulating factor IFN-γ, interferon γ; NCF, neutrophil chemotactic factor, TNF-α, tumor necrosis factor α. (From Libby P. Molecular bases of the acute coronary syndromes. *Circulation*. 1995;91:2844-2850.)

Endothelial Dysfunction

More than three decades ago, Ludmer and colleagues reported that a paradoxical reaction occurred when acetylcholine was administered intracoronary to patients with atherosclerosis.[50] Rather than the expected vasodilatory effect normally observed in epicardial coronary arteries, the investigators observed vasoconstriction in patients with atherosclerosis, even in territories without significant luminal narrowing. Acetylcholine had previously been identified as working through an endothelial-dependent mechanism,[51] and hence, the concept of clinical endothelial dysfunction was born.

The endothelium is a monolayer of cells derived from the embryonic mesoderm that form a continuous layer on the intimal surface of the entire cardiovascular system, including the arteries, veins, and chambers of the heart (endocardium); the capillary walls consist solely of endothelial cells. The endothelial cell has a variety of functions that play important roles in the maintenance of vascular integrity, including the regulation of vascular tone, vascular permeability, vessel wall inflammation, and thromboresistance through the expression of anticoagulants such as heparin sulfate and enzymes that destroy them.[52,53] Given these properties, it is important for the endothelium to undergo rapid repair when damaged and for apoptotic cells to be quickly replaced by circulating endothelial progenitor cells (EPCs), which are also central to angiogenesis throughout our lifespan.[54]

Vascular tone is regulated by numerous factors whose counterbalance maintains normal vascular tone and responds to various physiologic stimuli. Nitric oxide (NO), generated from L-arginine by the

Coronary Artery Cross Sections

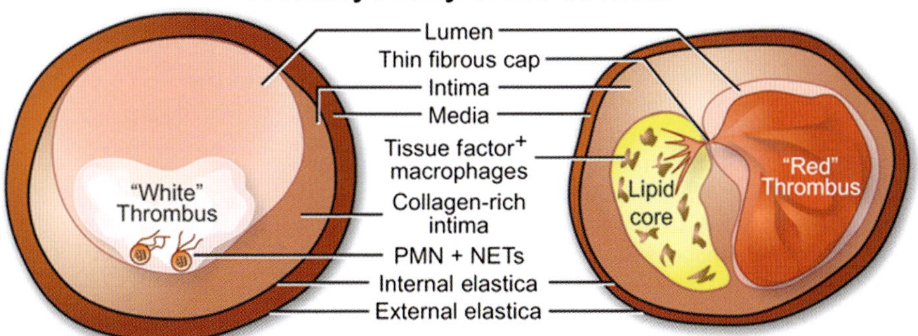

Thrombosis due to Erosion	Thrombosis due to Rupture
Fibrous cap thick & intact	Thin fibrous cap with fissure
"White" platelet-rich thrombus	"Red" fibrin-rich thrombus
Collagen trigger	Tissue factor trigger
Smooth muscle cells prominent	Macrophages prominent
Often sessile, nonocclusive thrombus	Often occlusive thrombus
Usually less remodelled outward	Usually expansively remodelled
Neutrophil extracellular traps (NETs) involved	Less NET involvement?
More frequent in non-STEMI?	More frequently cause STEMI?

FIGURE 1.6 Illustration of differences between plaque erosion and plaque rupture as causes of presentation with acute coronary syndrome. NETs, neutrophil extracellular traps; Non-STEMI, non-ST-segment elevation myocardial infarction; PMN, polymorphonuclear neutrophils; STEMI, ST-segment elevation myocardial infarction. (From Libby P. Superficial erosion and the precision management of acute coronary syndromes: not one-size-fits-all. *Eur Heart J.* 2017;38(11):801-803, by permission of Oxford University Press.)

action of endothelial NO synthase (eNOS) in the presence of cofactors such as tetrahydrobiopterin, diffuses to the vascular SMCs and activates guanylate cyclase, which results in cyclic guanosine monophosphate-dependent vasodilation.[55] The endothelium also mediates the hyperpolarization of vascular smooth muscle cells via a NO-independent pathway, which increases K^+ conductance and subsequently propagates the depolarization of vascular SMCs, maintaining vascular tone through the production of endothelium-derived hyperpolarizing factors (EDHFs).[56] Some vasoconstrictive molecules such as endothelin 1 lead to vasoconstriction and proliferation through the activation of endothelin ETA receptors and are known to be expressed in active plaque.[57,58] Thromboxane A_2, serotonin, and angiotensin II also play similar roles while inducing SMC proliferation. Vascular permeability and cell-to-cell communication are controlled by endothelial proteins such as vascular endothelial cadherin.[59] All these factors interact to maintain vascular tone in a variety of physiologic states.

Atherogenic stimuli activate cell signaling and therefore modulate cellular function in endothelial cells. The interaction between endothelial cells and immune cells is augmented in response to atherogenic stimuli by an upregulated expression of adhesion molecules. Vascular smooth muscle function is also modified through the altered production of vasoactive substances by endothelial cells.[60] A dysfunctional endothelium is an early marker of the development of atherosclerotic changes and can also contribute to cardiovascular events.[61] Vascular reactivity tests represent the most widely used methods of clinical assessment of endothelial function given the limited ability to visualize vessels <500 μm in diameter. The aim of these tests is to activate or block endothelial cell function while measuring consequent changes in vascular tone in selected vascular districts and are thus functional assessments of the microcirculation.[62] These methods include coronary flow reserve (CFR) and coronary blood flow (CBF). It is also important to note that there are also noninvasive methods for evaluating endothelial dysfunction, although a thorough discussion of these is beyond the scope of this chapter.

CFR is defined as the ratio of near-maximal to basal myocardial flow in response to maximal hyperemia. It is an amalgamated measure of CBF through both epicardial coronary arteries and the coronary microcirculation. A decrease in CFR could be attributed to both, and thus in the absence of epicardial vessel obstruction, it reflects solely on the microcirculation.[63]

Acetylcholine produces primarily a vasodilator response in patients with normal coronaries. In contrast, in patients with coronary artery disease or endothelial dysfunction, acetylcholine causes dose-dependent vasoconstriction.[64] Adenosine acts predominantly on vessels measuring less than 150 μm in diameter via stimulation of adenosine A_2 receptors on the SMCs and thus reflects changes in resistance as reflected in changes in flow.[65] These are two distinct mechanisms, of which the former is endothelial dependent, and the latter is endothelial independent. An increase >50% in CBF above the baseline in response to a acetylcholine and a CFR ratio of >2.5 (2.0-2.4, gray zone) in response to adenosine is considered normal.[65] An abnormal response to both acetylcholine and adenosine indicates dysfunction in epicardial and resistance vessels involving endothelium-dependent and endothelium-independent mechanisms. An abnormal response to adenosine with normal response to acetylcholine indicates endothelial-independent dysfunction, while an abnormal response to acetylcholine suggests an endothelial-dependent dysfunction.[65]

Endothelial dysfunction has been associated with stable angina, as well as unstable angina and MI, and is frequently categorized under the clinical umbrella of ischemia with nonobstructive coronary arteries (INOCAs). Marks et al. followed patients with chest pain/ischemic cardiac disease and normal coronary angiograms over a mean period of 8.5 years and noted a nearly threefold higher mortality for those patients with an abnormal CFR (20% vs 7%; P = .016).[66]

Britten et al., who followed up patients with angiographically normal or minimally diseased coronary arteries over an average of 6.5 years, noted a more than threefold higher cardiovascular event rate in patients in the lowest tertile than those in the highest tertile of CFR (18% vs 5%, P = .019), with 36% of all events related to acute coronary syndrome.[67] In one of the largest studies investigating the risk of endothelial dysfunction to date, Rubinshtein et al.[68] evaluated the relationship between the Framingham risk score (FRS) and the presence of coronary risk factors to coronary microcirculatory vasodilator function in patients with early coronary atherosclerosis. The authors included 1063 patients (age: 50 ± 12 years, 676 (64%) females) without significant narrowing (<30%) on coronary angiography who underwent invasive assessment of coronary endothelial function. CBF in response to the endothelium-dependent vasodilator acetylcholine was evaluated, as well as the microvascular (endothelium-independent) CFR in response to intracoronary adenosine. CBF and CFR were analyzed in relation to the FRS and the presence of traditional and novel risk factors. The authors concluded that in patients without obstructive coronary disease, a higher FRS was an independent predictor of reduced CFR, as was female sex and family history of coronary artery disease.[68]

The principles of the management of INOCA include establishing a diagnosis, evaluating the pathophysiological mechanisms (coronary macrovascular vs microvascular dysfunction), targeted treatment, lifestyle changes, and avoiding exacerbating factors.[69,70] Current management focuses on lifestyle modification and cardiac rehabilitation,[71] lipid-lowering agents that could improve dysfunction through their anti-inflammatory and anti-oxidant properties, and the ability to restore vascular NO availability,[61] angiotensin-converting enzyme inhibitors and angiotensin rennin blockers,[72] β-blockers,[73] L-arginine,[74] ranolazine,[75] xanthine derivatives,[76] and enhanced external counterpulsation.[77]

The COronary MICrovasvcular Angina (CorMicA) trial evaluated stratified medical therapy with an interventional diagnostic procedure that included an assessment of CFR followed by vasoreactivity testing with acetylcholine versus standard care with sham procedure in 151 patients with INOCA.[78] The authors found that the stratified medical therapy approach following an interventional diagnostic procedure was feasible and improved angina severity at 6 months in patients with INOCA.[78] Marked improvements in angina and overall quality of life persisted at 1 year.[79] Tailored therapy in CorMicA included calcium channel blockers and long-acting nitrates for those with vasospasm documented; beta-blockers, ACEi, and statins for those with coronary microvascular dysfunction; and discontinuation of antianginal therapy for those with normal testing. Two large ongoing follow-up randomized trials in INOCA populations, iCorMicA and the Women's Ischemia Trial to Reduce Events in Non-obstructive Coronary Artery Disease (WARRIOR),[80] are ongoing and should provide further insights into the optimal management of these patients. The agents used routinely as coronary vasodilators in the cath lab can be classified as endothelial dependent or independent and are included in **Table 1.2**.

TABLE 1.2 Endothelium-Independent and Endothelium-Dependent Vasodilators

Endothelium Independent
- Direct nitric oxide (NO) donors
  - NO gas
  - Sodium (Na) nitroprusside
  - Na Trioxodinitrate
- NO donors requiring metabolism
  - Nitroglycerin
  - Isosorbide dinitrate
  - Amyl nitrate
  - Nicorandil
- Smooth muscle cell relaxers
  - Calcium channel blockers

Endothelium Dependent
- Acetylcholine
- 5-Hydroxytryptamine
- Bradykinin

MEDICAL THERAPY OF ATHEROSCLEROSIS

Medical therapy of atherosclerosis centers around the control of risk factors, symptom control with antianginal agents, and a special emphasis on lipid lowering. First-line antianginal therapies include beta-blockers and calcium-channel blockers in conjunction with short-acting nitrates for breakthrough symptoms, with long-acting nitrates and ranolazine also being staples of therapy. Lipid-lowering with 3-hydroxy-3-methyl-glutaryl-CoA reductase inhibitors (statins) is the foundation of atherosclerotic treatment, with multiple randomized trials demonstrating the safety and efficacy of statins in both primary and secondary prevention populations.[81-83]

The improvement of cardiovascular outcomes via lipid lowering with non-statin therapies has been an active area of research in recent years. The IMPROVE-IT (Ezetimibe Added to Statin Therapy after Acute Coronary Syndromes) trial randomized 18,144 patients who had been hospitalized for acute coronary syndrome to a combination of simvastatin 40 mg and ezetimibe 10 mg versus simvastatin 40 mg alone, demonstrating an improvement in the composite primary cardiovascular endpoint.[84] Monoclonal antibodies inhibiting proprotein convertase subtilisin-kexin type 9 (PCSK9) have demonstrated dramatic lipid lowering while also improving cardiovascular outcomes in randomized trials. The FOURIER (Further Cardiovascular Outcomes Research with PCSK9 Inhibition in Subjects with Elevated Risk) trial evaluated the clinical efficacy of evolocumab when added to statin therapy in stable patients with clinically evident atherosclerotic cardiovascular disease, finding a significant reduction in the primary efficacy of cardiovascular composite with the evolocumab treatment.[85] The ODYSSEY OUTCOMES (Alirocumab and Cardiovascular Outcomes after Acute Coronary Syndrome) trial similarly investigated the safety and efficacy of alirocumab in reducing cardiovascular events in patients with an acute coronary syndrome within the prior 12 months, demonstrating a significant reduction in the primary endpoint of major ischemic cardiovascular events with alirocumab treatment.[86]

Many have postulated that the profound impact of statin therapy on reduction of coronary events is not just limited to the direct effects of LDL lowering but also the possible anti-inflammatory and pleiotropic effects of statins that confer benefits beyond lowering the lesion levels of cholesterol. The clearest link between inflammation and statins comes from the JUPITER (Justification for the Use of Statins in Prevention: an Intervention Trial Evaluating Rosuvastatin) trial.[87] This trial tested the hypothesis that in patients with relatively normal levels of cholesterol (LDL cholesterol < 130 mg/dL), patients with higher levels of inflammation as measured by high-sensitivity CRP (>2.0 mg/dL) would benefit from statin therapy.

In patients randomized to rosuvastatin, there was a 44% reduction in the primary endpoint, a composite of cardiovascular death, nonfatal MI, nonfatal stroke, hospitalization for unstable angina, or arterial revascularization. Modification of inflammatory risk in patients with underlying atherosclerosis remains with novel agents and is an active area of ongoing investigation.

CONCLUSIONS

Over the past decades, the molecular and cellular pathophysiology of atherosclerosis and related arteriopathies has been extensively studied. A more complete understanding of these processes has led to increasingly effective therapies for the treatment of atherosclerosis and acute coronary syndromes. Much remains to be determined, however, regarding the molecular mechanisms of atherosclerosis, the identification of high-risk plaques prone to inducing acute coronary syndrome, and novel therapeutic agents.

Key Points

- The molecular and cellular pathophysiology of atherosclerosis and related arteriopathies has revealed that hyperlipidemia is an inflammatory state. The metabolism of lipoproteins in the vessel wall and subsequent interaction with inflammatory cells initiate the process of atherosclerotic plaque formation.
- The identification of plaques prone to rupture focuses on processes of lipid accumulation, fibrous cap degradation, and vascular smooth muscle proliferation.
- The treatment of atherosclerosis and acute coronary syndrome is multifactorial and relies on therapies directed at reducing thrombotic risk and circulation and plaque lipids and inflammation.

For further review and interactivities, please see the chapter-based multiple choice questions and videos accessible in the complimentary eBook bundled with this text. Access instructions are located in the inside front cover.

References

1. Pothineni NVK, Subramany S, Kuriakose K, et al. Infections, atherosclerosis, and coronary heart disease. *Eur Heart J*. 2017;38(43):3195-3201. doi:10.1093/eurheartj/ehx362
2. Lusis AJ, Fogelman AM, Fonarow GC. Genetic basis of atherosclerosis: part I—new genes and pathways. *Circulation*. 2004;110(13):1868-1873. doi:10.1161/01.CIR.0000143041.58692.CC
3. Ridker PM, Rifai N, Rose L, Buring JE, Cook NR. Comparison of C-reactive protein and low-density lipoprotein cholesterol levels in the prediction of first cardiovascular events. *N Engl J Med*. 2002;347(20):1557-1565. doi:10.1056/NEJMoa021993
4. Brennan ML, Penn MS, Van Lente F, et al. Prognostic value of myeloperoxidase in patients with chest pain. *N Engl J Med*. 2003;349(17):1595-1604. doi:10.1056/NEJMoa035003
5. Ferrucci L, Fabbri E. Inflammageing: chronic inflammation in ageing, cardiovascular disease, and frailty. *Nat Rev Cardiol*. 2018;15(9):505-522. doi:10.1038/s41569-018-0064-2
6. Nayor M, Brown KJ, Vasan RS. The molecular basis of predicting atherosclerotic cardiovascular disease risk. *Circ Res*. 2021;128(2):287-303. doi:10.1161/CIRCRESAHA.120.315890
7. Chellan B, Sutton NR, Hofmann Bowman MA. S100/RAGE-Mediated inflammation and modified cholesterol lipoproteins as mediators of osteoblastic differentiation of vascular smooth muscle cells. *Front Cardiovasc Med*. 2018;5:163. doi:10.3389/fcvm.2018.00163
8. Cybulsky MI, Gimbrone MA Jr. Endothelial expression of a mononuclear leukocyte adhesion molecule during atherogenesis. *Science*. 1991;251(4995):788-791. doi:10.1126/science.1990440
9. Ridker PM. Intercellular adhesion molecule (ICAM-1) and the risks of developing atherosclerotic disease. *Eur Heart J*. 1998;19(8):1119-1121. doi: 10.1053/euhj.1998.1101
10. Rollins BJ. Chemokines. *Blood*. 1997;90(3):909-928.
11. Webb LM, Ehrengruber MU, Clark-Lewis I, Baggiolini M, Rot A. Binding to heparan sulfate or heparin enhances neutrophil responses to interleukin 8. *Proc Natl Acad Sci U S A*. 1993;90(15):7158-7162. doi:10.1073/pnas.90.15.7158
12. Libby P. Molecular bases of the acute coronary syndromes. *Circulation*. 1995;91(11):2844-2850. doi: 10.1161/01.cir.91.11.2844
13. Walpola PL, Gotlieb AI, Cybulsky MI, Langille BL. Expression of ICAM-1 and VCAM-1 and monocyte adherence in arteries exposed to altered shear stress. *Arterioscler Thromb Vasc Biol*. 1995;15(1):2-10. doi: 10.1161/01.atv.15.1.2
14. Matsuzaki K, Udagawa N, Takahashi N, et al. Osteoclast differentiation factor (ODF) induces osteoclast-like cell formation in human peripheral blood mononuclear cell cultures. *Biochem Biophys Res Commun*. 1998;246(1):199-204. doi:10.1006/bbrc.1998.8586
15. Sutton NR, Malhotra R, St Hilaire C, et al. Molecular mechanisms of vascular health: insights from vascular aging and calcification. *Arterioscler Thromb Vasc Biol*. 2023;43(1):15-29. doi:10.1161/ATVBAHA.122.317332
16. Hansson GK, Libby P, Schonbeck U, Yan ZQ. Innate and adaptive immunity in the pathogenesis of atherosclerosis. *Circ Res*. 2002;91(4):281-291. doi:10.1161/01.res.0000029784.15893.10
17. Bobryshev YV. Dendritic cells in atherosclerosis: current status of the problem and clinical relevance. *Eur Heart J*. 2005;26(17):1700-1704. doi:10.1093/eurheartj/ehi282
18. Gratchev A, Guillot P, Hakiy N, et al. Alternatively activated macrophages differentially express fibronectin and its splice variants and the extracellular matrix protein betaIG-H3. *Scand J Immunol*. 2001;53(4):386-392. doi:10.1046/j.1365-3083.2001.00885.x
19. Gratchev A, Schledzewski K, Guillot P, Goerdt S. Alternatively activated antigen-presenting cells: molecular repertoire, immune regulation, and healing. *Skin Pharmacol Appl Skin Physiol*. 2001;14(5):272-279. doi:10.1159/000056357
20. Brocheriou I, Maouche S, Durand H, et al. Antagonistic regulation of macrophage phenotype by M-CSF and GM-CSF: implication in atherosclerosis. *Atherosclerosis*. 2011;214(2):316-324. doi:10.1016/j.atherosclerosis.2010.11.023
21. Packard RR, Lichtman AH, Libby P. Innate and adaptive immunity in atherosclerosis. *Semin Immunopathol*. 2009;31(1):5-22. doi:10.1007/s00281-009-0153-8
22. Amento EP, Ehsani N, Palmer H, Libby P. Cytokines and growth factors positively and negatively regulate interstitial collagen gene expression in human vascular smooth muscle cells. *Arterioscler Thromb*. 1991;11(5):1223-1230.
23. Saigusa R, Winkels H, Ley K. T cell subsets and functions in atherosclerosis. *Nat Rev Cardiol*. 2020;17(7):387-401. doi:10.1038/s41569-020-0352-5
24. Perschinka H, Mayr M, Millonig G, et al. Cross-reactive B-cell epitopes of microbial and human heat shock protein 60/65 in atherosclerosis. *Arterioscler Thromb Vasc Biol*. 2003;23(6):1060-1065. doi:10.1161/01.ATV.0000071701.62486.49
25. Giachelli C, Bae N, Lombardi D, Majesky M, Schwartz S. Molecular cloning and characterization of 2B7, a rat mRNA which distinguishes smooth muscle cell phenotypes in vitro and is identical to osteopontin (secreted phosphoprotein I, 2aR). *Biochem Biophys Res Commun*. 1991;177(2):867-873. doi:10.1016/0006-291x(91)91870-i
26. Bostrom K, Watson KE, Horn S, Wortham C, Herman IM, Demer LL. Bone morphogenetic protein expression in human atherosclerotic lesions. *J Clin Invest*. 1993;91(4):1800-1809. doi:10.1172/JCI116391

27. Shanahan CM, Cary NR, Metcalfe JC, Weissberg PL. High expression of genes for calcification-regulating proteins in human atherosclerotic plaques. *J Clin Invest*. 1994;93(6):2393-2402. doi:10.1172/JCI117246
28. Libby P, Folco E. Tension in the plaque: hypoxia modulates metabolism in atheroma. *Circ Res*. 2011;109(10):1100-1102. doi:10.1161/RES.0b013e31823bdb84
29. Moulton KS. Plaque angiogenesis and atherosclerosis. *Curr Atheroscler Rep*. 2001;3:225-233. doi:10.1007/s11883-001-0065-0
30. Gossl M, Versari D, Hildebrandt HA, et al. Segmental heterogeneity of vasa vasorum neovascularization in human coronary atherosclerosis. *JACC Cardiovasc Imaging*. 2010;3(1):32-40. doi:10.1016/j.jcmg.2009.10.009
31. Kolev K, Skopal J, Simon L, Csonka E, Machovich R, Nagy Z. Matrix metalloproteinase-9 expression in post-hypoxic human brain capillary endothelial cells: H_2O_2 as a trigger and NF-kappaB as a signal transducer. *Thromb Haemost*. 2003;90(3):528-537. doi:10.1160/TH03-02-0070
32. Deguchi JO, Yamazaki H, Aikawa E, Aikawa M. Chronic hypoxia activates the Akt and beta-catenin pathways in human macrophages. *Arterioscler Thromb Vasc Biol*. 2009;29(10):1664-1670. doi:10.1161/ATVBAHA.109.194043
33. Burke B, Giannoudis A, Corke KP, et al. Hypoxia-induced gene expression in human macrophages: implications for ischemic tissues and hypoxia-regulated gene therapy. *Am J Pathol*. 2003;163(4):1233-1243. doi:10.1016/S0002-9440(10)63483-9
34. Hulten LM, Levin M. The role of hypoxia in atherosclerosis. *Curr Opin Lipidol*. 2009;20(5):409-414. doi:10.1097/MOL.0b013e3283307be8
35. Parathath S, Mick SL, Feig JE, et al. Hypoxia is present in murine atherosclerotic plaques and has multiple adverse effects on macrophage lipid metabolism. *Circ Res*. 2011;109(10):1141-1152. doi:10.1161/CIRCRESAHA.111.246363
36. Bostrom P, Magnusson B, Svensson PA, et al. Hypoxia converts human macrophages into triglyceride-loaded foam cells. *Arterioscler Thromb Vasc Biol*. 2006;26(8):1871-1876. doi:10.1161/01.ATV.0000229665.78997.0b
37. Gibbons GH, Dzau VJ. The emerging concept of vascular remodeling. *N Engl J Med*. 1994;330(20):1431-1438. doi:10.1056/NEJM199405193302008
38. Gonzalo N, Rodriguez V, Broyd CJ, Jimenez-Quevedo P, Escaned J. Remodeling of epicardial coronary vessels. In: Escaned J, Davies J, eds. *Physiological Assessment of Coronary Stenoses and the Microcirculation*. Springer London; 2017:55-63.
39. Galis ZS, Khatri JJ. Matrix metalloproteinases in vascular remodeling and atherogenesis: the good, the bad, and the ugly. *Circ Res*. 2002;90(3):251-262.
40. Fuster V, Badimon L, Badimon JJ, Chesebro JH. The pathogenesis of coronary artery disease and the acute coronary syndromes (2). *N Engl J Med*. 1992;326(5):310-318. doi:10.1056/NEJM199201303260506
41. Tonino PA, De Bruyne B, Pijls NH, et al; FAME Study Investigators. Fractional flow reserve versus angiography for guiding percutaneous coronary intervention. *N Engl J Med*. 2009;360(3):213-224. doi:10.1056/NEJMoa0807611
42. Lacolley P, Regnault V, Nicoletti A, Li Z, Michel JB. The vascular smooth muscle cell in arterial pathology: a cell that can take on multiple roles. *Cardiovasc Res*. 2012;95(2):194-204. doi:10.1093/cvr/cvs135
43. Ambrose JA, Winters SL, Arora RR, et al. Coronary angiographic morphology in myocardial infarction: a link between the pathogenesis of unstable angina and myocardial infarction. *J Am Coll Cardiol*. 1985;6:1233-1238. doi:10.1016/s0735-1097(85)80207-2
44. Stone GW, Maehara A, Lansky AJ, et al; PROSPECT Investigators. A prospective natural-history study of coronary atherosclerosis. *N Engl J Med*. 2011;364(3):226-235. doi:10.1056/NEJMoa1002358
45. Seshiah PN, Kereiakes DJ, Vasudevan SS, et al. Activated monocytes induce smooth muscle cell death: role of macrophage colony-stimulating factor and cell contact. *Circulation*. 2002;105(2):174-180. doi:10.1161/hc0202.102248
46. Muller JE, Stone PH, Turi ZG; et al. Circadian variation in the frequency of onset of acute myocardial infarction. *N Engl J Med*. 1985;313(21):1315-1322. doi:10.1056/NEJM198511213132103
47. Leor J, Kloner RA. The Northridge earthquake as a trigger for acute myocardial infarction. *Am J Cardiol*. 1996;77(14):1230-1232. doi:10.1016/s0002-9149(96)00169-5
48. Lee RT, Schoen FJ, Loree HM, Lark MW, Libby P. Circumferential stress and matrix metalloproteinase 1 in human coronary atherosclerosis. Implications for plaque rupture. *Arterioscler Thromb Vasc Biol*. 1996;16(8):1070-1073. doi:10.1161/01.atv.16.8.1070
49. Smith SC Jr. Risk-reduction therapy: the challenge to change. Presented at the 68th scientific sessions of the American Heart Association November 13, 1995 Anaheim, California. *Circulation*. 1996;93(12):2205-2211. doi:10.1161/01.cir.93.12.2205
50. Ludmer PL, Selwyn AP, Shook TL, et al. Paradoxical vasoconstriction induced by acetylcholine in atherosclerotic coronary arteries. *N Engl J Med*. 1986;315(17):1046-1051. doi: 10.1056/NEJM198610233151702
51. Furchgott RF, Zawadzki JV. The obligatory role of endothelial cells in the relaxation of arterial smooth muscle by acetylcholine. *Nature*. 1980;288(5789):373-376. doi:10.1038/288373a0
52. de Agostini AI, Watkins SC, Slayter HS, Youssoufian H, Rosenberg RD. Localization of anticoagulantly active heparan sulfate proteoglycans in vascular endothelium: antithrombin binding on cultured endothelial cells and perfused rat aorta. *J Cell Biol*. 1990;111(3):1293-1304. doi:10.1083/jcb.111.3.1293
53. Kanthi YM, Sutton NR, Pinsky DJ. CD39: interface between vascular thrombosis and inflammation. *Curr Atheroscler Rep*. 2014;16(7):425. doi:10.1007/s11883-014-0425-1
54. Urbich C, Dimmeler S. Endothelial progenitor cells functional characterization. *Trends Cardiovasc Med*. 2004;14(8):318-322. doi:10.1016/j.tcm.2004.10.001
55. Forstermann U, Munzel T. Endothelial nitric oxide synthase in vascular disease: from marvel to menace. *Circulation*. 2006;113(13):1708-1714. doi:10.1161/CIRCULATIONAHA.105.602532
56. Busse R, Edwards G, Feletou M, Fleming I, Vanhoutte PM, Weston AH. EDHF: bringing the concepts together. *Trends Pharmacol Sci*. 2002;23(8):374-380. doi:10.1016/s0165-6147(02)02050-3
57. Kinlay S, Behrendt D, Wainstein M, et al. Role of endothelin-1 in the active constriction of human atherosclerotic coronary arteries. *Circulation*. 2001;104(10):1114-1118. doi:10.1161/hc3501.095707
58. Hasdai D, Holmes DR Jr, Garratt KN, Edwards WD, Lerman A. Mechanical pressure and stretch release endothelin-1 from human atherosclerotic coronary arteries in vivo. *Circulation*. 1997;95(2):357-362. doi:10.1161/01.cir.95.2.357
59. Dejana E, Tournier-Lasserve E, Weinstein BM. The control of vascular integrity by endothelial cell junctions: molecular basis and pathological implications. *Dev Cell*. 2009;16(2):209-221. doi:10.1016/j.devcel.2009.01.004
60. Hirase T, Node K. Endothelial dysfunction as a cellular mechanism for vascular failure. *Am J Physiol Heart Circ Physiol*. 2012;302(3):H499-H505. doi:10.1152/ajpheart.00325.2011
61. Bonetti PO, Lerman LO, Lerman A. Endothelial dysfunction: a marker of atherosclerotic risk. *Arterioscler Thromb Vasc Biol*. 2003;23(2):168-175. doi:10.1161/01.atv.0000051384.43104.fc
62. Virdis A, Taddei S. How to evaluate microvascular organ damage in hypertension: assessment of endothelial function. *High Blood Press Cardiovasc Prev*. 2011;18(4):163-167. doi:10.2165/11593630-000000000-00000
63. Gould KL, Lipscomb K, Hamilton GW. Physiologic basis for assessing critical coronary stenosis. Instantaneous flow response and regional distribution during coronary hyperemia as measures of coronary flow reserve. *Am J Cardiol*. 1974;33(1):87-94. doi:10.1016/0002-9149(74)90743-7
64. Vrints CJ, Bult H, Hitter E, Herman AG, Snoeck JP. Impaired endothelium-dependent cholinergic coronary vasodilation in patients with angina and normal coronary arteriograms. *J Am Coll Cardiol*. 1992;19(1):21-31. doi:10.1016/0735-1097(92)90046-p
65. Hasdai D, Cannan CR, Mathew V, Holmes DR Jr, Lerman A. Evaluation of patients with minimally obstructive coronary artery disease and angina. *Int J Cardiol*. 1996;53(3):203-208. doi:10.1016/0167-5273(95)02548-0
66. Marks DS, Gudapati S, Prisant LM, et al. Mortality in patients with microvascular disease. *J Clin Hypertens*. 2004;6:304-309. doi:10.1111/j.1524-6175.2004.03254.x
67. Britten MB, Zeiher AM, Schachinger V. Microvascular dysfunction in angiographically normal or mildly diseased coronary arteries predicts adverse cardiovascular long-term outcome. *Coron Artery Dis*. 2004;15(5):259-264. doi:10.1097/01.mca.0000134590.99841.81
68. Rubinshtein R, Yang EH, Rihal CS, et al. Coronary microcirculatory vasodilator function in relation to risk factors among patients without obstructive

coronary disease and low to intermediate Framingham score. *Eur Heart J*. 2010;31(8):936-942. doi:10.1093/eurheartj/ehp459

69. Beltrame JF, Tavella R, Jones D, Zeitz C. Management of ischaemia with non-obstructive coronary arteries (INOCA). *BMJ*. 2021;375:e060602. doi:10.1136/bmj-2021-060602
70. Kunadian V, Chieffo A, Camici PG, et al. An EAPCI expert consensus document on ischaemia with non-obstructive coronary arteries in collaboration with European Society of Cardiology Working Group on coronary pathophysiology & microcirculation endorsed by coronary vasomotor disorders International Study Group. *Eur Heart J*. 2020;41(37):3504-3520. doi:10.1093/eurheartj/ehaa503
71. Eriksson BE, Tyni-Lenne R, Svedenhag J, et al. Physical training in Syndrome X: physical training counteracts deconditioning and pain in Syndrome X. *J Am Coll Cardiol*. 2000;36(5):1619-1625. doi:10.1016/s0735-1097(00)00931-1
72. Tiefenbacher CP, Friedrich S, Bleeke T, Vahl C, Chen X, Niroomand F. ACE inhibitors and statins acutely improve endothelial dysfunction of human coronary arterioles. *Am J Physiol Heart Circ Physiol*. 2004;286(4):H1425-H1432. doi:10.1152/ajpheart.00783.2003
73. Kaski JC, Rosano GM, Collins P, Nihoyannopoulos P, Maseri A, Poole-Wilson PA. Cardiac syndrome X: clinical characteristics and left ventricular function. Long-term follow-up study. *J Am Coll Cardiol*. 1995;25(4):807-814. doi:10.1016/0735-1097(94)00507-M
74. Palloshi A, Fragasso G, Piatti P, et al. Effect of oral L-arginine on blood pressure and symptoms and endothelial function in patients with systemic hypertension, positive exercise tests, and normal coronary arteries. *Am J Cardiol*. 2004;93(7):933-935. doi:10.1016/j.amjcard.2003.12.040
75. Deshmukh SH, Patel SR, Pinassi E, et al. Ranolazine improves endothelial function in patients with stable coronary artery disease. *Coron Artery Dis*. 2009;20(5):343-347. doi:10.1097/MCA.0b013e32832a198b
76. Emdin M, Picano E, Lattanzi F, L'Abbate A. Improved exercise capacity with acute aminophylline administration in patients with syndrome X. *J Am Coll Cardiol*. 1989;14(6):1450-1453. doi:10.1016/0735-1097(89)90380-x
77. Kronhaus KD, Lawson WE. Enhanced external counterpulsation is an effective treatment for Syndrome X. *Int J Cardiol*. 2009;135(2):256-257. doi:10.1016/j.ijcard.2008.03.022
78. Ford TJ, Stanley B, Good R, et al. Stratified medical therapy using invasive coronary function testing in angina: the CorMicA trial. *J Am Coll Cardiol*. 2018;72(23 pt A):2841-2855. doi:10.1016/j.jacc.2018.09.006
79. Ford TJ, Stanley B, Sidik N, et al. 1-Year outcomes of angina management guided by invasive Coronary Function testing (CorMicA). *JACC Cardiovasc Interv*. 2020;13(1):33-45. doi:10.1016/j.jcin.2019.11.001
80. Handberg EM, Merz CNB, Cooper-Dehoff RM, et al. Rationale and design of the women's ischemia trial to reduce events in nonobstructive CAD (WARRIOR) trial. *Am Heart J*. 2021;237:90-103. doi:10.1016/j.ahj.2021.03.011
81. Grundy SM, Stone NJ, Bailey AL, et al. 2018 AHA/ACC/AACVPR/AAPA/ABC/ACPM/ADA/AGS/APhA/ASPC/NLA/PCNA guideline on the management of blood cholesterol: a report of the American College of Cardiology/American Heart Association task force on clinical practice guidelines. *Circulation*. 2019;139(25):e1082-e1143. doi:10.1161/CIR.0000000000000625
82. Cholesterol Treatment Trialists' CTT Collaboration; Fulcher J, O'Connell R, Voysey M, et al. Efficacy and safety of LDL-lowering therapy among men and women: meta-analysis of individual data from 174,000 participants in 27 randomised trials. *Lancet*. 2015;385(9976):1397-1405. doi:10.1016/S0140-6736(14)61368-4
83. Cholesterol Treatment Trialists' CTT Collaboration; Baigent C, Blackwell L, Emberson J, et al. Efficacy and safety of more intensive lowering of LDL cholesterol: a meta-analysis of data from 170,000 participants in 26 randomised trials. *Lancet*. 2010;376(9753):1670-1681. doi:10.1016/S0140-6736(10)61350-5
84. Cannon CP, Blazing MA, Giugliano RP, et al. Ezetimibe added to statin therapy after acute coronary syndromes. *N Engl J Med*. 2015;372:2387-2397. doi:10.1056/NEJMoa1410489
85. Sabatine MS, Giugliano RP, Keech AC, et al; FOURIER Steering Committee and Investigators. Evolocumab and clinical outcomes in patients with cardiovascular disease. *N Engl J Med*. 2017;376(18):1713-1722. doi:10.1056/NEJMoa1615664
86. Schwartz GG, Steg PG, Szarek M, et al; ODYSSEY OUTCOMES Committees and Investigators. Alirocumab and cardiovascular outcomes after acute coronary syndrome. *N Engl J Med*. 2018;379(22):2097-2107. doi:10.1056/NEJMoa1801174
87. Ridker PM, Danielson E, Fonseca FA, Genest J, Gotto AM Jr, Nordestgaard BG, Shepherd J, Willerson JT, Glynn RJ, Kastelein JJ, Koenig W, Libby P, Lorenzatti AJ, MacFadyen JG; JUPITER Study Group. Rosuvastatin to prevent vascular events in men and women with elevated C-reactive protein. *N Engl J Med*. 2008;359(21):2195-2207. doi:10.1056/NEJMoa0807646

Restenosis

David A. Zidar

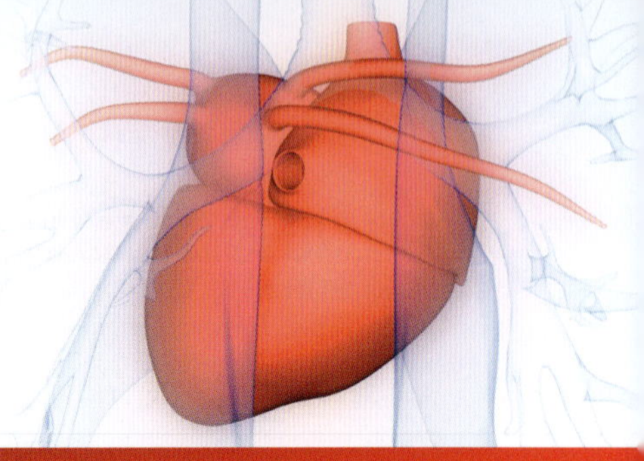

Despite remarkable technological improvements, restenosis, or re-narrowing of the artery, remains an important limitation to the long-term patency after interventional procedures.[1,2] Compared to balloon angioplasty, bare-metal stents (BMSs) decreased restenosis rates to approximately 30%,[3] and drug-eluting stents (DESs) have further reduced restenosis rates to 5% to 18% depending on the population.[4-7] First-generation DESs were accompanied by the risk of late (>1 month) and very late (>1 year) stent thrombosis (ST), a low frequency but devastating safety issue necessitating a more comprehensive understanding of device-related vascular healing. Iterative improvements subsequent in DES have yielded in a current generation of newer DES with ST rates lower than BMS, and further reductions in 1 year target lesion failure (TLF) rates compared to first-generation DES.

Yet, even with current-generation DESs, stent failure rates remain higher than de novo atherosclerotic event rates, and the goal of long-term durability over decades has not yet been achieved.[8] The aim of this chapter is to review the lessons from basic, translational, and clinical research that contributes to our current understanding of restenosis. We will discuss this remarkable progress, highlight the gaps in our current understanding of restenosis, and hope to motivate future discovery. Of particular importance has been the cross talk between basic mechanistic discovery efforts and adequately powered randomized clinical trials. This bidirectional flow of insights along the T0 to T4 spectrum exemplifies how device-related outcomes need to be continuously optimized in a rigorous, data-driven manner.

DEFINITIONS AND CLINICAL SEQUELAE OF RESTENOSIS

For most clinical trials, restenosis is defined by the binary endpoint of a reduction of 50% of the luminal diameter compared to the reference vessel.[9] This arbitrary definition endeavors to separate clinically important lesions from those without sequelae. Restenosis can also be described in continuous terms, which is helpful in understanding the pathophysiology of the process. For example, late lumen loss (LLL) is defined as the continuous angiographic measure of lumen deterioration and is calculated by subtracting minimal lumen diameter (MLD) at immediate follow-up from late-post-procedural MLD. This parameter has been used as a surrogate marker for the effects of different anti-restenotic therapies and to determine BMS and DES outcomes.[10,11] Importantly, when viewing restenosis as a continuous variable, it can be noted that virtually all patients suffer some degree of restenosis in a typical Gaussian distribution. However, it is only the few patients who have severe *symptomatic* in-stent restenosis (ISR) (usually with a lesion severity of >70%).

The average amount of LLL is 0.8 to 1.0 mm after implantation of a BMS, regardless of the size of the original vessel lumen. This is of critical significance, especially for smaller vessels. A 4-mm-diameter vessel would lose 44% of lumen area, with a loss of 1 mm in diameter. If a vessel with a 2-mm diameter experiences the same 1 mm of LLL, there is a 75% loss of lumen area and angiographic restenosis. Therefore, LLL and angiographic restenosis are related to the diameter of the reference vessel.[12] One of the most important concepts to understand is that restenosis rates vary greatly, depending on the particular definition used in any given study.

Discordance between the degree of LLL, binary restenosis, and symptoms is common. Although LLL has been very useful as a surrogate marker for the effectiveness of a given drug to prevent clinical restenosis, the relationship between LL and binary restenosis is nonlinear and is characterized by a curvilinear function (**Fig. 2.1**).[13] Especially in large diameter arteries, substantial LLL can be observed without clear clinical significance.

In a meta-analysis of all patients with angiographic ISR from the BENESTENT I, BENESTENT II pilot, BENESTENT II, MUSIC, WEST 1, DUET, FINESS 2, FLARE, SOPHOS, and ROSE studies that recruited 2690 patients who underwent percutaneous revascularization, restenosis (>50% diameter stenosis) occurred in 607 patients and was clinically silent in almost half of them.[14]

Although many patients present with stable exertional symptoms, unstable angina is also frequent presentation (26%-53%) and acute myocardial infarction (MI) has been described in 3.5% to 20% of patients.[15,16] DES restenosis has similar presentations. In one series, the rates of unstable angina and MI (18% and 2%, respectively) were comparable between the two groups.[17]

In contrast to atherosclerosis, the time course of restenosis following balloon angioplasty or BMS implantation is accelerated, typically apparent by 6 months,[18-20] and generally not progressive after 9 to 12 months. Routine follow-up angiography is no longer recommended.[21-23]

RISK FACTORS FOR RESTENOSIS

Clinical Risk Factors

Diabetes Mellitus (DM) is among the strongest and most consistently identified clinical predictor of restenosis. This may be due to metabolic alterations that promote endothelial dysfunction, accelerate intimal hyperplasia, and increase platelet aggregability and thrombogenicity.[24] Several studies suggest the relationship between diabetes and restenosis extends to DES, although the choice of DES may be relevant. The Swedish Coronary Angiography and Angioplasty Registry (SCAAR) involving >35,000 patients studied outcomes after four different types of DES (Endeavor, SES, Taxus Express, and Liberte) in real-world practice. At 2-year follow-up, restenosis rates were significantly higher in zotarolimus and sirolimus-eluting stents, whereas DM did not predict restenosis in patients receiving paclitaxel-eluting stents.[25]

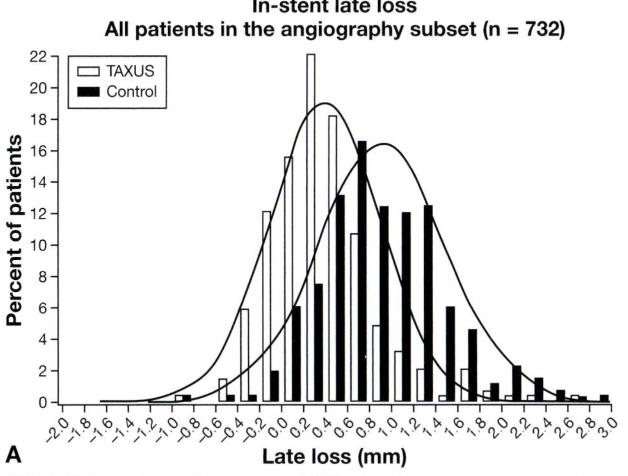

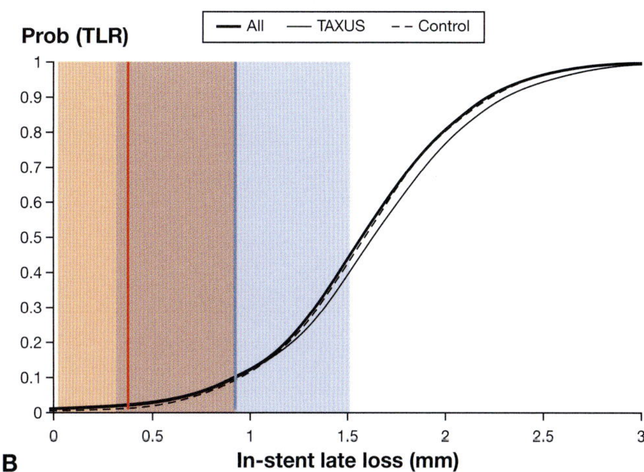

FIGURE 2.1 Data from the TAXUS IV trial shows the in-stent late loss (LL) for the Taxus and control bare-metal stent (BMS) in panel **(A)**. Panel **(B)** shows the probability of target lesion revascularization (TLR) as a function of in-stent LL, revealing a curvilinear distribution. Superimposed are the mean and standard deviations for the Taxus stent LL (*red*) and the control BMS (*blue*). The distribution of the Taxus stent LL falls along the relatively flat portion of the curve, whereas the distribution for the BMS falls along the steeper portion of the curve where there is greater correlation between LL and TLR. (From Ellis SG, Popma JJ, Lasala JM, et al. Relationship between angiographic LL and TLR after coronary stent implantation: analysis from the TAXUS-IV trial. *J Am Coll Cardiol*. 2005;45:1193-1200.)

Biologic Risk Factors

Evidence also suggests that some patients may be genetically predisposed to restenosis. Genetic abnormalities previously linked to restenosis include polymorphisms in genes with biologic relevance such as angiotensin-converting enzyme,[26,27] glycoprotein receptor IIIa,[28] and IL-8.[29] However, other studies have failed to validate these findings[30,31] and whether genetic testing can assist clinical decision making remains uncertain.

Attempts have been made to identify markers of inflammation and/or its sequalae, which predict an increased risk of ISR. A strong correlation exists between the number of macrophages in tissue samples obtained at the time of directional atherectomy and the propensity for restenosis.[32] Some,[33] but not all[34] blood studies have observed linkage between monocyte chemoattractant protein-1 (MCP-1) and restenosis. Similarly, levels of C-reactive protein (CRP) have been occasionally linked to restenosis.[35-37] Alterations in circulating matrix metalloproteinases (MMPs) may also have value in identifying those at higher-risk post-PCI.[38] However, there remains a substantial knowledge gap as to how to anticipate a pathologic injury response leading to restenosis risk at the time of index procedure.

Procedural Associations

Angiographic and intravascular imaging studies have demonstrated that a major determinant of clinical restenosis is the lumen size achieved at the end of the procedure.[39,40] Long lesion lengths is also a strong determinant of BMS restenosis risk, but appears less important after DES.[41] Stent underexpansion, malposition, or edge dissection can also increase the risk of restenosis as well as stent thrombosis. Some studies suggested that incomplete expansion also affects drug delivery (NIH).[42,43] The concept of geographical miss, referring to an area exposed to balloon injury but not covered with stent struts, has emerged as an important preventable mechanism of restenosis in the DES era.[44] Other anatomical features that increase the likelihood of restenosis include saphenous vein graft disease and chronic total occlusions.[45-49] A less common mechanical association is stent fracture, defined as complete or partial separation of a stent at follow-up that was contiguous after the original stent implantation.[50] The incidence of stent fracture with DES has been reported as 1% to 8%.[51-53] With stent fracture, additional vascular trauma may occur and drug delivery may also be impaired.[54]

PATTERNS OF IN-STENT RESTENOSIS

Mehran et al. developed an angiographic classification of ISR according to the geographic distribution of intimal hyperplasia in reference to the implanted stent (**Fig. 2.2**).[55] Four classes were defined as the following:

- Class I: Focal ISR group. Lesions are <10 mm in length and are positioned at the unscaffolded segment (ie, articulation or gap), the body of the stent, the proximal or distal margin (but not both), or a combination of these sites (multifocal ISR).
- Class II: "Diffuse intrastent" ISR. Lesions are >10 mm in length and are confined to the stent(s), without extending outside the margins of the stent(s).
- Class III: "Diffuse proliferative" ISR. Lesions are >10 mm in length and extend beyond the margin(s) of the stent(s).
- Class IV: ISR with "total occlusion." Lesions have a thrombolysis in myocardial infarction (TIMI) flow grade of 0.

BMS and DES have different patterns of in-segment restenosis (ISR), with a diffuse pattern more likely with the DES and a more focal pattern seen with BMS. Of interest, patients presenting with MI are likely to present with a diffuse pattern when compared to a non-MI presentation.[17,20]

PATHOGENESIS OF RESTENOSIS

The pathogenesis of restenosis is also significantly different from that of atherogenesis with respect to both their content of the lesion. Forrester proposed a paradigm for restenosis and suggested three phases: (1) the inflammatory phase, (2) a granulation or cellular proliferation phase, and (3) a remodeling phase involving extracellular matrix (ECM) protein synthesis.[56] Anatomically, restenosis is the net result of several inter-related processes, each

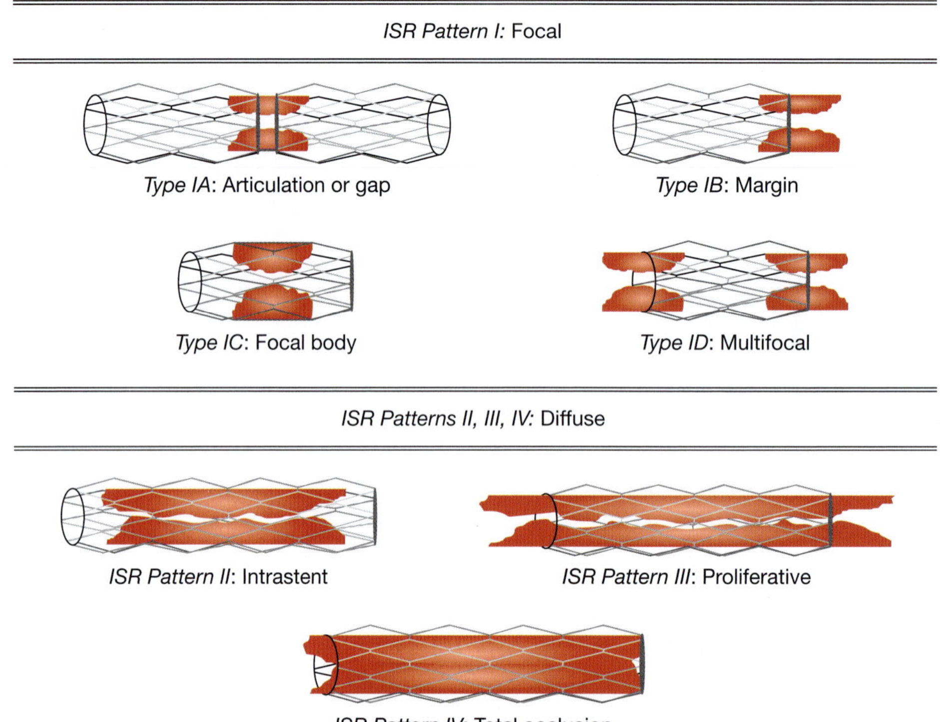

FIGURE 2.2 Common patterns of in-stent restenosis. (From Mehran R, Dangas G, Abizaid AS, et al. Angiographic patterns of in-stent restenosis: classification and implications for long-term outcome. *Circulation.* 1999; 100(18):1872-1878.)

leading to a reduction in luminal area. Elastic recoil is an acute process that is observed within a few minutes after balloon deflation, resulting in an inward collapse of the vessel wall. The recoil force can result in up to a 50% loss of cross-sectional area and a 33% loss in luminal diameter.[57] Negative remodeling is a second restenotic process that results from delayed contraction of the external elastic laminae weeks to months after injury. Neointimal hyperplasia (NIH) is a third mechanism of restenosis, initiated by this acute injury response but coupled to smooth muscle cell migration/proliferation and excessive ECM production.[58,59] More recently, Park and others have described in-stent neoatherosclerosis, especially after DES, with histologic findings similar to de novo coronary atherosclerosis.[60]

Acute Injury Response and Leukocyte Activation

When a balloon and stent contact the vessel, a series of events are initiated (**Fig. 2.3**). The initial injury immediately following stent placement includes de-endothelialization, often with dissection into the tunica media and occasionally the adventitia, resulting in stretching of the entire artery. A layer of platelets and fibrin are deposited at this site of injury.[61-63] Activated platelets on the surface expressing adhesion molecules, such as P-selectin and (glycoprotein) GP Ibα, attach to circulating leukocytes via platelet receptors such as P-selectin glycoprotein ligand (PSGL-1) and begin a process of rolling along the injured surface. Leukocytes then bind tightly to the surface and stop rolling (mediated through the leukocyte integrin [ie, Mac-1] class of adhesion molecules) via direct attachment to platelet receptors such as GP Ibα and through cross-linking with fibrinogen to the GP IIb/IIIa receptor. Migration of leukocytes across the platelet-fibrin layer and diapedesis into the tissue is driven by chemical gradients of cytokines released from smooth muscle cells and resident inflammatory cells. The β_2 integrin molecule Mac-1 (CD11b/CD18) is present on both neutrophils and monocytes and appears to be of central importance in leukocyte recruitment following vascular injury. In addition to promoting the accumulation of leukocytes at the sites of vascular injury, the binding of platelets to neutrophils amplifies the inflammatory response by inducing neutrophil activation, upregulating cell adhesion molecule expression, and generating signals that promote integrin activation and chemokine synthesis. These processes of activation may be mediated through the release of soluble CD40 ligand, a proinflammatory molecule stored most abundantly in platelets.

Farb et al investigated stented arteries from pathologic samples of 116 stents from 87 patients with greater than 90 days postprocedure. They found a statistically significant association between the extent of medial damage, inflammation, and restenosis.[64] Also linking leukocytes and restenosis is data by Moreno et al, in tissue retrieved from directional atherectomy at the time of angioplasty showing a strong positive correlation between the number of macrophages in the tissue and subsequent risk of restenosis.[32] Systemic markers of inflammation following angioplasty may also correlate with these local injury responses and restenosis risk.[65-68]

In several experimental animal models, cell adhesion molecules critical for leukocyte recruitment have been found to be upregulated by an atherogenic diet,[69-71] induction of diabetes,[72] and increased shear stress.[73] After balloon endothelial denudation in a rabbit model, vascular cell adhesion molecule-1, intracellular cell adhesion molecule-1, and MHC class II antigens, all have been shown to be upregulated in a sustained fashion.[74] Stent implants also lead to a brisk early inflammatory response with abundant surface-adherent leukocytes of both monocyte and granulocyte lineage.[75,76] Days and weeks later, macrophages invade and contribute to NIH, often clustering around stent struts.

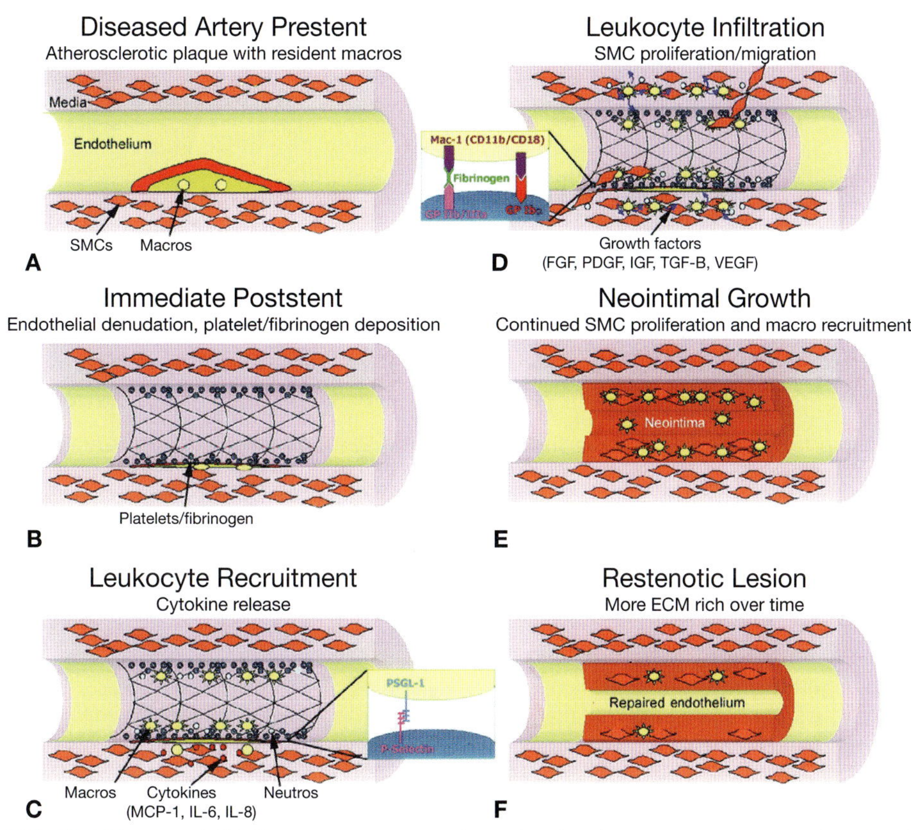

FIGURE 2.3 Panel **(A)** illustrates a mature atherosclerotic plaque prior to intervention. Panel **(B)** illustrates the immediate result of stent placement with endothelial denudation and platelet/fibrinogen deposition. Panels **(C)** and **(D)** illustrate leukocyte recruitment, infiltration, and smooth muscle cell (SMC) proliferation and migration in the days following the injury. Panel **(E)** demonstrates neointimal thickening in the weeks following the injury, with continued SMC proliferation and monocyte recruitment. Panel **(F)** illustrates the long-term (weeks to months) change from a predominantly cellular to a less cellular and more ECM-rich plaque. ECM, extracellular matrix; MCP-1, monocyte chemoattractant protein-1; IL-6, IL-8, interleukin-6; interleukin-8; VEGF, vascular endothelial growth factor. (From Welt FG, Rogers C. Inflammation and restenosis in the stent era. *Arterioscler Thromb Vasc Biol*. 2002;22:1769-1776.)

Preclinical evidence suggests that blocking early monocyte recruitment with anti-inflammatory agents reduces neointimal thickening.[76-78] Activated macrophages may influence vascular repair through various mechanisms, including production of a variety of mediators, such as members of the interleukin family, tumor necrosis factors (TNFs), monocyte chemoattractant protein-1, and growth factors such as platelet-derived growth factors, basic fibroblast growth factors, and heparin-binding epidermal growth factors.[79]

Several studies have also shown infiltration of neutrophils within the arterial wall following vascular injury.[80-82] As with macrophages, a concomitant reduction in neutrophil number and smooth muscle proliferation can be seen with administration of anti-inflammatory agents, resulting in less neointimal growth.[75] Neutrophils are also known to secrete cytokines, including IL-1, TNF-α, and IL-6,[83] and they also release reactive oxygen species and proteases.[79]

Ultimately, both balloon angioplastied and stented arteries tend to experience re-endothelialization that completes the acute stage of vessel healing from vascular injury. However, growth factors released from platelets, leukocytes, and tissue-resident cells can initiate a secondary phase leading to the proliferation and migration of smooth muscle cells leading to negative remodeling and NIH as described in the following.

NEGATIVE REMODELING

Remodeling is a change in the arterial size following vascular injury.[84] This process is primarily responsible for luminal loss after angioplasty and atherectomy.[85] The process of negative remodeling may be observed 1 to 6 months after balloon angioplasty and accounts for about 60% to 65% of luminal loss observed by intravascular ultrasound (IVUS).[84,86] The adventitia plays a crucial role in both the proliferation and concentric compression of the external elastic lamina (negative remodeling).[87] Three days after balloon injury in animals, a large number of proliferating cells were located in the adventitia, with significantly fewer positive cells found in the media and lumen. Seven days after injury, proliferating cells were found primarily in the NIH, extending along the luminal surface. In situ hybridization for PDGF A-chain and β-receptor mRNAs revealed that the expression of these two genes was closely correlated with the sites of proliferation at each time point.[87,88] On vessel injury, inflammatory cells stimulate conversion of adventitial fibroblasts to myofibroblasts that express α-smooth muscle actin and secrete ECM, leading to constriction of the vessel and the formation of a fibrotic scar within the adventitia surrounding the site of injury. Wilcox used antibodies against α-smooth muscle actin, myosin, and desmin to demonstrate the proliferation of myofibroblasts in the NIH and the adventitia.[88] Other studies demonstrated that using intracoronary radiation was effective in slowing this process when directed toward the adventitia, suggesting that the adventitia is not a passive player in restenosis.

VASCULAR SMOOTH MUSCLE CELL PROLIFERATION

Vascular smooth muscle cell (VSMC) proliferation and migration can be triggered after acute vascular injury and this process is central to NIH. The two major cascades that regulate the function of VSMC are the tyrosine kinase cascade and the cyclic-adenosine monophosphate (AMP) pathway. Growth factors bind to the receptors and activate tyrosine kinase that leads to a phosphorylation cascade, eventually activating *ras* proteins. This stimulates *raf* proteins to activate mitogen-activated protein kinase kinase (MAPKK), resulting in intranuclear activation of transcription factors that induce proliferation and migration of VSMC. The cyclic-AMP pathway leads to the activation of protein kinase A (PKA), which phosphorylates and activates the transcription factor cAMP responsive element binding protein (CREB). In addition, PKA phosphorylates *raf*, inhibiting the other major pathway involved in the activation of VSMC.[89] In vitro and in vivo studies demonstrate that the inactivation of *ras* and the activation of the cyclic-AMP pathway leads to a >50% reduction in neointimal formation at 14 days postballoon injury in rat carotid arteries. A similar effect on NIH formation is observed with inhibiting MAPKK by the dominant inhibitor mutant gene.[90-92]

Downstream from these events, other molecular processes regulate the progression of the cell through the cell cycle. The progression from the G_0 to G_1 phase is regulated by cyclin-dependent kinases (CDK), particularly cyclin D-CDK and cyclin E-CDK-2. Endogenous inhibitors of CDK (CKI) such as $p21^{cip1}$, $p27^{kip1}$, and INK4 families regulate the process of entering G_1 and keep VSMC in the G_0 phase. Vascular inflammation and injury decreases the level of $p27^{kip1}$, thereby promoting cell division. On the contrary, activation of cAMP leads to an increase in $p27^{kip1}$, thus promoting the proliferating cells to enter a quiescent phase.[89] This matrix of balanced events and intracellular signals leads to the conversion of VSMC to myofibroblasts and migration to the site of injury. Histologic analysis in the porcine model demonstrates that these actin (+) cells colonize the residual thrombus, which forms a cap across the thrombus and proliferates toward the tunica media. The myofibroblasts then degrade the thrombus and replace it with ECM, leading to the formation of the neointimal mass.[93] The amount of NIH produced appears to be influenced by the degree of inflammation generated during acute phase of vascular injury.[94]

DIFFERENCES BETWEEN BALLOON AND STENT INJURY

Angiographic analysis of the pivotal stent studies (the Stent Restenosis Study [STRESS] and Belgian Netherlands Stent Study [BENESTENT]) revealed major quantitative and qualitative differences between angioplasty-induced injury and injuries associated with stent placement. The initial luminal gain with stents is greater as scaffolding prevents recoil of the vessel. In addition, late negative remodeling is also abrogated by the presence of the rigid frame of the stent. However, stented vessels illicit greater NIH.[95,96] Hoffman et al compared stented and nonstented lesions using serial IVUS studies, confirming the observation that the main mechanism of ISR is due to NIH rather than negative remodeling.[97] Therefore, stents reduce restenosis rates in part because they are often able to achieve a larger initial lumen and prevent late remodeling despite inducing more LLL via NIH (**Fig. 2.4**).

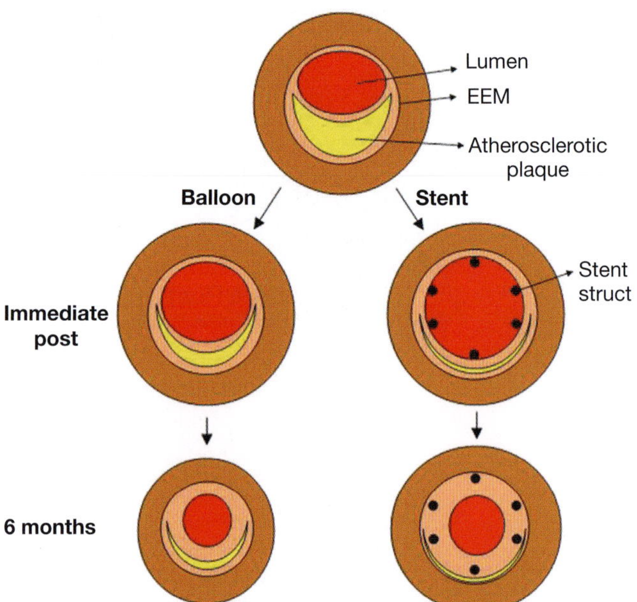

FIGURE 2.4 Illustration of differences in mechanisms of restenosis between plain balloon angioplasty and stenting. In balloon angioplastied vessels, restenosis is caused by a combination of neointimal growth and negative remodeling. Stented arteries have lower rates of restenosis despite incurring greater neointimal growth due to their ability to achieve a larger initial lumen size, and the elimination of negative remodeling. EEM, external elastic membrane.

The vascular injury and inflammation induced by balloons and stents also differ. Inoue et al. used flow cytometry to measure CD11b (a member of the integrin family of adhesion molecules) expression on neutrophils following PCI and found substantially higher levels in those undergoing stent implantation, as compared to balloon angioplasty alone. This increased inflammatory response may help explain the larger neointimal growth seen in stented arteries.[98] Kornowski et al, using a porcine model, demonstrated that stent strut perforation of the internal and external elastic lamina resulted in greater histologic inflammation and a larger volume of neointimal formation.[99] Contact allergy to metals including nickel and molybdenum may also stimulate inflammation via a delayed-type hypersensitivity response in a small subset of individuals.[100] A study was conducted in Germany on 131 patients after stent implantation, who underwent cutaneous patch testing to investigate the relation between nickel and molybdenum hypersensitivity and ISR. All 10 patients with a positive test result had restenosis (P = .03), requiring target vessel revascularization (TVR).[100]

NEOATHEROSCLEROSIS

In a subset of patients, a lesion develops within the stented segment that more closely resembles a native atherosclerotic plaque rather than NIH.[101] This has been termed neoatherosclerosis (**Fig. 2.5**). Histologically, in-stent neoatherosclerosis is manifested by the

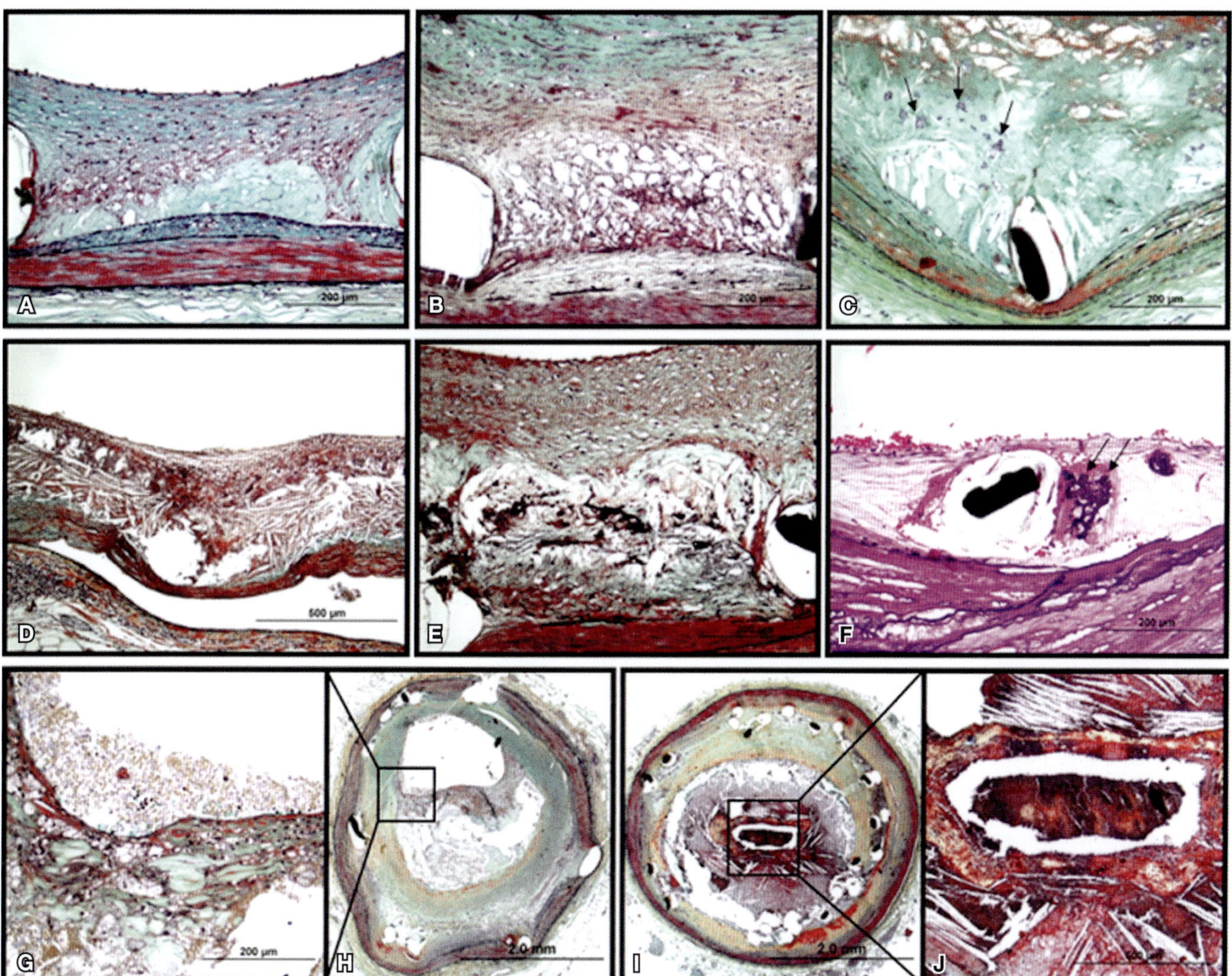

FIGURE 2.5 Representative images of various stages of newly formed atherosclerotic changes within neointima after stent implantation. **A:** Foamy macrophage clusters in the peristrut region of sirolimus-eluting stents (SESs) implanted for 13 months antemortem is seen. **B:** Fibroatheroma with foamy macrophage-rich lesion and early necrotic core formation in SES of 13 months' duration. **C:** Fibroatheroma with peristrut early necrotic core, cholesterol clefts, surface foamy macrophages, and early calcification (*arrows*) in SES at 13 months. **D:** Peristrut late necrotic core in the neointima, characterized by large aggregate of cholesterol cleft in SES at 17 months. **E:** Fibroatheroma with calcification in the necrotic core in SES of 10 months' duration. **F:** A peristrut calcification (*arrows*) with fibrin in SES of 7 months' duration. **G and H:** A low-power magnification image (**H**) of a severely narrowed bare-metal stent (BMS) implanted 61 months, with a thin-cap fibroatheroma. Note macrophage infiltration and a discontinuous thin fibrous cap in a high-power magnification image (**G**). **I:** A low-power magnification image shows a plaque rupture with an acute thrombus that has totally occluded the lumen in BMS implanted for 61 months antemortem. **J:** A high-power magnification image shows a discontinuous thin-cap with occlusive luminal thrombus. (From: Nakazawa G, Otsuka F, Nakano M, et al. The pathology of neoatherosclerosis in human coronary implants bare-metal and drug-eluting stents. *J Am Coll Cardiol.* 2011;57:1314-1322.)

accumulation of lipid-laden foamy macrophages, which start in the peri-strut area or adjacent to the luminal surface and then progress to a typical appearing fibroatheroma. This process may be associated with necrotic core formation and calcification.[101]

In-stent neoatherosclerosis occurs more frequently in DES than BMS, possibly due to polymer coating-induced inflammation, with an infiltration of macrophages, lymphocytes, and giant cells.[102] An autopsy study published by Nakazawa and others[101] showed that the prevalence of neoatherosclerosis is significantly higher in lesions with first-generation DES compared to BMS (31% vs 16%, respectively). Otsuka et al[103] demonstrated no significant difference in the prevalence of neoatherosclerosis in ***cobalt-chromium*** (CoCr)-everolimus-eluting stent (EES) and first-generation SES and paclitaxel-eluting stent (PES) with implant durations of 30 days to 3 years. An autopsy stent registry of 384 cases and 614 stented lesions (266 lesions with BMS, 285 with first-generation DES, and 63 with second-generation DES) were analyzed histologically for neoatherosclerosis.[104] The prevalence of neoatherosclerosis for implant duration <1 year was similar in the first- and second-generation DES (13% vs 17%, respectively) but higher than BMS (0%). Similar results were found when the lesions were assessed for the duration of implant >1 year and <3 years (51% for first-generation DES, 48% for second-generation DES, and 6% for BMS).

The mechanism of neoatherosclerosis is still poorly understood but may stem from delayed endothelial coverage of the stented segments. Furthermore, antiproliferative effects of the eluted drugs in DES also lead to reduced production of nitric oxide and antithrombotic molecules.[105-107]

EARLY ATTEMPTS TO PREVENT RESTENOSIS

There have been multiple proposed technical approaches and pharmacologic agents identified in preclinical studies that failed when tested in large-scale clinical trials. It was not until agents directed against smooth muscle cell proliferation were married with local delivery techniques that significant reduction in restenosis was observed.

EARLY MECHANICAL STRATEGIES

Mechanical strategies applied to reduce the frequency of ISR have included: (i) IVUS-guided, high-pressure deployment to achieve larger mean luminal diameter (MLD), (ii) debulking therapy, and (iii) avoidance of predilation with "direct" stenting. These strategies may achieve some reduction in restenosis rates in certain cases; however, large randomized controlled trials have failed to support these techniques as a general strategy.[108-110]

BARE-METAL STENTS

Bare-metal stents were developed as a mechanical scaffolding of the arterial wall for the primary reduction of restenosis. The BENESTENT study was the earliest randomized controlled study that assessed long-term outcomes after BMS implantation. The study was conducted in 520 patients with stable coronary disease, who were randomly assigned to a Palmaz-Schatz stent versus balloon angioplasty. There was a 30% reduction of the primary endpoint between the two groups in favor of the BMS. The primary clinical endpoints included death, MI, cerebrovascular events, the need for coronary artery bypass grafting (CABG), or a second PCI involving the previously treated lesion. The primary angiographic end-point was the minimal luminal diameter at follow-up. The clinical and angiographic outcomes were statistically better in the stent group in comparison to the angioplasty group, mainly with respect to restenosis rates (22% vs 32%, respectively).[3]

ANTITHROMBOTIC THERAPY

Heparin has been the archetypal modulator of vascular repair in animal models and has been shown to reduce neointimal proliferation and restenosis following vascular injury.[111,112] However, the maximum inhibition of NIH is noted with continued infusion for the duration of the experiment rather than intermittent use.[113] This effect was also witnessed in the Subcutaneous Heparin and Angioplasty Restenosis Prevention (SHARP) trial, which randomized 339 patients to subcutaneous therapy versus no therapy. The 4-month follow-up showed no difference in the outcome or restenosis.[114] Low-molecular-weight heparin has been evaluated in multiple studies and demonstrated no reduction in restenosis.[115,116] Hirudin, a small molecule direct thrombin inhibitor, showed promising results in animal femoral arteries with reductions in restenosis rates; however, subsequent clinical randomized studies showed no difference in restenosis when compared to heparin.[117-119]

The Antiplatelet Trialist Collaboration Investigators demonstrated a reduction of 25% of platelet aggregation with the addition of Ticlopidine to aspirin. Interestingly, this additive antiplatelet effect reduced the rates of thrombosis, but had no effect on restenosis.[120] Dipyridamole, another platelet inhibitor, similarly failed to reduce restenosis in combination with aspirin.[121] The addition of sulotroban to aspirin also showed no reduction in the rates of restenosis either.[122] Other antiplatelet agents, thromboxane inhibitors, and prostacyclin analogues have showed similar disappointing results.[123] Glycoprotein IIb with IIIa form the platelet fibrinogen receptor, the final step in the cascade of platelet aggregation. Despite promising in vitro and preclinical data,[124,125] human studies interrupting this pathway have also failed to reduce restenosis in human trials.

CILOSTAZOL

Cilostazol was approved by the US Food and Drug Administration (FDA) in 1998 for the treatment of intermittent claudication, and has been in use in other countries since 1988 for related indications. The pharmacologic effects of cilostazol are largely a result of selective inhibition of phosphodiesterase-3 (PDE3). In PDE3-rich cells, such as platelets and VSMCs, inhibition of PDE3 increases intracellular levels of cyclic-AMP, which activates PKA and ultimately results in phosphorylation of PKA substrates. These substrates mediate the potent antiplatelet effect of cilostazol, increase VSMCs relaxation and cardiac contractility, and inhibit VSMC proliferation.[126] Initial nonrandomized studies showed evidence that cilostazol affects restenosis in both patients who underwent either balloon angioplasty or stenting.[127]

Cilostazol for Restenosis (CREST) trial was a randomized study that sought to test the efficacy of cilostazol in preventing restenosis after BMS implantation in native coronary arteries.[128] The study enrolled 705 patients undergoing stenting at 19 sites who were randomized to therapy with cilostazol 200 mg/day (n = 354) or placebo (n = 351). At 6 months, in-segment restenosis was observed in 22.01% of patients receiving cilostazol and in 34.46% of patients receiving a placebo (P = .002). Reductions in the rates of ISRs were particularly large in patients with diabetes (17.7% vs 37.7%, for cilostazol and placebo, respectively; P = .01). Meta-analysis of 10 randomized studies has also been used to support the use of cilostazol for the reduction of BMS restenosis.[129]

ANTI-INFLAMMATORY AGENTS

Immune cell activation in the context of vascular injury may play a key role in initiating and amplifying the processes ultimately leading to VSMC proliferation and restenosis. Therefore, there has been great interest in anti-inflammatory agents as therapies to prevent restenosis. Broadly speaking, the classic anti-inflammatory agents such as corticosteroids and colchicine, a metaphase inhibitor, have shown little to no benefit in clinical trials.[130,131]

CALCIUM CHANNEL BLOCKERS

The Coronary Angioplasty Study Amlodipine Restenosis (CAPARES) randomized 635 patients to Amlodipine versus placebo in patients undergoing coronary intervention. The treatment was started 2 weeks prior to the procedure and continued for 4 months. There was no difference in minimum lumen diameter measured by quantitative angiography, but the incidence of repeat Percutaneous transluminal coronary angioplasty (PTCA) and the composite major adverse clinical events were significantly reduced during the 4-month follow-up period after PTCA with amlodipine, as compared with a placebo.[132]

Individual trials using Nifedipine, Verapamil, and Diltiazem were not able to demonstrate an effect either.[133-135] Although meta-analysis data demonstrated that patients treated with calcium channel blockers had a 32% reduction in angiographic restenosis compared to controls, the practice of routine use of these agents was never solidified, mostly due to concerns about increased incidence of ischemic events following MI.[136]

FIRST-GENERATION DESS

Local drug delivery has several important advantages in the treatment of restenosis. Most importantly, potentially toxic drugs can be delivered in sufficiently high doses locally to have an effect without systemic toxicity.[137] However, the efficacy of local drug delivery is complex and governed by the dose and rate of release of the agent, tissue retention, and the inherent properties of the drug. Low doses may be ineffective, whereas higher doses can lead to tissue death and fibrin deposition, leading to increased rates of thrombosis with delayed healing.[138,139] Release rates must be determined empirically to match the biologic processes.

Interestingly, with sirolimus as opposed to paclitaxel, fast release is just as effective in comparison to slow release in reduction of LLL.[140] The drug can be delivered by the stent through a variety of media that play a role in the rate of restenosis. Some drugs can be linked to the stent directly through processes of quaternary binding. However, most drugs require a polymer to harbor the drug and allow timed release. In this process, nonerodable polymers had to be developed with minimal inflammatory stimuli. Polymer release kinetics plays a critical role in the prevention of restenosis. The Paclitaxel In-Stent Controlled Elution Study (PISCES) trial 3 demonstrated this principle, involving the use of the Conor stent with six different polymer-drug release formulations. The duration of the drug release had a far greater effect on the inhibition of NIH than the dose of drug delivered. For example, 10 µg of paclitaxel released over 10 days following DES implantation appeared to have little effect on NIH formation, whereas the same dosage of drug released over a 30-day period led to a profound reduction in NIH, with more than half (57%) the reduction of the LLL, whereas 30 µg of the same drug released over a 10-day period also was less effective.[141] Molecular biology studies have suggested that the genes responsible for the proliferative response potentially remain active for a period of up to 21 days after vessel injury. These findings highlight the complexities of DES developmental programs.[142]

Sirolimus

Sirolimus (rapamycin) is a natural macrocyclic lactone with potent immunosuppressive and antimitotic action produced by a fungus, *Streptomyces hygroscopicus*. The agent binds intracellularly to the FKBP-12 forming the immunosuppressive complex that inhibits the mTOR, a key regulatory kinase. This leads to an increase in the levels of p27^{kip1}, which inhibits the cyclin-CDK complex, blocking the G_1-S transition and thereby restricting proliferation of VSMC.[143]

There have been four pivotal trials conducted with sirolimus-eluting stents (SESs) that led to FDA approval in April 2003. After initial impressive results from the First in Man (FIM)[140] experience, a double-blind, randomized, controlled trial was launched. The Randomized Study with the Sirolimus-Eluting Velocity Balloon-Expandable Stent (RAVEL) randomized 238 patients to either a single SES or the same single BMS.[144] The SES was prepared for release similar to the slow-release method from the FIM study. One-half of the patients presented with unstable angina. All patients received heparin during PCI, clopidogrel, or ticlopidine for 8 weeks after the procedure, and aspirin (100 mg or more/day) indefinitely. About 10% of patients also received GP IIb-IIIa inhibitors. At 6 months, there was a significant reduction of in-stent LLL, intimal hyperplasia, and restenosis for patients receiving the SES compared with the BMS. The significant reduction of in-stent loss was also evident when the proximal and distal edges were evaluated (in-segment loss). During a follow-up period of up to 1 year, the overall rate of major cardiac events was 5.8% in the sirolimus-stent group and 28.8% in the standard-stent group ($P < .001$). The RAVEL study was limited to noncomplex lesions. The SIRIUS trial,[11] comparing sirolimus DES stents with BMS, recruited patients in the United States who had more multivessel disease (40.7%) compared to RAVEL (29%). The study included more patients with DM (26% in SIRIUS vs 19% in RAVEL), longer lesions (mean 14.4 mm), and 60% of patients received GP IIb-IIIa inhibitors, compared with only 10% of patients in RAVEL. Patients treated with SESs had lower rates of binary (>50% diameter stenosis) angiographic restenosis within the segment (8.9% vs 36.3% with the BMS; $P < .001$) and within the stent (3.2% vs 35.4% with the BMS; $P < .001$). SESs were associated with significantly less LLL within the treated segment, within the stent, and within its 5-mm proximal and distal edges (all $P < .001$). The reduction of restenosis with the SES was consistent in patients at risk for restenosis, including those with small vessels, long lesions, and DM.[145]

Paclitaxel

Paclitaxel is a compound isolated from the bark of the Pacific yew tree of the northwestern US (*Taxus brevifolia*). Paclitaxel exerts its pharmacologic effect by inhibiting microtubule depolymerization, resulting in the formation of numerous decentralized and unorganized microtubules during cell division. This results in the inhibition of cellular replication at the G_0/G_1 and G_1/M phase and stops cytokine-mediated induction of cell proliferation and migration.

PES efficacy was demonstrated in the TAXUS II and TAXUS IV trials, which examined patients with low-risk lesions or previously untreated coronary stenosis, who randomly received BMS or PES with either a slow or a moderate drug-release rate. All trials resulted in reduction of ISR and TLR.[146-149] Furthermore, TAXUS IV demonstrated that these benefits were maintained in subgroups, including patients with vessels <2.5 mm in diameter, those with lesions >20 mm in length, and those with renal insufficiency or diabetes. Pooled and long-term analysis also revealed a reduction in CV events.

SES Versus PES Trials

The TAXi trial was the first prospective, randomized trial that compared the efficacy of SES (CYPHER) versus PES (TAXUS). Two hundred and two patients with similar demographics were randomized into two groups: the SES ($n = 102$) and the PES ($n = 100$) groups. Although the data showed no significant difference in MACE between SES and PES at 6 months, the trial was limited in its sample size to determine any clinical superiority between the two DESs.[5]

This was followed by the REALITY trial, a large prospective, randomized trial that compared the polymer-coated Cypher SES to the polymer-coated Taxus PES in terms of safety and efficacy. The study randomized 1353 patients with similar angiographic and clinical variables into SES (n = 684) and PES (n = 669) groups, with the primary endpoint of the in-lesion restenosis rate at 8 months. At the 8-month angiographic follow-up, significant differences were found in in-stent MLD, percentage diameter stenosis, LLL, and LLL index, all favoring the SES. These observations indicate a significantly greater degree of suppression of NIH achieved by the SES, particularly considering the smaller mean vessel diameter measured immediately after the implantation of the SES. However, the significant differences in several continuous angiographic variables, most importantly LLL, did not translate into significant differences in in-lesion binary restenosis or in TLR.[150] Other studies such as SIRTAX suggested superiority of SES to PES, with lower rates of TVR.[151] SES also proved superior to PES in suppression of NIH when evaluated by IVUS imaging.[152] Long-term follow-up of SIRTAX showed no difference between the two groups, likely attributed to the loss of initial release kinetics of SES compared to PES.[153]

NEWER-GENERATION DESS

Although first-generation DES provided unambiguous proof that the local delivery of cell cycle inhibitors could dramatically reduce restenosis rates, these devices had important limitations as exemplified by the rare but potentially catastrophic occurrence of late and very late stent thrombosis. First-generation scaffolds were also bulky to deliver to complex lesions. Rates of major adverse cardiac events at 5 years remained high (~20%). Several newer-generation DES have now been FDA approved with important refinements in the stent scaffold, different antiproliferative agents, and changes to the original polymer coatings (**Table 2.1**). In head-to-head randomized clinical trials vs first-generation DES, newer designs maintain low LLL, but result in substantially lower rates of clinically driven ***toll-like receptors*** (TLRs) and are associated with significantly lower risk of stent thrombosis.

Scaffold Design

Early-generation BMS and DES were mounted on stainless steel platforms with relatively large strut sizes. For instance, the Cypher stent utilized 316 L stainless steel with a strut thickness of 140 μm. The first-generation Taxus was also manufactured with 316 L stainless steel and had a strut thickness of 132 μm. Preclinical studies suggest that restenotic responses may be affected by the architecture, composition, and strut thickness of the scaffold.[154,155] The discovery of cobalt chromium and platinum alloys that enable thin strut scaffolds with preserved radial strength allowed this hypothesis to be tested in humans.[156]

Several randomized trials support the notion that stent characteristics, particularly strut size, affects the risk of restenosis.[157,158] The ISAR-STEREO trial showed that a thin strut (50 μm) RX multilink BMS design resulted in marked reduction in binary restenosis and TVR (12.3% vs 21.9%) compared to the thick strut (140 μm) BX velocity.[158] Contemporary DES have taken advantage of newer scaffolds and this may account in part for improved outcomes associated with newer DES compared to their first-generation counterparts.

Fully bioresorbable stent scaffolds have also been brought to market. For instance, the Absorb Bioresorbable Vascular Scaffold (BVS, Abbott Laboratories, Abbott Park, IL) has a backbone of

TABLE 2.1 Characteristics of Selected Drug-Eluting Stents

DES	MANUFACTURER	FDA APPROVAL	ANTI-PROLIFERATIVE	POLYMER	DRUG ELUTION PERIOD	STRUT COMPOSITION	STRUT THICKNESS	PIVITOL TRIALS/ PROGRAM
Cypher	Johnson & Johnson/ Cordis	2003	Sirolimus (1.4 μg/ mm^2)	67/33% PEVA-PBMA	80% in 30 d	316 L stainless steel	140 μm	RAVEL, SIRIUS
Taxus Express/ Liberte	Boston Scientific	2004	Paclitaxel (1.0 μg/ mm^2)	SIBS (Translute)	10% in 30 d	316 L stainless steel	132 μm/97 μm	TAXUS II
Xience V/ Promus	Abbott/Boston Scientific	2008	Everolimus (1.0 μg/mm^2)	Fluoropolymer (PBMA)	80% in 28 d	Cobalt chromium (L605)	81 μm	SPIRIT
Endeavor	Medtronic	2008	Zotarolimus (1.6 μg/mm^2)	Phosphorylcholine	98% in 14 d	Cobalt nickel (MP35N)	91 μm	ENDEAVOR
Promus Element	Boston Scientific	2011	Everolimus (1.0 μg/mm^2)	Fluoropolymer (PBMA)	80% in 28 d	Platinum chromium	81 μm	PLATINUM
Resolute/ Onyx	Medtronic	2012	Zotarolimus (1.6 μg/mm^2)	Biolinx (C10, C19, PVP polymers)	85% in 60 d	Cobalt nickel (MP35N)	91 μm	RESOLUTE-AC
Synergy	Boston Scientific	2015	Everolimus (1.0 μg/mm^2)[a]	Poly-DL-lactide-co-glycolide(PLGA)[b]	99% in 90 d	Platinum chromium	74 μm	EVOLVE II
Orsiro	Biotronik	2019	Sirolimus (1.4 μg/ mm^2)	Poly-L-lactide (PLLA)[b]	80% in 90 d	Cobalt chromium (L605)	60 μm/80 μm	BIOFLOW-V
BioFreedom	Biosensors	2022	Umirolimus (15.6 μg/mm)	None	98% in 28 d	316 L Stainless steel	112 μm	LEADERS

PBMA: poly n-butyl methacrylate; PEVA, polyethylene-co-vinyl acetate; SIBS: poly (styrene-b-isobutylene-b-styrene).
[a]abluminal surface only
[b]bioabsorbable polymer

poly-L-lactide and a strut thickness of 150 μm, which degrades to water and carbon dioxide within 3 years.[159] This BVS was approved by the USFDA in 2016 based on the 1st year results from the ABSORB III trial.[160] However, it was subject to a class 1 device recall by the FDA and pulled from the worldwide market in 2017 due to increased rates of adverse events between years 1 and 3.[161]

Anti-proliferative Drug Development

Newer-generation DES use derivatives of sirolimus, some with pharmacokinetic differences but similar mechanisms of action. For instance, zotarolimus (used in Endeavor, Resolute, and Onyx stents) differs from sirolimus at the carbon 40 position wherein a tetrazole substitution is made in place of the hydroxyl group. This modification leads to more lipophilicity and a shorter half-life, but does not substantially alter VSMC effects compared to sirolimus.[162] Xience, Promus, and Synergy DES elute Everolimus, a sirolimus analogue with a 2-hydroxyethyl substitution at position 40. This compound has decreased in vitro potency but similar in vivo efficacy in immunosuppression and transplant models.[163,164] Umirolimus is a sirolimus derivative with replacement of hydrogen at position 40 with an alkoxy-alkyl group, leading to greater lipophilicity (10-fold greater) and a longer half-life in arterial tissue.[165]

Polymer and Elution Kinetics

Preclinical studies indicate that the prevention of restenosis typically requires weeks of drug delivery.[146,166] Polymers attach drug to the stent but also control the elution kinetics. The polymer design used in the Cypher DES consisted a primer layer of Parylene C, a middle layer of 67% polyethylene-co-vinyl acetate (PEVA) and a third layer of 33% poly n-butyl methacrylate (PBMA) dissolved in the organic solvent *Tetrahydrofuran* (THF). This system leads to controlled elution of sirolimus over 30 to 60 days.[167] The Taxus stent had a polymer composed of polystyrene-b-isobutylene-b-styrene (SIBS, Translute), which eluted as an initial burst within the first 48 hours, followed by slower release over 10 to 90 days.

The Xience V/Promus stent was designed to capitalize on the biocompatibility of fluorinated surfaces.[168] This polymer is a single-phase layer of 7.8 μm consisting of a 83%/17% mixture of the semi-crystalline poly(vinylidene fluoride-co-hexafluoropropylene) (PVDF-HFP) and everolimus, leading to elution over the course of 4 months (25% released within the first day and an additional 50% over the first month.[169] In a rabbit model, this Xience V stent design had improved re-endothelialization compared to first-generation DES.[105] The Promus Element DES uses the same fluoropolymer/everolimus combination on a platinum chromium platform.

The polymer used for the Endeavor (Medtronic, Minneapolis MN) stent system is based on biomimicry of phosphorylcholine (PC), a phospholipid found on red blood cells, to optimize the biocompatibility of the surface coating. Biocompatibility testing in porcine coronary arteries shows no differences in endothelialization or inflammatory changes after PC-coated stent implantation compared to uncoated stents.[170-172] This system results in more rapid drug elution as 98% of zotarolimus elutes from the Endeavor DES within 14 days.[173]

In contrast to the Endeavor system, the zotarolimus used in Resolute stents elutes via the BioLinx polymer, resulting in more delayed elution—85% of zotarolimus elutes from the Resolute DES within 60 days and the remainder elutes by 180 days.[174] BioLinx is relatively inert in vitro due to its hydrophilic surface.[175] This formulation of three copolymers consists of a hydrophilic C19 polymer, polyvinylpyrrolidone (PVP), and a hydrophobic C10 polymer, combined in a ratio of 63%/10%/27%.

The Synergy (Boston Scientific, Marlborough, MA) stent (S-EES) uses bioabsorbable polymer attached to the abluminal surface of the stent, leaving the luminal surface polymer free. Everolimus is delivered via a polymer composed of poly-D,L-lactide-co-glycolide (PLGA). PLGA everolimus dissolution in this formulation is near complete resorption by 3 to 4 months.[176,177] The BioFreedom stent is a polymer-free construct in which the scaffold has a selectively micro-structured surface (SMS) on the abluminal side that creates greater surface area and allows umrolimus to be directly coated to the stent.

Clinical Trials of First-Generation Versus Newer DES

Trials of newer-generation DES have shown lower TLR reduced stent thrombosis rates compared with first-generation DES designs. For instance, in SPIRIT IV, the Xience V Everolimus eluting stent (X-EES) was compared to the Paclitaxel eluting stent (PES) in 3687 patients with stable CAD.[178] One year event rates were significantly lower with X-EES, including TLF (4.2% vs 6.8%; RR = 0.62, 95% CI, 0.46-0.82), MI (1.9% vs 3.1%, $P = .02$), and stent thrombosis (0.17% vs 0.85%, $P = .004$).

The COMPARE trial tested X-EES versus PES in higher-risk patients (60% had ACS and 25% had segment elevation myocardial infarction [STEMI]) and more complex lesions (45% had type C lesions).[179] The composite primary endpoint of all-cause mortality, myocardial infarction, and target vessel revascularization at 12 months was lower with X-EES (6% vs 9%, $P = 0{\cdot}02$), TLR was reduced (2% vs 5%, $P = .0002$) as was definite and probable ST (0.7% vs 3%, $P = .002$). These advantages also held up after 2 years for the primary endpoint (9.0% vs 13.7%, $P = .0016$) and definite/probable ST (0.9% vs 3.9%, $P < .0001$).[180] Rates of late ST between years 1 and 2 were also low with the X-EES (0.3% vs 1.5%, $P = .02$) despite the fact that only 13% of this high-risk population continued dual antiplatelet therapy beyond 1 year.

Clinical Trials Among Newer DES

Head-to-head trials comparing newer-generation DES have often used a noninferiority design. For instance, the Resolute All Comers trial was a noninferiority trial, powered for clinical events, comparing the Resolute zotarolimus-eluting stent (R-ZES) system to X-EES in 2292 patients (over 50% presented with ACS).[181] Rates of TLF were similar for both stents (8.2% for R-ZES vs 8.3%, $P < .001$ for non-inferiority). In-stent LLL was not statistically different between the two stents (0.27 ± 0.43 mm for R-ZES vs 0.19 ± 0.40 for X-EES, $P = .08$). Rates of definite, probable, or possible ST were similar for both stents (2.3% vs 1.5% X-EES, $P = .17$). These findings were confirmed in the TWENTE trial.[182] Patients treated with R-ZES had a TVF rate of 8.2% compared to 8.1% in patients treated with X-EES (difference 0.1%, CI: −2.8% to 3.0%, $P = .001$ for non-inferiority). Rates of definite-or-probable ST rates were similar for both stents (0.9% and 1.2% for X-EES, $P = .59$).

The Synergy (S-EES) stent was compared to the Promus Element in the EVOLVE II trial ($n = 1684$). This showed similar rates of the primary end point of 12-month target lesion failure (6.7% with Synergy; 6.5% Promus Element). Definite/probable stent thrombosis rates were also similarly low (0.4% vs 0.6%; $P = .50$).

The LEADER-FREE trial tested the BioFreedom DES versus the Gazelle BMS in those at high bleeding risk (HBR) using a background of 1 month DAPT ($n = 2466$). This trial showed superiority of this polymer-free DES compared to BMS for the primary safety end point (composite of cardiac death, myocardial infarction, and stent thrombosis) (9.4% vs 12.9%; hazard ratio, 0.71; 95% CI,

0.56-0.91; *P* < .001 for noninferiority and *P* = .005 for superiority) at 390 days. Clinically driven target-lesion revascularization was 5.1% in the drug-coated–stent group and 9.8% (hazard ratio, 0.50; 95% CI, 0.37-0.69; *P* < .001).

A recent network analysis of pooled data from 19 stent trials (*n* = 25,032) analyzed early and late events in patients receiving BMS, first-generation DES, and current-generation DES.[8] During the first year, rates of TLF were 17.8%, 8.1%, and 5.0% after BMS, first-generation DES, and current DES, respectively. However, less difference was observed in events that accrued after year 1. Between years 1 and 5, TLF rates were 7.7%, 9.5%, and 7.7% in patients receiving BMS, first-generation DES, and current DES, respectively. During this period between year 1 and 5 post-PCI, up to 40% of clinical events appear to be stent-related.[183] Thus, in contemporary PCI, TLF between years 2 and 5 exceeds the risk within the first year. Notably, in this study, there was no evidence of plateau between years 2 and 5, suggesting that TLF may still be expected to occur in ~25% to 50% of patients who live 10 to 20 years after PCI.

TREATMENT OF RESTENOSIS

DES as Therapy for ISR

The treatment for restenosis often includes a selection of procedures (intravascular imaging, various debulking options, brachytherapy, balloon angioplasty with or without a drug-coated balloon, and/or repeat stenting) that typically depend on angiographic features, clinical factors, and prior coronary procedure history.[184] Intravascular imaging is often a first step to evaluate for stent expansion or fracture and assess the degree of NIH. Such findings may factor into decisions about the need for debulking and whether to implant an additional DES. For example, focal ISR at an area of stent underexpansion may necessitate high-pressure balloon angioplasty alone.

In general, however, studies suggest repeat DES should be considered for treating the first occurrence of restenosis, especially when there is substantial residual NIH burden and/or the lesion extends outside the stented area. ISAR-DESIRE was a prospective, randomized, controlled trial that assessed the efficacy of DES in the treatment of ISR in comparison to conventional balloon angioplasty. Three hundred patients with documented angiographic ISR were randomized to receive either SES (*n* = 100), PES (*n* = 100), or balloon angioplasty (*n* = 100). Angiographic analysis preformed in 275 (92%) patients showed a significant decrease in rates of restenosis in both DES cohorts in comparison to balloon angioplasty at 9 months. A secondary analysis comparing the two DES cohorts showed a significant decrease in LLL (*P* = .004) and in-stent % DS (*P* = .004) in the SES versus the PES group. There were lower rates of in-stent, in-lesion restenosis, and MACE that did not reach significance in the SES group. There was no significant difference in the incidence of death or MI across all three groups.[185]

Brachytherapy

Intravascular brachytherapy has been shown to reduce neointimal proliferation and ISR in multiple randomized clinical trials.[186-188] The treatment was particularly successful in diabetic patients.[189] With the introduction of DES, brachytherapy has become very uncommon. The practical difficulty in scheduling the procedure with radiation oncologists and the catheterization lab, specialized availability at tertiary centers, and increased rates of subacute thrombosis have limited the wide acceptance of intracoronary radiation into clinical practice.[190,191]

Drug-Coated Balloon

Several studies suggest balloon angioplasty with a drug-coated balloon (DCB) may be an important tool for the treatment of restenosis. A study by Scheller et al showed patients with BMS ISR randomized to DCB had lower rates of restenosis and MACE (31% vs 4%, *P* = .01) compared to uncoated balloon angioplasty.[192] A paclitaxel DCB has been shown to yield similar results to restenting with a paclitaxel DES.[193] In RIBS V, BMS ISR patients randomized to DCB versus EES had inferior angiographic results but similarly low rates of TVR and MACE at 1 year.[194] In the PEPCAD-DES Study, the paclitaxel-coated balloon angioplasty arm had less LLL, lower binary restenosis rates, and 30% lower clinical events compared to uncoated balloon angioplasty for treatment of DES restenosis. Thus, coronary DCB is a promising treatment that has been approved in Europe but has yet to gain FDA approval.

CONCLUSION

Restenosis has been a limiting factor for the clinical success of PCI. The mechanism stems from an aberrant response to vascular injury including an inflammatory phase, a granulation or cellular proliferation phase, and a phase of remodeling involving ECM protein synthesis. Inflammation and cell recruitment after PCI is a complex cascade involving the aggregation of platelets and the release of chemotactic agents recruiting leukocytes, macrocytes, and monocytes. These processes stimulate smooth muscle cells to transition from a quiescent phase to active phase. The combination of a scaffold to prevent recoil and local drug delivery of an antiproliferative agent to minimize negative remodeling and NIH has proven to be a successful strategy to limit restenosis.

Iterative improvements in DES technology have led to thinner struts and optimized drug-elution strategies. Randomized clinical trials document these alterations to correspond with significant reductions in the rates of restenosis and adverse clinical events. PCI is now a durable treatment option for most patients with symptomatic CAD. Despite these advances, restenosis rates in the first year are 5% to 15% using contemporary devices in real-world populations. After 1 year, stent failure rates continue at ~2% annually without evidence of a plateau. Thus, PCI durability remains a major global health problem, requiring an even deeper understanding of the biologic mechanisms involved in vascular healing and arterial injury responses.

Key Points

- Restenosis is a pathologic form of vascular healing and occurs in three phases: an inflammatory response, granulation and cellular proliferation, and ECM protein synthesis.
- The mechanism of inflammation and cell recruitment is a complex cascade, with the aggregation of platelets and the release of chemotactic agents recruiting leukocytes prior to re-endothelialization.
- Inflammatory cells stimulate muscular SMCs from the quiescent phase to the active phase.

- The local drug delivery of antiproliferative agents has been a successful strategy in limiting restenosis.
- 1 year TLF rates for BMS, first-gen DES, and current-generation DES are approximately 18%, 8%, and 5% respectively, and 2%/year thereafter between years 1 and 5.
- The treatment of restenosis often includes repeat DES placement, but rigorous investigation of newer strategies including DCB is warranted.

References

1. Dotter CT, Judkins MP. Transluminal treatment of arteriosclerotic obstruction. description of a new technic and a preliminary report of its application. *Circulation*. 1964;30:654-670.
2. Gruntzig AR, Senning A, Siegenthaler WE. Nonoperative dilatation of coronary-artery stenosis: percutaneous transluminal coronary angioplasty. *N Engl J Med*. 1979;301(2):61-68.
3. Serruys PW, de Jaegere P, Kiemeneij F, et al. A comparison of balloon-expandable-stent implantation with balloon angioplasty in patients with coronary artery disease. Benestent Study Group. *N Engl J Med*. 1994;331(8):489-495.
4. Abbott JD, Voss MR, Nakamura M, et al. Unrestricted use of drug-eluting stents compared with bare-metal stents in routine clinical practice: findings from the National Heart, Lung, and Blood Institute Dynamic Registry. *J Am Coll Cardiol*. 2007;50(21):2029-2036.
5. Goy JJ, Stauffer JC, Siegenthaler M, Benoît A, Seydoux C. A prospective randomized comparison between paclitaxel and sirolimus stents in the real world of interventional cardiology: the TAXi trial. *J Am Coll Cardiol*. 2005;45(2):308-311.
6. Simonton CA, Brodie B, Cheek B, et al. Comparative clinical outcomes of paclitaxel- and sirolimus-eluting stents: results from a large prospective multicenter registry—STENT Group. *J Am Coll Cardiol*. 2007;50(13):1214-1222.
7. Cosgrave J, Melzi G, Corbett S, et al. Comparable clinical outcomes with paclitaxel- and sirolimus-eluting stents in unrestricted contemporary practice. *J Am Coll Cardiol*. 2007;49(24):2320-2328.
8. Madhavan MV, Kirtane AJ, Redfors B, et al. Stent-related adverse events >1 year after percutaneous coronary intervention. *J Am Coll Cardiol*. 2020;75(6):590-604. doi:10.1016/j.jacc.2019.11.058
9. Roubin GS, King SB III, Douglas JS Jr. Restenosis after percutaneous transluminal coronary angioplasty: the Emory University Hospital experience. *Am J Cardiol*. 1987;60(3):39B-43B.
10. Mehilli J, Kastrati A, Wessely R, et al. Randomized trial of a nonpolymer-based rapamycin-eluting stent versus a polymer-based paclitaxel-eluting stent for the reduction of late lumen loss. *Circulation*. 2006;113(2):273-279.
11. Morice MC, Serruys PW, Sousa JE, et al. A randomized comparison of a sirolimus-eluting stent with a standard stent for coronary revascularization. *N Engl J Med*. 2002;346(23):1773-1780.
12. Dobesh PP, Stacy ZA, Ansara AJ, Enders JM. Drug-eluting stents: a mechanical and pharmacologic approach to coronary artery disease. *Pharmacotherapy*. 2004;24(11):1554-1577.
13. Pocock SJ, Lansky AJ, Mehran R, et al. Angiographic surrogate end points in drug-eluting stent trials: a systematic evaluation based on individual patient data from 11 randomized, controlled trials. *J Am Coll Cardiol*. 2008;51(1):23-32.
14. Ruygrok PN, Webster MW, de Valk V, et al. Clinical and angiographic factors associated with asymptomatic restenosis after percutaneous coronary intervention. *Circulation*. 2001;104(19):2289-2294.
15. Bossi I, Klersy C, Black AJ, et al. In-stent restenosis: long-term outcome and predictors of subsequent target lesion revascularization after repeat balloon angioplasty. *J Am Coll Cardiol*. 2000;35(6):1569-1576.
16. Chen MS, John JM, Chew DP, Lee DS, Ellis SG, Bhatt DL. Bare metal stent restenosis is not a benign clinical entity. *Am Heart J*. 2006;151(6):1260-1264.
17. Rathore S, Kinoshita Y, Terashima M, et al. A comparison of clinical presentations, angiographic patterns and outcomes of in-stent restenosis between bare metal stents and drug eluting stents. *EuroIntervention*. 2010;5(7):841-846.
18. Serruys PW, Luijten HE, Beatt KJ, et al. Incidence of restenosis after successful coronary angioplasty: a time-related phenomenon. A quantitative angiographic study in 342 consecutive patients at 1, 2, 3, and 4 months. *Circulation*. 1988;77(2):361-371.
19. Ellis SG, Shaw RE, Gershony G, et al. Risk factors, time course and treatment effect for restenosis after successful percutaneous transluminal coronary angioplasty of chronic total occlusion. *Am J Cardiol*. 1989;63(13):897-901.
20. Nayak AK, Kawamura A, Nesto RW, et al. Myocardial infarction as a presentation of clinical in-stent restenosis. *Circ J*. 2006;70(8):1026-1029.
21. Meliga E, Garcia-Garcia HM, Valgimigli M, et al. Longest available clinical outcomes after drug-eluting stent implantation for unprotected left main coronary artery disease: the DELFT (Drug Eluting stent for LeFT main) Registry. *J Am Coll Cardiol*. 2008;51(23):2212-2219.
22. Buszman PP, Bochenek A, Konkolewska M, et al. Early and long-term outcomes after surgical and percutaneous myocardial revascularization in patients with non-ST-elevation acute coronary syndromes and unprotected left main disease. *J Invasive Cardiol*. 2009;21(11):564-569.
23. Serruys PW, Morice MC, Kappetein AP, et al. Percutaneous coronary intervention versus coronary-artery bypass grafting for severe coronary artery disease. *N Engl J Med*. 2009;360(10):961-972.
24. Aronson D, Bloomgarden Z, Rayfield EJ. Potential mechanisms promoting restenosis in diabetic patients. *J Am Coll Cardiol*. 1996;27(3):528-535.
25. Frobert O, Lagerqvist B, Carlsson J, Lindbäck J, Stenestrand U, James SK. Differences in restenosis rate with different drug-eluting stents in patients with and without diabetes mellitus: a report from the SCAAR (Swedish Angiography and Angioplasty Registry). *J Am Coll Cardiol*. 2009;53(18):1660-1667.
26. Ribichini F, Steffenino G, Dellavalle A, et al. Plasma activity and insertion/deletion polymorphism of angiotensin I-converting enzyme: a major risk factor and a marker of risk for coronary stent restenosis. *Circulation*. 1998;97(2):147-154.
27. Gürlek A, Güleç S, Karabulut H, et al. Relation between the insertion/deletion polymorphism of the angiotensin I converting enzyme gene and restenosis after coronary stenting. *J Cardiovasc Risk*. 2000;7(6):403-407. doi:10.1177/204748730000700602
28. Kastrati A, Schömig A, Seyfarth M, et al. Pl^A polymorphism of platelet glycoprotein IIIa and risk of restenosis after coronary stent placement. *Circulation*. 1999;99(8):1005-1010. doi:10.1161/01.CIR.99.8.1005
29. Vogiatzi K, Apostolakis S, Voudris V, Thomopoulou S, Kochiadakis GE, Spandidos DA. Interleukin 8 gene polymorphisms and susceptibility to restenosis after percutaneous coronary intervention. *J Thromb Thrombolysis*. 2010;29(1):134-140.
30. Koch W, Kastrati A, Mehilli J, Böttiger C, von Beckerath N, Schömig A. Insertion/deletion polymorphism of the angiotensin I-converting enzyme gene is not associated with restenosis after coronary stent placement. *Circulation*. 2000;102(2):197-202. doi:10.1161/01.cir.102.2.197
31. Ferrari M, Mudra H, Grip L, et al. Angiotensin-converting enzyme insertion/deletion polymorphism does not influence the restenosis rate after coronary stent implantation. *Cardiology*. 2002;97(1):29-36. doi:10.1159/000047416
32. Moreno PR, Bernardi VH, López-Cuéllar J, et al. Macrophage infiltration predicts restenosis after coronary intervention in patients with unstable angina. *Circulation*. 1996;94(12):3098-3102.
33. Cipollone F, Marini M, Fazia M, et al. Elevated circulating levels of monocyte chemoattractant protein-1 in patients with restenosis after coronary angioplasty. *Arterioscler Thromb Vasc Biol*. 2001;21(3):327-334.
34. Ikeda U, Shimada K. Elevated circulating levels of monocyte chemoattractant protein-1 in patients with restenosis after coronary angioplasty. *Arterioscler Thromb Vasc Biol*. 2001;21(6):1090-1091. doi:10.1161/01.ATV.21.6.1090
35. Segev A, Kassam S, Buller CE, et al. Pre-procedural plasma levels of C-reactive protein and interleukin-6 do not predict late coronary angiographic restenosis after elective stenting. *Eur Heart J*. 2004;25(12):1029-1035.

36. Yip HK, Hung WC, Yang CH, et al. Serum concentrations of high-sensitivity C-reactive protein predict progressively obstructive lesions rather than late restenosis in patients with unstable angina undergoing coronary artery stenting. *Circ J*. 2005;69(10):1202-1207.
37. Skowasch D, Jabs A, Andrié R, Lüderitz B, Bauriedel G. Progression of native coronary plaques and in-stent restenosis are associated and predicted by increased pre-procedural C reactive protein. *Heart*. 2005;91(4):535-536.
38. Katsaros KM, Wiesbauer F, Speidl WS, et al. High soluble Fas and soluble Fas ligand serum levels before stent implantation are protective against restenosis. *Thromb Haemost*. 2011;105(5):883-891.
39. de Feyter PJ, Kay P, Disco C, Serruys PW. Reference chart derived from post-stent-implantation intravascular ultrasound predictors of 6-month expected restenosis on quantitative coronary angiography. *Circulation*. 1999;100(17):1777-1783.
40. Serruys PW, Kay IP, Disco C, Deshpande NV, de Feyter PJ. Periprocedural quantitative coronary angiography after Palmaz-Schatz stent implantation predicts the restenosis rate at six months: results of a meta-analysis of the BElgian Netherlands Stent study (BENESTENT) I, BENESTENT II Pilot, BENESTENT II and MUSIC trials. Multicenter Ultrasound Stent in Coronaries. *J Am Coll Cardiol*. 1999;34(4):1067-1074.
41. Mauri L, O'Malley AJ, Popma JJ, et al. Comparison of thrombosis and restenosis risk from stent length of sirolimus-eluting stents versus bare metal stents. *Am J Cardiol*. 2005;95(10):1140-1145. doi:10.1016/j.amjcard.2005.01.039
42. Hwang CW, Wu D, Edelman ER. Physiological transport forces govern drug distribution for stent-based delivery. *Circulation*. 2001;104(5):600-605.
43. Takebayashi H, Mintz GS, Carlier SG, et al. Nonuniform strut distribution correlates with more neointimal hyperplasia after sirolimus-eluting stent implantation. *Circulation*. 2004;110(22):3430-3434.
44. Costa MA, Angiolillo DJ, Tannenbaum M, et al. Impact of stent deployment procedural factors on long-term effectiveness and safety of sirolimus-eluting stents (final results of the multicenter prospective STLLR trial). *Am J Cardiol*. 2008;101(12):1704-1711. doi:doi:10.1016/j.amjcard.2008.02.053
45. Hirshfeld JW Jr, Schwartz JS, Jugo R, et al. Restenosis after coronary angioplasty: a multivariate statistical model to relate lesion and procedure variables to restenosis. The M-HEART Investigators. *J Am Coll Cardiol*. 1991;18(3):647-656.
46. Foley DP, Melkert R, Serruys PW. Influence of coronary vessel size on renarrowing process and late angiographic outcome after successful balloon angioplasty. *Circulation*. 1994;90(3):1239-1251.
47. Violaris AG, Melkert R, Serruys PW. Long-term luminal renarrowing after successful elective coronary angioplasty of total occlusions. A quantitative angiographic analysis. *Circulation*. 1995;91(8):2140-2150.
48. Kastrati A, Schomig A, Elezi S, et al. Predictive factors of restenosis after coronary stent placement. *J Am Coll Cardiol*. 1997;30(6):1428-1436.
49. Kastrati A, Elezi S, Dirschinger J, Hadamitzky M, Neumann FJ, Schomig A. Influence of lesion length on restenosis after coronary stent placement. *Am J Cardiol*. 1999;83(12):1617-1622.
50. Doi H, Maehara A, Mintz GS, et al. Classification and potential mechanisms of intravascular ultrasound patterns of stent fracture. *Am J Cardiol*. 2009;103(6):818-823.
51. Aoki J, Nakazawa G, Tanabe K, et al. Incidence and clinical impact of coronary stent fracture after sirolimus-eluting stent implantation. *Catheter Cardiovasc Interv*. 2007;69(3):380-386.
52. Lee MS, Jurewitz D, Aragon J, Forrester J, Makkar RR, Kar S. Stent fracture associated with drug-eluting stents: clinical characteristics and implications. *Catheter Cardiovasc Interv*. 2007;69(3):387-394.
53. Umeda H, Gochi T, Iwase M, et al. Frequency, predictors and outcome of stent fracture after sirolimus-eluting stent implantation. *Int J Cardiol*. 2009;133(3):321-326.
54. Dangas GD, Claessen BE, Caixeta A, Sanidas EA, Mintz GS, Mehran R. In-stent restenosis in the drug-eluting stent era. *J Am Coll Cardiol*. 2010;56(23):1897-1907.
55. Mehran R, Dangas G, Abizaid AS, et al. Angiographic patterns of in-stent restenosis: classification and implications for long-term outcome. *Circulation*. 1999;100(18):1872-1878.
56. Forrester JS, Fishbein M, Helfant R, Fagin J. A paradigm for restenosis based on cell biology: clues for the development of new preventive therapies. *J Am Coll Cardiol*. 1991;17(3):758-769.
57. Rensing BJ, Hermans WR, Beatt KJ, et al. Quantitative angiographic assessment of elastic recoil after percutaneous transluminal coronary angioplasty. *Am J Cardiol*. 1990;66(15):1039-1044.
58. Violaris AG, Serruys PW. New technologies in interventional cardiology. *Curr Opin Cardiol*. 1994;9(4):493-502.
59. Mintz GS, Popma J, Pichard A, et al. Intravascular ultrasound assessment of the mechanisms and predictors of restenosis following coronary angioplasty. *J Invasive Cardiol*. 1996;8:1-14.
60. Park SJ, Kang SJ, Virmani R, Nakano M, Ueda Y. In-stent neoatherosclerosis: a final common pathway of late stent failure. *J Am Coll Cardiol*. 2012;59(23):2051-2057.
61. Marcus AJ. Thrombosis and inflammation as multicellular processes: significance of cell–cell interactions. *Semin Hematol*. 1994;31(4):261-269.
62. Diacovo TG, Roth SJ, Buccola JM, Bainton DF, Springer TA. Neutrophil rolling, arrest, and transmigration across activated, surface-adherent platelets via sequential action of P-selectin and the beta 2-integrin CD11b/CD18. *Blood*. 1996;88(1):146-157.
63. Yeo EL, Sheppard JA, Feuerstein IA. Role of P-selectin and leukocyte activation in polymorphonuclear cell adhesion to surface adherent activated platelets under physiologic shear conditions (an injury vessel wall model). *Blood*. 1994;83(9):2498-2507.
64. Farb A, Weber DK, Kolodgie FD, Burke AP, Virmani R. Morphological predictors of restenosis after coronary stenting in humans. *Circulation*. 2002;105(25):2974-2980.
65. Inoue T, Sakai Y, Morooka S, Hayashi T, Takayanagi K, Takabatake Y. Expression of polymorphonuclear leukocyte adhesion molecules and its clinical significance in patients treated with percutaneous transluminal coronary angioplasty. *J Am Coll Cardiol*. 1996;28(5):1127-1133.
66. Inoue T, Uchida T, Yaguchi I, Sakai Y, Takayanagi K, Morooka S. Stent-induced expression and activation of the leukocyte integrin Mac-1 is associated with neointimal thickening and restenosis. *Circulation*. 2003;107(13):1757-1763.
67. Pietersma A, Kofflard M, de Wit LE, et al. Late lumen loss after coronary angioplasty is associated with the activation status of circulating phagocytes before treatment. *Circulation*. 1995;91(5):1320-1325.
68. Gaspardone A, Crea F, Versaci F, et al. Predictive value of C-reactive protein after successful coronary-artery stenting in patients with stable angina. *Am J Cardiol*. 1998;82(4):515-518.
69. Cybulsky MI, Gimbrone MA Jr. Endothelial expression of a mononuclear leukocyte adhesion molecule during atherogenesis. *Science*. 1991;251(4995):788-791.
70. Li H, Cybulsky MI, Gimbrone MA Jr, Libby P. An atherogenic diet rapidly induces VCAM-1, a cytokine-regulatable mononuclear leukocyte adhesion molecule, in rabbit aortic endothelium. *Arterioscler Thromb*. 1993;13(2):197-204.
71. Li H, Cybulsky MI, Gimbrone MA Jr, Libby P. Inducible expression of vascular cell adhesion molecule-1 by vascular smooth muscle cells in vitro and within rabbit atheroma. *Am J Pathol*. 1993;143(6):1551-1559.
72. Richardson M, Hadcock SJ, DeReske M, Cybulsky MI. Increased expression in vivo of VCAM-1 and E-selectin by the aortic endothelium of normolipemic and hyperlipemic diabetic rabbits. *Arterioscler Thromb*. 1994;14(5):760-769.
73. Walpola PL, Gotlieb AI, Cybulsky MI, Langille BL. Expression of ICAM-1 and VCAM-1 and monocyte adherence in arteries exposed to altered shear stress. *Arterioscler Thromb Vasc Biol*. 1995;15(1):2-10.
74. Tanaka H, Sukhova GK, Swanson SJ, et al. Sustained activation of vascular cells and leukocytes in the rabbit aorta after balloon injury. *Circulation*. 1993;88(4 pt 1):1788-1803.
75. Welt FG, Edelman ER, Simon DI, Rogers C. Neutrophil, not macrophage, infiltration precedes neointimal thickening in balloon-injured arteries. *Arterioscler Thromb Vasc Biol*. 2000;20(12):2553-2558.
76. Rogers C, Welt FG, Karnovsky MJ, Edelman ER. Monocyte recruitment and neointimal hyperplasia in rabbits. Coupled inhibitory effects of heparin. *Arterioscler Thromb Vasc Biol*. 1996;16(10):1312-1318.
77. Rogers C, Edelman ER, Simon DI. A mAb to the beta2-leukocyte integrin Mac-1 (CD11b/CD18) reduces intimal thickening after

angioplasty or stent implantation in rabbits. *Proc Natl Acad Sci U S A*. 1998;95(17):10134-10139.
78. Mori E, Komori K, Yamaoka T, et al. Essential role of monocyte chemoattractant protein-1 in development of restenotic changes (neointimal hyperplasia and constrictive remodeling) after balloon angioplasty in hypercholesterolemic rabbits. *Circulation*. 2002;105(24):2905-2910.
79. Libby P, Schwartz D, Brogi E, Tanaka H, Clinton SK. A cascade model for restenosis. A special case of atherosclerosis progression. *Circulation*. 1992;86(6 suppl):III47-III52.
80. Kockx MM, De Meyer GR, Jacob WA, Bult H, Herman AG. Triphasic sequence of neointimal formation in the cuffed carotid artery of the rabbit. *Arterioscler Thromb*. 1992;12:1447-1457.
81. Jørgensen L, Grøthe AG, Groves HM, Kinlough-Rathbone RL, Richardson M, Mustard JF. Sequence of cellular responses in rabbit aortas following one and two injuries with a balloon catheter. *Br J Exp Pathol*. 1988;69(4):473-486.
82. Richardson M, Hatton MW, Buchanan MR, Moore S. Wound healing in the media of the normolipemic rabbit carotid artery injured by air drying or by balloon catheter de-endothelialization. *Am J Pathol*. 1990;137(6):1453-1465.
83. Lloyd AR, Oppenheim JJ. Poly's lament: the neglected role of the polymorphonuclear neutrophil in the afferent limb of the immune response. *Immunol Today*. 1992;13(5):169-172.
84. Mintz GS, Popma JJ, Pichard AD, et al. Arterial remodeling after coronary angioplasty: a serial intravascular ultrasound study. *Circulation*. 1996;94(1):35-43.
85. Lansky AJ, Mintz GS, Popma JJ, et al. Remodeling after directional coronary atherectomy (with and without adjunct percutaneous transluminal coronary angioplasty): a serial angiographic and intravascular ultrasound analysis from the Optimal Atherectomy Restenosis Study. *J Am Coll Cardiol*. 1998;32(2):329-337.
86. Kimura T, Nobuyoshi M. Remodelling and restenosis: intravascular ultrasound studies. *Semin Interv Cardiol*. 1997;2(3):159-166.
87. Scott NA, Cipolla GD, Ross CE, et al. Identification of a potential role for the adventitia in vascular lesion formation after balloon overstretch injury of porcine coronary arteries. *Circulation*. 1996;93(12):2178-2187.
88. Wilcox JN, Waksman R, King SB, Scott NA. The role of the adventitia in the arterial response to angioplasty: the effect of intravascular radiation. *Int J Radiat Oncol Biol Phys*. 1996;36(4):789-796.
89. Indolfi C, Mongiardo A, Curcio A, Torella D. Molecular mechanisms of in-stent restenosis and approach to therapy with eluting stents. *Trends Cardiovasc Med*. 2003;13(4):142-148.
90. Indolfi C, Avvedimento EV, Di Lorenzo E, et al. Activation of cAMP-PKA signaling in vivo inhibits smooth muscle cell proliferation induced by vascular injury. *Nat Med*. 1997;3(7):775-779.
91. Indolfi C, Avvedimento EV, Rapacciuolo A, et al. Inhibition of cellular ras prevents smooth muscle cell proliferation after vascular injury in vivo. *Nat Med*. 1995;1(6):541-545.
92. Indolfi C, Avvedimento EV, Rapacciuolo A, et al. In vivo gene transfer: prevention of neointima formation by inhibition of mitogen-activated protein kinase kinase. *Basic Res Cardiol*. 1997;92(6):378-384.
93. Schwartz RS, Henry TD. Pathophysiology of coronary artery restenosis. *Rev Cardiovasc Med*. 2002;3(suppl 5):S4-S9.
94. Grewe PH, Deneke T, Machraoui A, Barmeyer J, Müller KM. Acute and chronic tissue response to coronary stent implantation: pathologic findings in human specimen. *J Am Coll Cardiol*. 2000;35(1):157-163.
95. Breeman A, Serruys PW, van den Brand MJ, Deckers JW, van Herwerden LA, Roelandt JR. Complications shortly after transluminal angioplasty or following coronary surgery in 183 comparable patients with multi-vessel coronary disease. *Ned Tijdschr Geneeskd*. 1994;138(21):1074-1080.
96. Fischman DL, Leon MB, Baim DS, et al. A randomized comparison of coronary-stent placement and balloon angioplasty in the treatment of coronary artery disease. Stent Restenosis Study Investigators. *N Engl J Med*. 1994;331(8):496-501.
97. Hoffmann R, Mintz GS, Dussaillant GR, et al. Patterns and mechanisms of in-stent restenosis. A serial intravascular ultrasound study. *Circulation*. 1996;94(6):1247-1254.
98. Inoue T, Sohma R, Miyazaki T, Iwasaki Y, Yaguchi I, Morooka S. Comparison of activation process of platelets and neutrophils after coronary stent implantation versus balloon angioplasty for stable angina pectoris. *Am J Cardiol*. 2000;86(10):1057-1062.
99. Kornowski R, Hong MK, Tio FO, Bramwell O, Wu H, Leon MB. In-stent restenosis: contributions of inflammatory responses and arterial injury to neointimal hyperplasia. *J Am Coll Cardiol*. 1998;31(1):224-230.
100. Koster R, Vieluf D, Kiehn M, et al. Nickel and molybdenum contact allergies in patients with coronary in-stent restenosis. *Lancet*. 2000;356(9245):1895-1897.
101. Nakazawa G, Otsuka F, Nakano M, et al. The pathology of neoatherosclerosis in human coronary implants bare-metal and drug-eluting stents. *J Am Coll Cardiol*. 2011;57(11):1314-1322.
102. Nakazawa G, Ladich E, Finn AV, Virmani R. Pathophysiology of vascular healing and stent mediated arterial injury. *EuroIntervention*. 2008;4(suppl C):C7-C10.
103. Otsuka F, Vorpahl M, Nakano M, et al. Pathology of second-generation everolimus-eluting stents versus first-generation sirolimus- and paclitaxel-eluting stents in humans. *Circulation*. 2014;129(2):211-223.
104. Otsuka F, Sakakura K, Yahagi K. Contribution of in-stent neoatherosclerosis to late stent failure following bare metal and 1st- and 2nd-generation drug-eluting stent placement: an autopsy study. *J Am Coll Cardiol*. 2014;64:B190-B191.
105. Joner M, Nakazawa G, Finn AV, et al. Endothelial cell recovery between comparator polymer-based drug-eluting stents. *J Am Coll Cardiol*. 2008;52(5):333-342.
106. Nakazawa G, Nakano M, Otsuka F, et al. Evaluation of polymer-based comparator drug-eluting stents using a rabbit model of iliac artery atherosclerosis. *Circ Cardiovasc Interv*. 2011;4(1):38-46.
107. Otsuka F, Finn AV, Yazdani SK, Nakano M, Kolodgie FD, Virmani R. The importance of the endothelium in atherothrombosis and coronary stenting. *Nat Rev Cardiol*. 2012;9(8):439-453.
108. Fitzgerald PJ, Oshima A, Hayase M, et al. Final results of the Can Routine Ultrasound Influence Stent Expansion (CRUISE) study. *Circulation*. 2000;102(5):523-530.
109. Bittl JA, Chew DP, Topol EJ, Kong DF, Califf RM. Meta-analysis of randomized trials of percutaneous transluminal coronary angioplasty versus atherectomy, cutting balloon atherotomy, or laser angioplasty. *J Am Coll Cardiol*. 2004;43(6):936-942.
110. Martinez-Elbal L, Ruiz-Nodar JM, Zueco J, et al. Direct coronary stenting versus stenting with balloon pre-dilation: immediate and follow-up results of a multicentre, prospective, randomized study. The DISCO trial. DIrect Stenting of COronary Arteries. *Eur Heart J*. 2002;23(8):633-640.
111. Clowes AW, Clowes MM. Kinetics of cellular proliferation after arterial injury. II. Inhibition of smooth muscle growth by heparin. *Lab Invest*. 1985;52(6):611-616.
112. Clowes AW, Clowes MM. Kinetics of cellular proliferation after arterial injury. IV. Heparin inhibits rat smooth muscle mitogenesis and migration. *Circ Res*. 1986;58(6):839-845.
113. Edelman ER, Karnovsky MJ. Contrasting effects of the intermittent and continuous administration of heparin in experimental restenosis. *Circulation*. 1994;89(2):770-776.
114. Brack MJ, Ray S, Chauhan A, et al. The Subcutaneous Heparin and Angioplasty Restenosis Prevention (SHARP) trial. Results of a multicenter randomized trial investigating the effects of high dose unfractionated heparin on angiographic restenosis and clinical outcome. *J Am Coll Cardiol*. 1995;26(4):947-954.
115. Grassman ED, Leya F, Fareed J, et al. A randomized trial of the low-molecular-weight heparin certoparin to prevent restenosis following coronary angioplasty. *J Invasive Cardiol*. 2001;13(11):723-728.
116. Dangas G, Iakovou I. The end of systemic anticoagulation therapy for restenosis prevention. *J Invasive Cardiol*. 2001;13(11):729-731.
117. Sarembock IJ, Gertz SD, Gimple LW, Owen RM, Powers ER, Roberts WC. Effectiveness of recombinant desulphatohirudin in reducing restenosis after balloon angioplasty of atherosclerotic femoral arteries in rabbits. *Circulation*. 1991;84(1):232-243.
118. Serruys PW, Herrman JP, Simon R, et al. A comparison of hirudin with heparin in the prevention of restenosis after coronary angioplasty. Helvetica Investigators. *N Engl J Med*. 1995;333(12):757-763.
119. Burchenal JE, Marks DS, Tift Mann J, et al. Effect of direct thrombin inhibition with Bivalirudin (Hirulog) on restenosis after coronary angioplasty. *Am J Cardiol*. 1998;82(4):511-515.

120. Leon MB, Baim DS, Popma JJ, et al. A clinical trial comparing three antithrombotic-drug regimens after coronary-artery stenting. Stent Anticoagulation Restenosis Study Investigators. *N Engl J Med.* 1998;339(23):1665-1671.
121. Schwartz L, Bourassa MG, Lespérance J, et al. Aspirin and dipyridamole in the prevention of restenosis after percutaneous transluminal coronary angioplasty. *N Engl J Med.* 1988;318(26):1714-1719.
122. Savage MP, Goldberg S, Bove AA, et al. Effect of thromboxane A2 blockade on clinical outcome and restenosis after successful coronary angioplasty. Multi-Hospital Eastern Atlantic Restenosis Trial (M-HEART II). *Circulation.* 1995;92(11):3194-3200.
123. Rensing BJ, Hermans WR, Vos J, et al. Luminal narrowing after percutaneous transluminal coronary angioplasty. A study of clinical, procedural, and lesional factors related to long-term angiographic outcome. Coronary Artery Restenosis Prevention on Repeated Thromboxane Antagonism (CARPORT) Study Group. *Circulation.* 1993;88(3):975-985.
124. Welt FG, Rogers C. Inflammation and restenosis in the stent era. *Arterioscler Thromb Vasc Biol.* 2002;22(11):1769-1776.
125. Blindt R, Bosserhoff AK, Zeiffer U, Krott N, Hanrath P, vom Dahl J. Abciximab inhibits the migration and invasion potential of human coronary artery smooth muscle cells. *J Mol Cell Cardiol.* 2000;32(12):2195-2206.
126. Liu Y, Shakur Y, Yoshitake M, Kambayashi Ji J. Cilostazol (pletal): a dual inhibitor of cyclic nucleotide phosphodiesterase type 3 and adenosine uptake. *Cardiovasc Drug Rev.* 2001;19(4):369-386.
127. Tsutsui M, Shimokawa H, Higuchi S, et al. Effect of cilostazol, a novel anti-platelet drug, on restenosis after percutaneous transluminal coronary angioplasty. *Jpn Circ J.* 1996;60(4):207-215.
128. Douglas JS Jr, Holmes DR Jr, Kereiakes DJ, et al. Coronary stent restenosis in patients treated with cilostazol. *Circulation.* 2005;112(18):2826-2832.
129. Tamhane U, Meier P, Chetcuti S, et al. Efficacy of cilostazol in reducing restenosis in patients undergoing contemporary stent based PCI: a meta-analysis of randomised controlled trials. *EuroIntervention.* 2009;5(3):384-393.
130. Pepine CJ, Hirshfeld JW, Macdonald RG, et al. A controlled trial of corticosteroids to prevent restenosis after coronary angioplasty. M-HEART Group. *Circulation.* 1990;81(6):1753-1761.
131. Freed M, Safian RD, O'Neill WW, Safian M, Jones D, Grines CL. Combination of lovastatin, enalapril, and colchicine does not prevent restenosis after percutaneous transluminal coronary angioplasty. *Am J Cardiol.* 1995;76(16):1185-1188.
132. Schonbeck U, Sukhova GK, Graber P, Coulter S, Libby P. Augmented expression of cyclooxygenase-2 in human atherosclerotic lesions. *Am J Pathol.* 1999;155(4):1281-1291.
133. Whitworth HB, Roubin GS, Hollman J, et al. Effect of nifedipine on recurrent stenosis after percutaneous transluminal coronary angioplasty. *J Am Coll Cardiol.* 1986;8(6):1271-1276.
134. Hoberg E, Kubler W. Calcium-antagonists in preventing restenosis following coronary angioplasty. *Cardiologia.* 1991;36(12 suppl 1):225-227.
135. O'Keefe JH Jr, Giorgi LV, Hartzler GO, et al. Effects of diltiazem on complications and restenosis after coronary angioplasty. *Am J Cardiol.* 1991;67(5):373-376.
136. Hillegass WB, Ohman EM, Leimberger JD, Califf RM. A meta-analysis of randomized trials of calcium antagonists to reduce restenosis after coronary angioplasty. *Am J Cardiol.* 1994;73(12):835-839.
137. Suzuki T, Kopia G, Hayashi S, et al. Stent-based delivery of sirolimus reduces neointimal formation in a porcine coronary model. *Circulation.* 2001;104(10):1188-1193.
138. Farb A, Heller PF, Shroff S, et al. Pathological analysis of local delivery of paclitaxel via a polymer-coated stent. *Circulation.* 2001;104(4):473-479.
139. Park SJ, Shim WH, Ho DS, et al. A paclitaxel-eluting stent for the prevention of coronary restenosis. *N Engl J Med.* 2003;348(16):1537-1545.
140. Sousa JE, Costa MA, Abizaid A, et al. Lack of neointimal proliferation after implantation of sirolimus-coated stents in human coronary arteries: a quantitative coronary angiography and three-dimensional intravascular ultrasound study. *Circulation.* 2001;103(2):192-195.
141. Serruys PW, Sianos G, Abizaid A, et al. The effect of variable dose and release kinetics on neointimal hyperplasia using a novel paclitaxel-eluting stent platform: the Paclitaxel In-Stent Controlled Elution Study (PISCES). *J Am Coll Cardiol.* 2005;46(2):253-260.
142. Tanner FC, Yang ZY, Duckers E, Gordon D, Nabel GJ, Nabel EG. Expression of cyclin-dependent kinase inhibitors in vascular disease. *Circ Res.* 1998;82(3):396-403.
143. Poon M, Marx SO, Gallo R, Badimon JJ, Taubman MB, Marks AR. Rapamycin inhibits vascular smooth muscle cell migration. *J Clin Invest.* 1996;98(10):2277-2283.
144. Moses JW, Leon MB, Popma JJ, et al. Sirolimus-eluting stents versus standard stents in patients with stenosis in a native coronary artery. *N Engl J Med.* 2003;349(14):1315-1323.
145. Popma JJ, Leon MB, Moses JW, et al. Quantitative assessment of angiographic restenosis after sirolimus-eluting stent implantation in native coronary arteries. *Circulation.* 2004;110(25):3773-3780.
146. Colombo A, Drzewiecki J, Banning A, et al. Randomized study to assess the effectiveness of slow- and moderate-release polymer-based paclitaxel-eluting stents for coronary artery lesions. *Circulation.* 2003;108(7):788-794.
147. Halkin A, Stone GW. Polymer-based paclitaxel-eluting stents in percutaneous coronary intervention: a review of the TAXUS trials. *J Interv Cardiol.* 2004;17(5):271-282.
148. Stone GW, Ellis SG, Cox DA, et al. One-year clinical results with the slow-release, polymer-based, paclitaxel-eluting TAXUS stent: the TAXUS-IV trial. *Circulation.* 2004;109(16):1942-1947.
149. Stone GW, Ellis SG, Cox DA, et al. A polymer-based, paclitaxel-eluting stent in patients with coronary artery disease. *N Engl J Med.* 2004;350(3):221-231.
150. Morice MC, Colombo A, Meier B, et al. Sirolimus-vs paclitaxel-eluting stents in de novo coronary artery lesions: the REALITY trial—a randomized controlled trial. *JAMA.* 2006;295(8):895-904.
151. Windecker S, Remondino A, Eberli FR, et al. Sirolimus-eluting and paclitaxel-eluting stents for coronary revascularization. *N Engl J Med.* 2005;353(7):653-662.
152. Ohlmann P, Mintz GS, Kim SW, et al. Intravascular ultrasound findings in patients with restenosis of sirolimus- and paclitaxel-eluting stents. *Int J Cardiol.* 2008;125(1):11-15.
153. Raber L, Serruys PW. Late vascular response following drug-eluting stent implantation. *JACC Cardiovasc Interv.* 2011;4(10):1075-1078.
154. Garasic JM, Edelman ER, Squire JC, Seifert P, Williams MS, Rogers C. Stent and artery geometry determine intimal thickening independent of arterial injury. *Circulation.* 2000;101(7):812-818. doi:10.1161/01.cir.101.7.812
155. Rogers C, Edelman ER. Endovascular stent design dictates experimental restenosis and thrombosis. *Circulation.* 1995;91(12):2995-3001. doi:10.1161/01.cir.91.12.2995
156. Stone GW, Teirstein PS, Meredith IT, et al. A prospective, randomized evaluation of a novel everolimus-eluting coronary stent: the PLATINUM (A prospective, randomized, multicenter trial to assess an everolimus-eluting coronary stent system [PROMUS element] for the treatment of up to two de novo coronary artery lesions) trial. *J Am Coll Cardiol.* 2011;57(16):1700-1708. doi:10.1016/j.jacc.2011.02.016
157. Hoffmann R, Mintz GS, Haager PK, et al. Relation of stent design and stent surface material to subsequent in-stent intimal hyperplasia in coronary arteries determined by intravascular ultrasound. *Am J Cardiol.* 2002;89(12):1360-1364. doi:10.1016/s0002-9149(02)02347-0
158. Pache J, Kastrati A, Mehilli J, et al. Intracoronary stenting and angiographic results: strut thickness effect on restenosis outcome (ISAR-STEREO-2) trial. *J Am Coll Cardiol.* 2003;41(8):1283-1288. doi:doi:10.1016/s0735-1097(03)00119-0
159. Giacchi G, Ortega-Paz L, Brugaletta S, Ishida K, Sabaté M. Bioresorbable vascular scaffolds technology: current use and future developments. *Med Devices.* 2016;9:185-198. doi:10.2147/MDER.S90461
160. Ellis SG, Kereiakes DJ, Metzger DC, et al. Everolimus-eluting bioresorbable scaffolds for coronary artery disease. *N Engl J Med.* 2015;373(20):1905-1915. doi:10.1056/NEJMoa1509038
161. Kereiakes DJ, Ellis SG, Metzger C, et al. 3-Year clinical outcomes with everolimus-eluting bioresorbable coronary scaffolds: the ABSORB III trial. *J Am Coll Cardiol.* 2017;70(23):2852-2862. doi:10.1016/j.jacc.2017.10.010
162. Chen YW, Smith ML, Sheets M, et al. Zotarolimus, a novel sirolimus analogue with potent anti-proliferative activity on coronary smooth muscle cells and reduced potential for systemic immunosuppression. *J Cardiovasc Pharmacol.* 2007;49(4):228-235. doi:10.1097/FJC.0b013e3180325b0a

163. Schuler W, Sedrani R, Cottens S, et al. SDZ RAD, a new rapamycin derivative: pharmacological properties in vitro and in vivo. *Transplantation.* 1997;64(1):36-42.
164. Sedrani R, Cottens S, Kallen J, Schuler W. Chemical modification of rapamycin: the discovery of SDZ RAD. *Transplant Proc.* 1998;30(5):2192-2194. doi:10.1016/s0041-1345(98)00587-9
165. Tada N, Virmani R, Grant G, et al. Polymer-free biolimus a9-coated stent demonstrates more sustained intimal inhibition, improved healing, and reduced inflammation compared with a polymer-coated sirolimus-eluting cypher stent in a porcine model. *Circ Cardiovasc Interv.* 2010;3(2):174-183. doi:10.1161/circinterventions.109.877522
166. Lansky AJ, Costa RA, Mintz GS, et al. Non-polymer-based paclitaxel-coated coronary stents for the treatment of patients with de novo coronary lesions: angiographic follow-up of the DELIVER clinical trial. *Circulation.* 2004;109(16):1948-1954. doi:10.1161/01.cir.0000127129.94129.6f
167. Sousa JE, Costa MA, Abizaid AC, et al. Sustained suppression of neointimal proliferation by sirolimus-eluting stents: one-year angiographic and intravascular ultrasound follow-up. *Circulation.* 2001 2001;104(17):2007-2011. doi:10.1161/hc4201.098056
168. Guidoin R, Marois Y, Zhang Z, et al. The benefits of fluoropassivation of polyester arterial prostheses as observed in a canine model. *Am Soc Artif Intern Organs J.* 1994;40(3):M870-M879.
169. Sheiban I, Villata G, Bollati M, Sillano D, Lotrionte M, Biondi-Zoccai G. Next-generation drug-eluting stents in coronary artery disease: focus on everolimus-eluting stent (Xience V). *Vasc Health Risk Manag.* 2008;4(1):31-38.
170. Whelan DM, van der Giessen WJ, Krabbendam SC, et al. Biocompatibility of phosphorylcholine coated stents in normal porcine coronary arteries. *Heart.* 2000;83(3):338-345.
171. Lewis AL, Tolhurst LA, Stratford PW. Analysis of a phosphorylcholine-based polymer coating on a coronary stent pre- and post-implantation. *Biomaterials.* 2002;23(7):1697-1706. doi:10.1016/s0142-9612(01)00297-6
172. Malik N, Gunn J, Shepherd L, Crossman DC, Cumberland DC, Holt CM. Phosphorylcholine-coated stents in porcine coronary arteries: in vivo assessment of biocompatibility. *J Invasive Cardiol.* 2001;13(3):193-201.
173. Pinto Slottow TL, Waksman R. Overview of the 2007 Food and drug administration circulatory system devices panel meeting on the endeavor zotarolimus-eluting coronary stent. *Circulation.* 2008;117(12):1603-1608. doi:10.1161/circulationaha.107.752261
174. Meredith IT, Worthley S, Whitbourn R, et al. The next-generation Endeavor Resolute stent: 4-month clinical and angiographic results from the Endeavor Resolute first-in-man trial. *EuroIntervention.* 2007;3(1):50-53.
175. Hezi-Yamit A, Sullivan C, Wong J, et al. Novel high throughput polymer biocompatibility screening designed for SAR (Structure-Activity relationship): application for evaluating polymer coatings for cardiovascular drug-eluting stents. *Comb Chem High Throughput Screen.* 2009;12(7):664-676. doi:10.2174/138620709788923674
176. Bennett J, Dubois C. A novel platinum chromium everolimus-eluting stent for the treatment of coronary artery disease. *Biologics.* 2013;7:149-159. doi:10.2147/BTT.S34939
177. Wilson GJ, Marks A, Berg KJ, et al. The SYNERGY biodegradable polymer everolimus eluting coronary stent: porcine vascular compatibility and polymer safety study. *Catheter Cardiovasc Interv.* 2015;86(6):E247-E257. doi:10.1002/ccd.25993
178. Stone GW, Midei M, Newman W, et al; SPIRIT III Investigators. Comparison of an everolimus-eluting stent and a paclitaxel-eluting stent in patients with coronary artery disease: a randomized trial. *JAMA.* 2008;299(16):1903-1913.
179. Kedhi E, Joesoef KS, McFadden E, et al. Second-generation everolimus-eluting and paclitaxel-eluting stents in real-life practice (COMPARE): a randomised trial. *Lancet.* 2010;375(9710):201-209. doi:10.1016/s0140-6736(09)62127-9
180. Smits PC, Kedhi E, Royaards KJ, et al. 2-Year follow-up of a randomized controlled trial of everolimus- and paclitaxel-eluting stents for coronary revascularization in daily PracticeCOMPARE (comparison of the everolimus eluting XIENCE-V stent with the paclitaxel eluting TAXUS LIBERTÉ stent in all-comers: a randomized open label trial). *J Am Coll Cardiol.* 2011;58(1):11-18. doi:10.1016/j.jacc.2011.02.023
181. Serruys PW, Silber S, Garg S, et al. Comparison of zotarolimus-eluting and everolimus-eluting coronary stents. *N Engl J Med.* 2010;363(2):136-146. doi:10.1056/NEJMoa1004130
182. von Birgelen C, Basalus MWZ, Tandjung K, et al. A randomized controlled trial in second-generation zotarolimus-eluting Resolute stents versus everolimus-eluting Xience V stents in real-world patients: the TWENTE trial. *J Am Coll Cardiol.* 2012;59(15):1350-1361. doi:10.1016/j.jacc.2012.01.008
183. Sabaté M, Mack M. Very late outcomes after stent implantation: it is time to target the nontarget sites. *J Am Coll Cardiol.* 2020;75(6):605-607. doi:10.1016/j.jacc.2019.12.018
184. Giustino G, Colombo A, Camaj A, et al. Coronary in-stent restenosis: JACC state-of-the-art review. *J Am Coll Cardiol.* 2022;80(4):348-372. doi:10.1016/j.jacc.2022.05.017
185. Kastrati A, Mehilli J, von Beckerath N, et al. Sirolimus-eluting stent or paclitaxel-eluting stent vs balloon angioplasty for prevention of recurrences in patients with coronary in-stent restenosis: a randomized controlled trial. *JAMA.* 2005;293(2):165-171.
186. Raizner AE, Oesterle SN, Waksman R, et al. Inhibition of restenosis with beta-emitting radiotherapy: report of the Proliferation Reduction with Vascular Energy Trial (PREVENT). *Circulation.* 2000;102(9):951-958.
187. Sabate M, Pimentel G, Prieto C, et al. Intracoronary brachytherapy after stenting de novo lesions in diabetic patients: results of a randomized intravascular ultrasound study. *J Am Coll Cardiol.* 2004;44(3):520-527.
188. Coen V, Serruys P, Sauerwein W, et al. Reno, a European postmarket surveillance registry, confirms effectiveness of coronary brachytherapy in routine clinical practice. *Int J Radiat Oncol Biol Phys.* 2003;55(4):1019-1026.
189. Baumgart D, Bonan R, Naber C, et al. Successful reduction of in-stent restenosis in long lesions using beta-radiation—subanalysis from the RENO registry. *Int J Radiat Oncol Biol Phys.* 2004;58(3):817-827.
190. Amols HI, Zaider M, Weinberger J, Ennis R, Schiff PB, Reinstein LE. Dosimetric considerations for catheter-based beta and gamma emitters in the therapy of neointimal hyperplasia in human coronary arteries. *Int J Radiat Oncol Biol Phys.* 1996;36(4):913-921.
191. Sabate M, Costa MA, Kozuma K, et al. Methodological and clinical implications of the relocation of the minimal luminal diameter after intracoronary radiation therapy. Dose Finding Study Group. *J Am Coll Cardiol.* 2000;36(5):1536-1541.
192. Scheller B, Hehrlein C, Bocksch W, et al. Treatment of coronary in-stent restenosis with a paclitaxel-coated balloon catheter. *N Engl J Med.* 2006;355(20):2113-2124. doi:10.1056/NEJMoa061254
193. Unverdorben M, Vallbracht C, Cremers B, et al. Paclitaxel-coated balloon catheter versus paclitaxel-coated stent for the treatment of coronary in-stent restenosis. *Circulation.* 2009;119(23):2986-2994. doi:10.1161/circulationaha.108.839282
194. Alfonso F, Perez-Vizcayno MJ, Cardenas A, et al. A randomized comparison of drug-eluting balloon versus everolimus-eluting stent in patients with bare-metal stent-in-stent restenosis: the RIBS V Clinical Trial (Restenosis Intra-stent of Bare Metal Stents—paclitaxel-eluting balloon vs. everolimus-eluting stent). *J Am Coll Cardiol.* 2014;63(14):1378-1386. doi:10.1016/j.jacc.2013.12.006

Platelet Inhibitor Agents

Salvatore Giordano and Francesco Franchi

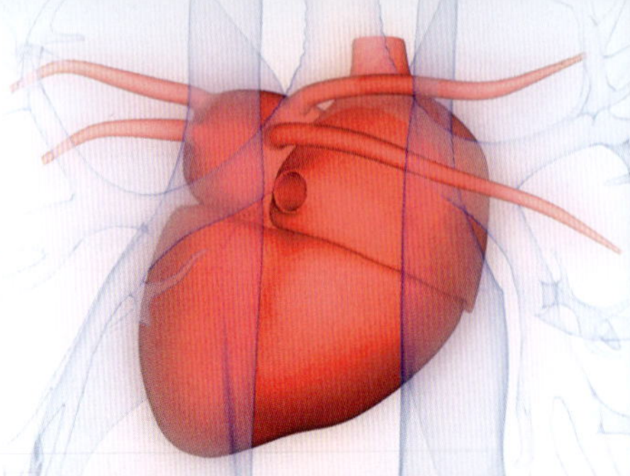

The rupture or erosion of an atheromatous plaque and subsequent thrombus formation is the main mechanism leading to an acute coronary syndrome (ACS). The rupture of an atherosclerotic plaque may also be iatrogenic, as occurs in the setting of percutaneous coronary interventions (PCIs). The exposure of subendothelial collagen after a plaque rupture or erosion prompts platelet adhesion, activation, and aggregation at the site of vessel injury. In addition, exposure of tissue factor triggers the extrinsic pathway of the coagulation cascade.[1,2] This is a dynamic process that results in thrombus formation (**Fig. 3.1**). Advances in the understanding of these complex mechanisms have been pivotal for the development of safer and more efficacious antithrombotic and antiplatelet therapies.[1] This chapter is aimed to review currently available antiplatelet therapies in the setting of PCI.

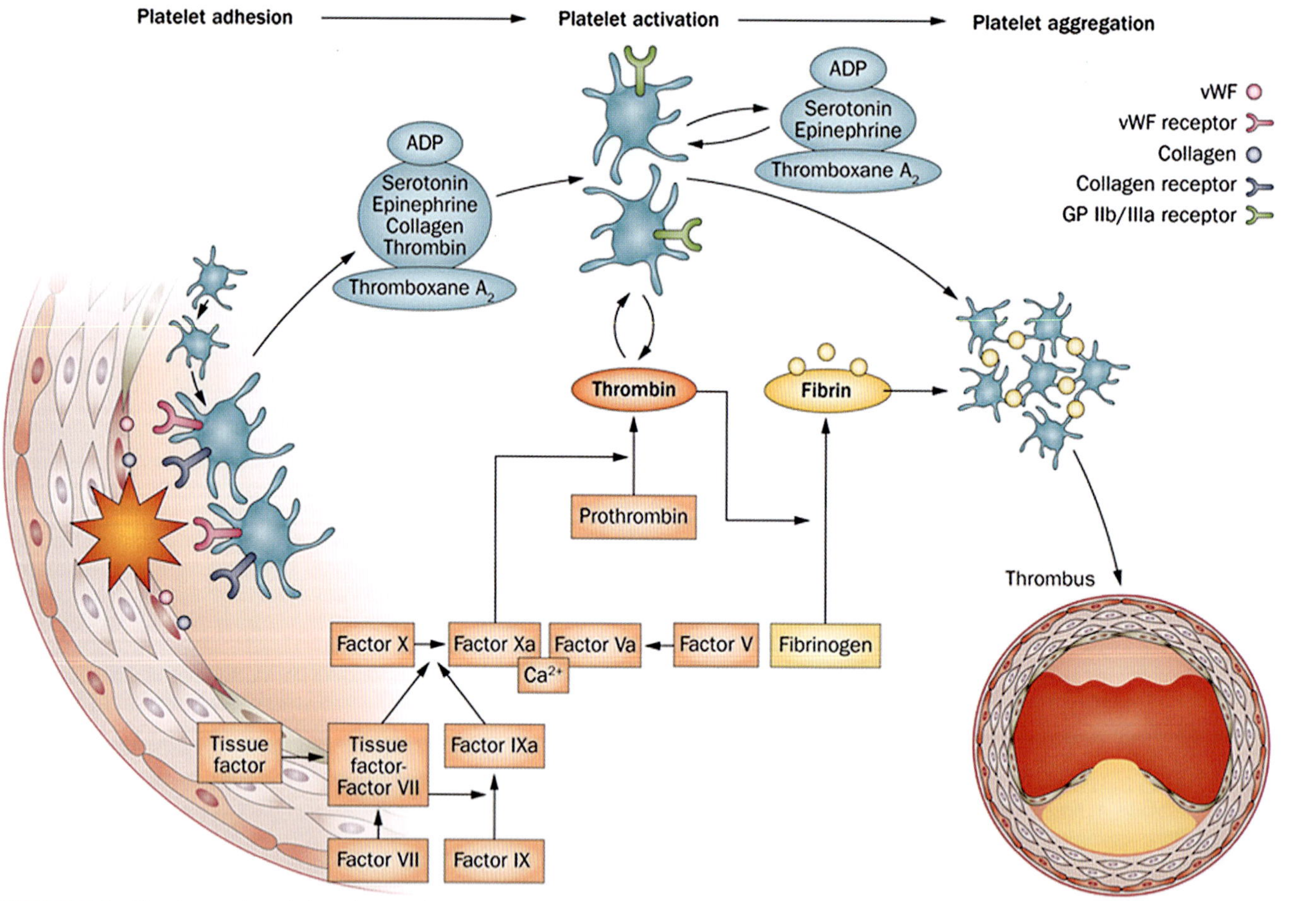

FIGURE 3.1 Platelet-mediated thrombosis. Plaque rupture exposes subendothelial components. Platelet adhesion during the rolling phase is mediated by interactions between vWF and GP Ib/V/IX receptor complexes located on the platelet surface and between platelet collagen receptors (GP VI and GP Ia) and collagen exposed at the site of vascular injury. Binding of collagen to GP VI induces the release of activating factors (ADP, thromboxane A_2, serotonin, epinephrine, and thrombin), which promote interactions between adherent platelets, as well as further recruitment and activation of circulating platelets. Platelet activation leads to changes in platelet shape, expression of proinflammatory molecules, platelet procoagulant activity, and activation of platelet integrin GP IIb/IIIa. Activated GP IIb/IIIa binds to the extracellular ligands fibrinogen and vWF, leading to platelet aggregation and thrombus formation. Vascular injury also exposes subendothelial tissue factor, which forms a complex with factor VIIa and sets off a chain of events that culminates in formation of the prothrombinase complex. Prothrombin is converted to thrombin, which subsequently converts fibrinogen to fibrin, generating a fibrin-rich clot, and further activates platelets through binding to PAR-1 and PAR-4 receptors. ADP, adenosine diphosphate; GP, glycoprotein; PAR, protease-activated receptor; vWF, von Willebrand factor. (Adapted with permission from: Franchi F, et al. Novel antiplatelet agents in acute coronary syndrome. *Nat Rev Cardiol.* 2015;12:30-47.)

ANTIPLATELET THERAPY

Currently, there are three families of antiplatelet agents for the treatment and prevention of recurrent events in patients undergoing PCI.[1] These include cyclooxygenase-1 (COX-1) inhibitors, adenosine diphosphate (ADP) $P2Y_{12}$ receptor inhibitors, and glycoprotein IIb/IIIa inhibitors (GPIs). Other agents with antiplatelet properties are available, such as vorapaxar, cilostazol, dipyridamole, and pentoxifylline. Vorapaxar is a protease-activated receptor-1 antagonist indicated in secondary prevention for the reduction of thrombotic cardiovascular events as an adjunct to aspirin and/or clopidogrel in patients with a history of myocardial infarction or with peripheral arterial disease.[1] The other mentioned agents do not have a clinical indication for prevention of recurrent ischemic events in patients with coronary artery disease (CAD).

ASPIRIN

Mechanisms of Action

Aspirin is an irreversible inhibitor of COX activity of prostaglandin H (PGH) synthase 1 and synthase 2, also known as COX-1 and COX-2, respectively.[3] These isoenzymes catalyze the conversion of arachidonic acid to PGH_2. The latter serves as a substrate for the generation of several prostanoids, including thromboxane A_2 (TXA_2) and prostacyclin (PGI_2). TXA_2, an amplifier of platelet activation and a vasoconstrictor, is mainly derived from platelet COX-1 and is highly sensitive to inhibition by aspirin.

Vascular PGI_2, a platelet inhibitor and a vasodilator, is derived largely from COX-2 and is less susceptible to inhibition by low doses of aspirin (**Fig. 3.2**). Only high doses of aspirin can inhibit COX-2, which has anti-inflammatory and analgesic effects, while low doses of aspirin are sufficient to inhibit COX-1 activity, leading to antiplatelet effects.[3] Plain aspirin is rapidly absorbed in the upper gastrointestinal tract and leads to platelet inhibition within 60 minutes. The plasma half-life of aspirin is ~20 minutes; peak plasma levels of aspirin are achieved within 30 to 40 minutes. Enteric-coated aspirin delays absorption up to approximately 3 to 4 hours. Because aspirin induces an irreversible COX-1 blockade, COX-mediated TXA_2 synthesis is prevented for the entire life span of the platelet (7-10 days).[1,3]

Indications

Aspirin is currently the mainstay of antiplatelet therapy for secondary prevention of recurrent ischemic events.[3] In high-risk patients, particularly those with ACS and undergoing PCI, a loading dose (LD) of aspirin followed by daily maintenance dose (MD) should be given as promptly as possible.[4-6] According to current guidelines, aspirin should be continued indefinitely after PCI (class I recommendation, level of evidence: B). The optimal maintenance dose of aspirin for prevention of cardiovascular events has been a subject of controversy. Registry data have shown oral aspirin

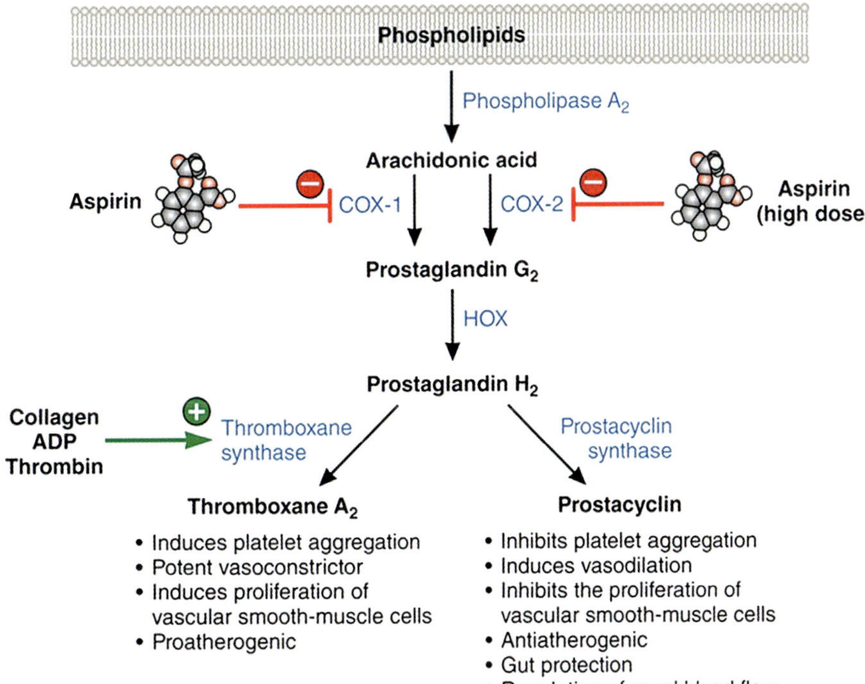

FIGURE 3.2 Mechanism of action of aspirin. Aspirin acts by irreversibly blocking the COX activity of the prostaglandin H synthases 1 and 2, also known as COX-1 and COX-2, respectively. This effect is achieved by acetylating a serine residue (serine 529 in COX-1 and serine 516 in COX-2), which prevents arachidonic acid from reaching the COX catalytic site of the enzyme. This causes the upstream block of prostanoid biosynthesis and, ultimately, inhibition of TXA_2 and prostacyclin generation. Mature platelets express only COX-1, whereas vascular endothelial cells express both COX-1 and COX-2 and represent the main site of prostacyclin generation. Low-dose aspirin selectively inhibits COX-1 activity, whereas higher doses inhibit both COX-1 and COX-2. ADP, adenosine diphosphate; COX, cyclooxygenase; HOX, hydroperoxidase; TXA_2, thromboxane A_2. (Reproduced with permission from: Capodanno D, Angiolillo DJ. Aspirin for primary cardiovascular risk prevention and beyond in diabetes mellitus. *Circulation.* 2016;134:1579-1594.)

doses of 75 to 150 mg/d to be as effective as higher doses for long-term prevention of ischemic events.[3,7] Importantly, higher doses of aspirin (>150 mg) do not offer greater protection from recurrent ischemic events, whereas bleeding events, in particular gastrointestinal bleeding, are significantly increased.[3,7] Results from the recent pragmatic ADAPTABLE (Aspirin Dosing: A Patient-Centric Trial Assessing Benefits and Long-term) trial have shown no differences between 325 and 81 mg dosing on cardiovascular events or major bleeding, with enhanced patient adherence to the lower dose. Hence, current guidelines endorse the use of 75 to 100 mg MD of aspirin only.[4-6,8,9]

Side Effects

The side effects of aspirin are primarily gastrointestinal and are dose related. Using low doses (75-162 mg/d) reduces these side effects.[3] Aspirin use can lead to gastric erosions, hemorrhage, and ulcers that can contribute to anemia. The mechanism of gastrointestinal toxicity includes a direct action of acetylsalicylic acid on gastric mucosa; hence, different formulations have been developed to bypass the stomach and deliver aspirin directly into the intestine. These formulations include enteric-coated (ie, with cellulose or silicon) aspirin,[10] which resists disintegration in the stomach, and phospholipid-aspirin liquid–filled capsules (PL-ASA), which are designed to reduce gastrointestinal injury by limiting direct contact with the stomach lining and release acetylsalicylic acid when in contact with higher duodenal pH.[11,12] Notably, while the absorption of enteric-coated aspirin is delayed, PL-ASA provides faster and more complete aspirin absorption and more prompt and potent platelet inhibition compared with enteric-coated aspirin, with a pharmacokinetic/pharmacodynamic profile very similar to that of plain aspirin, both with the 325-mg and 81-mg dose.[11,12]

Other interactions and side effects related to aspirin include those due to concomitant treatment with some nonsteroidal anti-inflammatory drugs, such as naproxen and ibuprofen.[3] These drugs in fact compete for the COX-1 active site and thus can interfere with the action of aspirin when administered concomitantly, resulting in attenuation of its antiplatelet effects.[3]This may contribute to a reduction in the cardioprotective effects of aspirin. Finally, three types of aspirin sensitivity have been described: respiratory sensitivity (asthma and/or rhinitis), cutaneous sensitivity (urticaria and/or angioedema), and systemic sensitivity (anaphylactoid reaction).[13] Desensitization using escalating doses of oral aspirin can be considered in these patients.[13]

$P2Y_{12}$ INHIBITORS

ADP is one of the main platelet-activating factors, and its effect is mainly mediated by the $P2Y_{12}$ receptor.[1] The $P2Y_{12}$ is a G-coupled receptor, which, once stimulated by ADP, leads to sustained platelet aggregation and stabilization of the platelet aggregate. Inhibition of the $P2Y_{12}$ signaling pathway is critical, particularly in the setting of PCI, as emerged from seminal studies with ticlopidine, a first-generation thienopyridine. In fact, the combination of aspirin and ticlopidine showed association with better outcomes—in particular, the prevention of thrombotic complications—compared with aspirin monotherapy or aspirin plus warfarin in patients undergoing coronary stenting.[14]

Ticlopidine has two major disadvantages: (a) it has a limited safety profile with nondepreciable rates of agranulocytosis, rash, and gastrointestinal effects; (b) it achieves antiplatelet effects slowly, given that the drug cannot be given under a loading dose because of risk of toxicity. Other oral and intravenous $P2Y_{12}$ receptor inhibitors with more favorable safety and/or efficacy profiles have been developed and are available for clinical use (**Table 3.1**).

Clopidogrel, a second-generation thienopyridine, has shown to have a more favorable safety profile than that of ticlopidine.[15] Because of this, clopidogrel has become the drug of choice in the setting of PCI in patients with stable CAD.[4-6,8] Clopidogrel has been evaluated in a large number of clinical investigations over the past 2 decades, supporting its role in the setting of ACS and PCI[1] (**Table 3.2**). Clopidogrel has limitations, however, the most important of which is its broad range in interindividual antiplatelet drug effects.[16] In particular, a considerable number of patients persist with high platelet reactivity despite clopidogrel therapy, exposing them to an increased risk of recurrent ischemic events, including stent thrombosis (ST).[16] This has set the basis for the development of newer-generation oral $P2Y_{12}$ receptor inhibitors. These include prasugrel, a third-generation thienopyridine, and ticagrelor, a first-in-class cyclopentyltriazolopyrimidine (CPTP).[1] In addition, cangrelor, an adenosine triphosphate (ATP) analogue, is the first intravenous $P2Y_{12}$ antagonist available, which is

TABLE 3.1 Pharmacologic Properties of Currently Approved $P2Y_{12}$ Receptor Inhibitors

	CLOPIDOGREL	PRASUGREL	TICAGRELOR	CANGRELOR
Group	Thienopyridine	Thienopyridine	CPTP	ATP analogue
Receptor blockade	Irreversible	Irreversible	Reversible	Reversible
Administration	Oral	Oral	Oral	IV
Dosage	Once daily	Once daily	Twice daily	Bolus plus infusion
Prodrug	Yes	Yes	No[a]	No
Onset of action[b]	2-8 h	30 min-4 h[b]	30 min-4 h[b]	2 min
Offset of action	7-10 d	7-10 d	3-5 d	~60 min
Approved settings	Stable CAD, ACS, PCI	ACS undergoing PCI	ACS (full spectrum), high-risk stable CAD	$P2Y_{12}$ receptor inhibitors-naïve patients undergoing PCI

[a]Although ticagrelor is direct acting, approximately 30% to 40% of its antiplatelet effects are attributed to an active metabolite (AR-C124910XX).
[b]Depending on clinical setting (for oral agents).
ACS, acute coronary syndrome; ATP, adenosine triphosphate; CAD, coronary artery disease; CPTP, cyclopentyltriazolopyrimidine; IV, intravenous; PCI, percutaneous coronary intervention.

TABLE 3.2 Large-Scale Randomized Clinical Trials Evaluating the Efficacy of Dual Antiplatelet Therapy With Aspirin and Clopidogrel in ACS/PCI Patients

TRIAL	PATIENTS (N)	SETTING	TREATMENT ARMS[a]	PRIMARY ENDPOINT	RESULTS[b]
CURE	12,562	UA/NSTE-ACS	Aspirin + clopidogrel vs aspirin	CV death, nonfatal MI or stroke at 1 y	9.3% vs 11.4% HR: 0.80 (0.72-0.90)
PCI-CURE	2658	PCI patients from CURE	Aspirin + clopidogrel vs aspirin	CV death, MI, or revascularization within 30 d	4.5% vs 6.4% RR: 0.70 (0.50-0.97)
CREDO	2116	Elective PCI	Aspirin + clopidogrel vs aspirin	CV death, MI, or stroke at 1 y	8.5% vs 11.5% RRR: 26.9% (3.9%-44.4%)
COMMIT	45,852	Acute MI (93% STEMI)	Aspirin + clopidogrel vs aspirin	Death, reinfarction, or stroke at 28 d	9.2% vs 10.1% OR: 0.91 (0.86-0.97)
CLARITY	3491	STEMI with fibrinolysis	Aspirin + clopidogrel vs aspirin	Occluded infarct-related artery, death, or recurrent MI before angiography	15.0% vs 21.7% OR: 0.64 (0.53-0.76)
PCI-CLARITY	1863	PCI patients from CLARITY	Aspirin + clopidogrel vs aspirin	CV death, recurrent MI, or stroke at 30 d	3.6% vs 6.2% OR: 0.54 (0.35-0.85)
CURRENT-OASIS 7	25,087	ACS patients referred invasive strategy	Aspirin + double-dose clopidogrel vs aspirin + standard-dose clopidogrel	CV death, MI, or stroke at 30 d	4.2% vs 4.4% HR: 0.94 (0.83-1.06)
CURRENT-OASIS 7 (PCI cohort)	17,263	PCI patients from CURRENT-OASIS 7	Aspirin + double-dose clopidogrel vs aspirin + standard-dose clopidogrel	CV death, MI, or stroke at 30 d	3.9% vs 4.5% HR: 0.86 (0.74-0.99)

[a]Clopidogrel was given as a 300-mg loading dose and then 75 mg daily in CURE, PCI-CURE, CREDO, COMMIT, and CLARITY. In CURRENT-OASIS 7, double-dose clopidogrel was defined as a 600-mg loading dose and 150 mg once daily for 7 d, followed by 75 mg once daily; standard-dose clopidogrel was defined as a 300-mg loading dose, followed by 75 mg once daily. Patients were also randomized to receive low-dose (75-100 mg/d) or high-dose (300-325 mg/d) aspirin.

[b]Results are expressed as % of events and association measure (95% confidence interval).

ACS, acute coronary syndrome; CLARITY, clopidogrel as adjunctive reperfusion therapy trial; COMMIT, clopidogrel and metoprolol in myocardial infarction trial; CREDO, clopidogrel for the reduction of events during observation trial; CURE, clopidogrel in unstable angina to prevent recurrent events trial; CURRENT-OASIS-7, clopidogrel optimal loading dose usage to reduce recurrent events/optimal antiplatelet strategy for intervention trial; CV, cardiovascular; HR, hazard ratio; MI, myocardial infarction; NSTE-ACS, non-ST-segment elevation acute coronary syndrome; OR, odds ratio; PCI, percutaneous coronary intervention; RR, relative risk; RRR, relative risk reduction; STEMI, ST-segment elevation myocardial infarction; UA, unstable angina.

approved by the Food and Drug Administration (FDA) for use in patients with CAD undergoing PCI[17] (**Tables 3.1** and **3.3**).

The interindividual response to clopidogrel (which exposes nonresponder subjects to an increased ischemic risk) and the increased risk of bleeding associated with the use of potent $P2Y_{12}$ inhibitors raised the interest toward the use of platelet function and genetic testing to guide the choice of the antiplatelet treatment.[18] A large number of studies linking guided antiplatelet therapy to clinical outcomes have been conducted over the course of the years. Although the initial trials failed to show a benefit of a guided approach in reducing ischemic complications, recent clinical trials and meta-analyses showed that a platelet function– or genotype-guided approach seems to confer a favorable efficacy/safety profile compared with a standard approach.[18-23] However, routine platelet function and genetic testing are not currently recommended by practice guidelines.

Mechanisms of Action

Thienopyridines (ticlopidine, clopidogrel, and prasugrel) are oral prodrugs and thus need to be metabolized by the hepatic cytochrome P450 (CYP) system to give rise to an active metabolite that irreversibly inhibits the $P2Y_{12}$ receptor (**Fig. 3.3**).[1,16] Clopidogrel is a second-generation thienopyridine, which requires a two-step oxidation by the CYP system to generate an active metabolite.[1,16] However, ~85% of the prodrug is hydrolyzed by prehepatic esterases to an inactive carboxylic acid derivative and only ~15% of the prodrug is metabolized by the CYP system into an active metabolite. Multiple CYP enzymes are involved in this process. Among these, CYP2C19 is pivotal because it is involved in both metabolic steps of clopidogrel. This explains why genetic variants associated with loss-of-function alleles and reduced metabolic activity of the CYP2C19 enzyme or drugs interfering with its activity, such as certain proton pump inhibitors (PPIs), can reduce the antiplatelet effects of clopidogrel.[1,16] Prasugrel is a third-generation thienopyridine, which has a more efficient metabolism than clopidogrel.[1,24] After oral ingestion, the prodrug is exposed to hydrolysis by carboxyesterases, mainly in the intestine, giving rise to an intermediate thiolactone, which then requires only a single-step hepatic metabolism (**Fig. 3.3**). In turn, the active metabolite is generated more rapidly and effectively.[1,24] This more favorable pharmacokinetic profile translates into better pharmacodynamic effects, showing faster onset, more potent platelet inhibition, and lower interindividual variability than clopidogrel, even when the latter is used at a high dose (>600 mg).[1,24] Although clopidogrel and prasugrel active metabolites have a half-life of only ~8 hours, they have an irreversible effect on platelets, which lasts for their life span (7-10 days).[1]

TABLE 3.3 Large-Scale Randomized Clinical Trials Evaluating the Efficacy of Dual Antiplatelet Therapy With Aspirin and New-Generation $P2Y_{12}$ Receptor Inhibitors in ACS/PCI Patients

TRIAL	PATIENTS (N)	SETTING	TREATMENT ARMS	PRIMARY ENDPOINT	RESULTS[a]
TRITON-TIMI 38	13,608	ACS patients undergoing PCI	Aspirin + prasugrel vs aspirin + clopidogrel	CV death, nonfatal MI or nonfatal stroke up to 15 mo	9.9% vs 12.1% HR: 0.81 (0.73-0.90)
ACCOAST	4033	NSTEMI scheduled for angiography	Pretreatment with prasugrel 30 mg vs placebo	CV death, MI, stroke, GPI bailout, or urgent revascularization at 7 d	10.0% vs 9.8% HR: 1.02 (0.84-1.25)
PLATO	18,624	ACS	Aspirin + ticagrelor vs aspirin + clopidogrel	Death from vascular causes, MI, or stroke at 12 mo	9.8% vs 11.7% HR: 0.84 (0.77-0.92)
PLATO invasive cohort	13,408	ACS with planned invasive strategy	Aspirin + ticagrelor vs aspirin + clopidogrel	Death from vascular causes, MI, or stroke at 12 mo	9.0% vs 10.7% HR: 0.84 (0.75-0.94)
CHAMPION PHOENIX	11,145	Stable angina or ACS undergoing PCI	Aspirin + cangrelor[c] vs aspirin + clopidogrel	Death from any cause, MI, IDR, and stent thrombosis at 48 h	4.7% vs 5.9% OR: 0.78 (0.66-0.93)
CHAMPION pooled analysis[b]	24,910	Patients undergoing PCI	Aspirin + cangrelor[d] vs aspirin + clopidogrel	Death from any cause, MI, IDR, and stent thrombosis at 48 h	3.8% vs 4.7% OR: 0.81 (0.71-0.91)
ISAR-REACT 5	4018	ACS with planned invasive strategy	Aspirin + ticagrelor vs Aspirin + prasugrel	Composite of death, myocardial infarction, or stroke at 1 y after randomization	9.3% vs 6.9% HR: 1.36 (1.09-1.70)

[a]Results are expressed as % of events and association measure (95% confidence interval).
[b]Pooled analysis of patient-level data from three CHAMPION trials (CHAMPION-PCI, CHAMPION-PLATFORM, and CHAMPION-PHOENIX) using the PHOENIX definition of MI.
[c]In CHAMPION PHOENIX, patients received 600 mg of clopidogrel at the end of cangrelor infusion; patients in the control arm received 300 or 600 mg of clopidogrel at the time of PCI (before or immediately after PCI, at the discretion of the site investigator).
[d]In CHAMPION PCI, clopidogrel loading dose (600 mg) was administered within 30 min before the procedure, whereas in CHAMPION PLATFORM, clopidogrel (600 mg) was administered at the end of PCI. In both trials, patients randomized to cangrelor received their loading dose of clopidogrel (600 mg) after stopping cangrelor infusion in order to avoid any possible interaction.
ACCOAST, a comparison of prasugrel at PCI or time of diagnosis of non-ST elevation myocardial infarction; ACS, acute coronary syndrome; CHAMPION, cangrelor versus standard therapy to achieve optimal management of platelet onhibition; CV, cardiovascular; GPI, glycoprotein IIb/IIIa inhibitor; HR, hazard ratio; IDR, ischemia-driven revascularization; MI, myocardial infarction; NSTE, non-ST-elevation; OR, odds ratio; PCI, percutaneous coronary intervention; PLATO, platelet inhibition and outcomes; TRITON, trial to assess improvement in therapeutic outcomes by optimizing platelet inhibition with prasugrel.

Ticagrelor is the first nonthienopyridine forming part of a new class of $P2Y_{12}$ inhibitors called CPTP approved for clinical use.[1,25] Ticagrelor is orally administered and direct acting, with reversible binding to the $P2Y_{12}$ receptor (**Fig. 3.3**).[1,25] Although ticagrelor has direct-acting effects (no metabolism required), ~30% to 40% of its effects are attributed to a metabolite generated by the CYP system, in particular by the CYP3A4 isoenzyme. Ticagrelor is rapidly absorbed and exerts its effects on $P2Y_{12}$-mediated signaling, acting as a noncompetitive ADP antagonist and inhibiting platelet inhibition via allosteric modulation of the receptor. Also, ticagrelor has shown faster, more potent, and less variable platelet inhibition than clopidogrel. Ticagrelor has a half-life of 7 to 12 hours, requiring twice-daily dosing. Although the slope of offset of ticagrelor is rapid, approximately 5 days are needed after ticagrelor withdrawal to return to baseline platelet function because of the profound platelet inhibition during treatment.[1,25]

Cangrelor is the first developed intravenous $P2Y_{12}$ antagonist available for clinical use. After being modified from ATP, the final molecule of cangrelor (2-trifluoropropylthio, N-[2-(methylthio) ethyl]-b, g-dichloromethylene ATP) has great affinity for the $P2Y_{12}$ receptor, being directly active after infusion (no metabolic activation into an active metabolite required). Cangrelor has an almost immediate onset of action, reaching steady-state concentrations within a few minutes, and a dose-dependent and very potent effect, achieving a very high degree of platelet inhibition (>90% of the $P2Y_{12}$ signaling pathway). In addition, this compound has a fast offset of action, due to its extremely short half-life (3-5 minutes) caused by a rapid deactivation by plasmatic ectonucleotidases, which allows platelet function to return to the baseline within 60 minutes after stopping the infusion.[17,26] The recommended dose of cangrelor is a 30-µg/kg bolus, followed by a 4-µg/kg/min infusion for at least 2 hours or the duration of the PCI, whichever is longer (the infusion may be continued for up to 4 hours).

Indications

Adding $P2Y_{12}$ receptor inhibitors to aspirin has shown to be particularly beneficial in the settings of PCI and across the spectrum of ACS manifestations (**Tables 3.2** and **3.3**).[1] Pivotal issues surrounding the optimal use of $P2Y_{12}$-receptor-inhibiting therapy in patients undergoing PCI include timing of treatment, dosing, and duration of therapy.

Although the optimal timing of the administration of $P2Y_{12}$ antagonists is still a matter of discussion, a loading dose of a $P2Y_{12}$ receptor inhibitor should be given in patients undergoing PCI with stenting.[4-6,8] In patients with stable CAD, there is no compelling evidence to support routine pretreatment with a $P2Y_{12}$ inhibitor before coronary angiography when the coronary anatomy is not known.[5,27] In patients with non-ST-segment elevation ACS, in contemporary times, with most patients with ACS undergoing early angiography, a strategy of loading with a $P2Y_{12}$ inhibitor after the anatomy is known appears to offer similar benefit to preloading. Of

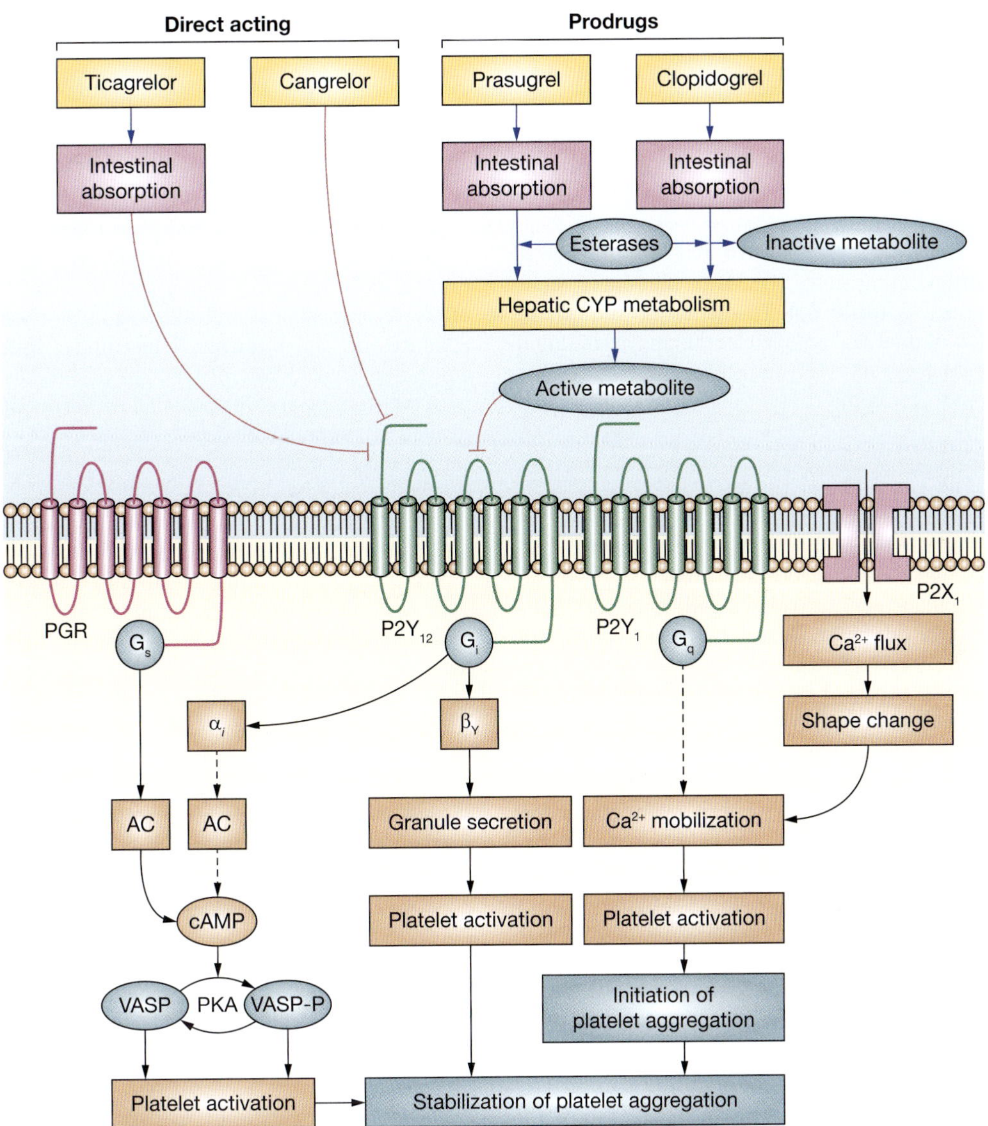

FIGURE 3.3 Mechanisms of action of $P2Y_{12}$ inhibiting agents. Clopidogrel is an oral prodrug, and after intestinal absorption, approximately 85% of clopidogrel is hydrolyzed by carboxylase to an inactive metabolite. The remaining approximately 15% is rapidly metabolized by hepatic cytochrome (CYP) P450 isoenzymes in a two-step oxidation process, with the generation of a highly unstable active metabolite. Prasugrel is also an oral prodrug with a similar intestinal absorption process. Nevertheless, in contrast to clopidogrel, prasugrel is oxidized more efficiently to its active metabolite via a single CYP-dependent step. Direct-acting antiplatelet agents (cangrelor and ticagrelor) have reversible effects and do not require hepatic metabolism for achieving pharmacodynamic activity. Ticagrelor is orally administered and, after intestinal absorption, directly inhibits platelet activation by allosteric modulation of the $P2Y_{12}$ receptor, binding to a site on the receptor distinct from the ADP-binding site. Cangrelor is intravenously administered and directly inhibits the $P2Y_{12}$ receptor, bypassing intestinal absorption. Platelets express at least two purinergic G protein–coupled receptors: $P2Y_1$ and $P2Y_{12}$. The activation of $P2Y_{12}$ inhibits AC, causing a decrease in the cAMP level, and the activation of $P2Y_1$ causes an increase in the intracellular Ca^{2+} level, leading to platelet aggregation through the change in the ligand-binding properties of the glycoprotein IIb/IIIa receptor. Clopidogrel, prasugrel, ticagrelor, and cangrelor bind to the $P2Y_{12}$ receptor and ultimately inhibit platelet activation and aggregation processes by modulating intraplatelet levels of cAMP and VASP-P. *Solid black arrows* indicate activation. *Dotted black arrows* indicate inhibition. AC, adenylyl cyclase; ADP, adenosine diphosphate; cAMP, cyclic adenosine monophosphate; CYP, cytochrome P450; PKA, protein kinases A; VASP, vasodilator-stimulated phosphoprotein; VASP-P, phosphorylation of VASP. (Adapted with permission from: Angiolillo DJ, et al. Optimizing platelet inhibition in clopidogrel poor metabolizers: therapeutic options and practical considerations. *JACC Cardiovasc Interv.* 2011;4:411-414.)

note, treatment with prasugrel is not recommended for "upfront" therapy in patients with non-ST-elevation ACS.[4-6,8,27] An important trade-off of starting therapy prior to knowing coronary anatomy is that patients will need to suspend therapy (at least 5-7 days for clopidogrel, 7 days for prasugrel, and 5 days for ticagrelor) if surgical revascularization is needed in order to minimize the risk of bleeding complications.[4-6,8,27] Guidelines outlining the recommended loading and maintenance dosing regimens of $P2Y_{12}$ inhibitors in patients with and without ACS who are undergoing PCI treated with drug-eluting stents (DESs) or bare-metal stents (BMSs) are summarized in **Table 3.4**. This table also summarizes the optimal duration of dual oral antiplatelet therapy according to the clinical setting (ACS vs non-ACS) and stent type used (DES vs BMS). Overall, clopidogrel is the drug of choice in patients with stable ischemic heart disease undergoing PCI, whereas a potent $P2Y_{12}$ inhibitor (prasugrel or ticagrelor) should be preferred over clopidogrel when a PCI is performed in the context of ACS.[4-6,8] Ticagrelor, preferably at the lower dose (60 mg bid), can also be considered in selected stable patients with ischemic heart disease undergoing PCI at high risk of myocardial infarction or stroke, especially those with diabetes.[28] In patients with ACS, the choice between prasugrel and ticagrelor should be made taking into account patients' clinical characteristics, drugs' contraindications, drug-drug interactions, expected adherence to treatment, and affordability. Recently, the ISAR-REACT 5 (Intracoronary Stenting and Antithrombotic Regimen: Rapid Early Action for Coronary Treatment 5) trial showed that, in patients with ACS, with or without ST-segment elevation, the incidence of death, myocardial infarction, or stroke was significantly lower in those treated with prasugrel than among those receiving ticagrelor, with an incidence of major bleeding, which did not significantly differ between the two groups.[29] Notably, results were consistent in the subgroup of patients who were treated with PCI.[30] Cangrelor has received FDA approval as an adjunct to PCI for reducing the risk of periprocedural myocardial infarction, repeat coronary revascularization, and stent thrombosis in patients who have not been treated with a $P2Y_{12}$ platelet inhibitor and are not being given a GPI. These recommendations stem from the CHAMPION (Cangrelor vs Standard Therapy to Achieve Optimal Management of Platelet Inhibition) PHOENIX trial, where the use of cangrelor followed by clopidogrel was associated with a reduction of peri-PCI ischemic events as compared with clopidogrel alone. Notably, no clinical trial has yet tested the effect of cangrelor in association with ticagrelor or prasugrel. However, pharmacodynamics studies showed that combining cangrelor with a potent oral $P2Y_{12}$ inhibitor enhances platelet inhibition.[31,32]

Side Effects

Bleeding complications remain the main concern in patients treated with $P2Y_{12}$ receptor inhibitors.[1] Bleeding events are increased with dual antiplatelet therapy (DAPT), rather than with aspirin alone. Other rare complications of thienopyridine use include neutropenia (0.1%) and thrombotic thrombocytopenic purpura, which have been shown mainly with clopidogrel.[1]

Spontaneous bleeding is further increased with the more potent $P2Y_{12}$ receptor antagonists prasugrel and ticagrelor.[1,18,24,25] With prasugrel and ticagrelor, the risk of spontaneous bleeding increases over time, and these drugs are contraindicated in patients at high risk of bleeding. In particular, there was no net clinical benefit of prasugrel, because it was offset by the increased bleeding risk, in low-weight (<60 kg) and elderly (>75 years) patients, which might suggest the need for dose modifications in these settings (eg, 5 mg).[1] The safety of the 5-mg dose has not been prospectively studied, however, and this dose derives from pharmacokinetic findings.[1] Importantly, patients with prior stroke or transient ischemic attack had net clinical harm from prasugrel, which therefore is contraindicated in these patients.[1] Prasugrel clinical profile has been shown to be unaffected by aspirin doses.

In comparison with clopidogrel, ticagrelor was not associated with a significant increase in overall bleeding events; it was, however, associated with a higher rate of spontaneous noncoronary artery bypass grafting–related major bleeding, including more instances of fatal intracranial bleeding.[25] Ticagrelor is therefore contraindicated in patients at high risk of bleeding and in those with a history of prior intracranial hemorrhage; it is also contraindicated in patients with severe hepatic dysfunction. Also, ticagrelor should be used with low-dose aspirin (<100 mg), as higher doses may limit its efficacy.[1,4-6,8] Other nonbleeding adverse events have been shown to be higher with ticagrelor than with clopidogrel. These include dyspnea, ventricular pauses, and an increase in serum uric acid and serum creatinine, which have been associated with high rates of treatment discontinuation.[1,25] In patients treated with ticagrelor, coadministration of strong CYP3A4 inhibitors (eg, ketoconazole, itraconazole, voriconazole, clarithromycin, nefazodone, ritonavir, saquinavir, nelfinavir, indinavir, atazanavir, and telithromycin) and strong CYP3A4 inducers (eg, rifampin, dexamethasone, phenytoin, carbamazepine, and phenobarbital) is not recommended.[1,25] Also, simvastatin and lovastatin doses of >40 mg should be avoided in ticagrelor-treated patients, and digoxin levels need to be monitored with initiation of, or any change in, ticagrelor therapy. Ultimately, because ticagrelor is administered twice daily, guidelines recommend cautionary use in patients with a history of poor compliance.[4-6,8]

Drug-regulating agencies prompted a boxed warning for clopidogrel-treated patients, which was mainly based on post hoc analyses and pharmacodynamic studies showing a drug interaction between PPIs, mainly omeprazole and esomeprazole (because they interfere with CYP2C19 activity), and clopidogrel, as well as the presence of reduced antiplatelet effects among patient carriers of loss-of-function alleles (mainly from CYP2C19).[18,33] Nevertheless, it is unclear whether the pharmacokinetic interaction between PPIs and clopidogrel translates into worse clinical outcomes.[34] These drug interactions and genetic modulating effects have not been demonstrated with prasugrel and ticagrelor.[1] Guidelines recommend that PPIs should be used in patients with a history of prior gastrointestinal bleeding or at increased risk of gastrointestinal bleeding who require DAPT, and in these patients, clinicians should choose to use a PPI that interferes less with CYP2C19 activity, such as pantoprazole (class I recommendation, level of evidence: C).[5]

In patients with atrial fibrillation requiring oral anticoagulation and DAPT due to PCI (triple therapy), the risk of bleeding is significantly increased. In these cases, whenever possible, a direct oral anticoagulant should be chosen over warfarin. Triple therapy should be used only in the peri-PCI period, and then dual antithrombotic therapy, consisting of an oral anticoagulant and a $P2Y_{12}$ inhibitor, preferably clopidogrel, should be continued up to 12 months, followed by the oral anticoagulant alone. This default approach can be, however, modified in intensity and duration based on the individual thrombotic and bleeding risk of the patient.[35] Prasugrel and ticagrelor use in patients treated with drugs associated with increased bleeding potential, including fibrinolytics and oral anticoagulant therapy, may result in an excessive risk of hemorrhages and is therefore discouraged.[1,4-6,8]

TABLE 3.4 ACC/AHA Guideline Recommendations for the Use of Oral and Intravenous Antiplatelet Therapy for Patients With Stable Ischemic Heart Disease, NSTE-ACS, or STEMI Undergoing PCI

RECOMMENDATIONS	CLASS AND LOE
Stable Ischemic Heart Disease and Acute Coronary Syndromes	
Oral Therapy	
In patients treated **with DAPT, a daily aspirin dose of 81 mg** (range, 75 to 100 mg) is recommended	I B-NR
In patients undergoing PCI, a **loading dose of aspirin**, followed by daily dosing, is recommended to reduce ischemic events	I B-R
In patients undergoing PCI within 24 h after **fibrinolytic therapy, a loading dose of 300 mg of clopidogrel**, followed by daily dosing, is recommended to reduce ischemic events	I C-LD
In selected patients undergoing PCI, **shorter-duration DAPT (1-3 mo)** is reasonable, with subsequent **transition to $P2Y_{12}$ inhibitor monotherapy** to reduce the risk of bleeding events	IIa A
In patients **<75 y of age** undergoing PCI within 24 h **after fibrinolytic therapy, ticagrelor may be a reasonable alternative to clopidogrel** to reduce ischemic events	IIb B-R
Prasugrel should not be administered to patients with a prior history of stroke or TIA	III: Harm B-R
Intravenous Therapy	
In patients undergoing PCI who are $P2Y_{12}$ inhibitor naïve, **intravenous cangrelor** may be reasonable to reduce periprocedural ischemic events	IIb B-R
Atrial Fibrillation and Anticoagulation	
In patients with atrial fibrillation who are undergoing PCI and are taking oral anticoagulant therapy, it is recommended to **discontinue aspirin treatment after 1 to 4 wk while maintaining $P2Y_{12}$ inhibitors** in addition to a direct oral anticoagulant (rivaroxaban, dabigatran, apixaban, or edoxaban) or warfarin to reduce the risk of bleeding	I B-R
In patients with atrial fibrillation who are undergoing PCI, are taking oral anticoagulant therapy, and are treated with DAPT or a $P2Y_{12}$ inhibitor monotherapy, **it is reasonable to choose a direct oral anticoagulant over warfarin to reduce the risk of bleeding**	IIa B-R
Stable Ischemic Heart Disease	
Oral Therapy	
In patients with SIHD treated with **DAPT after BMS implantation**, $P2Y_{12}$ inhibitor therapy (clopidogrel) should be given for a minimum of 1 mo	I A
In patients with SIHD treated with **DAPT after DES implantation**, $P2Y_{12}$ inhibitor therapy (clopidogrel) should be given for at least 6 mo	I B-R [SR]
In patients with SIHD undergoing PCI, a **loading dose of clopidogrel, followed by daily dosing**, is recommended to reduce ischemic events	I C-LD
In patients with SIHD treated with DAPT after BMS or DES implantation who have tolerated DAPT without a bleeding complication and who are not at high bleeding risk (eg, prior bleeding on DAPT, coagulopathy, oral anticoagulant use), **continuation of DAPT with clopidogrel for longer than 1 mo in patients treated with BMS or longer than 6 mo in patients treated with DES may be reasonable**	IIb A [SR]
In patients with SIHD treated with DAPT after DES implantation who develop a high risk of bleeding (eg, treatment with oral anticoagulant therapy), are at high risk of severe bleeding complication (eg, major intracranial surgery), or develop significant overt bleeding, **discontinuation of $P2Y_{12}$ inhibitor therapy after 3 mo may be reasonable**	IIb C-LD
Intravenous Therapy	
In patients with SIHD undergoing PCI, the **routine** use of an intravenous **glycoprotein IIb/IIIa inhibitor agent is not recommended**	III: No Benefit B-R
ACS (NSTE-ACS and STEMI)	
Oral Therapy	
In patients with ACS undergoing PCI, a **loading dose of $P2Y_{12}$ inhibitor, followed by daily dosing**, is recommended to reduce ischemic events	I B-R
In patients with ACS (NSTE-ACS or STEMI) treated with DAPT after BMS or DES implantation, $P2Y_{12}$ inhibitor therapy (clopidogrel, prasugrel, or ticagrelor) should be given for **at least 12 mo**	I B-R
In patients with ACS (NSTE-ACS or STEMI) treated with DAPT after coronary stent implantation, it is reasonable to use **ticagrelor in preference to clopidogrel** for maintenance $P2Y_{12}$ inhibitor therapy	IIa B-R
In patients with ACS (NSTE-ACS or STEMI) treated with DAPT after coronary stent implantation who are not at high risk for bleeding complications and who do not have a history of stroke or TIA, it is reasonable to choose **prasugrel over clopidogrel** for maintenance $P2Y_{12}$ inhibitor therapy	IIa B-R

(*continued*)

TABLE 3.4 ACC/AHA Guideline Recommendations for the Use of Oral and Intravenous Antiplatelet Therapy for Patients With Stable Ischemic Heart Disease, NSTE-ACS, or STEMI Undergoing PCI (*Continued*)

RECOMMENDATIONS	CLASS AND LOE
In patients with ACS (NSTE-ACS or STEMI) treated with coronary stent implantation who have tolerated DAPT without a bleeding complication and who are not at high bleeding risk (eg, prior bleeding on DAPT, coagulopathy, oral anticoagulant use), continuation of **DAPT** (clopidogrel, prasugrel, or ticagrelor) **for longer than 12 mo may be reasonable**	IIb A [SR]
In patients with ACS treated with DAPT after DES implantation who develop a high risk of bleeding (eg, treatment with oral anticoagulant therapy), are at high risk of severe bleeding complication (eg, major intracranial surgery), or develop significant overt bleeding, **discontinuation of $P2Y_{12}$ inhibitor therapy after 6 mo may be reasonable**	IIb C-LD
Intravenous Therapy	
In patients with ACS undergoing PCI with large thrombus burden, no-reflow, or slow flow, intravenous glycoprotein IIb/IIIa inhibitor agents are reasonable to improve procedural success	IIa C-LD

ACC, American College of Cardiology; ACS, acute coronary syndrome; AHA, American Heart Association; BMS, bare-metal stent; DAPT, dual antiplatelet therapy; DES, drug-eluting stent; GP, glycoprotein; LOE, level of evidence; NSTE-ACS, non-ST-segment elevation acute coronary syndrome; PCI, percutaneous coronary intervention; SIHD, stable ischemic heart disease; STEMI, ST-elevation myocardial infarction; TIA, transient ischemic attack.

Cangrelor is usually administered for a short period of time and has a rapid offset of action, which provides this agent with a good safety profile despite achieving very potent platelet inhibition. Nevertheless, the incidence of bleeding is slightly higher with cangrelor compared with clopidogrel (mainly driven by the occurrence of hematomas at the access site), and cangrelor is contraindicated in patients with significant active bleeding.[17,26] Nonbleeding adverse reactions include hypersensitivity, renal function impairment, and dyspnea (1.3%). In addition, caution must be taken when transitioning from cangrelor to thienopyridines in order to minimize the risk of having a gap in platelet inhibition due to drug-drug interaction that could result in thrombotic complications.[36] In particular, clopidogrel and prasugrel should be administered at the end of cangrelor infusion. On the other hand, no interaction has been shown with ticagrelor, which can be administered any time before, during, or after cangrelor infusion.[17,31,32,36]

Strategies to Reduce the Risk of Bleeding

While the risk of bleeding is chronically elevated in subjects on DAPT (especially on prasugrel or ticagrelor), the ischemic benefit is greater during the early phase after ACS/PCI. Several strategies have been tested to minimize the risk of bleeding while maintaining protection against ischemic events, including reducing DAPT intensity (eg, de-escalation) and shortening DAPT duration (eg, shortening $P2Y_{12}$ treatment, shortening aspirin treatment).[37]

De-escalation consists in switching from a potent $P2Y_{12}$ inhibitor to clopidogrel or reducing the dose of the potent $P2Y_{12}$ inhibitor and is mainly reserved for patients with ACS. De-escalation by switching can be guided by platelet function and genetic tests, which aim to detect poor clopidogrel responders, with the selective use of prasugrel or ticagrelor in those deemed to be likely poor responders. Alternatively, de-escalation can be clinically guided (ie, performed without knowing the patient's response to clopidogrel), which may expose clopidogrel nonresponders to increased risk of ischemic events and should be performed no sooner than 1 month from PCI. According to current guidelines, de-escalation should not be routinely performed and may represent an option in subjects at high bleeding risk.[36]

Shortening DAPT duration consists in either stopping the $P2Y_{12}$ inhibitor and continuing with aspirin monotherapy (ie, shortening $P2Y_{12}$ treatment) or stopping aspirin and continuing with $P2Y_{12}$ inhibitor monotherapy (ie, shortening aspirin treatment) prior to standard timing recommended by guidelines. Both strategies have proven to be beneficial in reducing bleeding risk and are endorsed by guidelines as strategies to employ in subjects with increased risk of bleeding (**Table 3.4**).[5,38]

GLYCOPROTEIN IIB/IIIA INHIBITORS

Mechanisms of Action

The GP IIb/IIIa receptor is an integrin, a heterodimer consisting of noncovalently associated alpha (αIIb) and beta (β3) subunits.[39] By competing with fibrinogen and von Willebrand factor for GP IIb/IIIa binding, GPIs interfere with platelet cross-linking and platelet-derived thrombus formation. Because the GP IIb/IIIa receptor represents the final common pathway leading to platelet aggregation, these agents are very potent platelet inhibitors. The lack of benefit, including increased mortality, in patients with ACS or in those undergoing PCI shown by the oral GPI stopped their investigations, and only parenteral forms are available for clinical use.[39]

There are three parenteral GPIs approved for clinical use: abciximab, eptifibatide, and tirofiban (**Table 3.5**). Abciximab is a large chimeric monoclonal antibody with a high binding affinity that results in a prolonged pharmacologic effect.[39] In particular, it is a Fab (antigen-binding fragment) of a chimeric human-mouse genetic reconstruction of 7E3. The specific binding site of abciximab is the β3 subunit. Its plasma half-life is biphasic, with an initial half-life of <10 minutes and a second-phase half-life of ~30 minutes. Because of its high affinity for the GP IIb/IIIa receptor, it has a biologic half-life of 12 to 24 hours, and because of its slow clearance from the body, it has a functional half-life of up to 7 days; platelet-associated abciximab can be detected for >14 days after treatment discontinuation.[39]

Eptifibatide and tirofiban, also called "small-molecule agents," do not induce immune response and have a lower affinity for the GP IIb/IIIa receptor compared with abciximab. Eptifibatide is a reversible and highly selective heptapeptide, which has a rapid onset and a short plasma half-life of 2 to 2.5 hours. After discontinuation of the infusion, the recovery of platelet aggregation occurs within 4 hours.[39] Tirofiban is a tyrosine-derived nonpeptide inhibitor that functions as a mimic of the RGD sequence and is highly specific for the GP IIb/IIIa receptor.[39] Tirofiban has a rapid onset and short duration of action, with a plasma half-life of ~2 hours.

TABLE 3.5 Pharmacologic Properties and Dosing of Currently Approved Glycoprotein IIb/IIIa Antagonists

	ABCIXIMAB	TIROFIBAN	EPTIFIBATIDE
Molecular structure	Fab of a monoclonal antibody	Nonpeptide synthetic molecule	Synthetic cyclic heptapeptide
Molecular mass	47.615 Da	495 Da	832 Da
Reversibility	Yes[a]	Yes	Yes
Affinity	Very high	High	Intermediate
Specificity	No[b]	Yes	Yes
Plasmatic half-life	Biphasic: <10 min and ~30 min	~2 h	~2.5 h
Duration of antiplatelet effect after discontinuation	Platelet life-span	~4–8 h	~4 h
PCI dosing	Bolus: 0.25 mg/kg Infusion: 0.125 µg/kg/min (maximum 10 µg/min)	Bolus: 25 µg/kg Infusion: 0.15 µg/kg/min	Bolus: 180 µg/kg + second 180 µg/kg bolus 10 min after the first one Infusion: 2 µg/kg/min
Renal adjustment	No	In patients with CrCl <30 mL/min, reduce infusion by 50%	In patients with CrCl <50 mL/min, reduce infusion by 50%

[a]Often reported as irreversible due to its great affinity for the receptor.
[b]It also binds to the vitronectin receptor on vascular cells and to the activated MAC-1 receptor on leukocytes.
CrCl, creatinine clearance; Da, Dalton; Fab, antigen-binding fragment; PCI, percutaneous coronary intervention.

Similar to eptifibatide, tirofiban has significant recovery of platelet aggregation within 4 hours of completion of infusion.[39]

Indications

Numerous clinical trials have been conducted over the past decades, and, currently, these agents are indicated only in the setting of PCI for ACS.[4-6] Clinical trial data, indeed, showed no benefit in using these agents in the setting of patients with stable CAD undergoing elective PCI, in particular if pretreated with clopidogrel.[39] In addition, clinical trials have failed to show any benefit with routine upstream use of these agents over ad hoc GP IIb/IIIa inhibition in patients with ACS undergoing PCI,[40] and thus, this approach is no longer recommended. GPI, however, has shown to be of benefit in the setting of patients with ACS undergoing PCI.[41] While no renal adjustments are required for abciximab, eptifibatide and tirofiban require dose adjustments in renal dysfunction (**Table 3.5**).[4-6] Guideline recommendations for the use of GPI are summarized in **Table 3.4**, which limit their selective use as bailout in patients with large thrombus burden, no-reflow, or slow flow. The main limiting factor for the use of GPI in clinical practice is the risk of bleeding complications. In addition, the reduced utilization of GPI in clinical practice is also attributed to the encouraging outcomes associated with bivalirudin, which has shown to significantly reduce bleeding without a trade-off in ischemic events (see Chapter: Anticoagulant and Fibrinolytic Agents for NSTE-ACS, PCI, and STEMI), and cangrelor.[4-6,8]

Side Effects

Bleeding is the primary adverse effect of GPI[39] and is increased in elderly patients and in those with chronic kidney disease. This has been frequently attributed to overdosing, underscoring the need for dose adjustments in these settings. In addition, adjusting heparin dosing (50-70 IU/kg) is pivotal to reduce bleeding complications in PCI patients treated with GPI.

Thrombocytopenia is also an undesired side effect of GPI, which is more common with abciximab than with eptifibatide and tirofiban. Thrombocytopenia in patients undergoing PCI is associated with more ischemic events, bleeding complications, and transfusions and warrants immediate cessation of therapy.[39] Finally, it is important to remember that readministration of abciximab, but not eptifibatide and tirofiban, is associated with a slightly increased risk of thrombocytopenia, which is considered to be an immune-related process; thus, its use should be avoided or small-molecule agents should be used in its place.

CONCLUSIONS

Platelets play a key role in ischemic complications in patients with ACS and in those undergoing PCI, underscoring the importance of platelet-inhibiting agents. DAPT with aspirin and a $P2Y_{12}$ receptor inhibitor is the mainstay of short- and long-term secondary prevention treatment of ACS and PCI patients. Clopidogrel is currently the most utilized $P2Y_{12}$ receptor inhibitor and is indicated in both ACS and non-ACS settings. Prasugrel and ticagrelor are newer and more potent oral $P2Y_{12}$ inhibitors, which are used mostly in patients with ACS. Although they are associated with an increased risk of bleeding complications, these agents have shown to reduce ischemic complications, including stent thrombosis, compared with clopidogrel, and should therefore be considered the first choice in patients with ACS. In this setting, clopidogrel use should be considered only when both prasugrel and ticagrelor are contraindicated or not available or in case of high bleeding risk. Cangrelor is a potent intravenous $P2Y_{12}$ antagonist that is approved for use in PCI patients not pretreated with an oral $P2Y_{12}$ inhibitor and not receiving a GPI for reducing the risk of ischemic adverse events, where it has been proven superior to clopidogrel. GPIs (abciximab, eptifibatide, and tirofiban) are available for parenteral administration, and their use is currently limited to the acute management of high-risk patients with ACS undergoing PCI. The elevated rates of bleeding complications with GPI, as well as the more favorable safety profiles of other antithrombotic agents, have led to a reduced utilization of these agents in clinical practice.

Key Points

- Platelets play a key role in ischemic complications in patients with ACS and in those undergoing PCI, underscoring the importance of platelet-inhibiting agents.
- Oral antiplatelet therapy is a pivotal component of secondary prevention of acute and long-term events in the settings of ACS and PCI. Dual antiplatelet therapy with aspirin and $P2Y_{12}$ receptor inhibitor is the mainstay of treatment of ACS and PCI patients.
- Clopidogrel is currently the most utilized $P2Y_{12}$ receptor inhibitor and is indicated in both ACS and non-ACS settings. Prasugrel and ticagrelor are newer and more potent $P2Y_{12}$ inhibitors that are mainly used in patients with ACS.
- Cangrelor is a potent intravenous $P2Y_{12}$ receptor antagonist indicated as an adjunct to PCI in patients who have not been treated with a $P2Y_{12}$ platelet inhibitor and are not being given a GPI.
- GPIs include abciximab, eptifibatide, and tirofiban. These agents are available for intravenous and intracoronary administration, and their use is limited for the acute management of high-risk ACS settings.

For further review and interactivities, please see the chapter-based multiple choice questions and videos accessible in the complimentary eBook bundled with this text. Access instructions are located in the inside front cover.

References

1. Franchi F, Angiolillo DJ. Novel antiplatelet agents in acute coronary syndrome. *Nat Rev Cardiol*. 2015;12(1):30-47. doi:10.1038/nrcardio.2014.156
2. Davi G, Patrono C. Platelet activation and atherothrombosis. *N Engl J Med*. 2007;357(24):2482-2494. doi:10.1056/NEJMra071014
3. Patrono C, Garcia Rodriguez LA, Landolfi R, Baigent C. Low-dose aspirin for the prevention of atherothrombosis. *N Engl J Med*. 2005;353(22):2373-2383. doi:10.1056/NEJMra052717
4. O'Gara PT, Kushner FG, Ascheim DD, et al. 2013 ACCF/AHA guideline for the management of ST-elevation myocardial infarction: a report of the American College of Cardiology Foundation/American Heart Association Task Force on Practice Guidelines. *J Am Coll Cardiol*. 2013;61(4):e78-e140. doi:10.1016/j.jacc.2012.11.019
5. Lawton JS, Tamis-Holland JE, Bangalore S, et al. 2021 ACC/AHA/SCAI guideline for coronary artery revascularization: executive summary—a report of the American College of Cardiology/American Heart Association Joint Committee on Clinical Practice Guidelines. *Circulation*. 2022;145(3):e4-e17. doi:10.1161/CIR.0000000000001039
6. Amsterdam EA, Wenger NK, Brindis RG, et al. 2014 AHA/ACC guideline for the management of patients with non-ST-elevation acute coronary syndromes: a report of the American College of Cardiology/American Heart Association Task Force on Practice Guidelines. *J Am Coll Cardiol*. 2014;64(24):e139-e228. doi:10.1016/j.jacc.2014.09.017
7. Antithrombotic Trialists' ATT Collaboration; Baigent C, Blackwell L, et al. Aspirin in the primary and secondary prevention of vascular disease: collaborative meta-analysis of individual participant data from randomised trials. *Lancet*. 2009;373(9678):1849-1860. doi:10.1016/S0140-6736(09)60503-1
8. Levine GN, Bates ER, Bittl JA, et al. 2016 ACC/AHA guideline focused update on duration of dual antiplatelet therapy in patients with coronary artery disease: a report of the American College of Cardiology/American Heart Association Task Force on Clinical Practice Guidelines. *J Am Coll Cardiol*. 2016;68(10):1082-1115. doi:10.1016/j.jacc.2016.03.513
9. Jones WS, Mulder H, Wruck LM, et al. Comparative effectiveness of aspirin dosing in cardiovascular disease. *N Engl J Med*. 2021;384(21):1981-1990. doi:10.1056/NEJMoa2102137
10. Kedir HM, Sisay EA, Abiye AA. Enteric-coated aspirin and the risk of gastrointestinal side effects: a systematic review. *Int J Gen Med*. 2021;14:4757-4763. doi:10.2147/IJGM.S326929
11. Angiolillo DJ, Bhatt DL, Lanza F, et al. Pharmacokinetic/pharmacodynamic assessment of a novel, pharmaceutical lipid-aspirin complex: results of a randomized, crossover, bioequivalence study. *J Thromb Thrombolysis*. 2019;48(4):554-562. doi:10.1007/s11239-019-01933-7
12. Franchi F, Schneider DJ, Prats J, et al. Pharmacokinetic and pharmacodynamic profiles of a novel phospholipid-aspirin complex liquid formulation and low dose enteric-coated aspirin: results from a prospective, randomized, crossover study. *J Thromb Thrombolysis*. 2022;54(3):373-381. doi:10.1007/s11239-022-02687-5
13. Rossini R, Angiolillo DJ, Musumeci G, et al. Aspirin desensitization in patients undergoing percutaneous coronary interventions with stent implantation. *Am J Cardiol*. 2008;101(6):786-789. doi:10.1016/j.amjcard.2007.10.045
14. Leon MB, Baim DS, Popma JJ, et al. A clinical trial comparing three antithrombotic-drug regimens after coronary-artery stenting. Stent anticoagulation restenosis study investigators. *N Engl J Med*. 1998;339(23):1665-1671. doi:10.1056/NEJM199812033392303
15. Bertrand ME, Rupprecht HJ, Urban P, Gershlick AH, CLASSICS Investigators. Double-blind study of the safety of clopidogrel with and without a loading dose in combination with aspirin compared with ticlopidine in combination with aspirin after coronary stenting: the clopidogrel aspirin stent international cooperative study (CLASSICS). *Circulation*. 2000;102(6):624-629. doi:10.1161/01.cir.102.6.624
16. Angiolillo DJ, Fernandez-Ortiz A, Bernardo E, et al. Variability in individual responsiveness to clopidogrel: clinical implications, management, and future perspectives. *J Am Coll Cardiol*. 2007;49(14):1505-1516. doi:10.1016/j.jacc.2006.11.044
17. Franchi F, Rollini F, Park Y, Angiolillo DJ. A safety evaluation of cangrelor in patients undergoing PCI. *Expert Opin Drug Saf*. 2016;15(2):275-285. doi:10.1517/14740338.2016.1133585
18. Sibbing D, Aradi D, Alexopoulos D, et al. Updated expert consensus statement on platelet function and genetic testing for guiding P2Y(12) receptor inhibitor treatment in percutaneous coronary intervention. *JACC Cardiovasc Interv*. 2019;12(16):1521-1537. doi:10.1016/j.jcin.2019.03.034
19. Galli M, Benenati S, Capodanno D, et al. Guided versus standard antiplatelet therapy in patients undergoing percutaneous coronary intervention: a systematic review and meta-analysis. *Lancet*. 2021;397(10283):1470-1483. doi:10.1016/S0140-6736(21)00533-X
20. Franchi F, Rollini F. Genotype-guided antiplatelet therapy in patients with coronary artery disease. *JACC Cardiovasc Interv*. 2021;14(7):751-753. doi:10.1016/j.jcin.2021.02.005
21. Claassens DMF, Vos GJA, Bergmeijer TO, et al. A genotype-guided strategy for oral P2Y(12) inhibitors in primary PCI. *N Engl J Med*. 2019;381(17):1621-1631. doi:10.1056/NEJMoa1907096
22. Sibbing D, Aradi D, Jacobshagen C, et al. Guided de-escalation of antiplatelet treatment in patients with acute coronary syndrome undergoing percutaneous coronary intervention (TROPICAL-ACS): a randomised, open-label, multicentre trial. *Lancet*. 2017;390(10104):1747-1757. doi:10.1016/S0140-6736(17)32155-4
23. Galli M, Benenati S, Franchi F, et al. Comparative effects of guided vs. potent P2Y12 inhibitor therapy in acute coronary syndrome: a network meta-analysis of 61 898 patients from 15 randomized trials. *Eur Heart J*. 2022;43(10):959-967. doi:10.1093/eurheartj/ehab836
24. Wiviott SD, Braunwald E, McCabe CH, et al. Prasugrel versus clopidogrel in patients with acute coronary syndromes. *N Engl J Med*. 2007;357(20):2001-2015. doi:10.1056/NEJMoa0706482

25. Wallentin L, Becker RC, Budaj A, et al. Ticagrelor versus clopidogrel in patients with acute coronary syndromes. *N Engl J Med.* 2009;361(11):1045-1057. doi:10.1056/NEJMoa0904327
26. Bhatt DL, Stone GW, Mahaffey KW, et al. Effect of platelet inhibition with cangrelor during PCI on ischemic events. *N Engl J Med.* 2013;368(14):1303-1313. doi:10.1056/NEJMoa1300815
27. Capodanno D, Angiolillo DJ. Pretreatment with antiplatelet drugs in invasively managed patients with coronary artery disease in the contemporary era: review of the evidence and practice guidelines. *Circ Cardiovasc Interv.* 2015;8(3):e002301. doi:10.1161/CIRCINTERVENTIONS.114.002301
28. Bhatt DL, Steg PG, Mehta SR, et al. Ticagrelor in patients with diabetes and stable coronary artery disease with a history of previous percutaneous coronary intervention (THEMIS-PCI): a phase 3, placebo-controlled, randomised trial. *Lancet.* 2019;394(10204):1169-1180. doi:10.1016/S0140-6736(19)31887-2
29. Schupke S, Neumann FJ, Menichelli M, et al. Ticagrelor or prasugrel in patients with acute coronary syndromes. *N Engl J Med.* 2019;381(16):1524-1534. doi:10.1056/NEJMoa1908973
30. Coughlan JJ, Aytekin A, Lahu S, et al. Ticagrelor or prasugrel for patients with acute coronary syndrome treated with percutaneous coronary intervention: a prespecified subgroup analysis of a randomized clinical trial. *JAMA Cardiol.* 2021;6(10):1121-1129. doi:10.1001/jamacardio.2021.2228
31. Franchi F, Ortega-Paz L, Rollini F, et al. Cangrelor in patients with coronary artery disease pretreated with ticagrelor: the switching antiplatelet (SWAP)-5 study. *JACC Cardiovasc Interv.* 2023;16(1):36-46. doi:10.1016/j.jcin.2022.10.034
32. Franchi F, Rollini F, Rivas A, et al. Platelet inhibition with cangrelor and crushed ticagrelor in patients with ST-segment-elevation myocardial infarction undergoing primary percutaneous coronary intervention. *Circulation.* 2019;139(14):1661-1670. doi:10.1161/CIRCULATIONAHA.118.038317
33. Angiolillo DJ, Gibson CM, Cheng S, et al. Differential effects of omeprazole and pantoprazole on the pharmacodynamics and pharmacokinetics of clopidogrel in healthy subjects: randomized, placebo-controlled, crossover comparison studies. *Clin Pharmacol Ther.* 2011;89(1):65-74. doi:10.1038/clpt.2010.219
34. Bhatt DL, Cryer BL, Contant CF, et al. Clopidogrel with or without omeprazole in coronary artery disease. *N Engl J Med.* 2010;363(20):1909-1917. doi:10.1056/NEJMoa1007964
35. Angiolillo DJ, Bhatt DL, Cannon CP, et al. Antithrombotic therapy in patients with atrial fibrillation treated with oral anticoagulation undergoing percutaneous coronary intervention: a North American perspective—2021 update. *Circulation.* 2021;143(6):583-596. doi:10.1161/CIRCULATIONAHA.120.050438
36. Angiolillo DJ, Rollini F, Storey RF, et al. International expert consensus on switching platelet P2Y(12) receptor-inhibiting therapies. *Circulation.* 2017;136(20):1955-1975. doi:10.1161/CIRCULATIONAHA.117.031164
37. Capodanno D, Morice MC, Angiolillo DJ, et al. Trial design principles for patients at high bleeding risk undergoing PCI: JACC Scientific Expert Panel. *J Am Coll Cardiol.* 2020;76(12):1468-1483. doi:10.1016/j.jacc.2020.06.085
38. Valgimigli M, Frigoli E, Heg D, et al. Dual antiplatelet therapy after PCI in patients at high bleeding risk. *N Engl J Med.* 2021;385(18):1643-1655. doi:10.1056/NEJMoa2108749
39. Muniz-Lozano A, Rollini F, Franchi F, Angiolillo DJ. Update on platelet glycoprotein IIb/IIIa inhibitors: recommendations for clinical practice. *Ther Adv Cardiovasc Dis.* 2013;7(4):197-213. doi:10.1177/1753944713487781
40. Giugliano RP, White JA, Bode C, et al. Early versus delayed, provisional eptifibatide in acute coronary syndromes. *N Engl J Med.* 2009;360(21):2176-2190. doi:10.1056/NEJMoa0901316
41. Kastrati A, Mehilli J, Neumann FJ, et al. Abciximab in patients with acute coronary syndromes undergoing percutaneous coronary intervention after clopidogrel pretreatment: the ISAR-REACT 2 randomized trial. *JAMA.* 2006;295(13):1531-1538. doi:10.1001/jama.295.13.joc60034

Anticoagulant and Fibrinolytic Agents for NSTE-ACS, PCI, and STEMI

Vivian G. Ng and Ajay J. Kirtane

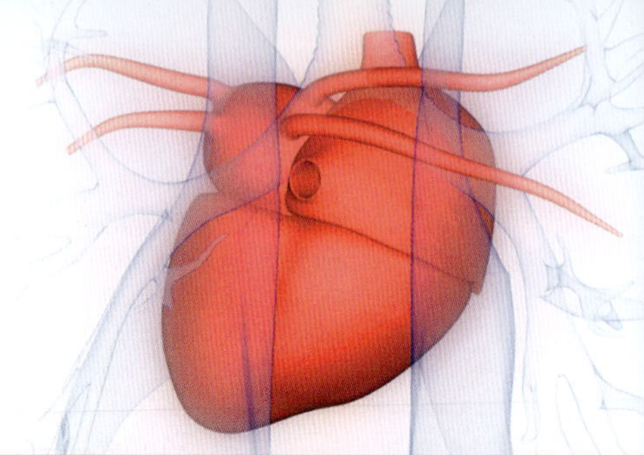

Acute coronary syndromes (ACSs) are typically characterized by thrombosis superimposed over rupture, erosion, or mechanical disruption of a thin fibrous cap overlying lipid-laden plaque within a culprit coronary artery. Exposure of plaque contents to the bloodstream initiates the activation and upregulation of various mediators of the thrombotic cascade, which further contribute to luminal compromise, resulting in worsening ischemia and reinfarction. Anticoagulant and antiplatelet therapies help minimize and placate the thrombotic process, which is the hallmark of ACS. As such, these agents are the cornerstones of adjunctive pharmacology for ACS. Additionally, anticoagulant and antiplatelet agents can more safely facilitate mechanical therapies such as percutaneous coronary intervention (PCI), which, while aiming to mechanically stabilize the plaque responsible for ACS, are at the same time prothrombotic and constitute an iatrogenic form of plaque rupture similar to natively occurring ACS. This chapter covers the indications and usage of various anticoagulant therapies in the setting of non–ST-segment acute coronary syndromes (NSTE-ACSs) and ST-segment elevation myocardial infarction (STEMI) and during PCI. This chapter also briefly touches upon the interventional aspects of fibrinolytic therapy, when administered to patients with STEMI.

OVERVIEW OF ACC/AHA/SCAI GUIDELINE RECOMMENDATIONS FOR NSTE-ACS

Anticoagulants in NSTE-ACS

The updated American College of Cardiology/American Heart Association (ACC/AHA) guidelines[1] summarizing the recommendations for the use of anticoagulant therapy in patients with NSTE-ACS first discuss the use of antithrombotic therapies for patients with definite or likely ACS. Once the diagnosis of ACS has been made, patients should be immediately started on anticoagulant therapy, regardless of the management strategy—a class I recommendation in the ACC/AHA guidelines (**Table 4.1**). The notable exception to this is for those patients whose ACS is not a consequence of an atherothrombotic process but is rather a secondary event (eg, as a result of severe blood loss, trauma, or sepsis, ie, type 2 infarction).

Several classes of anticoagulants have been shown to be effective in treating patients with ACS: unfractionated heparin (UFH), low-molecular-weight heparins (LMWHs), direct thrombin inhibitors, and factor Xa inhibitors. The primary function of these agents is to inhibit the coagulation cascade, thereby preventing or minimizing thrombosis in order to alleviate the ischemic effects of ACS. A critical management issue related to the use of anticoagulant agents in ACS is the potential trade-off of more potent anticoagulation (aimed at maximizing anti-ischemic efficacy) for an increase in bleeding complications. The association between ischemic events and late mortality has been recognized historically and well described in studies of ACS; in fact, this is one of the fundamental principles behind the use of anticoagulant therapy in ACS. More recently, a strong linkage between nonfatal bleeding events and subsequent mortality has also emerged in both randomized clinical trials and observational studies on ACS.[2-4] Thus, the treating physician must be acutely aware of the joint importance of both ischemic and bleeding complications when selecting the optimal anticoagulant strategy for patients with NSTE-ACS.

Initial Anticoagulant Use in Patients With Definite NSTE-ACS

In patients with definite NSTE-ACS, parenteral anticoagulation is recommended for all patients regardless of the choice of treatment strategy (early invasive vs ischemia-guided management). Options include enoxaparin, bivalirudin, fondaparinux, or UFH. Dosing is described in **Table 4.2**.

TABLE 4.1 ACC/AHA Guideline Recommendations for NSTE-ACS

RECOMMENDATION	CLASS OF RECOMMENDATION	LEVEL OF EVIDENCE
SC enoxaparin for duration of hospitalization or until PCI is performed	I	A
Bivalirudin until diagnostic angiography or PCI is performed in patients with early invasive strategy only	I	B
SC fondaparinux for the duration of hospitalization or until PCI is performed	I	B
Administer additional anticoagulant with anti-IIa activity if PCI is performed while patient is on fondaparinux	I	B
IV UFH for 48 h or until PCI is performed	I	B
IV fibrinolytic treatment not recommended in patients with NSTE-ACS	III	A

ACC/AHA, American College of Cardiology/American Heart Association; IV, intravenous; NSTE-ACS, non-ST-segment acute coronary syndrome; PCI, percutaneous coronary intervention; SC, subcutaneous; UFH, unfractionated heparin.

TABLE 4.2 Dosing of Anticoagulant Agents in NSTE-ACS

	UPSTREAM THERAPY FOR NSTE-ACS	DURING PCI (IF UPSTREAM THERAPY GIVEN FOR NSTE-ACS)	DURING PCI (NO UPSTREAM THERAPY GIVEN OR ELECTIVE PCI)
Bivalirudin	0.1-mg/kg IV bolus, 0.25-mg/kg/h IV infusion	0.5-mg/kg IV bolus, increase infusion to 1.75 mg/kg/h If UFH was given, discontinue UFH, wait for 30 min, then give 0.75-mg/kg IV bolus, 1.75-mg/kg/h IV infusion	0.75-mg/kg IV bolus, 1.75-mg/kg/h IV infusion
Unfractionated heparin (UFH)	Loading dose of 60 U/kg (max 4000 U) as IV bolus Maintenance IV infusion of 12 U/kg/h (max 1000 U/h) to maintain aPTT at 1.5-2.0 times control (approximately 50-70 s)	IV GP IIb/IIIa planned: IV bolus doses with target ACT 200–250 s No IV GP IIb/IIIa planned: IV bolus doses with target ACT 250-300 s for HemoTec; 300-350 s for Hemochron	IV GP IIb/IIIa planned: 50- to 70-U/kg IV bolus with target ACT 200–250 s No IV GP IIb/IIIa planned: 70- to 100-U/kg IV bolus to achieve target ACT of 250-300 s for HemoTec; 300-350 s for Hemochron
Enoxaparin	Loading dose of 30 mg IV may be given in selected patients Maintenance of 1 mg/kg SC every 12 h Extend dosing interval to 1 mg/kg SC every 24 h if estimated CrCl <30 mL/min	Last SC dose within 8 h: no additional therapy Last SC dose 8–12 h prior or if <2 therapeutic SC doses administered: 0.3-mg/kg IV bolus	0.5- to 0.75-mg/kg IV bolus
Fondaparinux	2.5 mg SC once daily Avoid for CrCl <30 mL/min	Use another agent with anti-IIa activity considering whether GP IIb/IIIa planned	N/A (use other agent if no prior exposure to fondaparinux)

ACT, activated clotting time; aPTT, activated partial thromboplastin time; CrCl, creatinine clearance; GP, glycoprotein; IV, intravenous; NSTE-ACS, non-ST-segment acute coronary syndrome; PCI, percutaneous coronary intervention; SC, subcutaneous.

Anticoagulant Use With an Early Invasive Management Strategy

Patients presenting with NSTE-ACS who are being treated with an early invasive management strategy are usually started on anticoagulant therapy at the time of diagnosis and typically taken to the catheterization laboratory within 48 hours of presentation. Anticoagulant agents that have been shown to be effective in this setting include intravenous bivalirudin, intravenous UFH, subcutaneously administered fondaparinux, or subcutaneously administered enoxaparin. There are limited comparative data among the various class I agents in this setting, and across-study comparative assessments based upon historical data are often confounded by changes in adjunctive therapies (eg, antiplatelet agents) over time. Thus, the specific choice of an anticoagulant agent may be a physician- or an institution-dependent decision, modified by patient-specific factors.

Patients with NSTE-ACS undergoing PCI frequently require uptitration of anticoagulant dosing at the time of PCI in order to minimize the additional thrombogenicity associated with the procedure (**Table 4.2**). Consistency in anticoagulant choice should be maintained in most circumstances, given that several studies have demonstrated an associated increased risk of bleeding when switching anticoagulant agents, particularly if enoxaparin is used as the initial anticoagulant.[5] In rare cases (eg, in the treatment of intraprocedural thrombotic complications), patients may require the use of more than one anticoagulant agent during PCI. Additionally, because of an increased rate of catheter-related thrombotic complications observed during PCI performed with fondaparinux,[2] intraprocedural treatment with an additional anticoagulant should be administered at the time of PCI.[6]

Anticoagulant therapy is typically discontinued immediately following PCI because continued administration has demonstrated limited additional anti-ischemic benefits and an increased risk of bleeding.

Anticoagulant Use With an Ischemia-Guided Management Strategy

The goal of anticoagulant therapy in patients with NSTE-ACS is first to placate the activated prothrombotic state. Appropriate patients can then be further risk stratified with noninvasive testing, which may lead to a more selective use of angiography and/or revascularization. Patients with NSTE-ACS receiving ischemia-guided management may be treated with various anticoagulants, including UFH, enoxaparin, or fondaparinux. According to the current ACC/AHA guidelines, bivalirudin is not considered part of the armamentarium for an ischemia-guided management strategy because of the limited data with this agent in these patients.

There are limited data regarding the exact duration of anticoagulant therapy in patients receiving ischemia-guided therapy. It is recommended that enoxaparin and fondaparinux should be continued for the duration of the hospitalization or until PCI is performed. In contrast, UFH is usually continued for only 48 hours or until PCI is performed.

Anticoagulants During PCI

Anticoagulation is generally administered during PCI in order to suppress the thrombotic process that may be precipitated by the introduction of foreign objects into the coronary vasculature (ie, catheters, wires, balloons, stents). Furthermore, anticoagulants can help suppress activation of the thrombotic cascade following vessel injury during PCI. There are several classes of anticoagulants that have been shown to be effective in treating patients undergoing PCI, including UFH; enoxaparin, an LWMH; and direct thrombin inhibitors such as bivalirudin.

Anticoagulants are typically not administered during diagnostic catheterization procedures with the exception of transradially performed diagnostic procedures. If the radial artery is chosen as the access site for angiography, it is recommended that parenteral anticoagulation be started promptly after the arterial sheath is placed, in order to reduce the risk of radial artery occlusion. Spaulding et al. demonstrated a correlation between the dose of UFH therapy used following transradial access and the rate of radial artery occlusion post procedure in 415 patients; occlusion occurred in 71% of patients with no UFH therapy, 24% in patients treated with 2000 to 3000 U of UFH, and 4.3% in those treated with 5000 U of UFH.[7] Whether the use of more modern hydrophilic sheaths, smaller catheter sizes, and shorter procedure times can completely mitigate this effect is unknown.

Once the decision is made to pursue PCI (irrespective of the access site), the ACC/AHA/Society for Cardiovascular Angiography and Interventions (SCAI) guidelines give a class I recommendation to administer additional parenteral anticoagulation at the time of the procedure.[8] Specific recommendations regarding the choice of agent depend upon the clinical scenario. For patients not previously on parenteral anticoagulants, an anticoagulant agent is chosen and typically administered as a parenteral bolus, with an infusion lasting for the duration of the PCI. For patients with NSTE-ACS treated with upstream therapy, the dose of anticoagulation is typically higher during PCI than during maintenance upstream therapy, and several therapies used upstream are not indicated for PCI; thus, specific decisions regarding switching anticoagulants, further bolus dosing, and/or increasing the dose of infusion are required (**Table 4.2**). Of the anticoagulants used during PCI, UFH is one agent for which intraprocedural monitoring of levels of anticoagulant activity is recommended.

In general, anticoagulant therapy is discontinued immediately following PCI. Decisions regarding management of the vascular access site depend upon several factors: the site of access (eg, femoral vs radial), whether use of a vascular closure device is planned, and the particular anticoagulant used. For femoral access, if use of a vascular closure device is planned, it is typically deployed immediately after PCI. For manual compression of a femoral access site, sheaths are usually removed when the activated clotting time (ACT) falls below 150 to 180 seconds in patients treated with UFH; for patients treated with bivalirudin, sheaths are typically removed 2 hours after termination of the infusion. For radial access, sheath removal is typically performed immediately after PCI by applying nonocclusive pressure, typically with a specialized pressure device to achieve patient hemostasis in order to preserve flow in the radial artery.

SPECIFIC ANTICOAGULANTS

Unfractionated Heparin

UFH is a mixture of polysaccharide chains with molecular weights ranging from 3000 to 30,000 Da, which exerts its major anticoagulant effect by indirectly inactivating thrombin and the coagulation cascade. UFH facilitates activation of antithrombin III, which then inactivates factors IIa (thrombin), IXa, and Xa. Bioavailability of UFH varies from patient to patient because of its nonspecific binding to plasma proteins and cells. As a consequence, the anticoagulant response to UFH varies among patients and necessitates the monitoring of the activated partial thromboplastin time (aPTT) or ACT in order to achieve the optimally desired level of anticoagulation.

Summary of Trial Data

NSTE-ACS

One of the oldest anticoagulants used to treat ACS, UFH has been studied in numerous trials involving patients with NSTE-ACS. In a meta-analysis comparing the effect of aspirin plus UFH with that of UFH alone, aspirin plus UFH was shown to reduce early ischemic events, with borderline significance noted in the reduction of early death or myocardial infarction (MI) (**Fig. 4.1**).[9] It should be noted that the effects of UFH regarding the endpoint of death/MI were not significant in any of the individual trials included in this meta-analysis. Furthermore, antiplatelet agents such as adenosine diphosphate (ADP) receptor blockers, which provide an additional anti-ischemic effect, were not included in these trials, so the "true" effect of UFH when used in conjunction with more potent antiplatelet agents compared with no UFH is poorly understood from clinical trials (**Fig. 4.1**).

Elective PCI

UFH was the sole anticoagulant used in PCI for many years, and because of its widespread and early acceptance, there are limited trial data examining its efficacy and safety compared with a background of no UFH. Clinical experience with the use of UFH suggests that the optimal intensity of anticoagulation is generally greater in patients undergoing PCI than in those with ACS who are being medically managed. Early on in the PCI experience, UFH was given at the beginning of the procedure as a standard dose of 10,000 U intravenously, with further bolus doses administered hourly. Nevertheless, because of variable anticoagulant effects observed with these fixed dosing regimens of UFH, as well as the observation of an increased rate of bleeding complications in patients treated with UFH plus potent antiplatelet agents such as glycoprotein (GP) IIb/IIIa inhibitors, the measurement of ACT has become integrated as part of the PCI procedure (see later discussion).

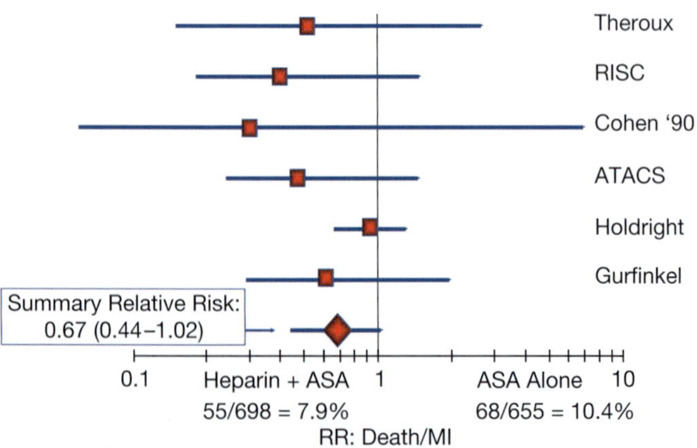

FIGURE 4.1 Meta-analysis of UFH plus aspirin versus aspirin alone in ACS. ACS, acute coronary syndrome; ASA, aspirin; MI, myocardial infarction; RR, relative risk; UFH, unfractionated heparin. (Adapted from Oler A, Whooley MA, Grady D. Adding heparin to aspirin reduces the incidence of myocardial infarction and death in patients with unstable angina. A meta-analysis. *JAMA*. 1996;276:811-815, with permission.)

Unfractionated Heparin: Dosing Strategies and Therapeutics

NSTE-ACS

In ACS, UFH is administered as an intravenous bolus followed by a continuous intravenous infusion. Traditionally, UFH is given as a 5000-U bolus followed by a 1000-U/h infusion, with further adjustments made according to the aPTT. Nevertheless, more predictable anticoagulation can be effected through weight-based dosing, which is the current recommendation in the ACC/AHA guidelines. These guidelines recommend an intravenous bolus dose of UFH (60 U/kg not to exceed 4000 U), followed by an initial 12-U/kg/h infusion (not to exceed 1000 U/h). Further dosing is dictated by monitoring of the aPTT or ACT (the latter for patients undergoing PCI).

Measurement of the aPTT can vary from institution to institution, so it is important to implement an institution-specific nomogram and/or protocol for UFH. Ideally, patients maintained on UFH should have a target aPTT in the range of 1.5 to 2.0 times control. This dosing is thought to optimize the anti-ischemic effects of UFH while minimizing bleeding that can occur at higher achieved levels of anticoagulation.[10] For patients undergoing PCI, additional intravenous boluses are typically administered.

The ACC/AHA guidelines recommend the administration of UFH up until the time of angiography for those patients undergoing an early invasive management strategy, but the optimal duration of UFH in patients with ACS beyond angiography is unknown. Patients who undergo PCI should have UFH discontinued after PCI; those undergoing coronary artery bypass grafting (CABG) should continue UFH. Patients being treated medically or those not undergoing an invasive management strategy are typically treated with UFH through their hospitalization (at least 48 hours), at which point it can be discontinued.

UFH is a reversible anticoagulant whose effect dissipates over time when the infusion is stopped. In more emergent settings, protamine sulfate can be administered for rapid reversal. A test dose is usually given prior to administering a full dose of protamine to prevent anaphylaxis-type reactions, which have been known to occur in patients with prior exposure to long-acting insulins.

During PCI

For PCI, UFH is administered as an intravenous bolus with therapeutic levels monitored by ACT. Because the intensity of anticoagulation during PCI is greater than during upstream medical therapy, heparin infusions are typically discontinued 30 minutes prior to PCI and full dosing of UFH is given at the time of PCI. Weight-based dosing should be employed, using doses of 50 to 70 U/kg with a target ACT of 200 to 250 seconds if GP IIb/IIIa inhibitors are used and 70 to 100 U/kg with a target ACT of 300 to 350 seconds if no GP IIb/IIIa inhibitors are used (**Table 4.2**). In rare cases, such as in retrograde PCI procedures, the current clinical standard is to maintain ACT at the higher end of this scale so as to mitigate against catheter thrombosis within a large ischemic territory. Patients undergoing PCI with UFH should have the anticoagulant stopped at the end of the procedure.

Chew and colleagues pooled the results from the UFH-only arms of six randomized control trials enrolling 5216 patients who were primarily treated with balloon angioplasty alone and then examined the association between ACT and outcomes after PCI.[11] In this analysis, patients with ACT values ranging from 350 to 375 seconds had the lowest ischemic event rates (**Fig. 4.2**, left panel); however, major or minor bleeding rates were lowest with ACT values between 300 and 350 seconds (**Fig. 4.2**, right panel). A pooled analysis of four more recent randomized trials, which included patients treated primarily with stents and GP IIb/IIIa inhibitors, demonstrated no significant correlation between maximal ACT and ischemic complications, with a monotonically increasing risk of bleeding at increasing levels of ACT.[12] Based upon these and other studies, current guidelines recommend ACT-based titration of UFH during PCI, with lower levels of ACT for patients treated with concomitant potent antiplatelet therapies.

Adverse Consequences

As an anticoagulant, UFH is associated with bleeding complications, which must be weighed against the potential anti-ischemic effects of the agent. While bleeding complications can occur despite a therapeutic range aPTT, higher aPTT values are associated with increased bleeding complications. Appropriate dosing and monitoring of UFH should be performed in order to maximize UFH's

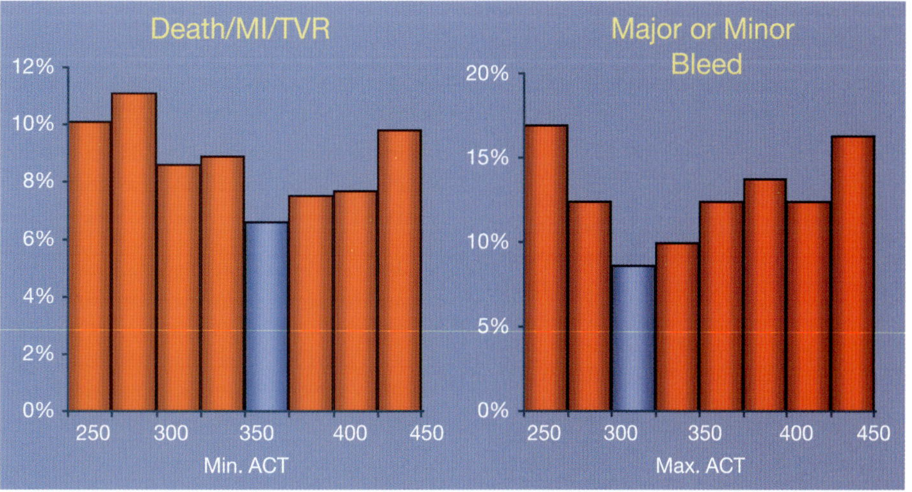

FIGURE 4.2 Optimal levels of anticoagulation with UFH based upon ACT. ACT, activated clotting time; MI, myocardial infarction; TVR, target vessel revascularization; UFH, unfractionated heparin. (Adapted from Chew DP, Bhatt DL, Lincoff AM, et al. Defining the optimal activated clotting time during percutaneous coronary intervention: aggregate results from 6 randomized, controlled trials. *Circulation*. 2001;103:961-966, with permission.)

risk-benefit ratio, as higher doses of both the bolus and infusion have been associated with adverse outcomes.[13] In a large observational registry of patients with ACS, excess dosing of UFH was found in almost one-third of patients.[14]

In addition to bleeding complications, exposure to UFH has also been associated with the development of heparin-induced thrombocytopenia, which can occur with or without thrombosis.[6,15] Mild thrombocytopenia may occur in 10% to 20% of patients, whereas significant thrombocytopenia (platelet count <100,000) occurs in 1% to 5% of patients and typically appears after several days of therapy. Discontinuation of UFH usually resolves the thrombocytopenia. Immune-mediated heparin-induced thrombocytopenia is a more rare complication of UFH treatment (<0.2%) and requires abrupt withdrawal of UFH and active treatment with a direct thrombin inhibitor to prevent the thrombotic sequelae of the syndrome. Finally, excess thrombin generation (the so-called rebound effect) has additionally been described following cessation of UFH; the actual adverse clinical sequelae of this effect are largely unknown, particularly in the era of more potent antiplatelet therapies.[16]

Low-Molecular-Weight Heparins

LWMHs, ranging from 1000 to 10,000 Da, are derived from UFH via chemical or enzymatic depolymerization. Similar to UFH, LMWH forms a complex with antithrombin III, converting it from a slow to a rapid inactivator of clotting factors. LMWHs are potent inactivators of factor Xa and factor IIa (thrombin). In addition, LMWHs exhibit less binding to plasma proteins and cells and have a longer half-life. This facilitates more predictable dose responses to LMWH compared with UFH and allows LMWH to be administered via subcutaneous administration with twice-daily dosing or daily dosing in those with renal impairment (creatinine clearance [CrCl] <30 mL/min).

Summary of Trial Data

NSTE-ACS

The FRISC study was the only large randomized trial that compared LMWH with placebos. It randomized 1506 patients with ACS and showed that the addition of dalteparin to aspirin reduced the risk of early death or MI (in the first 6 days) from 4.8% to 1.8% (*P* = .001) compared with aspirin alone.[17] This study primarily enrolled medically managed patients with ACS, and it should be noted that, among patients randomized to dalteparin, therapy was continued for several weeks.

Comparisons of LMWH Versus UFH

The majority of data with LMWH in ACS consist of randomized trials comparing the use of LMWH with UFH on a background of aspirin antiplatelet therapy. Although different preparations of LMWH have been studied (including dalteparin and nadroparin), the most positive results have been observed using enoxaparin.

Early data from the TIMI 11B and ESSENCE trials demonstrated reductions in the composite of death, MI, or recurrent ischemia with enoxaparin compared with UFH. These trials supported the use of LMWH in patients with ACS managed predominantly with an ischemia-guided strategy rather than with an invasive strategy.[18]

These favorable results led to the design of trials comparing the use of LMWH with UFH in invasively managed patients with ACS. In the 10,027-patient SYNERGY trial, the rate of the composite ischemic endpoint of death or MI was 14.0% with enoxaparin versus 14.5% with UFH (nonstatistically different); however, bleeding complications were more frequent with enoxaparin.[19] The use of enoxaparin in this trial was in addition to aspirin and, in approximately half of enrolled patients, GP IIb/IIIa inhibitors. In the smaller A-to-Z trial in which patients were randomized to enoxaparin or UFH groups on a background of aspirin and routine GP IIb/IIIa inhibition, treatment with enoxaparin was associated with a nonsignificantly lower rate of death, MI, or recurrent ischemia at 30 days (8.4% vs 9.4%), with numerically greater rates of bleeding compared with UFH.[20] In A-to-Z, however, only half of the patients were managed with an early invasive strategy and a post hoc subgroup analysis demonstrated that the benefit of enoxaparin was largely confined to patients managed using an ischemia-guided strategy.

A meta-analysis of all enoxaparin versus UFH trials in ACS has been conducted, which demonstrates an approximately 10% reduction in death or MI with enoxaparin over UFH, with no significant differences in major bleeding outcomes.[5] It should be noted that this meta-analysis included a number of patients who were managed using an ischemia-guided strategy and that higher rates of bleeding outcomes were observed with enoxaparin compared with UFH in the SYNERGY trial, the largest trial of invasively managed patients with ACS. A post hoc analysis of the SYNERGY trial showed that the higher rates of bleeding in the enoxaparin arm might have been a consequence of the use of either multiple anticoagulants or the switching of agents in the study. It remains unclear whether maintaining consistency in the use of anticoagulants could have minimized bleeding complications in this trial.[21]

Elective PCI

While the use of enoxaparin in PCI is not common in the United States, enoxaparin has a class IIb indication in the ACC/AHA/SCAI guidelines for elective PCI, largely on the basis of the randomized STEEPLE trial. STEEPLE enrolled over 3000 patients and compared three intravenously administered anticoagulant regimens in patients undergoing elective PCI: enoxaparin 0.5 mg/kg, enoxaparin 0.75 mg/kg, or UFH 70 to 100 U/kg adjusted for ACT (if GP IIb/IIIa inhibitors were used, then UFH was decreased to 50-70 U/kg).[22] The trial demonstrated a statistically significant reduction in the primary endpoint of non-CABG bleeding with enoxaparin 0.5 mg/kg compared with UFH (5.9% vs 8.5%, *P* = .01) but no statistically significant difference between enoxaparin 0.75 mg/kg and UFH. The incidence of minor bleeding was significantly reduced in both enoxaparin groups compared with UFH, and there were no statistically significant differences in the rates of death, MI, or urgent target vessel revascularization between study arms.

Differentiation Between LMWHs

Different formulations of LMWH have varying ratios of anti–factor Xa to anti–factor IIa activity. It is unclear, however, whether these differences have any clinically meaningful effects. Very few trials have directly compared the various LMWHs. Indirect comparisons between agents suggest that enoxaparin is likely the most clinically useful agent, and there is one small randomized trial comparing enoxaparin versus tinzaparin in patients with unstable angina (UA). In the EVET trial, patients treated with enoxaparin had significantly lower rates of ischemic outcomes compared with those treated with tinzaparin, with similar rates of bleeding outcomes.[23]

Dosing Strategies

NSTE-ACS

The ACC/AHA guidelines recommend the administration of LMWH up to the time of diagnostic angiography for patients treated according to an invasive management strategy. Patients who undergo PCI should have LWMH discontinued after PCI; those undergoing CABG should discontinue LMWH 12 to 24 hours prior to CABG. Patients being treated medically or those not undergoing an invasive management strategy should be treated with LMWH through hospitalization, at which point the agent can be discontinued.

The anticoagulant effect of LMWH can be measured directly by assessing factor Xa activity. The aPTT is not a reliable indicator of anticoagulant effect. Because of the predictable effects of LMWH, it is not necessary in clinical practice to monitor the level of anticoagulant effect, making LMWH easier to use compared with intravenously dosed UFH. Caution should be used when administering LMWH in patients with renal dysfunction; a dose reduction to once a day is recommended in patients with CrCl of <30 mL/min. LWMH can also be administered intravenously, which can be useful for PCI, particularly in patients who have not received prior doses of LWMH.

During PCI

Patients who have not received any prior anticoagulant therapy should be loaded with 0.5 to 0.75 mg/kg intravenous (IV) loading dose of enoxaparin. Patients who are being treated initially with subcutaneously administered enoxaparin and undergo PCI within 8 hours of the last dose do not need to have any additional anticoagulant given. Nevertheless, if PCI is undertaken in the 8- to 12-hour period after the last dose of subcutaneous enoxaparin, or if patients have received only one dose of enoxaparin, the guidelines recommend that they be given additional enoxaparin (0.3 mg/kg IV) at the time of PCI (**Table 4.2**). Those patients undergoing PCI more than 12 hours after the last dose of enoxaparin are typically treated as if they have not received upstream therapy. Once the procedure is completed, further anticoagulation should be stopped.

It is also reasonable to administer intravenous enoxaparin to those patients presenting for elective PCI who have not been given any prior anticoagulation. While direct assessment of factor Xa levels is possible, this test is rarely indicated because of the predictability of enoxaparin's effect. The initial intravenous dose given should be 30 mg. ACT levels are not reliable indicators of anticoagulant effect in patients who were administered enoxaparin.

Adverse Consequences of LMWH

LMWH agents, likely UFH, are associated with bleeding complications, which must be weighed against potential anti-ischemic benefits. In a large observational series of patients with ACS, excess dosing of LMWH agents occurred 13.6% of the time and was associated with increased rates of bleeding.[14] Thus, careful attention must be paid to optimal weight-based dosing and dose adjustments based on renal dysfunction for those agents that are primarily renally cleared in order to minimize bleeding complications.

LMWH have been associated with heparin-associated thrombocytopenia, but with a much lower frequency compared with UFH.[15] Additionally, LMWH causes less platelet activation and aggregation than UFH. The use of LMWH during PCI has been associated with a low but notable rate of episodes of catheter-related thrombotic complications, despite adequate inhibition of factor Xa.[24] This complication requires treatment with either UFH or a direct thrombin inhibitor. While a "rebound" phenomenon has been observed with cessation of LMWH therapy, LMWH, unlike UFH, can stimulate the release of tissue factor pathway inhibitors, which enhance anti–factor Xa activity and can attenuate the rebound hypercoagulability that has been observed with UFH.[25]

Direct Thrombin Inhibitors

Direct thrombin inhibitors offer advantages over UFH and LMWH in that they inhibit thrombin directly, rather than through activation of antithrombin III. Additionally, direct thrombin inhibitors can inhibit both free as well as clot-bound thrombin, provide a very stable level of anticoagulation, and do not cause thrombocytopenia. Hirudin, a naturally occurring anticoagulant derived from the medicinal leech, is made commercially by recombinant DNA technology in a number of formulations (including lepirudin, desirudin) and was used in early studies of ACS. Bivalirudin, another direct thrombin inhibitor, is an analogue of hirudin and binds reversibly to thrombin with a short half-life, inhibiting thrombin's activity. Bivalirudin is the most widely studied direct thrombin inhibitor in the contemporary management of ACS and patients undergoing PCI. Argatroban is another monovalent direct thrombin inhibitor that is approved for the treatment of heparin-induced thrombocytopenia, but it is not indicated for the treatment of ACS following negative studies with this agent in STEMI.

Summary of Trial Data

NSTE-ACS

Several early trials evaluated recombinant hirudin versus UFH for patients with ACS. The largest of these trials was GUSTO IIb, enrolling 12,142 patients with both NSTE-ACS and STEMI, including patients treated with fibrinolytic therapy. In this trial, although the 24-hour endpoint of death or MI favored hirudin, the 30-day rate of death or MI was not significantly lower with hirudin compared with UFH and the rate of moderate bleeding was higher with hirudin.[26] Further evaluation of hirudin continued in the 10,141-patient OASIS-2 trial, which again demonstrated improved ischemic outcomes with hirudin (but nonsignificantly so) and higher rates of bleeding.[27] Pooling of all the major hirudin trials has demonstrated an overall reduction, ~20%, in ischemic events (death or MI) with hirudin over UFH, but at the cost of an excess of bleeding complications.[27,28] Notably, these early trials were conducted on an antiplatelet background of aspirin alone.

Bivalirudin, a synthetic analogue of hirudin, was first studied in the BAT trial, a trial of bivalirudin versus UFH in 4098 patients undergoing PCI for UA or postinfarction angina. In this trial, bivalirudin did not significantly reduce the incidence of the composite primary ischemic endpoint (a combination of early death, MI, abrupt vessel closure, or clinical deterioration) compared with UFH but was associated with a reduction in bleeding.[29] A subsequent reevaluation of the data from this trial with a more contemporary ischemic endpoint of death, MI, or repeat revascularization demonstrated the benefit of using bivalirudin over UFH (6.2% vs 7.9%, $P = .039$), with lower rates of bleeding.[30] These data and other emerging favorable data for bivalirudin in PCI patients led to a reassessment of the use of bivalirudin for ACS in the ACUITY trial.

ACUITY randomly assigned 13,819 patients with moderate- to high-risk ACS to one of three antithrombotic regimens: UFH (or enoxaparin) plus a GP IIb/IIIa inhibitor, bivalirudin plus a GP IIb/IIIa inhibitor, or bivalirudin monotherapy.[31] Patients were managed with an early invasive strategy. In this trial, bivalirudin monotherapy was associated with a similar rate of composite ischemia (7.8% vs 7.3%, $P = .32$) and significantly reduced major bleeding (3.0% vs 5.7%, $P < .001$), compared with UFH/enoxaparin plus a GP IIb/IIIa inhibitor (**Fig. 4.3**). While these results were consistent in most major subgroups of the trial, the 30-day composite ischemic event rate was notably higher with bivalirudin

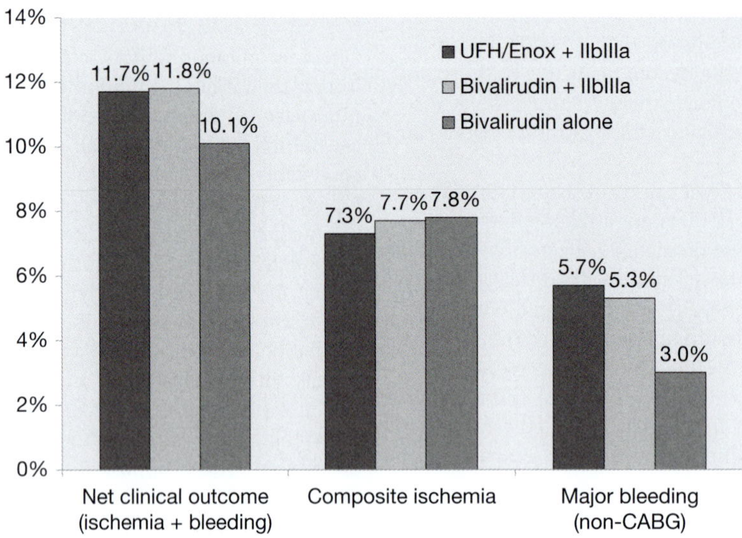

FIGURE 4.3 Thirty-day outcomes from the ACUITY Trial of bivalirudin in acute coronary syndromes. CABG, coronary artery bypass grafting; UFH, unfractionated heparin.

monotherapy than with UFH plus GP IIb/IIIa inhibition among patients not pretreated with an ADP-receptor antagonist (9.1% vs 7.1%, P = .05 for interaction). In ACUITY, treatment with bivalirudin plus routine GP IIb/IIIa inhibition resulted in similar rates of 30-day death, MI, or unplanned revascularization for recurrent ischemia compared with UFH/enoxaparin plus GP IIb/IIIa inhibitors (7.7% vs 7.3%, P = .39) and similar rates of major bleeding (5.3% vs 5.7%, P = .38).

Because both BAT and ACUITY employed invasive management strategies and in the case of ACUITY the time from admission to angiography was short (19.6 hours), current guidelines stress that, for patients experiencing more significant delays to catheterization, or patients with recurrent ischemia following the initial treatment strategy, consideration should be given to further escalation of the antithrombotic regimen (eg, through the addition of a GP IIb/IIIa inhibitor). In fact, some have questioned whether the potential benefits of bivalirudin over UFH alone could be replicated by more aggressive oral antiplatelet therapy (such as ADP-receptor blockade) in conjunction with UFH monotherapy (without a GP IIb/IIIa inhibitor). In the ISAR-REACT 3 study, this strategy was tested among patients undergoing PCI either electively or for UA.[32] In this trial on 4570 patients pretreated with 600 mg of clopidogrel, the rates of ischemic outcomes were similar for patients treated with bivalirudin or UFH, but bivalirudin-treated patients had a significantly lower rate of bleeding complications (3.1% vs 4.6%, P = .008). Further validation of the ACUITY results, however, has occurred in the ISAR-REACT-4 trial, a trial randomizing 1721 patients in a double-blind manner to abciximab plus UFH versus bivalirudin. The primary composite endpoint of death, MI, major bleeding, and urgent target-vessel revascularization was similar in both arms, with an increased risk of major bleeding observed with abciximab plus UFH compared with bivalirudin alone (4.6% vs 2.6%, P = .02).[33]

More recently, there have been conflicting data regarding whether the benefits of bivalirudin therapy persist when compared with heparin therapy alone and GP IIb/IIIA inhibitor use is reserved as a bailout therapy. For example, in the MATRIX study, 7213 patients with ACS were randomized to receive either UFH or bivalirudin. Thirty-day major adverse cardiovascular events (MACEs) rates (composite of death, MI, or stroke) were similar among patients receiving bivalirudin or heparin (10.3% vs 10.9%, P = .44).[34] Furthermore, in the NSTE-ACS patient subset, there was no significant difference in MACE rates between patients receiving bivalirudin or heparin (15.9% vs 16.5%, P = .74).[35] In contrast, bivalirudin was associated with fewer net adverse clinical events at 30 days compared with heparin (8.8% vs 13.2%, P = .008) in the BRIGHT trial, which included 2194 patients with acute myocardial infarction (AMI). Moreover, patients receiving bivalirudin had lower rates of 30-day bleeding compared with those receiving heparin (4.1% vs 7.5%, P < .001).[36] Additional large randomized controlled studies are needed to address this clinical question.

Elective PCI

Early trials such as BAT (see earlier) and REPLACE-1[37] were conducted to study the use of bivalirudin as an alternative anticoagulant for PCI. REPLACE-1 randomized 1056 patients undergoing elective or urgent PCI to bivalirudin versus UFH; the majority of patients were pretreated with clopidogrel, and 72% of patients received a GP IIb/IIIa inhibitor. Compared with UFH, bivalirudin was associated with a similar rate of death, MI, or repeat revascularization, with a similar frequency of major bleeding complications. The larger REPLACE-2 trial was designed to further test the use of bivalirudin in 6000 patients undergoing urgent or elective PCI; the majority of patients were pretreated with a thienopyridine platelet antagonist.[38] Patients were randomized to either bivalirudin and provisional GP IIb/IIIa inhibition (with either eptifibatide or abciximab) or UFH plus routine GP IIb/IIIa inhibition. There were no significant differences in the occurrence of the primary study endpoint of death, MI, urgent revascularization, or in-hospital major bleeding between study arms. Nevertheless, there was a significant reduction of major bleeding events (using a more sensitive bleeding scale) with bivalirudin compared with UFH (2.4% vs 4.1%; P < .001).

Direct Thrombin Inhibitors

The two direct thrombin inhibitors best studied in ACS are bivalirudin and hirudin. Hirudin and argatroban have limited ischemic efficacy and are presently only approved for those patients who have developed heparin-induced thrombocytopenia. The best-studied agent for use in PCI is bivalirudin. Argatroban can be used during PCI, but given the widespread availability of bivalirudin, its use is limited. Argatroban can be considered in patients with renal insufficiency because of its hepatic clearance. In these cases, the usual dose is an intravenous infusion of 2 μg/kg/min, which is adjusted to maintain an aPTT 1.5 to 3 times baseline (but not >100 seconds).

NSTE-ACS

Bivalirudin is given a class I recommendation from ACC/AHA for the treatment of invasively managed patients with NSTE-ACS, but it is not currently indicated for patients with NSTE-ACS receiving ischemia-guided management. Bivalirudin is administered as an intravenous bolus followed by an infusion (**Table 4.2**). Owing to its excellent bioavailability, there is no need for monitoring of therapeutic effect. Patients undergoing PCI should receive an additional bolus and an increased rate of infusion; dose adjustments should be made for those with CrCl < 30 mL/min. The bivalirudin infusion is typically discontinued immediately following cardiac catheterization (and/or PCI), although some have advocated a longer duration of therapy, particularly for patients not adequately treated with thienopyridines. Patients treated with bivalirudin who are medically managed following diagnostic angiography can have the bivalirudin stopped or continued for up to 72 hours at the treating physician's discretion. Patients scheduled to undergo CABG should have the bivalirudin stopped 3 hours prior to CABG and can then be treated with UFH if necessary.

During PCI

For patients undergoing elective PCI (or those with NSTE-ACS not on prior anticoagulation), an intravenous weight-based bolus of 0.75 mg/kg is administered, followed by an intravenous infusion of 1.75 mg/kg/h (**Table 4.2**). In patients who have already received UFH, the bolus and intravenous infusion rates should be started after the UFH has been stopped for 30 minutes. In patients who have already been started on a bivalirudin infusion, an additional 0.5 mg/kg loading dose should be given and the intravenous infusion rate should be increased to 1.75 mg/kg/h during PCI. Switching from another anticoagulant (eg, enoxaparin or UFH) to bivalirudin during PCI has not been associated with adverse outcomes.[39] Owing to bivalirudin's excellent bioavailability, there is no need for intraprocedural monitoring. Dose adjustments to the infusion should be made for those patients with a CrCl < 30 mL/min. Once the PCI procedure is complete, the infusion is typically discontinued.

Adverse Events

Bleeding complications are the primary adverse effects that need to be monitored in anticoagulated patients who are being treated with this agent. Unlike UFH, direct thrombin inhibitors cannot be reversed, and bleeding complications that arise need to be managed supportively until the anticoagulant effect has diminished. Despite this, bivalirudin is associated with lower bleeding complications compared with UFH and LMWH, particularly when the latter are coadministered with GP IIb/IIIa inhibitors. This makes bivalirudin an attractive agent to consider in patients who are at higher risk for bleeding complications.

Factor Xa Inhibition With Fondaparinux

Factor Xa inhibitors exert their anticoagulant effect more proximally in the coagulation cascade and have demonstrated promise in the treatment of ACS. The synthetic pentasaccharide fondaparinux is the best-studied parenteral factor Xa inhibitor used for patients with ACS. Fondaparinux is structurally similar to the antithrombin-binding portion of UFH (and LMWH), and by reversibly binding to antithrombin III, it indirectly inhibits factor Xa.

Summary of Trial Data

NSTE-ACS

The largest trial of fondaparinux in NSTE-ACS was the OASIS-5 trial. This trial randomized 20,078 patients with ACS to fondaparinux versus enoxaparin; both agents were administered subcutaneously for a mean of 6 days.[2] Patients in this trial were managed more conservatively compared with other contemporary ACS trials: overall, approximately two-thirds of patients underwent diagnostic coronary angiography. Patients undergoing PCI received additional anticoagulant therapy depending on the duration from the last administered study dose (in some cases in the fondaparinux arm, patients received additional intravenously administered fondaparinux). The rate of the primary composite endpoint of death, MI, or refractory ischemia was similar to that of fondaparinux and enoxaparin (5.8% vs 5.7%), but bleeding events were significantly decreased with the use of fondaparinux (2.2% vs 4.1%, $P < .001$) (**Fig. 4.4**). These benefits persisted at 30 days; in

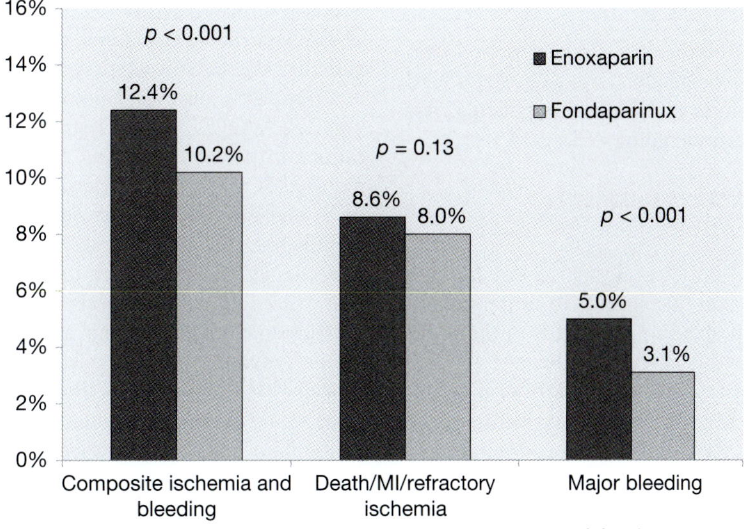

FIGURE 4.4 Thirty-day outcomes from the OASIS-5 Trial of fondaparinux in ACS. ACS, acute coronary syndrome; MI, myocardial infarction.

fact, 30-day mortality was lower with fondaparinux compared with enoxaparin (2.9% vs 3.5%, $P = .02$).

In the subset of patients undergoing PCI in OASIS-5, fondaparinux was associated with an increased risk of catheter-related thrombus (0.9% vs 0.3% for enoxaparin), a finding that was also confirmed in the OASIS-6 trial of fondaparinux for STEMI. As a result, operators were permitted to use open-label UFH during PCI for patients already treated with fondaparinux. A subsequent trial, FUTURA/OASIS-8, has examined the effects of UFH dosing during PCI for 2026 patients treated with fondaparinux for ACS.[40] In this trial, there was no difference in outcomes using a low dose of UFH versus a higher dose.

Elective PCI

Fondaparinux has been studied in patients with ACS but has not been studied in patients undergoing elective PCI.

Dosing Strategies and Adverse Events

Fondaparinux has minimal binding to plasma proteins other than antithrombin.[41] Thus, it is readily absorbed, with plasma concentrations peaking at around 2 hours. Its long elimination half-life of approximately 17 hours allows for once daily dosing, and there is no need for monitoring. Given that it is renally cleared, fondaparinux is contraindicated in patients with a CrCl < 30 mL/min.

The optimal duration of fondaparinux therapy in patients with ACS is unknown, but the ACC/AHA guidelines recommend continuing dosing up to the time of diagnostic angiography for patients undergoing an invasive management strategy. Patients who undergo PCI should have fondaparinux discontinued after PCI. Additional UFH should be given particularly during the performance of PCI in fondaparinux-treated patients to avoid the occurrence of catheter-related thrombus formation. Patients undergoing CABG should discontinue fondaparinux 24 hours prior to CABG. Patients being treated medically or those not undergoing an invasive management strategy should be treated with fondaparinux throughout their hospitalization, at which point it can be discontinued.

Other adverse events, such as bleeding complications, have been associated with treatment with fondaparinux, but these were less frequently observed in the OASIS-5 trial compared with enoxaparin, leading to the recommendation in the ACC/AHA guidelines for the use of this agent in patients managed using an ischemia-guided strategy at risk for bleeding.

Owing to the occurrence of catheter-related thrombus during PCI with fondaparinux anticoagulation, the ACC/AHA/SCAI guidelines for PCI give fondaparinux as a sole anticoagulant a class III (harm) indication for patients undergoing PCI.

Warfarin and Other Oral Anticoagulants for NSTE-ACS

While warfarin and other oral anticoagulants do not provide sufficient levels of anticoagulation for patients to undergo PCI, these agents have been studied as adjunctive add-on therapies for patients with ACS. It is of historical significance to note that early in the stent experience, anticoagulation with warfarin was used as a means of trying to prevent stent thrombosis. The use of warfarin following stent implantation dramatically decreased after several trials demonstrated that dual antiplatelet therapy (DAPT) with aspirin plus the thienopyridine ticlopidine was superior to aspirin plus warfarin following stent implantation.[42]

Warfarin in NSTE-ACS

Warfarin is an oral anticoagulant whose effect is mediated by inhibiting the formation of vitamin K–dependent coagulation factors (factors II, VII, IX, X, and proteins C and S). The anticoagulant activity of warfarin is variable, and the agent has a relatively narrow therapeutic window, which requires close monitoring of the prothrombin time/international normalized ratio in order to assure the optimal level of anticoagulation.

Oral anticoagulation with warfarin post ACS has been examined in several trials, with the rationale that prolonged treatment might extend the benefit of early anticoagulation in NSTE-ACS. The warfarin substudy of the OASIS-2 trial subrandomized 3712 patients to continued warfarin or standard therapy, including aspirin, following initial presentation and treatment for ACS.[43] In this trial, there were no significant differences in the rate of the composite of death, MI, or stroke with either therapy, but major bleeding was increased with warfarin therapy (2.7% vs 1.3%, $P = .004$). Subanalyses of the OASIS-2 data based upon countries with greater adherence to warfarin therapy (>70% compliance with the therapy at 35 days) demonstrated significant anti-ischemic benefits of warfarin among countries with greater adherence to warfarin therapy, but higher relative risks of bleeding complications. Similar data have been reported from other smaller trials, including patients at potentially higher risk, such as STEMI. In the WARIS-2 trial, which randomized 3630 post-MI patients to aspirin alone, warfarin alone, or aspirin plus warfarin, treatment with the combination of aspirin and warfarin was associated with the lowest rate of death, MI, or thromboembolic stroke (15.0% with aspirin plus warfarin vs 16.7% with warfarin alone vs 20% for aspirin alone, $P < .001$).[44] Nevertheless, the incidence of nonfatal bleeding was increased in both warfarin groups compared with that in aspirin alone.

Notable caveats to these early studies are that they largely excluded patients undergoing early revascularization and were conducted prior to more widespread use of DAPT. Oral antiplatelet agents such as $P2Y_{12}$ receptor antagonists have been demonstrated to reduce ischemic outcomes over therapy with aspirin alone and are recommended as the standard of care in virtually all patients with NSTE-ACS. Because the combination of warfarin plus aspirin alone has been associated with increased bleeding, and the combination of aspirin, a $P2Y_{12}$ receptor antagonist, and warfarin increases bleeding to an even greater extent, the role of "triple therapy" is generally limited to patients with other indications for warfarin anticoagulation (eg, mechanical valve, atrial fibrillation, stroke, ventricular thrombus, venous thromboembolism). In these patients, the benefit of preventing thromboembolic events and recurrent ischemic events must be balanced with the risk of bleeding. The WOEST trial investigated the use of antiplatelet medications in patients requiring oral anticoagulant medications who required PCI. This study contained 563 patients (25% with NSTE-ACS) and randomized them to single antiplatelet treatment with clopidogrel or to DAPT with aspirin and clopidogrel. Patients on anticoagulation randomized to clopidogrel alone had significantly fewer bleeding complications than those randomized to DAPT.[45] Furthermore, there was no significant difference in thrombotic events between the two treatment arms. Thus, when possible, shorter durations of triple therapy are recommended. Although there are no prospective data suggesting decreasing the target international normalized ratio to between 2.0 and 2.5 improves bleeding complication rates, it is currently a class IIb recommendation that this may be reasonable in patients requiring triple therapy.

While the data on triple therapy using clopidogrel are limited, even fewer data are available regarding the use of newer $P2Y_{12}$

inhibitors such as prasugrel and ticagrelor in patients requiring oral anticoagulation. These medications are associated with more potent platelet activation and may be associated with increased bleeding.[46] In the TRITON-TIMI 38 study, 13,608 patients with ACS undergoing PCI were randomized to either prasugrel or clopidogrel. Patients who received prasugrel had reduced rates of ischemic events, including death from cardiovascular causes, nonfatal myocardial infarction, or nonfatal stroke (9.9% vs 12.1%; $P < .001$). Nevertheless, they had an increased risk of major bleeding (2.4% vs 1.8%, $P = .01$), including life-threatening bleeding (1.4% vs 0.9%, $P = .01$).[46] Thus, it is recommended that these agents be used with caution in patients who require triple therapy.

Other Oral Factor Xa Inhibitors in NSTE-ACS

There is great interest in the use of oral factor Xa inhibitors for the treatment of ACS. It is theorized that many of the post-ACS/PCI cardiovascular events that occur despite aspirin and ADP-receptor antagonist administration may result from increased levels of thrombin generation precipitated by the initial event.[47] As stated earlier, anticoagulants targeting factor Xa have shown great promise in further downmodulating the thrombotic activation in patients with ACS. Rivaroxaban, a direct oral factor Xa inhibitor, was studied in the double-blind placebo-controlled ATLAS-TIMI 51 study, which enrolled over 15,000 patients.[48] In this trial, stabilized patients with recent ACS in whom the initial management strategy (eg, revascularization) had already been completed were randomized to rivaroxaban 2.5 mg twice daily, 5 mg twice daily, or a placebo. Treatment with rivaroxaban was associated with a reduction in the primary study endpoint of death from cardiovascular causes, MI, or stroke compared with a placebo for both the 2.5-mg dose (9.1% vs 10.7% with placebo, $P = .02$) and the 5-mg dose (8.8% vs 10.7% with placebo, $P = .03$). Despite these benefits, however, there was an increase in the rates of non-CABG-related major bleeding (2.1% vs 0.6%, $P < .001$) and intracranial hemorrhage (0.6% vs 0.2%, $P = .009$) in patients treated with rivaroxaban compared with a placebo, although bleeding complications were less frequent with the 2.5-mg dose of rivaroxaban compared with the 5-mg dose. Notably, the 2.5-mg dose of rivaroxaban was associated with a reduction in all-cause mortality compared with a placebo (2.9% vs 4.5%, $P = .002$), although the trial was underpowered for this comparison. Furthermore, the PIONEER AF-PCI trial demonstrated that the use of rivaroxaban in patients requiring triple therapy may be safer than the use of warfarin. This study randomized 2124 patients with atrial fibrillation undergoing PCI to either low-dose rivaroxaban (15 mg once daily), very-low-dose rivaroxaban (2.5 mg twice daily), or standard therapy with warfarin. Patients receiving either a low dose or very low dose of rivaroxaban had significantly lower rates of bleeding compared with patients receiving warfarin (16.8% vs 18.0% vs 26.7%, $P < .001$). Furthermore, the rates of death from cardiovascular causes, MI, or stroke were similar between all treatment groups.[49] These data suggest the safety of using these newer agents with DAPT; however, larger trials are needed. Furthermore, the role of this therapy as a third agent in the treatment of patients with ACS already on more potent DAPTs such as prasugrel or ticagrelor (see Chapter 17) is at present unstudied.

Apixaban, another oral factor Xa inhibitor, was similarly studied to determine its efficacy in reducing post-ACS cardiovascular events in the APPRAISE-2 trial, a randomized double-blind placebo-controlled trial comparing apixaban 5 mg twice daily with a placebo on a background of aspirin or aspirin plus clopidogrel.[50] While the trial managed to enroll over 7000 patients, the study was stopped early, after review of the data demonstrated an increase in major bleeding events with apixaban compared with the placebo (1.3% vs 0.5%, $P = .001$), without a counterbalancing reduction in ischemic events. More recently, the AUGUSTUS trial, randomly assigned patients with atrial fibrillation and who had ACS undergoing PCI in a 2 × 2 factorial fashion to apixaban versus vitamin K antagonist and to aspirin versus placebo for 6 months. The study found that major or clinically relevant nonmajor bleeding was less among patients receiving apixaban compared with those receiving vitamin K antagonist (10.5% vs 14.7%, $P < .001$). Furthermore, patients who received apixaban had a lower incidence of death or hospitalization than those who received vitamin K antagonist (23.5% vs 27.4%, $P = .002$). Patients assigned to aspirin had similar rates of death or hospitalization and rates of ischemic events compared with the placebo group. Thus, this study concluded that patients with ACS with atrial fibrillation receiving PCI who received apixaban without aspirin had fewer bleeding events without a significant difference in ischemic events compared with patients who received vitamin K or triple therapy with aspirin.[51]

PCI in Patients on Oral Anticoagulants

It is not unusual to be presented in the catheterization laboratory with a patient fully therapeutic on warfarin or another oral anticoagulant prescribed for another indication (eg, for stroke prevention in atrial fibrillation). In this scenario, as a general rule, it is recommended that the oral anticoagulant be discontinued (if possible and not contraindicated), and patients can then undergo angiography and/or PCI using standard techniques, including parenterally administered anticoagulation for PCI. For example, for patients undergoing elective PCI who are therapeutic on warfarin, it is recommended to stop warfarin therapy 2 to 3 days prior to the procedure, and once the procedure is complete (using standard parenteral anticoagulation if PCI is needed), patients can resume their home dose of medication. Patients being treated with the oral direct thrombin inhibitor dabigatran should have their medication stopped 1 to 2 days (if CrCl >50 mL/min) or 3 to 5 days (if CrCl < 50 mL/min) prior to the procedure; patients being treated with rivaroxaban or apixaban should have their medication stopped a day before the procedure. In low-risk patients, oral anticoagulants can typically be resumed after completion of the procedure.

For patients with mechanical valves or other indications requiring "bridging therapy," oral anticoagulation is typically converted to a parenteral agent such as UFH, which is typically maintained through the periprocedural period (and at a higher dose if PCI is required). Once the procedure is complete, the oral agent is typically resumed and the patient maintained on parenteral anticoagulation, until the oral agent has taken effect. Patients in whom the indication for angiography and/or PCI is more urgent can proceed with these procedures while orally anticoagulated, particularly if a transradial approach is utilized.

OVERVIEW OF ACC/AHA/SCAI GUIDELINE RECOMMENDATIONS FOR STEMI

Fibrinolytic Therapy in STEMI

While there is no role for fibrinolytic therapy in patients with UA/NSTEMI,[6] fibrinolytic therapy plays a critical role in patients with STEMI for whom the time delay to achieve successful reperfusion through primary PCI is too great. Fibrinolytic agents activate plasminogen by cleaving it into its active form plasmin, which

TABLE 4.3 Absolute Contraindications to Fibrinolytic Therapy

a. Previous hemorrhagic stroke
b. Ischemic stroke within 3 mo (unless within 3 h)
c. Closed-head trauma within 3 mo
d. Intracranial neoplasm or AVM
e. Active internal bleeding (not menses)
f. Suspected aortic dissection

AVM, arteriovenous malformation.

promotes fibrin degradation. Fibrinolytic therapy is recommended when patients with STEMI present to a non-PCI-capable hospital and patients are unable to be transferred to a PCI-capable facility within an anticipated first medical contact to PCI reperfusion time of 120 minutes.[52] In addition, current guidelines recommend that fibrinolytic therapy should be administered within 30 minutes of patient presentation. There are specific contraindications to fibrinolytic therapy that should be noted (**Table 4.3**). Despite the benefits of fibrinolytic therapy in terms of improving reperfusion, fibrinolytic therapy is associated with a constant risk of major bleeding complications, including the most feared complication of intracranial hemorrhage, which occurs in <1% of patients, but with variability based upon patient characteristics (eg, age).

The use of fibrinolytic therapy in patients with STEMI has been well established as a reperfusion strategy (especially for patients with delays to primary PCI). The GISSI-1 trial, containing 11,712 patients with STEMI, demonstrated that mortality rates at 21 days were significantly lower in patients treated with streptokinase compared with control patients (10.7% vs 13%, P = .0002).[53] In the ISIS-2 trial, 17,187 patients were randomized to streptokinase alone, aspirin alone, and streptokinase with aspirin or placebo. Patients who received streptokinase with aspirin had lower rates of death (8.0% vs 13.2%, P < .001) and reinfarction (1.8% vs 2.9%, P < .001) compared with patients who received a placebo.[54] Furthermore, in the ASSET trial, which randomized 8307 patients with AMI to either tissue-type plasminogen activator (t-PA) with heparin or heparin alone, patients receiving t-PA had lower rates of 1 month mortality (relative reduction 26%).[55]

In addition, patients with STEMI who present within the first 1 to 2 hours of symptom onset may benefit the most from immediate fibrinolytic therapy. In the CAPTIM trial, 840 patients were randomized to either primary PCI or prehospital fibrinolysis with immediate transfer to PCI-capable facilities. At 30 days, there were no significant differences in outcomes between the two groups. Long-term follow-up at 5 years found that all-cause mortality was similar between the two groups; however, patients treated within 2 hours of symptom onset with fibrinolysis had lower rates of all-cause mortality than the primary PCI group (5.8% vs 11.1%, P = .04).[56]

Choice of Fibrinolytic Agent

The ACC/AHA guidelines recommend that fibrin-specific fibrinolytic agents (tenecteplase, reteplase, alteplase) be used over non-fibrin-specific agents (streptokinase) when available.[52] Fibrin-specific agents deplete fibrinogen to a lesser extent than non-fibrin-specific agents, potentially improving the safety profile of these agents. The doses of fibrinolytic agents are detailed in **Table 4.4**. Multiple trials have compared the use of different thrombolytic therapies.[57-61] Early studies demonstrated the superiority of t-PA compared with streptokinase. For example, the

TABLE 4.4 Dosing of Fibrinolytic Agents in STEMI

FIBRINOLYTIC AGENT	DOSE
Tenecteplase	Single weight-based bolus <60 kg: 30 mg 60-69 kg: 35 mg 70-79 kg: 40 mg 80-89 kg: 45 mg >90 kg: 50 mg
Reteplase	10-U plus 10-U IV boluses given 30 min apart
Alteplase	90 min weight-based infusion Bolus 15 mg, infusion 0.75 mg/kg for 30 min (max 50 mg) then 0.5 mg/kg (max 35 mg) over next 60 min; total dose not to exceed 100 mg
Streptokinase	1.5 million units IV given over 30-60 min

IV, intravenous; STEMI, ST-segment elevation myocardial infarction.

GUSTO investigators compared the use of t-PA with streptokinase in 41,021 patients with STEMI. Patients receiving t-PA with UFH had lower 30-day mortality rates (6.3% vs 7.4%, P = .001) and death or disabling stroke rates (6.9% vs 7.8%, P = .006) compared with streptokinase with UFH.[57] In addition, the rate of infarct-related artery patency at 90 minutes was higher in patients receiving t-PA with intravenous UFH compared with patients receiving streptokinase with UFH (81% vs 60%, P < .001).[59] These findings suggested the superiority of t-PA over streptokinase.

Subsequent trials comparing recombinant plasminogen activator (rPA) and tenecteplase (TNK-tPA) with t-PA failed to show superiority of these agents over t-PA. For example, the GUSTO III trial compared rPA with t-PA in 15,059 patients with STEMI. Mortality rates were similar between these two therapies at 30 days (4.5% vs 7.2%, p = NS) and 1 year (11.2% vs 11.1%, p = NS).[61] Similarly, the ASSENT-2 trial compared TNK-tPA with t-PA and found no significant difference in mortality between the two randomized groups (6.2% vs 6.2%, p = NS).[60]

Anticoagulants in STEMI

The ACC/AHA guidelines summarizing the recommendations for the use of anticoagulant therapy in patients with STEMI separate anticoagulant management of these patients on the treatment strategy: for primary PCI, as an adjunct to fibrinolytic therapy, or support for PCI after administration of fibrinolytic therapy. Support for PCI after fibrinolytic therapy can occur during a rescue PCI strategy (PCI after a patient demonstrates signs or symptoms of failed reperfusion after fibrinolytic therapy) or as part of a pharmacoinvasive strategy (after fibrinolytic therapy the patient is transferred to a PCI-capable hospital for early coronary angiography and PCI when appropriate). Treatment strategies for STEMI are discussed in depth in Chapter 19.

Similar to NSTE-ACS, several classes of anticoagulants have been shown to be effective in treating patients with STEMI: UFH, enoxaparin, and direct thrombin inhibitors. Rapid reperfusion in patients with STEMI is of utmost importance, and delays to reperfusion are associated with higher mortality rates.[62] Thus, the need for rapid reperfusion drives the choice of reperfusion strategy and likely trumps the actual anticoagulant strategy chosen.[52]

Anticoagulation in patients with STEMI is generally administered during PCI in order to suppress the ongoing thrombotic process or any additional thrombosis that may be precipitated by equipment and vessel injury during PCI. In addition, anticoagulants are used to maintain vessel patency after fibrinolytic therapy.

Anticoagulant Use in Primary PCI

Primary PCI is the recommended reperfusion method when it can be performed within 120 minutes of the patient's presentation to a medical facility.[52] In fact, immediate transfer to a PCI-capable hospital for primary PCI is preferred for patients with STEMI when a first medical contact to reperfusion time is anticipated to be less than 120 minutes. For patients with STEMI undergoing primary PCI, ACC/AHA guidelines recommend supportive anticoagulation with either UFH or bivalirudin (class I indication). In contrast, fondaparinux should not be used as a sole anticoagulant in these patients (class III indication) for reasons of possible increased catheter thrombosis as described earlier.

Choice of Anticoagulant

UFH during primary PCI for STEMI has been routinely used and has been widely accepted. As a result, there are limited trial data examining its efficacy and safety compared with a background of no UFH. The HORIZONS-AMI trial demonstrated the effectiveness of bivalirudin use in patients with STEMI[63] by randomizing 3602 patients with STEMI undergoing primary PCI to either heparin with GP IIb/IIIa therapy or to bivalirudin alone. Patients treated with bivalirudin had similar rates of MACEs (5.4% vs 5.5%, $P = .95$) compared with patients receiving heparin; however, patients treated with bivalirudin had significantly lower rates of major bleeding (4.9% vs 8.3%, $P < .001$). Thus, bivalirudin is a possible alternative for anticoagulation during primary PCI, especially in patients who are at higher risk of bleeding.

While bivalirudin has been established as an anticoagulant choice in patients with STEMI, the optimal anticoagulant therapy has not been established. Prior studies compared the use of bivalirudin with heparin with routine GP IIb/IIIa inhibition. Recent studies have provided conflicting data regarding whether patients receiving bivalirudin have better outcomes compared with heparin when both patient populations receive GP IIb/IIIa only as a bailout therapy and GP IIb/IIIa is not a mandated therapy. The first study to investigate this question was the single-center HEAT-PPCI trial, which randomized 1829 patients with STEMI in a single center to either bivalirudin or heparin therapy. At 28 days, patients receiving bivalirudin had higher rates of the composite primary endpoint (all-cause mortality, cerebrovascular accidents, reinfarction, or unplanned target lesion revascularization) compared with patients receiving heparin (8.7% vs 5.7%, $P = .01$).[64] Stent thrombosis was also increased with the bivalirudin-only regimen. Since HEAT-PPCI, additional multicenter trials such as MATRIX and BRIGHT have investigated this clinical question and have provided conflicting results as described in the NSTE-ACS section. Postulated reasons for these differences in outcomes have included the following: differences between the practice patterns captured within single-center versus multicenter studies, differences in included patient populations across studies, type of access (femoral vs radial) used, doses of anticoagulant, and the duration of anticoagulation (with longer durations of the bivalirudin infusion seeming to mitigate the acute stent thrombosis seen with bivalirudin monotherapy). The VALIDATE-SWEDEHEART trial was a multicenter, prospective, randomized, registry-based, controlled clinical trial of patients with AMI designed to investigate whether bivalirudin use in patients receiving contemporary DAPT (ticagrelor, prasugrel, or cangrelor) has improved outcomes compared with patients receiving heparin.[65] Patients receiving bivalirudin had similar rates of the 6-month primary endpoint (composite of death from any cause, myocardial infarction, or major bleeding) compared with those receiving heparin (12.3% vs 12.8%, $P = .54$). There were similar rates of major bleeding between the two treatment groups.[66] Thus, the prior bleeding benefit seen with bivalirudin in earlier studies can likely be attributed to the higher rates of GP IIb/IIIa usage and lower rates of radial access.

There are limited data on the role of enoxaparin use in patients with STEMI receiving primary PCI. In the ATOLL study, in which 910 patients were randomized to receive either enoxaparin or UFH, treatment with enoxaparin had similar rates of the composite primary endpoint, including death, complication of MI, procedure failure, or major bleeding (28% vs 34%, $P = .06$).[67] Furthermore, there were no differences in the rates of the individual component events. As a result, enoxaparin is not a recommended anticoagulant for patients with STEMI undergoing primary PCI.

Dosing Strategy

Dosing of UFH during primary PCI is dependent on whether GP IIb/IIIa use is planned (**Table 4.5**). When GP IIb/IIIa use is not anticipated, a bolus of 70 to 100 U/kg heparin is given to achieve a recommended ACT target of 250 to 300 seconds (HemoTec device) or 300 to 350 seconds (Hemochron device). With GP IIb/IIIa use, a lower initial bolus of UFH is given (50- to 70-U/kg IV bolus) with a goal ACT between 200 and 250 seconds.

For primary PCI, bivalirudin is given as a 0.75-mg/kg IV bolus followed by a 1.75-mg/kg/h infusion regardless of prior treatment with UFH. An additional bolus of 0.3 mg/kg may be given if needed. Because this medication is renally cleared, the bivalirudin infusion should be reduced to 1 mg/kg/h if the patient has a CrCl < 30 mL/min.

Anticoagulant Use With Fibrinolytic Therapy

Regardless of the choice of fibrinolytic agent, patients who have received fibrinolytic therapy should receive additional anticoagulation for the duration of the hospitalization (up to 8 days or until revascularization is performed) and for a minimum of 48 hours. In these cases, anticoagulation is used to maintain coronary vessel patency after clot lysis with fibrinolytic therapy. After fibrinolytic therapy, recurrent clot formation may occur as a result of increased thrombin activity, which can lead to recurrent coronary thrombosis.[68] This may be suppressed by UFH, enoxaparin, or fondaparinux.

Choice of Anticoagulant

Early studies demonstrated that concurrent treatment with heparin in patients receiving fibrinolytic therapy resulted in improved coronary patency rates. In a study containing 84 patients, patients were randomized to receiving tissue plasminogen activator with and without heparin anticoagulation. All patients underwent coronary angiography 3 days after fibrinolytic therapy to document vessel patency. Patients who received concurrent heparin had higher rates of vessel patency after fibrinolytic therapy (71% vs 43%, $P = .015$).[69] Furthermore, in the HART trial, 205 patients were randomized to either aspirin or heparin after fibrinolysis with t-PA. Patients underwent angiography 7 to 24 hours after fibrinolysis. Patients receiving heparin had higher rates of infarct-related

TABLE 4.5 Dosing of Anticoagulant Agents in STEMI

	DURING PRIMARY PCI	AFTER FIBRINOLYTIC THERAPY	DELAYED PCI AFTER FIBRINOLYTIC THERAPY
Bivalirudin	0.75-mg/kg IV bolus then 1.75-mg/kg/h infusion with or without prior UFH treatment. Additional 0.3-mg/kg bolus if needed. Reduce infusion to 1 mg/kg/h if CrCl <30 mL/min.	NA	NA
Unfractionated heparin (UFH)	IV GP IIb/IIIa planned: 50- to 70-U/kg IV bolus to achieve target ACT 200-250. No IV GP IIb/IIIa planned: 70- to 100-U/kg bolus to achieve target ACT 250-300	Weight-adjusted IV bolus and infusion to obtain activated partial thromboplastin time 1.5-2.0 times the control. 60-U/kg (max 4000 U) IV bolus followed by 12-U/kg/h infusion (max 1000 U).	Continue through PCI with additional doses to achieve therapeutic ACT
Enoxaparin	NA	If age <75 y, 30-mg IV bolus followed in 15 min by 1 mg/kg SC injection every 12 h (max 100 mg for the first two doses). If age >75 y, 0.75 mg/kg SC every 12 h (max 75 mg for the first two doses). Regardless of age, if CrCl < 30 mL/min, use 1 mg/kg SC every 12 h	Last dose within 8 h: no additional dose required. Last dose 8–12 h earlier: 0.3-mg/kg IV bolus
Fondaparinux	Should not be used as sole agent	Initial 2.5-mg IV dose followed by 2.5 mg SC injections in 24 if CrCl > 30 mL/min	Should not be used as sole agent

ACT, activated clotting time; CrCl, creatinine clearance; GP, glycoprotein; IV, intravenous; PCI, percutaneous coronary intervention; SC, subcutaneous; STEMI, ST-segment elevation myocardial infarction.

artery patency compared with patients only receiving aspirin (82% vs 52%, $P < .0001$).[70]

The use of enoxaparin after fibrinolytic therapy has been studied against heparin therapy. In the ASSENT-3 trial, containing 6095 patients with STEMI receiving fibrinolytic therapy, patients receiving enoxaparin had lower rates of the composite 30-day endpoint of mortality, in-hospital reinfarction, or in-hospital refractory ischemia compared with patients receiving heparin (11.4% vs 15.4%, $P = .0002$).[71] In addition, patients receiving enoxaparin had lower rates of in-hospital intracranial hemorrhage or major bleeding complications (13.7% vs 17.0%, $P = .0037$). As a result of these findings, enoxaparin is recommended after fibrinolytic therapy and is the preferred anticoagulation therapy over heparin after 48 hours.

A subgroup analysis of the OASIS-6 trial demonstrated the benefit of using fondaparinux in patients with STEMI undergoing fibrinolytic therapy.[72] Of the 5436 patients included in this analysis, 2692 patients received fondaparinux. Treatment with fondaparinux was associated with lower rates of death and MI at 30 days (hazard ratio [HR] 0.79 [95% confidence interval (CI): 0.68-0.92]) compared with patients receiving UFH. Furthermore, the risk of severe bleeding was reduced among patients receiving fondaparinux (HR 0.62 [95% CI: 0.40-0.94]).

Dosing Strategy

For patients receiving fibrinolytic therapy, UFH should be administered as a weight-adjusted IV bolus and infusion to obtain an aPTT of 1.5 to 2.0 times the control for 48 hours or until revascularization (**Table 4.5**), an IV bolus of 60 U/kg (maximum 4000 U) followed by an infusion of 12 U/kg/h (maximum 1000 U). Enoxaparin should be given as an IV bolus, followed in 15 minutes by a subcutaneous (SC) injection. If the patient's age is <75 years, a 30-mg IV bolus is administered, followed in 15 minutes by 1 mg/kg subcutaneously every 12 hours (maximum 100 mg for the first two doses). If the patient's age is >75 years, a bolus is not given and only a 0.75 mg/kg SC injection every 12 hours (maximum 75 mg for the first two doses) is administered. If the patient has impaired renal function (CrCl < 30 mL/min), only a 1-mg/kg SC injection every 24 hours of enoxaparin should be administered, regardless of the patient's age. Fondaparinux should be administered with an initial intravenous dose, followed by daily SC injections if the patient's CrCl is greater than 30 mL/min. An initial dose of fondaparinux 2.5 mg IV, and then 2.5 mg SC daily starting the following day, may be used for the duration of the hospitalization up to 8 days or until revascularization.

Anticoagulant Use With Delayed PCI after Fibrinolytic Therapy

Despite appropriate doses of fibrinolytic therapy, a proportion of patients will still require PCI because of evidence of failed reperfusion or reocclusion of the target vessel. In these situations, anticoagulation should be continued uninterrupted from the time after fibrinolytic therapy to the time of the PCI procedure. Patients may be switched from UFH to bivalirudin for PCI. In addition, if the last dose of enoxaparin was >12 hours prior to PCI, the patient may be switched to either UFH or bivalirudin.

There are limited data comparing anticoagulation strategies in patients with STEMI undergoing PCI after receiving fibrinolytic therapy. The EXTRACT-TIMI 25 trial compared the use of enoxaparin with UFH in 20,479 patients with STEMI undergoing PCI after fibrinolytic therapy. Patients who received enoxaparin had lower rates of death or recurrent MI through 30 days compared with patients receiving UFH (10.7% vs 13.8%, $P < .001$), and there were no differences in major bleeding. Thus, enoxaparin use is an effective anticoagulant strategy in these patients.

Dosing Strategy

ACT monitoring should be performed on patients receiving UFH undergoing PCI after fibrinolytic therapy. Additional boluses of heparin should be administered in order to achieve appropriate ACT targets, depending on whether concomitant GP IIb/IIIa receptor antagonists are administered (**Table 4.5**). Patients receiving enoxaparin prior to PCI do not need additional anticoagulation dosing if the PCI is performed within 8 hours of the last enoxaparin administration. If PCI is performed 8 to 12 hours after the last dose of enoxaparin, an additional enoxaparin 0.3-mg/kg IV bolus should be administered.

FUTURE DIRECTIONS

Because of their antithrombotic effects, anticoagulants remain a cornerstone of therapy for patients with NSTE-ACS and STEMI. Despite an abundance of trial data on the use of anticoagulants for ACS and PCI, further trials are ongoing in an attempt to bring to market newer anticoagulants that will help improve the management and treatment of high-risk patients with atherothrombotic disease. Several of these agents are within the classes of agents discussed earlier, and other agents belong to novel classes of agents, with different mechanisms of action. Clearly affecting the development of novel anticoagulants is the increasing recognition of the complementary importance of both ischemic and bleeding events. The development of novel anticoagulant agents has therefore focused upon attempts to either provide incremental gains in anti-ischemic benefits without further increases in bleeding risk or preserve the anti-ischemic benefits of current agents while incrementally lowering bleeding risks. In light of the decreasing event rates in clinical trials of antithrombotic therapy because of the advances already made in this space, the margins through which these potential incremental clinical benefits can be measured are slim and the clinical trial sizes required to demonstrate these gains with statistical confidence often can be daunting. Nonetheless, further study of novel anticoagulant agents remains an area of active interest and investigation.

Key Points

- All patients with NSTE-ACS and STEMI (without contraindications) should be started on an anticoagulant as soon as possible after presentation (class I). Similarly, all PCI patients should be started on a parenteral anticoagulant at the time of PCI (class I).
- The duration of anticoagulation for patients undergoing PCI is up until (but not after) the PCI is performed.
- Four different agents are recommended as class I upstream options for patients with UA/NSTEMI being managed with an invasive strategy: UFH, enoxaparin, bivalirudin, or fondaparinux.
- At the time of PCI, agents with class I recommendations include bivalirudin and UFH in patients with NSTE-ACS and STEMI.
- Use of fondaparinux alone as an anticoagulant during PCI is contraindicated. Patients treated with upstream fondaparinux who require PCI should be treated with UFH at the time of the PCI to avoid catheter-related thrombus.
- The benefits and risks of triple antithrombotic therapy with aspirin, clopidogrel, and warfarin in NSTE-ACS have not been clearly established. Such therapy should be selected for clear indications for extended duration of oral anticoagulation, and given for the shortest duration of time, at the minimally effective doses necessary to achieve protection.
- Time to reperfusion in patients with STEMI is of upmost importance and may be more important than reperfusion strategy (primary PCI vs fibrinolytic therapy).
- Fibrin-specific agents (tenecteplase, reteplase, alteplase) are preferred agents over non-fibrin-specific fibrinolytics (streptokinase) in patients with STEMI undergoing fibrinolysis.
- Three different anticoagulant agents are recommended as class I options for patients with STEMI receiving fibrinolytic therapy: UFH, enoxaparin, or fondaparinux.

References

1. Lawton JS, Tamis-Holland JE, Bangalore S, et al. 2021 ACC/AHA/SCAI guideline for coronary artery revascularization: executive summary—a report of the American College of Cardiology/American Heart association joint committee on clinical practice guidelines. *Circulation*. 2022;145:e4-e17.
2. Fifth Organization to Assess Strategies in Acute Ischemic Syndromes Investigators; Yusuf S, Mehta SR, Choralavicius S, et al. Comparison of fondaparinux and enoxaparin in acute coronary syndromes. *N Engl J Med*. 2006;354(14):1464-1476.
3. Rao SV, Eikelboom JA, Granger CB, Harrington RA, Califf RM, Bassand JP. Bleeding and blood transfusion issues in patients with non-ST-segment elevation acute coronary syndromes. *Eur Heart J*. 2007;28(10):1193-1204.
4. Mehran R, Pocock SJ, Stone GW, et al. Associations of major bleeding and myocardial infarction with the incidence and timing of mortality in patients presenting with non-ST-elevation acute coronary syndromes: a risk model from the ACUITY trial. *Eur Heart J*. 2009;30(12):1457-1466.
5. Petersen JL, Mahaffey KW, Hasselblad V, et al. Efficacy and bleeding complications among patients randomized to enoxaparin or unfractionated heparin for antithrombin therapy in non-ST-Segment elevation acute coronary syndromes: a systematic overview. *JAMA*. 2004;292(1):89-96.
6. Amsterdam EA, Wenger NK, Brindis RG, et al. 2014 AHA/ACC guideline for the management of patients with non-ST-elevation acute coronary syndromes: a report of the American College of Cardiology/American Heart Association Task Force on Practice Guidelines. *J Am Coll Cardiol*. 2014;64(24):e139-e228.
7. Spaulding C, Lefèvre T, Funck F, et al. Left radial approach for coronary angiography: results of a prospective study. *Cathet Cardiovasc Diagn*. 1996;39(4):365-370.
8. Levine GN, Bates ER, Blankenship JC, et al. 2011 ACCF/AHA/SCAI guideline for percutaneous coronary intervention: executive summary—a report of the American College of Cardiology Foundation/American Heart Association Task Force on practice guidelines and the society for cardiovascular angiography and interventions. *Catheter Cardiovasc Interv*. 2012;79(3):453-495.
9. Oler A, Whooley MA, Oler J, Grady D. Adding heparin to aspirin reduces the incidence of myocardial infarction and death in patients with unstable angina. A meta-analysis. *JAMA*. 1996;276(10):811-815.
10. Anand SS, Yusuf S, Pogue J, Ginsberg JS, Hirsh J; Organization to Assess Strategies for Ischemic Syndromes Investigators. Relationship of activated partial thromboplastin time to coronary events and bleeding in

patients with acute coronary syndromes who receive heparin. *Circulation.* 2003;107(23):2884-2888.
11. Chew DP, Bhatt DL, Lincoff AM, et al. Defining the optimal activated clotting time during percutaneous coronary intervention: aggregate results from 6 randomized, controlled trials. *Circulation.* 2001;103(7):961-966.
12. Brener SJ, Moliterno DJ, Lincoff AM, Steinhubl SR, Wolski KE, Topol EJ. Relationship between activated clotting time and ischemic or hemorrhagic complications: analysis of 4 recent randomized clinical trials of percutaneous coronary intervention. *Circulation.* 2004;110(8):994-998.
13. Melloni C, Alexander KP, Chen AY, et al. Unfractionated heparin dosing and risk of major bleeding in non-ST-segment elevation acute coronary syndromes. *Am Heart J.* 2008;156(2):209-215.
14. Alexander KP, Chen AY, Roe MT, et al. Excess dosing of antiplatelet and antithrombin agents in the treatment of non-ST-segment elevation acute coronary syndromes. *JAMA.* 2005;294(24):3108-3116.
15. Arepally GM, Ortel TL. Clinical practice. Heparin-induced thrombocytopenia. *N Engl J Med.* 2006;355(8):809-817.
16. Granger CB, Miller JM, Bovill EG, et al. Rebound increase in thrombin generation and activity after cessation of intravenous heparin in patients with acute coronary syndromes. *Circulation.* 1995;91(7):1929-1935.
17. Low-molecular-weight heparin during instability in coronary artery disease, Fragmin during Instability in Coronary Artery Disease (FRISC) study group. *Lancet.* 1996;347:561-568.
18. Antman EM, Cohen M, Radley D, et al. Assessment of the treatment effect of enoxaparin for unstable angina/non-Q-wave myocardial infarction. TIMI 11B-ESSENCE meta-analysis. *Circulation.* 1999;100(15):1602-1608.
19. Ferguson JJ, Califf RM, Antman EM, et al. Enoxaparin vs unfractionated heparin in high-risk patients with non-ST-segment elevation acute coronary syndromes managed with an intended early invasive strategy: primary results of the SYNERGY randomized trial. *JAMA.* 2004;292(1):45-54.
20. Blazing MA, de Lemos JA, White HD, et al. Safety and efficacy of enoxaparin vs unfractionated heparin in patients with non-ST-segment elevation acute coronary syndromes who receive tirofiban and aspirin: a randomized controlled trial. *JAMA.* 2004;292(1):55-64.
21. Drouet L, Bal dit Sollier C, Martin J. Adding intravenous unfractionated heparin to standard enoxaparin causes excessive anticoagulation not detected by activated clotting time: results of the STACK-on to ENOXaparin (STACKENOX) study. *Am Heart J.* 2009;158(2):177-184.
22. Montalescot G, Gallo R, White HD, et al. Enoxaparin versus unfractionated heparin in elective percutaneous coronary intervention 1-year results from the STEEPLE (SafeTy and efficacy of enoxaparin in percutaneous coronary intervention patients, an international randomized evaluation) trial. *JACC Cardiovasc Interv.* 2009;2(11):1083-1091.
23. Michalis LK, Katsouras CS, Papamichael N, et al. Enoxaparin versus tinzaparin in non-ST-segment elevation acute coronary syndromes: the EVET trial. *Am Heart J.* 2003;146(2):304-310.
24. Dana A, Nguyen CM, Cloutier S, Barbeau GR. Macroscopic thrombus formation on angioplasty equipment following antithrombin therapy with enoxaparin. *Catheter Cardiovasc Interv.* 2007;70(6):847-853.
25. Gori AM, Fedi S, Pepe G, et al. Tissue factor and tissue factor pathway inhibitor levels in unstable angina patients during short-term low-molecular-weight heparin administration. *Br J Haematol.* 2002;117(3):693-698.
26. Global Use of Strategies to Open Occluded Coronary Arteries (GUSTO) IIb investigators. A comparison of recombinant hirudin with heparin for the treatment of acute coronary syndromes. *N Engl J Med.* 1996;335:775-782.
27. Effects of recombinant hirudin (lepirudin) compared with heparin on death, myocardial infarction, refractory angina, and revascularisation procedures in patients with acute myocardial ischaemia without ST elevation: a randomised trial. Organisation to Assess Strategies for Ischemic Syndromes (OASIS-2) Investigators. *Lancet.* 1999;353:429-438.
28. Direct Thrombin Inhibitor Trialists' Collaborative Group. Direct thrombin inhibitors in acute coronary syndromes: principal results of a meta-analysis based on individual patients' data. *Lancet.* 2002;359(9303):294-302.
29. Bittl JA, Strony J, Brinker JA, et al. Treatment with bivalirudin (Hirulog) as compared with heparin during coronary angioplasty for unstable or postinfarction angina. Hirulog Angioplasty Study Investigators. *N Engl J Med.* 1995;333(12):764-769.
30. Bittl JA, Chaitman BR, Feit F, Kimball W, Topol EJ. Bivalirudin versus heparin during coronary angioplasty for unstable or postinfarction angina: final report reanalysis of the Bivalirudin Angioplasty Study. *Am Heart J.* 2001;142:952-959.
31. Stone GW, McLaurin BT, Cox DA, et al. Bivalirudin for patients with acute coronary syndromes. *N Engl J Med.* 2006;355(21):2203-2216.
32. Kastrati A, Neumann FJ, Mehilli J, et al. Bivalirudin versus unfractionated heparin during percutaneous coronary intervention. *N Engl J Med.* 2008;359(7):688-696.
33. Kastrati A, Neumann FJ, Schulz S, et al. Abciximab and heparin versus bivalirudin for non-ST-elevation myocardial infarction. *N Engl J Med.* 2011;365(21):1980-1989.
34. Valgimigli M, Frigoli E, Leonardi S, et al. Bivalirudin or unfractionated heparin in acute coronary syndromes. *N Engl J Med.* 2015;373(11):997-1009.
35. Leonardi S, Frigoli E, Rothenbühler M, et al. Bivalirudin or unfractionated heparin in patients with acute coronary syndromes managed invasively with and without ST elevation (MATRIX): randomised controlled trial. *BMJ.* 2016;354:i4935.
36. Han Y, Guo J, Zheng Y, et al. Bivalirudin vs heparin with or without tirofiban during primary percutaneous coronary intervention in acute myocardial infarction: the BRIGHT randomized clinical trial. *JAMA.* 2015;313(13):1336-1346.
37. Lincoff AM, Bittl JA, Kleiman NS, et al. Comparison of bivalirudin versus heparin during percutaneous coronary intervention (the Randomized Evaluation of PCI Linking Angiomax to Reduced Clinical Events [REPLACE]-1 trial). *Am J Cardiol.* 2004;93(9):1092-1096.
38. Lincoff AM, Bittl JA, Harrington RA, et al. Bivalirudin and provisional glycoprotein IIb/IIIa blockade compared with heparin and planned glycoprotein IIb/IIIa blockade during percutaneous coronary intervention: REPLACE-2 randomized trial. *JAMA.* 2003;289(7):853-863.
39. Gibson CM, Ten Y, Murphy SA, et al. Association of prerandomization anticoagulant switching with bleeding in the setting of percutaneous coronary intervention (A REPLACE-2 analysis). *Am J Cardiol.* 2007;99(12):1687-1690.
40. FUTURA/OASIS-8 Trial Group; Steg PG, Jolly SS, Mehta SR, et al. Low-dose vs standard-dose unfractionated heparin for percutaneous coronary intervention in acute coronary syndromes treated with fondaparinux: the FUTURA/OASIS-8 randomized trial. *JAMA.* 2010;304(12):1339-1349.
41. Paolucci F, Claviés MC, Donat F, Necciari J. Fondaparinux sodium mechanism of action: identification of specific binding to purified and human plasma-derived proteins. *Clin Pharmacokinet.* 2002;41(suppl 2):11-18.
42. Leon MB, Baim DS, Popma JJ, et al. A clinical trial comparing three antithrombotic-drug regimens after coronary-artery stenting. Stent Anticoagulation Restenosis Study Investigators. *N Engl J Med.* 1998;339(23):1665-1671.
43. Effects of long-term, moderate-intensity oral anticoagulation in addition to aspirin in unstable angina. The Organization to Assess Strategies for Ischemic Syndromes (OASIS) investigators. *J Am Coll Cardiol.* 2001;37:475-484.
44. Hurlen M, Abdelnoor M, Smith P, Erikssen J, Arnesen H. Warfarin, aspirin, or both after myocardial infarction. *N Engl J Med.* 2002;347(13):969-974.
45. Dewilde WJ, Oirbans T, Verheugt FWA, et al. Use of clopidogrel with or without aspirin in patients taking oral anticoagulant therapy and undergoing percutaneous coronary intervention: an open-label, randomised, controlled trial. *Lancet.* 2013;381(9872):1107-1115.
46. Wiviott SD, Braunwald E, McCabe CH, et al. Prasugrel versus clopidogrel in patients with acute coronary syndromes. *N Engl J Med.* 2007;357(20):2001-2015.
47. Merlini PA, Bauer KA, Oltrona L, et al. Persistent activation of coagulation mechanism in unstable angina and myocardial infarction. *Circulation.* 1994;90(1):61-68.
48. Mega JL, Braunwald E, Wiviott SD, et al. Rivaroxaban in patients with a recent acute coronary syndrome. *N Engl J Med.* 2012;366(1):9-19.
49. Gibson CM, Mehran R, Bode C, et al. Prevention of bleeding in patients with atrial fibrillation undergoing PCI. *N Engl J Med.* 2016;375(25):2423-2434.
50. Alexander JH, Lopes RD, James S, et al. Apixaban with antiplatelet therapy after acute coronary syndrome. *N Engl J Med.* 2011;365(8):699-708.
51. Lopes RD, Heizer G, Aronson R, et al. Antithrombotic therapy after acute coronary syndrome or PCI in atrial fibrillation. *N Engl J Med.* 2019;380(16):1509-1524.
52. O'Gara PT, Kushner FG, Ascheim DD, et al. 2013 ACCF/AHA guideline for the management of ST-elevation myocardial infarction: executive

summary—a report of the American College of Cardiology Foundation/American Heart Association Task Force on practice guidelines—developed in collaboration with the American College of emergency physicians and society for cardiovascular angiography and interventions. *Catheter Cardiovasc Interv*. 2013;82(1):E1-E27.

53. Effectiveness of intravenous thrombolytic treatment in acute myocardial infarction. Gruppo Italiano per lo Studio della Streptochinasi nell'Infarto Miocardico (GISSI). *Lancet*. 1986;1:397-402.
54. Randomised trial of intravenous streptokinase, oral aspirin, both, or neither among 17,187 cases of suspected acute myocardial infarction: ISIS-2. ISIS-2 (Second International Study of Infarct Survival) Collaborative Group. *Lancet*. 1988;2:349-360.
55. Wilcox RG, von der Lippe G, Olsson CG, Jensen G, Skene AM, Hampton JR. Trial of tissue plasminogen activator for mortality reduction in acute myocardial infarction. Anglo-Scandinavian Study of Early Thrombolysis (ASSET). *Lancet*. 1988;2(8610):525-530.
56. Bonnefoy E, Steg PG, Boutitie F, et al. Comparison of primary angioplasty and pre-hospital fibrinolysis in acute myocardial infarction (CAPTIM) trial: a 5-year follow-up. *Eur Heart J*. 2009;30(13):1598-1606.
57. GUSTO investigators. An international randomized trial comparing four thrombolytic strategies for acute myocardial infarction. *N Engl J Med*. 1993;329(10):673-682.
58. Bode C, Smalling RW, Berg G, et al. Randomized comparison of coronary thrombolysis achieved with double-bolus reteplase (recombinant plasminogen activator) and front-loaded, accelerated alteplase (recombinant tissue plasminogen activator) in patients with acute myocardial infarction. The RAPID II Investigators. *Circulation*. 1996;94(5):891-898.
59. The GUSTO Angiographic Investigators. The effects of tissue plasminogen activator, streptokinase, or both on coronary-artery patency, ventricular function, and survival after acute myocardial infarction. *N Engl J Med*. 1993;329:1615-1622.
60. Assessment of the Safety and Efficacy of a New Thrombolytic ASSENT-2 Investigators; Van De Werf F, Adgey J, Ardissino D, et al. Single-bolus tenecteplase compared with front-loaded alteplase in acute myocardial infarction: the ASSENT-2 double-blind randomised trial. *Lancet*. 1999;354(9180):716-722.
61. Topol EJ, Ohman EM, Armstrong PW, et al. Survival outcomes 1 year after reperfusion therapy with either alteplase or reteplase for acute myocardial infarction: results from the Global Utilization of Streptokinase and t-PA for Occluded Coronary Arteries (GUSTO) III Trial. *Circulation*. 2000;102(15):1761-1765.
62. Rathore SS, Curtis JP, Chen J, et al. Association of door-to-balloon time and mortality in patients admitted to hospital with ST elevation myocardial infarction: national cohort study. *BMJ*. 2009;338:b1807.
63. Stone GW, Witzenbichler B, Guagliumi G, et al. Bivalirudin during primary PCI in acute myocardial infarction. *N Engl J Med*. 2008;358(21):2218-2230.
64. Shahzad A, Kemp I, Mars C, et al. Unfractionated heparin versus bivalirudin in primary percutaneous coronary intervention (HEAT-PPCI): an open-label, single centre, randomised controlled trial. *Lancet*. 2014;384(9957):1849-1858.
65. Erlinge D, Koul S, Eriksson P, et al. Bivalirudin versus heparin in non-ST and ST-segment elevation myocardial infarction-a registry-based randomized clinical trial in the SWEDEHEART registry (the VALIDATE-SWEDEHEART trial). *Am Heart J*. 2016;175:36-46.
66. Erlinge D, Omerovic E, Fröbert O, et al. Bivalirudin versus heparin monotherapy in myocardial infarction. *N Engl J Med*. 2017;377(12):1132-1142.
67. Montalescot G, Zeymer U, Silvain J, et al. Intravenous enoxaparin or unfractionated heparin in primary percutaneous coronary intervention for ST-elevation myocardial infarction: the international randomised open-label ATOLL trial. *Lancet*. 2011;378(9792):693-703.
68. Eisenberg PR. Role of heparin in coronary thrombolysis. *Chest*. 1992;101(4 suppl):131S-139S.
69. Bleich SD, Nichols TC, Schumacher RR, Cooke DH, Tate DA, Teichman SL. Effect of heparin on coronary arterial patency after thrombolysis with tissue plasminogen activator in acute myocardial infarction. *Am J Cardiol*. 1990;66(20):1412-1417.
70. Hsia J, Hamilton WP, Kleiman N, Roberts R, Chaitman BR, Ross AM. A comparison between heparin and low-dose aspirin as adjunctive therapy with tissue plasminogen activator for acute myocardial infarction. Heparin-Aspirin Reperfusion Trial (HART) Investigators. *N Engl J Med*. 1990;323(21):1433-1437.
71. Assessment of the Safety and Efficacy of a New Thrombolytic Regimen (ASSENT)-3 Investigators. Efficacy and safety of tenecteplase in combination with enoxaparin, abciximab, or unfractionated heparin: the ASSENT-3 randomised trial in acute myocardial infarction. *Lancet*. 2001;358:605-613.
72. Peters RJ, Joyner C, Bassand JP, et al. The role of fondaparinux as an adjunct to thrombolytic therapy in acute myocardial infarction: a subgroup analysis of the OASIS-6 trial. *Eur Heart J*. 2008;29(3):324-331.

Vasoactive and Antiarrhythmic Drugs in the Catheterization Laboratory

Nathaniel Smilowitz

VASOACTIVE DRUGS

Vasodilators

Coronary vasodilators are generally classified into endothelium dependent or endothelium independent based on their mode of action (**Table 5.1**). The endothelium-dependent drugs act via a healthy endothelium to convert L-arginine into nitric oxide, which in turn relaxes the vascular smooth muscle cells (VSMCs), causing vasodilation. The endothelium-independent drugs bypass the endothelium and act directly on the VSMCs to convert guanosine-5′-triphosphate into cyclic guanosine monophosphate (GMP), leading to vascular smooth muscle relaxation and subsequent vasodilation.[1]

Nitroglycerin

Nitroglycerin is metabolized in the VSMCs into nitric oxide, which is in turn converted to S-nitrosothiol that activates guanylate cyclase and generates cyclic GMP, resulting in vascular smooth muscle relaxation and vasodilatation. Nitroglycerin has a more pronounced effect on the venous compared with the arterial circulation. In patients with angina, nitroglycerin's anti-ischemic effect is more related to venodilatation and preload reduction, which reduces myocardial wall stress, which in turn decreases myocardial oxygen demand and indirectly improves subendocardial myocardial flow and collateral flow when present. Nitroglycerin also dilates both normal and diseased coronary arteries, although this action is of uncertain clinical importance except in patients who have vasospastic angina.

Nitroglycerin has a rapid onset of action and a short duration. It can be administered via the sublingual, intra-arterial (IA), intravenous (IV), and intracoronary (IC) routes. Nitroglycerin is generally used in the catheterization laboratory to prevent or treat arterial spasm and is used during coronary angiography or percutaneous coronary interventions (PCIs) to improve coronary flow, prevent or alleviate coronary spasm, provoke myocardial bridging, relieve angina, or reduce preload in patients with elevated filling pressures.[1]

Prophylactic administration of IC nitroglycerin is commonly used before intravascular imaging or coronary atherectomy. Nitroglycerin is also used in the pharmacologic cocktail given via the radial artery to prevent or treat radial artery spasm during transradial procedures. Sublingual nitroglycerin is administered as a 0.4-mg tablet or spray. IV, IA, or IC nitroglycerin is commonly administered in 50- to 400-µg boluses. Higher doses can result in hypotension and reflex tachycardia without further augmentation in coronary vasodilation. Nitroglycerin should not be administered to patients with a systolic blood pressure of <90 mm Hg or to patients who have taken phosphodiesterase-5 inhibitors within 24 (sildenafil [Viagra or Revatio], avanafil [Stendra or Spedra] and vardenafil [Levitra]) to 48 hours (tadalafil [Cialis or Adcirca]).[4] It should be administered cautiously to patients with severe aortic stenosis, hypertrophic cardiomyopathy, severe left main disease, right ventricular infarction, volume depletion, or volume-dependent pathology (such as restrictive cardiomyopathy) due to increased risk of an exaggerated and deleterious hypotensive response.[1,5,6] Hypotension caused by the administration of nitroglycerin can be treated with administration of IV fluids or vasopressors.

Nitroprusside

Nitroprusside is a direct nitric oxide donor that activates guanylate cyclase and generates cyclic GMP, resulting in smooth muscle relaxation

TABLE 5.1 Properties and Hemodynamic Effects of the Adrenergic Agonists[1-3]

	RECEPTOR				EFFECT		
	DOPAMINE	ALPHA ADRENERGIC	B1 ADRENERGIC	B2 ADRENERGIC	BP	CI	HR
Dopamine							
Low (<3 µg/kg/min)	++	0	+	0	0	0-↑	0-↑
Medium (3-7 µg/kg/min)	++	++	++	+	↑	↑	↑
High (>7 µg/kg/min)	++	++++	++++	+	↑↑	↑↑	↑↑
Dobutamine	0	0/+	++++	+++	0-↓	↑↑↑	↑
Epinephrine	0	++++	++++	++	↑↑↑	↑↑	↑↑↑
Norepinephrine	0	++++	++++	+	↑↑↑	↑↑	↑↑
Phenylephrine	0	++++	0	0	↑↑	0	0
Isoproterenol	0	0	++++	++++	0-↓	↑↑↑	↑↑↑

BP, blood pressure; CI, cardiac index; HR, heart rate.

From Zoghbi G. Vasoactive and antiarrhythmic drugs in the catheterization laboratory. In: Kern M, ed. *SCAI Interventional Board Review*. 2nd ed. Philadelphia, PA: Lippincott Williams & Wilkins; 2014:49-56; Holmes CL. Vasoactive drugs in the intensive care unit. *Curr Opin Crit Care*. 2005;11:413-417; and Overgaard CB, Dzavik V. Inotropes and vasopressors: review of physiology and clinical use in cardiovascular disease. *Circulation*. 2008;118:1047-1056.

and subsequent vasodilatation of the various venous and arterial beds. Unlike nitroglycerin, nitroprusside has a more potent effect on the arterial beds compared with the venous beds. Nitroprusside can be used to treat hypertensive crisis and acute heart failure, particularly due to acute mitral regurgitation. The IV nitroprusside dose starts at 0.25 to 0.3 µg/kg/min and can be titrated by 0.5 µg/kg/min every few minutes to achieve the desired hemodynamic effects (maximum dose of 10 µg/kg/min). Nitroprusside has been used to treat slow flow or no-reflow during PCIs and is given in 25- to 200-µg IC boluses with a quick saline flush of up to 1000 µg.[1,7]

Calcium Channel Blockers

Calcium channel blockers inhibit the L-type calcium channel on VSMCs and the slow-responding myocardial cells. Calcium channel blockers are classified as either dihydropyridines or nondihydropyridines. Dihydropyridines (such as amlodipine, felodipine, isradipine, nicardipine, and nifedipine) have a predominant vasodilator effect with very little or no effect on cardiac contractility or conduction. In contrast, nondihydropyridines (such as verapamil and diltiazem) have a lesser vasodilator effect and a more pronounced effect on reducing cardiac contractility and atrioventricular (AV) nodal conduction. In general, calcium channel blockers decrease peripheral vascular resistance (PVR), decrease blood pressure, alleviate coronary spasm, and increase coronary blood flow. Calcium channel blockers can be used in the catheterization laboratory to treat supraventricular and atrial arrhythmias (nondihydropyridines), hypertensive crisis (nicardipine), radial or coronary spasm, and slow flow or no-reflow (nondihydropyridines and nicardipine). Common side effects include hypotension, reflex tachycardia (dihydropyridines), negative inotropy (more pronounced with the nondihydropyridines), and bradycardia due to conduction disturbances such as AV nodal blocks or sinus arrest (nondihydropyridines). The nondihydropyridines are generally contraindicated in patients with left or right ventricular dysfunction due to their negative inotropic effects (more pronounced with verapamil compared with diltiazem).[1,7-10]

1. Diltiazem: IV bolus of 0.25 mg/kg (15-20 mg) over 2 minutes, followed by a maintenance rate of 5 to 20 mg/h for supraventricular tachycardia (SVT)/atrial tachycardias; 2.5- to 5-mg IA for prophylactic treatment or treatment of radial artery spasm; 0.5- to 2-mg IC boluses for treatment of slow flow or no-reflow.
2. Verapamil: IV bolus of 2.5 to 5 mg over 2 minutes; second dose of 5 to 10 mg (~0.15 mg/kg) may be given 15 to 30 minutes later (for SVT/atrial tachycardias); 2.5 to 5 mg IA for prophylactic treatment or treatment of radial artery spasm; 50- to 200-µg slow IC boluses, for 2 to 4 boluses, if needed for treatment of slow flow or no-reflow (60%-100% success).
3. Nicardipine: Nicardipine is the only dihydropyridine that can be given IV or IA. IV infusion of 5 mg/h (maximum dose of 15-20 mg/h) for treating hypertension; 200-µg IC boluses, for 2 to 4 boluses, for the treatment of slow flow or no-reflow (99% success in one study; some benefit in prophylactic administration to prevent no-reflow in saphenous vein graft [SVG] PCIs and rotational atherectomy); 2.5 to 5 mg IA for prophylactic treatment or treatment of radial artery spasm during transradial procedures.

Adenosine Agonists

Adenosine is a nonselective adenosine receptor agonist. Adenosine binding to the A2A receptors on arteriolar smooth muscle cells (SMCs) increases the production of cyclic adenosine monophosphate (AMP), which leads to SMC relaxation and arteriolar vasodilation.[11] Adenosine produces coronary hyperemia and has been used in conjunction with nuclear myocardial perfusion imaging and for assessing fractional flow reserve (FFR), coronary flow reserve (CFR), and microvascular resistance in the catheterization laboratory.[11] Adenosine can be administered as an IC bolus (50-100 µg for the right coronary artery [RCA] and 100-200 µg for the left coronary artery [LCA]) or IV infusion (140 µg/kg/min) over 2 to 3 minutes for FFR or CFR evaluation.

A dose-response study of adenosine demonstrated that an IC adenosine bolus injection of 100 µg in the RCA and 200 µg in the LCA induced maximal hyperemia with minimal side effects.[12] The peak hyperemic effect of IC adenosine is achieved within a few seconds of its bolus administration, with a sustained plateau of hyperemia of around 5 seconds. The peak hyperemic effect of IV adenosine is reached within 2 minutes of its administration and lasts for <30 seconds from its termination. IV adenosine permits measuring a pullback FFR and has been shown in one study to cause more hyperemia than IC adenosine.[13] Adenosine has also been used in the catheterization laboratory in vasodilator challenge testing in patients with pulmonary hypertension, where IV adenosine is initially infused at 50 µg/kg/min and is increased by 50 µg/kg/min every 2 minutes to a maximum dose of 250 µg/kg/min.[14] IC adenosine boluses of 24 to 60 µg with a quick saline flush have been used to treat slow flow or no-reflow during coronary and SVG PCIs, with a 90% success rate.

Regadenoson is a selective adenosine A2A receptor agonist that is administered as a single 0.4-mg IV bolus and is used as a stress agent in conjunction with nuclear myocardial perfusion imaging. Peak hyperemia is reached within seconds of its administration and lasts for around 2 minutes from its administration. Regadenoson single IV bolus of 0.4 mg was compared with an IV adenosine infusion at 140 µg/kg/min for evaluation of coronary stenoses using FFR.[15,16] Regadenoson was as effective as adenosine in measuring FFR, with a strong linear correlation with adenosine and similar frequency in detecting FFR <0.8, a similar hemodynamic response, more rapid hyperemia, more ease of use, and an excellent side-effect profile.[15,16]

Common side effects of adenosine include bronchospasm, chest pain, dyspnea, flushing, AV block, modest hypotension, and modest increases in heart rate. The side effects are short lived and can be reversed with 50 to 100 mg of IV aminophylline if they become severe and prolonged. Adenosine is contraindicated in patients with heart transplantation or in patients with second- or third-degree heart block in the absence of a functional pacemaker. Adenosine should be used cautiously in patients with bronchospastic lung disorders due to the risk of adenosine-induced bronchoconstriction.[1,11,12,15,17-20]

Papaverine

Papaverine is a potent arterial vasodilator, whose mechanism of action is thought to be due to inhibition of a phosphodiesterase enzyme that results in increasing cyclic AMP in SMCs, with resultant smooth muscle relaxation and arterial vasodilatation. IC papaverine is used to induce coronary hyperemia for assessment of CFR or FFR. Its onset of action is within 10 to 30 seconds and its duration is for 45 to 60 seconds from time of administration. Commonly used IC bolus doses are 8 mg for the RCA and 12 mg for the LCA. Papaverine can prolong the QT segment and cause torsades de pointes. Papaverine can cause crystallization when combined with some of the ionic contrast agents and can also increase coronary venous lactate production, which may cause myocardial ischemia.[1,13,18,21-23]

Coronary Vasoconstrictors

Acetylcholine

Acetylcholine is an endogenous neurotransmitter that stimulates muscarinic receptors on endothelial cells and causes endothelial-dependent vasodilatation via release of nitric oxide and other vasoactive substances in the presence of a normal endothelium and causes vasoconstriction via direct activation of receptors on SMCs.[1] The balance of these actions determines the response to intracoronary acetylcholine; in normal coronary arteries with a healthy endothelium, the net effect of acetylcholine is a mild vasodilation or no change in vessel caliber. In patients with endothelial dysfunction, acetylcholine can lead to vasoconstriction or coronary spasm. Acetylcholine has been used to diagnose vasospastic angina, particularly in patients who have normally apparent coronary arteries on coronary angiography.

Acetylcholine has also been used to assess epicardial and microvascular vasomotor responses, which can lead to ischemia in patients with stable angina who have normal or minimal coronary artery disease.[1] In one study of patients with stable angina and normal or minimal coronary artery disease, two-thirds of the patients had an abnormal test where 45% of the patients had epicardial spasm (>75% coronary narrowing with symptom production) and 55% of the patients had microvascular spasm (symptom reproduction with ischemic electrocardiogram [ECG] changes and no epicardial spasm).[24] IC incremental doses of acetylcholine of 20, 50, and 80 µg are usually injected into the RCA and of 20, 50, 100, and 200 µg are injected into the LCA. Spasm is defined as a ≥90% coronary narrowing after acetylcholine administration associated with clinical evidence of ischemia. Spasm caused by low doses of acetylcholine is usually more proximal and focal. Spasm caused by higher acetylcholine doses is associated with more distal and diffuse spasm. Acetylcholine-induced coronary spasm can be reversed with intracoronary nitroglycerin.

Acetylcholine is very short acting and rapidly inactivated. Continuous infusions of 0.02 to 2.2 µg (10^{-8}, 10^{-7}, 10^{-6} M) have been used to identify normal endothelial coronary artery function with mild vasodilatation and an augmentation of coronary blood flow. Side effects of acetylcholine can include marked bradycardia, heart block, and profound vasospasm, and temporary pacing is recommended during its administration in the RCA. In a large meta-analysis of 16 studies with 12,585 patients, intracoronary acetylcholine was associated with a 0.5% (95% confidence interval: 0.0%-1.3%) incidence of major complications, without any reports of death.[25]

Ergonovine

Ergonovine is an ergot derivative that causes SMC contraction and is commonly used to induce uterine contractions to treat or prevent postpartum hemorrhage. It can also be used in the coronary tree to provoke coronary spasm and evaluate patients with angina pectoris who have normal coronaries or minimal coronary artery disease on coronary angiography.[1] Ergonovine can be administered IC as an infusion of 10 µg/min over 4 minutes for a maximal dose of 40 µg in the RCA and as 16 µg/min over 4 minutes for a total dose of 64 µg in the LCA.[26] Alternatively, ergonovine can be administered by slow IC injections over 1 minute each of sequential doses of 1, 5, 10, and 30 µg at 3- to 5-minute intervals with a maximum cumulative dose of 50 µg.[27] An ECG is obtained at the end of each interval or if the patient develops angina symptoms.

Angiography of the right and left coronary arteries should be promptly performed when angina symptoms occur. Diffuse coronary narrowing is a physiologic response to ergonovine, whereas a severe focal coronary narrowing (>75% narrowing in some studies and >90% in others) is indicative of coronary spasm when associated with ischemic ECG changes or typical symptoms.[26] Ergonovine-induced spasm can be reversed with the administration of IC nitroglycerine. In one study, IC acetylcholine-induced spasm (873 patients) was compared with IC ergonovine-induced spasm (635 patients). Acetylcholine was more likely to provoke spasm in patients without fixed stenosis than ergonovine (36.2% vs 25.5%). In this series, complications occurred in 1.4% of patients with the acetylcholine test, and in 0.2% of patients with the ergonovine test, with no occurrence of any myocardial infarction or death with either test.[1,26]

Vasopressors and Inotropes

Vasopressor drugs generally cause peripheral vasoconstriction, leading to an increase in systemic vascular resistance (SVR) and mean arterial pressure (MAP). Inotropic drugs, on the other hand, increase cardiac contractility and chronotropy. Some of the vasopressor drugs have both vasopressor and inotropic effects, depending on the receptors they stimulate.[1] Stimulation of peripheral α1 receptors causes vasoconstriction, and stimulation of cardiac α1 receptors augments inotropy. Stimulation of β1 receptors (located mainly on myocytes) augments inotropy and chronotropy. Stimulation of the β2 receptors (located mainly in the vasculature) augments vasodilatation. Stimulation of the dopaminergic receptors DA1 causes vasodilatation in the renal, splanchnic cerebral, and coronary beds.[1-3,28] Drugs acting on these receptors can be used in the catheterization laboratory depending on the clinical scenario and the desired hemodynamic effect (**Table 5.1**).[1-3]

Phenylephrine (Neosynephrine)

Phenylephrine is a pure α receptor agonist. Its main effect is peripheral vasoconstriction, with minimal cardiac inotropy and minimal effect on cardiac output. Phenylephrine is used in hypotension with low SVR, such as sepsis, neurologic disorders, and anesthesia- or medication-induced hypotension. It is commonly used in the catheterization laboratory to correct medication-related hypotension (eg, from nitroglycerin or nitroprusside) or transient hypotension related to ischemia or during carotid stenting. It is also used in patients with severe aortic valve stenosis or hypertrophic obstructive cardiomyopathy who develop hypotension. It can be given as 50- to 200-µg rapid boluses to correct sudden-onset hypotension or as an IV drip (**Table 5.2**). Phenylephrine can cause marked increase in blood pressure (especially in patients on nonselective β blockers), reflex-mediated bradycardia, and severe peripheral and visceral vasoconstriction.[1-3]

Norepinephrine (Levophed)

Norepinephrine predominantly stimulates the α1 and β1 receptors, with less effect on the β2 receptors. It has a significant vasoconstrictor effect and minimal inotropic and chronic effects and as such is used to treat severe cardiogenic shock, septic shock, or shock refractory to other pressors, particularly in low-SVR states. Norepinephrine can cause peripheral ischemia and arrhythmias and increase SVR and blood pressure (especially in patients with non-selective β blockers) (**Table 5.2**).[1-3]

Epinephrine

Epinephrine has equipotent effects on the α1 and β1 receptors and modest effects on the β2 receptors. At lower doses, epinephrine increases cardiac output with a minimal decrease in SVR and

TABLE 5.2 Indications and Doses of the Various Vasopressors and Inotropes[1,3,29,30]

DRUG	INDICATION AND DOSE
Epinephrine	ACLS/cardiac arrest: 1 mg (1:10,000) IV/IO q 3-5 min; 2-2.5 mg (1:1000) ET tube q 3-5 min Symptomatic bradycardia or heart block unresponsive to atropine or pacing/shock (cardiogenic/vasodilatory): 2-10 μg/min IV maintenance Anaphylaxis/bronchospasm: 0.1-0.5 mg (1:1000) SC/IM q 5-15 min or 0.1-0.25 mg (1:10,000) IV q 5-15 min
Norepinephrine	Shock (vasodilatory/cardiogenic): Start 0.5-1 μg/min IV, maintenance 2-12 μg/min up to 30 g/min
Phenylephrine	Shock (vagally mediated/medication induced), hypotension in aortic valve stenosis, and HOCM: 100-500 μg IV bolus q 10-15 min, maintenance 40-60 μg/min IV infusion up to 200 μg/min
Isoproterenol	Bradyarrhythmias (especially in torsades des pointes and Brugada syndrome): 20-60 μg IV bolus, 2-10 μg/min IV maintenance
Dopamine	Heart failure: 1-3 μg/kg/min Symptomatic bradycardia unresponsive to atropine or pacing: 2-10 μg/kg/min Shock (cardiogenic/vasodilatory): 2-20 μg/kg/min (up to 50 μg/kg/min for refractory shock)
Dobutamine	Low cardiac output (decompensated heart failure, cardiogenic shock, sepsis-induced myocardial dysfunction)/symptomatic bradycardia unresponsive to atropine or pacing: 2-10 μg/kg/min (up to 20 μg/kg/min)
Milrinone	Low cardiac output (decompensated heart failure/post cardiotomy): 50 μg/kg IV bolus followed by 0.375-0.75 μg/kg/min (decrease dose based on Cr clearance)
Vasopressin	ACLS/cardiac arrest: 40 units IV × 1; 80-100 units ET tube Shock (vasodilatory/cardiogenic): 0.01-0.10 units/min IV maintenance

ACLS, advanced cardiac life support; Cr, creatinine; ET, endotracheal; HOCM, hypertrophic obstructive cardiomyopathy; IM, intramuscular; IO, intraosseous; IV, intravenous; SC, subcutaneous.

From Zoghbi G. Vasoactive and antiarrhythmic drugs in the catheterization laboratory. In: Kern M, ed. *SCAI Interventional Board Review.* 2nd ed. Philadelphia, PA: Lippincott Williams & Wilkins; 2014:49-56; Overgaard CB, Dzavik V. Inotropes and vasopressors: review of physiology and clinical use in cardiovascular disease. *Circulation.* 2008;118:1047-1056; Field JM, Hazinski MF, Sayre MR, et al. Part 1: executive summary—2010 American Heart Association Guidelines for cardiopulmonary resuscitation and emergency cardiovascular care. *Circulation.* 2010;122(18 suppl 3):S640-S656; and Hazinski MF, Nolan JP, Billi JE, et al. Part 1: executive summary—2010 international consensus on cardiopulmonary resuscitation and emergency cardiovascular care science with treatment recommendations. *Circulation.* 2010;122(16 suppl 2):S250-S275.

variable effect on MAP (due to equal stimulation of α1 and β2 receptors). At higher doses, stimulation of the α1 receptors predominates over β2 receptor stimulation, resulting in more peripheral vasoconstriction than vasodilatation and increases in SVR. Epinephrine is the first-line drug used in cardiac arrest (asystole, pulseless electrical activity, and ventricular fibrillation [VF]) and anaphylactic shock and is a second-line drug for treating severe cardiogenic shock. It is commonly used to treat hypotension following cardiac surgery (**Table 5.2**). Epinephrine can cause tachycardia, ventricular arrhythmias, increased oxygen demand, cardiac ischemia, increased SVR, and severe hypertension that can cause cerebrovascular hemorrhage.[1-3]

Dopamine

Dopamine stimulates various receptors and produces its effects in a dose-dependent manner. At a low dose of 1 to 2 μg/kg/min, it activates the dopamine receptors (renal DA1 and peripheral DA2 receptors) with resultant vasodilatation in the renal, splanchnic, coronary, and cerebral circulations. Low-dose dopamine augments renal blood flow and may assist with natriuresis. Medium-dose dopamine (2-7 μg/kg/min) stimulates the β1 receptors and has variable effects on SVR and blood pressure, depending on the balance of peripheral vasodilatation and the increased cardiac output. High-dose dopamine (>7-10 μg/kg/min) predominantly stimulates the α1 receptors, resulting in vasoconstriction and increases in SVR and MAP. Dopamine is occasionally used to treat hypotension due to nonprofound septic or cardiogenic shocks, poor tissue perfusion states (oliguria, anuria, altered level of consciousness), or symptomatic bradycardia, particularly in patients without central venous access. Dopamine, particularly at high doses, can cause tachycardia, arrhythmias, renal vasoconstriction, and tissue ischemia at high doses (**Table 5.2**).[1-3]

Dobutamine

Dobutamine is a predominant β1 receptor agonist with less effect on the β2 receptor, and as such it is an inotrope rather than a pressor drug. Dobutamine is mainly used to treat low cardiac output congestive heart failure (CHF) by augmenting cardiac output and decreasing SVR and cardiac filling pressures. It has no effect on or causes a minimal decrease in MAP. It can cause tachycardia, an increase in ventricular response in atrial arrhythmias, ventricular arrhythmias, cardiac ischemia, and occasionally hypotension (**Table 5.2**).[1-3]

Isoproterenol (Isuprel)

Isoproterenol is a pure β1 and β2 agonist with predominant chronotropic effect and a lesser effect on inotropy and peripheral vasodilatation. It is mainly used in the electrophysiology laboratory to induce tachycardia and to stimulate the sinus node in some situations of resistant bradycardia unresponsive to atropine and dopamine, as well as in hypotension related to bradycardia or post-cardiac transplantation. Continuous IV isoproterenol infusion can cause a significant increase in heart rate and inotropy, a decrease in diastolic blood pressure and SVR, and increased myocardial work. It can also cause ventricular arrhythmias, cardiac ischemia, and hypertension or hypotension (**Table 5.2**).[1-3]

Phosphodiesterase Inhibitors

Phosphodiesterase inhibitors such as milrinone are inotropes that inhibit phosphodiesterase III and increase intracellular cyclic AMP, independent of the β-adrenergic receptors. Milrinone has equipotent inotropic effects and both a more potent central and peripheral vasodilator effect and a lesser chronotropic effect compared with dobutamine. It is used to treat low cardiac output heart failure. It can cause ventricular arrhythmias, hypotension, cardiac ischemia, and torsades des pointes (**Table 5.2**).[1-3]

Vasopressin

Vasopressin is an antidiuretic hormone that has vasopressor effects. It stimulates V1 receptors on VSMCs and V2 receptors in the renal collecting duct system. It can be used as a second-line drug for catecholamine-refractory septic or anaphylactic shock or as a first-line drug during cardiac arrest instead of epinephrine. It can cause arrhythmias, hypertension, cardiac ischemia, decreased cardiac output (at high doses), and severe peripheral ischemia leading to splanchnic and skin vasoconstriction (**Table 5.2**).[1-3,31]

Side Effects

The vasopressors and inotropes have potential serious complications. Stimulation of the α receptors can cause significant peripheral vasoconstriction and decreased perfusion with resultant limb ischemia, renal hypoperfusion and renal ischemia, mesenteric ischemia, gastritis, and shock liver. Stimulation of the β1 receptor augments chronotropy that can result in sinus tachycardia and atrial or ventricular arrhythmias. Chronotropic and inotropic augmentation can also lead to myocardial ischemia, particularly in patients with underlying coronary artery disease. Extravasation of vasopressors into surrounding skin and connective tissue can cause local vasoconstriction with subsequent skin and tissue necrosis.[1,3]

ANTIARRHYTHMIC DRUGS

Antiarrhythmic drugs are classified based on their predominant mechanism of action, such as with the modified Vaughn-Williams classification.[32,33] **Table 5.3** summarizes the different antiarrhythmic drugs, with their properties, indications, and side effects. The antiarrhythmic drugs commonly used in cardiac catheterization are those needed to treat or control acute ventricular or supraventricular arrhythmias.[1]

Procainamide

Procainamide is a class IA antiarrhythmic drug with electrophysiologic properties similar to those of quinidine, but without the vagolytic and α receptor effects. Procainamide has a ganglionic blocker effect that accounts for some of the hypotension noted with its IV administration. *N*-acetyl procainamide (NAPA) is a major procainamide metabolite that also blocks the K channel, similar to the parent drug. Procainamide is hepatically metabolized to NAPA, and both the parent compound and its metabolite are renally excreted. The significant side-effect profile of procainamide precludes its long-term use. Procainamide is indicated for hemodynamically stable monomorphic VT or preexcited atrial fibrillation. The loading dose is infused at 20 to 50 mg/min or 100 mg every 5 minutes until the arrhythmia is controlled, hypotension occurs, the QRS widens by 50% of its original width, or a total of 17 mg/kg is given. The maintenance infusion is 1 to 4 mg/min. Procainamide should not be administered if the QT is prolonged or if the patient has CHF.[1,29,30,32,33]

Lidocaine

Lidocaine is a class IB antiarrhythmic drug that has minimal effect on the QT compared with other class I drugs. Lidocaine's suppressive effects are mainly on the depolarized myocardium, and it is used to treat ventricular arrhythmias induced by ischemia. Lidocaine is metabolized in the liver into two metabolites that have less antiarrhythmic effects than the parent drug. Lidocaine levels should be monitored closely to prevent toxicities, particularly in patients with CHF or liver dysfunction. In the catheterization laboratory, lidocaine can be given as an IV bolus of 50 to 100 mg before ventriculography to suppress ventricular ectopy or to treat ischemia-induced ventricular arrhythmias during cardiac catheterization or PCI. Lidocaine is indicated for VF or pulseless VT if amiodarone is not available and for hemodynamically stable VT. Lidocaine is administered as a 1- to 1.5-mg/kg IV bolus, with a repeat bolus of 0.5 to 0.75 mg/kg every 5 to 10 minutes (the maximum cumulative dose is 3 mg/kg) for refractory VF or pulseless VT, followed by a maintenance infusion of 1 to 4 mg/min.[1,29,30,32,33]

Amiodarone

Amiodarone is a class III antiarrhythmic drug that also has class I, II, and IV effects. Desethylamiodarone, the main metabolite of amiodarone, is a potent Na channel blocker. Amiodarone requires a solvent (polysorbate 80) for its IV administration. The solvent, as well as the β and calcium channel blocker effects of amiodarone, can decrease the heart rate and reduce the blood pressure, particularly during IV bolus administration. Amiodarone is metabolized in the liver, with minimal renal elimination and a very long elimination half-life (mean of 54 days). Amiodarone can decrease the hepatic or renal clearance of other antiarrhythmic drugs such as flecainide, procainamide, and quinidine. Concomitant use of amiodarone with other antiarrhythmic drugs (mexiletine, propafenone, quinidine, disopyramide, procainamide), tricyclic antidepressants, and some of the antipsychotic drugs can prolong the QT interval and induce torsades de pointes. Warfarin and digoxin doses should be reduced by half when used long term with amiodarone. Amiodarone should be used with caution in conjunction with antihypertensives, β blockers, or calcium channel blockers. Amiodarone is indicated for VF or pulseless VT and is given as a 300-mg IV bolus, with a supplemental 150-mg IV bolus dose if VF or pulseless VT continues after defibrillation, or if it recurs. Amiodarone is infused at 1 mg/min for 6 hours followed by 0.5 mg/min for 18 hours after the return of spontaneous circulation. Amiodarone is also indicated for stable VT or for pharmacologic conversion or rate control of supraventricular or atrial arrhythmias. A 150-mg IV bolus is infused over 10 minutes, followed by a maintenance dose infused at 1 mg/min for 6 hours followed by 0.5 mg/min for 18 hours.[1,29,30,32,33]

β Blockers

β Blockers belong to class II antiarrhythmic drugs. β Blockers can be used in the catheterization laboratory for rate control of fast supraventricular or atrial arrhythmias, as well as for suppression of ventricular arrhythmias, particularly with long-term use. Metoprolol (Lopressor) can be administered as 2.5- to 5-mg IV boluses every 2 to 5 minutes for a maximum of 15 mg. Esmolol is the β blocker of choice for a maintenance IV infusion. Esmolol is given as a 500-µg/kg bolus over 1 minute, followed by a maintenance infusion at 50 µg/kg/min that can be titrated upward in 50-µg/kg/min increments every 4 minutes, to a maximum of 200 µg/kg/min.[1]

Calcium Channel Blockers

The nondihydropyridine calcium channel blockers belong to class IV antiarrhythmic agents. Similar to the β blockers, they can be used in the catheterization laboratory for rate control of fast supraventricular or atrial arrhythmias (discussed in the "Vasodilators" section earlier).

TABLE 5.3 Classification and Properties of Antiarrhythmic Drugs[1,32,33]

	ACTION	USE	SIDE EFFECTS
Class IA	Na channel blocker; slows conduction velocity, prolongs action potential duration		
Quinidine	Na and K channel blocker, α blocker, vagolytic activity	Conversion of Afib, Aflutter and maintenance of sinus rhythm, life-threatening ventricular arrhythmias	Proarrhythmias, QT prolongation, torsades de pointes, GI intolerance, tinnitus, headache, thrombocytopenia, SLE, worsening myasthenia gravis, hypotension, and sinus tachycardia with IV use or high oral dose
Procainamide	Na and K channel blocker, ganglionic blocker	Ventricular arrhythmias, reentrant SVT, Afib or Aflutter associated with WPW	QT prolongation, drug-induced lupus, rash, arthralgia, fever, pericardial and pleural effusions, bone marrow aplasia, agranulocytosis, hypotension with IV dose or high serum levels
Disopyramide	Na and K channel blocker, vagolytic activity of primary metabolite	Ventricular arrhythmias, SVT, HCM (reduce LVOT gradient)	Anticholinergic effects, constipation, urinary retention, dry mouth, GERD, glaucoma exacerbation, worsening CHF (negative inotropic effect)
Class IB	Na channel blocker, no effect on conduction velocity		
Lidocaine	Shortens action potential, minimal effect on QT	Ischemia-induced ventricular arrhythmias or recurrent ventricular arrhythmias	CNS symptoms such as tremor, paresthesias, hearing abnormalities, slurred speech, depressed mentation, seizure, coma, and nausea
Mexilitine	Derivative of lidocaine with similar properties	Refractory ventricular arrhythmias	CNS symptoms such as tremor, dizziness, dysphoria, and GI intolerance
Class IC	Slows conduction velocity, minimal prolongation of action potential duration		
Flecainide	Late opening Na channels, delayed rectifier K channel and calcium channel blocker; prolong action potential at fast rates, no effect on QT	Prevention of PAF and SVT in patients without structural heart disease, prevention of life-threatening ventricular arrhythmias	Blurred vision and dry eyes, CHF exacerbation with abnormal LV function
Propafenone	Fast Na channel blocker, decrease membrane excitability and spontaneous automaticity, β blocker activity	SVT, Afib in patients without structural heart disease, ventricular arrhythmias	Metallic taste, GI intolerance, dizziness, blurred vision, fatigue, hepatotoxicity, lupus, blood dyscrasias, bronchospasm, proarrhythmia in patients with depressed LV function or history of ventricular arrhythmias
Class II	β Blockers, β1 receptor blocker, sinus rate and AV nodal slowing, decreased contractility	SVT, rate control of Afib and Aflutter, ventricular arrhythmias	
Class III	Delayed K rectifier channel blocker; prolong action potential duration, no effect on conduction velocity	Suppress atrial and ventricular arrhythmias	QT prolongation, torsades de pointes
Amiodarone	Class I, II, and IV action	Suppressing and preventing ventricular and supraventricular arrhythmias to maintain sinus rhythm, tolerated in patients with depressed LV function	GI intolerance, hypotension and phlebitis (IV administration), pulmonary and hepatotoxicities, hyper- or hypothyroidism, peripheral neuropathy, skin discoloration, and corneal deposits
Dronedarone	Similar to amiodarone	Preventing Afib, maintain sinus rhythm	Similar to amiodarone, contraindicated in patients with permanent Afib, or history of or current heart failure or LV dysfunction
Sotalol	β Blockade	Ventricular arrhythmias, conversion of Afib, and maintain sinus rhythm	Proarrhythmias, QT prolongation, torsades de pointes, close monitoring during initiation
Ibutilide	Analogue of sotalol, IV administration only	Conversion of Afib or Aflutter	Proarrhythmias, QT prolongation, torsades de pointes

(continued)

TABLE 5.3 Classification and Properties of Antiarrhythmic Drugs[1,32,33] *(Continued)*

	ACTION	USE	SIDE EFFECTS
Dofetilide	Prolong repolarization	Conversion of Afib, maintain sinus rhythm	Proarrhythmias, QT prolongation, torsades de pointes, close monitoring during initiation and in patients with renal dysfunction
Class IV	Nondihydropyridine calcium channel blockers; slow Ca channel blockers in sinus and AV nodes; negative inotropic effects	Acute and chronic treatment of SVT, rate control of Afib and Aflutter	Caution in patients with LV dysfunction and patients with WPW

Afib, atrial fibrillation; Aflutter, atrial flutter; AV, atrioventricular; CHF, congestive heart failure; CNS, central nervous system; GERD, gastroesophageal reflux disorder; GI, gastrointestinal; HCM, hypertrophic cardiomyopathy; IV, intravenous; LV, left ventricular; LVOT, left ventricular outflow tract; PAF, paroxysmal atrial fibrillation; SLE, systemic lupus erythematosus; SVT, supraventricular tachycardia; WPW, Wolff-Parkinson-White syndrome.

From Zoghbi G. Vasoactive and antiarrhythmic drugs in the catheterization laboratory. In: Kern M, ed. *SCAI Interventional Board Review.* 2nd ed. Philadelphia, PA: Lippincott Williams & Wilkins; 2014:49-56; Kowey PR. Pharmacological effects of antiarrhythmic drugs. Review and update. *Arch Intern Med.* 1998;158:325-332; and Kowey PR, Marinchak RA, Rials SJ, Bharucha DB. Classification and pharmacology of antiarrhythmic drugs. *Am Heart J.* 2000;140(1):12-20.

Adenosine

Adenosine (Adenocard) is indicated for pharmacologic conversion of AV nodal reentrant SVT. Adenosine has a very short half-life of a few seconds. Adenosine is administered as a rapid IV bolus of 6 mg that can be repeated in 1 to 2 minutes as a 12-mg rapid IV bolus if the first dose was ineffective.[1]

Key Points

- Nitroglycerin causes more venous than arterial vasodilatation. It improves coronary flow, prevents or alleviates coronary spasm, provokes myocardial bridging, relieves angina, reduces preload in patients with elevated filling pressures, and prevents or treats radial artery spasm.
- Nitroprusside, a direct nitric oxide donor, can be used to treat hypertensive emergencies, acute heart failure particularly due to acute mitral regurgitation, and no-reflow during PCIs.
- Dihydropyridines calcium channel blockers (such as amlodipine, felodipine, isradipine, nicardipine, and nifedipine) have a predominant vasodilator effect, with very little or no effect on cardiac contractility or conduction.
- Nondihydropyridines calcium channel blockers (such as verapamil and diltiazem) have a lesser vasodilator effect and a more pronounced effect on reducing cardiac contractility and conduction.
- Calcium channel blockers decrease PVR, decrease blood pressure, alleviate coronary spasm, and increase coronary blood flow.
- Calcium channel blockers can be used to treat supraventricular and atrial arrhythmias (nondihydropyridines). They are also used in prophylactic treatment or treatment of radial or coronary spasm and no-reflow (nondihydropyridines and nicardipine).
- Adenosine, a nonselective adenosine receptor agonist, produces coronary hyperemia for assessing CFR and FFR. It can also be used for vasodilator testing in patients with pulmonary hypertension.
- Regadenoson, a selective adenosine A2A receptor agonist, is administered as a single 0.4-mg IV bolus for assessing CFR and FFR.
- Papaverine, a potent arterial vasodilator, can also be used to induce coronary hyperemia for assessment of CFR or FFR.
- Acetylcholine, an endogenous neurotransmitter, causes endothelial-dependent vasodilatation via the release of nitric oxide and other vasoactive substances in the presence of a normal endothelium and causes vasoconstriction via direct activation of receptors on SMCs in the presence of an abnormal endothelium.
- IC acetylcholine administration constricts diseased coronary arteries (endothelial dysfunction or atherosclerosis) and vasodilates normal coronary arteries (normal endothelial function). It is used to assess epicardial and microvascular vasomotor responses and to diagnose vasospastic angina.
- Ergonovine, an ergot derivative, is an alternative to acetylcholine that also causes SMC contraction and is used to provoke coronary spasm and evaluate patients with angina pectoris who have normal coronaries or minimal coronary artery disease on coronary angiography.
- Phenylephrine, a pure α receptor agonist, produces peripheral vasoconstriction with minimal cardiac inotropy and minimal effect on cardiac output. Phenylephrine is used to treat hypotension with low SVR, medication-related hypotension, or transient hypotension related to ischemia or carotid stenting.
- Norepinephrine predominantly stimulates the $\alpha 1$ and $\beta 1$ receptors, with less effect on the $\beta 2$ receptors, and is used to treat septic shock or severe cardiogenic shock. Epinephrine has equipotent effects on the $\alpha 1$ and $\beta 1$ receptors and modest effects on the $\beta 2$ receptors. It is used as a first-line drug in cardiac arrest and anaphylactic shock and as a second-line drug for treating septic shock or severe cardiogenic shock, or when treating hypotension following cardiac surgery.
- Dopamine's effects depend on its infusion dose. Medium to high dopamine doses further stimulate the $\alpha 1$ receptors, in addition to the $\beta 1$ receptors, and are used to treat septic or cardiogenic shock or symptomatic bradycardia.

- Dobutamine is a predominant β1 receptor agonist with less effect on the β2 receptor. It is used as an inotrope to treat low cardiac output CHF.
- Isoproterenol is a pure β1 and β2 agonist with a predominant chronotropic effect and a lesser effect on inotropy and peripheral vasodilatation. It is mainly used to induce tachycardia during electrophysiology studies, to treat hypotension related to bradycardia, or to stimulate the sinus node postcardiac transplantation.
- Phosphodiesterase inhibitors, such as milrinone, are inotropes that inhibit phosphodiesterase III and increase intracellular cyclic AMP, independent of the β adrenergic receptors.
- Vasopressin, an antidiuretic hormone, is used as a second-line drug for catecholamine-refractory septic or anaphylactic shock or as a first-line drug instead of epinephrine during cardiac arrest.

References

1. Zoghbi G. Vasoactive and antiarrhythmic drugs in the catheterization laboratory. In: Kern M, ed. *SCAI Interventional Board Review*. 2nd ed. Lippincott Williams & Wilkins; 2014:49-56.
2. Holmes CL. Vasoactive drugs in the intensive care unit. *Curr Opin Crit Care*. 2005;11(5):413-417.
3. Overgaard CB, Dzavik V. Inotropes and vasopressors: review of physiology and clinical use in cardiovascular disease. *Circulation*. 2008;118(10):1047-1056.
4. Kloner RA. Cardiovascular effects of the 3 phosphodiesterase-5 inhibitors approved for the treatment of erectile dysfunction. *Circulation*. 2004;110(19):3149-3155.
5. Abrams J. Hemodynamic effects of nitroglycerin and long-acting nitrates. *Am Heart J*. 1985;110(1 Pt 2):216-224.
6. Chen Z, Zhang J, Stamler JS. Identification of the enzymatic mechanism of nitroglycerin bioactivation. *Proc Natl Acad Sci U S A*. 2002;99(12):8306-8311.
7. Wong DT, Puri R, Richardson JD, Worthley MI, Worthley SG. Myocardial 'no-reflow': diagnosis, pathophysiology and treatment. *Int J Cardiol*. 2013;167(5):1798-1806.
8. Fischell TA, Haller S, Pulukurthy S, Virk IS. Nicardipine and adenosine "flush cocktail" to prevent no-reflow during rotational atherectomy. *Cardiovasc Revasc Med*. 2008;9(4):224-228.
9. Huang RI, Patel P, Walinsky P, et al. Efficacy of intracoronary nicardipine in the treatment of no-reflow during percutaneous coronary intervention. *Catheter Cardiovasc Interv*. 2006;68(5):671-676.
10. Caputo RP, Tremmel JA, Rao S, et al. Transradial arterial access for coronary and peripheral procedures: executive summary by the Transradial Committee of the SCAI. *Catheter Cardiovasc Interv*. 2011;78(6):823-839.
11. Zoghbi GJ, Iskandrian AE. Coronary artery disease detection: pharmacologic stress SPECT. In: Zaret BL, Beller GA, eds. *Clinical Nuclear Cardiology: State of the Art and Future Directions*. Mosby Elsevier; 2010:225-266.
12. Adjedj J, Toth GG, Johnson NP, et al. Intracoronary adenosine: dose-response relationship with hyperemia. *JACC Cardiovasc Interv*. 2015;8(11):1422-1430.
13. De Bruyne B, Pijls NHJ, Barbato E, et al. Intracoronary and intravenous adenosine 5'-triphosphate, adenosine, papaverine, and contrast medium to assess fractional flow reserve in humans. *Circulation*. 2003;107(14):1877-1883.
14. McLaughlin VV, Archer SL, Badesch DB, et al. ACCF/AHA 2009 expert consensus document on pulmonary hypertension: a report of the American College of Cardiology Foundation Task Force on Expert Consensus Documents and the American Heart Association developed in collaboration with the American College of Chest Physicians; American Thoracic Society, Inc.; and the Pulmonary Hypertension Association. *J Am Coll Cardiol*. 2009;53(17):1573-1619.
15. Nair PK, Marroquin OC, Mulukutla SR, et al. Clinical utility of regadenoson for assessing fractional flow reserve. *JACC Cardiovasc Interv*. 2011;4(10):1085-1092.
16. Prasad A, Zareh M, Doherty R, et al. Use of regadenoson for measurement of fractional flow reserve. *Catheter Cardiovasc Interv*. 2014;83(3):369-374.
17. Casella G, Leibig M, Schiele TM, et al. Are high doses of intracoronary adenosine an alternative to standard intravenous adenosine for the assessment of fractional flow reserve? *Am Heart J*. 2004;148(4):590-595.
18. McGeoch RJ, Oldroyd KG. Pharmacological options for inducing maximal hyperaemia during studies of coronary physiology. *Catheter Cardiovasc Interv*. 2008;71(2):198-204.
19. Assali AR, Sdringola S, Ghani M, et al. Intracoronary adenosine administered during percutaneous intervention in acute myocardial infarction and reduction in the incidence of "no reflow" phenomenon. *Catheter Cardiovasc Interv*. 2000;51(1):27-32.
20. Fischell TA, Carter AJ, Foster MT, et al. Reversal of "no reflow" during vein graft stenting using high velocity boluses of intracoronary adenosine. *Cathet Cardiovasc Diagn*. 1998;45(4):360-365.
21. Kapoor N, Fahsah I, Karim R, Jevans AJ, Leesar MA. Physiological assessment of renal artery stenosis: comparisons of resting with hyperemic renal pressure measurements. *Catheter Cardiovasc Interv*. 2010;76(5):726-732.
22. Subramanian R, White CJ, Rosenfield K, et al. Renal fractional flow reserve: a hemodynamic evaluation of moderate renal artery stenoses. *Catheter Cardiovasc Interv*. 2005;64(4):480-486.
23. van der Voort PH, van Hagen E, Hendrix G, van Gelder B, Bech JW, Pijls NH. Comparison of intravenous adenosine to intracoronary papaverine for calculation of pressure-derived fractional flow reserve. *Cathet Cardiovasc Diagn*. 1996;39(2):120-125.
24. Ong P, Athanasiadis A, Borgulya G, Mahrholdt H, Kaski JC, Sechtem U. High prevalence of a pathological response to acetylcholine testing in patients with stable angina pectoris and unobstructed coronary arteries: the ACOVA Study (Abnormal COronary VAsomotion in patients with stable angina and unobstructed coronary arteries). *J Am Coll Cardiol*. 2012;59(7):655-662.
25. Takahashi T, Samuels BA, Li W, et al. Safety of provocative testing with intracoronary acetylcholine and implications for standard protocols. *J Am Coll Cardiol*. 2022;79(24):2367-2378. doi:10.1016/j.jacc.2022.03.385
26. Sueda S, Kohno H, Fukuda H, et al. Clinical impact of selective spasm provocation tests: comparisons between acetylcholine and ergonovine in 1508 examinations. *Coron Artery Dis*. 2004;15(8):491-497.
27. Coma-Canella I, Castano S, Macías A, Calabuig J, Artaiz M. Ergonovine test in angina with normal coronary arteries. Is it worth doing it? *Int J Cardiol*. 2006;107(2):200-206.
28. Diamond LM. Cardiopulmonary resuscitation and acute cardiovascular life support—a protocol review of the updated guidelines. *Crit Care Clin*. 2007;23(4):873-880.
29. Field JM, Hazinski MF, Sayre MR, et al. Part 1: executive summary—2010 American Heart Association Guidelines for cardiopulmonary resuscitation and emergency cardiovascular care. *Circulation*. 2010;122(18 suppl 3):S640-S656.
30. Hazinski MF, Nolan JP, Billi JE, et al. Part 1: executive summary—2010 international consensus on cardiopulmonary resuscitation and emergency cardiovascular care science with treatment recommendations. *Circulation*. 2010;122(16 suppl 2):S250-S275.
31. Leone M, Martin C. Vasopressor use in septic shock: an update. *Curr Opin Anaesthesiol*. 2008;21(2):141-147.
32. Kowey PR. Pharmacological effects of antiarrhythmic drugs. Review and update. *Arch Intern Med*. 1998;158(4):325-332.
33. Kowey PR, Marinchak RA, Rials SJ, Bharucha DB. Classification and pharmacology of antiarrhythmic drugs. *Am Heart J*. 2000;140(1):12-20.

Secondary Prevention: Lipid Management, SGLT2 Inhibition

Raghava S. Velagaleti

Atherosclerotic cardiovascular disease (ASCVD) continues to be a major cause of morbidity and mortality in the United States. Patients with established ASCVD constitute a particular high-risk subset for recurrent cardiovascular (CV) events and CV death, therefore warranting secondary prevention strategies.[1] A plethora of approaches to address secondary prevention are available to cardiologists; this chapter will focus on lipid modulation and sodium-glucose cotransporter 2 inhibition. The chapter will emphasize the rich body of randomized clinical trials (RCTs) that have evaluated both these approaches and form the base for clinical practice guidelines. These RCTs have used composite outcomes defined variously; in this chapter, where the phrase "CV event(s)" is used, it refers to one or a combination of the following outcomes of interest for patients and physicians: coronary heart disease (CHD) or CV death, nonfatal myocardial infarction (MI), hospitalization for unstable angina, hospitalization or urgent treatment for heart failure (HF), coronary revascularization, and nonfatal ischemic stroke or transient ischemic attack that is not of embolic origin (the specific composite outcome for each RCT is provided in the tables). The narrower term "major adverse cardiovascular events" (MACE) refers to the combination of CV death, nonfatal MI, and nonfatal stroke.

THERAPEUTIC LIFESTYLE CHANGES AND CARDIAC REHABILITATION

A comprehensive approach to lifestyle management is indicated for all ASCVD patients and extensively emphasized in clinical practice guidelines. The individual components of lifestyle management include (a) heart-healthy diet, (b) at least moderate-intensity exercise, (c) weight loss where indicated, and (d) smoking cessation where relevant. Lifestyle changes can help with simultaneous management of multiple CV risk factors and thus form the base of both primary and secondary prevention efforts. Enrollment in a cardiac rehabilitation program is indicated for all patients with ASCVD. Apart from the physiological benefits of cardiac rehabilitation, enrollment in these programs can help facilitate successfully adopting (and sustaining) lifestyle changes with better efficacy than clinic-based advice alone.

SECONDARY PREVENTION OF ASCVD VIA LIPID MANAGEMENT

Reduction in low-density lipoprotein cholesterol (LDL-C) levels is the cornerstone of secondary prevention strategies in ASCVD patients. All patients irrespective of baseline LDL-C should receive high-intensity statin therapy (see below) with atorvastatin or rosuvastatin as tolerated. Some patients may need initiation at lower doses and progressive titration to a high-intensity or maximally tolerated dosage. Lipid profiles can be remeasured 6 to 8 weeks after these drugs have been titrated to maximum (or maximally tolerated) doses, and the need for adding additional agents is determined by residual LDL-C levels and the patient risk profile.

Statins

Inhibitors of 3-hydroxy 3-methyl glutaryl coenzyme A (HMG-CoA inhibitors, commonly referred to as statins) are the mainstay of lipid-modulation therapy in patients with ASCVD. They have an excellent efficacy[2] and safety[3] profile and are largely well tolerated. Of the several congeners in this class, two agents (atorvastatin and rosuvastatin) can achieve LDL-C reduction >50% at maximal doses. Therefore, atorvastatin at 40 to 80 mg/d and rosuvastatin at 20 to 40 mg/d are considered "high-intensity" statin therapy. These statins at lower doses, or all other statins at various doses, are considered low- to moderate-intensity statin therapy. Statins other than atorvastatin and rosuvastatin achieve lesser degrees of LDL-C reduction and are typically used when the aforementioned two drugs are not tolerated, with the caveat that additional non-statin drugs are typically necessary to achieve secondary prevention LDL-C targets.

Multiple RCTs demonstrated the efficacy of statins in terms of both LDL-C reduction and decreases in major adverse CV events. Key RCTs forming the basis for high-intensity statin therapy for secondary prevention are presented in **Table 6.1**.[4-10] These clinical trials enrolled patients with varying degrees of baseline risk for recurrent events and presentation with both chronic and acute coronary syndromes (ACS). When compared with placebo, treatment with many statins is associated with a significant reduction in CV events (**Table 6.1A**). In addition, high-intensity statin therapy leads to further reductions in CV events compared with low- to moderate-intensity statin therapy (**Table 6.1B**). While the impact of statin therapy on CHD/CV death has been inconsistently noted in individual RCTs, metanalyses of statin trials have clearly shown that aggressive LDL-C-lowering reduces mortality, with similar effects in men and women.[2,11,12] Cumulatively, these data form the basis for the strong recommendation in the guidelines from cardiology societies that patients with established ASCVD be initiated and maintained on high-intensity statin, unless not tolerated.[13,14] The goal for all ASCVD patients is to achieve at least a 50% lowering of LDL-C and to a level less than 70 mg/dL.

Use of Non-Statin Drugs for LDL-C Lowering

There are three key settings for the use of non-statin LDL-C-lowering drugs, instead of or in addition to statins, for lipid modulation in ASCVD patients:

1. Patients on high-intensity statin therapy, or maximally tolerated doses of statins, who have not achieved LDL-C <70 mg/dL.
2. Patients who are intolerant of statins.
3. Patients who have achieved LDL-C of 70 mg/dL on maximally tolerated statin doses but are candidates for additional LDL-C lowering owing to having a "very high risk" of recurring CV events.

TABLE 6.1 Important RCTs Demonstrating the Efficacy of Statins for Secondary Prevention

	STUDY POPULATION[a]	TREATMENT ARMS AND RANDOMIZED NUMBERS[b]	PRIMARY ENDPOINT AND MAIN RESULTS[c]	OTHER KEY ASPECTS[d]
A. Comparisons of Statin Therapy to Placebo				
SSSS[4]	Age 35-70 y h/o angina pectoris or MI No revascularization planned	Simvastatin 20-40 mg – 2221 (82% men) Placebo – 2223 (81% men)	All-cause mortality 8.2% vs 11.5%; RR 0.70 (0.58-0.85), *P* = .0003	Coronary death RR 0.58 (0.46-0.73) Key secondary endpoint of cardiac death, MI, resuscitated cardiac arrest RR 0.66 (0.59-0.75), *P* < 00001
CARE[5]	Age 21 – 75 y Men and post-menopausal women TC < 240 mg/dL MI within prior 3-20 mo EF > 25% and no HF	Pravastatin 40 mg - 2081 (86% men) Placebo - 2078 (86% men)	CHD death, MI 10.2% vs 13.2%; RRR 24% (9-36), *P* = .003	Also decreases in MI, stroke, and revascularization rates of ~25%
LIPID[6]	Age 31-75 MI or UA hospitalization in preceding 3-36 mo TC 155-271 mg/dL	Pravastatin 40 mg - 4512 (83% men) Placebo - 4502 (83% men)	CHD death 6.4% vs 8.3%; RRR 24% (12-35), *P* < .001	Similar magnitude reductions in all-cause and CV death and MI
MIRACL[7]	Age > 18 y NSTEACS admission with no planned revascularization TC < 240 mg/dL	Atorvastatin 80 mg – 1538 (65% men) Placebo – 1548 (66% men)	Death, MI, resuscitated cardiac arrest, hospitalization for ischemia. 14.8% vs 17.4%; HR 0.84 (0.70-1.0), *P* = .48	Short duration of follow-up (16 wk) Reduction in ischemia hospitalization ~26% Marked reduction in stroke ~50%
B. Comparisons of High-Intensity Statin Therapy to Low-Moderate Intensity Statin Therapy.				
PROVE IT-TIMI 22[8]	Age >18 y Recent (<10 d) ACS hospitalization TC < 240 mg/dL	Atorvastatin 80 mg – 2099 (78% men) Pravastatin 40 mg – 2063 (78% men)	All-cause death, MI, stroke, UA hospitalization, revascularization. 22.4% vs 26.3%; RRR 16% (5-26), *P* = .005	Reduction in UA hospitalization ~29% and revascularization ~14%
TNT[9]	Age 35 – 75 y h/o CHD	Atorvastatin 80 mg – 4995 (81% men) Atorvastatin 10 mg – 5006 (81% men)	CHD death, MI, stroke, resuscitated cardiac arrest. 8.7% vs 10.9%; HR 0.78 (0.69-0.89), *P* < .001	Any or major coronary events, stroke, and HF hospitalization also reduced ~20%
IDEAL[10]	Age <80 y h/o MI	Atorvastatin 80 mg – 4439 (% men) Simvastatin 20 mg – 4449 (78% men)	CHD death, MI, resuscitated cardiac arrest. 9.3% vs 10.4%; HR 0.89 (0.78-1.01), *P* = .07	16% reduction in any CHD events (primary endpoint + UA hospitalization + revascularization) 17% RRR in MI

ACS, acute coronary syndrome; CARE, Cholesterol and Recurrent Events; CHD, coronary heart disease; EF, ejection fraction; HF, heart failure; HR, hazards ratio; IDEAL, Incremental Decrease in End Points Through Aggressive Lipid Lowering; LIPID, Long-Term Intervention with Pravastatin in Ischemic Disease; MI, myocardial infarction; MIRACL, Myocardial Ischemia Reduction with Aggressive Cholesterol Lowering; NSTEACS, non-ST segment elevation acute coronary syndrome; PROVE IT-TIMI 22, Pravastatin or Atorvastatin Evaluation and Infection Therapy–Thrombolysis in Myocardial Infarction 22; RR, relative risk; RRR, relative risk reduction; SSSS, Scandinavian Simvastatin Survival Study; TC, total cholesterol; TNT, Treating to New Targets; UA, unstable angina.

[a]Patients included in the clinical trial.

[b]The intervention and control arms and the respective number (% men) randomized to each group.

[c]Primary endpoint and the results of the clinical trial with respect to this endpoint; event proportions are listed for interventional arm versus control arm in that order.

[d]Other aspects of the clinical trial of interest include important caveats, key secondary results, and so on.

In the aforementioned three scenarios, the addition or substitution of other lipid-lowering agents is indicated. While a variety of drugs and drug classes are available to reduce LDL-C, compelling data indicating consequent CV event reduction are limited to those discussed below.

Patients are considered to be at "very high risk" if (a) they have already experienced multiple major ASCVD events or (b) had one major ASCVD event and also have multiple "high-risk conditions." In this context, the following constitute a "major ASCVD event": a recent (within prior 12 months) ACS, history of MI(s) other than the recent ACS, history of ischemic stroke, presence of symptomatic peripheral artery disease, or revascularization(s) for peripheral artery disease or limb amputation(s). "High-risk conditions" include age >65 years, the presence of diabetes mellitus (DM), hypertension, current smoking or heterozygous familial hypercholesterolemia, a history of prior coronary artery bypass surgery or percutaneous coronary intervention performed in a context other than a major ASCVD event(s), history of HF, presence of chronic kidney disease with an estimated glomerular filtration rate of <60 mL/min/1.73 m^2, or persistently elevated LDL-C (LDL-C > 100 mg/dL despite maximally tolerated statin therapy and ezetimibe).

Non-Statin Drugs That Achieve Moderate Reductions in LDL-C

Two drugs achieve moderate reductions in LDL-C and have been studied in CV outcome RCTs: ezetimibe and bempedoic acid (**Table 6.2** lists the relevant RCTs). Ezetimibe reduces the intestinal absorption of cholesterol by targeting the Niemann–Pick C1–like 1 protein in the gut. It can be expected to reduce LDL-C an additional 20% when added to statin therapy. In the IMPROVE-IT trial (**Table 6.2A**),[15] ezetimibe, when added to maximally tolerated statin doses, additionally reduced CV events compared to

TABLE 6.2 Key RCTs of Non-Statin LDL-C-Lowering Drugs

	STUDY POPULATION[a]	TREATMENT ARMS AND RANDOMIZED NUMBERS[b]	PRIMARY ENDPOINT AND MAIN RESULTS[c]	OTHER KEY ASPECTS[d]
A. Moderate LDL-C-reducing agents.				
IMPROVE-IT[15]	Age >50 y Recent (<10 d) ACS hospitalization LDL >50 and <100 mg/dL Patients planned for CABG excluded	Simvastatin 40 mg + Ezetimibe 10 mg – 9067 (76% men) Simvastatin 40 mg – 9077 (76% men)	CV death, MI, stroke, UA hospitalization, revascularization. 32.7% vs 34.7%; HR 0.94 (0.89-0.99), *P* = .016	Achieved LDL-C 53.7 vs69.5 mg/dL. Reductions in MI and stroke ~13%
CLEAR Outcomes[16]	Age 18 – 85 y Statin intolerant 70% were secondary prevention population	Bempedoic acid 180 mg – 6992 (52% men) Placebo – 6978 (52% men)	CV death, MI, stroke, revascularization. 11.7% vs13.3%; HR 0.87 (0.79-0.96), *P* = .004	Also decrease in MI, revascularization. 23% of patients were taking low dose statin; 12% taking ezetimibe.
B. Strong LDL-C-reducing agents				
FOURIER[17]	Age 40 – 85 y Established ASCVD LDL-C ≥ 70 mg/dL	Evolocumab 140 mg q2weeks or 420 mg/month – 13784 (75% men) Placebo – 13780 (76% men)	CV death, MI, stroke, UA hospitalization, revascularization. 9.8% vs11.3%; HR 0.85 (0.79-0.92), *P* < .001	Also decrease in MACE and revascularization 70% were on baseline high intensity statin; 30% on moderate intensity statin
ODYSSEY Outcomes[18]	Age ≥40 y ACS within previous 1 – 12 mo LDL-C ≥ 70 mg/dL	Alirocumab 75 mg q2weeks – 9462 (75% men) Placebo – 9462 (75% men)	CHD death, MI, stroke, UA hospitalization. 9.5% vs11.1%; HR 0.85 (0.78-0.93), *P* < .001	Blinded dose adjustments allowed to keep LDL-C within 25-50 mg/dL. Also decrease in MACE and any CHD. 88.8% were on baseline high intensity statin

CHD, coronary heart disease; CLEAR, Cholesterol Lowering via Bempedoic Acid, an ACL-Inhibiting Regimen; CV, cardiovascular; FOURIER, Further Cardiovascular Outcomes Research with PCSK9 Inhibition in Subjects with Elevated Risk; HR, hazards ratio; IMPROVE-IT, Improved Reduction of Outcomes: Vytorin Efficacy International Trial; MACE, major adverse cardiovascular events, a combination of CV death, nonfatal myocardial infarction, and nonfatal stroke; MI, myocardial infarction; ODYSSEY, Occurrence of Cardiovascular Events in Patients Who Have Recently Experienced an Acute Coronary Syndrome; UA, unstable angina.

[a]Patients included in the clinical trial.

[b]The intervention and control arms and the respective number (% men) randomized to each group.

[c]Primary endpoint and the results of the clinical with respect to this endpoint; event proportions are listed for interventional arm versus control arm in that order.

[d]Other aspects of the clinical trial of interest include important caveats, key secondary results, and so on.

placebo. In addition, in patients who have difficulty tolerating high-intensity statin therapy, but are able to tolerate low-moderate intensity statin therapy, the addition of ezetimibe to low-dose statin achieves similar LDL-C reduction and clinical outcomes when compared to rosuvastatin alone at the 20-mg/d dose.[19] This regimen offers an alternative option for patients who have difficulty tolerating high-intensity statins.

Bempedoic acid is an inhibitor of adenosine triphosphate citrate lyase, an enzyme that acts upstream of HMG-CoA in the cholesterol biosynthesis pathway. It can be expected to achieve an additional 16% reduction in LDL-C levels when added to statins or up to 28% reduction when used without background statin therapy. In the recently reported CLEAR Outcomes trial (**Table 6.2A**) comprising statin-intolerant patients, bempedoic acid significantly reduced LDL-C levels and CV events compared with placebo.[16] In a prior RCT which evaluated the impact of this drug in patients on maximally tolerated statin therapy, bempedoic acid further reduced LDL-C levels by ~16%[20]; whether addition of bempedoic acid to high-dose statins also reduces CV events has yet to be demonstrated. While the aforementioned two drugs individually reduce LDL-C modestly, a combination formulation is now available and can reduce LDL-C ~ 40%[21] and can serve as an alternative in statin-intolerant patients.

Non-Statin Drugs That Achieve Large Reductions in LDL-C

Proprotein convertase subtilisin/kexin type 9 inhibitors (PCSK9i) are monoclonal antibodies that inhibit the PCSK9 enzyme. They lead to an increase in LDL receptor levels, which leads to increased scavenging of LDL-C and reduction in their circulating levels. Two agents, evolocumab and alirocumab, have been shown to reduce LDL-C markedly (>50% reduction)[21] and also reduce incident CV events in patients with established ASCVD[17,18] and are approved for secondary prevention. They are administered subcutaneously and have an excellent safety profile with injection-site reactions being the common side effect.[22] In a large RCT of patients with chronic CHD (**Table 6.2.B**), evolocumab reduced the combined endpoint of CV death, MI, stroke, unstable angina, or the need for revascularization by 15%.[17] The recently published extension study of the same trial also showed reductions individually in CHD death, MI and revascularization, and the event reduction sustained over 8 years of follow-up.[23] Similarly, in patients with a recent acute coronary event (Table 6.2B), alirocumab induced large reductions in LDL-C levels and reduced CV events (15%), including MACE (14%).[18]

Inclisiran is a small interfering ribonucleic acid that inhibits the synthesis of the PCSK9 enzyme in the liver, and thus works upstream of PCSK9i. Of note, it has not been studied in combination with them and should be considered only when a PCSK9i cannot be used. Its advantage is that it can be administered once every 6 months during maintenance therapy. It can induce LDL-C reduction of ~50% when added to maximally tolerated statin therapy.[24] It is approved for use in both familial hypercholesterolemia and secondary prevention settings. Evinacumab is a monoclonal antibody that inhibits angiopoietin-like 3 (ANGPTL3), a protein that inhibits lipoprotein lipase and endothelial lipase, thereby elevating cholesterol levels. It achieves LDL-C reduction of about ~50% at the maximum tested subcutaneous dose, when added to a multidrug lipid-lowering regimen that includes a PCSK9i.[25] It is currently approved as an adjunctive agent for treating patients with familial hypercholesterolemia. Outcome data are awaited for both these novel agents, and their role in the broader population of ASCVD patients with hyperlipidemia needs clarification. Patients who may need these agents should be considered for referral to a lipid specialist.

MODULATION OF LIPID SUBFRACTIONS OTHER THAN LDL-C

Therapy to Reduce Triglycerides

Results from older clinical trials evaluating fibrates and marine omega-3 carboxylic acids (n-3 CA) for triglyceride lowering have shown inconsistent results with respect to CV event reduction, but a metanalysis of these trials (along with niacin RCTs) indicated a benefit from triglyceride lowering.[26] That finding supported optimism in favor of a triglyceride-lowering approach for secondary prevention. However, a large recent trial of pemafibrate (**Table 6.3**) showed that the drug reduces triglyceride levels markedly but has no impact on CV outcomes.[29] Formulations of n-3 CA in various doses have been tested in RCTs, again with inconsistent results on CV event reduction. Most recently, the STRENGTH trial (**Table 6.3**) tested a high-dose formulation (4 gm/d) of n-3 CA; while there was a reduction in triglyceride levels, there was no impact on CV outcomes.[27] However, one highly purified form of eicosapentaenoic acid (icosapent ethyl [IPE]) has been shown to reduce CV events in the REDUCE-IT (Reduction of Cardiovascular Events with Icosapent Ethyl–Intervention; **Table 6.3**) trial.[28] There have been concerns expressed about the adverse biomarker profiles of the patients in the mineral oil placebo group in the trial and how that may drive the outcomes differences, whereas others have argued that the impact of mineral oil on outcomes would be modest and does not explain the trial results.[30,31] The magnitude of IPE-induced triglyceride lowering does not explain the outcome benefits, and putative alternate explanations for the benefit of IPE noted in the trial include pleiotropic effects of high-dose purified eicosapentaenoic acid.[32] Of concern, both STRENGTH and REDUCE-IT trials reported a prominent increase in atrial fibrillation incidence with the tested drug formulations. Thus, triglyceride reduction or n-3 CA supplementation as a strategy for secondary prevention continuous to be a subject of intense debate. The 2021 American College of Cardiology Expert Consensus Pathway[33] regarding triglyceride management offers a nuanced discussion of the issues involved and qualified support for the use of IPE in limited settings; practicing clinicians should consider these factors when identifying patients for IPE therapy.

Therapy to Increase High-Density Lipoprotein Cholesterol

Higher levels of high-density lipoprotein cholesterol (HDL-C) have been associated with lower incidence of CV events in observational studies. This finding drove interest in identifying therapies that increase HDL-C. Older data (prior to adoption of statins) indicated that niacin increases HDL-C and is associated with improved outcomes. However, two large RCTs, one testing extended-release

TABLE 6.3 Major RCTs Evaluating Triglyceride Modulation for CV Event Reduction

	STUDY POPULATION[a]	TREATMENT ARMS AND RANDOMIZED NUMBERS[b]	PRIMARY ENDPOINT AND MAIN RESULTS[c]	OTHER KEY ASPECTS[d]
STRENGTH[27]	Age ≥18 y LDL-C < 100 mg/dL TG = 180-500 mg/dL High risk for ASCVD events (56% of patients were secondary prevention population)	Omega-3 CA 4 gm – 6539 (65% men) Corn oil placebo – 6539 (65% men)	CV death, MI, stroke, UA hospitalization, revascularization. 12% vs 12.2%; HR 0.99 (0.90-1.09), *P* = .84	No reduction in any component or secondary endpoints Significant increase in AF with Omega-3 FA
REDUCE-IT[28]	Age ≥45 y and h/o ASCVD OR Age >50 y with diabetes and 2 other risk factors TG = 150 – 499 LDL-C = 41 - 100	Icosapent ethyl 4 gm – 4089 (72% men) Mineral oil placebo – 4090 (71% men)	CV death, MI, stroke, UA hospitalization, revascularization. 17.2% vs 22%; HR 0.75 (0.68-0.83), *P* = .001	71% were secondary prevention cohort; results same in them. 62% of patients were on moderate-intensity statin; 32% on high-intensity statin
PROMINENT[29]	Age ≥50 (men) or ≥55 y (women) without ASCVD OR Age ≥18 with ASCVD Diagnosis of type 2 DM TG – 200 – 499 mg/dL HDL-C ≤ 40 mg/dL	Pemafibrate 0.2 mg bid – 5240 (72% men) Placebo – 5257 (72% men)	CV death, MI, stroke, coronary revascularization 10.9% vs 10.7%; HR 1.03 (0.91-1.15), *P* = .67	69% were on high-intensity statin; 98% were on any statin. TG and VLDL reduced ~26% No effect on any clinical endpoint

CHD, coronary heart disease; CV, cardiovascular; EF, ejection fraction; HF, heart failure; HR, hazards ratio; MI, myocardial infarction; PROMINENT, Pemafibrate to Reduce Cardiovascular Outcomes by Reducing Triglycerides in Patients with Diabetes; REDUCE-IT, Reduction of Cardiovascular Events with Icosapent Ethyl–Intervention; STRENGTH, Long-Term Outcomes Study to Assess Statin Residual Risk with Epanova in High Cardiovascular Risk Patients with Hypertriglyceridemia; TG, triglycerides; UA, unstable angina.
[a]Patients included in the clinical trial.
[b]The intervention and control arms and the respective number (% men) randomized to each group.
[c]Primary endpoint and the results of the clinical with respect to this endpoint; events proportions are listed for interventional arm versus control arm in that order.
[d]Other aspects of the clinical trial of interest include important caveats, key secondary results, and so on.

niacin (**Table 6.4**; AIM-HIGH[34]) and another evaluating the combination of niacin and laropiprant (a drug that reduces niacin-related side effects; **Table 6.4**; HPS2-THRIVE[35]) failed to show any benefit from niacin therapy. Inhibitors of cholesteryl ester transfer protein (CETPi) markedly elevate HDL-C, and four congeners of this class were studied in large RCTs (**Table 6.4**). Torcetrapib was associated with harm,[36] and evacetrapib and dalcetrapib had a neutral effect on clinical outcomes.[38,39] Anacetrapib reduced CV events compared with placebo in the REVEAL[37] trial (**Table 6.4**), but the finding is likely explained by the modest LDL-C reduction associated with anacetrapib treatment, not the marked HDL-C elevation. At present, there is no role for targeting HDL-C for secondary prevention.

Key Points

- LDL-C lowering is the mainstay of lipid-modulating approaches to secondary prevention.
- All patients with ASCVD should receive high-intensity statin therapy. (In patients older than 75 years or those with untreated LDL-C < 50 mg/dL, starting with a moderate-intensity regimen may be considered.)
- Additional agents with proven efficacy for reducing CV events should be added to statin therapy as necessary to achieve LDL-C < 70 mg/dL.
- In select very-high-risk patients, targeting an LDL-C level less than 55 mg/dL is appropriate.
- Apart from statins, compelling outcome data demonstrating CV event reduction are available for ezetimibe, bempedoic acid, and the PCSK9i (evolocumab and alirocumab).
- Patients with hyperlipidemia refractory to agents with proven efficacy in reducing CV events should be considered for referral to a specialized lipid clinic or a lipidologist.

SGLT2 INHIBITION FOR SECONDARY PREVENTION

Observational studies have demonstrated that type 2 DM is a strong risk factor for incident ASCVD and for recurrent events after the onset of ASCVD. However, a clear benefit to normalizing blood glucose in terms of reducing CV events has been more difficult to

TABLE 6.4 Studies of Agents That Elevate HDL-C for CV Event Lowering in Patients With ASCVD

	STUDY POPULATION[a]	TREATMENT ARMS AND RANDOMIZED NUMBERS[b]	PRIMARY ENDPOINT AND MAIN RESULTS[c]	OTHER KEY ASPECTS[d]
AIM-HIGH[34]	Age ≥45 h/o ASCVD HDL < 40 mg/dL (men) HDL < 50 mg/dL (women) TG = 150 – 400 ng/dL LDL < 180 mg/dL	Niacin extended release 1500-2000 mg – 1718 (women 15%) Placebo – 1696 (women 15%)	CHD death, MI, stroke, ACS hospitalization, coronary or cerebral revascularization 16.4% vs 16.2%; HR 1.02 (0.87-1.21), *P* = .80	Results similar for components of primary endpoint and for secondary endpoints
HPS2-THRIVE[35]	Age 50-80 y h/o ASCVD Those receiving simvastatin 40 mg + ezetimibe 10 mg or equivalent were excluded	Niacin 2 g - Laropiprant 40 mg – 17,838 (women 17%) Placebo 12,835 (women 17%)	CHD death, MI, stroke, or any revascularization 13.2% vs 13.7%; RR 0.96 (0.90-1.03), *P* = .29	No improvement in any of the secondary end points
ILLUMINATE[36]	Age 45-75 and ASCVD or DM All received atorvastatin titrated to LDL <100 mg/dL	Torcetrapib 60 mg - 7533 (men 78%) Placebo - 7534 (men 78%)	CHD death, MI, stroke, UA hospitalization 6.2% vs 5.0%; HR 1.25 (1.09-1.44), *P* = .001	Increase in primary endpoint and all-cause mortality with torcetrapib
REVEAL[37]	Age >50 y with ASCVD Background atorvastatin titrated to achieve LDL-C < 77 mg/dL	Anacetrapib 100 mg – 15,225 (16% women) Placebo – 15,224 (women 16%)	Coronary death, MI, coronary revascularization 10.8% vs 11.8%; RR 0.91 (0.85-0.97), *P* = .004)	HDL-C increased by 43%; LDL-C reduced by 26% Reduced LDL-C likely explains results rather than HDL-C elevation

ACS, acute coronary syndrome; AIM-HIGH, Atherothrombosis Intervention in Metabolic Syndrome with Low HDL/High Triglycerides: Impact on Global Health Outcomes; CHD, coronary heart disease; EF, ejection fraction; HF, heart failure; HPS2-THRIVE, Heart Protection Study 2–Treatment of HDL to Reduce the Incidence of Vascular Events; HR, hazards ratio; ILLUMINATE, Investigation of Lipid Level Management to Understand its Impact in Atherosclerotic Events; MI, myocardial infarction; REVEAL, Randomized Evaluation of the Effects of Anacetrapib through Lipid Modification; RR, relative risk/rate ratio; TG, triglycerides; UA, unstable angina.
[a]Patients included in the clinical trial.
[b]The intervention and control arms and the respective number (% men) randomized to each group.
[c]Primary endpoint and the results of the clinical with respect to this endpoint; event proportions are listed for interventional arm versus control arm in that order.
[d]Other aspects of the clinical trial of interest include important caveats, key secondary results, and so on.

demonstrate, with earlier clinical trials showing either no improvement in macrovascular complications[40] or even potential harm with intensive glucose lowering.[41]

The recent development of sodium-glucose cotransporter 2 inhibitors (SGLT2i) and glucagon-like peptide 1 receptor agonists (GLP1ra) has thus revolutionized the management of DM patients because they have been shown to reduce CV events in patients with DM. In addition, the publication in short order of several RCTs that show the benefit of SGLT2i in patients with HF further increases the salience of these agents to cardiologists. This section will focus on the SGLT2i ("gliflozins"). The SGLT2 protein is located in the proximal convoluted tubule of the nephrons in the kidney and is responsible for reabsorption of glucose from the glomerular ultrafiltrate. By inhibiting this process, the SGLT2i induce glycosuria and osmotic diuresis and a reduction in blood glucose levels, intravascular volume, and a small reduction in blood pressure. Initially developed only for glycemic control in patients with DM, these agents have proven to be efficacious in achieving two important outcomes from a CV perspective: (1) In patients with DM with established ASCVD, these agents reduce MACE and (2) in patients with HF of any type with or without DM, they have been shown to consistently reduce the combined endpoint of CV death and HF hospitalization. Details of individual RCTs evaluating SGLT2i in these two settings are presented in **Tables 6.5** and **6.6**.

Several SGLT2i have been studied in dedicated CV outcome trials to evaluate their impact on CV events (**Table 6.5**), when used for glucose lowering in patients with DM.[42-44] The trials evaluating these drugs varied in the composition of the study population in terms of proportion with underlying ASVCD, duration of follow-up, other specific inclusion and exclusion criteria, and so on. The results of the studies therefore varied in terms of magnitude and type of CV event reduction. However, metanalyses of the SGLT2i demonstrate a reduction in all-cause mortality, CV mortality, and MACE, in patients with DM and established ASCVD.[49,50] In addition, although not all of the initial CV outcome RCTs were designed to evaluate SGLT2i impact on HF outcomes, an improvement was noted consistently. In terms of safety concerns, all agents in this class are associated with a small increase in urogenital infections and rarely diabetic ketoacidosis; canagliflozin is also associated with an increased risk of fractures

TABLE 6.5 Key SGLT2i Trials for Secondary Prevention in Patients With Type 2 Diabetes Mellitus

	STUDY POPULATION[a]	TREATMENT ARMS AND RANDOMIZED NUMBERS[b]	PRIMARY ENDPOINT AND MAIN RESULTS[c]	OTHER KEY ASPECTS[d]
EMPA-REG OUTCOME[42]	Age >18 y and DM and ASCVD	Empagliflozin 10 mg/25 mg - 4687 (71% men) Placebo - 2333 (72% men)	MACE 10.5% vs 12.1%; HR 0.86 (0.74-0.99), *P* = .04	All cause and CV mortality also reduced
CANVAS[43]	DM and age >30 with ASCVD OR DM and age >50 plus 2 or more other CV risk factors	Canagliflozin 100 mg/300 mg - 5795 (65% men) Placebo - 4347 (63% men)	MACE 26.9% vs 31.5%; HR 0.86 (0.75-0.97), *P* = .02	~70% with ASCVD Increased risk for fractures and amputations in canagliflozin arms
DECLARE-TIMI 58[44]	DM, age >40 y, and ASCVD OR multiple CV risk factors	Dapagliflozin 10 mg - 8582 (37% women) Placebo 8578 (38% women)	Co-primary endpoints of MACE: 8.8% vs 9.4%; HR 0.93 (0.84–1.03), *P* = .17 CV death + HF hospital-ization: 4.9% vs 5.8%; HR 0.83 (0.73–0.95), *P* = .005	Established CVD in 40% Separate sub-analysis showed MACE reduction in those with prior MI

CANVAS, Canagliflozin Cardiovascular Assessment Study; CV, cardiovascular; DECLARE-TIMI 58, Dapagliflozin Effect on Cardiovascular Events–Thrombolysis in Myocardial Infarction 58; DM, type 2 diabetes mellitus; EMPA-REG, Empagliflozin Cardiovascular Outcome Event Trial in Type 2 Diabetes Mellitus Patients–Removing Excess Glucose; HR, hazards ratio; HF, heart failure; MACE, major adverse cardiovascular events, a combination of CV death, nonfatal myocardial infarction, and non-fatal stroke; MI, myocardial infarction.

[a]Patients included in the clinical trial.

[b]The intervention and control arms and the respective number (% men) randomized to each group.

[c]Primary endpoint and the results of the clinical with respect to this endpoint; event proportions are listed for interventional arm versus control arm in that order.

[d]Other aspects of the clinical trial of interest include important caveats, key secondary results, and so on.

TABLE 6.6 SGLT2i for the Management of HF Patients

	STUDY POPULATION[a]	TREATMENT ARMS AND RANDOMIZED NUMBERS[b]	PRIMARY ENDPOINT AND MAIN RESULTS[c]	OTHER KEY ASPECTS[d]
DAPA-HF[45]	Age ≥18 y Class II, III, IV symptoms EF ≤ 40% NT-proBNP ≥ 600 pg/mL	Dapagliflozin 10 mg – 2373 (76% men) Placebo – 2371 (77% men)	CV death or worsening HF 16.3% vs 21.2%; HR 0.74 (0.65-0.85), *P* < .001	Individual components of the composite endpoint also reduced
EMPEROR-Reduced[46]	Age ≥18 y Class II, III, IV symptoms EF ≤ 40% EF specific NT-proBNP thresholds	Empagliflozin 10 mg – 1863 (76% men) Placebo – 1867 (76% men)	CV death or HF hospitalization 19.4% vs 24.7%; HR 0.75 (0.65-0.86), *P* < .001	Also reductions in total HF hospitalization and renal function decline
EMPEROR-Preserved[47]	Age ≥18 y Class II, III, IV symptoms EF > 40% NT-proBNP >300 pg/mL	Empagliflozin 10 mg – 2997 (45% women) Placebo – 2991 (45% women)	CV death or HF hospitalization 13.8% vs 17.1%; HR 0.79 (0.69-0.90), *P* < .001	Also reductions in total HF hospitalization and renal function decline
DELIVER[48]	Age ≥40 y Stable HF EF > 40% Evidence of structural heart disease Elevated natriuretic peptide levels	Dapagliflozin 10 mg – 3131 (44% women) Placebo – 3132 (44% women)	CV death or worsening HF 16.4% vs 19.5%; HR 0.82 (0.73-0.92), *P* < .001	Reductions in HF hospital-izations and HF symptom burden

CV, cardiovascular; DAPA-HF, Dapagliflozin and Prevention of Adverse Outcomes in Heart Failure; DELIVER, Dapagliflozin Evaluation to Improve the Lives of Patients with Preserved Ejection Fraction Heart Failure; EF, ejection fraction; EMPEROR-Preserved, Empagliflozin Outcome Trial in Patients with Chronic Heart Failure with Preserved Ejection Fraction; EMPEROR-Reduced, Empagliflozin Outcome Trial in Patients with Chronic Heart Failure and a Reduced Ejection Fraction; HR, hazards ratio; HF, heart failure; NT-proBNP, n terminal pro b-type natriuretic peptide.

[a]Patients included in the clinical trial.

[b]The intervention and control arms and the respective number (% men) randomized to each group.

[c]Primary endpoint and the results of the clinical with respect to this endpoint; event proportions are listed for interventional arm versus control arm in that order.

[d]Other aspects of the clinical trial of interest include important caveats, key secondary results, and so on.

and limb amputations. If hypoglycemia is a concern when starting these drugs in patients already receiving insulin or insulin secretagogues, the doses of the other drugs can be reduced to facilitate the introduction of SGLT2i.

The reduction in HF outcomes noted in the initial CV outcome trials spurred the conduct of dedicated RCTs (**Table 6.6**) to evaluate the benefit of these patients in HF with reduced EF,[45,46] HF with preserved EF populations,[47,48] and in patients with acute recent worsening of HF irrespective of underlying EF.[51] All these trials consistently showed a lowering of the combined endpoint of CV death and hospitalization for HF. Cumulatively, these RCTs demonstrate the benefit of SGLT2 inhibition across the full spectrum of EF in HF patients, and the outcome reductions are evident irrespective of the background HF therapy.[52] In addition, the benefits were equally prominent in patients without DM.[53] While individual trial outcomes were driven mainly by HF hospitalizations, metanalyses of these studies have shown that SGLT2i also significantly reduce CV mortality.[54]

These data from the CV outcome trials in patients with DM and the dedicated HF trials form the basis for the strong recommendations from the American Heart Association, the American Diabetes Association, and the American Association of Clinical Endocrinology for use of these agents in the management of patients with diabetes and ASCVD and those with HF with or without diabetes.[55-57]

Key Points

- In patients with DM who have ASCVD, SGLT2i are recommended to reduce the risk of MACE. Background DM therapy can be adjusted as appropriate to facilitate the introduction of SGLT2i.
- In patients with HF, SGLT2i are indicated to reduce CV death and HF hospitalization:
  - regardless of the presence/absence of DM and
  - irrespective of type of HF (preserved vs reduced).
- For either indication, there are no dose titrations or biomarker targets to achieve; the drugs are used at fixed doses that have been proven efficacious in the relevant RCTs.
- For the purpose of MACE reduction in patients with DM and ASCVD, agents proven efficacious for this purpose in the pivotal CV outcome RCTs are recommended.
- For the purpose of HF management, the clinical trials to date suggest that the benefit is a class effect; any of the drugs in this class can be used, taking into consideration the cost, availability, and side effect profiles.

References

1. Tsao CW, Aday AW, Almarzooq ZI, et al. Heart disease and stroke statistics-2023 update: a report from the American Heart Association. *Circulation*. 2023;147(8):e93-e621.
2. Cholesterol Treatment Trialists' CTT Collaboration; Baigent C, Blackwell L, Emberson J, et al. Efficacy and safety of more intensive lowering of LDL cholesterol: a meta-analysis of data from 170,000 participants in 26 randomised trials. *Lancet*. 2010;376(9753):1670-1681.
3. Collins R, Reith C, Emberson J, et al. Interpretation of the evidence for the efficacy and safety of statin therapy. *Lancet*. 2016;388(10059):2532-2561.
4. Randomised trial of cholesterol lowering in 4444 patients with coronary heart disease: the Scandinavian Simvastatin Survival Study (4S). *Lancet*. 1994;344:1383-1389.
5. Sacks FM, Pfeffer MA, Moye LA, et al. The effect of pravastatin on coronary events after myocardial infarction in patients with average cholesterol levels. Cholesterol and Recurrent Events Trial investigators. *N Engl J Med*. 1996;335(14):1001-1009.
6. Long-Term Intervention with Pravastatin in Ischaemic Disease Study Group. Prevention of cardiovascular events and death with pravastatin in patients with coronary heart disease and a broad range of initial cholesterol levels. *N Engl J Med*. 1998;339:1349-1357.
7. Schwartz GG, Olsson AG, Ezekowitz MD, et al. Effects of atorvastatin on early recurrent ischemic events in acute coronary syndromes: the MIRACL study—a randomized controlled trial. *JAMA*. 2001;285(13):1711-1718.
8. Cannon CP, Braunwald E, McCabe CH, et al. Intensive versus moderate lipid lowering with statins after acute coronary syndromes. *N Engl J Med*. 2004;350(15):1495-1504.
9. LaRosa JC, Grundy SM, Waters DD, et al. Intensive lipid lowering with atorvastatin in patients with stable coronary disease. *N Engl J Med*. 2005;352(14):1425-1435.
10. Pedersen TR, Faergeman O, Kastelein JJ, et al. High-dose atorvastatin vs usual-dose simvastatin for secondary prevention after myocardial infarction—the IDEAL study: a randomized controlled trial. *JAMA*. 2005;294(19):2437-2445.
11. Cannon CP, Steinberg BA, Murphy SA, Mega JL, Braunwald E. Meta-analysis of cardiovascular outcomes trials comparing intensive versus moderate statin therapy. *J Am Coll Cardiol*. 2006;48(3):438-445.
12. Cholesterol Treatment Trialists Collaboration; Fulcher J, O'Connell R, Voysey M, et al. Efficacy and safety of LDL-lowering therapy among men and women: meta-analysis of individual data from 174,000 participants in 27 randomised trials. *Lancet*. 2015;385:1397-1405.
13. Grundy SM, Stone NJ, Bailey AL, et al. 2018 AHA/ACC/AACVPR/AAPA/ABC/ACPM/ADA/AGS/APhA/ASPC/NLA/PCNA guideline on the management of blood cholesterol: a report of the American College of Cardiology/American Heart Association task force on clinical practice guidelines. *J Am Coll Cardiol*. 2019;73(24):e285-e350.
14. Visseren FLJ, Mach F, Smulders YM, et al. 2021 ESC Guidelines on cardiovascular disease prevention in clinical practice. *Eur Heart J*. 2021;42(34):3227-3337.
15. Cannon CP, Blazing MA, Giugliano RP, et al. Ezetimibe added to statin therapy after acute coronary syndromes. *N Engl J Med*. 2015;372:2387-2397.
16. Nissen SE, Lincoff AM, Brennan D, et al. Bempedoic acid and cardiovascular outcomes in statin-intolerant patients. *N Engl J Med*. 2023;388(15):1353-1364.
17. Sabatine MS, Giugliano RP, Keech AC, et al. Evolocumab and clinical outcomes in patients with cardiovascular disease. *N Engl J Med*. 2017;376(18):1713-1722.
18. Schwartz GG, Steg PG, Szarek M, et al. Alirocumab and cardiovascular outcomes after acute coronary syndrome. *N Engl J Med*. 2018;379(22):2097-2107.

19. Kim BK, Hong SJ, Lee YJ, et al. Long-term efficacy and safety of moderate-intensity statin with ezetimibe combination therapy versus high-intensity statin monotherapy in patients with atherosclerotic cardiovascular disease (RACING): a randomised, open-label, non-inferiority trial. *Lancet*. 2022;400(10349):380-390.
20. Ray KK, Bays HE, Catapano AL, et al. Safety and efficacy of bempedoic acid to reduce LDL cholesterol. *N Engl J Med*. 2019;380(11):1022-1032.
21. Toth PP, Bray S, Villa G, et al. Network meta-analysis of randomized trials evaluating the comparative efficacy of lipid-lowering therapies added to maximally tolerated statins for the reduction of low-density lipoprotein cholesterol. *J Am Heart Assoc*. 2022;11(18):e025551.
22. Li J, Du H, Wang Y, et al. Safety of proprotein convertase subtilisin/kexin 9 inhibitors: a systematic review and meta-analysis. *Heart*. 2022;108(16):1296-1302.
23. O'Donoghue ML, Giugliano RP, Wiviott SD, et al. Long-term evolocumab in patients with established atherosclerotic cardiovascular disease. *Circulation*. 2022;146(15):1109-1119.
24. Ray KK, Wright RS, Kallend D, et al. Two phase 3 trials of inclisiran in patients with elevated LDL cholesterol. *N Engl J Med*. 2020;382(16):1507-1519.
25. Rosenson RS, Burgess LJ, Ebenbichler CF, et al. Evinacumab in patients with refractory hypercholesterolemia. *N Engl J Med*. 2020;383(24):2307-2319.
26. Marston NA, Giugliano RP, Im K, et al. Association between triglyceride lowering and reduction of cardiovascular risk across multiple lipid-lowering therapeutic classes: a systematic review and meta-regression analysis of randomized controlled trials. *Circulation*. 2019;140(16):1308-1317.
27. Nicholls SJ, Lincoff AM, Garcia M, et al. Effect of high-dose omega-3 fatty acids vs corn oil on major adverse cardiovascular events in patients at high cardiovascular risk: the STRENGTH randomized clinical trial. *JAMA*. 2020;324(22):2268-2280.
28. Bhatt DL, Steg PG, Miller M, et al. Cardiovascular risk reduction with icosapent ethyl for hypertriglyceridemia. *N Engl J Med*. 2019;380(1):11-22.
29. Das Pradhan A, Glynn RJ, Fruchart JC, et al. Triglyceride lowering with pemafibrate to reduce cardiovascular risk. *N Engl J Med*. 2022;387:1923-1934.
30. Doi T, Langsted A, Nordestgaard BG. A possible explanation for the contrasting results of REDUCE-IT vs. STRENGTH: cohort study mimicking trial designs. *Eur Heart J*. 2021;42(47):4807-4817.
31. Steg PG, Bhatt DL. The reduction in cardiovascular risk in REDUCE-IT is due to eicosapentaenoic acid in icosapent ethyl. *Eur Heart J*. 2021;42(47):4865-4866.
32. Mason RP, Eckel RH. Mechanistic insights from REDUCE-IT STRENGTHen the case against triglyceride lowering as a strategy for cardiovascular disease risk reduction. *Am J Med*. 2021;134(9):1085-1090.
33. Virani SS, Morris PB, Agarwala A, et al. 2021 ACC Expert Consensus decision pathway on the management of ASCVD risk reduction in patients with persistent hypertriglyceridemia: a report of the American College of Cardiology solution set Oversight Committee. *J Am Coll Cardiol*. 2021;78(9):960-993.
34. AIM-HIGH Investigators; Boden WE, Probstfield JL, Anderson T, et al. Niacin in patients with low HDL cholesterol levels receiving intensive statin therapy. *N Engl J Med*. 2011;365(24):2255-2267.
35. HPS2-THRIVE Collaborative Group; Landray MJ, Haynes R, Hopewell JC, et al. Effects of extended-release niacin with laropiprant in high-risk patients. *N Engl J Med*. 2014;371(3):203-212.
36. Barter PJ, Caulfield M, Eriksson M, et al. Effects of torcetrapib in patients at high risk for coronary events. *N Engl J Med*. 2007;357(21):2109-2122.
37. Group HTRC, Bowman L, Hopewell JC, et al. Effects of anacetrapib in patients with atherosclerotic vascular disease. *N Engl J Med*. 2017;377:1217-1227.
38. Schwartz GG, Olsson AG, Abt M, et al.. Effects of dalcetrapib in patients with a recent acute coronary syndrome. *N Engl J Med*. 2012;367(22):2089-2099.
39. Lincoff AM, Nicholls SJ, Riesmeyer JS, et al. Evacetrapib and cardiovascular outcomes in high-risk vascular disease. *N Engl J Med*. 2017;376(20):1933-1942.
40. Group AC, Patel A, MacMahon S, et al. Intensive blood glucose control and vascular outcomes in patients with type 2 diabetes. *N Engl J Med*. 2008;358:2560-2572.
41. Ismail-Beigi F, Craven T, Banerji MA, et al. Effect of intensive treatment of hyperglycaemia on microvascular outcomes in type 2 diabetes: an analysis of the ACCORD randomised trial. *Lancet*. 2010;376(9739):419-430.
42. Zinman B, Wanner C, Lachin JM, et al. Empagliflozin, cardiovascular outcomes, and mortality in type 2 diabetes. *N Engl J Med*. 2015;373(22):2117-2128.
43. Neal B, Perkovic V, Mahaffey KW, et al. Canagliflozin and cardiovascular and renal events in type 2 diabetes. *N Engl J Med*. 2017;377(7):644-657.
44. Wiviott SD, Raz I, Bonaca MP, et al. Dapagliflozin and cardiovascular outcomes in type 2 diabetes. *N Engl J Med*. 2019;380(4):347-357.
45. McMurray JJV, Solomon SD, Inzucchi SE, et al. Dapagliflozin in patients with heart failure and reduced ejection fraction. *N Engl J Med*. 2019;381(21):1995-2008.
46. Packer M, Anker SD, Butler J, et al. Cardiovascular and renal outcomes with empagliflozin in heart failure. *N Engl J Med*. 2020;383(15):1413-1424.
47. Anker SD, Butler J, Filippatos G, et al. Empagliflozin in heart failure with a preserved ejection fraction. *N Engl J Med*. 2021;385(16):1451-1461.
48. Solomon SD, McMurray JJV, Claggett B, et al. Dapagliflozin in heart failure with mildly reduced or preserved ejection fraction. *N Engl J Med*. 2022;387(12):1089-1098.
49. Zelniker TA, Wiviott SD, Raz I, et al. SGLT2 inhibitors for primary and secondary prevention of cardiovascular and renal outcomes in type 2 diabetes: a systematic review and meta-analysis of cardiovascular outcome trials. *Lancet*. 2019;393(10166):31-39.
50. Marilly E, Cottin J, Cabrera N, et al. SGLT2 inhibitors in type 2 diabetes: a systematic review and meta-analysis of cardiovascular outcome trials balancing their risks and benefits. *Diabetologia*. 2022;65(12):2000-2010.
51. Bhatt DL, Szarek M, Steg PG, et al. Sotagliflozin in patients with diabetes and recent worsening heart failure. *N Engl J Med*. 2021;384(2):117-128.
52. Docherty KF, Jhund PS, Inzucchi SE, et al. Effects of dapagliflozin in DAPA-HF according to background heart failure therapy. *Eur Heart J*. 2020;41(25):2379-2392.
53. Zannad F, Ferreira JP, Pocock SJ, et al. SGLT2 inhibitors in patients with heart failure with reduced ejection fraction: a meta-analysis of the EMPEROR-Reduced and DAPA-HF trials. *Lancet*. 2020;396(10254):819-829.
54. Vaduganathan M, Docherty KF, Claggett BL, et al. SGLT-2 inhibitors in patients with heart failure: a comprehensive meta-analysis of five randomised controlled trials. *Lancet*. 2022;400(10354):757-767.

55. Blonde L, Umpierrez GE, Reddy SS, et al. American association of clinical endocrinology clinical practice guideline: developing a diabetes mellitus comprehensive care plan-2022 update. *Endocr Pract.* 2022;28:923-1049.
56. Davies MJ, Aroda VR, Collins BS, et al. Management of hyperglycemia in type 2 diabetes, 2022. A Consensus Report by the American Diabetes Association (ADA) and the European Association for the Study of Diabetes (EASD). *Diabetes Care.* 2022;45(11): 2753-2786.
57. Joseph JJ, Deedwania P, Acharya T, et al. Comprehensive management of cardiovascular risk factors for adults with type 2 diabetes: a scientific statement from the American Heart Association. *Circulation.* 2022;145(9): e722-e759.

Fundamentals of X-Ray Imaging, Radiation Safety, and Contrast Media

Jeremy D. Rier and Rhian E. Davies

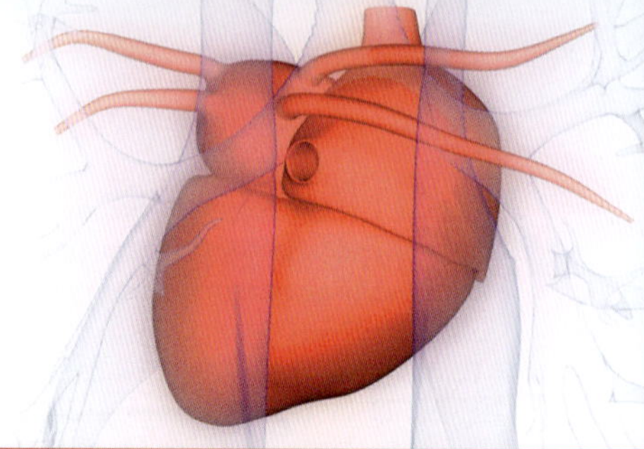

In interventional cardiology, X-ray radiation is used to perform a variety of procedures, including angiography, catheterization, angioplasty, and stent and valve placement. The use of contrast agents can enhance the visibility of blood vessels, chambers, and other structures during interventional procedures. Despite the benefits of X-ray radiation and contrast use, there are also potential risks associated with exposure to ionizing radiation and radiographic contrast agents. To minimize these risks, interventional cardiologists must be knowledgeable about the basics of radiation physics, operation of an X-ray Cine/Fluoroscopic Unit, contrast media (CM) agents, and complications of radiation/contrast use. To that end, this chapter is written as a concise schematic look at these intertwined issues of radiation and contrast management for the purposes of interventional cardiology board review with the additional hope to impact best practice.

FUNDAMENTALS OF IMAGING

The Physics of Imaging

The electromagnetic spectrum is a range of all frequencies of electromagnetic radiation. It is divided into seven regions, in order of decreasing wavelength and increasing energy and frequency. Ionizing electromagnetic waves, which include X-ray and gamma ray, have sufficient energy to ionize atoms or molecules by detaching electrons from them.[1] X-ray radiation has much more energy than visible light. X-rays have a wavelength that is about 1000 times shorter than that of visible light and an energy that is about 10,000 to 100,000 times greater.[2]

X-rays can be harnessed to generate image structures inside the body with the use of an X-ray source and an X-ray detector. As X-rays travel through the body, they are absorbed differentially depending on the radiologic density of the tissue they pass through. Radiologic density is determined by the atomic number (the number of protons in an atom's nucleus) of the material being imaged.[3] Finally, the radiation that exits the patient is composed of varying energies and interacts with the image receptor or detector to form the latent or invisible image and must be processed to create a visible image.[4] Bones contain calcium that has a higher atomic number than most other tissues. As a result, bones readily absorb X-rays and therefore produce high contrast on the X-ray detector. Fat and other soft tissues absorb less and appear gray. Air absorbs the least amount of X-ray and appears black. Fluoroscopy differs from X-ray imaging in that the images produced appear in real time, allowing evaluation of dynamic processes. Additionally, fluoroscopic images appear with an inverted grayscale (black/white is reversed) compared with standard radiographs.

Biologic Effects From X-Ray Exposure

Ionizing electromagnetic waves or ionizing radiation can be classified as directly or indirectly ionizing.[5] Direct ionization radiation produces charged particles that have enough energy to disrupt the atomic structure of the material strikes producing chemical and biological changes. X-rays and gamma rays are indirectly ionizing, meaning that when their uncharged particles are absorbed, they produce a variety of fast-moving particles that can ionize other atoms, which can break vital chemical bonds.[5]

The biologic effects due to the production of free radicals result from either a single-stranded break or a double-stranded DNA break. Single-stranded breaks are readily healed, with no cell death, but if they are incorrectly repaired, a mutation may occur. Double-stranded breaks are less common but more serious. If enough cell damage occurs to prevent normal function, necrosis occurs, appearing within days to months following the exposure. However, if DNA damage occurs without necrosis, carcinogenesis may occur, becoming evident many years following the exposure.[5]

Each of the body's organs has a variable susceptibility to radiation injury. In general, the more biologically active an organ the more susceptible is to radiation. The international commission on radiation units and measurements has suggested a tissue waiting factor for the various organs, and this generally corresponds to the organ's susceptibility to the effects of ionizing radiation[6] (**Table 7.1**).

Radiation-induced injury can be classified as deterministic and stochastic effects. Deterministic effects are dose-dependent direct health effects of radiation, for which a threshold exists, linear with threshold. These tissue reactions can cause cell necrosis, preventing normal function, including repair. If extensive enough damage occurs, clear tissue injury will occur.[8] Skin injury is the most common tissue reaction observed in cardiovascular imaging and may lead to significant tissue necrosis, typically presenting weeks after

TABLE 7.1 Tissue Weighting Factors According to ICRP 103 (ICRP 2007)[7]

TISSUE	TISSUE WEIGHTING FACTOR (WT)	ΣWT
(*) Remaining tissues: Adrenals, extrathoracic region, gall bladder, heart, kidneys, lymphatic nodes, muscle, oral mucosa, pancreas, prostate (♂), small intestine, spleen, thymus, uterus/cervix (♀)		
Bone marrow (red), colon, lung, stomach, breast, remaining tissues (*)	0.12	0.72
Gonads	0.08	0.08
Bladder, esophagus, liver, thyroid	0.04	0.16
Bone surface, brain, salivary glands, skin	0.01	0.04
	Total	1.00

[a]Accounts additional tissues/organs, such as adrenals, kidney, small and large intestine, muscle, pancreas, spleen, thymus, and uterus.

Modified from The 2007 recommendations of the International Commission on Radiological Protection. ICRP publication 103. *Ann ICRP*. 2007;37(2-4):1-332.

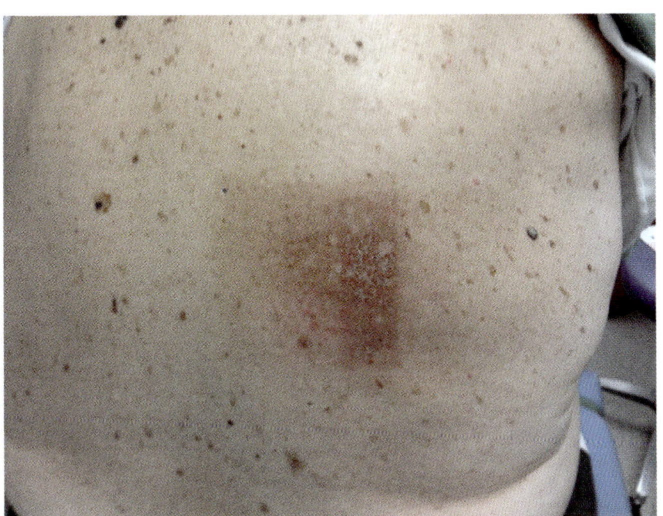

FIGURE 7.1 Tissue injury is seen 1 month following a complex PCI.[9] Notice the characteristic square configuration, as well as the variation in coloration. FT was 104 minutes with no dose recorded. This color variation represents variations in skin exposure produced by alterations in angles and/or collimation. This produced representative skin dose injury that is likely 5 Gy at the least intense coloration and exceeding 10 Gy at the most intense color changes. FT, fluoroscopic time; PCI, percutaneous coronary intervention. (From Kern MJ, Seto AH. Society of cardiac angiography and intervention. In: Kern MJ, Seto AH, eds. *SCAI Interventional Cardiology Review.* 3rd ed. Philadelphia: Wolters Kluwer Health; 2018:490.)

exposure (**Fig. 7.1**). Patient factors associated with skin injury include light-colored skin, smoking, poor nutrition, obesity, hyperthyroidism, diabetes, connective tissue disorders, chemotherapy, and recent radiation exposure or previous high-dose radiation tissue injury. Air kerma at the interventional reference point (IRP), $K_{a,r}$, is used to approximate the patient's entrance skin dose relating to skin injury listed (**Table 7.2**). Dose-dependent skin injury occurs with a time delay that can impede correct early recognition (**Table 7.3**). Therefore, all patients who receive a $K_{a,r}$ greater than 5 Gy should be told of potential skin injury and provided follow-up. X-ray-induced skin injuries are often best managed with good dermatologic care, without biopsy, if possible, to prevent further tissue damage that may not heal.[10]

Stochastic effects of radiation occur by chance in a population of exposed persons, for which no clear threshold exists. Probability is proportional to radiation dose, and the severity is independent of dose, linear, and nonthreshold. A stochastic injury occurs when there is nonfatal injury to the DNA backbone that does not properly heal itself, resulting in mutation, which leads to either cancer or a genetic abnormality.[5] The risk is related to the dose delivered and the volume of tissue exposed and requires time for one transformed cell to multiply into a malignancy with a latent period in years (average 20 years). Therefore, the stochastic risk from a given radiation exposure is greater in the young and, at a given age, greater in females than males. Knowing the individual's age and sex, as well as the organs at greatest risk, assists the operator in assessing individual patient risk. This may be inconsequential if the patient's expected survival is less than the latent period for the adverse effect to occur.[5,9]

Although stochastic effects are not dose dependent, higher doses increases the likelihood of stochastic effects. Models have been created to calculate coefficients that estimate the excess relative/absolute risk per sievert of exposure. The BEIR VII model for incidence and mortality for all solid cancers (excluding thyroid and nonmelanoma skin) lists the associated risk with a dose of one sievert.[11] The risk estimates for ages greater than 60 is limited by small sample sizes in the studied population. The data clearly demonstrate the direct age relationship for sensitivity to radiation-induced cancer. These are gender averaged and thus do not reflect differences between males and females.

Terminology: Quantifying Radiation Exposure

There are several interchangeable terms used throughout radiologic literature to describe radiation, absorption, and radiation exposure. The basic unit of radiation ionization is the roentgen (R). It is the amount of ionization that a defined mass of air undergoes when bombarded by X-rays or γ-rays. The amount of energy absorbed by material is the ***radiation absorbed dose (rad)*** and varies according to the type of radiation and atomic number

TABLE 7.2 Chronology and Severity Thresholds of Tissue Reactions From Single-Delivery Radiation Dose[10]

SINGLE SITE (GY)	PROMPT	EARLY	MID TERM	LONG TERM
ACUTE SKIN DOSE	<2 WK	2-8 WK	6-52 WK	>52 WK
0-2	No observable effects expected			
2-5	Transient erythema	Epilation	Recovery from hair loss	None expected
5-10	Transient erythema	Erythema, epilation	Recovery; high doses cause Prolonged erythema and Permanent partial epilation	Recovery; higher Dose cause dermal Atrophy/induration
10-15	Transient erythema	Erythema, epilation Dry/moist desquamation	Prolonged erythema Permanent epilation	Telangiectasia; dermal Atrophy/induration
>15	Transient erythema Very high-dose causes Edema/ulceration	Erythema, epilation Moist desquamation	Dermal atrophy with Secondary ulceration Late surgical repair likely	Telangiectasia; dermal Atrophy/induration Skin breakdown Surgical repair likely

Modified from Balter S, Schuler BA, Miller DL, et al. *NCRP Radiation Dose Management for Fluoroscopically Guided Interventional Medical Procedures.* National Council on Radiation Protection and Measures, NCRP Report No.168. NCRP; 2011. Available at: http://www.ncrppublications.org/Reports/168, with permission of the National Council on Radiation Protection and Measurements. http://NCRPonline.org

TABLE 7.3 Suggested Values for First and Subsequent Notifications and the Substantial Radiation Dose Level (SRDL)[10]

DOSE METRIC	FIRST NOTIFICATION	SUBSEQUENT NOTIFICATIONS (INCREMENTS)	SRDL
$D_{skin,max}$[a]	2 Gy	0.5 Gy	3 Gy
$K_{a,r}$[b]	3 Gy	1 Gy	5 Gy[b]
P_{KA}[c]	300 Gy cm[2d]	100 Gy cm[2d]	500 Gy cm[2d]
Fluoroscopy time	30 min	15 min	60 min

[a]$D_{skin,max}$ is peak skin dose, requiring calculations by physicist.
[b]$K_{a,r}$ is total air kerma at the reference point.
[c]P_{KA} is air kerma area product.
[d]Assuming a 100 cm^2 field at the patient's skin. For other field sizes, the P_{KA} values should be adjusted proportionally to the actual procedural field size (eg, for a field size of 50 cm^2, the SRDL value for P_{KA} would be 250 Gy cm^2).
Modified from Balter S, Schuler BA, Miller DL, et al. *NCRP Radiation Dose Management for Fluoroscopically Guided Interventional Medical Procedures*. National Council on Radiation Protection and Measures, NCRP Report No.168. NCRP; 2011. Available at: http://www.ncrppublications.org/Reports/168, with permission of the National Council on Radiation Protection and Measurements. http://NCRPonline.org

of the material. Radiation protection units are simply rads times some quality factor that is dependent on the type of radiation, and these units are called ***rems*** (Roentgen equivalent man, rem dose = rad dose × QF × other modifying factors). In cardiology, the quality factor is 1.0 for both X-rays and γ-rays, so rems and rads are equal. The units for rads are expressed in Gray (Gy) and for rems in Seiverts (Sv). One Sv equals 100 rem, or 1 rem equals 10 mSv. When one discusses radiation being delivered, Gy units are used. When one discusses radiation absorbed, then Sv are used (**Table 7.4**).

The following is a list of commonly used terms:

- *Exposure:* Exposure is rarely used as a quantity, with ***air kerma*** now preferred for measuring the amount of radiation present at a location. The Système Internationale (SI) units of the measurement of exposure are coulombs of charge produced per kilogram of air (C/kg). However, an older obsolete unit, the roentgen (abbreviated R and equal to 2.58×10^{-4} C/kg), is sometimes reported.
- *Kerma:* This is Kinetic Energy Released in Material, used to measure units of energy per mass in mGy.
- *Air kerma:* This is the above-defined kerma delivered to air.
- *Dose:* Radiologic ***dose*** is the local concentration of energy, extracted from a radiation field, when it interacts with matter. It refers to the absorption of energy in matter following interactions with ionizing radiation.
- *Absorbed dose:* This is energy absorbed per mass of material measured in mGy. It is directly related to the severity of reactions (skin effects).
- *Effective dose:* This is the hypothetical equivalent of ***whole-body dose*** that produces the same magnitude of cancer risk as dose from an actual absorbed/equivalent dose delivered to a limited portion of the body. The effective dose represents a sum of equivalent doses from different tissues adjusted for the radiation absorption capacity of each tissue.
- *Equivalent dose:* This is a term needed for dosimetry of neutrons. In cardiology, while equivalent dose for a specific organ exposed may be used interchangeably with absorbed dose, it often creates confusion due to different units/quantities of measure. *Therefore, caution is recommended in using this term in fluoroscopic imaging.*

Terminology: Quantifying Dose in Fluoroscopic Procedures

Because all fluoroscopic equipment sold in the United States since 2006 is required to measure and display dose parameters, current guidelines recommend recording all relevant patient procedure radiation dose data.[10,13,14] These measures include the following:

Total air kerma at the IRP ($K_{a,r}$, *Gy*) is the procedural cumulative air kerma (CAK, X-ray energy delivered to air) at the IRP. This point is 15 cm on the X-ray tube side of isocenter (**Fig. 7.2**), which is the primary X-ray beam intersection with the rotational axis of the "C" arm gantry. $K_{a,r}$ is used to monitor patient dose burden because it is associated with threshold-dependent deterministic skin effects. This is also referred to as CAK.

TABLE 7.4 Common Radiation Measures[12]

RADIATION QUANTITY	MOST USED UNIT	COMMENT
Equivalent dose	mSv	Allows to estimate risk in a tissue or organ
Effective dose (ED)	mSv	Allows to estimate global risk
Air kerma area product or dose-area product	Gy cm^2	Measured or calculated by the X-ray system (allows the calculation of overall risk, ie, conversion to ED)
Cumulative air kerma	mGy	Measured by the X-ray system (allows to estimate the skin dose)
Personal dose equivalent	mSv	Measured by the personal occupational dosimeters

Modified from Heidbuchel H, Wittkampf FHM, Vano E, Ernst S, Schilling R, Picano E, et al. Practical ways to reduce radiation dose for patients and staff during device implantations and electrophysiological procedures. *EP Europace*. 2014;16(7):946-964, by permission of Oxford University Press.

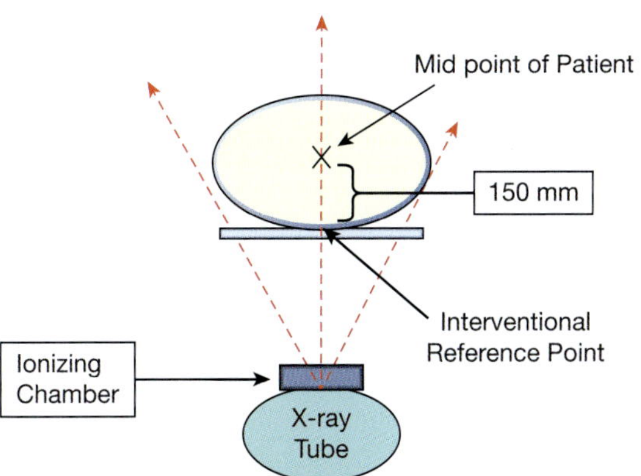

FIGURE 7.2 The dose-area product (DAP) and interventional reference point.[15] The total amount of radiation sent from the X-ray tube can be estimated by use of an ionizing box attached to the output of the X-ray system. This provides the DAP. The total amount, though, does not provide an accurate measurement of the patient's skin exposure. Short of a monitoring device on the skin, the dose to the skin of the patient can be estimated at about 15 cm from the patient's midpoint (150 mm) and calculating what the skin dose would be expected at that point, by applying in the inverse square law. (From Bashore TM. Fundamentals of X-ray imaging, radiation safety, and contrast media. Kern MJ, ed. *SCAI 2012 Interventional Cardiology Review Book*. 2nd ed. Wolters Kluwer; 2013:57-68.)

Air kerma area product (KAP) (P_{KA}, Gy cm^2) is the product of instantaneous air kerma and X-ray field area. Unlike $K_{a,r}$, P_{KA} is impacted by collimation because it includes the field exposed. P_{KA} is used to monitor the linear nonthreshold patient dose burden associated with potential stochastic/cancer effects. This is also referred to as dose-area product (DAP) and KAP.

Peak skin dose (*PSD, Gy*) is the maximum dose received by any area of a patient's skin. While some systems provide these estimates, the most accurate assessments of PSD are obtained by a qualified physicist if air kerma and X-ray geometry details are known.

Fluoroscopic time (*FT, min*), once a time-honored parameter to follow, is now recognized as not being a measure of procedural radiation, as are these other true dose parameters. This is time dependent, not dose dependent, and does not include cine imaging nor reflect dose changes with angulation or frame rate. Steeper angulations, larger patients, and patient extremities in the field of view will significantly increase dose without affecting FT. The operator who utilizes store fluoroscopy, minimizes angles, and reduces frame rate will decrease dose. However, when compared based on FT to other operators and labs, these improvements will not be seen.[16]

RADIATION SAFETY

Radiation Exposure for Patients

Most of the radiation an individual receives annually comes from background radiation. Natural radiation accounts for about 82% of the radiation we receive (radon accounts for 55% of the total background radiation dose) and man-made radiation for 18%. Though the numbers vary widely depending on location, altitude, and so forth, the average background radiation per year received in the United States is about 3.6 mSv.[17] Compare this with a patient's exposure from a routine chest X-ray being around 0.02 to 0.04 mSv. **Table 7.5** outlines the typical radiation effective doses of common cardiac procedures. The current exposure limit for the public recommended by the International Council for Radiation protection (ICRP) is an effect dose of 1 mSV in a year. The annual equivalent dose limits for eye and skin/hands/feet is 15 and 50 mSv, respectively.[17,19]

TABLE 7.5 Typical Effective Doses for Cardiac Procedures[18]

MODALITY	PROTOCOL	EFFECTIVE DOSE (MSV)
MDCT	CT angio.: prospective triggering	0.5-7
MDCT	CT angio.: high-pitch helical	<0.5-3
MDCT	CT angio., pre-TAVR (multiphase)	5-50
MDCT	Calcium scoring	1-5
SPECT	10/30 mi Ci 99m Tc sestamibi St/Rst	11
SPECT	10/30 mi Ci 99m Tc tetrofosmin St/Rst	9
SPECT	Dual isotope (3.5 mi Ci Tl/30 mi Ci Tc)	22-23
PET	50 mCi 82 Rb rest/50 mCi 82 Rb stress	4
Inv. Dx	Dx cath: coronaries and ventriculography	2-20
Inv. Inter.	PCI intervention, with or without Dx cath	5-57
TAVR	Early data (?):, transapical and transfemoral	12 ≥ 50?
EP	Diagnostic	0.1-3.2
EP	Ablation	1-25
EP	Device insertion	0.2-8

CT, computed tomography; MDCT, multidetector computed tomography; PET, positron emission tomography; TAVR, transcatheter aortic valve replacement.
Modified from Einstein AJ. Patient-centered imaging: shared decision making for cardiac imaging procedures exposure to ionizing radiation. *J Am Coll Cardiol*. 2014;63:1480-1489.

Previous increases in radiation from medical imaging have appropriately heightened concerns for radiation safety. In 2010, the Food and Drug Administration called for radiation reduction in medical imaging.[20] Equipment manufacturers responded with system modifications and best practice protocols in fluoroscopic imaging. Organization and societies have published their recommendations on radiation dose management in the cardiac catheterization laboratory.[10,13,14] With increasing awareness and improved practice patterns, there has been a 15% to 20% reduction in nontherapeutic medical radiation dose over the last 10 years.[21] The estimated average effective dose is approximately 2.16 mSv.[21] A minority of this is directly attributed to cardiac interventional fluoroscopy, which represents 6% of the effective dose.[21] Awareness of radiation safety has resulted in dose reduction to the patient, staff, and operators.

A successful cardiac catheterization laboratory must have a radiation safety program committed to reducing patient and staff radiation exposure to a level that reflects the ALARA principle.[22] Procedure justification and dose optimization are key concepts. The first step is avoiding unnecessary use of ionizing radiation by requiring justification for exposure. Recognizing the role for

Appropriate Use Criteria and preventing repetitive procedures is essential for all imaging modalities. Once justified, dose optimization is essential. The interventional imaging team, physicians, technologists, physicists, and other medical personnel should be responsible for developing protocols, implementing regular equipment quality control tests, and monitoring patients' radiation doses. This requires a quality assurance program emphasizing and monitoring best practices in radiation management.[10]

A procedure-based review of radiation dose management is essential, including preprocedure, procedure, and postprocedure best practice recommendations, outlined in **Table 7.6**.[10,13,14] Preprocedure planning includes identifying the high-risk patient (obese, complex disease, or fluoroscopic procedures needed within 30-60 days) and obtaining informed consent. It is recommended to screen women of reproductive age for pregnancy prior to procedures utilizing ionizing radiation per institutional protocol. During the case, the physician should manage dosage from the outset, monitoring key components of this optimal procedure. Dose management is reviewed below. Staff must provide periodic dose updates to assist the operator with radiation awareness. Postprocedure, all cardiac catheterization reports should include available radiation parameters: FT (min), $K_{a,r}$, (Gy), and PKA (Gy cm^2). Patient notification, chart documentation, and communication with the primary care provider should be routine for high-dose procedures. ($K_{a,r}$ > 5 Gy, PKA > 500 Gy cm^2). Patients should be educated regarding potential skin changes with a 2- to 4-week phone call follow-up or office visit as required. For $K_{a,r}$ > 10 Gy (PKA > 1000 Gy cm^2), a qualified physicist should promptly calculate PSD. The Joint Commission identifies PSD > 15 Gy as a sentinel event; hospital risk management and regulatory agencies should be contacted within 24 hours.[14]

TABLE 7.6 Components of Radiation Dose Management in PCI[9]

Preprocedure
Obtain patient's radiation history; check patient's skin if positive Hx
Extend radiation aspects of informed consent when appropriate especially for high-risk cases (chronic total occlusion)
Plan alternative beam orientations for forthcoming case when necessary
Time Out
Verify that fluoroscopic system settings are correct for the planned procedure
All staff should be wearing their personal radiation monitors (staff safety item)
All staff wearing their radiation and nonradiation personal protective equipment (staff safety item)
Ancillary radiation shielding devices present in lab (staff safety item)
During Procedure
Minimizing radiation exposure to the patient (Table 7.11)
Time, distance, and shielding for occupational dose reduction (see the *Text*)
Remember: Best practices to reduce patient dose benefit operator and staff
Regular radiation dose notification by staff with brief pause to assess benefit-risk
Postprocedure
Complete patient dosimetry recorded in medical record and case report
Substantial dose of radiation justified in medical record when appropriate
Patient notified if substantial dose of radiation was used; and given their initial follow-up processes
Patents receiving substantial doses followed as appropriate
Radiation safety issues must be a part of the Cardiac Catheterization Laboratory Quality Program

From Kern MJ, Seto AH. Society of cardiac angiography and intervention. In: Kern MJ, Seto AH, eds. *SCAI Interventional Cardiology Review*. 3rd ed. Philadelphia: Wolters Kluwer Health; 2018:490.

No system is currently in place to monitor an individual patients' cumulative lifetime radiation exposure. The availability and American College of Cardiology Foundation/American Heart Association/Society for Cardiovascular Angiography and Interventions-recommended reporting of all relevant patient procedure radiation dose data—including FT (minute), total air kerma at the IRP (Gy), and air KAP (Gy cm^2)—make such a monitoring system possible.[23] However, the dispersion of patient radiation exposures across multiple care sites with separate medical records will require a comprehensive program to document an individual patient's cumulative radiation exposure.

Radiation Exposure for Health Care Workers

Radiation exposure to the health care workers is usually measured with either a TLD (thermoluminescent dosimeter) badge or an OSL (optically simulated luminescent) badge. The TLD badge has a lithium fluoride crystal that absorbs X-rays. When heated, it releases light photons in proportion to the amount of X-ray absorbed. The OSL badge is similar, but the substrate is aluminum oxide doped with carbon, and it releases light in proportion to the amount of X-ray absorbed when struck with a laser. The badges have different filters to mimic attenuation for different parts of the body. The results are usually reported for shallow, lens, or deep dose exposure. It is an individual's responsibility to wear a dosimeter for personal benefit, although state regulations are in place to enforce this practice.

While a single dosimeter worn outside the collar can be used and is acceptable, two dosimeters, when properly worn (one under the garment and one at the collar outside the protective garment), is a better reflection of effective dose.[16,24] Real-time operator dose monitoring has been studied and shown to be effective in procedural dose reduction.[25] The pregnant worker should wear a dosimeter under the lead collar, as well as on the thyroid collar, with no more than 0.5 mSv (0.05 rem)/mo, not to exceed 5 mSv (0.5 rem) total exposures, once the pregnancy is declared. Legal precedent supports a pregnant worker remaining in the laboratory if she chooses, but counseling from the radiation safety officer is recommended.[17,26,27]

Maternal and fetal risks are reviewed in several multisocietal papers.[26,27] Radiation exposure to the fetus is particularly an issue during the first trimester. However, radiation exposure within 2 weeks of uterine implantation of the fertilized egg may be less critical, because all the cells at that point are pluripotent. The United Nations Scientific Committee on the Effects of Atomic Radiation (UNSCEAR) suggests that the risk of a fetal congenital malformation or a malignancy is about 0.0002% per mSv (0.002% per rem) exposure. A dose of 100 mSv (10 rem) during the most sensitive period (10 days to 26 weeks) is often regarded as the cutoff point for considering a therapeutic abortion. With appropriate safeguards, pregnancy in the cardiac catheterization laboratory is

TABLE 7.7 Recommended Fetal Radiation Dose Limits[29-31]

GOVERNING BODY	DOSE LIMIT
ACOG, NCRP	<0.5 mSv (50 mrem) per month <5 mSv (500 mrem) during gestation
ICRP	<1 mSv (100 mrem) during gestation

ACOG, American College of Obstetricians and Gynecologists; ICRP, International Commission on Radiological Protection; NCRP, National Council on Radiation Protection and Measurements.
Modified from Cheney AE, Vincent LL, McCabe JM, Kearney KE. Pregnancy in the cardiac catheterization laboratory: a safe and feasible endeavor. *Circ Cardiovasc Interv*. 2021;14(4):E009636.

both safe and feasible.[28] The recommended fetal dose limits, effects of fetal radiation exposure, and approaches to managing radiation safety in the pregnant interventional cardiologist are shown in **Tables 7.7-7.9**.

Compared to a patient, an operator's single procedure exposure is significantly less. Operator exposure is expressed as *equivalent dose* for organ-specific exposure and as *effective dose* for whole-body exposure. The effective dose represents a sum of equivalent doses from different tissues adjusted for the radiation absorption capacity of each tissue. Note that the total recommended maximal dose for an invasive cardiologist is 50 mSv (rem)/y, and the total accumulative dose is age × 10 mSv (age × total rems).[17] **Table 7.10** lists the National Council on Radiation Protection (NCRP) recommendations for occupational radiation dose limits. The ICRP has lowered their limits to 20 mSv not only for total body annual but also for the eye.[33] This is based upon concerns that eye injury occurs at doses lower than previously reported.

An interventional cardiologist, utilizing best practices for radiation protection, receives about 1 to 10 mSv/y,[34] dependent upon volume and case section. This is significantly below the US occupational dose limit of 50 mSv/y. However, a busy interventionalist doing complex cases may receive in excess of 50 mSv/y; this emphasizes the importance of personnel dosimeters and best practices for radiation safety. Nurses and technologists, dependent upon their role and location during the procedure, receive approximately 2 mSv/y. The cumulative additional risk for cancer in those exposed to occupational radiation is about 0.004% × mSv (or 0.04% × rem). If a busy interventionist receives 25 mSv/y and practices for 20 years, his or her total dose would be about 500 mSv (50 rem), with an added risk of 500 × 0.004% or 2%. This additional radiation exposure would increase the cancer risk 20% to 22% from baseline.[34]

TABLE 7.8 Effects of Gestational Age and Radiation Dose on Radiation-Induced Teratogenesis[32]

	EFFECTS	ESTIMATED THRESHOLD DOSE
Gestational Period		
Before implantation (0-2 wk after fertilization)	Death of embryo or no consequence	50-100 mGy
Organogenesis (2-8 wk after fertilization)	Congenital anomalies (skeleton, eyes, and genitals)	200 mGy
	Growth restriction	200-250 mGy
Fetal Period		
8-15 wk	Severe intellectual disability (high risk)	60-310 mGy
	Intellectual deficit	25 IQ point loss/1000 mGy
	Microcephaly	200 mGy
16-25 wk	Severe intellectual disability (low risk)	250-280 mGy

IQ, intelligence quotient.
Adapted from the ACOG Guidelines for Diagnostic Imaging During Pregnancy. Modified from Wagner LK, Hayman LA. Pregnancy and women radiologists. *Radiology*. 1982;145(2):559-562.

TABLE 7.9 Approach to Managing Radiation Safety in the Pregnant Interventionalist[28]

Obtain a fetal radiation badge (dosimeter)
Ensure protective garments provide at least 0.5 mm LE throughout the entire pregnancy
Minimize the weight of protective garments to avoid additional musculoskeletal strain
Pay close attention to fit of protective garments as fetus grows

LE, lead equivalency.
Modified from Cheney AE, Vincent LL, McCabe JM, Kearney KE. Pregnancy in the cardiac catheterization laboratory: a safe and feasible endeavor. *Circ Cardiovasc Interv*. 2021;14(4):E009636.

Basic Operation of an X-Ray Cine/Fluoroscopic Unit

Formation of the X-Ray Beam

The general concept of what happens between the generator and the X-ray tube when forming X-rays is shown in **Fig. 7.3**.[15] The X-ray tube is a vacuum tube with a cathode coil (or coils) facing a spinning anode. Electrons are sent to the cathode from the generator, and the cathode becomes white hot (about 3,000 °F). At this temperature, the electrons virtually boil off (thermionic emission). The generator also sets up a voltage potential across the X-ray tube. The electrons from the cathode cross from the cathode to the anode

TABLE 7.10 Recommended Dose Limits From the NCRP[5]

BACKGROUND RADIATION	3.6 MSV (0.36 REM)
Chest X-ray	0.02-0.04 mSv
Annual Dose Limits	
Stochastic effects	
Cumulative	10 mSv × age (rem × age)
Annual	50 mSv (5 rems)
Deterministic effects (annual)	
Eye	150 mSv/y (15 rem)
Skin	500 mSv/y (50 rem)
Embryo or fetus	0.5 mSv/mo (0.05 rem)

Adapted from Hall EJ. Radiation protection. In: Hall EJ, ed. *Radiobiology for the Radiologist*. Philadelphia, PA: Lippincott Williams & Wilkins; 2000:234-248; International Commission on Radiation Units and Measurements. *Recommendations. Report 60*. New York, NY: Pergamon Press; 1991; National Council on Radiation Protection and Measurement. *Recommendations for Limits on Exposure to Ionizing Radiation. Report 116*. Bethesda, MD: National Council on Radiation Protection and Measurement; 1993.

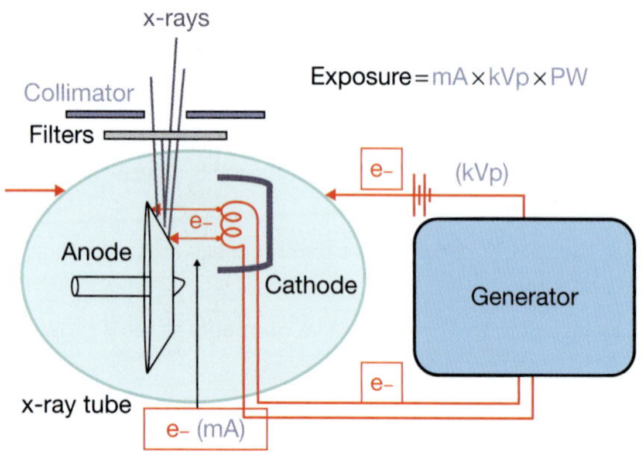

FIGURE 7.3 The X-ray tube is depicted.[9] A potential is set up across the X-ray tube that encourages electrons from the cathode inside the vacuum tube to jump to the anode. The peak voltage across the X-ray tube is referred to as the kVp of the system, and the number of electrons that jump is referred to as the mA. The exposure equation is defined as the mA × kVp × pulse width. Collimators and filters help shape and filter out unusable X-rays. (From Kern MJ, Seto AH. Society of cardiac angiography and intervention. In: Kern MJ, Seto AH, eds. *SCAI Interventional Cardiology Review.* 3rd ed. Philadelphia: Wolters Kluwer Health; 2018:490.)

as a result of this voltage potential. The maximal (peak) voltage across the X-ray tube is referred to as the kVp, representing the energy of the photons. The number of photons that cross from the cathode to the anode is mA (milliamperes). Radiation dose is determined by variations in mA and kVp and ultimately impacts image quality. Most of the electrons that cross from the cathode to the anode produce heat, with only a small percentage actually striking the anode to produce X-rays. Early generation X-ray tubes were limited due to the challenges of heat production. Current systems control the heat generated, with the anode rotating rapidly (3500-10,000 rpm) in conjunction with oil circulating around the X-ray tube to help cool it. Photons that strike the tungsten anode produce X-rays that emerge from a point source called the X-ray beam focal spot. Because low-frequency X-rays are not clinically useful and only contribute to noise, many of them are absorbed by copper and aluminum filters added at the output of the X-ray tube. Collimation helps shape the X-ray beam as it emerges as well as reduce scatter and decrease exposure. Scatter radiation from Compton interactions within the patient is directly related to dose, degrades image quality, and serves as the primary source of radiation exposure to the operator and staff.[35]

Basics of X-Ray Imaging Systems

To understand how an X-ray system creates an image, it is helpful to follow the flow of energy through the system. Electrons produced in the generator are sent to the X-ray tube, where they are converted to X-rays. These X-rays diverge immediately and travel through the table and the patient, where most are absorbed or scattered. A few then make it to an image detector (either image intensifier or flat panel). There they pass through a filter on the detector and strike a face layer of cesium-iodide phosphor, and a clump of light photons are emitted. From here, things differ depending on the imaging device.

"Flat-panel" detectors have replaced the image intensifier and television camera in traditional analog imaging chains for improved efficiency of the image formation process (**Fig. 7.4**). In a *flat-panel* system, the clumps of photons are converted to electrons by a layer of photodiodes. This technology incorporates detectors with a charge-coupled visible-light device that is in direct contact with the input phosphor. This signal is then digitized and sent directly from the panel to the monitor for display. This direct digital video signal is generated from the original visible-light fluorescence without an intervening stage. *The fewer steps in image transfer, the less the image is degraded. This results in enhanced image uniformity, uniform brightness, and dynamic range when compared to the multiple image transfer required in the image intensifier.* The avoidance of another conversion of energy to light, and then to electricity, improves the overall performance of the flat-panel system. Improved image quality through reduced image transfer allows for dose reduction. Although "analog" and "digital" systems share similar X-ray tube technologies, it is the "detector" that has fundamentally changed the way images are formed and processed.[36]

Flat-panel technology has significantly improved the prior challenges with dynamic range that resulted in blooming over denser bones, where more exposure was required, than the lungs. Patient characteristics, such as an obese patient, and procedure requirements, such as steep angulated views, require an increased dose to satisfy the exposure equation. Magnification increases dose, although to a lesser degree in the current era of flat-panel technology. These parameters are initially set by the manufacturer, with modification required based upon individual laboratory needs. Resolution is dependent upon field size. With small field-of-view imaging, the resolution may increase. However, with a larger field of view, image processing bundles pixels to achieve magnification. Because the image may actually lose resolution, an increase in X-ray dose is required to keep the signal-to-noise ratio satisfactory.[10]

Complete system operation is determined by the combination of operator-selectable parameters and feedback elements that stabilize system performance and imaging. The operator is the center for many of these control loops (**Fig. 7.5**).

Multiple imaging parameters influence exposure associated with a cine/fluoroscopic examination.[10,36] These include the following:

1. *X-ray image detector dose per pulse:* This is the dose for each X-ray pulse (typically measured in nanogray) that reaches the detector. It is important to note that the detector dose is considerably smaller than the subject dose, given that generally 5% or less of the incident radiation penetrates the subject and reaches the detector.
2. *X-ray unit framing (pulsing) rate:* This is the number of pulses the X-ray system generates per unit of time. It is an operator-selectable parameter that ranges between 4 and 30 pulses/s and is a determinant of image *temporal* resolution.
3. *Imaging field size:* This is the area of the X-ray beam that impinges on the subject. It is discussed in greater depth under "KAP" in the "Quantifying Dose in Fluoroscopic Procedures" section.
4. *X-ray beam filtration*: An X-ray tube produces a spectrum of X-ray photon energies. The lower-energy photons (photon energies <30 keV) have insufficient penetrating power to reach the detector and thus expose the subject without contributing to image formation. These "undesirable" photons are typically "filtered" out of the X-ray beam by interposing layers of aluminum and copper in the X-ray tube exit port.

Image Storage

While high-quality real-time fluoroscopic imaging is required for procedure performance, cineangiographic acquisition for postprocedure review, as well as long-term access, is similarly necessary. Digital imaging allows for high-resolution image data to be made immediately available. However, this increase in information content that

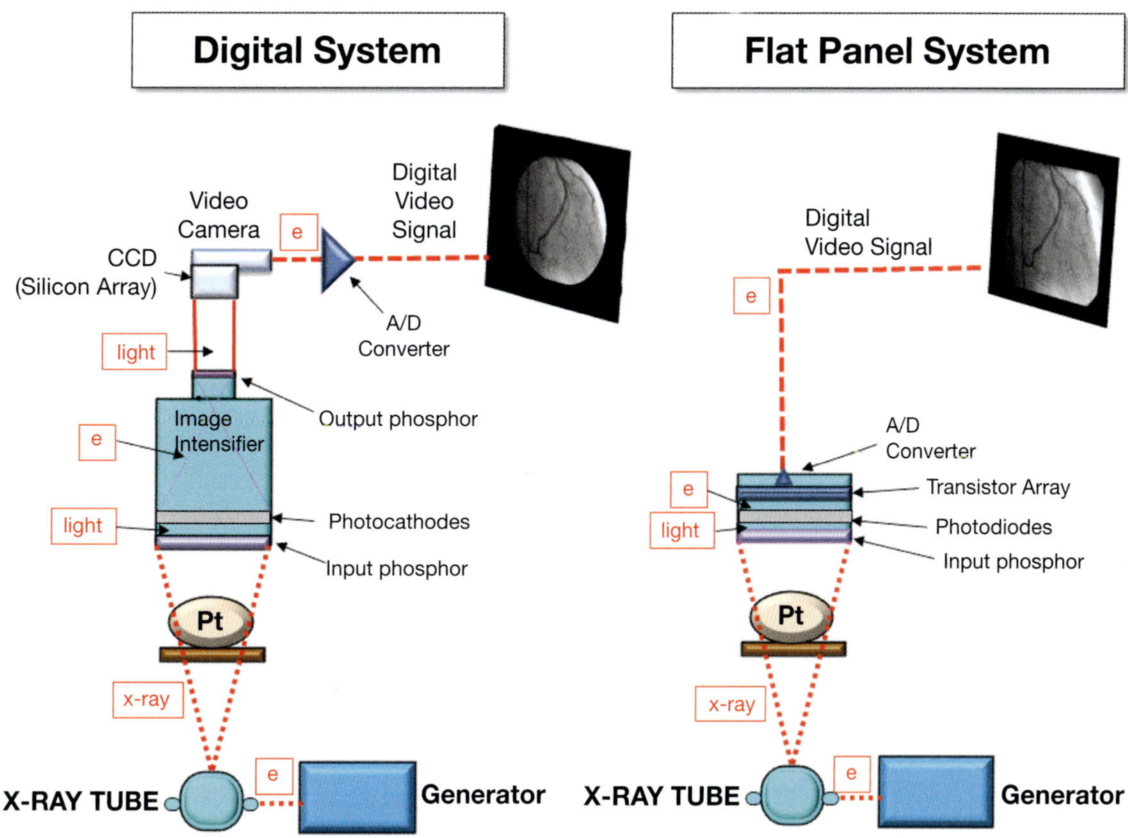

FIGURE 7.4 The left panel represents the older digital imaging system with the image intensifier.[9] The right panel illustrates the current flat-panel system. Electrons generated are converted to X-rays, pass through the patient, and are sensed on the input phosphor and converted to light in both systems. The limitation with the *image intensifier* is the multiple steps involved. Light photons are converted back to electrons, accelerated, and strike the output phosphor. The image is then picked up by the CCD chips, converted to a video signal, digitized in the A/D converter, and sent to the monitor. In the *flat-panel system*, the light is converted to electrons, sensed by a transistor array, digitized, and sent directly to the monitor. (From Kern MJ, Seto AH. Society of cardiac angiography and intervention. In: Kern MJ, Seto AH, eds. *SCAI Interventional Cardiology Review.* 3rd ed. Philadelphia: Wolters Kluwer Health; 2018:490.)

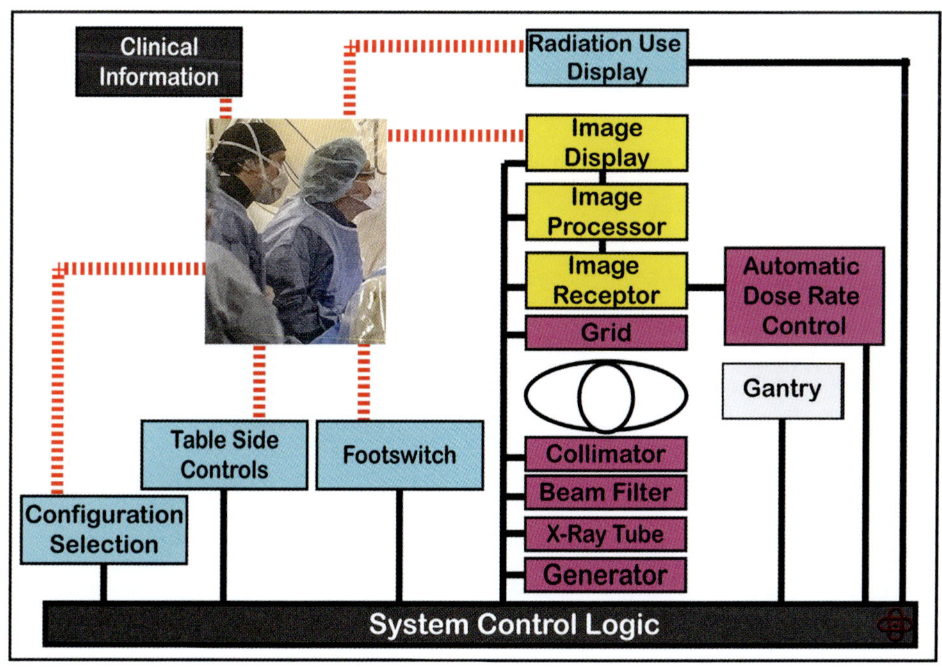

FIGURE 7.5 This is a diagrammatic representation of an X-ray fluoroscopy system illustrating the pathway from X-ray production through image formation.[9] This emphasizes the role of a knowledgeable physician recognizing the appropriate feedback loops in controlling radiation dose and image quality. (From Kern MJ, Seto AH. Society of cardiac angiography and intervention. In: Kern MJ, Seto AH, eds. *SCAI Interventional Cardiology Review.* 3rd ed. Philadelphia: Wolters Kluwer Health; 2018:490.)

occurs with digital imaging requires a significant increase in system "bandwidth" to facilitate "on-line" and postacquisition review and archiving of studies. All the newer systems have the system bandwidth for storage and transfer of large amounts of data. Once in a digital format, the data are then written to the disk using the DICOM (Digital Communication in Medicine) standard, established in the 1990s. This format provides for "seamless" image access of these digital data for viewing across internal and external network connections. Additionally, this provides a medium for short- and long-term image storage on a variety of archival media devices, including disaster recovery technology to prevent data loss. Initially limited by large expensive storage capabilities, the duration of digital image storage, previously defined in the film era as 7 years, was continued. However, as the cost of digital storage has dropped, with ready availability of terabytes for large media storage, the long-term availability of these cine images for case review has become less of a concern and has often been extended.[35]

RADIATION DOSE MANAGEMENT IN THE CATHETERIZATION LABORATORY

Training

The interventional cardiology board certification examination includes physics and radiation safety. Although only certain states mandate fluoroscopy training, everyone should receive radiation safety training commensurate to their responsibilities. This catheterization laboratory radiation safety education program should be coordinated in conjunction with the hospital radiation safety officer and include the following NCRP components[10]:

1. Initial didactic training that should include the following topics: physics of X-ray production; equipment technology with modes of operation; image quality in fluoroscopy; dosimetry, quantities and units; biological effects of radiation; principles of radiation safety; applicable federal, state, and local regulations; requirements and techniques to minimize patient and staff dose.
2. Periodic, annual, updates on radiation safety.
3. Hands-on training for newly hired operators and current operators on new equipment.

Keys to Optimal Procedural Dose Management

Operator dose is directly proportional to patient dose, thus reducing the dose to the patient will benefit the operator and staff. Developing good techniques is essential to minimize radiation dose through meticulous application of established best practices. A procedure-based review of radiation dose management is outlined in **Table 7.6**. Minimizing patient exposure benefits operator and staff (**Table 7.11**). It is important to use fluoroscopy only when looking at the monitor and limit cine imaging. Steep angles,[37] frame rate, collimation, protective shielding, and table and image receptor height are all important variables during the procedure. Operator and staff must maximize their distance from the X-ray tube (using the inverse square law). The greater the distance, the operator/staff can be from the radiation source and patient, the lesser the exposure. To the operator, most of the exposure occurs from the scatter from the entry side of the patient. When the X-ray tube is closest to the operator, the amount of radiation exposure to the operator is the greatest. Thus, in a cranial left anterior oblique view, with the X-ray tube on the same side of the table as the operator, operator exposure occurs six times more than in a caudal right anterior oblique, where the X-ray tube is on the opposite side of the table. All appendages of the operator and patient should be out of the imaging field (Box 7.1).

Three basic tenets for minimizing ***occupational exposure*** are ***time, distance, and shielding***. Keep the studies as short as possible. Although a minute of fluoroscopy may only result in one-tenth the dose of 1 minute of cineangiography, most of the radiation exposure in the laboratory is due to fluoroscopy. In fact, the operator typically receives about six times the dose from fluoroscopy than from cine. The table height and I.I. can have significant effects on radiation dose and exposure as a result of scatter (**Figs. 7.6** and **7.7**). In general, scatter radiation is lowest when the table height is higher and the I.I. is close to the patient. Stay as far from the X-ray source as possible. Use of extension tubing should be attached to catheters to allow operators to be farther from the X-ray source when possible. Distance may impact radial cases with increased operator dose, but this decreases with increased operator experience.[38]

TABLE 7.11 Minimizing Radiation Exposure to the Patient[9]

Minimizing Radiation Exposure to the Patient
Proper collimation
Minimize the beam "on-time"
Use filters at the output of the X-ray tube
Keep the kVp as high as possible to maintain good image contrast
Minimize mA
Use the minimal number of views
Keep the image intensifier as close to the patient as possible
Keep the source-to-image distance as narrow as possible
Use the lowest framing rate possible
Use pulsed fluoroscopy
Limit "high-dose" fluoroscopy
Keep the number of magnified views to a minimum
Use direct shielding of gonadal organs
Vary views to distribute radiation over a wider area

From Kern MJ, Seto AH. Society of cardiac angiography and intervention. In: Kern MJ, Seto AH, eds. *SCAI Interventional Cardiology Review.* 3rd ed. Philadelphia: Wolters Kluwer Health; 2018:490.

Box 7.1 The Acronym "DRAPED" Provides a Practical Approach to Reducing Radiation Exposure

D	Distance	Inverse square law; ie, utilize tubing extensions as needed Radiation exposure = 1/distance^2
R	Receptor	Keep image receptor close to patient and collimate
A	Angles	Avoid steep angles
P	Pedal	Keep foot off pedal except when looking at the monitor
E	Extremities	Keep patient and operator extremities out of the beam
D	Dose	Limit cine, adjust frame rate, wear personal dosimeter

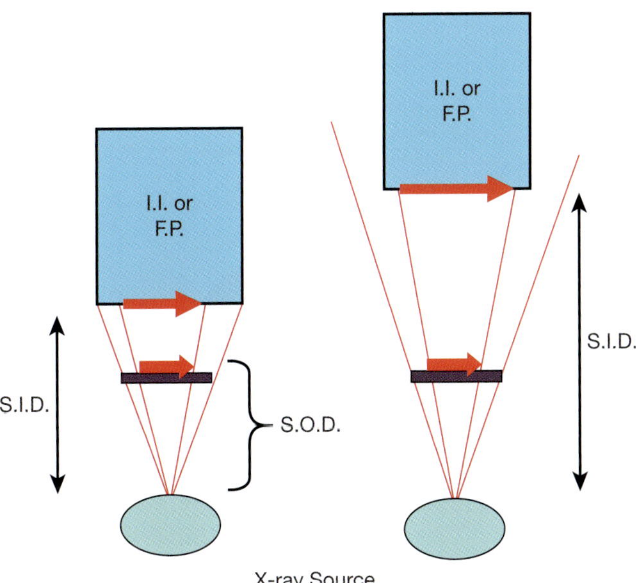

FIGURE 7.6 Magnification that occurs when the source-to-image distance is increased.[15] Increasing the source-to-image distance results in loss of X-rays owing to their divergence. The image appears larger, and to satisfy the exposure equation, the amount of X-ray dose increases. (From Bashore TM. Fundamentals of X-ray imaging, radiation safety, and contrast media. In: Kern MJ, ed. *SCAI 2012 Interventional Cardiology Review Book*. 2nd ed. Philadelphia, PA: Lippincott Williams & Wilkins; 2013:57-68.)

Operators and staff should routinely utilize all available personal protective apparel and in-room shielding. Protective garments and aprons with thyroid shielding stop approximately 95% of scatter radiation. Ceiling- and table-mounted shields are available and are effective in operator dose reduction. With posterior subcapsular cataract formation, a proven risk for those exposed to significant eye radiation, protective glasses are effective in reducing this risk but must fit properly, have 0.25-mm lead-equivalent protection, and additional side shielding.[39] Radiation caps, both disposable and reusable, are available as lead and lead-equivalent options and have been shown to reduce cranial radiation, but long-term benefits are less well established.[40] Sterile protective disposable drapes will decrease operator scatter but may increase patient dose.

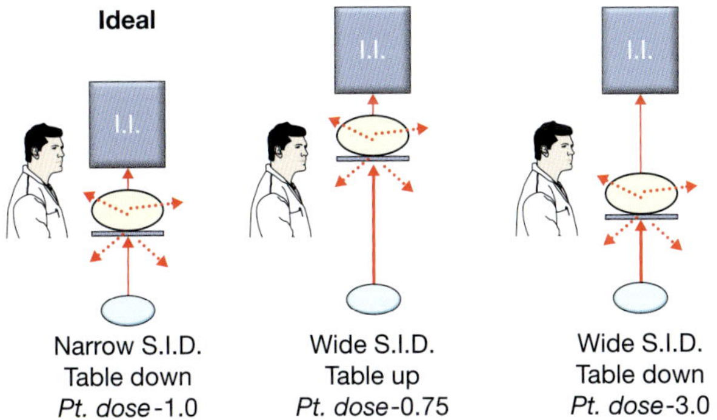

FIGURE 7.7 The effects of various relationships between the table and source-to-image distance heights.[15] In the first panel, the source-to-image distance is low to the patient, and he is a comfortable distance from the X-ray tube. In the middle panel, the image intensifier is close to the patient, but he is far from the X-ray tube. This increase in the source-to-image distance requires a greater X-ray dose and more exposure to the operator with less to the patient based on the inverse square law. In the right panel, the patient is at a comfortable distance from the X-ray tube, but the source-to-image distance is too wide. This increases the X-ray dose and results in an increased dose to the patient. (From Bashore TM. Fundamentals of X-ray imaging, radiation safety, and contrast media. In: Kern MJ, ed. *SCAI 2012 Interventional Cardiology Review Book*. 2nd ed. Philadelphia, PA: Lippincott Williams & Wilkins; 2013:57-68.)

Additional catheterization laboratory options have been developed to reduce operator dose. The development of floor mounted mobile lead shielding devices significantly reduce radiation and allow operators to possibly forgo wearing lead.[41,42] While mobile shielding devices offer significant protection, these systems lack of extra protection for personnel at the head of the bed and the left side of the table. Robotic systems offer a radiation-free environment for the operator in a remote/non-in-procedure room laboratory location.

While invasive/interventional cardiology is appropriately focused on patient outcomes, the risks to the profession have received far less attention and differ significantly from other medical disciplines. In addition to the potential radiation concerns, which include cataract formation,[43] brain tumors,[44] skin injury, and inheritable defects, orthopedic injuries from protective attire are frequent. These are often categorized as anecdotal and are thus underestimated.[45] Recognizing that techniques utilized to reduce patient dose will reduce operator dose, the interventional cardiologist should assess this benefit; that is, the risk analysis for the patient comes in understanding that operator and staff benefits must be considered in the context of maximal patient safety. As interventional cardiologists, we need to continue to strive for the safest environment for our patients, staff, and ourselves.

CONTRAST MEDIA

Background

The introduction of radiodinated contrast has been indispensable in the evaluation of cardiac structure and function in the cardiac catheterization laboratory. Although necessary, the use of contrast agents can result in complications that can be broadly categorized as hypersensitivity and chemotoxic reactions. Advances in the understanding of the structure and properties of CM have led to improvement in prevention and management of complications that result from contrast agents.[46]

Structure and Properties of the CM Agents

CM were first introduced for urinary tract visualization in 1923. All CM agents have a basic structure consisting of a benzene ring (one benzene ring—monomeric; two rings—dimeric), which has iodine (located at positions 2, 4, and 6) and side chains (located at positions 1, 3, and 5) that differentiate the various CM agents (**Figs. 7.8-7.10**).

Iodine is a particularly good absorber of the X-rays in the emitted energy range, and that is the reason why it is used as a contrast agent. The iodine absorption spectrum is shown superimposed on the X-ray spectrum (**Fig. 7.11**). Note that as the energy increases, the iodine absorbs fewer of the X-rays until suddenly there is marked absorption. This is the energy of the K-shell electron of the iodine and is referred to as the K edge. Progressively increasing the X-ray energy again results in progressively less absorption past this K edge.

The two major classifications of contrast agents for cardiovascular imaging are based on their ability to either dissociate into ionic particles in solution (ionic) or not dissociate (nonionic). The ionic agents were the first group developed, with sodium diatrizoate and iothalamate anions as the iodine carriers, such as Renografin, Hypaque, and Angiovist. Nonionic contrast agents began to impact

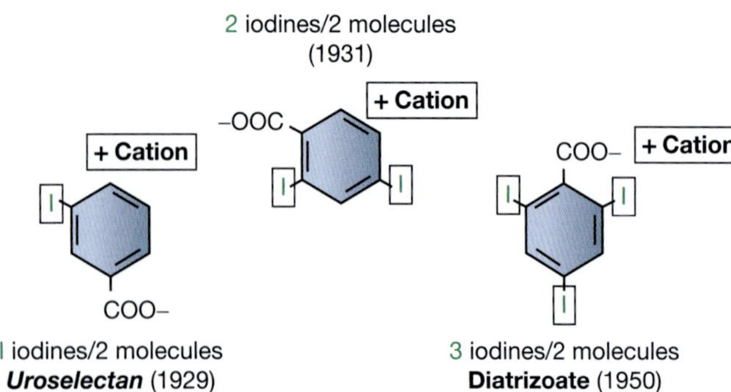

FIGURE 7.8 Ionic and high-osmolar contrast agents.[9] Each ring has a progressive increase in the number of iodines attached. The more iodines present per molecule, the fewer the number of molecules in solution and the lower the osmolality. (From Kern MJ, Seto AH. Society of cardiac angiography and intervention. In: Kern MJ, Seto AH, eds. *SCAI Interventional Cardiology Review.* 3rd ed. Philadelphia: Wolters Kluwer Health; 2018:490.)

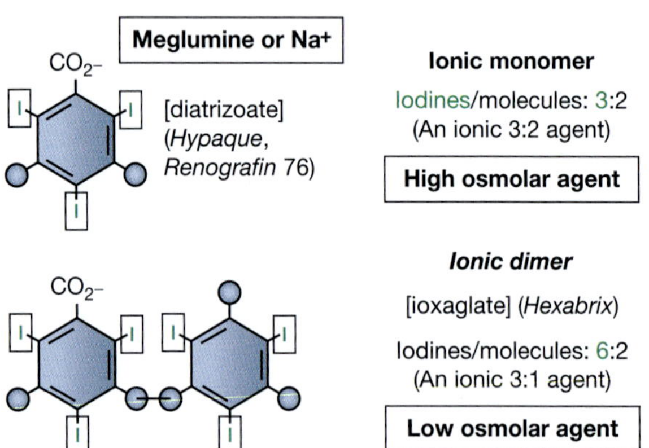

FIGURE 7.9 Ionic contrast agents.[9] The top represents the 3:2 agent, the high-osmolar diatrizoate. The bottom combines these two into a larger molecule that still ionizes, but now has six iodines per molecule (a 6:2 or 3:1 agent) ioxaglate. Because the combination results in fewer molecules in solution, it is referred to as a low-osmolar agent. (From Kern MJ, Seto AH. Society of cardiac angiography and intervention. In: Kern MJ, Seto AH, eds. *SCAI Interventional Cardiology Review.* 3rd ed. Philadelphia: Wolters Kluwer Health; 2018:490.)

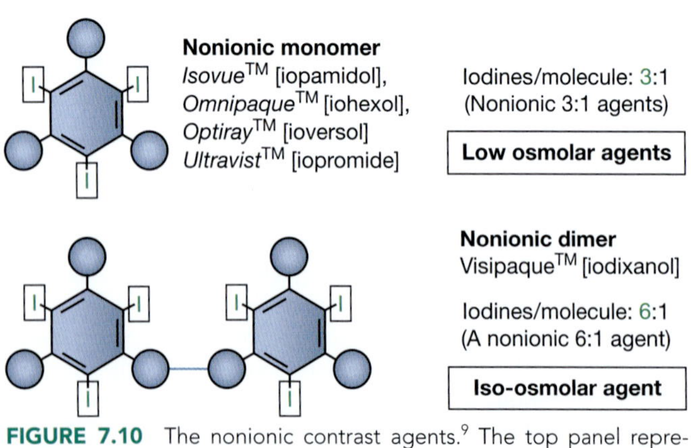

FIGURE 7.10 The nonionic contrast agents.[9] The top panel represents the nonionic agents, each with three iodines attached. Because there are fewer molecules in solution, these are considered low-osmolar agents. The bottom panel attaches two of these together and results in a 6:1 agent. Although a large molecule (increased viscosity), the number of molecules in solution is much lower and not too dissimilar to serum. It is referred to as an iso-osmolar agent. (From Kern MJ, Seto AH. Society of cardiac angiography and intervention. In: Kern MJ, Seto AH, eds. *SCAI Interventional Cardiology Review.* 3rd ed. Philadelphia: Wolters Kluwer Health; 2018:490.)

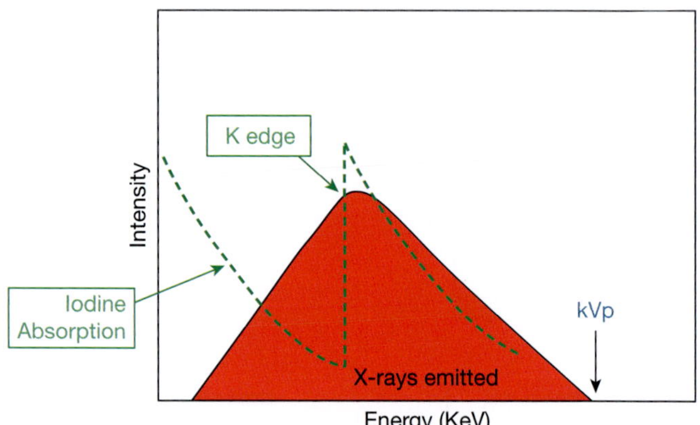

FIGURE 7.11 The X-ray spectrum and iodine absorption.[15] X-rays emitted from the X-ray tube are diverse in their energy levels with the maximal energy correlating with the kVp. When the iodine absorption curve overlies the energies sent from the X-ray tube, the dotted line is noted. Initially as the energy increases, the iodine absorbs less and then suddenly the energy from the K shell of the iodine is reached, and it absorbs much more of the X-ray energy. This is the K edge. This is the reason iodine is used to provide radiographic contrast. (From Bashore TM. Fundamentals of X-ray imaging, radiation safety, and contrast media. In: Kern MJ, ed. *SCAI 2012 Interventional Cardiology Review Book.* 2nd ed. Philadelphia, PA: Lippincott Williams & Wilkins; 2013:57-68.)

clinical practice in the 1980s and now are the contrast agent of choice.[47,48] While most are nonionic monomers, there are two dimeric compounds: one ionic dimer and one nonionic dimer.[46,48] These are listed in **Table 7.12**.

In addition to iconicity, contrast agents are characterized by two additional properties: osmolality and viscosity. Osmolality refers to the concentration of a solution expressed as the number of osmotically active molecules per fluid mass. CM are characterized most commonly by their osmolality in reference to the normal blood osmolality (280 mOsm/kg H_2O) and include high-osmolar, low-osmolar, and iso-osmolar contrast media (IOCM) agents. Ionic CM have anionic (usually a carboxyl group) and cationic (usually sodium) components that dissociate in solution resulting in a higher osmolality. Because nonionic CM do not ionize in solution, they have a lower osmolality (**Table 7.12**).[46] A nonionic agent may further increase their iodine carrying capacity/molecule and thereby further decrease there osmolality by becoming a dimer.[46] Viscosity refers to the resistance of the CM to flow. Viscosity is directly related to particle size and is inversely related to osmolality and temperature.[46]

High-osmolar contrast media (HOCM) are rarely used in the catheterization laboratory today.[39,40] HOCMs consist of ionic monomers (single benzene ring) and has an osmolality of >1400 mOsm/kg H_2O.[46] The HOCM agents have a ratio of three iodine atoms for every ion in solution (3:2) (**Fig. 7.8**). Many of the side effects, which include arrhythmic and hemodynamic side effects, are thought to result from the hypertonicity and ability to chelate calcium.[49] Low-osmolar contrast media (LOCM) have an osmolality of 500 to 1000 mOsm/kg H_2O, which is lower than the prior generation of CM but is hypertonic relative to normal blood plasma. The earliest developed LOCM agent, ioxaglate, is an ionic dimer. Ioxaglate has six iodines for every two molecules (6:2 or 3:1) (**Fig. 7.9**). Subsequent LOCM contrast agents (iopamidol, iohexol, ioxilan, ioversol, and iopromide) were developed and are nonionic monomers that have a 3:1 ratio of iodine per ion. The newest generation of CM agents is the IOCM. Iodixanol (Visipaque) is a nonionic dimer that has a 6:1 ratio of iodine per ion (**Fig. 7.10**). While its osmolality is similar to that of plasma, its larger molecular size results in a higher viscosity than that of the older-generation contrast agents. Warming the agent can reduce the viscosity of this agent.[46]

TABLE 7.12 Contrast Agents (Nonionic Both Monomeric and Dimeric)[9]

PRODUCT	TYPE OF CONTRAST AGENT	CONCENTRATION (MG/ML)	OSMOLALITY (MOSM/KG) OF WATER
Monomers			
Iohexol (Omnipaque)	Nonionic LOCM	350	844
Iopamidol (Isovue)	Nonionic LOCM	370	796
Ioxilan (Oxilan)	Nonionic LOCM	350	695
Iopromide (Ultravist)	Nonionic LOCM	370	774
Ioversol (Optiray)	Nonionic LOCM	350	792
Dimers			
Iodixanol (Visipaque)	Nonionic IOCM	320	290
Ioxaglate (Hexabrix)	Ionic LOCM	320	600

Ultravist is a registered trademark of Berlex Laboratories; Isovue is a registered trademark of Bracco Diagnostics; Omnipaque and Visipaque are registered trademarks of Nycomed, Inc; Optiray is a registered trademark of Mallinckrodt Medical, Inc; and Hexabrix is a registered trademark of Guerbet, S.A. IOCM, isosmolar contrast media; LOCM, low-osmolality contrast media.

From Kern MJ, Seto AH. Society of cardiac angiography and intervention. In: Kern MJ, Seto AH, eds. *SCAI Interventional Cardiology Review.* 3rd ed. Philadelphia: Wolters Kluwer Health; 2018:490.

Physiologic Effects of CM

Direct Cardiovascular Effects

CM can directly affect the cardiovascular system, which can manifest as impaired contractility/myocardial depression, peripheral vasodilation with hypotension, fluid overload, vasovagal response, and arrhythmias (bradycardia, atrioventricular conduction delay with heart block, QRS prolongation, and ventricular arrhythmias).[49] The increased osmolality and calcium-binding capacity of higher osmolality agents are thought to be responsible for these cardiovascular effects. These effects are transient and much less common with LOCM agents.[46]

Coagulation Issues

Both ionic and nonionic agents have anticoagulant and antiplatelet effects, these being pronounced with ionic agents. With the introduction of nonionic CM, there was a concern for potential thrombus formation in angiographic catheters. Initial in vitro and randomized clinical trials presented conflicting evidence regarding the procoagulant and antithrombotic effects of nonionic compared to ionic CM. However, further studies have identified no difference between ionic and nonionic agents regarding thrombotic complications of either type of agent.[50] Although minute thrombi may form when blood and nonionic contrast remain in a syringe, clinical sequelae have not been noted. In light of current anticoagulation regimens, possible differences in thrombogenic potential are likely negligible.[46]

Hyperthyroidism

Although the true incidence is unknown and likely very rare, the use of iodinated CM has been associated with both hyperthyroidism and hypothyroidism. The iodine load from CM is involved in the development of this pathologic state. The patients who are at the highest risk of developing thyrotoxicosis after contrast medium are patients with Graves disease, multinodular goiter, and patients living in areas of iodine deficiency.[51] The highest risk patients may benefit from an endocrinology evaluation.

COMPLICATIONS FROM THE USE OF CONTRAST AGENTS

CM adverse reactions are infrequent and range from 5% to 12% for HOCM and from 1% to 3% for LOCM.[49] When only serious adverse events are considered, the incidence for HOCM agents is estimated at about 1.0% compared with about 0.05% for LOCM agents. **Table 7.13** outlines the common complications associated with contrast agents in the cardiac catheterization laboratory. They include cardiovascular complications (both electrophysiologic and hemodynamic), hypersensitivity reactions (both acute and delayed), coagulation issues, hyperthyroidism, contrast-induced nephrotoxicity, and metformin-related lactic acidosis.[46]

Anaphylactoid Reactions

Immediate

Allergic reactions to iodinated CM occur in ≤1% of all procedures. Contrast reactions are not truly anaphylactic because they are not IgE mediated.[49,52,53] The best characterization is that they are anaphylactoid, in that they involve degranulation of mast cells and circulating basophils through direct complement activation. Therefore, CM reactions can occur even without previous exposure to contrast agents. These reactions are idiosyncratic, generally occur within 20 minutes of contrast administration, and are independent of contrast volume. This negates the potential benefits of "test dosing"

TABLE 7.13 Complications From Radiographic Contrast Media[9]

Hypersensitivity reactions
Anaphylactoid
Delayed
Direct cardiovascular effects
Hemodynamic and myocardial
Electrophysiologic
Potential coagulopathy
Contrast nephropathy
Others
Hyperthyroidism
Encephalopathy
Compartment syndrome (extravasation)

From Kern MJ, Seto AH. Society of cardiac angiography and intervention. In: Kern MJ, Seto AH, eds. *SCAI Interventional Cardiology Review.* 3rd ed. Philadelphia: Wolters Kluwer Health; 2018:490.

to determine potential reactivity. Hypersensitivity reactions occur at a higher incidence with HOCM compared to LOCM agents. Anaphylactoid reactions are more frequent in patients with a history of atopy (asthma, allergic rhinitis, atopic dermatitis, or food allergies) (three to five times), patients with previous reactions (four to six times), patients with cardiovascular and renal disease, and individuals on β-blockers.[52,53] It is a common misconception that shellfish allergies are associated with an allergy to iodinated CM. Although it was thought to be an "iodine" allergy, shellfish-specific tropomyosin is thought to be responsible for shellfish allergies.[54] Therefore, prophylaxis is not recommended in these patients.[23]

Although infrequent, serious contrast-mediated anaphylactoid reactions occur, so the symptoms and treatment are important to review (**Table 7.14**). The clinical presentation of anaphylactoid reactions may be mild (skin rash, itching, nasal discharge, nausea, and vomiting), moderate (persistence of mild symptoms, facial or laryngeal edema, bronchospasm, dyspnea, tachycardia, or bradycardia), or severe (life-threatening arrhythmias, hypotension, overt bronchospasm, laryngeal edema, pulmonary edema, seizure, syncope, and death). Severe reactions must be recognized and treated immediately with aggressive fluid resuscitation, antihistamines, and, if required, epinephrine (repeat boluses or infusion if necessary). Intubation may be necessary if there is evidence of airway compromise. Patients who are on β-blockers may not respond to epinephrine and should be treated with glucagon (boluses as needed every 5 minutes, followed by an infusion if necessary) if symptoms are refractory.[56]

Pretreatment for prevention of acute/immediate reactions is recommended for patients with a known prior allergy to contrast and potentially considered for the patient with a strong atopic history.[52,53] The recurrence rate of anaphylactoid reactions was initially estimated at 35%, a figure that originates from a single study in which a high-osmolar agent, Urografin, was used in aortic root injection. Several different treatment protocols exist, which may include glucocorticoids, H1 blockers, and H2 blockers (**Table 7.15**). Current regimens include oral prednisone 50 mg (13, 7, and 1 hour prior to the procedure) for nonurgent cases, often with the addition of H1 blockers (diphenhydramine, 50 mg). The benefit of H2 blocker therapy (cimetidine/ranitidine) is less well substantiated. With prophylaxis, recurrent reactions may occur but are unlikely. Limited data are available for emergent procedures in patients with known contrast-induced anaphylactoid reaction. Rapidly administering high-dose intravenous steroid or intravenous glucocorticoid (hydrocortisone or methylprednisolone) immediately upon recognizing the indication for the procedure, combined with the H1 blocker diphenhydramine, is an approach utilized when delaying the procedure is not an option.[55]

TABLE 7.14 Presentation and Treatment of Hypersensitivity Reactions[55]

SEVERITY	SYMPTOMS	MANAGEMENT
Mild	Urticarial rash Pruritus	Stop infusion Diphenhydramine 50 mg intravenous (IV) Observe for progression to severe
Severe	Hives Angioedema Laryngospasm causing stridor Bronchospasm with wheezing Respiratory distress Circulatory collapse (hypotension and tachycardia)	Stop contrast media infusion IM epinephrine 0.3-0.5 mg Intubation if clinically indicated Supplemental oxygen (at least 8-10 L) Normal saline boluses for hypotension Methyl prednisone 125 mg IV Diphenhydramine 50 mg IV Ranitidine 50 mg IV
Refractory symptoms	Patients with inadequate response to IM epinephrine and IV saline	Epinephrine continuous infusion, 2-10 μg/min Additional pressor if needed If patient on β-blockers and not responding to epinephrine: glucagon 1-5 mg IV over 5 min

From Klein LW. The use of radiographic contrast media during PCI: a focused review—a position statement of the Society of Cardiovascular Angiography and Interventions. *Catheter Cardiovasc Interv*. 2009;74:728-746.

TABLE 7.15 Prevention of Hypersensitivity Reactions From CM[55]

PATIENT STATUS	RECOMMENDED PROTOCOL
No previous history of contrast media reaction	Premedication not recommended
Previous history of adverse reaction (elective procedure)	Prednisone 50 mg orally 13, 7, and 1 h prior to procedure Diphenhydramine 50 mg PO 1 h prior to procedure
Previous history of adverse reaction (emergent procedure)	Hydrocortisone 200 mg intravenous (IV) once Diphenhydramine 50 mg IV

From Klein LW. The use of radiographic contrast media during PCI: a focused review—a position statement of the Society of Cardiovascular Angiography and Interventions. *Catheter Cardiovasc Interv*. 2009;74:728-746.

Delayed

The delayed reactions commonly occur within 2 days but can occur up to 5 days following contrast injection. Symptoms most commonly include rash, fever, fatigue, congestion, abdominal pain, diarrhea, constipation, and polyarthropathy.[49,52,53] These reactions are common (5%-8%) but frequently not identified due to the heterogeneous nature of their symptoms. Atopy has been well documented as an associated risk factor for the occurrence of both delayed and immediate reactions. Reactions such as the Koebner response, iodine sialadenitis, toxic epidermal necrolysis, and fatal acute vasculitis have all been reported as delayed reactions to CM. It is important to recognize this condition to prevent the unnecessary discontinuation of important medications, such as P2Y12 inhibitors, on the assumption the symptoms may be because of a new medication. Because these reactions are IgE and IgA mediated, they are generally self-limiting but often respond well to antihistamines. Steroids are rarely necessary. It is important to elicit any history of delayed contrast reaction, because these patients are at risk for immediate hypersensitivity on repeat exposure to contrast agents.[46]

Acute Kidney Injury: Contrast-Induced Nephropathy/ Contrast-Induced Acute Kidney Injury

Epidemiology

Acute kidney injury (AKI) is a major complication that may affect as many as 16% of patients undergoing cardiac catheterization.[57,58] While it is unclear if it is a marker of a patient's overall underlying disease severity, AKI after catheterization has been associated with worse outcomes, which include prolonged hospital stays, greater inpatient costs, short-term and long-term adverse outcomes.[59]

There are many potential etiologies of AKI after catheterization, including dehydration, hemodynamic instability, drug toxicity, atheroembolic disease/cholesterol embolization syndrome, and contrast-induced nephropathy (CIN), also referred to as contrast-induced acute kidney injury (CI-AKI).

The cause of CI-AKI has not been well defined. Direct cytotoxic effects to the renal tubules and ischemic injury to the renal medulla may develop secondary to the viscosity of contrast, vasoconstriction, or decreased vasodilation.[60] The loss of nitric oxide production secondary to oxidative stress may cause CI-AKI; this has been targeted in prevention.[61] The true incidence of CI-AKI after catheterization is unknown due to variations in definitions and populations studied. It is estimated to be around 3%.[62] CI-AKI has been defined as a rise in serum creatinine of at least 0.5 mg/dL or a 25% increase from baseline within 48 to 72 hours after contrast administration.[63] The Kidney Disease Improving Global Outcomes (KDIGO) working group has defined CI-AKI as any of the following: increase in serum creatinine by >0.3 mg/dL (>26.5 μmol/L) within 48 hours; increase in serum creatinine to >1.5 times baseline, which is known or presumed to have occurred within the prior 7 days; or urine volume <0.5 mL/kg/h for 6 hours.[64] The clinical course of CI-AKI is usually benign, with creatinine levels peaking approximately at 48 to 72 hours and returning to baseline within 1 to 2 weeks.[65] Occasionally, CI-AKI may progress, requiring hemodialysis in approximately 1% of patients who develop CI-AKI; this is higher in a patient with risk factors.[66,67]

Chronic kidney disease (CKD) is the most powerful predictor of subsequent CI-AKI. The risk of CI-AKI increases with the decrease in estimated glomerular filtration rate (eGFR), with increased risk defined as an eGFR <60 mL/min/1.73 m^2. Other important risk factors include presentation (acute coronary syndrome, heart failure, and cardiogenic shock), age, and history of diabetes mellitus, anemia, and volume of contrast used during the procedure.[46,59] Risk models (by Mehran et al, Gurm et al, and Tsai et al) have been developed to predict the risk of CI-AKI.[68-70] The amount of contrast used can also predict the risk of developing CI-AKI. A volume of contrast to creatinine clearance ratio (V/CrCl) of >3.7 is an independent predictor of increase in creatinine.[71] A maximal radiographic contrast dose has been defined as MRCD = 5 mL × body weight (kg)/serum creatinine (mg/dL). This formula, developed by Freeman et al,[66] represents the volume of contrast that predicts the risk of nephropathy requiring hemodialysis.

Prevention

With limited treatment options for CI-AKI, it is most important to reduce the risk with the goal to ultimately prevent its occurrence. However, despite significant advances in identification of risk, as well as therapeutic approaches for reduction of risk, CI-AKI is not preventable in the high-risk patient requiring contrast administration. Therefore, protocols must be in place to assure best practice for risk reduction and assessment of occurrence if prevention is not possible in the extremely high-risk patient.

Identification of the high-risk patient with assurance of adequate hydration is essential. Several prevention strategies that have been employed with negative or mixed results include increased diuresis (mannitol and furosemide), renal vasodilators (dopamine, theophylline, fenoldopam, calcium channel blockers, endothelin receptor antagonist, atrial natriuretic peptide, and prostacyclins), antioxidants (acetylcysteine, vitamin C, and trimetazidine), hypothermia, and IOCM (**Table 7.16**). Because of the risk for nephrogenic systemic fibrosis, gadolinium is not an alternative.[46,59]

The primary strategy that has yielded consistent results has been periprocedural hydration. Although several treatment regimens have been proposed, the CI-AKI Consensus Working Panel recommends intravenous volume expansion with isotonic crystalloid (1.0-1.5 mL/kg/h) for 3 to 12 hours preprocedurally and continuing for 6 to 24 hours postprocedurally.[72] Close observation is required in the patient with reduced ventricular function prone to heart failure. While there has been interest in encouraging oral hydration preprocedurally, results of trials have shown a potential increased risk of CI-AKI with only oral hydration.[73] However, appropriate reassessment of prolonged nothing by mouth periods preprocedure often need to be reassessed. In situations where there is evidence of inadequate periprocedural hydration, algorithms have been proposed for left ventricular end-diastolic pressure-guided periprocedural hydration rates.[74] Isotonic sodium bicarbonate results in alkalization, which may protect from free radical injury. While results of clinical trials evaluating sodium bicarbonate have shown some promise, meta-analysis suggests a limited additional benefit over intravenous saline.[75]

N-acetylcysteine (NAC) has been used as an antioxidant in the prevention of CI-AKI with conflicting results. Meta-analysis has not shown a significant benefit in reduction in CI-AKI with the use of NAC. Although this agent has not obviously shown a benefit, some advocate continued use for patients at the highest risk of developing nephropathy due to limited risk of therapy. Despite the fact that contrast is eliminated primarily via the kidneys, hemodialysis has not been shown to be effective in prevention of CI-AKI.

TABLE 7.16 Preventive Strategies for CIN[46]

PREVENTIVE STRATEGY	RECOMMENDATION
Hydration with normal saline	Strongly recommended for all patients
Hydration with sodium bicarbonate	No additional benefit over normal saline
Minimize amount of CM	Strongly recommended for all patients
Use of nonionic LOCM or IOCM	Recommended for all patients, especially if renal impairment is present
Hemodialysis	Not recommended
Continuous venovenous hemofiltration	Likely beneficial but not cost-effective
Systemic fenoldopam	Not recommended
Intrarenal fenoldopam	Further studies are required to establish effectiveness
Theophylline	Controversial—currently not recommended
N-acetylcysteine	No proven benefit Considering that it is safe and inexpensive, we do not recommend against its use
Ascorbic acid	Not recommended
Statins	Likely beneficial—further studies are required
RenalGuard System	Investigational device—not available for commercial use

CIN, contrast-induced nephropathy; IOCM, iso-osmolar contrast media; LOCM, low-osmolar contrast media.

Adapted from Georgios C, Baber U, Mehran R. In: Bhatt DL, ed. *Contrast Selection*, Vol. 2015. Philadelphia, PA: Saunders; 2016:105-112.

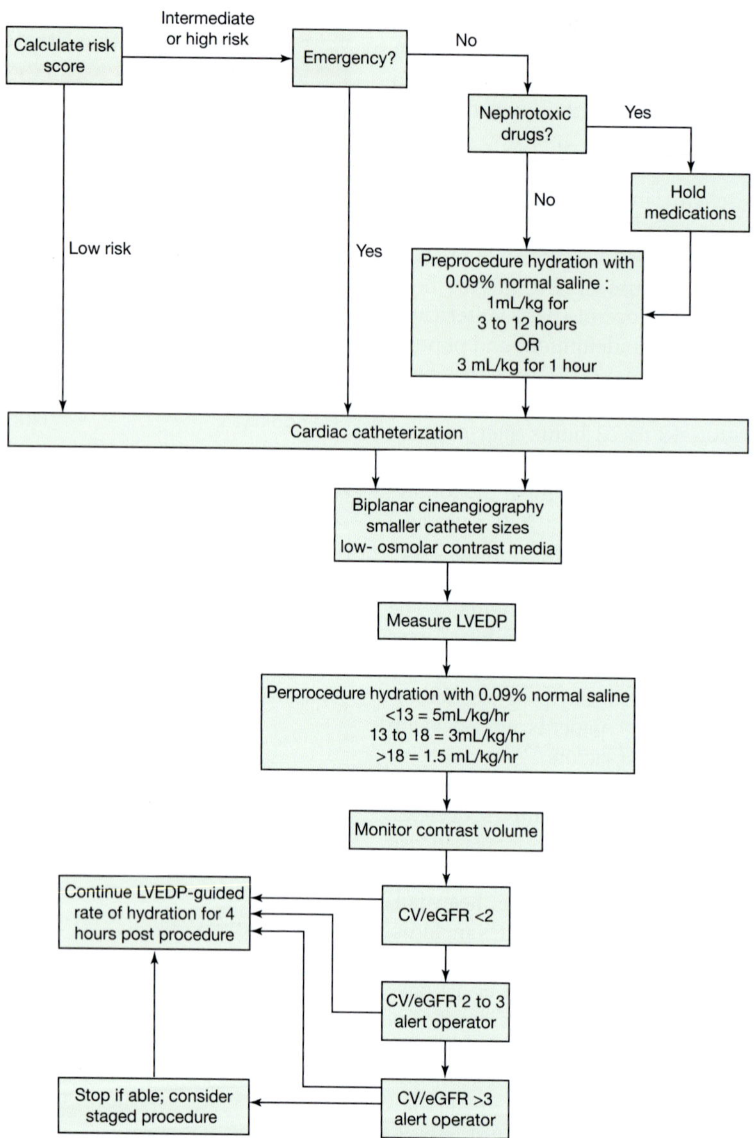

FIGURE 7.12 Algorithm for preventing/decreasing risk of CIN-AKI from contrast media.[9,59] AKI, acute kidney injury; CIN, contrast-induced nephropathy. (From Kern MJ, Seto AH. Society of cardiac angiography and intervention. In: Kern MJ, Seto AH, eds. *SCAI Interventional Cardiology Review.* 3rd ed. Philadelphia: Wolters Kluwer Health; 2018:490 and Allen SF, Nallamothu BK, Patel UD. Contrast-induced acute kidney injury and the role of chronic kidney disease in percutaneous coronary intervention. In: Topol EJ, Teirstein PS, eds. *Textbook of Interventional Cardiology.* 7th ed. 2015:108-117.)

Continuous venovenous hemofiltration has been shown to be protective against nephropathy but is invasive and arguably not cost-effective. High-dose statins have shown promise in prevention of CI-AKI,[76] although meta-analyses have questioned the benefit of statins in patients with baseline CKD,[77] with further studies needed to determine their role in therapy.

There are several strategies that can be employed to prevent CI-AKI. **Fig. 7.12** outlines the current approaches to reduce the incidence of contrast nephropathy.[23,78] Use of LOCM or IOCM agents has clearly resulted in decreased rates of CI-AKI. While theoretically more advantageous, the use of IOCM has not consistently reduced the rates of CI-AKI, although controversy still exists.[79] Limiting contrast volume is essential. Both before and during the procedure, the maximal contrast dose should be discussed with contrast dose management key. If available, biplane coronary angiography should be considered to reduce the contrast administered. Additionally, the contrast volume can be minimized by avoiding "test" injections, use of smaller French size catheters, careful selection of diagnostic imaging, and elimination of ventriculography/angiography.[59] Performing ad hoc percutaneous coronary intervention might not be best in the patient at risk for developing CI-AKI. If clinically appropriate, the patient should return for a "staged" procedure if there is concern about the volume of contrast administered. Staged procedures should allow for the 48- to 72-hour identification of possible CI-AKI and then deferred if needed until renal function recovers.[46,59] The catheterization laboratory quality improvement program should oversee local protocols for prevention and processes for patient follow-up.[23]

Metformin-Associated Lactic Acidosis

Metformin-associated lactic acidosis is a rare condition associated with renal failure in patients who take metformin. Although its onset occurs after the development of renal failure, *metformin is not related to CI-AKI*. It may have a mortality rate as high as 50%. Given that diabetics are at increased risk of developing CI-AKI, diabetic patients should not take their metformin on the day of the procedure and should resume it at 48 hours or when the creatinine has returned to a normal level.[80]

CONCLUSIONS

As a text for board review, the authors were asked to provide a basic understanding of radiation and contrast with facts and concepts more as a learning resource than as a practice tool. The physics of imaging and the biochemistry of contrast constitute a basic knowledge base required for the interventionist to intelligently manage the dose of these entities in the context of a multifaceted interventional procedure. The hope for this chapter is that it also provides the reader with the opportunity to incorporate this basic understanding of radiation and contrast, which is necessary for board review preparation but also to be applied as best practice in the catheterization laboratory.

Acknowledgments

Thank you, Dr Charles E. Chambers, MD, MSCAI for your mentorship and dedication to radiation safety and quality improvement in the field of interventional cardiology. This chapter could not have been completed without full access to the excellent prior chapter written by Dr Thomas Bashore. Additional thanks are extended to Dr Stephen Balter for his expertise in the field of radiation physics.

Key Points

X-Ray Formation

- Knowledge of the physics of imaging allows one to utilize the X-ray system to achieve the best image quality at the lowest dose through a balance of mA, kVp, and pulse width.
- Flat-panel image receptor technology provides for direct contact with the input phosphor, resulting in less image transfer creating the potential for improved image quality.
- Magnification in the flat-panel system differs from prior technology. Although now pixel based, it still requires increased dose to minimize noise and improve imaged quality.
- Understanding that image quality is directly related to dose allows the operator to accept the image quality required for the procedure to appropriately minimize radiation exposure.
- The current era of image acquisition and storage requires rapid Ethernet-transmission speeds for the acquiring images at mega-pixel resolution that are then "processed," "filtered," and presented for review, utilizing high-resolution monitors and cost-effective long-term terabyte capacity archival DICOM-based digital image storage with disaster recovery.

Radiation Safety

- Basic terminology requires an understanding of different kinds of assessments, appreciating that *absorbed* and *equivalent dose* is interchangeable in cardiac imaging and applies to the targeted organ, while *effective* dose extrapolates this to the potential total body doses.
- Fluoroscopy time is not an accurate assessment of dose because it does not account for cine, frame rate, patient size, image angulations, etc. Therefore, total air kerma at the IRP (CAK) and air KAP (DAP) should be measured and reported for all invasive interventional cardiac procedures.
- All ionizing radiations have the potential to produce breaks in the DNA backbone, single or double stranded, and either directly or indirectly result in two risk classifications.
- Deterministic events require a well-defined, linear, dose-dependent threshold effect resulting in tissue injury (ie, skin). Stochastic events (cancers, mutations) are probability based, linear to dose (the higher the radiation dose, the higher the probability of an event), but not threshold dependent (no specific dose for an individual to produce a defined event).
- Air KAP is a measure of the total radiation delivered to a body area and correlates more with stochastic injury. Total air kerma at the IRP is a point dose in space, approximating skin dose, and correlating with deterministic injury.
- Pre, during, and postcase dose management is required with initial patient assessment, in lab radiation dose management, and appropriate postcase follow-up when a high dose is utilized.
- Best practices in the laboratory require dose management from the outset of the case. Patient dose exposure can be minimized by using collimation, limiting magnified views, using the fewest number of frames, avoiding steep angles, keeping the image receptor close to the patient, spending the least amount of "on pedal time," and limiting unnecessary cine acquisition.
- Operator/staff exposure requires an understanding of time, distance, and shielding with best practices for the patient safety correlating to operator and staff safety.
- Personnel dosimeters should be worn by all for individual assessment of risk. While two badges, outside at collar and inside at waist, are often recommended, one badge at collar worn correctly is an adequate assessment and is better than two badges worn incorrectly.
- Pregnant women may continue to work in the catheterization laboratory as long as they see a radiation safety officer and wear an additional badge under their lead.
- The maximal dose of occupational radiation exposure is 50 mSv/y or your age × 10 mSv for a lifetime to reduce stochastic effects. The annual cutoff is 150 mSv/y for deterministic effects (eye); however, eye injury may be evident at lower exposure.

Contrast Media

- Osmolality relates to the number of molecules in solution, with the terms ionic and nonionic referring to whether they dissociate or do not dissociate in solution, respectively. By not ionizing, the three iodine benzene ring is a low-osmolar 3:1 agent (ie, iopamidol, iohexol). Creating a nonionic dimer produces a 6:1 agent (iodixanol) that is iso-osmolar to serum.
- The most clinically impactful complications from CM include immediate and delayed hypersensitivity and CI-AKI. These complications have decreased significantly since the introduction of LOCM.
- Treatment of anaphylactoid reactions includes generous fluid administration, epinephrine (severe reactions), and other supportive measures. Glucagon can be given if the patient is on β-blockers. These reactions are idiosyncratic and more

common in atopic individuals. Shellfish allergy invokes a separate allergen; therefore, pretreatment is not required.

- Pretreatment with steroids is effective in reducing the incidence of an anaphylactoid reaction but necessitates initiation of therapy at least 12 to 13 hours prior to contrast. H1 blockers are often combined with steroids. However, H2 blockers are often used but with little data.
- CIN, also known as CI-AKI, after administration of contrast agents is most seen in high-risk patients with baseline impaired renal function and diabetes. Protocols must be in place to assure these patients are identified preprocedure, with methods to reduce the risk employed.
- If AKI/CIN is not prevented, it is associated with worse outcomes, including increased morbidity and mortality, and/or prolonged hospital stays with associated costs.
- Methods to reduce and ideally prevent AKI/CIN are primarily focused on ensuring adequate hydration pre- and postprocedure, as well as limiting procedural contrast load. Because renal impairment is seldom evident until 48 to 72 hours postcontrast, a follow-up program should be in place to identify these high-risk patients.

References

1. Ionizing radiation, health effects and protective measures. 2023. Available at: https://www.who.int/news-room/fact-sheets/detail/ionizing-radiation-health-effects-and-protective-measures
2. *X-Ray—Fundamental Characteristics*. Britannica; 2023. Available at: https://www.britannica.com/science/X-ray/Fundamental-characteristics
3. Basics of X-ray physics—tissue densities. 2023. Available at: https://www.radiologymasterclass.co.uk/tutorials/physics/x-ray_physics_densities
4. Radiology-TIP—Database. Latent image. 2023. Available at: https://www.radiology-tip.com/serv1.php?type=db1&dbs=Latent%20Image
5. Hall E. *Radiobiology for the Radiologist*. 5th ed. Lippincott Williams and Wilkins; 2000:234-248.
6. Valentin J; International Commission on Radiation Protection. Managing patient dose in multi-detector computed tomography(MDCT). ICRP Publication 102. *Ann ICRP*. 2007;37(1):1-332.
7. Table 7.1: tissue weighting factors according to ICRP 103 (ICRP 2007)—Figures and Tables—European Commission. 2023. Available at: https://ec.europa.eu/health/scientific_committees/opinions_layman/security-scanners/en/figtableboxes/tissue-weighting-factors.htm
8. Balter S, Miller DL. Patient skin reactions from interventional fluoroscopy procedures. *AJR Am J Roentgenol*. 2014;202(4):W335-W342.
9. Kern MJ, Seto AH; Society of Cardiac Angiography and Intervention. In: Kern MJ, Seto AH, eds. *SCAI Interventional Cardiology Review*. 3rd ed. Wolters Kluwer Health; 2018:490. Available at: https://www.ncbi.nlm.nih.gov/nlmcatalog/101715986
10. Balter S. *NCRP Radiation Dose Management for Fluoroscopically Guided Interventional Medical Procedures*. National Council on Radiation Protection and Measures; 2015. Available at: http://www.ncrppublications.org/Reports/168
11. The National Academics of Sciences Engineering Medicine. *Health Risks From Exposure to Low Levels of Ionizing Radiation: BEIR VII Phase 2. Consensus Study Report*; 2010. Available at: http://www.nap.edu/catalog.php?record_id=11340#toc
12. Heidbuchel H, Wittkampf FHM, Vano E, et al. Practical ways to reduce radiation dose for patients and staff during device implantations and electrophysiological procedures. *Europace*. 2014;16(7):946-964.
13. Balter S. Administrative Policies for Managing Substantial Dose Procedures and Tissue Reactions Associated with Fluoroscopically Guided Interventions (FGI). NCRP; 2010.
14. Chambers CE, Fetterly KA, Holzer R, et al. Radiation safety program for the cardiac catheterization laboratory. *Catheter Cardiovasc Interv*. 2011;77(4):546-556.
15. Bashore TM. Fundamentals of X-ray imaging, radiation safety, and contrast media. In: Kern MJ, ed. *SCAI 2012 Interventional Cardiology Review Book*. 2nd ed. Wolters Kluwer publishers; 2013:57-68.
16. Chambers CE. Radiation dose monitoring in the cath lab: is fluoroscopy time enough? *Catheter Cardiovasc Interv*. 2013;82(7):1106-1107.
17. National Council on Radiation Protection and Measurement. Recommendations for limits on exposure to ionizing radiation. NCRP Report (116); 2015. Available at: http://www.ncrponline.org/Publications/Press_Releases/116press.html
18. Einstein AJ, Berman DS, Min JK, et al. Patient-centered imaging: shared decision making for cardiac imaging procedures with exposure to ionizing radiation. *J Am Coll Cardiol*. 2014;63(15):1480-1489.
19. 1990 Recommendations of the International Commission on Radiological Protection. *Ann ICRP*. 1991;21(1-3):1-201.
20. FDA Center for Devices and Radiologic Health. Initiative to Reduce Radiation Exposure from Medical Imaging. FDA Library Publication; 2019.
21. NCRP. Medical Radiation Exposure of Patients in the United States. Report No. 184. 2019;(18). Available at: https://ncrponline.org/shop/reports/report-no-184-medical-radiation-exposure-of-patients-in-the-united-states-2019/
22. Fetterly KA, Mathew V, Lennon R, Bell MR, Holmes DR Jr, Rihal CS. Radiation dose reduction in the invasive cardiovascular laboratory. Implementing a culture and philosophy of radiation safety. *JACC Cardiovasc Interv*. 2012;5(8):866-873.
23. Levine GL. ACCF/AHA/SCAI guidelines for percutaneous coronary intervention. *J Am Coll Cardiol*. 2011;58:44-122.
24. Duran A, Hian SK, Miller DL, Le Heron J, Padovani R, Vano E. Recommendations for occupational radiation protection in interventional cardiology. *Catheter Cardiovasc Interv*. 2013;82(1):29-42.
25. Christopoulos G, Papayannis AC, Alomar M, et al. Effect of a real-time radiation monitoring device on operator radiation exposure during cardiac catheterization: the radiation reduction during cardiac catheterization using real-time monitoring study. *Circ Cardiovasc Interv*. 2014;7(6):744-750.
26. Best PJ. SCAI consensus document on occupational radiation exposure to the pregnant cardiologist and technical personnel. *EuroIntervention*. 2011;77:232-241.
27. Dauer LT, Miller DL, Schueler B, et al. Occupational radiation protection of pregnant or potentially pregnant workers in IR: a joint guideline of the Society of Interventional Radiology and the Cardiovascular and Interventional Radiological Society of Europe. *J Vasc Interv Radiol*. 2015;26(2):171-181.
28. Cheney AE, Vincent LL, McCabe JM, Kearney KE. Pregnancy in the cardiac catheterization laboratory: a safe and feasible endeavor. *Circ Cardiovasc Interv*. 2021;14(4):E009636.
29. National Council on Radiation Protection and Measurement. Implementation of the principle of as low as reasonably achievable (Alara) for medical and dental personnel. NCRP report no 107. 1990:126. Available at: https://ncrponline.org/shop/reports/report-no-107-implementation-of-the-principle-of-as-low-as-reasonably-achievable-alara-for-medical-and-dental-personnel-1990/
30. Griffiths HJ. Radiation protection for medical and allied health personnel. NCRP report no. 105. *Radiology*. 1990;176(3):702. Available at: https://pubs.rsna.org/doi/10.1148/radiology.176.3.702
31. Kneale GW, Stewart AM. Mantel-haenszel analysis of Oxford data. II. Independent effects of fetal irradiation subfactors. *J Natl Cancer Inst*. 1976;57(5):1009-1014.
32. Wagner LK, Hayman LA. Pregnancy and women radiologists. *Radiology*. 1982;145(2):559-562.
33. International Commission on Radiation Units and Measurement; 2005. Available at: http://www.iaea.org/ns/tutorials/regcontrol/intro/resources.htm
34. Kim KP, Miller DL, Balter S, et al. Occupational radiation doses to operators performing cardiac catheterization procedures. *Health Phys*. 2008;94(3):211-227.
35. Hirshfeld JW Jr, Balter S, Brinker JA, et al. ACCF/AHA/HRS/SCAI clinical competence statement on physician knowledge to optimize patient safety and image quality in fluoroscopically guided invasive cardiovascular procedures: a report of the American College of Cardiology Foundation/American Heart Association/American College of Physicians Task Force on clinical competence and training. *Circulation*. 2005;111:511-532.

36. Chida K, Inaba Y, Saito H, et al. Radiation dose of interventional radiology system using a flat-panel detector. *AJR Am J Roentgenol*. 2009;193(6):1680-1685.
37. Agarwal S, Parashar A, Bajaj NS, et al. Relationship of beam angulation and radiation exposure in the cardiac catheterization laboratory. *JACC Cardiovasc Interv*. 2014;7(5):558-566.
38. Abdelaal E, Plourde G, MacHaalany J, et al. Effectiveness of low rate fluoroscopy at reducing operator and patient radiation dose during transradial coronary angiography and interventions. *JACC Cardiovasc Interv*. 2014;7(5):567-574.
39. Maeder M, Brunner-La Rocca HP, Wolber T, et al. Impact of a lead glass screen on scatter radiation to eyes and hands in interventional cardiologists. *Catheter Cardiovasc Interv*. 2006;67(1):18-23.
40. Karadag B, Ikitimur B, Durmaz E, et al. Effectiveness of a lead cap in radiation protection of the head in the cardiac catheterisation laboratory. *EuroIntervention*. 2013;9(6):754-756.
41. Scott H, Gallagher S, Abbott W, Talboys M. Assessment of occupational dose reduction with the use of a floor mounted mobile lead radiation protection shield. *J Radiol Prot*. 2022;42(3).
42. Dixon SR, Rabah M, Emerson S, Schultz C, Madder RD. A novel catheterization laboratory radiation shielding system: results of pre-clinical testing. *Cardiovasc Revasc Med*. 2022;36:51-55.
43. Ciraj-Bjelac O, Rehani M, Minamoto A, Sim KH, Liew HB, Vano E. Radiation-induced eye lens changes and risk for cataract in interventional cardiology. *Cardiology*. 2012;123(3):168-171.
44. Reeves RR, Ang L, Bahadorani J, et al. Invasive cardiologists are exposed to greater left sided cranial radiation: the BRAIN study (brain radiation exposure and attenuation during invasive cardiology procedures). *JACC Cardiovasc Interv*. 2015;8(9):1197-1206.
45. Klein LW, Tra Y, Garratt KN, et al. Occupational health hazards of interventional cardiologists in the current decade: results of the 2014 SCAI membership survey. *Catheter Cardiovasc Interv*. 2015;86(5):913-924.
46. Georgios C, Baber U, Mehran R. In: Bhatt DL, ed. *Contrast Selection*. In: *Braunwald's Heart Disease*. Vol. 2015. Saunders; 2016:105-112.
47. Siegle RL. Rates of idiosyncratic reactions. Ionic versus nonionic contrast media. *Invest Radiol*. 1993;28:S95-S99.
48. Solomon R. Contrast media: are there differences in nephrotoxicity among contrast media? *BioMed Res Int*. 2014;2014:934947.
49. Bottinor W, Polkampally P, Jovin I. Adverse reactions to iodinated contrast media. *Int J Angiol*. 2013;22(3):149-154.
50. Reiner JS. Contrast media and clotting: what is the evidence? *Catheter Cardiovasc Interv*. 2010;75(suppl 1):S35-S38.
51. Lee SY, Rhee CM, Leung AM, Braverman LE, Brent GA, Pearce EN. A review: radiographic iodinated contrast media-induced thyroid dysfunction. *J Clin Endocrinol Metab*. 2015;100(2):376-383.
52. Idee JM, Pinès E, Prigent P, Corot C. Allergy-like reactions to iodinated contrast agents. A critical analysis. *Fundam Clin Pharmacol*. 2005;19(3):263-281.
53. Brockow K, Ring J. Anaphylaxis to radiographic contrast media. *Curr Opin Allergy Clin Immunol*. 2011;11(4):326-331.
54. Huang SW. Seafood and iodine: an analysis of a medical myth. *Allergy Asthma Proc*. 2005;26(6):468-469.
55. Klein LW, Sheldon MW, Brinker J, et al. The use of radiographic contrast media during PCI: a focused review—a position statement of the Society of Cardiovascular Angiography and Interventions. *Catheter Cardiovasc Interv*. 2009;74(5):728-746.
56. Javeed N, Javeed H, Javeed S, Moussa G, Wong P, Rezai F. Refractory anaphylactoid shock potentiated by beta-blockers. *Cathet Cardiovasc Diagn*. 1996;39(4):383-384.
57. Fox CS, Muntner P, Chen AY, Alexander KP, Roe MT, Wiviott SD. Short-term outcomes of acute myocardial infarction in patients with acute kidney injury: a report from the national cardiovascular data registry. *Circulation*. 2012;125(3):497-504.
58. Tsai TT, Patel UD, Chang TI, et al. Contemporary incidence, predictors, and outcomes of acute kidney injury in patients undergoing percutaneous coronary interventions: insights from the NCDR Cath-PCI registry. *JACC Cardiovasc Interv*. 2014;7:1-9.
59. Allen SF, Nallamothu BK, Patel UD. Contrast-induced acute kidney injury and the role of chronic kidney disease in percutaneous coronary intervention. In: Topol EJ, Teirstein PS, eds. *Textbook of Interventional Cardiology*. 7th ed. Elsevier; 2015:108-117.
60. Persson PB, Tepel M. Contrast medium-induced nephropathy: the pathophysiology. *Kidney Int Suppl*. 2006;100:S8-S10.
61. Katholi RE, Woods WT Jr, Taylor GJ, et al. Oxygen free radicals and contrast nephropathy. *Am J Kidney Dis*. 1998;32(1):64-71.
62. Rihal CS, Textor SC, Grill DE, et al. Incidence and prognostic importance of acute renal failure after percutaneous coronary intervention. *Circulation*. 2002;105(19):2259-2264.
63. McCullough PA, Adam A, Becker CR, et al. Epidemiology and prognostic implications of contrast-induced nephropathy. *Am J Cardiol*. 2006;98(6A):5K-13K.
64. Kidney Disease Improving Global Outcomes (KDIGO) Acute Kidney Injury Work Group. KDIGO clinical practice guideline for acute kidney injury. *Kidney Inter*. 2012;2:1-138.
65. Thomsen HS, Morcos SK. Contrast media and the kidney: European Society of Urogenital Radiology (ESUR) guidelines. *Br J Radiol*. 2003;76(908):513-518.
66. Freeman RV, O'Donnell M, Share D, et al. Nephropathy requiring dialysis after percutaneous coronary intervention and the critical role of an adjusted contrast dose. *Am J Cardiol*. 2002;90(10):1068-1073.
67. Nikolsky E, Mehran R, Turcot D, et al. Impact of chronic kidney disease on prognosis of patients with diabetes mellitus treated with percutaneous coronary intervention. *Am J Cardiol*. 2004;94(3):300-305.
68. Mehran R, Aymong ED, Nikolsky E, et al. A simple risk score for prediction of contrast-induced nephropathy after percutaneous coronary intervention: development and initial validation. *J Am Coll Cardiol*. 2004;44(7):1393-1399.
69. Gurm HS, Seth M, Kooiman J, Share D. A novel tool for reliable and accurate prediction of renal complications in patients undergoing percutaneous coronary intervention. *J Am Coll Cardiol*. 2013;61(22):2242-2248.
70. Tsai TT, Patel UD, Chang TI, et al. Validated contemporary risk model of acute kidney injury in patients undergoing percutaneous coronary interventions: insights from the National Cardiovascular Data Registry Cath-PCI Registry. *J Am Heart Assoc*. 2014;3(6):e001380.
71. Laskey WK, Jenkins C, Selzer F, et al. Volume-to-creatinine clearance ratio: a pharmacokinetically based risk factor for prediction of early creatinine increase after percutaneous coronary intervention. *J Am Coll Cardiol*. 2007;50(7):584-590.
72. Caixeta A, Mehran R. Evidence-based management of patients undergoing PCI: contrast-induced acute kidney injury. *Catheter Cardiovasc Interv*. 2010;75(suppl 1):S15-S20.
73. Trivedi HS, Moore H, Nasr S, et al. A randomized prospective trial to assess the role of saline hydration on the development of contrast nephrotoxicity. *Nephron Clin Pract*. 2003;93(1):C29-C34.
74. Howe M, Gurm HS. A practical approach to preventing renal complications in the catheterization laboratory. *Interv Cardiol Clin*. 2014;3:429-439.
75. Subramaniam RM, Suarez-Cuervo C, Wilson RF, et al. Effectiveness of prevention strategies for contrast-induced nephropathy: a systematic review and meta-analysis. *Ann Intern Med*. 2016;164(6):406-416.
76. Leoncini M, Toso A, Maioli M, Tropeano F, Villani S, Bellandi F. Early high-dose rosuvastatin for contrast-induced nephropathy prevention in acute coronary syndrome: results from the PRATO-ACS Study (Protective effect of Rosuvastatin and antiplatelet therapy on contrast-induced acute kidney injury and myocardial damage in patients with Acute Coronary Syndrome. *J Am Coll Cardiol*. 2014;63(1):71-79.
77. Zhang BC, Li WM, Xu YW. High-dose statin pretreatment for the prevention of contrast-induced nephropathy: a meta-analysis. *Can J Cardiol*. 2011;27(6):851-858.
78. Amsterdam EA, Wenger NK, Brindis RG, et al. 2014 AHA/ACC guideline for the management of patients with non-ST-elevation acute coronary syndromes: a report of the American College of Cardiology/American Heart Association Task Force on Practice Guidelines. *J Am Coll Cardiol*. 2014;64(24):e139-e228.
79. Biondi-Zoccai G, Lotrionte M, Thomsen HS, et al. Nephropathy after administration of iso-osmolar and low-osmolar contrast media: evidence from a network meta-analysis. *Int J Cardiol*. 2014;172(2):375-380.
80. DeFronzo R, Fleming GA, Chen K, Bicsak TA. Metformin-associated lactic acidosis: current perspectives on causes and risk. *Metabolism*. 2016;65(2):20-29.

Coronary Angiography for Percutaneous Coronary Intervention

Morton J. Kern, Arnold H. Seto, and Nathaniel Smilowitz

Coronary angiography for percutaneous coronary intervention (PCI) should characterize vessel caliber, lesion location, length, morphology, and degree of calcification (or thrombus), as well as the relationship of atherosclerosis to side branches. Knowledge of optimal angiographic projections and coronary anatomy can guide catheter selection, visualize the target vessel course without significant foreshortening and estimate the true (maximally vasodilated) dimensions of the target vessel to facilitate optimal treatment.

Optimal definition of the ostial and proximal coronary segment is critical to guide PCI catheter selection. Assessment of calcium from angiography is less reliable than from intravascular ultrasound imaging (IVUS) or optical coherence tomographic imaging but still serves a useful purpose when considering plaque modification using rotational atherectomy, intravascular coronary lithotripsy, or use of an intracoronary laser.

Coronary angiography identifies anatomic features associated with prognosis and procedural risks and confirms successful coronary intervention.

For planned PCI in patients with chronic total vessel occlusion (CTO), angiography assesses the feasibility and limits of successful intervention. When CTO PCI is considered, the distal vessel should be visualized as clearly as possible. Adequate angiography requires cineangiography of sufficient duration to visualize late collateral vessel filling and the length of the occluded segment and may require the simultaneous "dual" injection of collateral supply arteries with a second catheter. A complete understanding of basic angiographic techniques, angulations, and access for PCI can be found elsewhere.[1-4]

Longer procedures engender more radiation exposure. PCI procedures are longer than diagnostic procedures.[5-7] Reducing radiation exposure without loss of good visualization should be the goal of all angiographic procedures. This goal requires continued awareness of the inverse square law of radiation propagation to reduce the exposure to patients, interventional operators, and cath lab teams. Obtaining quality angiographic images should not necessitate increasing the ordinary procedural radiation exposure to either the patient or catheterization personnel.

COMMON ANGIOGRAPHIC VIEWS FOR PCI

The nomenclature for angiographic views will be reviewed briefly here, emphasizing the optimal visualization of coronary anatomy to guide appropriate revascularization. Classic terminology for angiographic projections with regard to left and right anterior oblique, cranial and caudal angulation, and lateral projections is defined in previous discussions of diagnostic coronary angiography.

Anteroposterior Imaging

The image intensifier is positioned directly above the patient, with the beam perpendicular to the patient lying supine on the radiography table (**Fig. 8.1**). The anteroposterior (AP) view or shallow right anterior oblique (RAO) view displays ***the left main coronary artery*** in its entire perpendicular length. In this view, the branches of the left anterior descending (LAD) and left circumflex coronary artery branches overlap. In patients with acute coronary syndromes, starting with an AP view with caudal angulation can exclude left main or ostial LAD stenosis and will facilitate PCI. The AP cranial view is also excellent for visualizing the entire LAD, with septals moving to the left (on screen) and diagonals to the right, helping wire placement.

Right Anterior Oblique Imaging

The RAO caudal view shows the left main coronary artery bifurcation, providing excellent visualization of the origin and course of the circumflex/obtuse marginals, ramus intermediate branch, and proximal LAD segment. The LAD beyond the proximal segment is often obscured by overlapped diagonals. The RAO cranial or AP cranial views are used to open the diagonals along the mid- and distal LAD.

For the right coronary artery (RCA), the RAO view shows the mid-RCA and the length of the posterior descending artery and posterolateral branches. Patent ductus arteriosus (PDA) septals may show an occluded LAD via collaterals. The posterolateral branches overlap and may be best displayed with cranial angulation.

Left Anterior Oblique Imaging

The left anterior oblique (LAO) cranial view shows a foreshortened left main coronary artery and the full course of the LAD. Septal and diagonal branches are separated clearly. The circumflex and marginals are foreshortened and overlapped. Cranial angulation tilts the left main coronary artery down and permits visualization of the LAD/circumflex bifurcation.

For the RCA, the LAO cranial view shows the origin of the artery, its entire length, and the posterior descending artery bifurcation (crux). Cranial angulation tilts the posterior descending artery down to reduce foreshortening. A single angiogram in the LAO cranial view is often sufficient to provide a complete view of the RCA.

The LAO caudal view ("spider" view) shows a foreshortened left main coronary artery but excellent visualization of the bifurcation of the circumflex and LAD. Proximal and midportions of the circumflex and the origins of obtuse marginal branches are well seen. The LAD is markedly foreshortened in this view (**Fig. 8.2**).

A left lateral view shows the mid- and distal LAD best. This view is best to see coronary artery bypass graft (CABG) conduit anastomosis to the LAD. The LAD and circumflex are well separated. Diagonals usually overlap. The course of the (ramus) intermediate branch is also well visualized.

For the RCA, the lateral view also shows the origin (especially in those with more anteriorly oriented orifices) and the mid-RCA well. The posterior descending artery and posterolateral branches are foreshortened.

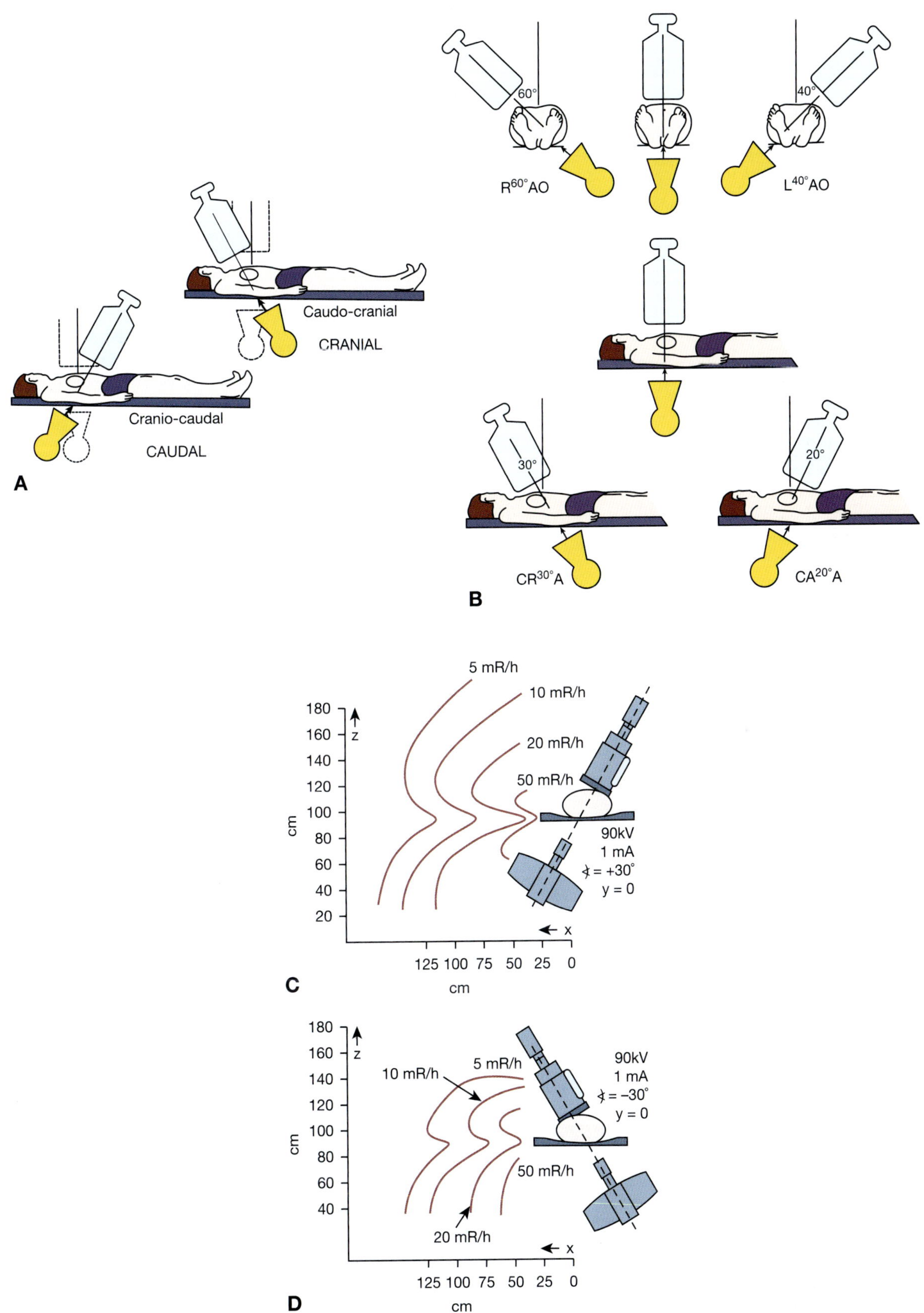

FIGURE 8.1 Diagrammatic view of image intensifier for common angiographic projections. Left Panel **A**, diagrams of cranial and caudal angulation. Center Panel **B**, positions for left and right anterior oblique (LAO, RAO) views and anteroposterior view. Right, radiation isobars showing field of exposure for LAO (Panel **C**) and RAO (Panel **D**) angulations. (From *Kern's Cath Lab Handbook*. 7th ed. Original figures modified from Paulin S. Terminology for radiographic projections in cardiac angiography. *Cathet Cardiovasc Diagn*. 1981;7:341.)

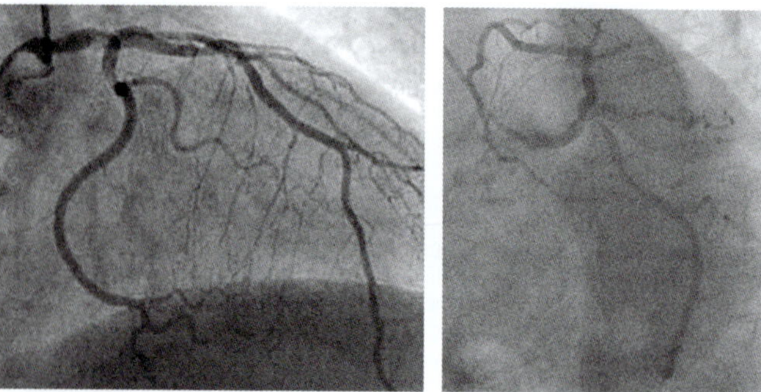

FIGURE 8.2 Frame from cineangiogram showing LM narrowing in RAO (*left*) and LAO caudal (*right*). Ostial CFX was not well seen until LAO caudal was reviewed. CFX, circumflex artery; LAO, left anterior oblique; LM, left main; RAO, right anterior oblique.

Angulations for Saphenous Bypass Grafts

Coronary artery saphenous vein grafts are visualized in at least two views (LAO and RAO). It is important to show the aortic anastomosis, the body of the graft, and the distal anastomosis. The distal runoff and continued flow or collateral channels are also critical. The graft vessel anastomosis is best seen in the view that depicts the native vessel best (**Figs. 8.3** and **8.4**; **Table 8.1**). The graft views can be summarized as follows:

1. RCA graft: LAO cranial/RAO, and lateral
2. LAD graft (or internal mammary artery): lateral, RAO cranial, LAO cranial, and AP (the lateral view is especially useful to visualize the anastomosis to the LAD)
3. Circumflex (and obtuse marginals) grafts: LAO and RAO caudal

General Strategy for Coronary Artery Bypass Graft Angiography

Following native LCA and RCA angiography and visualization of missing or reciprocally filled vessel segments, saphenous vein graft (SVG) angiography is performed using views known for specific coronary artery segments with contingency views for confusing or overlapped arteries.

SVG to RCA (lowest, see **Fig. 8.4**) is best engaged in an LAO projection. The graft travels downward, paralleling the RCA. A multipurpose catheter or Judkins right (JR) catheter is preferred with other options, which include a right coronary bypass graft catheter or an Amplatz right modified catheter. The best views for these grafts are LAO cranial, RAO, and AP cranial.

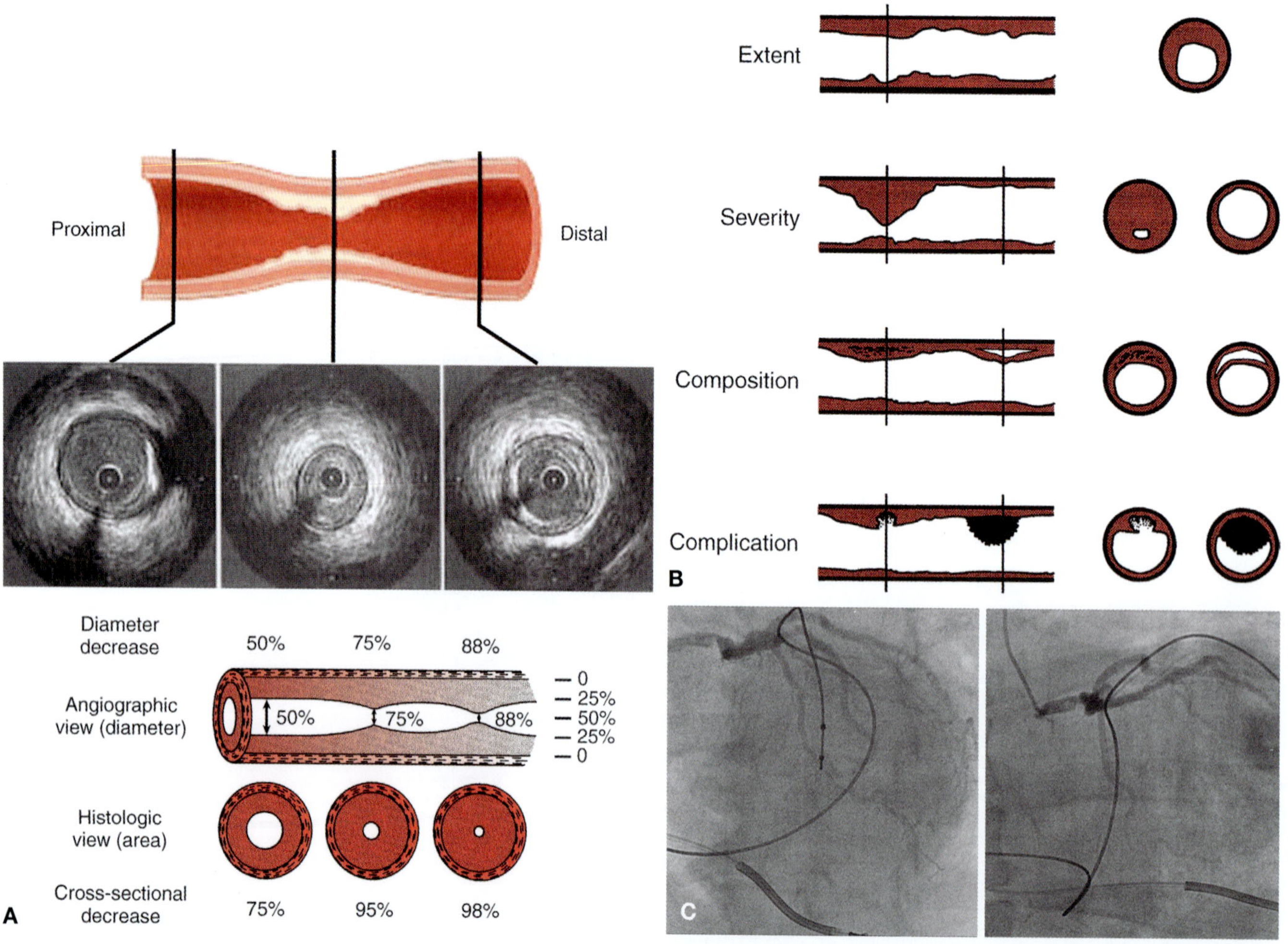

FIGURE 8.3 **A:** Diagram of coronary artery with stenosis (*top*) and corresponding intravascular ultrasound images demonstrating diffuse nature of coronary artery disease. The percent narrowing is compared only to the "normal"-appearing angiographic lumen, which may not be normal at all. **B:** Characteristics of different angiographic lesions. **C:** Frame from cineangiogram showing clot in left main segment as lucent filling defect. View best seen was RAO caudal.

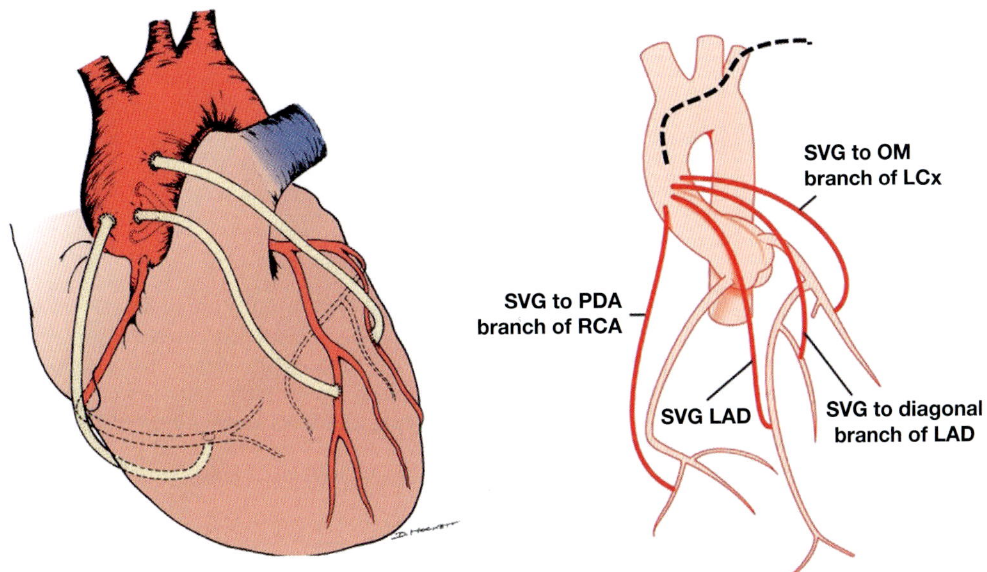

FIGURE 8.4 Saphenous vein graft (SVG) angiography. LAD, left anterior descending artery; LCx, left circumflex artery; OM, obtuse marginal; PDA, posterior descending artery; RAO, right anterior oblique; RCA, right coronary artery. Source, internet.

A. **SVG to LAD** (second lowest, above RCA): The LAD SVG graft typically originates from the anatomic leftward aspect of the anterior aorta and is best engaged in RAO using a JR4 (Judkins right, 4 cm), left coronary bypass (LCB), or Amplatz left (AL) catheter. The best views for a LAD graft are lateral, RAO cranial, LAO cranial, and AP (the lateral view is especially useful to visualize the anastomosis to the LAD).
B. **SVG to diagonal:** Diagonal SVGs also are best visualized in the RAO projection and using the same catheters as those used for SVG to LAD. Often, a slight clockwise rotation from an inferior graft permits the JR4 to engage this graft. The best views for SVGs to diagonal are LAO cranial and RAO cranial.
C. **SVG to obtuse marginal** (highest SVG on the aorta): SVG marginal grafts are best engaged in RAO projections using a JR4, LCB, or AL catheter. The best views for an SVG to obtuse marginal are caudal (LAO to RAO).
D. **LIMA to the LAD**: The left internal mammary artery (LIMA) is best approached from the left arm or leg with an internal mammary artery (IMA) curved catheter. The right internal mammary artery (RIMA) can be cannulated in the same way via the right arm or leg. The best view to see the LIMA-LAD anastomosis is the left lateral projection.

Right Gastroepiploic Artery

Because of the strong patency of arterial grafts, some surgeons graft the RCA or PDA using the right gastroepiploic artery (GEA). The right GEA, a branch of the gastroduodenal artery, originates from the common hepatic artery, which is one of the main three branches from the celiac trunk. If the operative report is not available, use of this graft should be considered if median sternotomy extends inferiorly into the abdominal cavity or numerous surgical clips extend up from the abdominal cavity to the inferior wall of the heart. Selective angiography of these grafts requires special technique. It is recommended that only operators familiar with peripheral anatomy and angiography perform GEA angiography because it requires knowledge of the vessel anatomy and selective canalization of the GEA. First, the celiac trunk (located anterior and inferiorly directed) must be engaged using specialized peripheral catheters, such as the Cobra (Cook Medical, Bloomington, IN) or Simmons Sidewinder. Anticoagulation with heparin or bivalirudin is recommended, given the need for subbranch vessel wiring. Once the celiac trunk is engaged, an angioplasty-style wire (typically 0.018 or 0.014 inches) should be passed through the common hepatic to the gastroduodenal and then to the GEA using "roadmap imaging". Over this wire, a smaller 4-F or 5-F catheter (Terumo straight glide catheter) or transit catheter (0.035-inch Quick-Cross [Spectranetics]) can be advanced to perform selective GEA graft angiography. Care must be exerted not to cause vessel dissection. The prophylactic administration of nitroglycerin should prevent vessel spasm.

Angiographic TIMI Classification of Blood Flow

The Thrombolysis in Myocardial Infarction (TIMI) group's system of flow grading has been used to assess, in a qualitative fashion, the degree of perfusion before and after thrombolysis or angioplasty in patients with acute myocardial infarction. **Table 8.2** provides descriptions used to assign TIMI flow grades.

Classification of Distal Angiographic Contrast Runoff

The distal runoff is classified into four stages (also known as TIMI grade):

- TIMI 3: Brisk antegrade flow into the entire vessel, with normal distal runoff and rapid clearance.
- TIMI 2: Contrast opacifies entire vessel but perceptibly more slowly than noninvolved territories.
- TIMI 1: Contrast passes into vessel of interest slowly, hangs up, and fails to opacify entire artery, with poor distal runoff.
- TIMI 0: No perfusion or distal runoff.

TIMI flow grades 0 to 3 have become a standard description of coronary blood flow in clinical trials. TIMI grade 3 flows have been associated with improved clinical outcomes.

TIMI Frame Count

Contrast runoff can be performed quantitatively by using cine frame counts. The number of cine frames from the introduction of dye in the coronary artery to a predetermined distal landmark is counted. The TIMI frame count (TFC) for each major vessel is thus

TABLE 8.1 Recommended "Key" Angiographic View for Specific Coronary Artery Segments

CORONARY SEGMENT	ORIGIN/ BIFURCATION	COURSE/BODY
Left main	AP caudal	Caudal
	LAO cranial	LAO cranial
	LAO caudal[a]	
Proximal LAD	LAO cranial	LAO cranial
	RAO caudal	RAO caudal
Mid LAD	LAD cranial	
	RAO cranial	
	Lateral	
Distal LAD	AP	
	RAO cranial	
	Lateral	
Diagonal	LAO cranial	RAO cranial, caudal, or straight
	RAO cranial	
Proximal circumflex	RAO caudal	LAO caudal
	LAO caudal	
Intermediate	RAO caudal	RAO caudal
	LAO caudal	Lateral
Obtuse marginal	RAO caudal	RAO caudal
	LAO caudal	
	RAO cranial (distal marginals)	
	Proximal RCA	LAO
	Lateral	
Mid RCA	LAO	LAO
	Lateral	Lateral
	RAO	RAO
Distal RCA	LAO cranial	LAO cranial
	Lateral	Lateral
PDA	LAO cranial	RAO
Posterolateral	LAO cranial	RAO cranial
	RAO cranial	RAO cranial

[a]Horizontal hearts.

AP, anteroposterior; LAD, left anterior descending artery; LAO, left anterior oblique; PDA, posterior descending artery (from RCA); RAO, right anterior oblique; RCA, right coronary artery.

Adapted from Kern MJ, ed. *The Cardiac Catheterization Handbook*. St Louis, MO: Mosby; 1995:286.

standardized according to specific distal landmarks.[8] The method uses cineangiography with 6F catheters. Traditionally, TFCs are obtained with cineangiography at 30 frames/s, although correction can be applied for images obtained at lower frame rates.

Typically, a normal contrast frame count reflecting normal flow is 24 ± 10 frames. The TFC can further be corrected for the length of the LAD. The TFC in the LAD requires normalization or correction for comparison with the two other major arteries. This is called corrected TIMI frame count (CTFC). High TFC (ie, slow blood flow) may be associated with resting microvascular dysfunction despite an open epicardial artery, although associations between CTFC and wire-based quantitative measures are suboptimal and the role of CTFC in clinical management is not well established. A CTFC of <20 frames has been associated with a low risk for adverse events in patients following myocardial infarction. The TFC method provides valuable information relative to clinical response after coronary intervention.

TIMI Myocardial Blush Grades

Washout of contrast from the microvasculature in the patient with acute infarction is coupled to prognosis. Improved blush scores indicate a larger amount of myocardial salvage, while failure to improve the myocardial blush grade (MBG) suggests microvascular dysfunction or occlusion. The MBG scoring system is shown in **Table 8.2**.

Angiographic Classification of Collateral Flow

Collateral flow can be seen and classified angiographically. The late opacification of a totally or subtotally (99%) occluded vessel through antegrade or retrograde channels will assist in correct guidewire placement, lesion localization, and a successful coronary intervention. The collateral circulation is graded angiographically, as established by Rentrop:

- Grade 0: No collateral branches seen.
- Grade 1: Very weak (ghostlike) opacification.
- Grade 2: Opacified segment is less dense than the source vessel and fills slowly.
- Grade 3: Opacified segment is as dense as the source vessel and filling rapidly.

Collateral visualization may help establish the size of the recipient vessel for the purposes of selecting an appropriately sized balloon but may underestimate the true size of the vessel because it is underpressurized and therefore underfilled. Determining whether the collateral circulation is ipsilateral (eg, proximal RCA to distal RCA collateral supply) or contralateral (eg, circumflex to distal RCA collateral supply) and exactly which region will be affected should collateral supply be disrupted is important to be able to gauge procedural risk. Grade 0 and 1 collaterals provide minimal protection from ischemia, whereas grade 2 and 3 collaterals may be sufficient to prevent angina.

Assessment of Coronary Stenoses

The degree of an angiographic narrowing (stenosis) is reported as the estimated percentage lumen reduction of the most severely narrowed segment compared with the adjacent angiographically normal reference vessel segment, as seen in the radiographic projection that creates the most severely narrowed appearance. Visual estimation yields an approximate stenosis severity; exact evaluation of the minimal luminal diameter requires intravascular imaging. There is a ±20% variation between readings of two or more experienced angiographers. Stenosis severity alone should not always be assumed to be associated with abnormal physiology (flow) and ischemia.

Moreover, coronary artery disease (CAD) is a diffuse process and thus minimal luminal irregularities on angiography may represent significant, albeit nonobstructive, CAD at the time of angiography. The stenotic segment lumen is compared with a nearby lumen that does not appear to be obstructed but that may have diffuse atherosclerotic disease. This explains why postmortem examinations, as well

TABLE 8.2 Thrombolysis in Myocardial Infarction (TIMI) Flow: Grade and Blush Scores

TIMI FLOW GRADE	DESCRIPTION
Grade 3 (complete reperfusion)	Anterograde flow into the terminal coronary artery segment through a stenosis is as prompt as anterograde flow into a comparable segment proximal to the stenosis. Contrast material clears as rapidly from the distal segment as from an uninvolved, more proximal segment.
Grade 2 (partial reperfusion)	Contrast material flows through the stenosis to opacify the terminal artery segment. Nevertheless, contrast enters the terminal segment perceptibly more slowly than more proximal segments. Alternatively, contrast material clears from a segment distal to a stenosis noticeably more slowly than from a comparable segment not preceded by a significant stenosis.
Grade 1 (penetration with minimal perfusion)	A small amount of contrast flows through the stenosis but fails to fully opacify the artery beyond.
Grade 0 (no perfusion)	There is no contrast flow through the stenosis.

Myocardial Blush Grade.
0: No myocardial blush or contrast density. Myocardial blush persisted ("staining").
1: Minimal myocardial blush or contrast density.
2: Moderate myocardial blush or contrast density but less than that obtained during angiography of a contralateral or ipsilateral noninfarct-related coronary artery.
3: Normal myocardial blush or contrast density, comparable with that obtained during angiography of a contralateral or ipsilateral noninfarct-related coronary artery.
Modified from Sheehan F, et al. The effect of intravenous thrombolytic therapy on left ventricular function: a report on tissue-type plasminogen activator and streptokinase from the Thrombolysis in Myocardial Infarction (TIMI) Phase I Trial. *Circulation*. 1987;72:817-829.

as IVUS, describe much more plaque than is seen on angiography (**Fig. 8.3**). Because coronary arteries normally taper as they travel to the apex, proximal segments are always larger than distal segments, often explaining the large disparity between several observers' estimates of stenosis severity. *Area stenosis* is always greater than *diameter stenosis* and assumes the lumen is circular, whereas the lumen is usually eccentric. Assessment of the ischemic impact of a coronary stenosis requires objective evidence acquired from stress testing, measurement of fractional flow reserve (FFR), or nonhyperemic pressure ratios (eg, instantaneous wave-free ratio (iFR)).

Quantitative Coronary Angiography

The degree of coronary stenosis reported from the cineangiogram in clinical practice is a visual estimation of the percentage of diameter narrowing. While widely used in clinical practice, visual assessment is often inadequate for PCI research studies. Modern quantitative coronary angiography systems now generate three-dimensional reconstructions of the coronary anatomy from cineangiography views and using computational fluid dynamics models, can predict the FFR of a stenosis.

Coronary Lesion Descriptions for PCI

There are at least three different major classifications of lesion characteristics (**Table 8.3**), which were derived from large studies in which the characteristics of the lesions were associated with different clinical outcomes and used to assess the risk for adverse cardiac events in the performance of PCI.

General characteristics of the lesion and of the artery proximal to the lesion are as follows:

1. Tortuosity:
   None/mild = straight proximal segment or only one bend of >60°.
   Moderate = two bends of 60° or more proximal to the lesion.
   Severe = three or more bends of 60° or more proximal to the lesion.
2. Arterial calcification:
   Light = proximal artery wall calcification (not necessarily the lesion) seen as thin line(s).
   Moderate = contrast visible on one side of the coronary vessel.
   Heavy = easily seen calcification on both sides of the coronary vessel.

TABLE 8.3 Major Classifications of Lesion Characteristics

ACC/AHA LESION-SPECIFIC CHARACTERISTICS		
TYPE A—LOW RISK	**TYPE B—MEDIUM RISK**	**TYPE C—HIGH RISK**
Discrete (<10 mm length) Concentric Readily accessible Nonangulated segment <45° Smooth contour Little or no calcification Less than totally occlusive Not ostial in location No major branch involvement Absence of thrombus	Tubular (10-20 mm length) Eccentric Moderate tortuosity of proximal segment Moderately angulated segment, 45°-90° Irregular contour Moderate to heavy calcification Ostial in location Bifurcation lesions requiring double guidewires Some thrombus present Total occlusion <3 months old	Diffuse (length >2 cm) Excessive tortuosity of proximal segment Extremely angulated segments >90° Total occlusions >3 months old ± bridging collaterals Inability to protect major side branches Degenerated vein grafts with friable lesions

Note: If more than two medium-risk factors are present, lesion is classified as type B2 and is considered complex.
ACC/AHA, American College of Cardiology/American Heart Association.

3. Arrangement of the lesion(s):
   Tandem = two lesions separated by one balloon length (ie, both lesions can be covered during a single balloon inflation).
   Sequential = two lesions located at a distance longer than the balloon.
4. Length:
   Discrete = <10 mm in length.
   Tubular = 10 to 20 mm in length.
   Diffuse = >20 mm in length.
5. Eccentricity:
   Concentric = lumen axis is located along the long axis of the artery or on either side of it, but by no more than 25% of the normal arterial diameter.
6. Contour: Smooth, irregular, or ulcerated.
7. Thrombus:
   Definite = intraluminal, round filling defect, visible in two views, largely separated from the vessel wall, and/or documentation of embolization of this material.
   Possible = other filling defects not associated with calcification, lesion haziness, irregularity with ill-defined borders, intraluminal staining at the total occlusion site.

The SYNTAX Score

A quantitative score based on angiographically defined coronary anatomy was developed for the 2009 SYNTAX trial, which compared multivessel PCI (including patients with left main CAD) with CABG (9-11). The SYNTAX score, which can range from 0 to 60, was used in the SYNTAX trial to stratify CAD complexity. The results of this randomized study demonstrated that patients with high SYNTAX scores (>34) had improved clinical outcomes with CABG compared with PCI, while in patients with lower SYNTAX scores, PCI and CABG were associated with a similar risk of major adverse cardiac events.

The SYNTAX score is the sum of the points assigned to each individual coronary lesion with >50% diameter narrowing in vessels >1.5 mm diameter. The coronary tree is divided into 16 segments according to the American Heart Association classification (**Fig. 8.5A**; **Table 8.4**). Each segment is given a score of 1 or 2 based on the presence of disease, and this score is then weighted based on the amount of myocardium at risk, with values ranging from 3.5 for the proximal LAD artery to 5.0 for the left main and 0.5 for smaller branches. Branches <1.5 mm in diameter, despite having severe lesions, are not included in the SYNTAX score. The percent diameter stenosis is not a consideration in the SYNTAX score, only the presence of a stenosis from 50% to 99% diameter, <50% diameter narrowing, or the total occlusion. A multiplication factor of 2 is used for nonocclusive lesions, while 5 is used for occlusive lesions, reflecting the difficulty of PCI. The SYNTAX score also considers complex lesions including bifurcations, thrombus, calcification, and small diffuse disease.

Table 8.4 summarizes the SYNTAX grade categories. The SYNTAX score remains a useful tool to guide decisions about modes of revascularization for multivessel CAD. High SYNTAX scores confer the poorest prognosis for revascularization with PCI compared with CABG surgery. In patients with lower SYNTAX scores, either PCI or CABG may be considered as a strategy with equivalent anticipated outcomes (**Fig 8.5**).

Radiographic Contrast Media for PCI

The contrast material is selected from several commercially available solutions with varying features of osmolarity, viscosity, and sodium content found to be appropriate for the specific procedure to be conducted. The most common contrast medium for PCI is nonionic, low-osmolar contrast agents because of safety, patient tolerance, and cost. Selection of a specific nonionic, low-osmolar contrast agent for the particular interventional procedure is, to a large extent, a matter of personal preference. Iso-osmolar agents (iodixanol) may be better tolerated in peripheral vascular procedures and in patients with prior contrast reactions but carry an equal risk of contrast nephropathy.

Renal Arteriography

Nonselective renal arteriography (eg, aortic flush) is used to evaluate the renal artery origins and vasculature. The origins of the arteries usually arise at the L1 vertebra (just below the T12 ribs). Selective renal arterial injections provide the most detail. The LAO projection often provides the best view of the renal artery ostia in a majority of patients. Acutely angled origins of the renal artery may require specially shaped catheters or an upper extremity arterial approach. Atherosclerotic disease of the renal artery usually involves the proximal one-third of the renal artery and is seldom present without abdominal atherosclerotic plaques.

Aortography of the thoracic and abdominal aorta is used to assess disease, dissections, and the course of the vessel in order to perform and plan interventions. In high-risk PCI, abdominal aortography with visualization of common iliac arteries may be useful prior to insertion of intra-aortic balloon pump or left ventricular support devices, and as part of evaluation for percutaneous aortic valvuloplasty or replacement.

Lower Extremity Angiography

Angiography of the lower extremities is typically performed with small-diameter (5F–6F) catheters and reduced contrast volumes (10-20 mL over 1-2 seconds), which are injected, panning down and following the artery course to the most distal locations. Angulated views may be necessary to open bifurcations and overlying vessels that obscure the vessel origin. Even with the imaging equipment to the side of the patient, the ability to pan down to the ankle should be tested before injection. Digital subtraction techniques are commonly used for peripheral vascular imaging but preclude the use of panning.

The distal superficial femoral artery in the abductor canal is the vascular territory most frequently affected by peripheral atherosclerotic disease of the lower extremity (**Fig. 8.6**). The calf (tibial) and knee (popliteal) arteries are the next most commonly involved vessels after the superficial femoral artery. Disease in the deep femoral artery (femoral profunda) is rare. Pathways of collateralization are often rich and varied in patients with chronic distal femoral artery disease, especially in total occlusion of the superficial femoral artery that reconstitutes at or below the knee, close to the branching trifurcation of the tibial and deep peroneal arteries. Magnified images focusing on the area of interest are frequently needed.

Left dominance

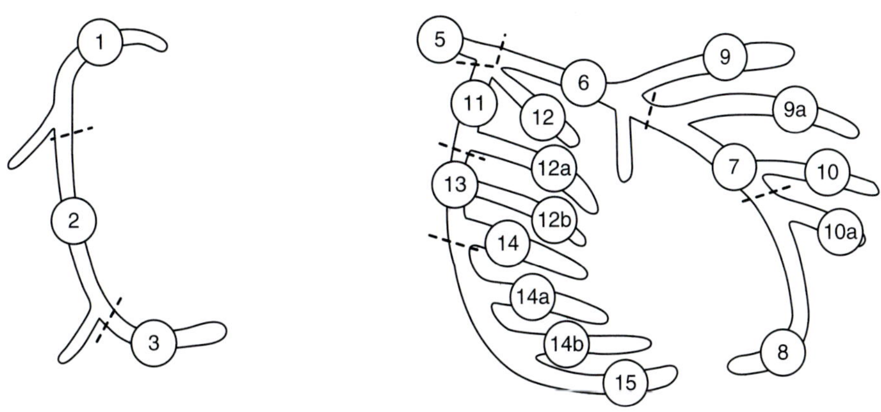

Right dominance

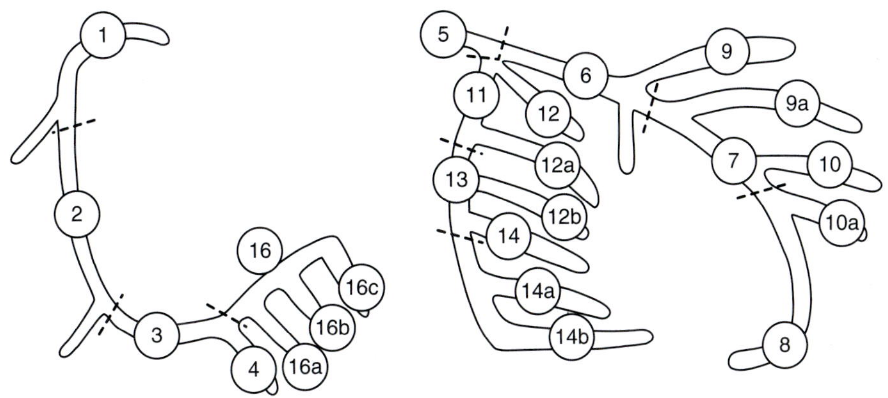

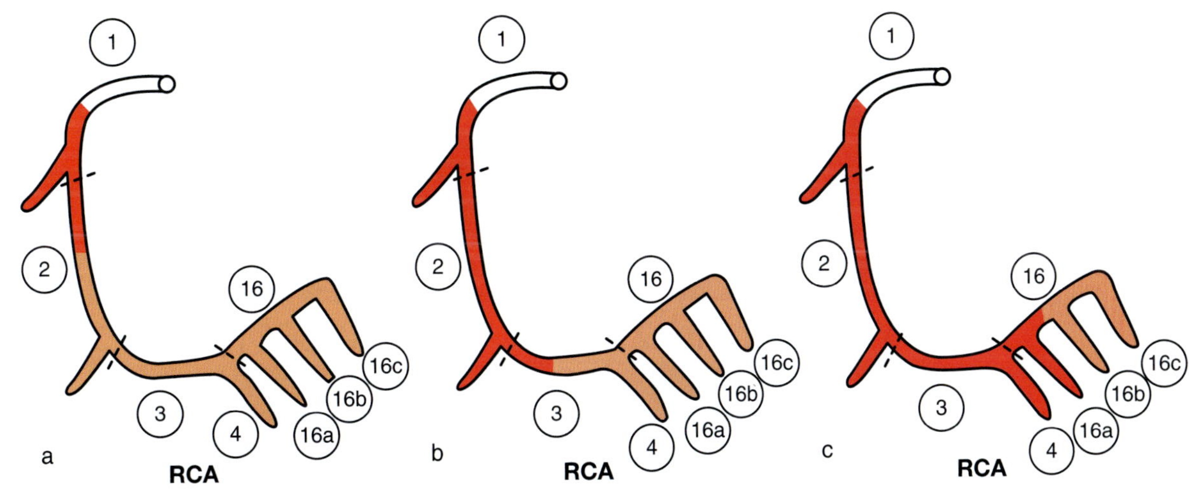

Patent segment

Occluded segment

A Segement distal from the occlusion filed with collateral flow (visualized by contrast)

FIGURE 8.5 *(continued)*

Definition of the coronary tree segments

1. RCA proximal: From the ostium to one half the distance to the acute margin of the heart.
2. RCA mid: From the end of the first segment to the acute margin of the heart.
3. RCA distal: From the acute margin of the heart to the origin of the posterior descending artery.
4. Posterior descending artery: Running in the posterior interventricular groove.
5. Left main: From the ostium of the LCA through bifurcation into the left anterior descending and left circumflex branches.
6. LAD proximal: Proximal to and including first major septal branch.
7. LAD mid: LAD immediately distal to origin of first septal branch and extending to the point where LAD forms an angle (RAO view). If this angle is not identifiable, this segment ends at one half the distance from the first septal to the apex of the heart.
8. LAD apical: Terminal portion of LAD, beginning at the end of the previous segment and extending to or beyond the apex.
9. First diagonal: The first diagonal originating from segment 6 or 7.

9a. First diagonal a: Additional first diagonal originating from segment 6 or 7, before segment 8.

10. Second diagonal: Originating from segment 8 or the transition between segments 7 and 8.

10a. Second diagonal a: Additional second diagonal originating from segment 8.

11. Proximal circumflex artery: Main stem of the circumflex, from its origin of the left main, and including the origin of its first obtuse marginal branch.
12. Intermediate/anterolateral artery: Branch from the trifurcating left main other than the proximal LAD or LCX. It belongs to the circumflex territory.

12a. Obtuse marginal a: First side branch of the circumflex, running in general to the area of the obtuse margin of the heart.

12b. Obtuse marginal b: Second additional branch of the circumflex, running in the same direction as 12.

13. Distal circumflex artery: The stem of the circumflex distal to the origin of the most distal obtuse marginal branch, and running along the posterior left atrioventricular groove. The caliber may be small or the artery absent.
14. Left posterolateral: Running to the posterolateral surface of the left ventricle. May be absent or a division of obtuse marginal branch.

14a. Left posterolateral a: Distal from 14 and running in the same direction.

14b. Left posterolateral b: Distal from 14 and 14a and running in the same direction.

15. Posterior descending: Most distal part of the dominant left circumflex when present. It gives origin to septal branches. When this artery is present, segment 4 is usually absent. (From: Sianos G, Morel MA, Kappetein AP, et al. The SYNTAX score: an angiographic tool grading the complexity of coronary artery disease. *EuroInterv.* 2005;1:219–227.)
16. Posterolateral branch from RCA: The posterolateral branch originating from the distal coronary artery distal to the crux.

16a. Posterolateral branch from RCA: The first posterolateral branch from segment 16.

16b. Posterolateral branch from RCA: The second posterolateral branch from segment 16.

16c. Posterolateral branch from RCA: The third posterolateral branch from segment 16.

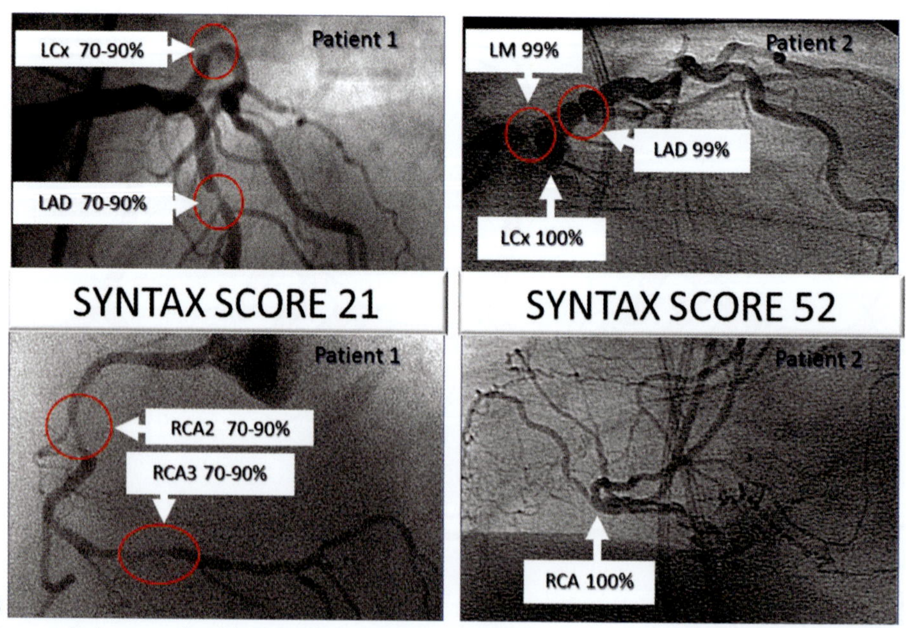

FIGURE 8.5 **A:** SYNTAX diagram. **B:** An example of the SYNTAX score and the specific angiographic anatomy. LAD, left anterior descending; LCx, left circumflex artery; LM, left main; RCA, right coronary artery.

TABLE 8.4 The SYNTAX Score Algorithm

1. Dominance
2. Number of lesions
3. Segments involved per lesion, with lesion characteristics
4. Total occlusions with subtotal occlusions:
   a. Number of segments
   b. Age of total occlusions
   c. Blunt stumps
   d. Bridging collaterals
   e. First segment beyond occlusion visible by antegrade or retrograde filling
   f. Side branch involvement
7. Trifurcation, number of segments diseased
8. Bifurcation type and angulation
9. Aorto-ostial lesion
10. Severe tortuosity
11. Lesion length
12. Heavy calcification
13. Thrombus
14. Diffuse disease, with number of segments

Angiography of Common Coronary Anomalies

Anomalous origin of the coronary arteries is a common challenge in the catheterization laboratory. Although locating the ostium can be difficult, it is an error to assume that a vessel is occluded if it has not been selectively engaged. Once the anomalous ostium has been identified, even experienced angiographers may have difficulty delineating the true course of the vessel. Computed tomography coronary angiography is generally superior to invasive angiography to determine the true course of anomalous coronary vessels and should be considered in most cases. **Fig. 8.7** diagrams five pathways of anomalous coronary arteries.

Separate Origins of the LAD and LCx

Separate but adjacent ostia of the LAD and left circumflex (LCx) coronary arteries in the left sinus of Valsalva is the most common benign abnormality, observed in ~0.4% of individuals. Selective engagement of each coronary ostia required for coronary angiography may be difficult, and in some cases, two different catheters are required, typically with a smaller catheter used to cannulate the LAD.

Anomalous Origin of the Left Main Coronary Artery From the Right Sinus of Valsalva

When the LMCA arises from the right sinus of Valsalva or the proximal RCA, it may follow one of four pathways (**Figs. 8.8** and **8.9**; **Table 8.5**):

1. Septal course (benign variant). The LMCA runs an intramuscular course through the septum along the floor of the right ventricular outflow tract.
2. Anterior free wall course (benign variant). The LMCA crosses the anterior free wall of the right ventricle and then divides at the midseptum into the LAD and circumflex arteries.
3. Retroaortic course (benign course). The LMCA passes posteriorly around the aortic root to its normal position on the anterior surface of the heart. (It is also seen with anomalous origin of circumflex from the right sinus.)
4. Interarterial course (malignant). The LMCA courses between the aorta and PA to its normal position on the anterior surface of the heart. During RAO ventriculography, aortography, or coronary angiography, the LMCA is seen "on end," anterior to the aorta, and appears as a radiopaque dot to the left of the aortic root.

The interarterial course of the LMCA originating from the right sinus of Valsalva has been associated with exertional angina, syncope, and sudden death at a young age. The mechanism causing myocardial ischemia appears to be the slit-like opening in the aortic wall that narrows further during activity with dynamic compression of the obliquely arising LMCA ostium as it courses between the aortic root and the root of the pulmonary trunk. When this anomaly is identified in patients with myocardial ischemia, coronary revascularization (especially with surgical "unroofing" or bypass) is indicated. The need for revascularization in older or asymptomatic patients with this anomaly is less clear. A decision for revascularization should be based on the severity of concomitant obstructive coronary disease and inducible myocardial ischemia. **Fig. 8.10** summarizes the methods and techniques used to assess the anomalous LMCA.

Anomalous Origin of the Circumflex Coronary Artery

The most common coronary anomaly is the circumflex artery arising from the proximal RCA (**Fig. 8.11**). This feature is often suggested during left coronary angiography when a long LMCA segment is present with a small or trivial circumflex branch. When the circumflex coronary artery arises from the right coronary cusp or the proximal RCA, it invariably follows a retroaortic course and passes posteriorly around the aortic root to its normal position. During RAO ventriculography, aortography, or coronary angiography, the circumflex artery is seen on end, appearing as a radiopaque dot posterior to the aorta.

Anomalous Origin of the RCA From the Left Sinus of Valsalva

When the RCA arises from the left coronary cusp or the proximal LMCA, it generally follows only one path, although other courses are theoretically possible. The RCA courses between the aorta and PA to its normal position. During RAO ventriculography, aortography, or coronary angiography, the RCA is seen on end, anterior to the aorta, and appears as a radiopaque dot. This coronary anomaly has been associated with symptoms of myocardial ischemia, particularly when the RCA is dominant. Coronary revascularization should be considered when this anomaly is associated with symptoms of myocardial ischemia.

Anomalous RCA Above the Sinus of Valsalva or From the Anterior Aortic Wall

The RCA may arise from an anterior location or high above the sinus of Valsalva. Aortic root flush injection helps locate the ostium for proper, subselective catheter selection (eg, Amplatz left 2 or multipurpose). This variant is benign.

LAD and Circumflex Coronary Arteries From Separate Ostia in the Left Aortic Sinus

When the LAD and circumflex coronary arteries arise from separate ostia in the left coronary cusp, the normal proximal course is followed. Also, a conus branch has a separate ostium arising from the right coronary cusp.

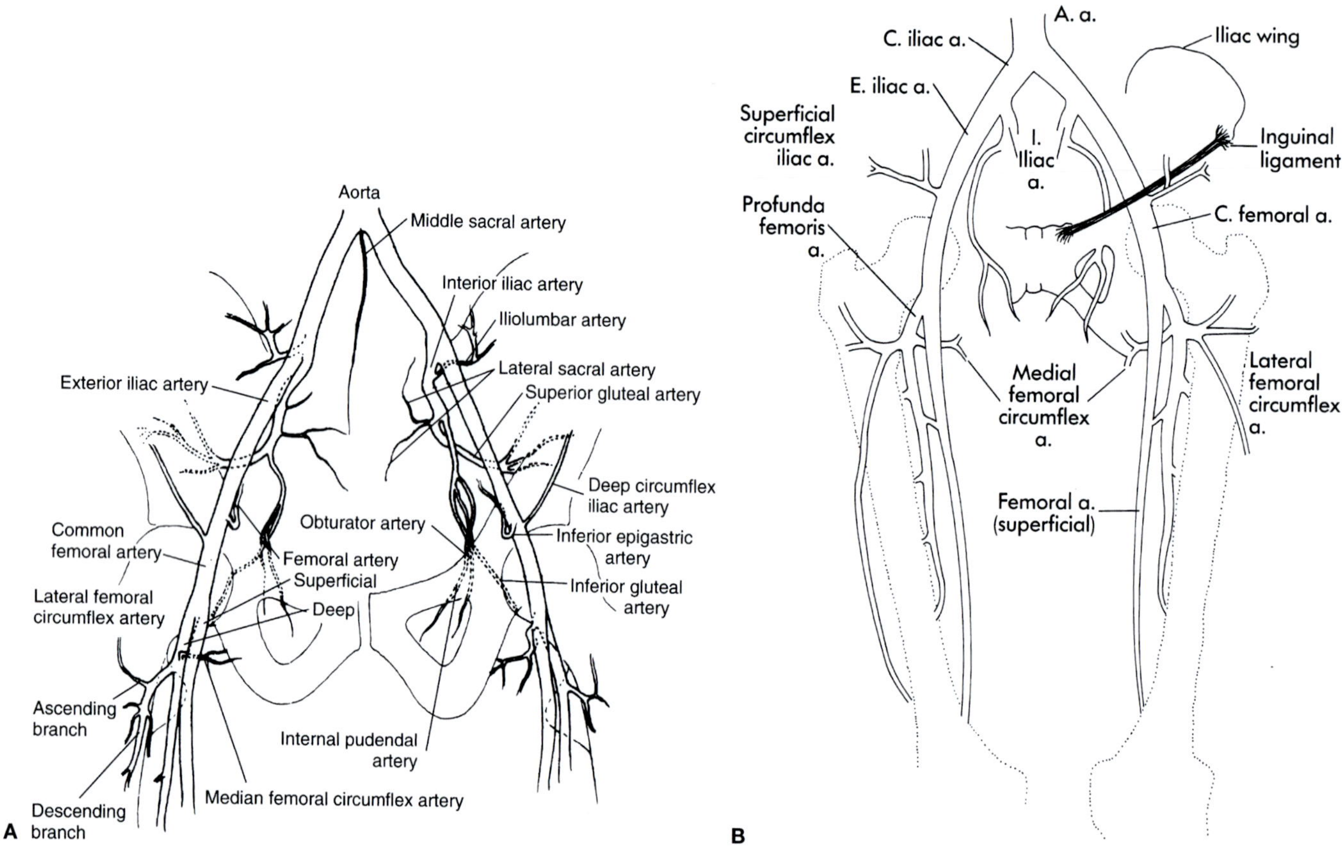

Aorta
Middle sacral artery
Interior iliac artery
Iliolumbar artery
Exterior iliac artery
Lateral sacral artery
Superior gluteal artery
Deep circumflex iliac artery
Common femoral artery
Obturator artery
Inferior epigastric artery
Femoral artery
Superficial
Deep
Inferior gluteal artery
Lateral femoral circumflex artery
Ascending branch
Internal pudendal artery
Descending branch
Median femoral circumflex artery
A
A. a.
C. iliac a.
Iliac wing
E. iliac a.
Superficial circumflex iliac a.
I. Iliac a.
Inguinal ligament
Profunda femoris a.
C. femoral a.
Medial femoral circumflex a.
Lateral femoral circumflex a.
Femoral a. (superficial)
B

FIGURE 8.6 **A** and **B:** Pelvic and proximal femoral arterial branches. (From Johnsrude IS, et al. *A Practical Approach to Angiography*. 2nd ed. Boston, MA: Little, Brown & Co.; 1987.)

PV
Proximal course can be intramural (within aortic wall) or not intramural
Ao
MV
TV
Left
Right
Prepulmonic
Interarterial
Subpulmonic
Retroaortic
Retrocardiac

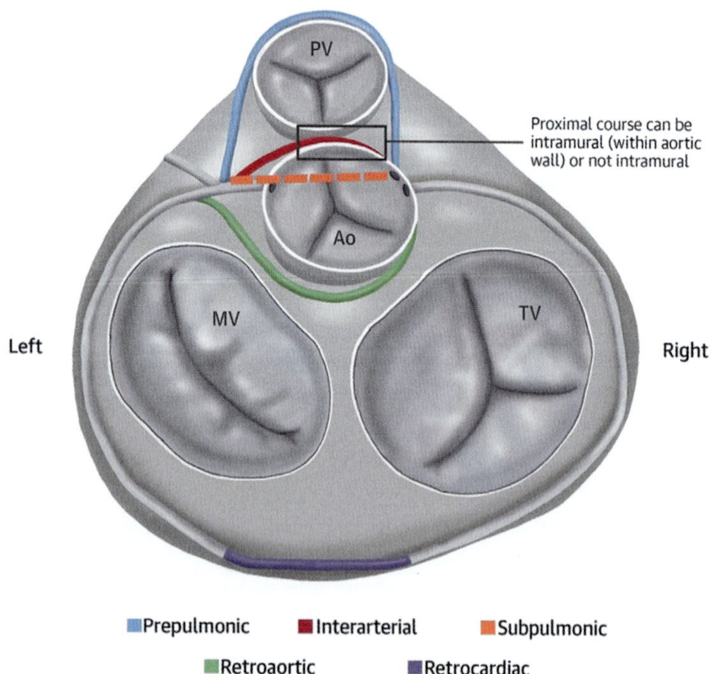

FIGURE 8.7 Pathways of the anomalous coronary arteries. (From Cheezum MK, Liberthson RR, Shah NR, et al. Anomalous aortic origin of a coronary artery from the inappropriate sinus of Valsalva. *J Am Coll Cardiol*. 2017;69:1592-1608.)

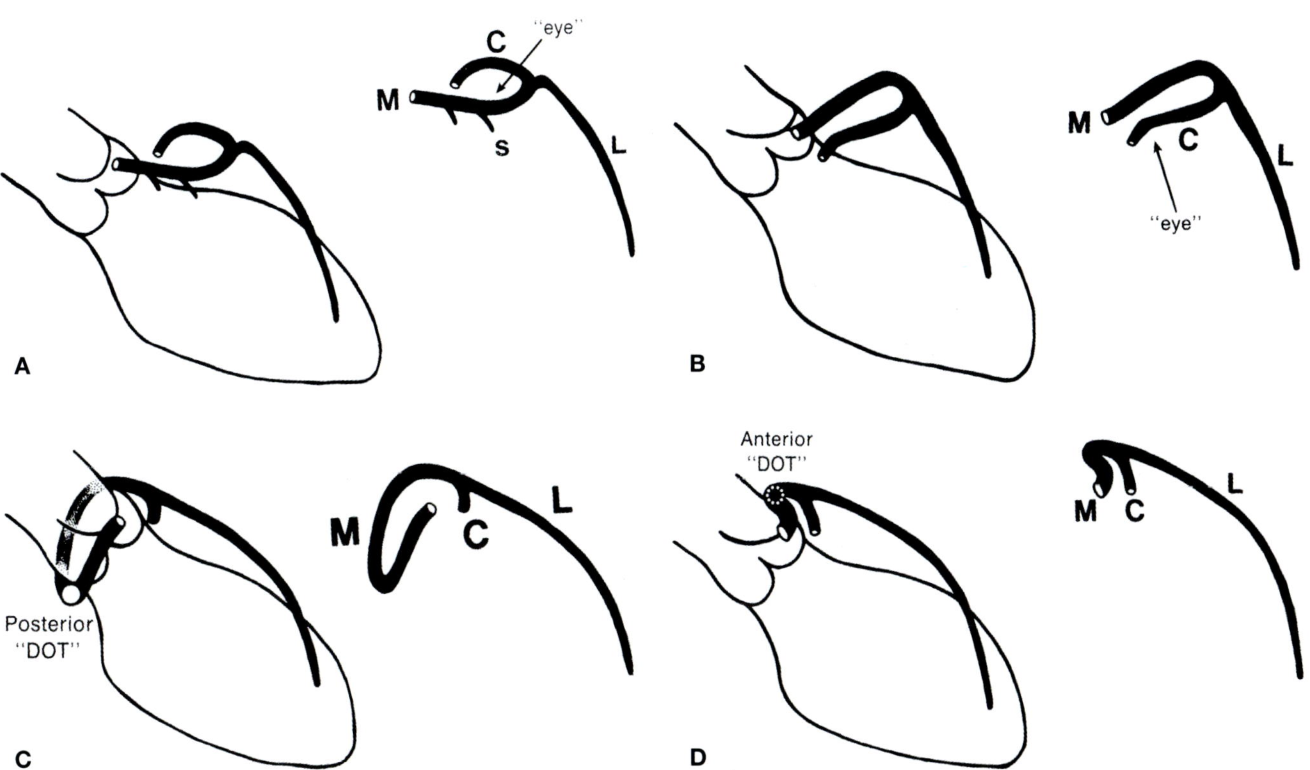

FIGURE 8.8 Diagram of four courses of the anomalous left coronary artery as viewed in the right anterior oblique projection. Panel **A:** Septal course. Panel **B:** Anterior course. Panel **C:** Retro-aortic course. Panel **D:** Inter-arterial course. M, left main; C, circumflex; L, left anterior descending artery; S, septal.

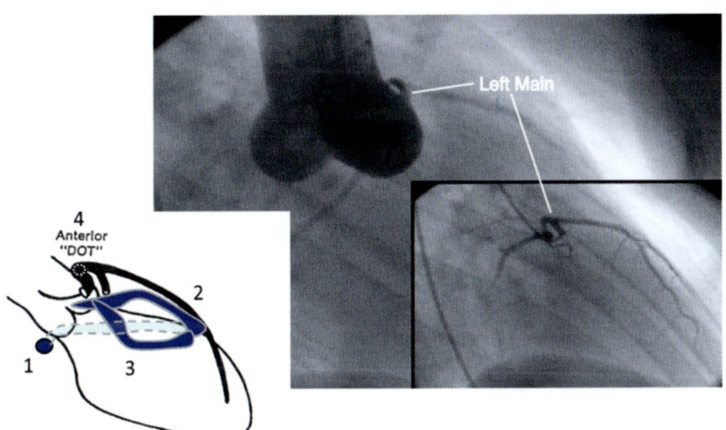

FIGURE 8.9 Four pathways of the anomalous left main coronary artery from the right sinus of Valsalva (ALMCA-R). 1, retroaortic; 2, anterior; 3, subcristal or septal; 4, interarterial.

TABLE 8.5 Radiographic Appearance of Anomalous Origin of the Left Main Coronary Artery From the Right Sinus of Valsalva

COURSE OF ANOMALOUS	RAO AORTOGRAPHY OR VENTRICULOGRAPHY			
Left main				
Coronary	Dot	Eye	LAD length	Septal branches arising from LMCA
Septal (lower LMCA)	–	+ (upper CFX)	Short	Yes
Anterior (lower CFX)	–	+ (upper LMCA)	Short	No
Retroaortic	+ (posterior)	–	Normal	
Interarterial	+ (anterior)	–	Normal	No

+, Present; –, absent. Posterior and anterior are in reference to the aorta root.
CFX, circumflex coronary artery; LAD, left anterior descending coronary artery; LMCA, left main coronary artery.

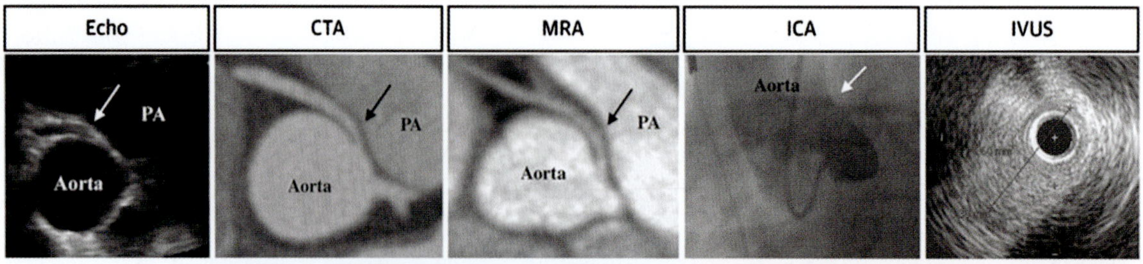

	Echo	CTA	MRA	ICA	IVUS
Indication for AAOCA Imaging	-	Class I	Class I	Class IIa	Class IIa
Spatial Resolution	0.8 × 1.5 mm (4-MHz transducer)	0.5 mm (isotropic)	1.0 mm (volumetric)	0.3 mm	0.15 × 0.25 mm
Temporal Resolution	30 msec	75-175 msec	60 - 120 msec	7-20 msec	Variable
Visualize surround structures	Limited	✔✔	✔	X	X
Dynamic imaging	Limited	Limited	Limited	✔ (Limited at ostium)	✔✔
Strengths	✓ Noninvasive, rapid ✓ Widely available ✓ Low cost	✓ Noninvasive, rapid ✓ Visualize takeoff + course + surrounding structures ✓ Evaluate CAD ✓ Examine multiple AAOCA features *	✓ Noninvasive ✓ Visualize takeoff + course + surrounding structures ✓ Evaluate cardiac function, perfusion and prior MI ✓ Avoid radiation & iodinated contrast	✓ Availability ✓ Improved spatial and temporal resolution ✓ Ancillary techniques (IVUS, OCT, FFR)	✓ Dynamic imaging ✓ Evaluation of proximal narrowing
Limitations	× Limited accuracy for detection of AAOCA × Dependent on body habitus and operator technique	× Limited availability × Iodinated contrast × Radiation (low dose, e.g. 2-8 mSv now routine)	× Limited availability × Cost and scan-time increased vs. CTA × Spatial resolution decreased vs. CTA	× Invasive; Cost × Contrast and radiation × Limited visualization of ostium, proximal course, surrounding structures	× Invasive × Cost × Difficulty engaging anomalous vessel

FIGURE 8.10 Methods and techniques to assess the anomalous coronary artery. AAOCA, anomalous aortic origin of the coronary artery; CAD, coronary artery disease; FFR, fractional flow reserve; IVUS, intravascular ultrasound imaging; OCT, optical coherence tomography. (From Cheezum MK, Liberthson RR, Shah NR, et al. Anomalous aortic origin of a coronary artery from the inappropriate sinus of Valsalva. *J Am Coll Cardiol.* 2017;69:1592-1608.)

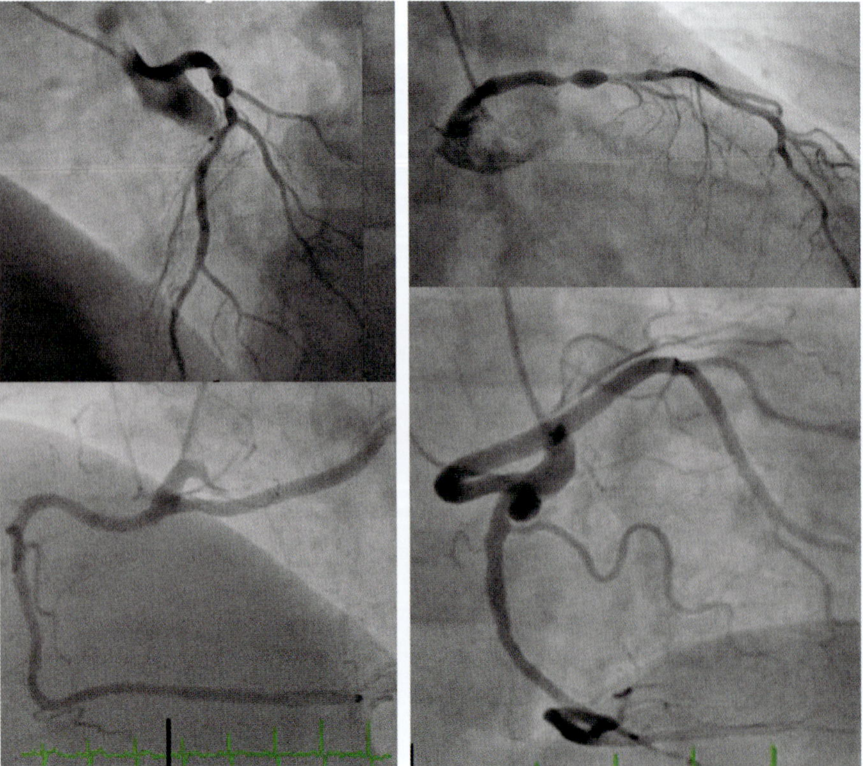

FIGURE 8.11 Frames from cineangiogram showing (*top, left and right*) the elongated LAD in the LAO cranial and RAO caudal views and (*bottom, left and right*) the right coronary artery with the circumflex originating in the RCA ostium in the LAO and RAO views. The retroaortic course is evident in the RAO view as a "dot" of density because the circumflex is in the viewer's plane as it runs behind the aorta. LAO, left anterior oblique; RAO, right anterior oblique; RCA, right coronary artery.

Key Points

- All lesions should be visualized in at least two angiographic views to establish severity.
- The working view should be selected to optimally visualize the lesion and guide the catheter and distal vessel, while minimizing vessel foreshortening.
- The presence and quality of collaterals affect the risk and potential benefits of PCI.
- Visual estimation of stenosis severity has a high interobserver variability and should not be considered a diagnostic of ischemia for intermediately narrowed lesions.
- Vessel and lesion characteristics, including tortuosity and calcification, in addition to clinical factors determine the risk of PCI.
- The SYNTAX score takes into account lesion characteristics and the myocardium at risk and is useful in choosing between multivessel PCI and CABG.
- Peripheral angiography requires specific techniques and equipment.
- Knowledge of typical coronary artery anomalies is important to determine whether a vessel is missing or merely anomalous in location. For the ALMCA-R the angiogram can help differentiate benign from a malignant pathway.

References

1. Kern MJ, Lim MJ, Sorraja P, eds. *The Interventional Cardiac Catheterization Handbook*. 5th ed. Elsevier; 2022:450-454.
2. Kern MJ, ed. *Kern's Cardiac Catheterization Handbook*. 7th ed. Elsevier-Saunders; 2018:145-218.
3. Balter S, Moses J. Managing patient dose in interventional cardiology. *Catheter Cardiovasc Interv*. 2007;70(2):244-249.
4. Hirshfeld JW Jr, Balter S, Brinker JA, et al. ACCF/AHA/HRS/SCAI clinical competence statement on physician knowledge to optimize patient safety and image quality in fluoroscopically guided invasive cardiovascular procedures. A report of the American College of Cardiology Foundation/American Heart Association/American College of Physicians Task Force on Clinical Competence and Training. *J Am Coll Cardiol*. 2004;44(11):2259-2282.
5. Valgimigli M, Serruys PW, Tsuchida K, et al. Cyphering the complexity of coronary artery disease using the SYNTAX score to predict clinical outcome in patients with three-vessel lumen obstruction undergoing percutaneous coronary intervention. *Am J Cardiol*. 2007;99(8):1072-1081.
6. Serruys PW, Morice MC, Kappetein AP, et al. Percutaneous coronary intervention versus coronary-artery bypass grafting for severe coronary artery disease. *N Engl J Med*. 2009;360(10):961-972.
7. White CJ, Jaff MR, Haskal ZJ, et al. Indications for renal arteriography at the time of coronary arteriography: a science advisory from the American Heart Association Committee on Diagnostic and Interventional Cardiac Catheterization, Council on Clinical Cardiology, and the Councils on Cardiovascular Radiology and Intervention and on Kidney in Cardiovascular Disease. *Circulation*. 2006;114(17):1892-1895.
8. Cheezum MK, Liberthson RR, Shah NR, et al. Anomalous aortic origin of a coronary artery from the inappropriate sinus of Valsalva. *J Am Coll Cardiol*. 2017;69(12):1592-1608.

Intravascular Ultrasound

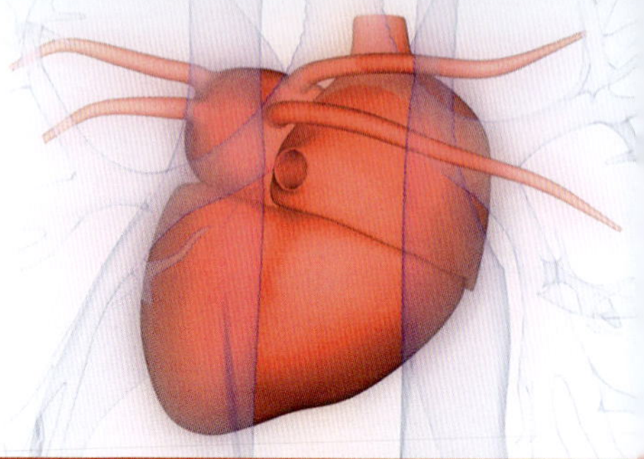

Yiannis Chatzizsis

INTRODUCTION

Since intravascular ultrasound (IVUS) was first performed in 1988, it has been instrumental in enhancing our understanding of coronary anatomy and pathophysiology and has allowed detailed evaluation of interventional procedures.[1] IVUS enables direct visualization of vascular anatomy during diagnostic catheterization. Unlike angiography, which mostly depicts a silhouette of the coronary lumen, IVUS provides a tomographic and cross-sectional perspective and allows direct measurements of the lumen dimensions, including the minimum and maximum diameter and cross-sectional area.[2] By employing an automated timed pullback, plaque length measures can also be obtained. Ultrasound-derived measurements are more accurate than quantitative angiographic dimensions.[3] Furthermore, IVUS is unique in imaging the full thickness of the arterial wall, enabling the characterization of plaque size, plaque distribution, and composition.[4] Finally, IVUS can effectively detect structural abnormalities of the vessel wall after mechanical interventions, including calcium fractures, stent underexpansion, malapposition, tissue protrusion, intramural hematoma, dissection, and perforation.

CLINICAL BENEFIT OF IVUS-GUIDED PERCUTANEOUS CORONARY INTERVENTIONS WITH DRUG-ELUTING STENTS

To date, 16 randomized controlled trials (RCTs), 28 observational studies, and 35 meta-analyses comparing the clinical outcomes of IVUS-guided percutaneous coronary intervention (PCI) with drug-eluting stent (DES) versus angiography-guided PCI have been published (**Table 9.1**). These studies have shown clearly that compared to angiography-guided PCI, IVUS-guided PCI is associated with a significant reduction (up to 50%) of adverse events, including all-cause mortality, cardiovascular mortality, myocardial infarction (MI), stent thrombosis (ST), target lesion revascularization, and target vessel revascularization.[5-7,9-11]

IVUS DEVICES

The available IVUS devices in the market as of January 2024 are summarized in **Table 9.2**. The quality of IVUS images depends on spatial resolution and depth. Spatial resolution is the minimum distance between two adjacent points that can be distinguished. Depth is the ability of IVUS to visualize the far field (tissue penetration). IVUS visualizes the arterial wall by using higher ultrasound frequencies (20-60 MHz) than standard echocardiography, providing an axial resolution that ranges between 20 and 150 µm, a lateral resolution of 200 to 250 µm, and tissue penetration (depth) of 6 to 12 mm.[12] High-definition IVUS with a transducer frequency of 60 MHz provides improved axial resolution of 20 to 40 µm. The IVUS systems require two components: (i) a catheter incorporating a miniaturized transducer and (ii) a console containing the necessary electronics to reconstruct the ultrasound image. IVUS catheters typically range in size from 2.9 to 3.6F (0.96-1.17 mm) and are compatible with 5F or 6F guide catheters. There are two types of transducer design: (i) mechanically rotated transducers and (ii) multielement electronic phased-array transducers.[13] In clinical practice, both transducer types provide sufficiently accurate information, although mechanical systems typically achieve higher resolution. IVUS systems use a monorail design to facilitate rapid catheter exchange.

TECHNIQUE AND SAFETY OF IVUS

The technique of IVUS is identical to that of introducing a PCI catheter. After heparin anticoagulation, a guide wire is introduced through a guide catheter to the ostial aortic position. The IVUS catheter is advanced over the guidewire distal to the target area of interest. Manual or motorized catheter pullback is performed to provide a longitudinal image for quantitation of the vessel characteristics. The technique is relatively safe.[14] Despite the relative safety of coronary ultrasound, any intracoronary instrumentation carries the potential risk of intimal injury or acute vessel dissection, and therefore, careful manipulations by the operators are recommended. The imaging transducer can transiently occlude the coronary artery when advanced into severe stenosis or a small distal vessel, but patients generally do not experience chest pain if the catheter is promptly withdrawn. Preinstrumentation intracoronary administration of nitroglycerine (50-200 µg) is highly recommended to prevent coronary spasm and induce maximal vasodilation. Adequate anticoagulation is required prior to catheter insertion; an activated clotting time of greater than 250 or 300 seconds (depending on the activated clotting time device) is recommended.

IVUS IMAGE INTERPRETATION

IVUS is considered a workhorse intracoronary imaging modality in the cardiac catheterization laboratory, and therefore, operators should be familiar with the performance and interpretation of IVUS.[15] Distinguishing between different types of plaque, accurately measuring lumen and plaque dimensions, and assessing the severity of stenosis depends on the operator's skills and knowledge of IVUS. IVUS provides detailed information about the various constituents of the coronary wall, including (**Fig. 9.1**)[16,17]:

(i) Blood/lumen: Flowing blood exhibits a characteristic pattern of echogenicity on IVUS, often observed as finely textured echoes moving in a swirling pattern. The pattern of blood echogenicity depends on blood flow velocity. Reduction in

TABLE 9.1 Summary of Studies Comparing the Clinical Outcomes of IVUS-Guided Versus Angiography-Guided Percutaneous Interventions With DESs

RCTS											
					IVUS- VS ANGIOGRAPHY-GUIDED PCI						
STUDY NAME	YEAR	STUDY DESIGN	DURATION OF STUDY	NUMBER OF PARTICIPANTS	ALL-CAUSE MORTALITY	CARDIOVASCULAR MORTALITY	MI	TVR	TLR	ST	MACE
Home DES IVUS	2010	RCT	18 mo	210	N/A	3% vs 2%	1% vs 4%	N/A	6% vs 6%	4% vs 6%	11% vs 12%
Excellent	2012	RCT	12 mo	1421	1.0% vs 0.6% HR = 1.56 *P* = .46	0.3% vs 0.4% HR = 0.87, *P* = .87	2.1% vs 0.7% HR = 2.77, *P* = .04	2.7% vs 2.9% HR = 0.96, *P* = .87	2.1% vs 2.2% HR = 0.93, *P* = .84	0.3% vs 0.6% HR = 0.52, *P* = .43	5.5% vs 3.9% HR = 1.43, *P* = .15
Reset	2013	RCT	12 mo	543	1.1% vs 0.7%, RR = 1.53, *P* = .64	0% vs 0.4%, *P* = 1.00	0% vs 0.7%, *P* = .50	4.5% vs 6.6% RR = 0.66, *P* = .28	N/A	0.4% vs 0.4%, *P* = 1.0	4.5% vs 7.3% RR = 0.59, *P* = .16
Avio	2013	RCT	24 mo	284	N/A	0% vs 1.4%	7.0% vs 8.5%	9.8% vs 15.5%	9.2% vs 11.9%	N/A	16.9% vs 23.2%
Wang et al	2014	RCT	12 mo	80	N/A	0% vs 0%	2.6% vs 0%	0% vs 4.70%	N/A	0.26% vs 4.7%	N/A
Mozart	2014	RCT	4 mo	83	N/A	4.2% vs 0%, *P* = .3	4.2% vs 3.3%, *P* > .9	N/A	N/A	0% vs 0%	N/A
Air-CTO	2015	RCT	24 mo	230	5.2% vs 6.1%, *P* = 0.78	2.6% vs 4.3%, *P* = .56	17.4 vs 13.0, *P* = .46	7.8 vs 12.2, *P* = .38	6.9% vs 10.4%, *P* = .48	2.6% vs 6.9%, *P* = .16	21.7% vs 25.2%, *P* = .64
CTO-IVUS	2015	RCT	12 mo	402	1.0% vs 1.5%, HR = 0.67, *P* = .66	0% vs 1% HR = N/A, *P* = .16	0% vs 1% HR = N/A, *P* = .16	2.6% vs 5.2% HR = 0.48, *P* = .19	2.6% vs 4.1% HR = 0.62, *P* = .40	0% vs 1.5% HR = N/A, *P* = .11	2.6% vs 7.1% HR = 0.35, *P* = .035
Tan et al	2015	RCT	24 mo	123	N/A	3.3% vs 4.8%, *P* = .65	1.6% vs 3.2%, *P* = .58	N/A	9.1% vs 24%, *P* = .045	1.6% vs 3.2%, *P* = .57	12.8% vs 27.3%, *P* = .05
Zhang et al	2016	RCT	12 mo	84	N/A	0% vs 0%	2.4% vs 4.8%, *P* = 1.0	4.8 vs 16.7%, *P* = .078	N/A	N/A	N/A
Liu et al	2019	RCT	12 mo	336	N/A	1.8% vs 5.9%, *P* = .05	11.4% vs 13.6%, *P* = .48	4.2% vs 8.9%, *P* = .07	1.2% vs 3.0%, *P* = .24	1.2% vs 3%, *P* = .24	13.2% vs 21.9%, *P* = .03
IVUS-XPL	2020	RCT	60 mo	1400	N/A	0.9% vs 2.2% HR = 0.43, *P* = .074	0.6% vs 0.9% HR = 0.67, *P* = .52	N/A	4.8% vs 8.4% HR = 0.54, *P* = .007	0.3 vs 0.3% HR = 1.0, *P* = 1.00	5.6 vs 10.7% HR = 0.50, *P* = 0.001

(*continued*)

ILUMIEN III	2021	RCT	12 mo	278	0 vs 0%	N/A	2.2% vs 2.3%	2.2% vs 1.4%	2.9% vs 1.4%	0% vs 0%	9.1% vs 7.9%
ULTIMATE	2021	RCT	36 mo	1423	4.3% vs 4.4% HR = 0.99 P = .98	1.8% vs 2.7% HR = 0.68 P = .28	1.0% vs 2.1% HR = 0.46 P = .09	4.5% vs 6.9% HR = 0.64, P = .05	3.8% vs 6.3% HR = 0.59, P = .03	0.1% vs 1.1% HR = 0.12, P = .02	5.9% vs 10.2% HR = 0.57, P = .003
iSIGHT	2021	RCT	30 mo	150	N/A	0% vs 2%, P = .91	2.0% vs 4.1%, P = .21	2.0% vs 4.1%, P = .36	0.0% vs 0.0%	0.0% vs 0.0%	4.0% vs 6.1%, P = .77
RENOVATE-COMPLEX-PCI[a]	2023	RCT	25 mo	1639	5.3% vs 6.4%, HR = 0.74	1.7% vs 3.8%, HR = 0.47	4.4% vs 6.2%, HR = 0.78	3.4% vs 5.5%, HR = 0.69	2.6% vs 4.4%, HR = 0.66	0.1% vs 0.7%, HR = 0.25	9.2% vs 7.7%, HR = 0.64
OBSERVATIONAL STUDIES											
STUDY NAME	**YEAR**	**STUDY DESIGN**	**DURATION OF STUDY**	**NUMBER OF PARTICIPANTS**	**IVUS- VS ANGIOGRAPHY-GUIDED PCI**						
					ALL-CAUSE MORTALITY	**CARDIOVASCULAR MORTALITY**	**MI**	**TVR**	**TLR**	**ST**	**MACE**
Roy et al	2008	Observational	12 mo	1768	5.7% vs 7.1%, OR = 0.83, P = .24	1.9% vs 2.8% OR = 0.66, P = .19	2.1% vs 3.1% OR = 0.69, P = .12	8.5% vs 9.1% OR = 0.94, P = .67	5.1% vs 7.2% OR = 0.69, P = .07	0.7% vs 2.0%, P = .01	14.5% vs 16.2% OR = 0.72, P = .33
Park et al (MAIN-Compare)	2009	Retrospective observational	36 mo	975	2.5% vs 9.0% HR = 0.39, P = .05	3.0% vs 10.4%	7.4% vs 12% HR = 0.83, P = .56	11.3% vs 9.4% HR = 0.80, P = .62	N/A	N/A	15% vs 33.7% HR = 0.64, P = .074
Maluenda et al	2010	Prospective observational	12 mo	905	6.4% vs 5.1% RR = 1.26 P = .44	2.1% vs 1.6% RR = 1.37 P = .55	7.8% vs 8.9%	11.8% vs 11% RR = 1.08 P = .69	7.3% vs 8%, P = .72	0 vs 1%, P = .08	14.5% vs 14.3% RR = 1.02 P = .94
Kinoshita et al	2010	Retrospective observational	24 mo	454	0.8% vs 3.5% RR-0.25	0.8% vs 3.5%, P = .054	N/A	9.8% vs 17.8%, P < .001	N/A	N/A	N/A
Youn et al	2011	Prospective observational	36 mo	341	3.7% vs 0.8%, RR = 0.23, P = 1.6	N/A	3.7% vs 2.4% RR= N/A P = .752	13.4% vs 12% RR = 0.89 P = .741	7.9% vs 8% RR = N/A P = 1.0	1.4% vs 2.4% RR = N/A P = .673	18.1% vs 12.8% RR = 0.71 P = .224
Kim et al	2011	Observational	36 mo	974	3.1% vs 3.6%, HR = 0.58, P = .30	3.8% vs 7.8%, HR = 0.32, P = .03	0.7% vs 1.6% HR = 0.32, P = .09	N/A	7.4% vs 6.7% HR = 0.91, P = .76	0.2% vs 0.6% HR = 0.33, P = .34	10.9% vs 12.1% HR = 0.73, P = .20

TABLE 9.1 Summary of Studies Comparing the Clinical Outcomes of IVUS-Guided Versus Angiography-Guided Percutaneous Interventions With DESs (*Continued*)

OBSERVATIONAL STUDIES											
STUDY NAME	YEAR	STUDY DESIGN	DURATION OF STUDY	NUMBER OF PARTICIPANTS	IVUS- VS ANGIOGRAPHY-GUIDED PCI						
					ALL-CAUSE MORTALITY	CARDIOVASCULAR MORTALITY	MI	TVR	TLR	ST	MACE
Claessen et al	2011	Observational	24 mo	1504	3% vs 4.5%, HR = 0.89, *P* = .68	1.2% vs 1.9%, HR = 0.63 *P* = .03	2.1% vs 5.1%, HR = 0.43, *P* ≤ 0.01	11.1% vs 12.8%, *P* = .25	N/A	0.5% vs 0.9%, *P* = .16	13.4% vs 17%, HR = 0.81, *P* = .15
Ahmed et al	2011	Retrospective observational	12 mo	7710	1.0% vs 2.0%, RR = 0.49 *P* = .01	0.3% vs 1.3% RR = 0.24, *P* = .003	1.4% vs 0.8%, *P* = .02	0.4% vs 0.7% RR = 0.63, *P* = .17	2.0% vs 1.5%, *P* = .56	N/A	6.6% vs 6.1% RR = 1.07, *P* = .29
Wakabayashi et al	2012	Retrospective observational	12 mo	1984	5.9% vs 8.4%, *P* = .077	1.9% vs 4.4%, *P* = .01	2.0% vs 2.8%, *P* = .36	9.2% vs 10.6%, *P* = .42	5.5% vs 7.5%, *P* = .17	1.6% vs 1.7%, *P* = .83	11.0% vs 15.6%, *P* = .017
Hur et al	2013	Retrospective observational	36 mo	8371	HR = 0.49 *P* < .001	N/A	HR = 0.48 *P* = .04	HR = 1.15, *P* = .25	N/A	HR = 0.89, *P* = .61	HR = 0.85, *P* = .07
Chen et al	2013	Observational	12 mo	628	2.2% vs 3.9%, *P* = .24	0.9% vs 3.3% OR = 0.27, *P* = .049	4.6% vs 8.9% OR = 0.50, *P* = .038	10.2% vs 15.5% OR = 0.62, *P* = .05	8.6% vs 13.5% OR = 0.61, *P* = .05	1.2% vs 6.9% OR = 0.17, *P* < .001	15.7% vs 19.7% OR = 0.33, *P* = .21
Yoon et al	2013	Observational	12 mo	1574	0.2% vs 0.8% HR = 0.19 *P* = .12	0.2% vs 0.4% HR = 0.34, *P* = .34	0.2% vs 0.3% HR = 0.45, *P* = .45	2.1 vs 1.5% HR = 1.34, *P* = .44	N/A	0.2% vs 0.2% HR = 0.68, *P* = .75	2.3% vs 2.1% HR = 1.06, *P* = .87
Ahn et al	2013	Observational	24 mo	85	N/A	6.1% vs 5.6%, *P* = 1.0	2.0% vs 13.9%, *P* = .08	N/A	0% vs 27.8%, *P* < .001	2.0% vs 11.1%, *P* = .16	8% vs 33.3%, *P* = .005
Gao et al	2014	Observational	12 mo	1016	N/A	1.8% vs 6.2% OR = 0.32 *P* = .002	11.3% vs 17.2% OR = 0.79, *P* = .013	3.3% vs 11.8%, OR = 0.32, *P* < .001	2.4% vs 9.4%, OR = 0.31, *P* < .001	0.6% vs 2.7% OR = 0.14, *P* = 0.02	14.8% vs 27.7% OR = 0.58, *P* < .001
de la Torre Hernandez et al	2014	Observational	36 mo	1010	7.4% vs 13%, OR = 0.57 *P* = .01	3.3% vs 6% OR = 0.55, *P* = .07	4.5% vs 6.5% OR = 0.68, *P* = .4	N/A	7.7% vs 6.3% OR = 1.24, *P* = .7	0.6% vs 2.2%, OR = 0.27, *P* = .04	11.7% vs 16.0%, OR = 0.73, *P* = .04
Hong et al	2014	Observational	24 mo	534	1.9% vs 3.4%, *P* = .33	1.0% vs 2.4% OR = 0.62, *P* = .22	8.3% vs 7.6% OR = 1.1, *P* = .87	1.0% vs 3.7% OR = 0.26, *P* = .06	10.2% vs 10.4% OR = 0.98, *P* = .94	0% vs 2.1% OR = 0.10, *P* = .05	8.7% vs 9.5% OR = 0.68, *P* = .78

(*continued*)

Witzebbichler et al	2014	Prospective observational	12 mo	8583	1.8% vs 2.0% HR = 0.87 *P* = .4	0.8% vs 1.2% HR = 0.71 *P* = .12	2.5% vs 3.7% HR = 0.67 *P* = .002	2.4% vs 4% HR = 0.60 *P* < .001	1.5% vs 2.4% HR = 0.64 *P* = .007	0.6% vs 1% HR = 0.53 *P* = .02	3.1% vs 4.7% HR = 0.67 *P* < .001
Nakatsuma et al	2016	Retrospective observational	60 mo	3028	13% vs 16% HR = 0.87 *P* = .15	N/A	5.2% vs 6.6% HR = 0.81 *P* = .21	22% vs 27% HR = 0.76 *P* < .001	N/A	1.2% vs 3.1% HR = 0.39 *P* = .003	34% vs 40% HR = 0.83 *P* = .003
Kim et al	2017	Prospective observational	36 mo	196	7% vs 22%, HR = 0.45, P = .01	3.3% vs 18%, HR = 0.37, *P* = .001	10% vs 3.6%, HR = 0.46, *P* = 0.09	25% vs 14%, HR = 0.7, *P* = .001	20% vs 6%, HR = 0.34, *P* = .006	N/A	43% vs 21%, HR = 0.63, *P* = .001
Tian et al	2017	Observational	36 mo	1899	2.9% vs 3.9% HR = 0.76 *P* = .29 7% vs 22%, *P* = .002	1.8% vs 2.7% HR = 0.67 *P* = .23	5.2% vs 6.8% HR = 0.76 *P* = .16	6% vs 6% HR = 1.01 *P* = .97	3.1% vs 3.3% HR = 0.94 *P* = .81	1.4% vs 1.7% HR = 0.83 *P* = .63	5.8% vs 7.7%, HR = 0.75, *P* = .12
Andell et al	2017	Retrospective observational	10 y	2468	12.0% vs 27.1% HR = 0.44 *P* ≤ .001	N/A	N/A	N/A	N/A	0.0% vs 0.4%, HR = N/A	N/A
Okura et al	2019	Prospective observational	In-hospital	2636	5.1% vs 10.4%, *P* < .01	N/A	N/A	N/A	N/A	N/A	18.2% vs 19.3%, *P* = .09
Choi et al	2019	Retrospective observational	64 mo	6005	17.1% vs 25.5 HR = 0.61, *P* < .001	10.2% vs 16.9% HR = 0.57, *P* < .001	4.8% vs 7.3% HR = 0.64, *P* = .003	N/A	8.3% vs 11.4% HR = 0.75, *P* = .02	3.1% vs 4.4% HR = 0.59, *P* = .006	18.5% vs 28.1% HR = 0.62, *P* < .001
Kim et al	2020	Prospective observational	12 mo	7572	4.4% vs 7.0% RR = 0.70, *P* < .001	3.3% vs 5.2% RR = 0.69, *P* < .001	1.5% vs 1.6%, *P* = .83	0.6% vs 0.7%, *P* = .55	1.7% vs 1.5%, *P* = .60	N/A	5.6% vs 8.5%, *P* = .66
Kang et al	2021	Retrospective observational	10 y	976	16.4% vs 31.0% HR = 0.54, *P* < .001	N/A	2.4% vs 2.7% HR = 0.74, *P* = .53	18.3% vs 21.8% HR = 1.16, *P* = .41	N/A	N/A	N/A
Cortese et al	2022	Retrospective observational	12 mo	730	5% vs 13.9% HR = 0.37	1.9% vs 4.5% HR = 0.41	3.2% vs 4.2% HR = 0.76	N/A	10.2% vs 11% HR = 0.92	1.9 vs 0.6%	N/A
Hannan et al	2022	Prospective observational	30 mo	44,305	7.6% vs 9.6% OR = 0.89	N/A	N/A	8.71% vs 10.54%, OR = 0.88	N/A	N/A	N/A
Roh et al	2023	Retrospective observational	36 mo	4070	8% vs 12.9% HR = 0.60, *P* < .001	4.8% vs 8.3% HR = 0.57, *P* = .001	2.8% vs 4.2% HR = 0.65, *P* = .049	N/A	2.0% vs 3.3% HR = 0.60, *P* = .048	0.5% vs 1.1% HR = 0.41, *P* = .088	17.3% vs 22.5% HR = 0.75, *P* = .001

TABLE 9.1 Summary of Studies Comparing the Clinical Outcomes of IVUS-Guided Versus Angiography-Guided Percutaneous Interventions With DESs (*Continued*)

META-ANALYSES											
STUDY NAME	YEAR	NUMBER OF STUDIES	NUMBER OF RCTS	NUMBER OF PARTICIPANTS	IVUS- VS ANGIOGRAPHY-GUIDED PCI						
					ALL-CAUSE MORTALITY	CARDIOVASCULAR MORTALITY	MI	TVR	TLR	ST	MACE
Zhang et al	2012	11	1	19,619	HR = 0.59 (0.48-0.73)	N/A	HR = 0.82 (0.63-1.06)	HR = 0.90 (0.77-1.05)	HR = 0.90 (0.73-1.11)	HR = 0.58 (0.44-0.77)	HR = 0.87 (0.78-0.96)
Zhang et al	2013	14	3	29,029	HR = 0.66 (0.55-0.78)	N/A	HR = 0.74 (0.62-0.90)	N/A	HR = 0.82 (0.68-0.97)	HR = 0.57 (0.44-0.73)	HR = 0.86 (0.77-0.95)
Klersy et al	2013	12	3	18,707	HR = 0.60 (0.48-0.74)	N/A	HR = 0.59 (0.44-0.80)	HR = 0.95 (0.82-1.09)	N/A	HR = 0.50 (0.32-0.80)	HR = 0.80 (0.71-0.89)
Jang et al	2014	15	3	24,849	HR = 0.64 (0.51-0.81)	N/A	HR = 0.57 (0.42-0.78)	HR = 0.81 (0.68-0.95)	HR = 0.76 (0.62-0.94)	HR = 0.59 (0.42-0.82)	HR = 0.79 (0.69-0.91)
Ahn et al	2014	17	3	26,503	HR = 0.61 (0.48-0.79)	N/A	HR = 0.57 (0.44-0.75)	HR = 0.82 (0.70-0.97)	HR = 0.81 (0.66-1.00)	HR = 0.59 (0.47-0.75)	HR = 0.74 (0.64-0.85)
Zhang et al	2015	20	3	29,068	HR = 0.62 (0.54-0.71)	N/A	HR = 0.64 (0.55-0.75)	HR = 0.86 (0.77-0.97)	HR = 0.81 (0.69-0.94)	HR = 0.59 (0.47-0.73)	HR = 0.77 (0.71-0.83)
Steinvil et al	2016	25	7	31,283	HR = 0.62 (0.54-0.72)	N/A	HR = 0.67 (0.56-0.80)	HR = 0.85 (0.76-0.95)	HR = 0.77 (0.67-0.89)	HR = 0.58 (0.47-0.73)	HR = 0.76 (0.70-0.82)
Elgendy et al	2016	7	7	3275	N/A	HR = 0.46 (0.21-1.00)	HR = 0.52 (0.26-1.02)	HR = 0.61 (0.41-0.91)	HR = 0.60 (0.43-0.84)	HR = 0.49 (0.24-0.99)	HR = 0.60 (0.46-0.77)
Shin et al	2016	3	3	2345	N/A	HR = 0.38 (0.10-1.42)	N/A	N/A	HR = 0.61 (0.40-0.93)	HR = 0.50 (0.13-0.99)	HR = 0.36 (0.13-0.99)
Nerlekar et al	2017	15	6	9313	N/A	HR = 0.55 (0.36-0.83)	HR = 0.67 (0.50-0.90)	HR = 0.79 (0.64-0.98)	HR = 0.66 (0.52-0.84)	HR = 0.52 (0.38-0.72)	HR = 0.73 (0.64-0.85)
Fan et al	2017	15	6	8084	HR = 0.52 (0.40-0.67)	N/A	HR = 0.70 (0.56-0.86)	HR = 0.53 (0.40-0.70)	HR = 0.69 (0.50-0.94)	HR = 0.31 (0.20-0.50)	HR = 0.63 (0.53-0.73)
Bavishi et al	2017	8	8	3276	HR = 1.00 (0.48-2.09)	HR = 0.51(0.23-1.12)	HR = 0.90 (0.58-1.41)	HR = 0.60 (0.26-1.23)	HR = 0.62 (0.45-0.86)	HR = 0.57 (0.26-1.23)	HR = 0.64 (0.51-0.80)
Buccheri et al	2017	31	17	17,882	HR = 0.74 (0.58-0.98)	HR = 0.47 (0.32-0.66)	HR = 0.72 (0.52-0.93)	N/A	HR = 0.74 (0.58-0.90)	HR = 0.42 (0.20-0.72)	HR = 0.79 (0.67-0.91)
Räber et al	2018	8	8	3276	N/A	HR = 0.51 (0.23-1.12)	HR = 0.61 (0.51-0.80)	N/A	HR = 0.60 (0.43-0.83)	N/A	HR = 0.64 (0.51-0.80)

(*continued*)

Di Mario et al	2018	9	9	4724	N/A	HR = 0.51 (0.27-0.96)	HR = 0.62 (0.36-1.05)	N/A	HR = 0.58 (0.43-0.78)	N/A	HR = 0.62 (0.51-0.77)
Gao et al	2019	9	9	4724	HR = 0.78 (0.46-1.31)	HR = 0.49 (0.26-0.92)	HR = 0.79 (0.54-1.17)	HR = 0.58 (0.42-0.80)	HR = 0.59 (0.44-0.80)	HR = 0.45 (0.23-0.87)	HR = 0.61 (0.49-0.74)
Elgendy et al	2019	10	10	5060	N/A	HR = 0.44 (0.26-0.75)	HR = 0.55 (0.32-0.94)	N/A	HR = 0.57 (0.42-0.77)	HR = 0.44 (0.24-0.79)	N/A
Kumar et al	2019	11	11	5352	N/A	HR = 0.45 (0.25-0.80)	HR = 0.83 (0.54-1.28)	N/A	HR = 0.56 (0.41-0.77)	HR = 0.47 (0.24-0.94)	N/A
Malik et al	2020	10	10	5007	N/A	HR = 0.51 (0.27-0.96)	HR = 0.86 (0.58-1.29)	HR = 0.59 (0.43-0.81)	HR = 0.59 (0.43-0.81)	HR = 0.50 (0.24-1.04)	HR = 0.63 (0.51-0.77)
Darmoch et al	2020	19	6	27,637	N/A	HR = 0.63 (0.54-0.73)	HR = 0.71 (0.58-0.86)	N/A	HR = 0.81 (0.70-0.94)	HR = 0.57 (0.41-0.79)	N/A
Pang et al	2020	18	10	62,197	HR = 0.88 (0.24-2.80)	N/A	HR = 1.0 (0.09-11.0)	N/A	N/A	N/A	HR = 0.45 (0.20-0.97)
Zhang et al	2021	20	3	24,783	HR = 0.79 (0.63-0.98)	HR = 0.62 (0.47-0.82)	HR = 0.68 (0.57-0.80)	HR = 0.74 (0.65-0.85)	HR = 0.67 (0.65-0.85)	HR = 0.47 (0.33-0.67)	HR = 0.65 (0.58-0.73)
Groenland et al	2022	9	1	838,902	HR = 0.70 (0.59-0.82)	HR = 0.62 (0.29-1.33)	N/A	HR = 0.83 (0.29-1.33)	N/A	N/A	HR = 0.86 (0.29-1.33)
Khan et al[a]	2023	20	20	11,698	AR = 0.81 (0.64-1.02)	AR = 0.53 (0.39-0.72)	AR = 0.81 (0.68-0.97)	AR = 0.74 (0.61-0.89)	AR = 0.71 (0.59-0.86)	AR = 0.44 (0.27-0.72)	N/A
Park et al[a]	2023	28	28	12,895	RR = 1.15 (0.85-1.56)	RR = 0.64(0.43-0.94)	RR = 0.82 (0.64-1.04)	RR = 0.64 (0.50-0.81)	RR = 0.68 (0.57-0.80)	RR = 0.61 (0.36-1.04)	RR = 0.74 (0.63-0.88)
Kuno et al[a]	2023	32	32	22,684	RR = 0.86(0.66-1.11)	RR = 0.56(0.42-0.75)	RR = 0.81(0.66-0.99)	N/A	RR = 0.75 (0.57-0.99)	RR = 0.48 (0.31-0.73)	RR = 0.72(0.62-0.82)
Sreenivasan et al[a]	2024	16	16	7814	RR = 0.81(0.61-1.07)	RR = 0.49, (0.34-0.71)	RR = 0.82 (0.62-1.07)	RR = 0.60, (0.45-0.80)	RR = 0.67 (0.49-0.91)	RR = 0.63 (0.40-0.99)	RR = 0.67 (0.55-0.82)
Stone et al	2024	22	22	15,964	RR = 0.76 (0.57-1.01)	RR = 0.56 (0.38-0.83)	RR = 0.89 (0.69-1.15)	RR = 0.68 (0.56-0.82)	RR = 0.70 (0.57-0.86)	RR = 0.63 (0.35-1.11)	N/A
Giacoppo et al	2024	24	24	15,489	OR = 0.77 (0.55-1.08)	OR = 0.57 (0.37-0.90)	OR = 0.91 (0.70-1.19)	OR = 0.65 (0.53-0.81)	OR = 0.69 (0.54-0.87)	OR = 0.60 (0.35-1.05)	OR = 0.67 (0.56-0.80)

TABLE 9.1 Summary of Studies Comparing the Clinical Outcomes of IVUS-Guided Versus Angiography-Guided Percutaneous Interventions With DESs (*Continued*)

LM PCI: IVUS- VS ANGIOGRAPHY-GUIDED											
STUDY NAME	YEAR	NUMBER OF STUDIES	NUMBER OF RCTS	NUMBER OF PARTICIPANTS	IVUS- VS ANGIOGRAPHY-GUIDED PCI						
					ALL-CAUSE MORTALITY	CARDIOVASCULAR MORTALITY	MI	TVR	TLR	ST	MACE
Ye et al	2017	10	1	6480	HR = 0.60 (0.47-0.75)	HR = 0.47 (0.33-0.66)	HR = 0.80 (0.61-1.06)	HR = 0.89 (0.66-1.20)	HR = 0.43 (0.25-0.73)	HR = 0.28 (0.12-0.67)	N/A
Wang et al	2018	7	1	4592	HR = 0.55 (0.42-0.71)	HR = 0.45 (0.32-0.62)	HR = 0.66 (0.55-0.80)	HR = 0.64 (0.26-1.56)	HR = 0.60 (0.31-1.18)	HR = 0.48 (0.27-0.84)	HR = 0.61 (0.53-0.70)
Elgendy et al	2019	9	2	4971	HR = 0.53 (0.40-0.70)	HR = 0.40 (0.28-0.59)	HR = 0.69 (0.50-0.96)	N/A	HR = 0.76 (0.50-1.16)	HR = 0.47 (0.32-0.70)	N/A
Elgendy et al	2020	11	2	15,083	HR = 0.59 (0.53-0.66)	HR = 0.39 (0.27-0.58)	HR = 0.66 (0.48-0.90)	N/A	HR = 0.51 (0.39-0.68)	HR = 0.38 (0.26-0.56)	N/A
Saleem et al	2021	14	2	18,944	HR = 0.57 (0.46-0.70)	HR = 0.37 (0.26-0.54)	HR = 0.80 (0.66-0.97)	N/A	HR = 0.63 (0.45-0.89)	HR = 0.57 (0.31-1.05)	N/A
Kwon et al[a]	2023	18	3	21,701	RR = 0.53 (0.49-0.59)	RR = 0.37 (0.26-0.53)	N/A	N/A	N/A	N/A	N/A

[a]Provides combined outcomes for IVUS and OCT.

AR, absolute risk; CTO, chronic total occlusion; DES, drug-eluting stent; HR, hazard ratio; IVUS, intravascular ultrasound; MACE, major adverse cardiovascular event; MI, myocardial infarction; N/A, not applicable; OR, odds ratio; PCI, percutaneous coronary intervention; RCT, randomized controlled trial; RR, risk ratio; ST, stent thrombosis; TLR, target lesion revascularization; TVR, target vessel revascularization.

Adapted from Refs. 5-8.

TABLE 9.2 Summary of Available IVUS Devices in the Market as of July 2023

CHARACTERISTICS	PHILIPS VOLCANO EAGLE EYE	PHILIPS VOLCANO REFINITY	PHILIPS VOLCANO REVOLUTION	TERUMO	BOSTON SCIENTIFIC OPTICROSS	ACIST KODAMA	IVUS/OCT	INFRAREDX IVUS-NIRS
Transducer frequency	20 MHz	45 MHz	45 MHz	40-60 MHz	40-60 MHz	60 MHz	IVUS: 40-45 MHz	IVUS: 35-65 MHz
Transducer type	Phased array	Mechanical	Mechanical	Mechanical	Mechanical	Mechanical	Mechanical IVUS combined with OCT	Mechanical
Catheter crossing profile	3.5 Fr	3.0 Fr	3.2 Fr	3.2 Fr	3.1 Fr	<3.4 Fr	3.0-3.6 Fr	3.2 Fr
Transducer to tip length	10 mm (2.5 mm for short-tip version)	20.5 mm	30 mm	8-30 mm	20 mm	20 mm	10-20 mm	20 mm
Guiding catheter compatibility	≥5 Fr	≥5 Fr	≥6 Fr	≥5 Fr	≥5 Fr	≥6 Fr	≥5 Fr	≥6 Fr
Axial resolution	<170 μm	50 μm	50 μm	<30-69 μm	22-38 μm	40 μm	10-20 μm	40 μm
Penetration depth	>5 mm	>5 mm	>5 mm	N/A	6 mm	3-8 mm	>5 mm	3-8 mm
Pullback length	150 mm	150 mm	150 mm	150 mm	100 mm	120 mm	75-150 mm	150 mm

IVUS, intravascular ultrasound; NIRS, near-infrared spectroscopy; OCT, optical coherence tomography.
Adapted from Refs. 12 and 13.

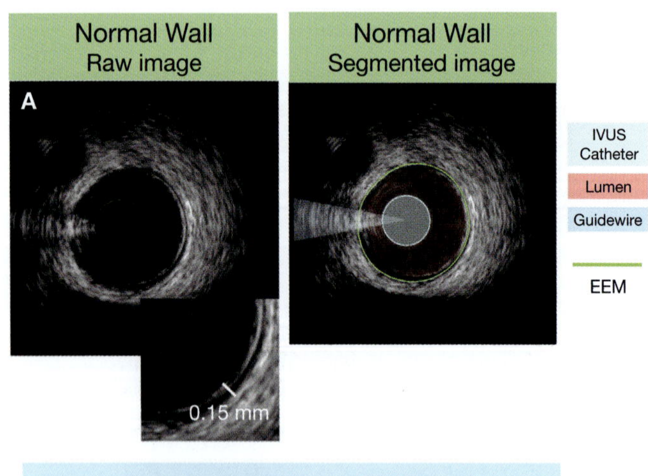

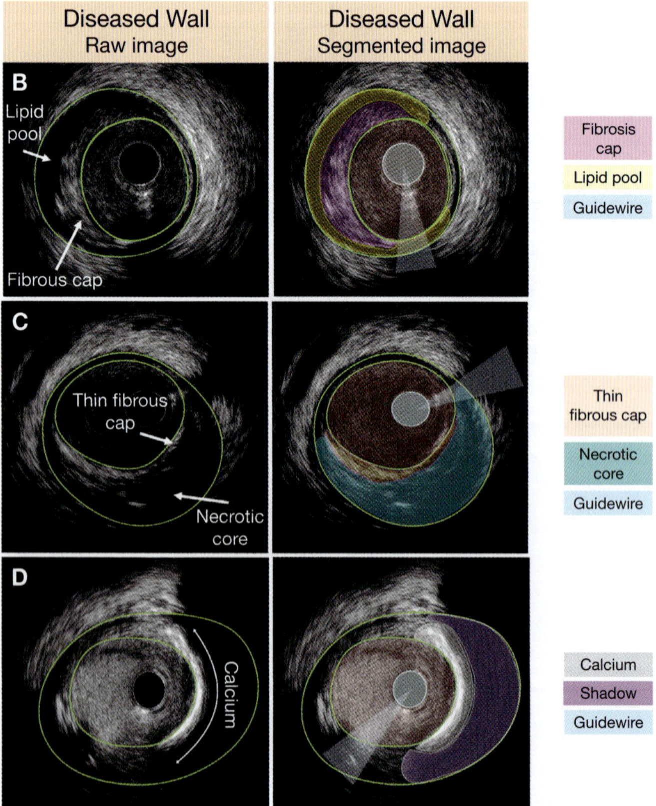

Plaque constituents by IVUS

- Lipid → Echolucent (dark/light grey)
- Necrotic core → Echolucent (black) behind an echodense leading edge (fibrous cap)
- Fibrous → Echodense (bright gray/white) without shadow
- Calcium → More echodense (bright white) than fibrous with shadow
- Thrombus → Fresh: Echolucent (black), Organized: Echodense (gray) without shadow

FIGURE 9.1 IVUS image interpretation. **A,** Normal wall; **B,** Fibroatheroma; **C,** Thin-cap fibroatheroma; **D,** Fibrocalcified plaque. IVUS, intravascular ultrasound.

blood flow leads to higher intensity and a coarser texture. Blood "speckle" is more prominent at higher imaging frequencies, which may interfere with the delineation of the blood-tissue interface. The lumen area is determined by the planimetry of the leading edge of the blood-intima acoustic interface.

(ii) Normal wall: IVUS can visualize all three layers of the arterial wall: intima, media, and adventitia. The intima appears as an echodense (gray) layer closest to the transducer. Outside the intima, the media layer appears as an echolucent (black) ring, exhibiting weak scattering due to the presence of smooth muscle cells mixed with only a small amount of collagen matrix. Media are surrounded by the adventitia, which appears as an echodense connective tissue layer. Adventitia produces the highest gray-level intensity due to greater scattering of the ultrasound waves.

(iii) Plaque constituents: The characteristic gray-level appearance of plaque constituents is defined by their brightness relative to that of adventitia.

Lipid tissue: Lipid-rich tissue within a plaque appears homogenously hypoechoic regions (black or light gray), often with irregular or poorly defined borders. Notably, necrotic core appears usually as a black region.

Fibrous tissue: Fibrous tissue is characterized by moderately echodense regions (mixture of gray and white; similarly bright to adventitia) of heterogeneous texture and without a shadow.

Calcium: Calcified tissue typically appears as a highly echodense region (bright white; brighter than adventitia) with complete distal acoustic shadowing.

Thrombus: Thrombus appears as a luminal mass with variable echogenicity. Fresh thrombus appears echolucent (black), while older or organized thrombus has a more heterogeneous echodense appearance (gray).

ARTIFACTS AND LIMITATIONS

IVUS, like any other imaging modality, has artifacts and limitations that can affect the quality and interpretation of the images (**Fig. 9.2**)[12,18]:

(i) Wire artifact: Most transducer designs position the guide wire external to the transducer, thereby introducing a "wire artifact," which looks like a gray or a black shade.

(ii) Shadow artifact: High-density structures, such as calcium deposits or stent struts, can cause shadowing artifacts, creating dark areas behind them. This can limit the visualization of structures located beyond the calcified or stent material.

(iii) Ringdown artifact: Transducer ringdown appears in virtually all medical ultrasound devices. This artifact arises from acoustic oscillations in the piezoelectric transducer material,

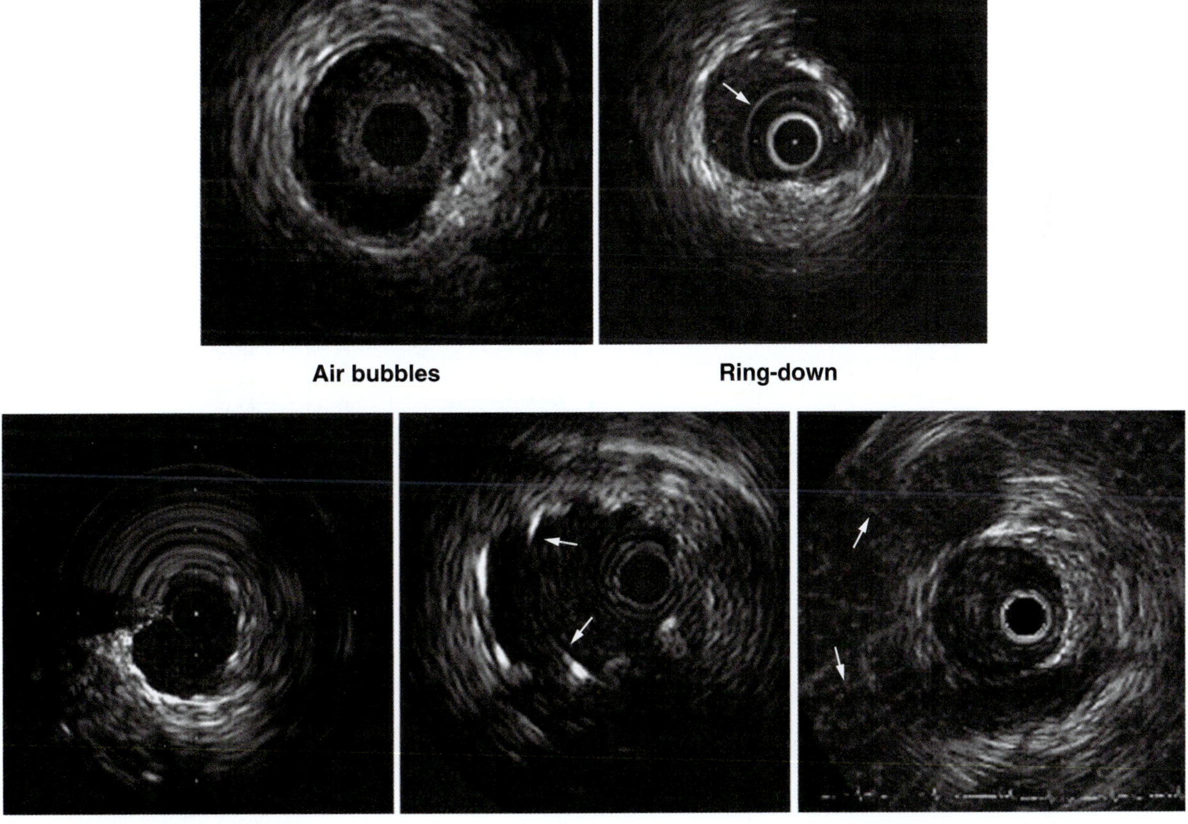

FIGURE 9.2 Common IVUS image artifacts. Air bubbles can cause a high echoic noise around the imaging catheter with image deterioration. Ring-down artifacts seen as a series of bright rings around the mechanical IVUS catheter (*arrow*) can also be caused by air bubbles, which need to be flushed out. Nonuniform rotational distortion (NURD) results in a wedge-shaped, smeared appearance in one or more segments of the image (between 9 and 4 o'clock in this example). White cap artifacts caused by side-lobe echoes (*arrows*) originate from a strong reflecting surface, such as metal stent struts or calcification. Smearing of the strut image can lead to the mistaken impression that the struts are protruding into the lumen. Radiofrequency noise (*arrows*) appears as alternating radial spokes or random white dots in the far-field. The interference is usually caused by other electrical equipment in the cardiac catheterization laboratory. IVUS, intravascular ultrasound. (From Honda Y, Fitzgerald PJ, Yock PG. Intravascular Imaging Techniques. In: Moscucci M, ed. *Grossman & Baim's Cardiac Catheterization, Angiography, and Intervention*. 9th ed. Wolters Kluwer; 2021:554-586. Figure 25.1.)

resulting in high-amplitude signals that obscure the near-field imaging. In mechanical systems, this artifact may be merged with the imaging sheath artifact. In electronic array catheters, this artifact may be largely removed by mask subtraction.

(iv) Reverberation artifact: Repetitive false echoes that occur when the IVUS beam encounters two parallel strong reflecting surfaces, such as calcium, metal stents, guide wires, and guide catheters. As a result, the IVUS waves are reflected back and forth repeatedly, causing the IVUS transducer to interpret the returning sound waves as deeper structures. Consequently, these reflections appear as multiple evenly spaced circumferential layers on the IVUS image.

(v) Nonuniform rotational distortion (NURD): Mechanical transducers may exhibit variations in rotational speed arising from a mechanical drag on the catheter driveshaft, creating NURD and producing visible distortion. NURD is most evident when the driveshaft is bent into a small radius of curvature by a tortuous vessel and is recognized as circumferential "stretching" of a portion of the image with "compression" of the contralateral vessel wall.

(vi) Attenuation artifact: Sound waves emitted by the IVUS probe may be attenuated as they pass through certain tissues or materials. This can decrease the image quality or penetration in areas with significant attenuation, such as heavily calcified or fibrotic plaques.

(vii) Geometric distortion: All IVUS imaging systems are subjected to geometric distortion produced by oblique imaging. Thus, when the ultrasound beam interrogates a plane that is not orthogonal to the vessel wall, the originally circular lumen appears elliptical in shape. This is particularly evident in the lumen imaging of the left main (LM) coronary artery.

CLINICAL APPLICATIONS OF IVUS

The 2021 American College of Cardiology/American Heart Association/Society for Cardiovascular Angiography and Interventions (ACC/AHA/SCAI) guidelines for PCI assign a class IIa recommendation for performing IVUS to define lesion severity and provide procedural guidance to reduce ischemic events, particularly for LM or complex coronary artery stenting.[19] There is also a IIa recommendation for IVUS use to determine the mechanism of stent failure.[19]

The clinical applications of IVUS extend from PCI planning to PCI optimization and follow-up (**Fig. 9.3**).[20]

PCI Planning

Lesion significance: The hemodynamic severity of ischemia across a stenosis is best assessed by physiologic studies. IVUS provides indirect information about the hemodynamic severity of a lesion; however, physiologic tests are still the gold standard and should not be substituted by IVUS.

Non-LM lesions: Ischemia across non-LM lesions has been shown to best correlate with the minimum lumen area (MLA) by

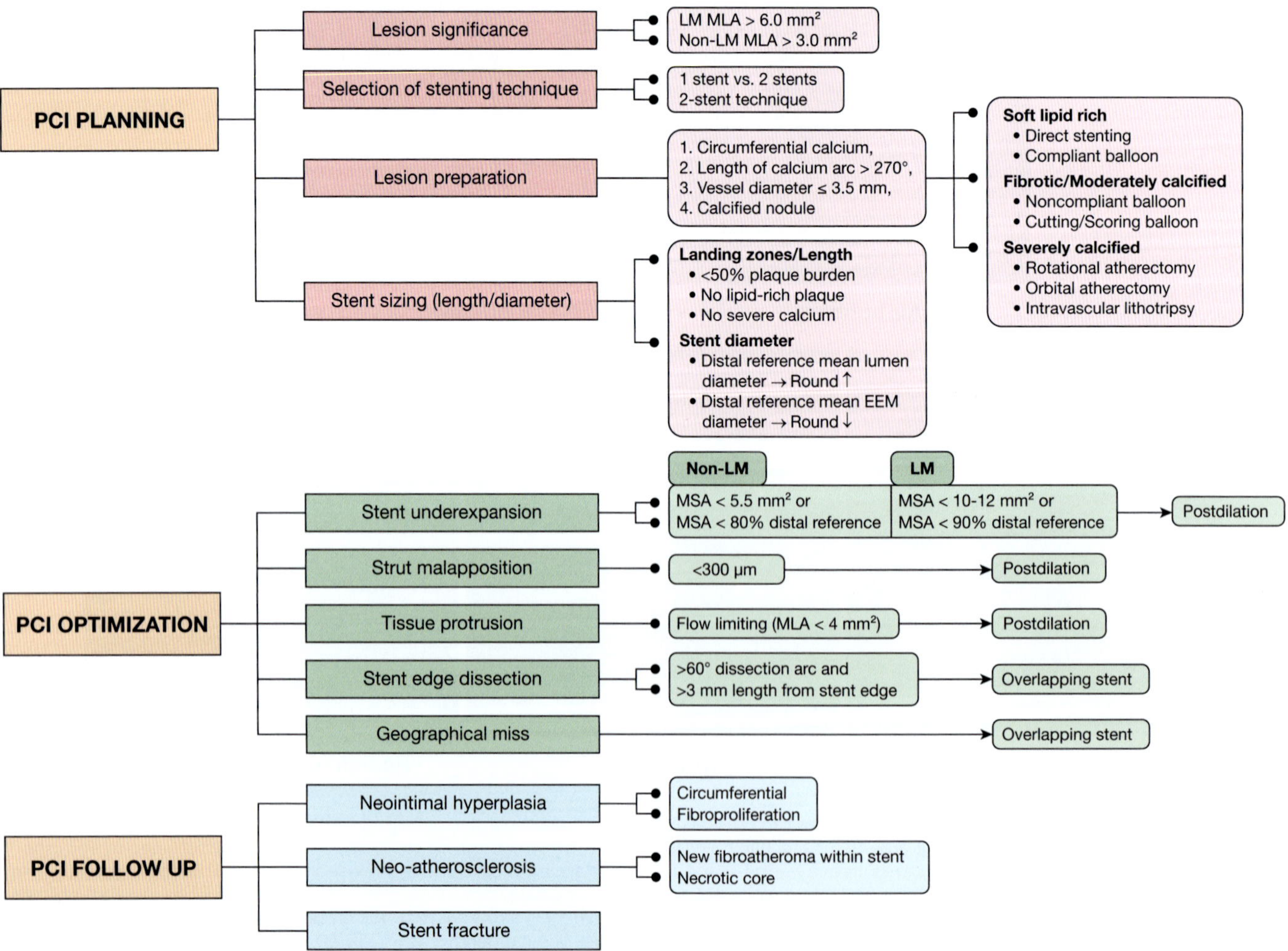

FIGURE 9.3 Summary of the clinical applications of IVUS. IVUS, intravascular ultrasound.

IVUS. In IVUS studies, MLA cutoffs ranged from 2.1 to 4.4 mm^2, with 3.0 mm^2 being the recommended cutoff by the meta-analyses (**Fig. 9.4**).[15] However, these cutoffs demonstrated relatively high negative predictive value, but low positive predictive value, suggesting a poor correlation between IVUS MLA and physiologic studies in assessing the hemodynamic significance of non-LM stenoses.[15] Overall, using an IVUS MLA cutoff to predict which non-LM lesions will result in stress-induced ischemia or low fractional flow reserve (FFR) should be avoided because other lesion characteristics, such as length, area stenosis, plaque burden, reference vessel size, and location, are important contributors to the hemodynamic significance of a lesion.[16,21]

LM lesions: Unlike non-LM coronary arteries, the LM has a reasonably high correlation between IVUS and FFR.[15] Studies have shown that patients with LM MLA > 6.0 mm^2 and deferred revascularization had similar outcomes to the revascularized group, whereas the outcomes in patients with LM MLA < 6.0 mm^2, who did not undergo revascularization, were significantly worse compared to the patients who had revascularization (**Fig. 9.4**).[15,22] According to the current recommendations, in LM lesions with MLA > 6.0 mm^2, revascularization can be safely deferred, in LM lesions with MLA < 4.5 mm^2, revascularization should be pursued, and in LM lesions with MLA between 4.5 and 6.0 mm^2, further evaluation with invasive or noninvasive physiologic studies should be considered.[18,22,23]

Lesion preparation: IVUS provides detailed plaque tissue characterization that can guide the lesion preparation strategy. Plaques that are predominantly lipid rich can be predilated with a compliant balloon or even stented directly. Predominantly fibrotic or moderately calcified plaques can be predilated with a noncompliant, high pressure, or cutting/scoring balloon. Severely calcified plaques warrant plaque modification using atherectomy devices (rotational, orbital) or intravascular lithotripsy. Calcium is frequent in target lesions (75%) but poorly detected by fluoroscopy or angiography (sensitivity only 40%).[5] Calcification markedly increases both the periprocedural risks (stent underexpansion, dissection, perforation, and acute lumen closure) and postprocedural outcomes. Calcified nodules have been associated with worse post-PCI outcomes and in-stent restenosis as they tend to lead to major stent underexpansion and protrusion of the calcified nodule through stent struts. Therefore, adequate preparation of these lesions appears to be critical.[24] IVUS provides accurate information about the severity of calcification based on the scoring system summarized in **Fig. 9.5** and subsequently guides the lesion preparation strategy according to the algorithm illustrated in **Fig. 9.6**.[25,26]

Stent sizing: IVUS offers distinct advantages over angiography in the identification of reference segments and stent sizing (**Fig. 9.7**). Traditionally, angiography (either eyeballing or quantitative coronary angiography) tends to underestimate the lumen dimensions compared to IVUS.[15,18] IVUS guidance results in larger stent diameter, greater angiographic mean lumen diameter (MLD), and minimum stent area (MSA), and implantation of more and longer stents compared to angiographically-guided stent implantation.[15,18]

Stent landing zones and length: Incomplete coverage of the lesion throughout its length (geographical miss) remains one of the most important predictors of stent failure and adverse clinical outcomes.[17] Stent length is based on the distance between the proximal and distal landing zone, which should have a plaque burden (percentage of mean external elastic membrane [EEM] area occupied by plaque) of less than 50% (ideally as close to normal as possible) and absence of lipid-rich material or severe calcification to minimize the risk of stent edge dissection and restenosis, respectively.[18,23,27]

Stent diameter: Stent underexpansion is a powerful predictor of ST and restenosis, and therefore, the selection of the correct stent diameter is of critical importance.[15,18] Stent diameter should be based on the distal landing zone, the site of the largest lumen distal to stenosis (ideally within the same segment with no intervening major branches). There are two different approaches for stent diameter (**Fig. 9.8**): The conservative approach advocates for stent diameter based on the MLD of distal reference rounded up to the closest available stent diameter quarter (eg, if the MLD at distal reference is 3.6 mm, then select a 3.75 mm stent). The less conservative approach considers the EEM diameter at the distal reference rounded down to the closest available stent diameter quarter (eg, if the mean EEM diameter at the distal reference is 3.9 mm, then select a 3.75 mm stent).[15,18]

PCI Optimization

Post PCI, IVUS imaging can be used to visualize fine abnormalities related to stent implantation,[15,18,23] which are summarized in **Fig. 9.7**: (i) stent underexpansion, (ii) strut malapposition, (iii) edge dissection, (iv) tissue protrusion, and (v) geographical miss. Stent underexpansion is a major predictor of stent restenosis. Early

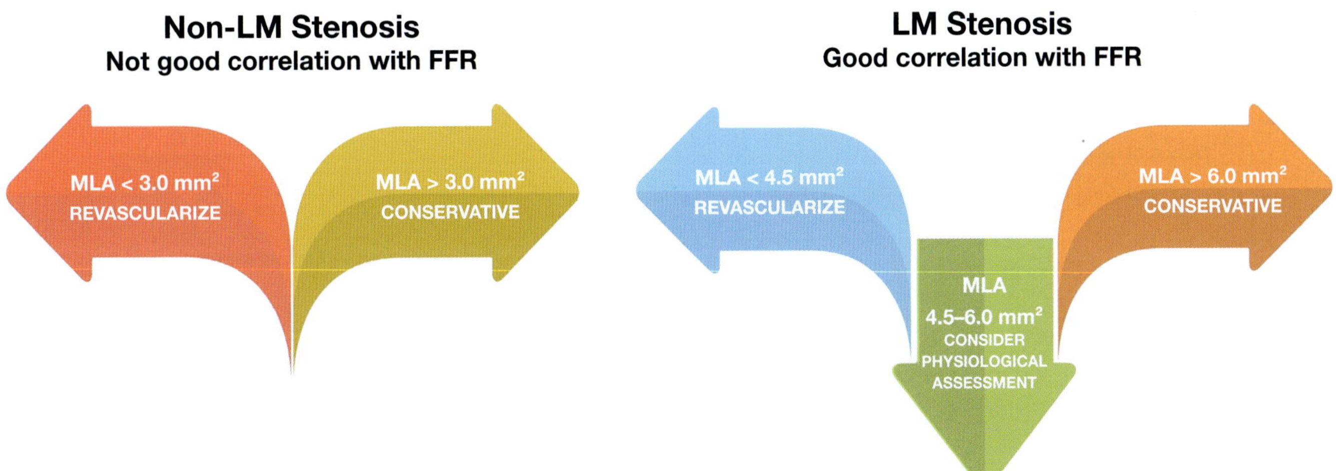

FIGURE 9.4 Role of IVUS in the assessment of functional significance of a stenosis. IVUS, intravascular ultrasound. (Adapted from Räber L, Mintz GS, Koskinas KC, et al. Clinical use of intracoronary imaging. Part 1: guidance and optimization of coronary interventions. An expert consensus document of the European Association of percutaneous cardiovascular interventions. *Eur Heart J.* 2018;39(35):3281-3300, by permission of Oxford University Press.)

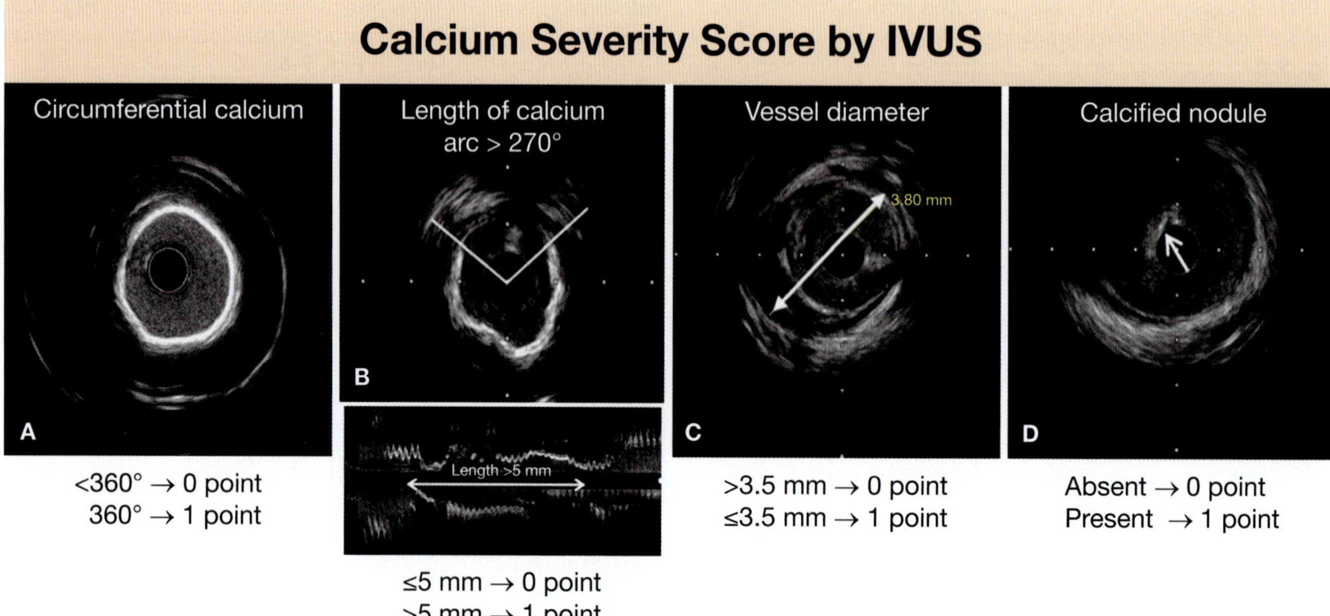

FIGURE 9.5 Calcium severity scoring based on IVUS imaging. **A,** Circumferential calcium; **B,** Length of calcium with arc >270°; **C,** Vessel diameter; and **D,** Protruding calcified nodules. The score ranges from 0 to 4. A score of ≥2 indicates severe calcium. IVUS, intravascular ultrasound. (Adapted by permission from Springer Karimi Galougahi K, Shlofmitz E, Jeremias A, et al. Therapeutic approach to calcified coronary lesions: disruptive technologies. *Curr Cardiol Rep*. 2021;23(4):33.)

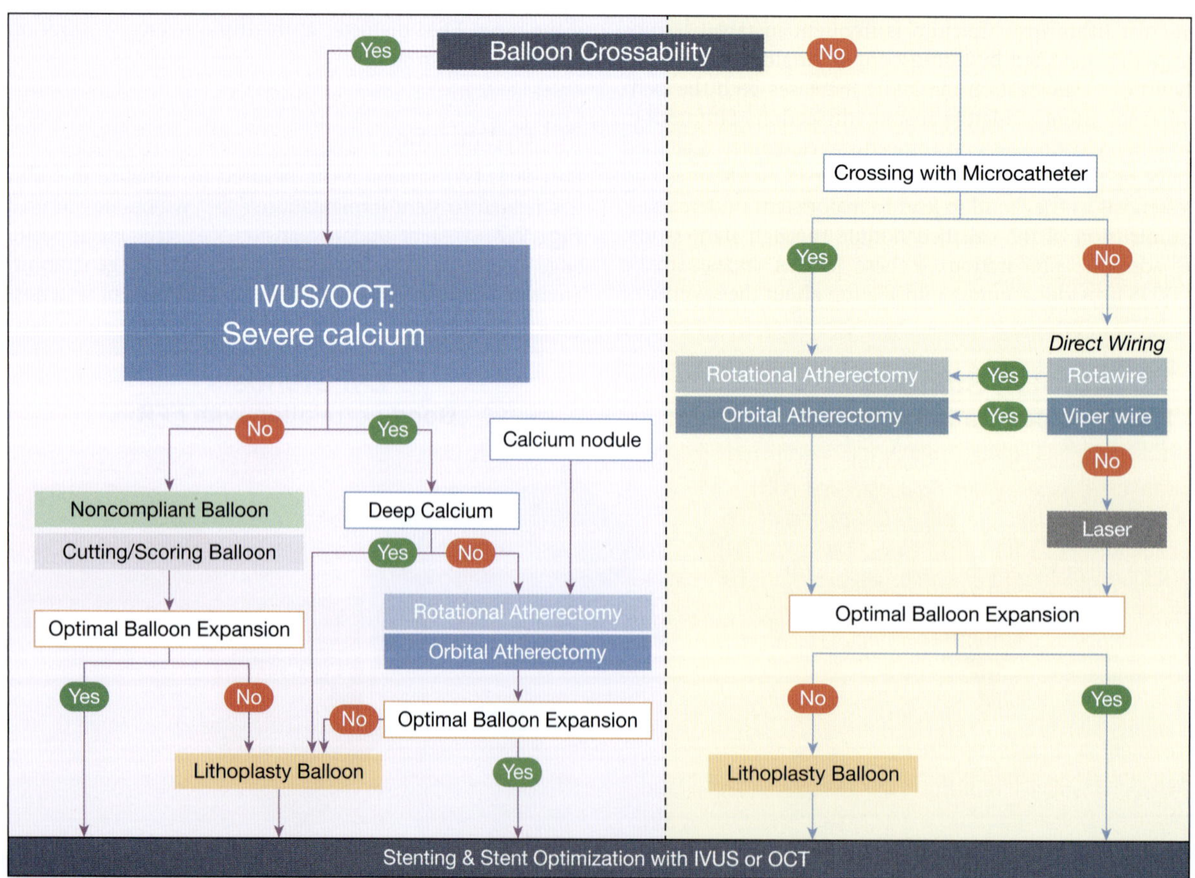

FIGURE 9.6 Intracoronary imaging-guided algorithmic approach for the preparation and optimal treatment of calcified coronary lesions. (Adapted from De Maria GL, Scarsini R, Banning AP. Management of calcific coronary artery lesions: is it time to change our interventional therapeutic approach? *JACC: Cardiovasc Interv*. 2019;12(15):1465-1478.)

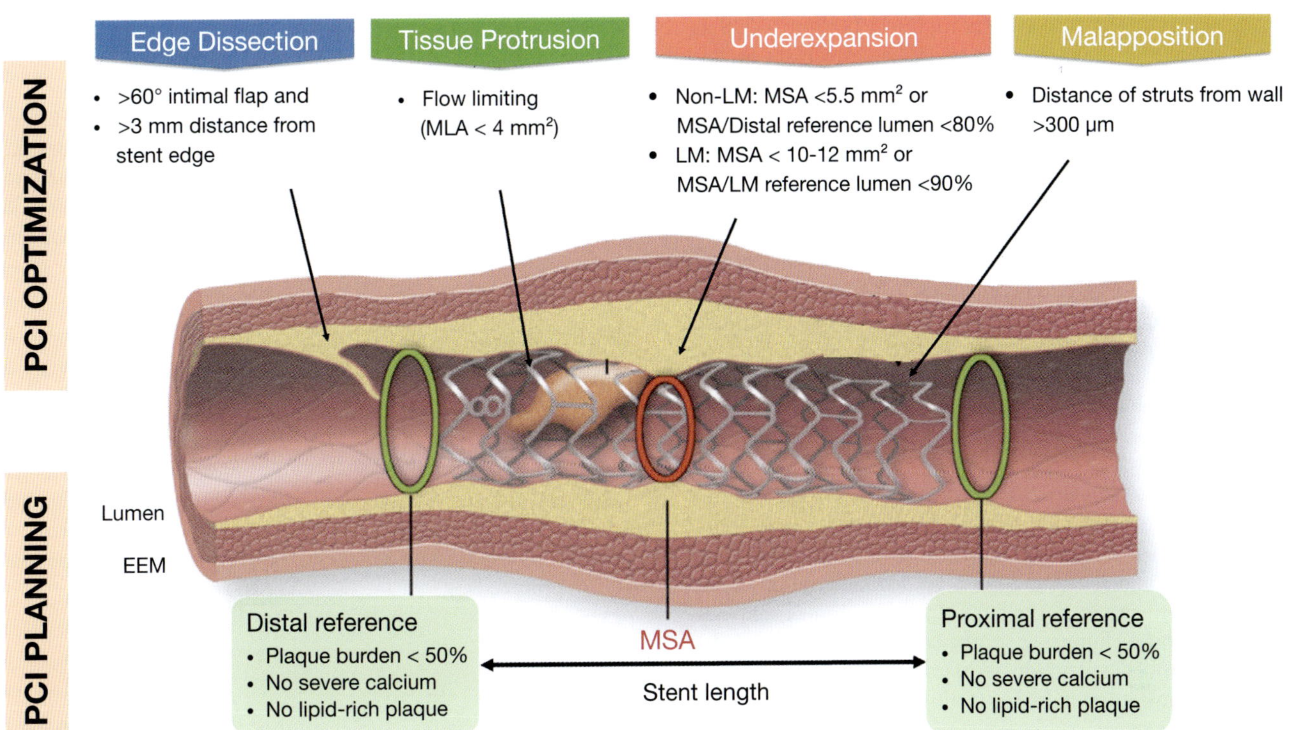

FIGURE 9.7 IVUS-guided PCI planning and optimization. IVUS, intravascular ultrasound; PCI, percutaneous coronary intervention. (Adapted from Räber L, Mintz GS, Koskinas KC, et al. Clinical use of intracoronary imaging. Part 1: guidance and optimization of coronary interventions. An expert consensus document of the European Association of Percutaneous Cardiovascular Interventions. *Eur Heart J.* 2018; 39(35):3281–3300, by permission of Oxford University Press.)

ST, occurring within 30 days after implantation, is primarily related to procedural issues, such as underexpansion, malapposition, and edge dissection. Late ST, occurring after 30 days, is associated with underexpansion, late stent malapposition, neoatherosclerosis, and uncovered stent struts.

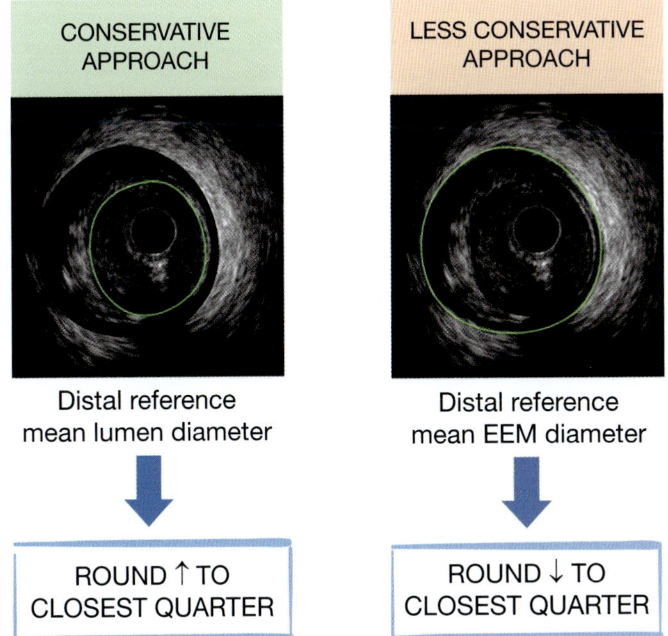

FIGURE 9.8 IVUS-guided approach for the selection of optimal stent diameter. IVUS, intravascular ultrasound.

PCI Follow Up—Assessment of Mechanism of Stent Failure

Certain findings on IVUS, such as MLA, plaque composition, and plaque burden, can predict restenosis after intervention.[23] Although stent placement abolishes negative remodeling and recoil after angioplasty, it stimulates neointimal hyperplasia, which is the primary mechanism of in-stent restenosis. The 2021 ACC/AHA/SCAI guidelines for PCI assign a class IIa recommendation for performing IVUS to identify the mechanism of stent restenosis (neointimal hyperplasia or neoatherosclerosis and rarely stent fracture) and guide subsequent therapy.[19]

ROLE OF IVUS IN SPECIAL CLINICAL SCENARIOS

(i) LM and bifurcation interventions: In both LM and non-LM bifurcation PCI, IVUS and intracoronary imaging in general are highly advised since they can inform on the complexity and extent of the disease, help with stenting strategy selection, and optimize PCI.[28] The recommended IVUS-based criteria of MSA to predict angiographic restenosis following LM PCI are <8.0 mm^2 at the LM (<10-12 mm2 in US population), <7.0 mm^2 at the polygon of confluence, <6.0 mm^2 at the LAD ostium, and <5.0 mm^2 at the LCX ostium.[29]

(ii) Cardiac allograft vasculopathy: Cardiac transplant patients may have diffuse vessel involvement making the diagnosis by coronary angiography challenging. Rapidly progressive vasculopathy detected by IVUS was found to be a powerful predictor of death and MI in cardiac transplant recipients.[30] For that reason, several transplant centers routinely perform IVUS as part of an annual catheterization in cardiac transplant recipients. The 2011 ACC/AHA/SCAI guidelines for PCI assigned a class IIa recommendation for performing IVUS at 4 to 6 weeks and at 1 year after cardiac transplantation to exclude donor coronary artery disease, detect rapidly progressive cardiac allograft vasculopathy, and provide prognostic information.[31]

(iii) Spontaneous coronary artery dissection (SCAD): IVUS is a valuable tool for the diagnosis of SCAD. IVUS visualizes the dissection flap, intramural hematoma, and true and false lumen.[32] Even though intervention to SCAD is not routinely recommended, when clinically needed, IVUS can confirm the location of the wire in the true lumen and prevent wiring the false lumen, which might result in perforation or distal propagation of the dissection.[33]

(iv) CTO: The CTO-IVUS trial showed a reduction in the composite of death/MI with IVUS-guided versus angiography-guided PCI optimization.[34] There are several scenarios where IVUS may be useful during CTO PCI: (i) identification of an ambiguous proximal cap and IVUS-guided penetration of the cap, (ii) identification of the subintimal position of the wire and facilitation of luminal re-entry, (iii) simplification of the reverse-controlled antegrade retrograde tracking maneuver, and (iv) optimization of the result after stent implantation.[34]

FUTURE DIRECTIONS

Table 9.3 summarizes the future directions in IVUS imaging focused on (i) software solutions that incorporate artificial intelligence tools to streamline the image acquisition and interpretation process and subsequent PCI guidance and (ii) hardware solutions, including hybrid IVUS catheters or higher resolution catheters.[13,15,35] From the educational standpoint, surveys indicate that only around 20% of interventional cardiology fellows feel adequately prepared to use IVUS or OCT in clinical practice, despite the skill being deemed "essential" by the Accreditation Council for Graduate Medical Education. The scientific community should work rigorously to train the next generation of interventional cardiologists on intracoronary imaging.[9]

TABLE 9.3 Future Directions in IVUS Imaging

SOFTWARE SOLUTION	HARDWARE SOLUTIONS
Artificial intelligence-driven plaque segmentation, characterization, and PCI guidance	Improved IVUS transducers • High-frequency transducers • Micromachined ultrasound transducers
IVUS-derived FFR	Miniature IVUS catheters
IVUS/angiography coregistration	IVUS with real-time distal pressure measurements
Fusion imaging • IVUS combined with MRI or CT	Hybrid IVUS systems • IVUS/OCT → commercially available • IVUS-NIRS → commercially available • IVUS-IVPA → not commercially available • IVUS-NIRF → not commercially available • IVUS-TRFS (FLIM) → not commercially available • IVUS-OCT-NIRF → not commercially available • IVUS-OCT-IVPA → not commercially available
	Guidewire-based IVUS

FFR, fractional flow reserve; FLIM, fluorescence lifetime imaging; IVPA, intravascular photoacoustic imaging; IVUS, intravascular ultrasound; NIRF, near infrared fluorescence imaging; NIRS, near-infrared spectroscopic imaging; OCT, optical coherence tomography; TRFS, time-resolved fluorescence spectroscopic imaging.

SUMMARY

IVUS adds significantly to day-to-day decision making in the cardiac catheterization laboratory. The clinical applications of IVUS extend from PCI planning to PCI optimization and PCI follow-up. IVUS is particularly useful in complicated anatomies, and long and bifurcated lesions. All interventional cardiologists should have a good working knowledge of IVUS to determine how it can be best used to optimize PCI.

Key Points

- Unlike angiography, which only depicts the silhouette of the coronary lumen, IVUS provides a cross-sectional perspective.
- IVUS is a workhorse intracoronary imaging modality in the cardiac catheterization laboratory, and therefore, operators should be familiar with the performance and interpretation of IVUS.
- More than 75 studies, including RCTs, observational studies, and meta-analyses, have demonstrated that compared to angiography-guided PCI, IVUS-guided PCI is associated with a significant reduction (up to 50%) of adverse events, including all-cause mortality or cardiovascular mortality.
- IVUS visualizes the arterial wall by using higher ultrasound frequencies (20-60 MHz) than that of standard echocardiography, providing an axial resolution that ranges between 20 and 150 µm, a lateral resolution of 200 to 250 µm, and tissue penetration (depth) of 6 to 12 mm.
- There are two types of transducer design: (i) mechanically rotated transducers and (ii) multielement electronic phased-array transducers.[13] In clinical practice, both transducer types provide sufficiently accurate information, although mechanical systems typically achieve higher resolution.
- IVUS imaging is safe, with no long-term untoward effects.
- IVUS provides information about the plaque constituents (ie, lipid, fibrous, fibrolipid, calcium, thrombus) based on their characteristic gray-level appearance relative to that of adventitia.
- IVUS, like any other imaging modality, has artifacts and limitations that can affect the quality and interpretation of the images, including ringdown artifact, wire artifact, shadow artifact, NURD, reverberation artifact, attenuation artifact, and geometric distortion.

- The 2021 ACC/AHA/SCAI guidelines for PCI assign a class IIa recommendation for performing IVUS to define lesion severity and provide procedural guidance to reduce ischemic events, particularly for LM or complex coronary artery stenting.
- The clinical applications of IVUS extend from PCI planning to PCI optimization and PCI follow-up. Regarding PCI planning, IVUS provides information about lesion significance, lesion preparation, and stent sizing. In terms of PCI optimization, IVUS provides information about stent underexpansion, strut malapposition, edge dissection, tissue protrusion, and geographical miss. In terms of PCI follow-up, IVUS provides information on the mechanism of stent restenosis (neointimal hyperplasia vs neoatherosclerosis).
- IVUS is useful in specific lesion subsets, such as bifurcation, LM lesions, cardiac allograft vasculopathy, spontaneous coronary artery dissection, and chronic total occlusions.
- Future directions in IVUS imaging are focused on improving the software and hardware as well as combining multiple imaging modalities to improve the image depth and resolution.

Acknowledgments

The author and editors acknowledge the authors of the prior version of this chapter, Drs Arnold H. Seto and Sonia R. Samtani, whose editing served as the basis for this updated chapter. Also, we acknowledge the significant contribution of Dr Akshat Banga in the writing of the chapter and of Dr Ruben Tapia Orihuela in the creation of figures.

Disclosures

Yiannis S. Chatzizisis: Speaker honoraria, advisory board fees, and research grant from Boston Scientific, Inc, advisory board fees and research grant from Medtronic, Inc, issued US patent (no.: 11,026,749) and international patent pending (application no.: PCT/US2020/057304) for the invention entitled "Computational simulation platform for the planning of interventional procedures"; Cofounder of ComKardia, Inc.

For further review and interactivities, please see the chapter-based multiple choice questions and videos accessible in the complimentary eBook bundled with this text. Access instructions are located in the inside front cover.

References

1. Schoenhagen P, Nissen SE. Coronary atherosclerotic disease burden: an emerging endpoint in progression/regression studies using intravascular ultrasound. *Curr Drug Targets Cardiovasc Haematol Disord*. 2003;3(3):218-226.
2. Mintz GS, Nissen SE, Anderson WD, et al. American College of Cardiology clinical expert consensus document on standards for acquisition, measurement and Reporting of Intravascular Ultrasound Studies (IVUS). A report of the American College of Cardiology task force on clinical expert consensus documents developed in collaboration with the European Society of Cardiology endorsed by the Society of cardiac angiography and interventions. *Eur J Echocardiogr*. 2001;2(4):299-313.
3. Jensen LO, Thayssen P, Mintz GS, et al. Comparison of intravascular ultrasound and angiographic assessment of coronary reference segment size in patients with type 2 diabetes mellitus. *Am J Cardiol*. 2008;101(5):590-595.
4. Stone GW, Maehara A, Lansky AJ, et al; PROSPECT Investigators. A prospective natural-history study of coronary atherosclerosis. *N Engl J Med*. 2011;364(3):226-235.
5. Giacoppo D, Laudani C, Occhipinti G, et al. Coronary angiography, intravascular ultrasound, and optical coherence tomography for guiding of percutaneous coronary intervention: a systematic review and network meta-analysis. *Circulation*. 2024;149(14):1065-1086.
6. Mintz GS, Bourantas CV, Chamié D. Intravascular imaging for percutaneous coronary intervention guidance and optimization: the evidence for improved patient outcomes. *J Soc Cardiovasc Angiogr Interv*. 2022;1(6):100413.
7. Stone GW, Christiansen EH, Ali ZA, et al. Intravascular imaging-guided coronary drug-eluting stent implantation: an updated network meta-analysis. *Lancet*. 2024;403(10429):824-837.
8. Kwon W, Lee JM, Yun KH, et al; RENOVATE COMPLEX-PCI Investigators. Clinical benefit of intravascular imaging compared with conventional angiography in left main coronary artery intervention. *Circ Cardiovasc Interv*. 2023;16(12):e013359.
9. Khan SU, Agarwal S, Arshad HB, et al. Intravascular imaging guided versus coronary angiography guided percutaneous coronary intervention: systematic review and meta-analysis. *BMJ*. 2023;383:e077848.
10. Kuno T, Kiyohara Y, Maehara A, et al. Comparison of intravascular imaging, functional, or angiographically guided coronary intervention. *J Am Coll Cardiol*. 2023;82(23):2167-2176.
11. Sreenivasan J, Reddy RK, Jamil Y, et al. Intravascular imaging–guided versus angiography-guided percutaneous coronary intervention: a systematic review and meta-analysis of randomized trials. *J Am Heart Assoc*. 2024;13(2):e031111.
12. Xu J, Lo S. Fundamentals and role of intravascular ultrasound in percutaneous coronary intervention. *Cardiovasc Diagn Ther*. 2020;10(5):1358-1370.
13. Peng C, Wu H, Kim S, Dai X, Jiang X. Recent advances in transducers for Intravascular Ultrasound (IVUS) imaging. *Sensors*. 2021;21(10):3540.
14. Mintz GS, Pichard AD, Popma JJ, et al. Determinants and correlates of target lesion calcium in coronary artery disease: a clinical, angiographic and intravascular ultrasound study. *J Am Coll Cardiol*. 1997;29(2):268-274.
15. Mintz GS, Matsumura M, Ali Z, Maehara A. Clinical utility of intravascular imaging: past, present, and future. *JACC Cardiovasc Imaging*. 2022;15(10):1799-1820.
16. Nissen SE, Yock P. Intravascular ultrasound: novel pathophysiological insights and current clinical applications. *Circulation*. 2001;103(4):604-616.
17. Papafaklis MI. Basic interpretation of intracoronary ultrasound and optical coherence tomography images: examples. *Continuing Cardiol Edu*. 2016;2(2):115-121.
18. Räber L, Mintz GS, Koskinas KC, et al; ESC Scientific Document Group. Clinical use of intracoronary imaging. Part 1: guidance and optimization of coronary interventions. An expert consensus document of the European Association of Percutaneous Cardiovascular Interventions. *Eur Heart J*. 2018;39(35):3281-3300.
19. Writing Committee Members; Lawton JS, Tamis-Holland JE, Bangalore S, et al. 2021 ACC/AHA/SCAI guideline for coronary artery revascularization: executive summary—a report of the American College of Cardiology/American Heart Association Joint Committee on clinical practice guidelines. *J Am Coll Cardiol*. 2022;79(2):197-215.
20. Truesdell AG, Alasnag MA, Kaul P, et al; ACC Interventional Council. Intravascular imaging during percutaneous coronary intervention: JACC state-of-the-art review. *J Am Coll Cardiol*. 2023;81(6):590-605.
21. Waksman R, Di Mario C, Torguson R, et al; LRP Investigators. Identification of patients and plaques vulnerable to future coronary events with near-infrared spectroscopy intravascular ultrasound imaging: a prospective, cohort study. *Lancet*. 2019;394(10209):1629-1637.
22. de la Torre Hernandez JM, Hernández Hernandez F, Alfonso F, et al; LITRO Study Group Spanish Working Group on Interventional Cardiology. Prospective application of pre-defined intravascular ultrasound criteria for assessment of intermediate left main coronary artery lesions: results from the multicenter LITRO study. *J Am Coll Cardiol*. 2011;58(4):351-358.
23. Johnson TW, Räber L, di Mario C, et al. Clinical use of intracoronary imaging. Part 2: acute coronary syndromes, ambiguous coronary angiography

findings, and guiding interventional decision-making—an expert consensus document of the European Association of Percutaneous Cardiovascular Interventions. *Eur Heart J*. 2019;40(31):2566-2584.

24. Sato T, Matsumura M, Yamamoto K, et al. Impact of eruptive vs noneruptive calcified nodule morphology on acute and long-term outcomes after stenting. *JACC Cardiovasc Interv*. 2023;16(9):1024-1035.
25. De Maria GL, Scarsini R, Banning AP. Management of calcific coronary artery lesions: is it time to change our interventional therapeutic approach? *JACC Cardiovasc Interv*. 2019;12(15):1465-1478.
26. Karimi Galougahi K, Shlofmitz E, Jeremias A, et al. Therapeutic approach to calcified coronary lesions: disruptive technologies. *Curr Cardiol Rep*. 2021;23(4):33.
27. Zhang J, Gao X, Kan J, et al. Intravascular ultrasound versus angiography-guided drug-eluting stent implantation: the ULTIMATE trial. *J Am Coll Cardiol*. 2018;72(24):3126-3137.
28. Mintz G.S, Lefèvre T, Lassen JF, et al. Intravascular ultrasound in the evaluation and treatment of left main coronary artery disease: a consensus statement from the European Bifurcation Club. *EuroIntervention*. 2018;14(4):e467-e474.
29. Park S, Park SJ, Park DW. Percutaneous coronary intervention for left main coronary artery disease: present status and future perspectives. *JACC Asia*. 2022;2(2):119-138.
30. Tuzcu EM, Kapadia SR, Sachar R, et al. Intravascular ultrasound evidence of angiographically silent progression in coronary atherosclerosis predicts long-term morbidity and mortality after cardiac transplantation. *J Am Coll Cardiol*. 2005;45(9):1538-1542.
31. Levine GN, Bates ER, Blankenship JC, et al. 2011 ACCF/AHA/SCAI guideline for percutaneous coronary intervention: a report of the American College of Cardiology Foundation/American Heart Association task force on practice guidelines and the Society for Cardiovascular Angiography and Interventions. *Circulation*. 2011;124(23):e574-e651.
32. Christian JMV. Spontaneous coronary artery dissection. *Heart*. 2010;96(10):801.
33. Nepal S, Bishop MA. *Spontaneous Coronary Artery Dissection—StatPearls—NCBI Bookshelf*; 2023.
34. Werner GS. *Use ofIntravascular Ultrasound in the Assessment of Chronic Total Occlusions*. RadcliffeCardiology.com. 2017.
35. Moon IT, Kim SH, Chin JY, et al. Accuracy of artificial intelligence–based automated quantitative coronary angiography compared to intravascular ultrasound: retrospective cohort study. *JMIR Cardio*. 2023;7:e45299.

Intracoronary Optical Coherence Tomography

Keyvan Karimi Galougahim, Doosup Shin,
Richard A. Shlofmitz, and Ziad A. Ali

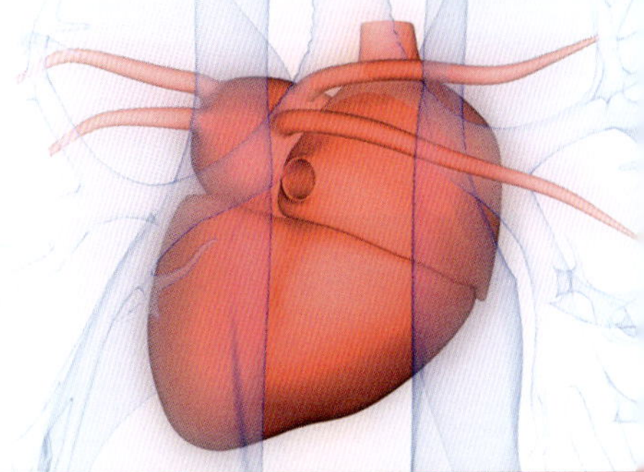

INTRODUCTION

The limitations of fluoroscopic angiography, which provides a lumenogram from two-dimensional projections of three-dimensional coronary tree, are established. By providing cross-sectional tomographic and longitudinal imaging of the coronary artery, intravascular imaging provides information that is complementary to angiography. Intravascular imaging thus aids in the accurate assessment of vessel dimension, disease morphology, and optimization of percutaneous coronary intervention (PCI).[1-7] The two commonly used intravascular imaging modalities in the cardiac catheterization laboratory are intravascular ultrasound (IVUS) and optical coherence tomography (OCT). The focus of this chapter is on the utility of OCT in PCI.

OCT IN PCI

Technology and Imaging Platforms

Intracoronary OCT is an imaging modality that utilizes near-infrared light to generate cross-sectional and three-dimensional volumetric images of the vessel structure. Compared with IVUS, OCT provides higher quality images due to greater axial resolution (10-20 vs 50-150 µm, respectively) but has lower penetration depth (1-2 vs 5-6 mm, respectively). OCT imaging can be affected by the presence of structures that absorb or attenuate the infrared light, such as thrombus, lipid necrotic core, or calcium.[8] Since blood also attenuates OCT signal by scattering the infrared light, flushing with radiocontrast, or sometimes saline, is required to displace blood from imaging field during OCT image acquisition.

Among the multiple intracoronary OCT image systems, the globally most commonly used is ILUMIEN OPTIS (Abbott, Santa Clara, CA). LUNAWAVE (Terumo, Tokyo, Japan) is used frequently in Japan but is not available in the United States. Some emerging OCT systems are incorporated with IVUS (Novasight Hybrid [Conavi Medical, Inc, Toronto, Canada] and Dual Sensor [Terumo, Tokyo, Japan]), near-infrared spectroscopy (HyperVue, SpectraWave, Bedford, MA), or near-infrared fluorescence (Canon Medical, Cambridge, MA) enabling simultaneous utilization of advantages of different imaging modalities. Recently, OCT-derived vessel geometries have been used to derive virtual fractional flow reserve by application of computational fluid dynamics, and this developing technology may allow for evaluation of both functional significance and morphological characteristics of plaque at the same time.

Practical Steps in OCT Image Acquisition

OCT imaging systems consist of an imaging catheter, a drive motor operating control, and software. The imaging catheter needs to be flushed with the same material planned to flush coronary artery during the image acquisition (mostly radiocontrast and occasionally saline). Appropriate guide catheter engagement is critical for optimal image acquisition to ensure optimal flushing of the coronary artery while avoiding ejection of the guide catheter. It is also recommended to give intracoronary nitroglycerin prior to the image acquisition to dilate the vessel and reduce catheter-induced coronary spasm.

The OCT imaging steps in sequence are position, purge, puff, and pullback. The OCT catheter is positioned approximately 10 mm distal to the target lesion over coronary guidewire and purged again. Then, a small puff is given through the guide catheter to ensure optimal guide catheter engagement and clearance of blood. If clearance is suboptimal, guide catheter position and engagement should be adjusted. Occasionally, a guide catheter extension is required to prevent reflux of flush medium into the aorta. Finally, automated pullback of the OCT catheter is activated. During the pullback, the contrast (or saline) can be injected manually or by an automated injector. The flush rate is most commonly set at 4 mL/s for a total volume of 14 to 16 mL for the left coronary artery and 3 mL/s for a total volume of 12 to 14 mL for the right coronary artery, with a pressure limit of 300 psi.[8] Larger volumes may be required for larger arteries. Cine angiography is performed during the pullback to facilitate OCT coregistration.

Interpretation of OCT Image

The bright-dark-bright trilaminar appearance of the normal coronary artery represents the light reflected from the three layers of the vessel corresponding to intima, media, and adventitia (**Fig. 10.1A**). In diseased vessels, there is a loss of this normal architecture, with morphologies observed on OCT that correlate with different types of atherosclerotic plaques. A simplified algorithm for OCT image interpretation of the most frequent pathological morphologies is shown in **Fig. 10.2**. These morphologies in the vessel wall include low-attenuating signal-rich (bright) lesions (fibrous plaques; **Fig. 10.1B**), high-attenuating signal-poor (dark) regions covered with a fibrous cap (lipid-rich plaques; **Fig. 10.1C**), and low-attenuating and sharply demarcated signal-poor regions (calcific plaques; **Fig. 10.1D**). In the lumen, high-attenuating red thrombus that casts a shadow on the vessel wall (**Fig. 10.1E**) or low-attenuating white thrombus (**Fig. 10.1F**) are the most common pathologies.

The high resolution of OCT also enables identification of culprit lesions of acute coronary syndrome (ACS), such as plaque rupture, erosion, and eruptive calcified nodule (**Fig. 10.3A-C**). The ability to identify different causes of ACS may have a potential role in the tailored management of ACS. OCT can also be helpful in evaluating patients with spontaneous coronary artery dissections or myocardial infarction (MI) with nonobstructive coronary arteries and resolving the ambiguity regarding the culprit lesions of non-ST segment elevation MI.[8] Last, OCT can also be helpful in identifying high-risk vulnerable plaques that are prone to rupture and cause ACS, such as thin-cap fibroatheroma (TCFA) (**Fig. 10.3D**), which will be further discussed in another chapter.

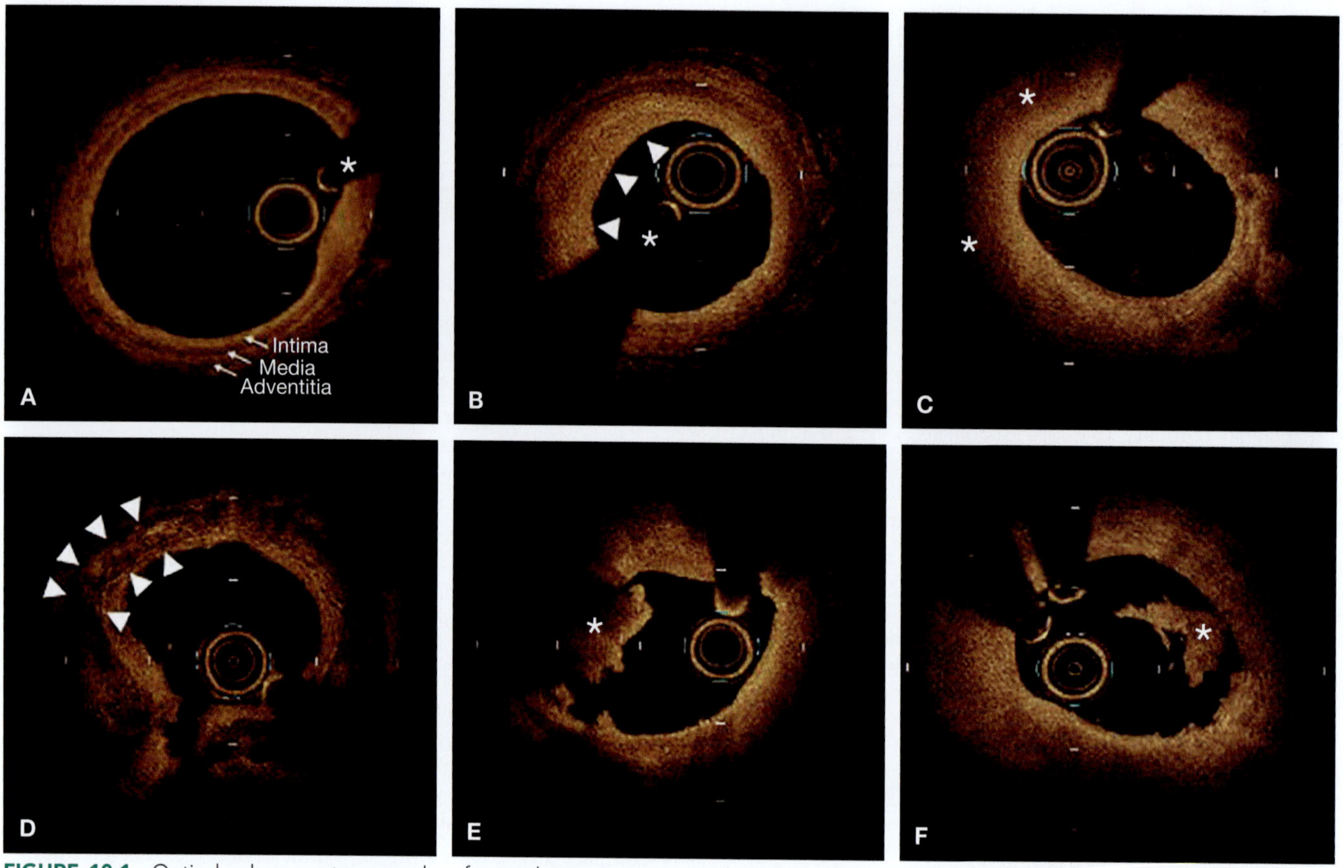

FIGURE 10.1 Optical coherence tomography of normal coronary artery and most common pathologies. **A,** The three vascular layers (intima, media, and adventitia, *arrows*) are visualized in a normal coronary artery. **B,** A fibrous plaque is visualized as a low-attenuating signal-rich region in the vessel wall (*arrowhead*). The three-layer structure is preserved and clearly visualized. **C,** Lipidic plaque is visualized as a high-attenuating signal-poor region (*asterisk*). Due to attenuation of light by lipid, the vessel structure beyond the lipid-rich plaque is poorly visualized. **D,** Calcific plaques are observed as a low-attenuating, sharply demarcated, and signal-poor structure (*arrowheads*). Here, the entire thickness of calcium is visualized. High-attenuating, red thrombus **(E)** and low-attenuating, platelet-rich white thrombus **(F)** are visualized within the lumen (*asterisk*). Note significant signal dropout in red thrombus but not in white thrombus.

PCI Guidance by OCT

PCI can be guided by OCT images using a standardized approach. Pre-PCI OCT images can be used to strategize the procedure by (1) assessing lesion morphology to determine appropriate lesion preparation strategies, (2) identifying proximal and distal stent landing zones with minimal or no disease, and (3) measuring vessel diameter to select balloon and stent sizes. Post-PCI, OCT images can be used to optimize the stents by assessing (1) medial edge dissection requiring additional stent implantation, (2) malapposition, and (3) underexpansion of the stents requiring further postdilation. This standardized approach can be summarized with the mnemonic MLD-MAX (pre-PCI, MLD: Morphology, Length, and Diameter; post-PCI, MAX: Medial dissection, Apposition, eXpansion).

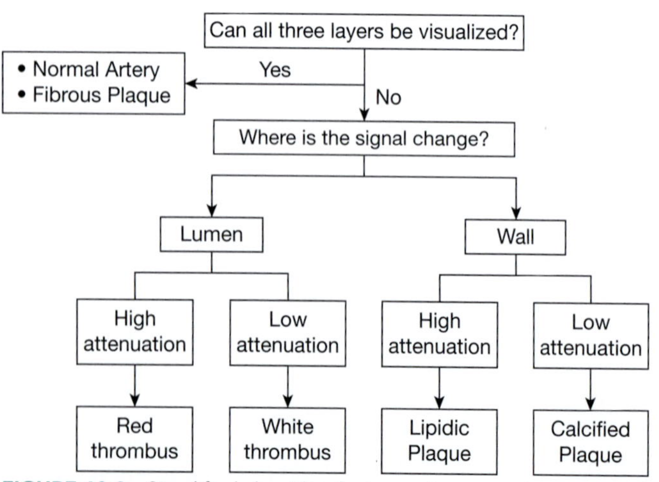

FIGURE 10.2 Simplified algorithm for image interpretation on optical coherence tomography.

Pre-PCI MLD: Strategize

Morphology: In the presence of predominantly fibrous or lipid-rich plaques, lesion preparation with an undersized balloon or direct stenting may be undertaken, whereas noncompliant balloon, cutting or scoring balloon, atherectomy, or intravascular lithotripsy (IVL) are recommended for moderate-severe or severely calcified plaques. OCT is particularly helpful in the presence of calcified plaques, since it allows more detailed assessment of calcium than IVUS. An OCT-based scoring system can be used to determine the need for advanced calcium modification with atherectomy or IVL (**Fig. 10.4**).[9,10] Since stent expansion was lowest in the presence of calcified plaques with maximum arc >50% of the circumference, maximum thickness >0.5 mm, and length >5 mm, atherectomy or IVL may be needed in those plaques ("rule of 5").

Length: To determine the lesion length, proximal and distal reference segments with minimal atherosclerotic disease and greatest

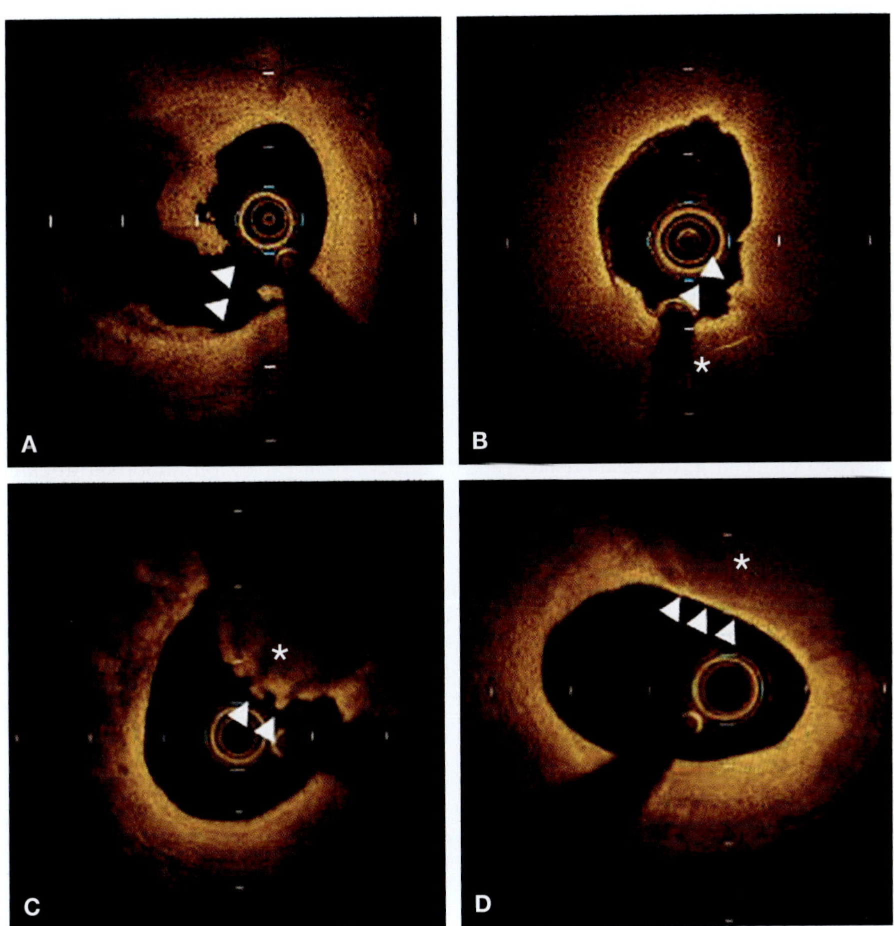

FIGURE 10.3 Culprit lesions for acute coronary syndrome and thin-cap fibroatheroma visualized by optical coherence tomography. **A,** Plaque rupture, the most common cause of acute coronary syndrome, is visualized as a disrupted fibrous cap (*arrowhead*) and a cavity with or without an overlying thrombus (here with white thrombus). **B,** Plaque erosion identified as a lipid-rich plaque (*asterisk*) with intact fibrous cap with overlying thrombus (*arrowhead*). Thrombus can be absent in plaque erosion. **C,** Eruptive calcified nodule is the least common cause of acute coronary syndrome and is visualized as a protruding nodule with disrupted fibrous cap. Note irregular surface and signal dropout due to protruding fractured calcium and overlying red thrombus. **D,** Thin-cap fibroatheroma is considered a "vulnerable" high-risk plaque, identified as a lipid-rich plaque (*asterisk*) with a thin fibrous cap (<65 μm in thickness; *arrowhead*).

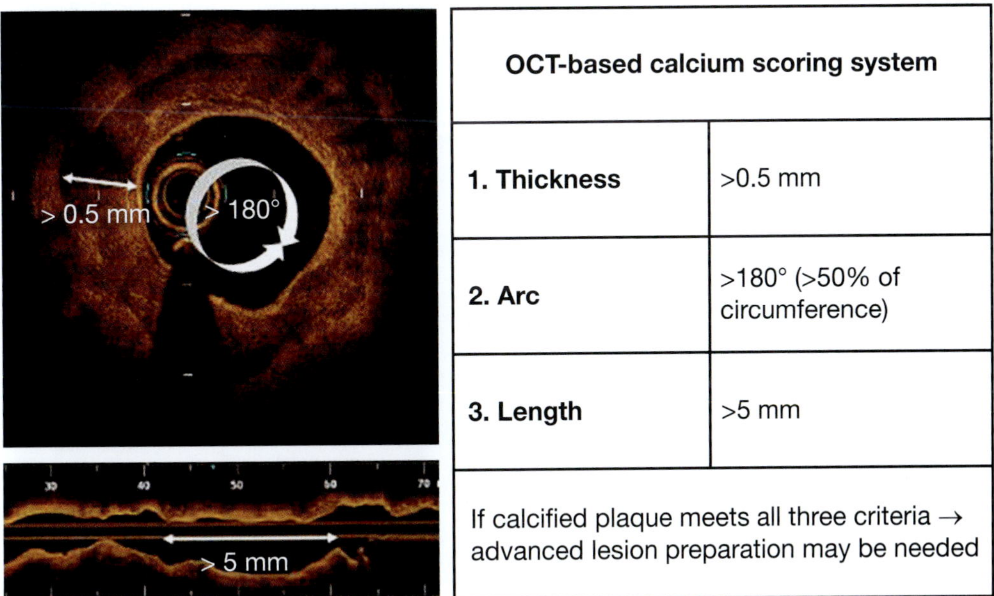

OCT-based calcium scoring system	
1. Thickness	>0.5 mm
2. Arc	>180° (>50% of circumference)
3. Length	>5 mm
If calcified plaque meets all three criteria → advanced lesion preparation may be needed	

FIGURE 10.4 Optical coherence tomography-based scoring system for coronary calcification. Volumetric analysis of calcified deposit is performed by breaking the volume down to calcium thickness, arc, and length. A combination of calcified plaque >0.5 mm in thickness, >50% of the arterial circumference, and >5 mm in length is associated with stent underexpansion, suggesting that advanced calcium modification may be needed to optimize stent expansion.

visibility of the vessel wall need to be selected. The length between the proximal and distal reference segments is automatically calculated by the imaging software, and the reference segments can be adjusted to make the lesion length correspond to the length of a commercially available drug-eluting stent. This strategy minimizes stent edge problems, including the presence of inflow and outflow disease or TCFA at the reference segments, which may lead to worse clinical outcomes.[11-16]

Diameter There are two methods to determine appropriate device sizes: external elastic lamina (EEL)- or lumen-guided strategies (**Fig. 10.5**). Compared with a lumen-guided strategy, an EEL-guided strategy is preferred if two measurements, at least one quadrant apart, can be obtained, since it leads to the use of a larger balloon or stent by ~0.5 mm, which can translate into a larger lumen area without increasing complications.[17-19] To determine the stent size, the EEL-based mean diameter of the distal reference is rounded down to the nearest available stent size.[20] If the EEL is not well visualized, often due to attenuation from plaque at the reference segments, the mean lumen diameter of the distal reference is rounded up to the next available stent size.[20] Postdilation balloon size can be determined based on the respective reference diameter measurements with the same strategies.

Post-PCI MAX: Optimize

Medial dissection: After PCI, the proximal and distal reference segments are assessed to check for medial dissection or intramural hematoma (**Fig. 10.6A**). Although OCT can identify post-PCI edge dissections in up to 40% of cases due to its high resolution,[18] most dissections detected by OCT heal without significant impact on clinical outcomes.[16,21] However, the presence of major edge dissection on OCT is considered to be a predictor of adverse clinical outcomes.[13-16] It has been recommended to place an additional stent if there was a major dissection involving ≥60° of the circumference and ≥3 mm in length extending into the media unless anatomically prohibitive.[20]

Apposition: Stent malapposition refers to the lack of contact between the stent struts and the vessel wall.[8,22] Although acute stent malapposition is commonly seen on OCT after stent implantation (≈50%),[15] it does not appear to increase the risk of stent failure or stent thrombosis.[14,23-25] However, if there is proximal malapposition that can later interfere with rewiring, large malapposition for >3 mm in length, or malapposition associated with stent underexpansion, further optimization should be considered (**Fig. 10.6B**). For this purpose, inflation of semicompliant balloon at nominal pressure is sufficient in most cases.

eXpansion: Stent expansion is a major predictor of stent failure and can be assessed by absolute (minimal stent area; MSA) or relative measures (MSA divided by the reference lumen area).[22] The current European consensus recommends optimal stent result as (1) MSA > 4.5 mm^2 on OCT for nonleft main lesions (absolute expansion) or (2) MSA > 80% of the mean of the proximal and distal reference lumen area (relative expansion). Although absolute stent expansion or MSA appears to be more important than relative stent expansion to predict adverse clinical outcomes, it may not always be possible to achieve this value in small vessels, which makes relative stent expansion important in clinical practice.[22] Amongst the multiple criteria to define adequate relative stent expansion, expansion goals are achieved in ≈50%.[26] When stent underexpansion is identified (**Fig. 10.6C**), high-pressure (≥18 atm) inflation of a noncompliant balloon should be undertaken in an attempt to achieve adequate expansion. If stent underexpansion persists, further optimization attempts should be balanced with the risk of complications such as perforation.

Limitations of OCT in PCI

There are several recognized limitations of OCT. First, it has limited role in assessing the aorto-ostial coronary segments, since it is difficult to clear the blood from the coronary ostia. Second, contrast use to clear blood during OCT image acquisition is prohibited in patients with advanced chronic kidney disease. Third, the caliber of the left main coronary artery may prohibit it from adequate flush clearance. Several alternative flushing agents including normal saline have been investigated, but issues with blood mixing and potential for risk of arrhythmia still exit.

Clinical Studies on OCT-Guided PCI

In the earliest studies, OCT was found to influence the procedural strategy. For example, post-PCI OCT identified adverse features that warranted additional intervention in 35% of cases in the

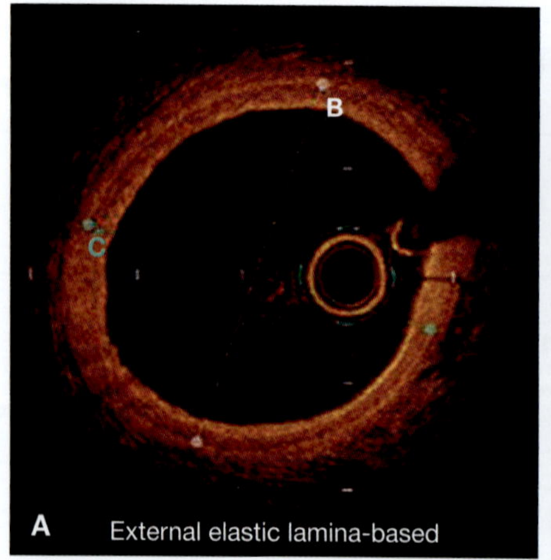

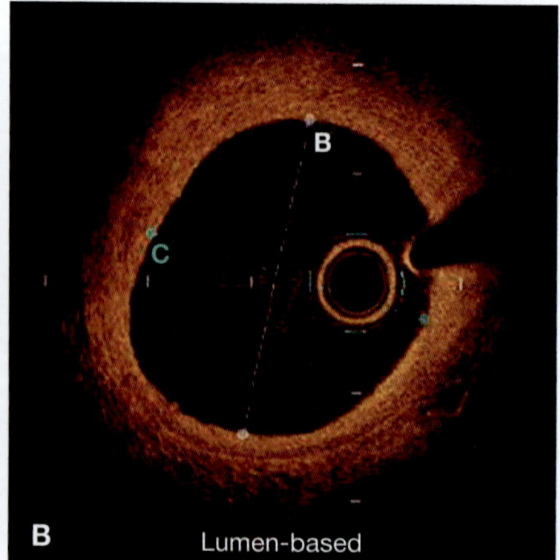

FIGURE 10.5 Lumen- and external elastic lamina-based measurement of vessel size on optical coherence tomography. Measurement of vessel diameter can be determined by two methods: external elastic lamia (EEL)- or lumen based. **A,** EEL-based measurement. For selection of balloons or stents, the mean EEL-based diameter is rounded down to the nearest available device size. **B,** If the EEL is not well visualized, the lumen-based diameter is measured and rounded up to the next available device size.

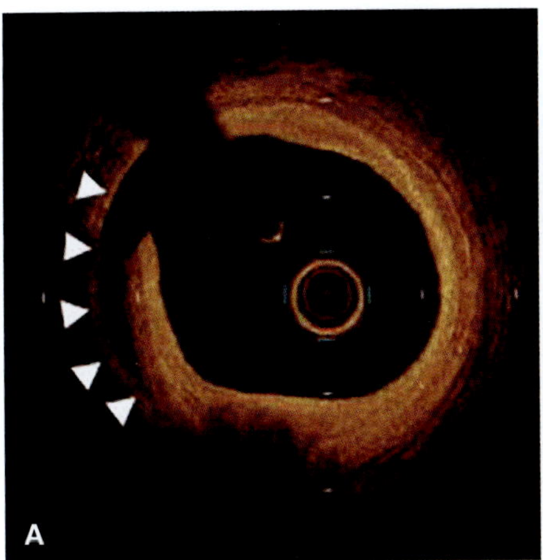

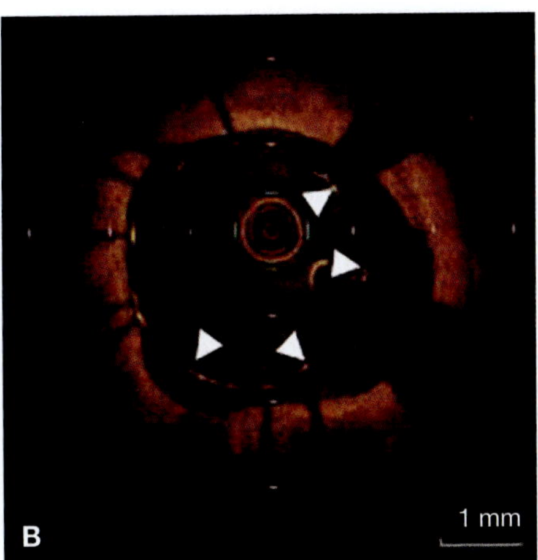

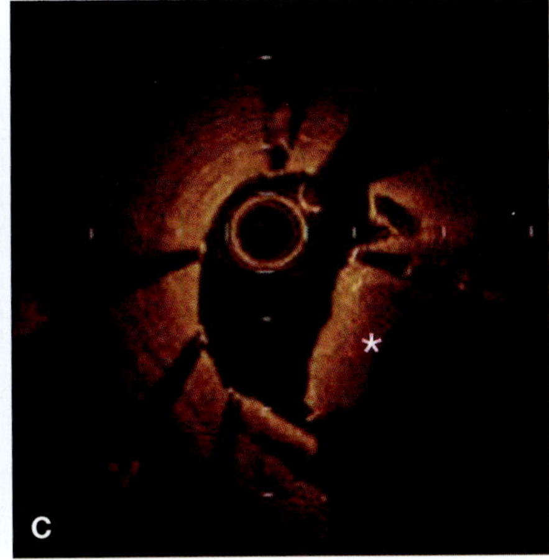

FIGURE 10.6 Evaluation of procedural results after stent implantation by optical coherence tomography. **A,** A distal edge dissection involving media (*arrowhead*), **(B)** malapposition of the stent struts (*arrowhead*), and **(C)** stent underexpansion in the presence of a calcified nodule (*asterisk*).

CLI-OPCI study.[27] Furthermore, OCT-guided PCI was associated with a reduced risk of MI or cardiac death at 1 year after adjusting for potential confounders. The OPINION trial[19] first compared clinical outcomes between OCT- and IVUS-guided PCI (n = 414 and 415, respectively) and did not show any significant difference in primary endpoint of target vessel failure at 1 year, demonstrating noninferiority of OCT guidance compared to IVUS guidance. In the ILUMIEN III trial,[18] OCT-guided PCI was noninferior to IVUS-guided PCI in terms of final MSA. A recent, large-scale, randomized controlled trial, the OCTIVUS trial,[28] demonstrated that OCT-guided PCI (n = 1005) was noninferior to IVUS-guided PCI (n = 1003) for a composite endpoint of cardiac death, target-vessel MI, or ischemia-driven target-vessel revascularization at 1 year.

The ILUMIEN IV trial[26] was a large-scale, global, multicenter, randomized controlled trial that compared clinical outcomes between OCT- and angiography-guided PCI (n = 1233 and 1254, respectively) in high-risk patients or those with high-risk lesions. In this trial, OCT guidance led to larger final MSA (5.72 ± 2.04 mm^2 vs 5.36 ± 1.87 mm^2; $P < .001$) and greater stent expansion compared with angiography guidance due to selection of larger stents and more frequent postdilation at higher pressures. Although there was no apparent difference in the primary clinical endpoint, a composite of cardiac death, target-vessel MI, or ischemia-driven target-vessel revascularization at 2 years, OCT-guided PCI significantly reduced stent thrombosis compared with angiography-guided PCI. The OCTOBER trial[29] was a randomized controlled trial, which compared clinical outcomes between OCT- and angiography-guided PCI (n = 600 and 601, respectively) in complex bifurcation lesions. In this trial, OCT-guided PCI significantly lowered the risk of a composite of cardiac death, target-lesion MI, or ischemia-driven target-vessel revascularization at 2 years. In RENOVATE-COMPLEX PCI trial,[30] intravascular imaging-guided PCI reduced the risk of a composite of cardiac death, target vessel-related MI, or clinically driven target vessel revascularization compared with angiography-guided PCI in patients with complex coronary lesions. In this trial, both IVUS (74.5%) and OCT (25.5%) were used, and the results were consistent in subgroup analysis according to the intravascular imaging device used.

In summary, clinical benefits of OCT- versus angiography-guided PCI are supported by multiple large-scale clinical trials, especially for high-risk patients or those with complex coronary lesions. In addition, there is no apparent difference in clinical outcomes between OCT- and IVUS-guided PCI.

CONCLUSION

Intravascular OCT is a relatively new imaging modality, which plays an important role in evaluating coronary anatomy and pathologies. OCT can be used to strategize and optimize PCI with acute and long-term clinical benefits over angiography-guided PCI that are supported by multiple large-scale clinical trials.

For further review and interactivities, please see the chapter-based multiple choice questions and videos accessible in the complimentary eBook bundled with this text. Access instructions are located in the inside front cover.

References

1. Maehara A, Mintz GS, Witzenbichler B, et al. Relationship between intravascular ultrasound guidance and clinical outcomes after drug-eluting stents. *Circ Cardiovasc Interv*. 2018;11:e006243.
2. Jones DA, Rathod KS, Koganti S, et al. Angiography alone versus angiography plus optical coherence tomography to guide percutaneous coronary intervention: outcomes from the Pan-London PCI cohort. *JACC Cardiovasc Interv*. 2018;11(14):1313-1321.
3. Park H, Ahn JM, Kang DY, et al. Optimal stenting technique for complex coronary lesions: intracoronary imaging-guided pre-dilation, stent sizing, and post-dilation. *JACC Cardiovasc Interv*. 2020;13(12):1403-1413.
4. Hong SJ, Mintz GS, Ahn CM, et al; IVUS-XPL Investigators. Effect of intravascular ultrasound-guided drug-eluting stent implantation: 5-year follow-up of the IVUS-XPL randomized trial. *JACC Cardiovasc Interv*. 2020;13(1):62-71.
5. Zhang J, Gao X, Kan J, et al. Intravascular ultrasound versus angiography-guided drug-eluting stent implantation: the ULTIMATE trial. *J Am Coll Cardiol*. 2018;72(24):3126-3137.
6. di Mario C, Koskinas KC, Räber L. Clinical benefit of IVUS guidance for coronary stenting: the ULTIMATE step toward definitive evidence? *J Am Coll Cardiol*. 2018;72(24):3138-3141.
7. Elgendy IY, Mahmoud AN, Elgendy AY, Mintz GS. Intravascular ultrasound-guidance is associated with lower cardiovascular mortality and myocardial

infarction for drug-eluting stent implantation—insights from an updated meta-analysis of randomized trials. *Circ J*. 2019;83(6):1410-1413.

8. Ali ZA, Karimi Galougahi K, Mintz GS, Maehara A, Shlofmitz RA, Mattesini A. Intracoronary optical coherence tomography: state of the art and future directions. *EuroIntervention*. 2021;17(2):e105-e123.
9. Fujino A, Mintz GS, Matsumura M, et al. A new optical coherence tomography-based calcium scoring system to predict stent underexpansion. *EuroIntervention*. 2018;13(18):e2182-e2189.
10. Ali ZA, Galougahi KK. Shining light on calcified lesions, plaque stabilisation and physiologic significance: new insights from intracoronary OCT. *EuroIntervention*. 2018;13(18):e2105-e2108.
11. Ino Y, Kubo T, Matsuo Y, et al. Optical coherence tomography predictors for edge restenosis after everolimus-eluting stent implantation. *Circ Cardiovasc Interv*. 2016;9(10):e004231.
12. Prati F, Kodama T, Romagnoli E, et al. Suboptimal stent deployment is associated with subacute stent thrombosis: optical coherence tomography insights from a multicenter matched study. From the CLI Foundation investigators—the CLI-THRO study. *Am Heart J*. 2015;169(2):249-256.
13. Prati F, Romagnoli E, Gatto L, et al. Clinical impact of suboptimal stenting and residual intrastent plaque/thrombus protrusion in patients with acute coronary syndrome: The CLI-OPCI ACS substudy (Centro per la Lotta Contro L'Infarto-optimization of percutaneous coronary intervention in acute coronary syndrome). *Circ Cardiovasc Interv*. 2016;9(12):e003726.
14. Prati F, Romagnoli E, La Manna A, et al. Long-term consequences of optical coherence tomography findings during percutaneous coronary intervention: the Centro Per La Lotta Contro L'infarto - optimization of Percutaneous Coronary Intervention (CLI-OPCI) LATE study. *EuroIntervention*. 2018;14(4):e443-e451.
15. Prati F, Romagnoli E, Burzotta F, et al. Clinical impact of OCT findings during PCI: the CLI-OPCI II study. *JACC Cardiovasc Imaging*. 2015;8(11):1297-1305.
16. van Zandvoort LJC, Tomaniak M, Tovar Forero MN, et al. Predictors for clinical outcome of untreated stent edge dissections as detected by optical coherence tomography. *Circ Cardiovasc Interv*. 2020;13(3):e008685.
17. Shlofmitz E, Jeremias A, Parviz Y, et al. External elastic lamina vs. luminal diameter measurement for determining stent diameter by optical coherence tomography: an ILUMIEN III substudy. *Eur Heart J Cardiovasc Imaging*. 2021;22(7):753-759.
18. Ali ZA, Maehara A, Genereux P, et al; ILUMIEN III OPTIMIZE PCI Investigators. Optical coherence tomography compared with intravascular ultrasound and with angiography to guide coronary stent implantation (ILUMIEN III: OPTIMIZE PCI)—a randomised controlled trial. *Lancet (London, England)*. 2016;388(10060):2618-2628.
19. Kubo T, Shinke T, Okamura T, et al; OPINION Investigators. Optical frequency domain imaging vs. intravascular ultrasound in percutaneous coronary intervention (OPINION trial): one-year angiographic and clinical results. *Eur Heart J*. 2017;38(42):3139-3147.
20. Ali Z, Landmesser U, Karimi Galougahi K, et al. Optical coherence tomography-guided coronary stent implantation compared to angiography: a multicentre randomised trial in PCI—design and rationale of ILUMIEN IV—OPTIMAL PCI. *EuroIntervention*. 2021;16(13):1092-1099.
21. Radu MD, Räber L, Heo J, et al. Natural history of optical coherence tomography-detected non-flow-limiting edge dissections following drug-eluting stent implantation. *EuroIntervention*. 2014;9:1085-1094.
22. Räber L, Mintz GS, Koskinas KC, et al. Clinical use of intracoronary imaging. Part 1: guidance and optimization of coronary interventions. An expert consensus document of the European Association of Percutaneous Cardiovascular Interventions. *EuroIntervention*. 2018;14(6):656-677.
23. Wang B, Mintz GS, Witzenbichler B, et al. Predictors and long-term clinical impact of acute stent malapposition: an assessment of dual antiplatelet therapy with drug-eluting stents (ADAPT-DES) intravascular ultrasound substudy. *J Am Heart Assoc*. 2016;5(12):e004438.
24. Steinberg DH, Mintz GS, Mandinov L, et al. Long-term impact of routinely detected early and late incomplete stent apposition: an integrated intravascular ultrasound analysis of the TAXUS IV, V, and VI and TAXUS ATLAS workhorse, long lesion, and direct stent studies. *JACC Cardiovasc Interv*. 2010;3(5):486-494.
25. Im E, Kim BK, Ko YG, et al. Incidences, predictors, and clinical outcomes of acute and late stent malapposition detected by optical coherence tomography after drug-eluting stent implantation. *Circ Cardiovasc Interv*. 2014;7(1):88-96.
26. Ali ZA, Landmesser U, Maehara A, et al. Optical coherence tomography-guided versus angiography-guided PCI. *N Engl J Med*. 2023;389:1466-1476.
27. Prati F, Di Vito L, Biondi-Zoccai G, et al. Angiography alone versus angiography plus optical coherence tomography to guide decision-making during percutaneous coronary intervention: the Centro per la Lotta contro l'Infarto-Optimisation of Percutaneous Coronary Intervention (CLI-OPCI) study. *EuroIntervention*. 2012;8(7):823-829.
28. Kang DY, Ahn JM, Yun SC, et al; OCTIVUS Investigators. Optical coherence tomography-guided or intravascular ultrasound guided percutaneous coronary intervention: the OCTIVUS randomized clinical trial. *Circulation*. 2023;148(16):1195-1206.
29. Holm NR, Andreasen LN, Neghabat O, et al; OCTOBER Trial Group. OCT or angiography guidance for PCI in complex bifurcation lesions. *N Engl J Med*. 2023;389(16):1477-1487.
30. Lee JM, Choi KH, Song YB, et al; RENOVATE-COMPLEX-PCI Investigators. Intravascular imaging-guided or angiography-guided complex PCI. *N Engl J Med*. 2023;388(18):1668-1679.

11 Vulnerable Plaque Imaging

Eric A. Osborn and Farouc A. Jaffer

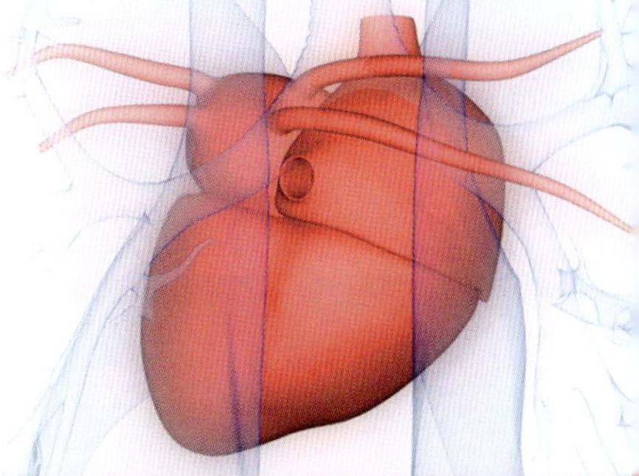

Complications related to atherosclerotic vascular disease remain a leading cause of cardiovascular morbidity and mortality in the United States and around the globe. While atherosclerosis is recognized as a systemic disease that mandates aggressive medical therapy and lifestyle changes, individual plaques exhibit differential risks spanning stable, quiescent plaques to unstable, "vulnerable" plaques at high risk of future complication due to thrombosis overlying plaque rupture of thin-capped fibroatheroma (TCFA), plaque erosion, and calcific nodules.[1] As high-risk atheroma (bulky, lipid-rich, inflamed) plaques underlie the majority of acute coronary syndrome (ACS) events, there remains substantial interest and resources focused on defining vulnerable plaque phenotypes. The potential to predict and prevent devastating ACS events arising from vulnerable plaques provides a strong rationale to pursue precomplication plaque imaging of high-risk features of human coronary arteries.

Several noninvasive and intravascular coronary artery–targeted imaging technologies have furnished new insights into the pathophysiology of vulnerable plaque complications. To date, the primary imaging focus revolves around assessing high-risk structural features, including the detection of large plaque burden, thin fibrous caps, lipid, and neovessels.[1] While coronary computed tomography angiography (CCTA) is a powerful approach to noninvasively image human coronary artery disease (CAD), due to spatiotemporal resolution constraints, the bulk of knowledge regarding high-risk plaques has been gleaned from structure-based high-resolution intravascular imaging including intravascular ultrasound (IVUS), optical coherence tomography (OCT), and near-infrared spectroscopy (NIRS). Structural imaging alone, however, appears insufficiently precise to identify vulnerable plaques,[2] motivating the continued development of new plaque-imaging approaches to uncover plaque pathophysiology and new structural phenotypes, such as near-infrared fluorescence (NIRF) imaging, fluorescence lifetime imaging (FLIm), and photoacoustic tomography (PAT).[3] This chapter showcases key concepts in vulnerable plaque imaging, focusing on clinically available and emerging intravascular imaging approaches.

DETECTING VULNERABLE PLAQUE

The predominant cause of atherosclerosis-based myocardial infarction, stroke, and sudden cardiac death is vulnerable plaque that undergoes plaque disruption and resultant atherothrombosis leading to a reduction in coronary blood flow.[4] As opposed to severely obstructive coronary lesions identified by coronary angiography that are the common targets for percutaneous or surgical revascularization in symptomatic patients, vulnerable plaques originate as subclinical and typically nonobstructive, mild-to-moderately stenotic lesions in asymptomatic patients.[5]

Although x-ray angiography, stress testing, and even invasive physiology measures such as fractional flow reserve (FFR) are often normal in patients harboring vulnerable plaques, a subset of these plaques can rapidly progress and cause cardiovascular events within an accelerated time frame.[6-8] Local biologic mediators and mechanical stressors can destabilize such vulnerable plaques, leading to ACS or progressive luminal stenosis that causes chronic coronary syndromes. At the time of ACS presentation, culprit plaques identified by coronary angiography may exhibit plaque ulcerations, lumen irregularities and haziness, contrast dye staining, and filling defects within the lumen indicating thrombus.

In contrast, angiography is highly insensitive for phenotyping subclinical (nonvulnerable and nonischemic) coronary vulnerable plaques. This limitation of angiography is due to its inability to directly image the arterial wall. Positively remodeled plaques can accumulate substantial plaque burden yet maintain relatively normal lumen dimensions and thus be overlooked by angiography alone (**Fig. 11.1**). These limitations of coronary angiography have motivated a new era of vulnerable plaque-imaging approaches to interrogate high-risk plaque features resident within the vessel wall, rather than focus solely on the severity of lumen stenosis.

VULNERABLE PLAQUE HISTOPATHOLOGY

Detailed autopsy studies of patients suffering sudden death have elucidated the histopathologic underpinnings of vulnerable atheroma (**Fig. 11.2**),[1] and thus the sphere of vulnerable plaque imaging targets. The prototypical vulnerable plaque is denoted as the TCFA, a structure comprised of a large, thrombogenic lipid-rich core with necrotic elements constrained by a thin fibrous cap measuring less than 65 μm in thickness.[9] TCFAs are the etiologic precursor in approximately two-thirds of ACS cases. In combination with local biomechanical forces, fibrous cap inflammation (characterized by infiltrating macrophages that liberate destabilizing tissue proteases) can promote plaque rupture, followed by extrusion of the lipid contents, and consequent atherothrombosis and ACS events. Geographically, TCFAs are most often located in the proximal one-third of the major epicardial coronary arteries,[10] and thus, they often subtend a large area of at-risk myocardium.

As outlined in **Table 11.1**, beyond the aforementioned features, vulnerable plaques may exhibit inflammatory cellular elements, leaky neovessels, intraplaque hemorrhage, microcalcifications, and penetrating cholesterol crystals (**Fig. 11.3**).[11] Developing intimal neovessels contain "leaky" endothelium, resulting in extravasation of blood cells and molecules, and may contribute to plaque progression and the development of complex lesion phenotypes. Calcified nodules near the luminal surface increase biomechanical stress of the plaque ultrastructure and may promote plaque disruption by hemodynamic forces exerted on the vessel wall.[12] Finally, inflammation promotes collagenolysis and fibrous cap weakening that can lead to subsequent plaque disruption,[13] as evidenced by a greater number of ACS events in patients with underlying chronic inflammatory disorders.[14] Many of these vulnerable features can

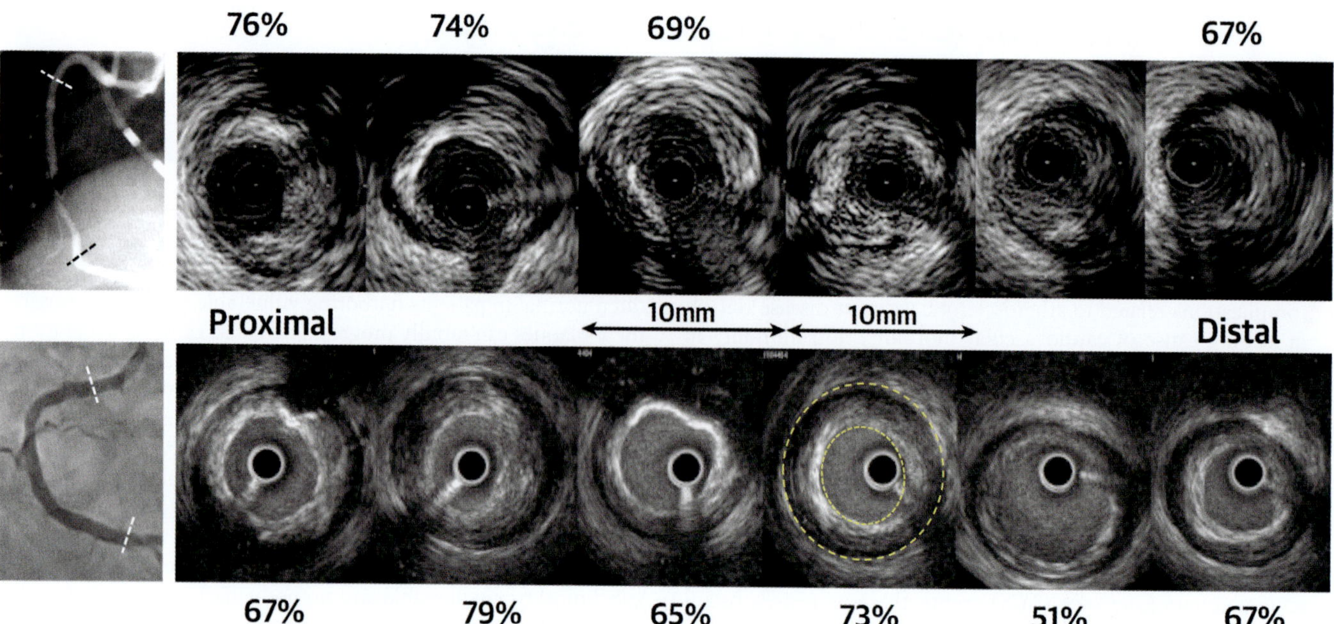

FIGURE 11.1 Intracoronary imaging identifies significant extraluminal coronary atherosclerosis not apparent by angiography. Intravascular ultrasound (IVUS) images from two different right coronary arteries, one with an angiographically significant stenosis (**top panels**) and another with no obstructive disease (**bottom panels**). The start and end points of the IVUS pullbacks are identified by the dashed lines on the angiograms. IVUS plaque burden is recorded above each cross-section, demonstrating 50% to 80% plaque burden in segments that appear visually normal by angiography. (Reprinted with permission from Mintz GS, Matsumura M, Ali Z et al. Clinical utility of intravascular imaging: past, present, and future. *JACC Cardiovasc Imaging*. 2022;15:1799-1820.)

occur in combination within an individual plaque and can evolve over time. The emerging field of intravascular NIRF molecular imaging aims to image specific molecules and cells within human CAD, to complement IVUS and OCT structural imaging and enhance the precision of vulnerable plaque detection.[3,15,16]

INTRAVASCULAR STRUCTURAL IMAGING OF VULNERABLE PLAQUE

As a result of its long-standing clinical use in percutaneous coronary intervention (PCI) and capability to image the entire coronary arterial wall through blood, IVUS remains the most utilized approach to assess vulnerable plaque features, namely plaque burden, in CAD patents. More recent intravascular optical imaging approaches such as high-resolution OCT and NIRS-IVUS have provided additional structural and chemical assessments of high-risk plaques, including fibrous cap thickness, lipid burden, subclinical thrombus, and eruptive calcific nodules. A summary of existing clinical intravascular plaque imaging technologies is presented in **Table 11.2**.

Intravascular Ultrasound/Virtual Histology

Conventional grayscale IVUS can delineate plaque structure, lumen dimensions, and stent complications in human coronary arteries. IVUS has several attributes including through-blood imaging without flushing, sensitive calcium detection, and outstanding tissue depth penetration, allowing determination of positive and negative plaque remodeling.[17] Importantly, IVUS can derive plaque burden, defined as (100% × [external elastic lamina (EEL) area − lumen area]/EEL area), a key plaque predictor of ACS[6-8,18,19] and the defining criteria behind the novel bioresorbable scaffold-preventive PCI trial PROSPECT-ABSORB.[20] The most predictive criteria for high-risk plaque defined by IVUS are those with ≥65% to 70% plaque burden, although other high-risk features can also be detected by IVUS (**Fig. 11.4**). In ACS patients, IVUS of unstable culprit plaques may demonstrate rupture with an empty cavity remnant indicating an extruded lipid core, an intimal flap, and/or luminal thrombus.

Nevertheless, the 100- to 200-μm moderate axial resolution of conventional IVUS limits the discrimination of finer plaque ultrastructural features, such as the fibrous cap thickness, especially in cases where the cap thickness is <65 μm, a classic criterion of histologic TCFA.[9] High-definition IVUS imaging systems with 50- to 100-μm resolution utilizing higher-frequency 60 MHz (as opposed to conventional 40 MHz) transducers have been developed,[21] allowing more precise structural assessment. However, while IVUS can sensitively detect plaque calcium, due to acoustic shadowing, it cannot quantify calcium thickness, which is a key factor in determining the need for calcium modification during PCI,[22] and could be potentially important in stratifying vulnerable plaques. In addition, IVUS struggles to resolve plaque components, such as lipid-rich versus fibrotic lesions, nor distinguish specific molecular or cellular inflammatory components that drive TCFA complications.

Given the limitations of standalone IVUS, imaging advancements have been developed to better discriminate plaque composition. Virtual histology (VH)-IVUS is an IVUS technology that employs radiofrequency signal backscatter spectral analysis to further atheroma tissue characterization.[23] Via postprocessing algorithms of the reflected ultrasound signal, VH-IVUS categorizes plaque constituents into four categories: fibrous, fibrofatty, necrotic core (NC), and dense calcium (**Fig. 11.5**). Each plaque tissue type is then color-coded for display purposes, allowing rapid ease of image interpretation. Of note, in recent years, the use of VH-IVUS has diminished.

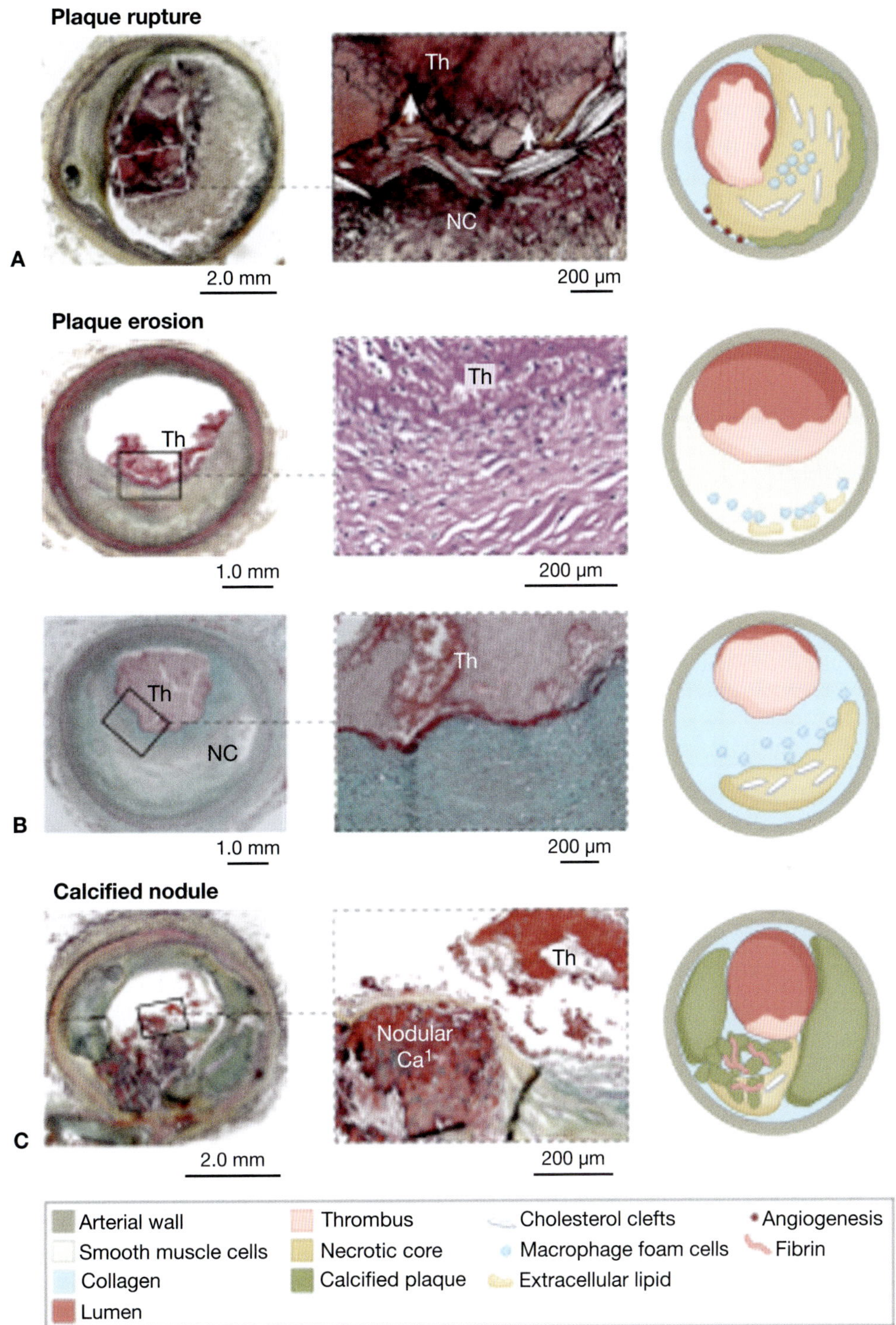

FIGURE 11.2 Atherosclerotic plaque-based mechanisms responsible for acute coronary syndromes. Paired histology and illustrations of the three main plaque types associated with thrombus (Th) formation in acute coronary syndrome: **(A)** plaque rupture, **(B)** plaque erosion, and **(C)** calcified nodule. In plaque rupture, a prototypical thin-cap fibroatheroma is characterized by a large necrotic core (NC), possibly with neovessels and intraplaque hemorrhage, situated beneath an overlying thin fibrous cap (arrowheads) that can harbor microcalcifications and inflammatory macrophages. Plaque erosion, more often observed in eccentric smooth muscle and collagen-rich lesions without substantial NC, may occur in lesions exhibiting pathological intimal thickening (**top panels**) or fibroatheroma (**bottom panels**). Eruptive calcified nodules disturb local blood flow patterns to promote Th by substantially protruding into the vessel lumen. (Reprinted with permission from Gaba P, Gersh BJ, Muller J et al. Evolving concepts of the vulnerable atherosclerotic plaque and the vulnerable patient: implications for patient care and future research. *Nat Rev Cardiol.* 2023;20:181-196.)

TABLE 11.1 Histopathologic Features Associated With Plaque Vulnerability

Large necrotic/lipid core
Fibrous cap covering the necrotic core
Thin cap (<65 µm)
High macrophage density
Few smooth muscle cells
Expansive remodeling preserving the lumen
Large plaque burden
Neovascularization from vasa vasorum
Intraplaque hemorrhage
Adventitial/perivascular inflammation
Spotty calcification
Penetrating cholesterol crystals

Reprinted with permission from Bentzon JF, Otsuka F, Virmani R et al. Mechanisms of plaque formation and rupture. *Circ Res.* 2014;114:1852-1866.)

Clinical Outcomes Studies

IVUS structural and VH-TCFA features were evaluated as predictors of future cardiovascular events in the landmark PROSPECT trial (Providing Regional Observations to Study Predictors of Events in the Coronary Tree), a natural history atherosclerosis clinical study of 697 ACS patients presenting to the cardiac catheterization laboratory.[7] The PROSPECT investigators performed three-vessel VH-IVUS in patients undergoing PCI of culprit lesions, with guideline-directed medical therapy (GDMT) for nonculprit lesions. Subjects were then followed up for subsequent cardiovascular outcomes over time to prospectively identify baseline VH-IVUS structural plaque characteristics linked to future events. A strength of the PROSPECT study is that most follow-up events were adjudicated by x-ray angiography, which was critical to assign plaque-specific outcomes. Over the 3.4-year median follow-up period, 20% of the enrolled subjects experienced 177 repeat adverse events, despite GDMT (albeit at less-stringent treatment targets than present day). Approximately one-half of events occurred due to nonculprit plaque progression, leading to primarily unstable angina and urgent revascularization, with very low (1%) rates of acute myocardial infarction, cardiac arrest, or cardiac death. The other half of events arose as culprit-lesion stent complications of restenosis (85%) or thrombosis (15%). By multivariate analysis, a nonculprit VH-TCFA significantly predicted an increased likelihood of subsequent events (hazard ratio [HR] 3.35), although events occurred in only 26 of 595 (4.4%) nonculprit VH-TCFA identified. In addition, IVUS morphologic measurements revealed that bulky (large plaque burden >70%; HR 5.03; strongest predictor) and stenotic (minimum lumen area [MLA] <4.0 mm^2; HR 3.21) lesions also significantly predicted a recurrent, nonculprit plaque-specific event. In combination, lesions exhibiting all three predictors (plaque burden >70%, lumen area <4.0 mm^2, and VH-TCFA morphology) portended the greatest future risk (HR 11.05). Nevertheless, in practice, few lesions exhibited all three VH-IVUS imaging high-risk features (4.2% prevalence), and yet such patients still only had an 18% recurrent event rate over 3.4 years, and thus limited the use of standalone IVUS/VH-IVUS for actionable treatment of vulnerable plaque. While subsequent prospective VH-IVUS studies (VIVA: VH-IVUS in Vulnerable Atherosclerosis; AtheroRemo: European Collaborative Project on Inflammation and Vascular Wall Remodeling in Atherosclerosis) confirmed the prognostic capacity of VH-TCFA for future cardiovascular events[18,19] and the incorporation of shear stress,[24] the overall low positive predictive value of pure IVUS-based methods has limited its clinical translation for vulnerable plaque detection.[25] Thus, while IVUS still serves a vital role assessing high-risk plaque features of large plaque burden >70% and small luminal area <4.0 mm^2, newer multimodal methods (IVUS-NIRS, IVUS-OCT, IVUS-based FLIm, IVUS-NIRF) incorporating microstructural, molecular, and flow-based interrogations are positioned to substantially improve the predictive capacity of intravascular imaging readouts.[3]

"Preventative PCI" In patients with nonobstructive coronary disease, it has been hypothesized that treatment of vulnerable plaques before they cause adverse events may offer a clinical advantage on top of contemporary medical therapy. Early data from the small pilot study SECRITT (Santorini Criteria for Investigating and Treating Thin Capped Fibroatheroma) using a self-expanding bare-metal stent to treat VH-TCFA demonstrated good procedural success and short-term clinical safety, with a 4-fold increase in OCT fibrous cap thickness 6 months after stent implantation.[26] The concept of preventative PCI was further assessed for non–flow-limiting, lipid-rich coronary atheromas with a large plaque burden in the multicenter study PROSPECT ABSORB (Providing Regional Observations to Study Predictors of Events in the Coronary Tree II Combined with a Randomized, Controlled, Intervention Trial).[20] From patients enrolled in PROSPECT II, 182 subjects found to have a nonobstructive lesion (median angiographic diameter stenosis 41.6%), with entry criteria of a large plaque burden >65% randomized to GDMT with or without adjunctive PCI with an everolimus-eluting bioabsorbable vascular scaffold (BVS). The primary effectiveness endpoint of IVUS-derived MLA at 25-month angiographic follow-up demonstrated a more than doubling of the MLA in the preventative PCI group (6.9 vs 3.0 mm^2 for GDMT alone; $P < .0001$). Importantly, a preventative PCI strategy appeared to be safe, with no difference in target lesion failure at 24 months (4.3% vs 4.5%; $P = .96$), representing a combination of cardiac death, target vessel-related myocardial infarction, or clinically driven target lesion revascularization. At 4-year follow-up, however, notably the outcome curves began to widen in favor of preventative PCI with numerically less lesion-based major adverse cardiac events in the BVS group (4.3% vs 10.7% for GDMT alone, OR 0.38; $P = .12$), suggesting the possibility of longer-term benefit (**Fig. 11.6**). Of note, PROSPECT ABSORB was not powered for clinical events. Thus, these data support larger, adequately powered randomized studies and with newer generations of thin-strut bioabsorbable scaffolds[27,28] that may diminish the inherent long-term risks of permanent metal stents, such as neoatherosclerosis and late-stent restenosis.

OPTICAL COHERENCE TOMOGRAPHY

OCT is a high-resolution optical intravascular imaging modality that has revolutionized visualization of intracoronary plaque and stent structures.[29] Utilizing reflected and backscattered near-infrared (NIR) light at ~1300 nm emanating from tissues of different optical density, OCT achieves 10- to 20-µm axial resolution, an approximate 10-fold increase compared to conventional grayscale IVUS imaging systems operating at 40 MHz.[30] OCT image datasets are rapidly collected in a few seconds during catheter pullback speeds of 20 to 100 mm/s, compared to the standard 0.5 to 1.0 mm/s pullback speed for IVUS catheters. In addition, OCT

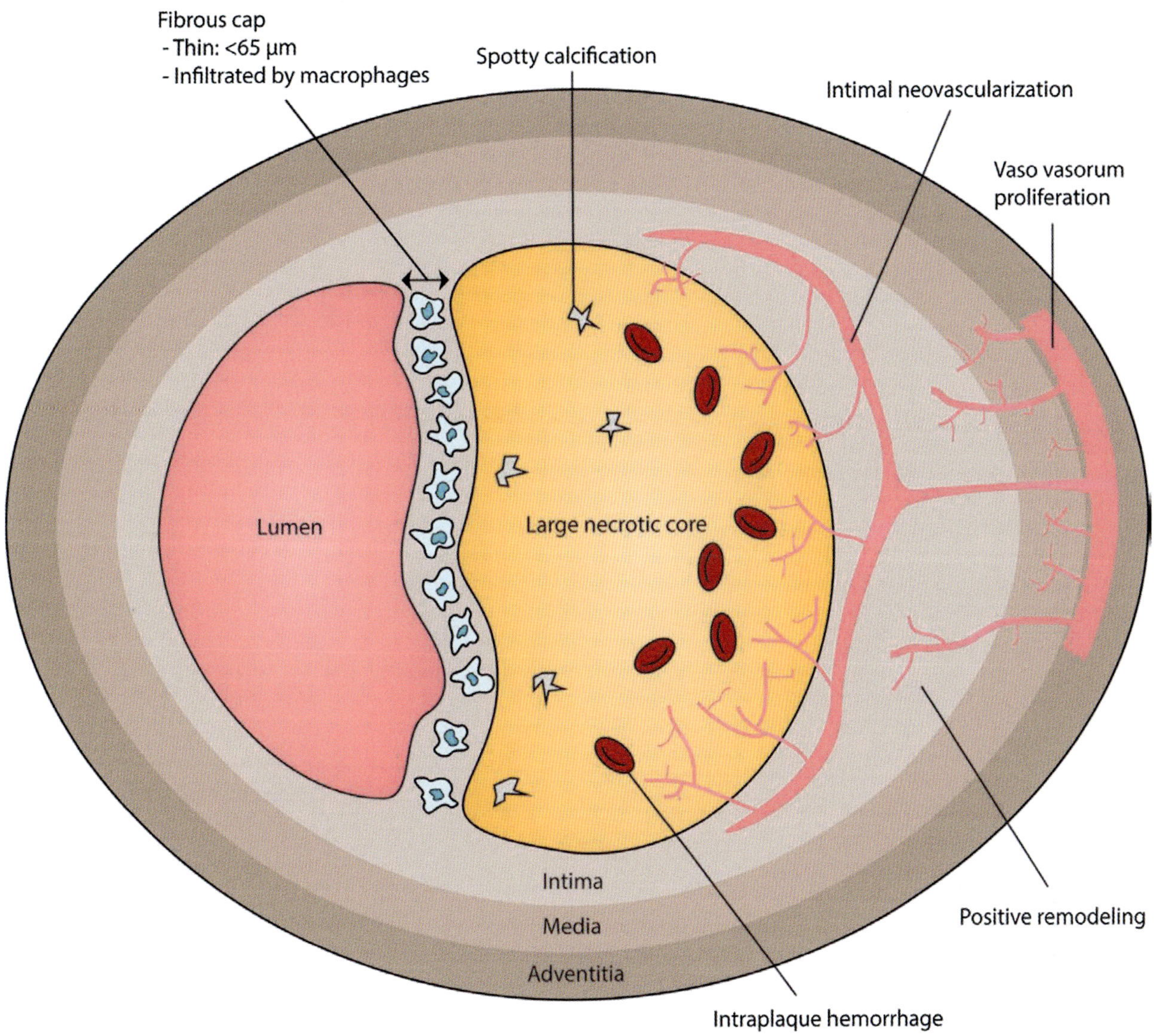

FIGURE 11.3 Illustration of common vulnerable plaque characteristics. A thin fibrous cap (<65 μm) with infiltrating inflammatory macrophages overlies a large, thrombogenic necrotic core beneath. To preserve lumen dimensions, the vessel tends to positively remodel outward by accumulating progressive plaque, that may also demonstrate spotty calcifications, within the vessel wall. Intimal neovascularization occurs via proliferation of the adventitial vasa vasorum, with the neovessels comprised of an incompetent endothelial barrier that can lead to progressive leakage of red blood cells resulting in intraplaque hemorrhage. (Reprinted with permission from Bom MJ, van der Heijden DJ, Kedhi E et al. Early detection and treatment of the vulnerable coronary plaque: can we prevent acute coronary syndromes? *Circ Cardiovasc Imaging.* 2017;10:e005973.)

catheter dimensions range from 1.8 to 2.7 French, and therefore are smaller-diameter devices than 3.1 to 3.5 French IVUS catheters. However, as the NIR light required for OCT does not penetrate through blood, OCT requires displacement of luminal blood from the imaging field in order to visualize the arterial wall. Blood displacement is typically achieved by manual or automated injection of iodinated contrast (or potentially saline or dextrose) through a properly engaged coronary artery guiding catheter, via manual or power injection. Contrast displacement is a limitation of OCT, both due to risk of kidney injury, as well challenges in displacing blood from the coronary ostia or larger vessels such as the proximal left main or saphenous vein grafts. More recent co-registration systems facilitate collection of OCT images at the same time as angiography, improving safety and procedural workflow efficiency.[31]

High-resolution OCT imaging provides superb intracoronary images of the luminal plaque surface in vivo, showing very good overall agreement (κ statistic 0.84) with histologic fibrous, fibrocalcific, and lipid-rich coronary plaques at autopsy.[32] In particular, OCT can visualize the thin fibrous caps of TCFA and provide quantitative measurements at near histological resolution. OCT is the current gold standard for detecting coronary plaque rupture, erosion, and spotty calcification that are otherwise unrecognized on x-ray angiography or IVUS imaging.[33] In addition, OCT can detect red (red blood cell-rich) and white (platelet-rich) thrombus and neovessels and potentially identify macrophage accumulations resident in plaques.[29] Mechanisms of ACS have been further elucidated by clinical intravascular OCT registries, revealing that plaque erosion, rather than rupture, may represent a significantly more frequent ACS etiology in non-ST-elevation myocardial infarction (NSTEMI), whereas the traditional plaque rupture paradigm remains dominant in ST-elevation myocardial infarction (STEMI; **Fig. 11.7**).[34] In ACS patients with OCT evidence of plaque erosion, data from 49 subjects in the EROSION (Effective Anti-Thrombotic Therapy Without Stenting: Intravascular Optical

TABLE 11.2 Comparison of Existing Intracoronary Imaging Modalities

IMAGING MODALITIES	FEATURES ASSOCIATED WITH INCREASED PLAQUE VULNERABILITY							FAST ANALYSIS	CURRENT STATUS
	LUMEN DIMENSIONS	PLAQUE BURDEN AND POSITIVE REMODELING	LIPID COMPONENT	CAP THICKNESS	NEO-ANGIOGENESIS	INFLAMMATION	ESS ASSESSMENT		
IVUS + x-ray	+++	+++	+	+	–	–	+++	–	Extensive applications in the study of the role of ESS in atherosclerotic evolution
OCT + x-ray	+++	+	++	+++	++	+	+++	–	Extensive applications in the study of the role of ESS in atherosclerotic evolution
IVUS + CTCA	+++	+++	+	+	–	–	+++	–	Implemented to evaluate the efficacy of CTCA in assessing plaque morphology
OCT + CTCA	+++	+	++	+++	++	+	+++	–	Limited applications in the study of the association between plaque characteristics and the local hemodynamic forces
NIRS-IVUS	+++	+++	+++	++	–	–	–	++	Commercially available
IVUS-OCT	+++	+++	++	+++	++	+	–	+	In vivo validation
OCT-NIRF	+++	+	++	+++	++	+++	–	NK	First in man studies
IVUS-NIRF	+++	+++	+	+	–	+++	–	NK	Under development
OCT-NIRS	+++	+	+++	+++	++	+	–	NK	Ex vivo validation
IVUS-IVPA	+++	+++	++	+	+	++	–	NK	Ex vivo validation
IVUS-FLIm	+++	+++	++	+++	–	++	–	NK	In vivo validation

Performance: +++, excellent; ++, moderate; +, poor; –, not currently possible; NK, not known.

CTCA, computed tomographic coronary angiography; ESS, endothelial shear stress; FLIm, fluorescence lifetime imaging; IVPA, intravascular photoacoustic imaging; IVUS, intravascular ultrasound; NIRF, near-infrared fluorescence; NIRS, near-infrared spectroscopy; OCT, optical coherence tomography.

Reprinted with permission from Bourantas CV, Jaffer FA, Gijsen FJ et al. Hybrid intravascular imaging: recent advances, technical considerations, and current applications in the study of plaque pathophysiology. *Eur Heart J.* 2016, by permission of Oxford University Press.

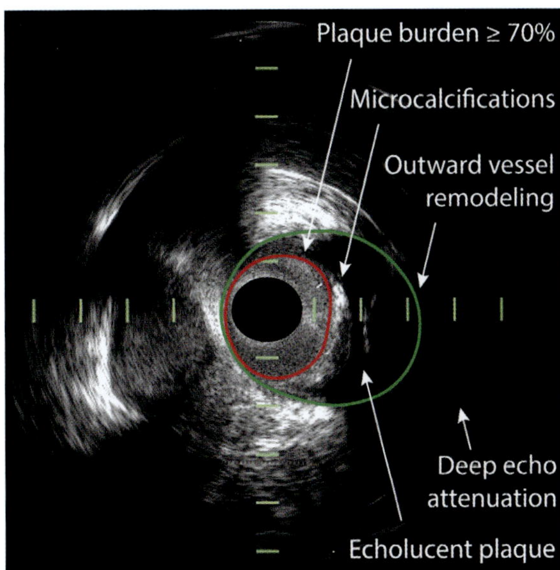

FIGURE 11.4 Vulnerable plaque features observed by intravascular ultrasound (IVUS). This IVUS cross-sectional image demonstrates plaque burden >70%, defined as (100% × [external elastic lamina (EEL) area − lumen area]/EEL area). Here, the EEL location is identified by the green line and the lumen border by the red line. The plaque further shows echolucency with deep attenuation, suggesting the possible presence of a large lipid-rich core. Additional features of positive (outward) vessel remodeling and microcalcifications are apparent. (Reprinted with permission from van Veelen A, van der Sangen NMR, Delewi R et al. Detection of vulnerable coronary plaques using invasive and non-invasive imaging modalities. *J Clin Med.* 2022;11(5):1361).

Coherence Tomography-Based Management in Plaque Erosion) study indicate that stent implantation may not always be required, as treatment with dual-antiplatelet therapy alone provided freedom from MACE at 1 year in 92.5% of subjects, with only 5.7% requiring subsequent PCI for exertional angina.[35] Furthermore, in 226 STEMI patients in EROSION III randomized to angiography or OCT-guided PCI, OCT guidance led to 15% less stent implantation than angiography alone and no difference in MACE at 1 year (composite of cardiac death, recurrent MI, TLR, and unstable angina-induced rehospitalization; $P = .67$), with most OCT-guided PCI subjects exhibiting plaque erosion (25 of 29 not stented) or calcified nodule (four of five not stented) treated medically.[36] OCT also can illuminate another less-appreciated ACS subtype, eruptive calcified nodules, that protrude through the overlying fibrous cap and are associated with luminal thrombosis and may offer additional new opportunities for lesion- and patient-tailored OCT-guided treatment decisions.[12]

Due to the inability of NIR light to penetrate the arterial wall more than 1 to 2 mm, OCT is limited in assessing important vulnerable plaque attributes such as plaque burden and positive (expansive) plaque remodeling, which are significant IVUS predictors of subsequent cardiovascular events.[6-8] Combination single-catheter IVUS-OCT consoles and catheters are now clinically available and could offer the best of both worlds through simultaneous IVUS and OCT imaging to allow broader vulnerable plaque assessment.

The first large OCT-based vulnerable plaque outcomes trial was the prospective CLIMA study. OCT was performed in the left anterior descending artery of 1003 patients, and 1-year follow-up was attained, with 3.7% of patients reaching the clinical primary endpoint. OCT analyses of 1776 lipid-rich plaques revealed that an MLA < 3.5 mm², fibrous cap thickness <75 μm, lipid arc >180°, and macrophages were linked to increased composite risk of death and target-segment myocardial infarction, with the highest clinical risk when all four OCT lesion characteristics were present together (HR 7.54, CI 3.1-18.6; **Fig. 11.8**).[37] In a prospective study of diabetic patients identified to have OCT-TCFA that were not flow limiting (FFR > 0.80), the COMBINE OCT-FFR trial found a nearly 5-fold greater incidence at 1.5 years of the composite primary endpoint (cardiac death, target vessel myocardial infarction, clinically driven target lesion revascularization, or unstable angina requiring hospitalization) compared to those without evidence of OCT-TCFA.[38] Additional natural history studies assessing OCT-vulnerable plaque features to predict subsequent events are eagerly awaited (NCT02316886, NCT05599061).

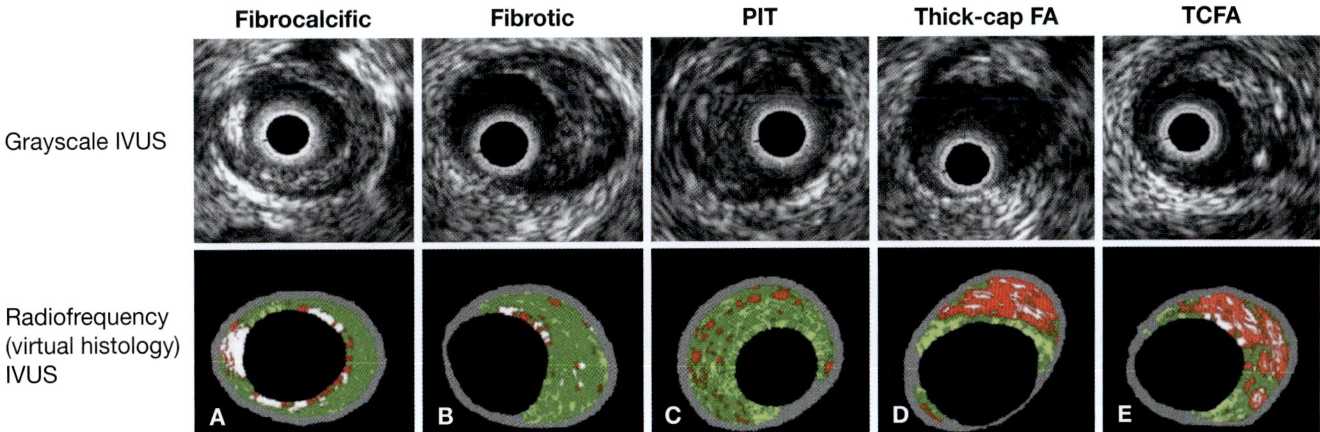

FIGURE 11.5 Virtual histology intravascular ultrasound (VH-IVUS) plaque classification. Radiofrequency VH-IVUS categorizes plaque constituents into fibrous (dark green), fibrofatty (light green), necrotic core (red), and dense calcium (white). Based on the local plaque composition, VH-IVUS can then distinguish five separate types of atheroma: **(A)** fibrocalcific, **(B)** fibrotic, **(C)** pathological intimal thickening (PIT), **(D)** thick-cap fibroatheroma (FA), and **(E)** thin-cap fibroatheroma (TCFA). Note that due to resolution constraints (150-250 μm), VH-IVUS cannot discriminate pathological <65 μm fibrous caps, and therefore, VH-TCFA are defined as a >30° necrotic core lesions abutting the lumen that lacks detectable overlying fibrous tissue on three consecutive cross-sectional slices. (Reprinted with permission from Gaba P, Gersh BJ, Muller J et al. Evolving concepts of the vulnerable atherosclerotic plaque and the vulnerable patient: implications for patient care and future research. *Nat Rev Cardiol.* 2023;20:181-196).

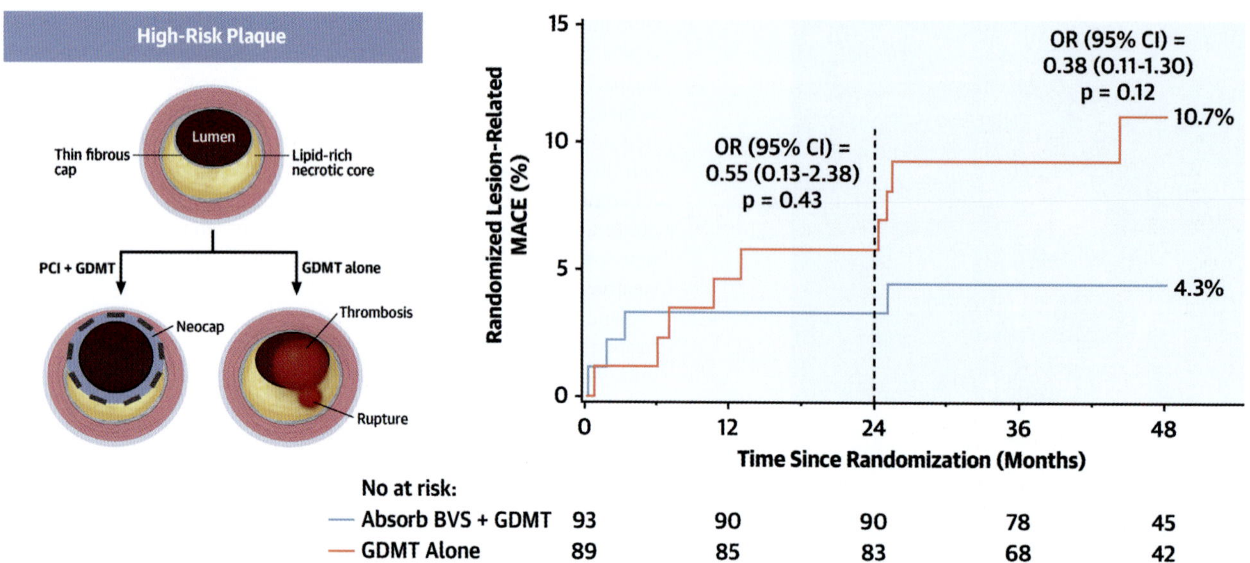

FIGURE 11.6 Prospect absorb and the concept of "preventative" percutaneous coronary intervention (PCI) for vulnerable plaques. **(Left panel)** A schematic of a high-risk vulnerable plaque consisting of a <65-μm-thin fibrous cap (blue) overlying a well-formed necrotic core (yellow) composed of cholesterol, inflammatory cells, and their remnants. Following "preventative" PCI, conceptually the lumen is enlarged by the stent struts (gray dashes), the local lipid content is reduced (via embolization or plaque translation), and there is subsequent formation of a thickened 100- to 200-μm fibrous tissue neocap. In contrast, with guideline-directed medical therapy (GDMT) alone, an uncovered vulnerable plaque may rupture, leading to vessel thrombosis and acute coronary syndrome. **(Right panel)** The randomized lesion-related major adverse cardiac events (MACE), defined as the composite of cardiac death, myocardial infarction, and unstable or progressive angina, are shown from the PROSPECT ABSORB trial over 4-year follow-up period. Routine angiographic follow-up was performed at 25 months, just after the 24-month timepoint (dotted line). BVS, bioresorbable vascular scaffold; CI, confidence interval; OR, odds ratio. (Adapted with permission from Stone GW, Maehara A, Ali ZA et al. Percutaneous coronary intervention for vulnerable coronary atherosclerotic plaque. *J Am Coll Cardiol*. 2020;76:2289-2301.)

NIR SPECTROSCOPY

Intravascular NIRS imaging is a sensitive method to detect lipid-core coronary plaques.[11,39] From a technical perspective, NIRS imaging employs an optical fiber integrated with a conventional rotational IVUS or OCT catheter (NIRS-IVUS, NIRS-OCT) that detects the specific chemical signature associated with plaque lipid NIR light absorption by cholesterol moieties. The spectroscopic NIRS signal is then decoded by the imaging software into a relative probability of lipid-rich plaque (LRP) being present at a particular coronary region and displayed as a pseudocolor lookup table ranging from red (low probability of lipid) to yellow (high-probability of lipid), termed a "chemogram" (**Fig. 11.9**). Beyond the local angular lipid content display on axial IVUS OR OCT images, a block chemogram is also presented on the long-view pullback image that sums the probability of a coronary lipid plaque being present for each 2-mm distance throughout the length of the catheter pullback. As NIRS images only lipid and is not depth-resolved, NIRS requires to be integrated with grayscale IVUS to provide simultaneous structural information that complements NIRS lipid data, and more recently with high-resolution OCT imaging.[39]

Following positive validation studies for NIRS lipid plaque detection in both cadaveric coronary plaques and in vivo ACS patients, several early clinical studies demonstrated poorer clinical outcomes associated with lipid-rich atheroma detected by NIRS. NIRS-identified LRP associated with an increased risk of periprocedural myocardial infarction during PCI.[40] Compared to patients with stable angina undergoing PCI, ACS patients were more likely to have LRPs at the culprit PCI location (84.4% vs 52.8%), as well as more nonculprit NIRS-positive plaques,[41] implying that NIRS reports on the systemic vulnerability of coronary disease in general. NIRS has also demonstrated that intensive lipid-lowering pharmacotherapy with rosuvastatin reduces intracoronary NIRS LRP content in patients after only 7 weeks,[42] supporting clinical trial data that statins can have a rapid stabilizing effect on vulnerable atheroma and reduce coronary events.

Clinical Outcomes Studies

In recent years, investigations examining the natural history of NIRS lipid-rich coronary atheroma and subsequent cardiac events have shed increasing light on the clinical risk that vulnerable NIRS lesions portend. The AtheroRemo-IVUS study, a prospective analysis of nonculprit plaques from a mix of approximately 200 stable angina and ACS patients imaged with standalone NIRS, showed that coronary atheroma with greater than the median positive NIRS signal (reported as the lipid core burden index) held a significantly increased 1 year risk of adverse cardiovascular events (HR 4.04), driven predominately by urgent revascularization.[43]

To further understand the ability of intracoronary NIRS imaging to detect vulnerable plaques, the natural history of nonculprit, nonobstructive, lipid-rich atheroma by combination NIRS-IVUS was evaluated in two landmark prospective studies, LRP (Lipid-Rich Plaque)[8] and PROSPECT II (Providing Regional Observations to Study Predictors of Events in the Coronary Tree II).[6] In LRP, a total of 1563 patients with suspected CAD planned for coronary angiography underwent three-vessel coronary imaging using NIRS-IVUS to assess the presence of nonobstructive lipid core plaque, defined by the maximal lipid-core burden index over 4-mm pullback length ($maxLCBI_{4mm}$; range 0-1000, equivalent to 0% to 100% yellow pixels in the region of interest). Over a 2-year follow-up period, subjects with significantly elevated plaque lipid composition ($maxLCBI_{4mm} > 400$) independently predicted greater nonculprit MACE, both on a per-patient (13% vs 6%, $P < .0001$) and per-plaque (3% vs 1%, $P < .0001$) basis.[8]

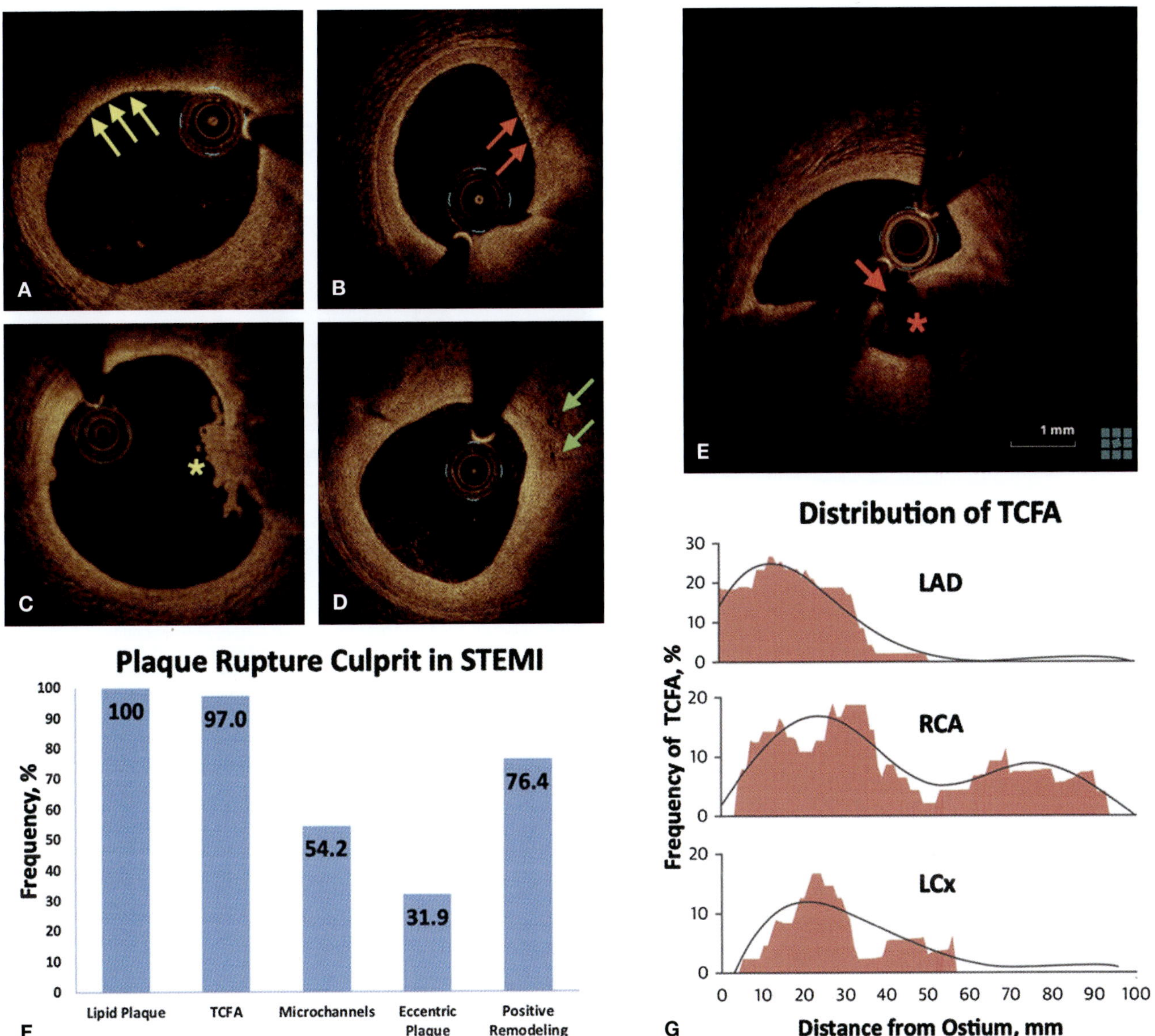

FIGURE 11.7 Thin-cap fibroatheroma (TCFA) and atherosclerotic plaque rupture identified by optical coherence tomography (OCT) imaging. Due to its high spatial resolution (10-20 μm), intracoronary OCT is able to identify multiple structural vulnerable plaque features including: **(A)** TCFA (yellow arrows), **(B)** fibrous cap with macrophage infiltration (red arrows), **(C)** luminal thrombus (yellow asterisk), and **(D)** intimal neovessel microchannels (green arrows). **(E)** Ruptured plaques discovered by OCT show interruption of the fibrous cap (red arrow) and are often associated with a cavity (red asterisk) where plaque constituents were extruded. **(F)** In patients suffering ST-elevation myocardial infarction (STEMI) due to plaque rupture at the culprit lesion, OCT frequently identifies vulnerable plaque features such as TCFA and neovessels. **(G)** As most OCT TCFA are found clustered in the proximal coronary segment, these vulnerable lesions frequently subtend a larger myocardial territory at risk. LAD, left anterior descending; LCx, left circumflex; RCA, right coronary artery. (Reprinted with permission from Aguirre AD, Arbab-Zadeh A, Soeda T et al. Optical coherence tomography of plaque vulnerability and rupture: JACC focus seminar part 1/3. *J Am Coll Cardiol*. 2021;78:1257-1265.)

In PROSPECT II, 898 patients with recent ACS underwent 3-vessel NIRS-IVUS to assess 3629 nonculprit lesions. Over 4 years, highly lipidic lesions ($maxLCBI_{4mm} > 325$) by NIRS at baseline predicted greater events, and when highly NIRS-positive plaques coincided with large PB lesions, higher MACE rates were observed in patient-level (13.2%) and lesion-level (7.0%) analyses.[6] While it remains unclear if intensified medical therapy alone, or with the addition of pre-emptive PCI such as that evaluated in the PROSPECT ABSORB study as discussed above or upcoming PREVENT trial (NCT02316886), will further reduce clinical risk, the positive results of these key trials led to US FDA approval of intracoronary NIRS as a diagnostic modality for detection of vulnerable patients and plaques. A current limitation of NIRS includes a lack of depth information on lipid content; however, future developments in NIRS technology, or the development of PAT, may bridge this gap.

Angioscopy

Intracoronary angioscopy utilizes an angioscope equipped with color fiber optic video bundle that directly illuminates the coronary artery wall. Angioscopy is mainly performed in Japan, and similar to light-based OCT, it requires displacement of blood from the imaging field (typically via saline injection). Angioscopy has provided important insights into coronary atherosclerosis pathophysiology,[44] where it can detect the presence of luminal thrombus

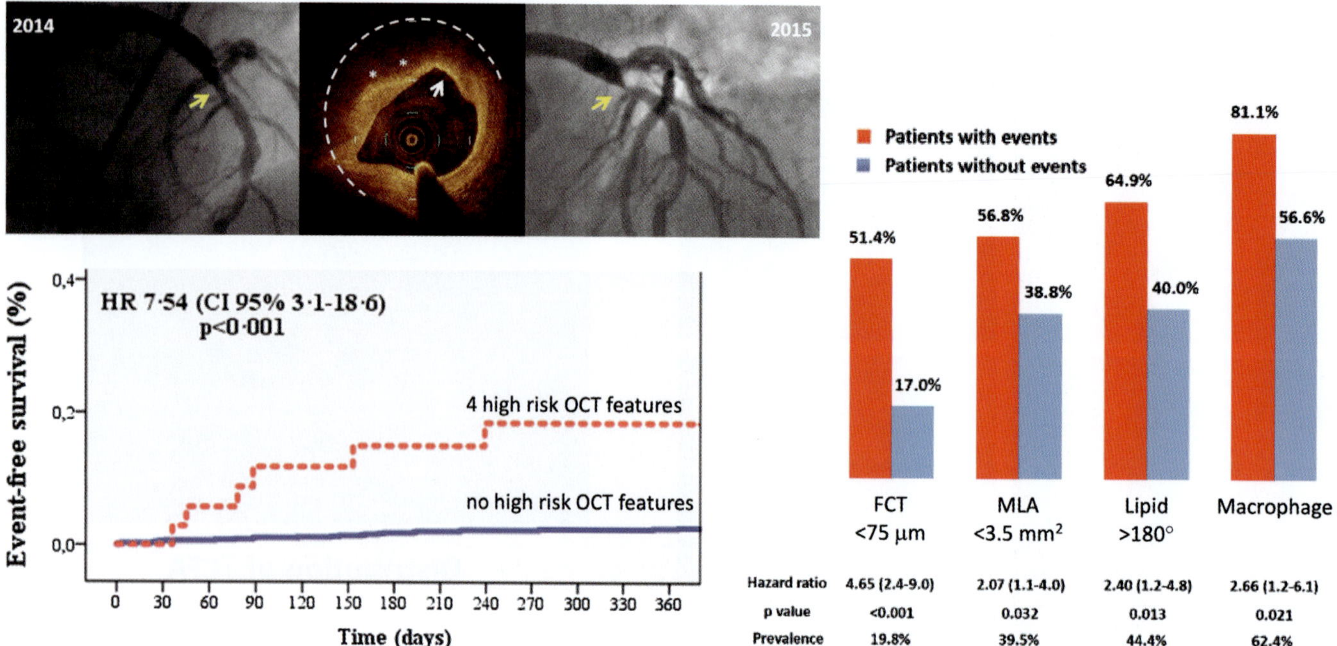

FIGURE 11.8 Associations between high-risk plaque features identified by optical coherence tomography (OCT) and subsequent cardiovascular events. **(Top panels)** A moderately stenotic proximal left anterior descending (LAD) lesion by angiography (yellow arrow) exhibits all four high-risk OCT imaging criteria: minimum lumen area (MLA) <3.5 mm^2, fibrous cap thickness (FCT) <75 µm (arrow), lipid arc >180° (dotted line), and inflammatory macrophage accumulations (asterisk). One year following the baseline study, the LAD plaque had significantly progressed angiographically (yellow arrow) leading to presentation with an acute coronary syndrome. **(Right panel)** Clinical event rates in the CLIMA study at 1 year stratified by OCT high-risk plaque features. **(Bottom panel)** Event-free survival from target-vessel myocardial infarction or cardiac death in subjects with or without high-risk proximal LAD coronary plaque features identified by OCT imaging. (Adapted with permission from Prati F, Romagnoli E, Gatto L et al. Relationship between coronary plaque morphology of the left anterior descending artery and 12 months clinical outcome: the CLIMA study. *Eur Heart J* 2020;41:383-391).

(red-blood-cell–enriched red thrombus or platelet-predominant white thrombus) and plaque ulcerations, or frank disruptions, as well as color variations in the surface of intact atheroma that indicate plaque lipid composition and fibrous cap thickness. White-colored plaques seen by angioscopy reflect plaques with high fibrous tissue content, whereas yellow hues signify LRPs with thinner overlying fibrous caps, a finding validated by intracoronary OCT, where in one study, plaques with the highest yellow coloration had a measured fibrous cap thickness of 40 ± 14 µm.[45] Angioscopic glistening yellow plaques are therefore considered equivalent to histologic TCFA and accordingly have been associated with an increased likelihood of ACS presentation at 1 year in a prospective clinical study of patients with baseline stable angina.[46] In comparison, subjects with white or nonglistening yellow angioscopic lesions had a lower frequency of ACS. The addition of color fluorescence plaque imaging with selective visible light wavelength filters may increase the detection capability of angioscopy for vulnerable plaque features, including collagen content and oxidized low-density lipoprotein (LDL).[44] Angioscopy thus holds promise for prospective vulnerable plaque identification, although due to the larger diameter, lack of motorized pullback, and requirement for blood displacement, it has not achieved the widespread adoption that could enable validation in larger patient populations.

FLUORESCENCE

Currently available clinical intravascular imaging modalities—IVUS, OCT, and NIRS—are able to interrogate vulnerable plaque structural features, but they lack the ability to report on important plaque biologic factors inherent in plaque instability. To address this unmet need, intravascular fluorescence imaging has been developed as a translatable coronary imaging approach for quantitative, high-resolution plaque and stent imaging (**Fig. 11.10**).[3,47,48] NIRF imaging, the primary approach used for molecular imaging, has several beneficial attributes for intracoronary applications, including through-blood imaging without the need for flushing, no ionizing radiation exposure, good tissue penetration in the NIR light wavelengths with low background tissue autofluorescence, and a high sensitivity for NIR fluorophore-labeled probes that leads to excellent signal-to-noise characteristics. In addition, because intracoronary optical imaging (ie, OCT, NIRS) is already routinely employed in many catheterization laboratories, intravascular fluorescence imaging is attractive clinically.

Fluorescence Lifetime Imaging

A recently developed promising clinical optical imaging approach is intravascular FLIm, which is a technique capable of measuring the autofluorescence decay rate of distinct plaque constituents following excitation with 355-nm ultraviolet light. FLIm detects wavelengths in the visible light range from 380 to 560 nm and then creates an image based on the various fluorescence lifetimes observed. One advantage of FLIm is that it can resolve multiple biochemical components according to each unique fluorescence lifetime—lipid, calcium, and fibrous tissues—even if the components fluoresce at the same wavelength. As with NIRS, however, FLIm has no depth or associated structural information, and therefore must be paired with IVUS or OCT in a multimodality catheter system to map FLIm plaque features onto local structural elements. As FLIm is entirely based on endogenous tissue autofluorescence

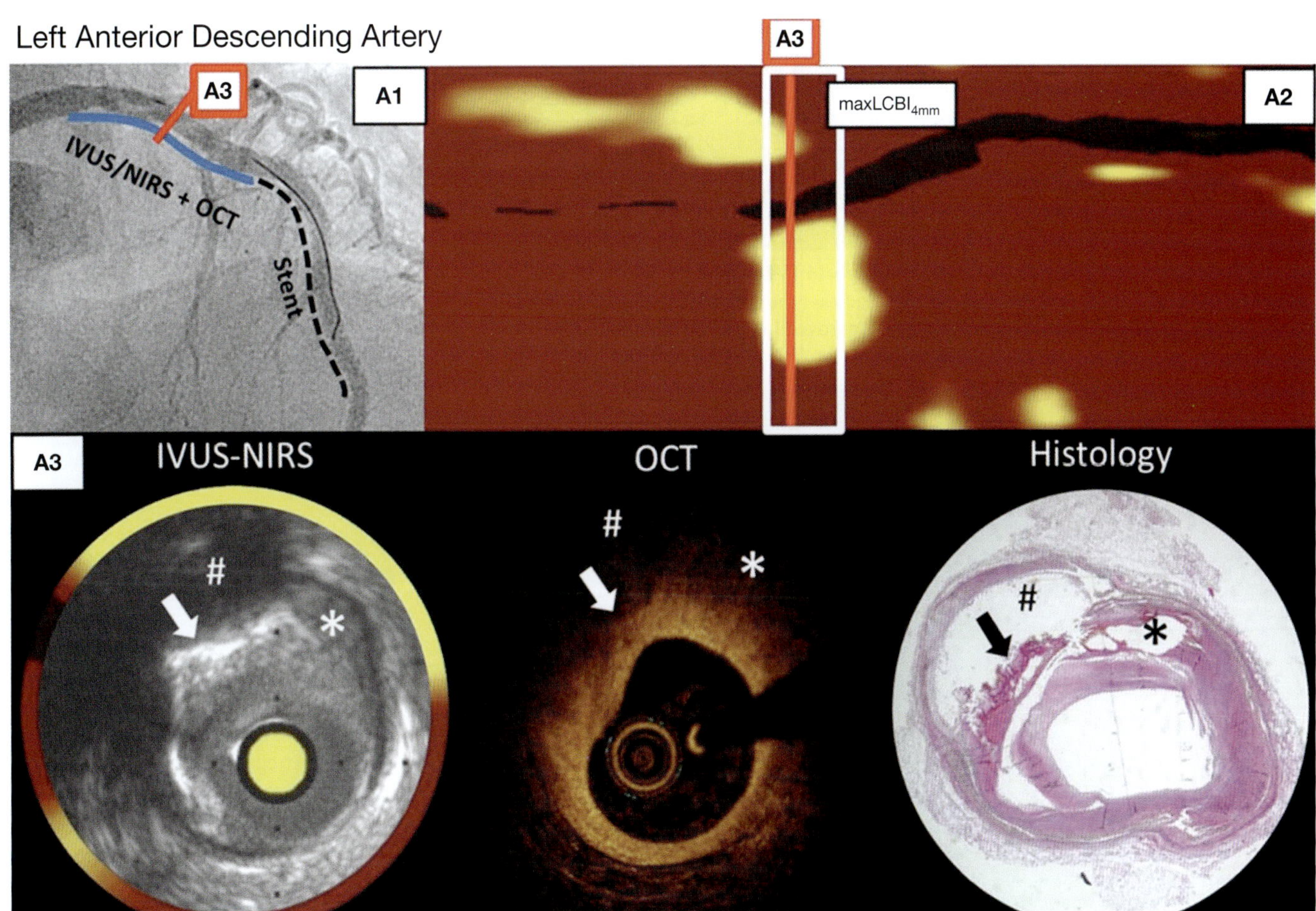

FIGURE 11.9 Multi-modality plaque imaging with near-infrared spectroscopy (NIRS), intravascular ultrasound (IVUS), and optical coherence tomography (OCT). (**A1**) Coronary angiogram demonstrating location of stent implantation (black dashed line) in the mid left anterior descending artery and the location of intracoronary imaging (blue solid line) with IVUS-NIRS and OCT proximal to the stent. (**A2**) IVUS-NIRS chemogram identifies a region with a large lipid deposit (white solid box). (**A3**) Cross-sectional imaging at the location of this lipid-rich plaque with IVUS-NIRS and OCT, confirmed by paired histopathology, reveals lipid core (hashtag), lipid pool (asterisk), and superficial calcification (arrow). (Reprinted with permission from Muller J, Madder R. OCT-NIRS imaging for detection of coronary plaque structure and vulnerability. *Front Cardiovasc Med.* 2020;7:90.)

properties, an advantage of this technique is that it does not rely on administration of intravenous fluorescent agents. In cadaveric human atherosclerotic plaques, IVUS-FLIm has been shown to delineate calcium, lipid, fibrous tissue, and macrophage accumulations with high agreement to histology.[49] Intracoronary OCT-FLIm has also been shown to improve macrophage detection over standalone OCT in a preclinical atherosclerosis swine model using a clinically translatable 2.9-French catheter[50] and is currently being studied in a first-in-human clinical trial (NCT04835467). Limitations of FLIm, and fluorescence imaging in general, are that the signal recorded is primarily obtained from the plaque surface due to diminished light penetration into deeper plaque structures. However, many vulnerable plaque features (such as TCFA) abut those of the lumen and thus are readily detectable by FLIm and other fluorescence-based molecular imaging techniques.

NIR Fluorescence Molecular Imaging

Fundamentally, atherosclerosis is an inflammatory disease orchestrated by activated macrophages that drive atherogenesis, plaque growth, structural/mechanical destabilization, and thrombus precipitation. Anti-inflammatory specific therapy reduces cardiac events.[51,52] Moreover, recent clinical studies demonstrate that residual systemic inflammation (measured by blood biomarkers such as high-sensitivity C-reactive protein and cathepsin S) predicts poorer outcomes for CAD and ACS patients—even with optimal LDL control.[53-56] At present, however, no clinical approaches exist for direct imaging of coronary plaque inflammation at high resolution in clinical subjects. While OCT, FLIm, and NIR autofluorescence are attractive as they do not require injection of an exogenous imaging agent, they are not specific for inflammatory activity, nor other key pathological processes such as apoptosis, ferroptosis, oxidative stress, or autophagy, known drivers of plaque complications.

To address this unmet need, intravascular NIRF molecular imaging is emerging clinically through the use of NIRF-OCT and NIRF-IVUS catheter technology.[57-59] After intravenous injection of a NIRF inflammation molecular imaging agent, a NIRF catheter is placed into the coronary artery to image the fluorescence signal generated by the molecular imaging agent that targets a specific cell (eg, macrophage) or molecule (eg, cathepsin protease or matrix metalloproteinase). Three significant steps forward in the field of NIRF molecular imaging have been completed recently. First, intracoronary NIRF-OCT, without the use of a contrast agent, has been performed in 12 clinical subjects to detect NIR autofluorescence, a marker of plaque ceroid and intraplaque hemorrhage.[60-63]

Atherosclerotic lesion
- Macrophage infiltration
- Accumulation of LDL
- Endothelial dysfunction
- Collagen degradation
- Calcification
- Intraplaque hemorrhage

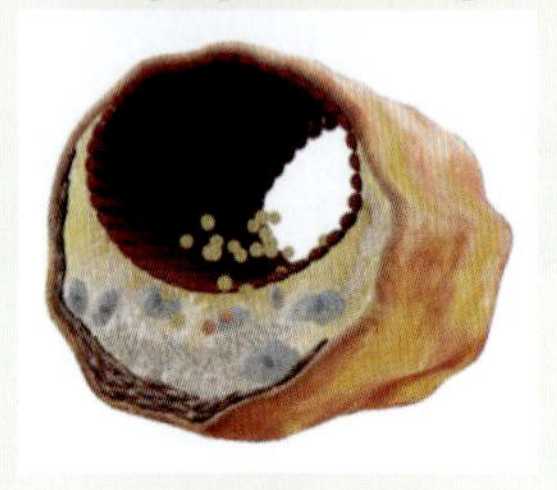

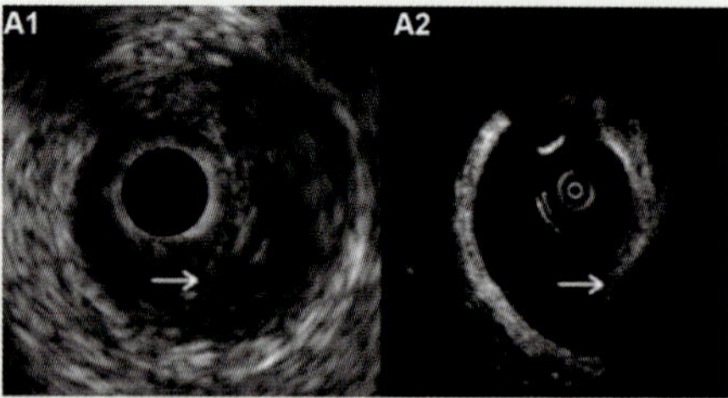

Hybrid IVUS-OCT
Increase the morphological information.
Approved for clinical use.

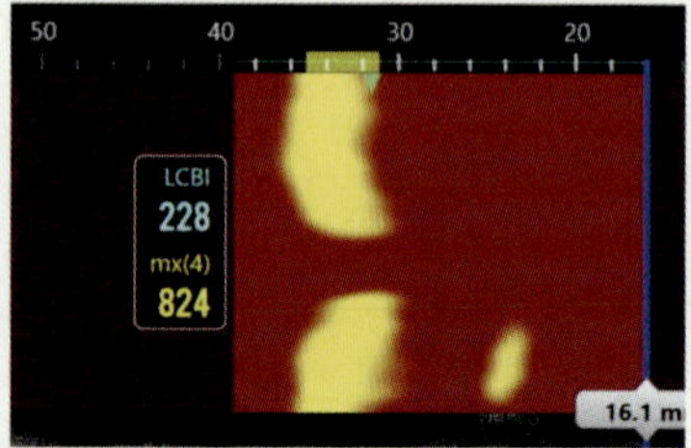

NIRS-IVUS
Visualize the intra-plaque lipid accumulation using near-infrared light.
Approved for clinical use.

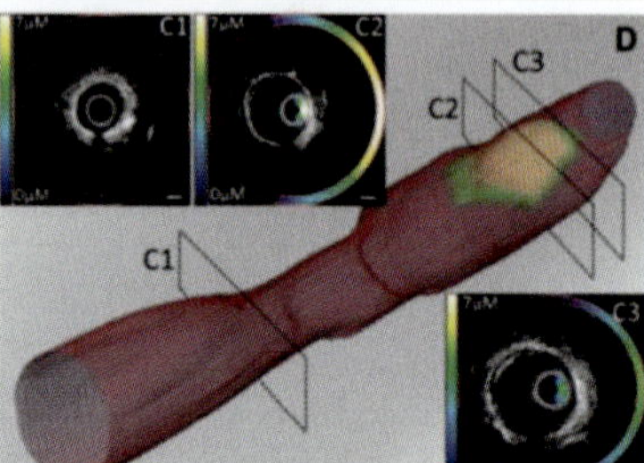

NIRF-IVUS/OCT
Visualize a wide range of biological processes using near-infrared light.
Not approved for clinical use.

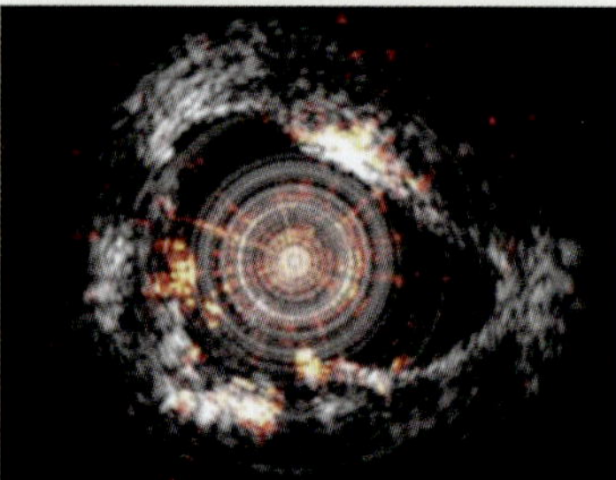

IVPA-IVUS
Visualize the plaque components using photoacoustic wave.
Not approved for clinical use.

FIGURE 11.10 Overview of emerging clinical intracoronary imaging modalities. Near-infrared fluorescence (NIRF) imaging utilizes illumination by near-infrared (NIR) light 600 to 900 nm, an efficient wavelength range for light to penetrate through blood. Clinically, NIR autofluorescence (NIRAF) has been detected in coronary artery disease patients using NIRF-OCT catheters at 630 nm and illuminates plaque ceroid (protein-lipid conglomerates formed in oxidative stress-rich environment) and intraplaque hemorrhage. For clinical vulnerable plaque molecular imaging that is on the horizon, a NIRF molecular imaging agent will be preinjected intravenously to target a specific molecule or cell (eg, macrophage), followed by NIRF-OCT or NIRF-IVUS imaging. This development will enable high-resolution quantitative imaging of coronary plaque inflammation in patients. IVPA, intravascular photoacoustic; IVUS, intravascular ultrasound; LDL, low-density lipoprotein; NIRS, near-infrared spectroscopy; OCT, optical coherence tomography. (Reprinted with permission from Seguchi M, Aytekin A, Lenz T et al. Intravascular molecular imaging: translating pathophysiology of atherosclerosis into human disease conditions. *Eur Heart J Cardiovasc Imaging.* 2022;24:e1-e16, by permission of Oxford University Press.)

TABLE 11.3 Guideline Recommendations on Intracoronary Imaging

2021 ACC/AHA/SCAI GUIDELINE FOR CORONARY ARTERY REVASCULARIZATION

Class 2a

- In patients with intermediate stenosis of the left main artery, IVUS is reasonable to help define lesion severity (Level of evidence: B)
- In patients undergoing coronary stent implantation, IVUS can be useful for procedural guidance, particularly in cases of left main or complex coronary artery stenting, to reduce ischemic events. (Level of evidence: B)
- In patients undergoing coronary stent implantation, OCT is a reasonable alternative to IVUS for procedural guidance, except in ostial left main disease. (Level of evidence: B)
- In patients with stent failure, IVUS or OCT is reasonable to determine the mechanism of stent failure. (Level of evidence: C)

ACC/AHA, American College of Cardiology/American Heart Association; IVUS, intravascular ultrasound; OCT, optical coherence tomography; SCAI, Society for Cardiovascular Angiography and Interventions.

Writing Committee M, Lawton JS, Tamis-Holland JE et al. 2021 ACC/AHA/SCAI guideline for coronary artery revascularization: a report of the American College of Cardiology/American Heart Association Joint Committee on Clinical Practice Guidelines. *J Am Coll Cardiol.* 2022;79:e21-e129.

Second, an FDA-approved NIRF imaging agent indocyanine green (ICG) has been found to serve as an atherosclerosis-targeting imaging agent and has been injected into patients undergoing carotid endarterectomy.[64,65] ICG targets plaque macrophages and lipids in areas of high plaque endothelial permeability. Third, a NIRF-OCT clinical study has been funded by the NIH to perform first-in-human coronary plaque inflammation imaging (R01HL165453). These developments position NIRF molecular imaging to be clinically viable within the next few years.

GUIDELINES FOR INTRAVASCULAR PLAQUE IMAGING

While society consensus guidelines provide Class IIa-IIb recommendations for the use of IVUS and OCT imaging in certain patients,[66] given the lack of currently available evidence supporting the clinical utility of vulnerable plaque imaging, routine use of intravascular imaging to identify vulnerable plaque features is of uncertain clinical significance and should not be performed. No present guidelines exist regarding the use of NIRS or the other emerging intravascular imaging modalities. **Table 11.3** provides a summary of available society guidelines and expert consensus statement recommendations. As intracoronary imaging continues to evolve rapidly, society guidelines are very likely to include new clinical trial data and new intravascular imaging technologies in future recommendations.

CONCLUSIONS

Due to the leading cause of death and disability attributable to CAD worldwide, vulnerable plaque imaging continues to generate significant interest from a clinical and research perspective in the cardiovascular and interventional community. The hypothesis driving vulnerable plaque imaging is predicated on the concept that early identification of specific structural and/or biologic high-risk plaque features will allow prediction and prevention of future major adverse cardiovascular events and personalized tailoring of anti-CAD therapeutics, including anti-inflammatory drugs. Through continued research and development of vulnerable plaque-imaging approaches, including the key benefits of merging imaging technologies with different strengths into multimodality intravascular catheter imaging systems, prospective vulnerable plaque detection offers hope for the development of new therapeutic strategies to treat plaque complications before they occur.

Key Points

- Autopsy studies of individuals suffering cardiac death demonstrate vulnerable plaque features, including thin fibrous caps, lipid-rich necrotic cores, neovessels, intraplaque hemorrhage, inflammation, and calcific nodules.
- Correlation between intracoronary imaging findings and gold-standard histopathology has in general been good, but the sensitivity and specificity of detecting individual vulnerable plaque feature varies.
- Each intracoronary vulnerable plaque-imaging modality has strengths and weaknesses, and no single imaging modality is currently able to detect all vulnerable plaque features. Multimodal approaches will provide greater clinical value.
- Intracoronary imaging with IVUS, VH-IVUS, OCT, NIRS, NIRAF, and FLIm are clinically studied intravascular imaging technologies that can characterize important structural features of vulnerable plaques.
- The PROSPECT trial revealed that nonculprit VH-IVUS TCFA, as well as plaque burden >70% and minimum lumen area <4 mm^2, were independent predictors of subsequent adverse cardiovascular events. Nevertheless, the low positive predictive value of these variables has limited clinical application of routine standalone IVUS vulnerable plaque imaging.
- The CLIMA study showed that OCT could predict LAD plaque complications at 1 year. However, standalone OCT does not have enough predictive power to justify nonculprit plaque imaging. NIRS-OCT is clinically emerging and may offer new predictive capabilities.
- The LRP and PROSPECT II trials revealed that lipid-rich plaque detected by NIRS was an independent predictor of clinical events in individual plaques and patients. Furthermore, lipid-rich NIRS plaque in combination with a large IVUS plaque burden portends a higher risk of future events. Yet, similar to standalone IVUS, NIRS-IVUS does not yet have the predictive power to justify routine intracoronary nonculprit plaque imaging.
- Emerging intracoronary NIRF molecular imaging (NIRF-OCT, NIRF-IVUS) offers a new approach to investigate in vivo plaque biology such as inflammation, as well as plaque autofluorescence (NIRAF) to detect plaque ceroid, intraplaque hemorrhage, and oxidative stress.
- Current society guideline recommendations do not support routine intravascular imaging to detect vulnerable plaque.
- PROSPECT Absorb showed that a preventative PCI strategy with BVS appears to be safe; however, additional studies examining preventative PCI of vulnerable plaque and cardiovascular outcomes are needed.

Disclosures

Dr. Jaffer received research funding from Canon, Siemens, Shockwave, Teleflex, Mercator, Boston Scientific, HeartFlow, and Neovasc and has consulting agreements with and/or receives speaker's fees from Boston Scientific, Siemens, Magenta Medical, Philips, Biotronik, Mercator, Abiomed, and Medtronic. Dr Jaffer holds equity in Intravascular Imaging Inc and DurVena. Massachusetts General Hospital has patent licensing arrangements with Terumo, Spectrawave, and Canon Corporation; Dr. Jaffer has rights to receive royalties through these licensing arrangements. Dr. Osborn received research funding from Dyad Medical, OpSens, Philips, and Zoll and has consulting agreements with Abbott Vascular, Gentuity, NuPulse, and Philips. Dr Osborn is on the Scientific Advisory Board of and holds equity in Dyad Medical.

Acknowledgments

This work was supported by NIH R01HL150538 and R01HL165453.

For further review and interactivities, please see the chapter-based multiple choice questions and videos accessible in the complimentary eBook bundled with this text. Access instructions are located in the inside front cover.

References

1. Gaba P, Gersh BJ, Muller J, Narula J, Stone GW. Evolving concepts of the vulnerable atherosclerotic plaque and the vulnerable patient: implications for patient care and future research. *Nat Rev Cardiol*. 2023;20(3):181-196.
2. Jaffer FA, Chandrashekhar Y. The ongoing quest to better detect high-risk coronary plaques. *JACC Cardiovasc Imaging*. 2020;13(4):1103-1105.
3. Seguchi M, Aytekin A, Lenz T, et al. Intravascular molecular imaging: translating pathophysiology of atherosclerosis into human disease conditions. *Eur Heart J Cardiovasc Imaging*. 2022;24(1):e1-e16.
4. Arbab-Zadeh A, Fuster V. From detecting the vulnerable plaque to managing the vulnerable patient: JACC state-of-the-art review. *J Am Coll Cardiol*. 2019;74(12):1582-1593.

5. Maddox TM, Stanislawski MA, Grunwald GK, et al. Nonobstructive coronary artery disease and risk of myocardial infarction. *JAMA*. 2014;312(17):1754-1763.
6. Erlinge D, Maehara A, Ben-Yehuda O, et al. Identification of vulnerable plaques and patients by intracoronary near-infrared spectroscopy and ultrasound (PROSPECT II): a prospective natural history study. *Lancet*. 2021;397(10278):985-995.
7. Stone GW, Maehara A, Lansky AJ, et al. A prospective natural-history study of coronary atherosclerosis. *N Engl J Med*. 2011;364(3):226-235.
8. Waksman R, Di Mario C, Torguson R, et al. Identification of patients and plaques vulnerable to future coronary events with near-infrared spectroscopy intravascular ultrasound imaging: a prospective, cohort study. *Lancet*. 2019;394(10209):1629-1637.
9. Virmani R, Burke AP, Farb A, Kolodgie FD. Pathology of the vulnerable plaque. *J Am Coll Cardiol*. 2006;47(8 Suppl):C13-C18.
10. Cheruvu PK, Finn AV, Gardner C, et al. Frequency and distribution of thin-cap fibroatheroma and ruptured plaques in human coronary arteries: a pathologic study. *J Am Coll Cardiol*. 2007;50(10):940-949.
11. Bom MJ, van der Heijden DJ, Kedhi E, et al. Early detection and treatment of the vulnerable coronary plaque: can we prevent acute coronary syndromes? *Circ Cardiovasc Imaging*. 2017;10(5):e005973.
12. Torii S, Sato Y, Otsuka F, et al. Eruptive calcified nodules as a potential mechanism of acute coronary thrombosis and sudden death. *J Am Coll Cardiol*. 2021;77(13):1599-1611.
13. Libby P, Tabas I, Fredman G, Fisher EA. Inflammation and its resolution as determinants of acute coronary syndromes. *Circ Res*. 2014;114(12):1867-1879.
14. Mason JC, Libby P. Cardiovascular disease in patients with chronic inflammation: mechanisms underlying premature cardiovascular events in rheumatologic conditions. *Eur Heart J*. 2015;36(8):482-9c.
15. Jaffer FA, Weissleder R. Molecular imaging in the clinical arena. *JAMA*. 2005;293(7):855-862.
16. Osborn EA, Jaffer FA. The advancing clinical impact of molecular imaging in CVD. *JACC Cardiovasc Imaging*. 2013;6(12):1327-1341.
17. Mintz GS, Matsumura M, Ali Z, Maehara A. Clinical utility of intravascular imaging: past, present, and future. *JACC Cardiovasc Imaging*. 2022;15(10):1799-1820.
18. Calvert PA, Obaid DR, O'Sullivan M, et al. Association between IVUS findings and adverse outcomes in patients with coronary artery disease: the VIVA (VH-IVUS in Vulnerable Atherosclerosis) Study. *JACC Cardiovasc Imaging*. 2011;4(8):894-901.
19. Cheng JM, Garcia-Garcia HM, de Boer SP, et al. In vivo detection of high-risk coronary plaques by radiofrequency intravascular ultrasound and cardiovascular outcome: results of the ATHEROREMO-IVUS study. *Eur Heart J*. 2014;35(10):639-647.
20. Stone GW, Maehara A, Ali ZA, et al. Percutaneous coronary intervention for vulnerable coronary atherosclerotic plaque. *J Am Coll Cardiol*. 2020;76(20):2289-2301.
21. Chin CY, Maehara A, Fall K, Mintz GS, Ali ZA. Imaging comparisons of coregistered native and stented coronary segments by high-definition 60-MHz intravascular ultrasound and optical coherence tomography. *JACC Cardiovasc Interv*. 2016;9(12):1305-1306.
22. Fujino A, Mintz GS, Matsumura M, et al. A new optical coherence tomography-based calcium scoring system to predict stent underexpansion. *EuroIntervention*. 2018;13(18):e2182-e2189.
23. Maehara A, Cristea E, Mintz GS, et al. Definitions and methodology for the grayscale and radiofrequency intravascular ultrasound and coronary angiographic analyses. *JACC Cardiovasc Imaging*. 2012;5(3 suppl):S1-S9.
24. Stone PH, Saito S, Takahashi S, et al. Prediction of progression of coronary artery disease and clinical outcomes using vascular profiling of endothelial shear stress and arterial plaque characteristics: the PREDICTION study. *Circulation*. 2012;126(2):172-181.
25. Kaul S, Diamond GA. Improved prospects for IVUS in identifying vulnerable plaques? *JACC Cardiovasc Imaging*. 2012;5(3 suppl):S106-S110.
26. Wykrzykowska JJ, Diletti R, Gutierrez-Chico JL, et al. Plaque sealing and passivation with a mechanical self-expanding low outward force nitinol vShield device for the treatment of IVUS and OCT-derived thin cap fibroatheromas (TCFAs) in native coronary arteries: report of the pilot study vShield evaluated at Cardiac hospital in Rotterdam for Investigation and Treatment of TCFA (SECRITT). *EuroIntervention*. 2012;8:945-954.
27. Haude M, Ince H, Abizaid A, et al. Safety and performance of the second-generation drug-eluting absorbable metal scaffold in patients with de-novo coronary artery lesions (BIOSOLVE-II): 6 month results of a prospective, multicentre, non-randomised, first-in-man trial. *Lancet*. 2016;387(10013):31-39.
28. Seguchi M, Baumann-Zumstein P, Fubel A, et al. Preclinical evaluation of the degradation kinetics of third-generation resorbable magnesium scaffolds. *EuroIntervention*. 2023;19(2):e167-e175.
29. Tearney GJ, Regar E, Akasaka T, et al. Consensus standards for acquisition, measurement, and reporting of intravascular optical coherence tomography studies: a report from the international working group for intravascular optical coherence tomography standardization and validation. *J Am Coll Cardiol*. 2012;59(12):1058-1072.
30. Maehara A, Matsumura M, Ali ZA, Mintz GS, Stone GW. IVUS-guided versus OCT-guided coronary stent implantation: a critical appraisal. *JACC Cardiovasc Imaging*. 2017;10(12):1487-1503.
31. Osborn EA, Johnson M, Maksoud A, et al. Safety and efficiency of percutaneous coronary intervention using a standardised optical coherence tomography workflow. *EuroIntervention*. 2023;18(14):1178-1187.
32. Yabushita H, Bouma BE, Houser SL, et al. Characterization of human atherosclerosis by optical coherence tomography. *Circulation*. 2002;106(13):1640-1645.
33. Kubo T, Imanishi T, Takarada S, et al. Assessment of culprit lesion morphology in acute myocardial infarction: ability of optical coherence tomography compared with intravascular ultrasound and coronary angioscopy. *J Am Coll Cardiol*. 2007;50(10):933-939.
34. Aguirre AD, Arbab-Zadeh A, Soeda T, Fuster V, Jang IK. Optical coherence tomography of plaque vulnerability and rupture: JACC focus seminar Part 1/3. *J Am Coll Cardiol*. 2021;78(12):1257-1265.
35. Xing L, Yamamoto E, Sugiyama T, et al. EROSION study (effective anti-thrombotic therapy without stenting: intravascular optical coherence tomography-based management in plaque erosion)—a 1-year follow-up report. *Circ Cardiovasc Interv*. 2017;10(12):e005860.
36. Jia H, Dai J, He L, et al. EROSION III: a multicenter RCT of OCT-guided reperfusion in STEMI with early infarct artery patency. *JACC Cardiovasc Interv*. 2022;15(8):846-856.
37. Prati F, Romagnoli E, Gatto L, et al. Relationship between coronary plaque morphology of the left anterior descending artery and 12 months clinical outcome: the CLIMA study. *Eur Heart J*. 2020;41(3):383-391.
38. Kedhi E, Berta B, Roleder T, et al. Thin-cap fibroatheroma predicts clinical events in diabetic patients with normal fractional flow reserve: the COMBINE OCT-FFR trial. *Eur Heart J*. 2021;42(45):4671-4679.
39. Muller J, Madder R. OCT-NIRS imaging for detection of coronary plaque structure and vulnerability. *Front Cardiovasc Med*. 2020;7:90.
40. Goldstein JA, Maini B, Dixon SR, et al. Detection of lipid-core plaques by intracoronary near-infrared spectroscopy identifies high risk of periprocedural myocardial infarction. *Circ Cardiovasc Interv*. 2011;4(5):429-437.
41. Madder RD, Smith JL, Dixon SR, Goldstein JA. Composition of target lesions by near-infrared spectroscopy in patients with acute coronary syndrome versus stable angina. *Circ Cardiovasc Interv*. 2012;5(1):55-61.
42. Kini AS, Baber U, Kovacic JC, et al. Changes in plaque lipid content after short-term intensive versus standard statin therapy: the YELLOW trial (reduction in yellow plaque by aggressive lipid-lowering therapy). *J Am Coll Cardiol*. 2013;62(1):21-29.
43. Oemrawsingh RM, Cheng JM, Garcia-Garcia HM, et al. Near-infrared spectroscopy predicts cardiovascular outcome in patients with coronary artery disease. *J Am Coll Cardiol*. 2014;64(23):2510-2518.
44. Uchida Y, Uchida Y, Kawai S, et al. Detection of vulnerable coronary plaques by color fluorescent angioscopy. *JACC Cardiovasc Imaging*. 2010;3(4):398-408.
45. Takano M, Jang IK, Inami S, et al. In vivo comparison of optical coherence tomography and angioscopy for the evaluation of coronary plaque characteristics. *Am J Cardiol*. 2008;101(4):471-476.
46. Uchida Y, Nakamura F, Tomaru T, et al. Prediction of acute coronary syndromes by percutaneous coronary angioscopy in patients with stable angina. *Am Heart J*. 1995;130(2):195-203.

47. Bourantas CV, Jaffer FA, Gijsen FJ, et al. Hybrid intravascular imaging: recent advances, technical considerations, and current applications in the study of plaque pathophysiology. *Eur Heart J.* 2017;38(6):400-412.
48. Khraishah H, Jaffer FA. Intravascular molecular imaging: near-infrared fluorescence as a new Frontier. *Front Cardiovasc Med.* 2020;7:587100.
49. Bec J, Vela D, Phipps JE, et al. Label-free visualization and quantification of biochemical markers of atherosclerotic plaque progression using intravascular fluorescence lifetime. *JACC Cardiovasc Imaging.* 2021;14(9):1832-1842.
50. Kim S, Nam HS, Lee MW, et al. Comprehensive assessment of high-risk plaques by dual-modal imaging catheter in coronary artery. *JACC Basic Transl Sci.* 2021;6(12):948-960.
51. Ridker PM, Everett BM, Thuren T, et al. Antiinflammatory therapy with canakinumab for atherosclerotic disease. *N Engl J Med.* 2017;377:1119-1131.
52. Tardif JC, Kouz S, Waters DD, et al. Efficacy and safety of low-dose colchicine after myocardial infarction. *N Engl J Med.* 2019;381(26):2497-2505.
53. Guedeney P, Claessen BE, Kalkman DN, et al. Residual inflammatory risk in patients with low LDL cholesterol levels undergoing percutaneous coronary intervention. *J Am Coll Cardiol.* 2019;73(19):2401-2409.
54. Kalkman DN, Aquino M, Claessen BE, et al. Residual inflammatory risk and the impact on clinical outcomes in patients after percutaneous coronary interventions. *Eur Heart J.* 2018;39(46):4101-4108.
55. Ridker PM, Bhatt DL, Pradhan AD, et al. Inflammation and cholesterol as predictors of cardiovascular events among patients receiving statin therapy: a collaborative analysis of three randomised trials. *Lancet.* 2023;401(10384):1293-1301.
56. Stamatelopoulos K, Mueller-Hennessen M, Georgiopoulos G, et al. Cathepsin S levels and survival among patients with non-ST-segment elevation acute coronary syndromes. *J Am Coll Cardiol.* 2022;80(10):998-1010.
57. Bozhko D, Osborn EA, Rosenthal A, et al. Quantitative intravascular biological fluorescence-ultrasound imaging of coronary and peripheral arteries in vivo. *Eur Heart J Cardiovasc Imaging.* 2017;18(11):1253-1261.
58. Kellnberger S, Wissmeyer G, Albaghdadi M, et al. Intravascular molecular-structural imaging with a miniaturized integrated near-infrared fluorescence and ultrasound catheter. *J Biophotonics.* 2021;14(10):e202100048.
59. Yoo H, Kim JW, Shishkov M, et al. Intra-arterial catheter for simultaneous microstructural and molecular imaging in vivo. *Nat Med.* 2011;17(12):1680-1684.
60. Albaghdadi MS, Ikegami R, Kassab MB, et al. Near-infrared autofluorescence in atherosclerosis associates with ceroid and is generated by oxidized lipid-induced oxidative stress. *Arterioscler Thromb Vasc Biol.* 2021;41(7):e385-e398.
61. Htun NM, Chen YC, Lim B, et al. Near-infrared autofluorescence induced by intraplaque hemorrhage and heme degradation as marker for high-risk atherosclerotic plaques. *Nat Commun.* 2017;8(1):75.
62. Kunio M, Gardecki JA, Watanabe K, et al. Histopathological correlation of near infrared autofluorescence in human cadaver coronary arteries. *Atherosclerosis.* 2022;344:31-39.
63. Ughi GJ, Wang H, Gerbaud E, et al. Clinical characterization of coronary atherosclerosis with dual-modality OCT and near-infrared autofluorescence imaging. *JACC Cardiovasc Imaging.* 2016;9(11):1304-1314.
64. Verjans JW, Osborn EA, Ughi GJ, et al. Targeted near-infrared fluorescence imaging of atherosclerosis: clinical and intracoronary evaluation of indocyanine green. *JACC Cardiovasc Imaging.* 2016;9:1087 1095.
65. Vinegoni C, Botnaru I, Aikawa E, et al. Indocyanine green enables near-infrared fluorescence imaging of lipid-rich, inflamed atherosclerotic plaques. *Sci Transl Med.* 2011;3(84):84ra45.
66. Writing Committee M, Lawton JS, Tamis-Holland JE, et al. 2021 ACC/AHA/SCAI guideline for coronary artery revascularization: a report of the American College of Cardiology/American Heart Association Joint Committee on clinical practice guidelines. *J Am Coll Cardiol.* 2022;79:e21-e129.
67. van Veelen A, van der Sangen NMR, Delewi R, Beijk MAM, Henriques JPS, Claessen BEPM. Detection of vulnerable coronary plaques using invasive and non-invasive imaging modalities. *J Clin Med.* 2022;11(5):1361.
68. Bentzon JF, Otsuka F, Virmani R, Falk E. Mechanisms of plaque formation and rupture. *Circ Res.* 2014;114(12):1852-1866.

Coronary Hemodynamics: Pressure and Flow

Morton J. Kern and Arnold H. Seto

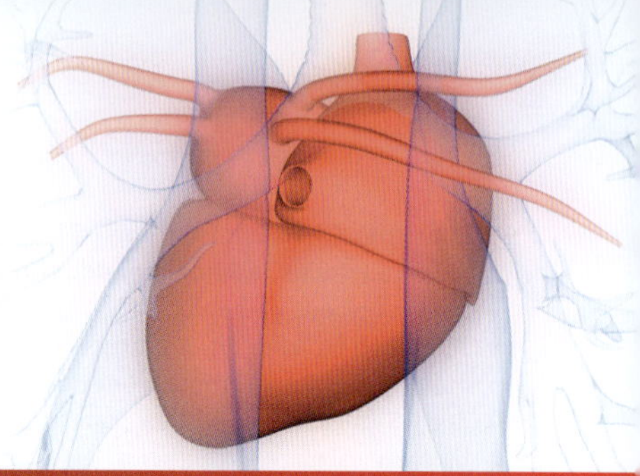

Coronary physiologic lesion assessment in the catheterization (cath) lab is required to overcome the inability of anatomy (either angiographic or intravascular ultrasound imaging) to accurately predict the ischemic potential of a coronary luminal narrowing. Measurements of coronary pressure and flow in the cath lab are now used in daily clinical practice and associated with improved clinical outcomes over angiographic decision making alone.

The rationale for using translesional coronary physiologic assessment is twofold[1]: for narrowings of an intermediate nature, coronary angiography cannot demonstrate the clinical significance of lesions (**Fig. 12.1**) that for revascularization decisions by either percutaneous coronary intervention (PCI) or coronary artery bypass graft (CABG) surgery, objective data of ischemia are required but may not be available based on clinical information or from noninvasive testing. **Table 12.1** lists the indices of coronary pressure and flow measurements.

CORONARY BLOOD FLOW AND RESISTANCE

As in any vascular bed, blood flow to the myocardium depends on the coronary artery driving (aortic) pressure and the resistance produced by the serial vascular components. Coronary vascular resistance, in turn, is regulated by several inter-related control mechanisms that include myocardial metabolism (metabolic control), endothelial (and other humoral) control, autoregulation, myogenic control, extravascular compressive forces, and neural control. These control mechanisms may be impaired in diseased states, thereby contributing to the development of myocardial ischemia.

Coronary arterial resistance (R, pressure/flow) is the summed resistances of the epicardial coronary conductance (R1), precapillary arteriolar (R2), and intramyocardial capillary (R3) resistance circuits (**Fig. 12.2**). Microvascular and macrovascular functions in coronary artery disease (CAD) are depicted in **Fig. 12.3**. Normal epicardial coronary arteries in humans typically taper gradually from the base of the heart to the apex. The epicardial vessels are >400 µm (R1) and do not offer significant resistance to blood flow in their normal nondiseased state. Epicardial vessel resistance (R1) is trivial until atherosclerotic obstructions develop. Coronary epicardial resistance would manifest as a pressure drop along the length of the epicardial arteries.[1]

Precapillary arterioles (R2) are small (100-400 µm in size) resistive vessels connecting epicardial arteries to myocardial capillaries and are the main controllers of coronary blood flow. Precapillary

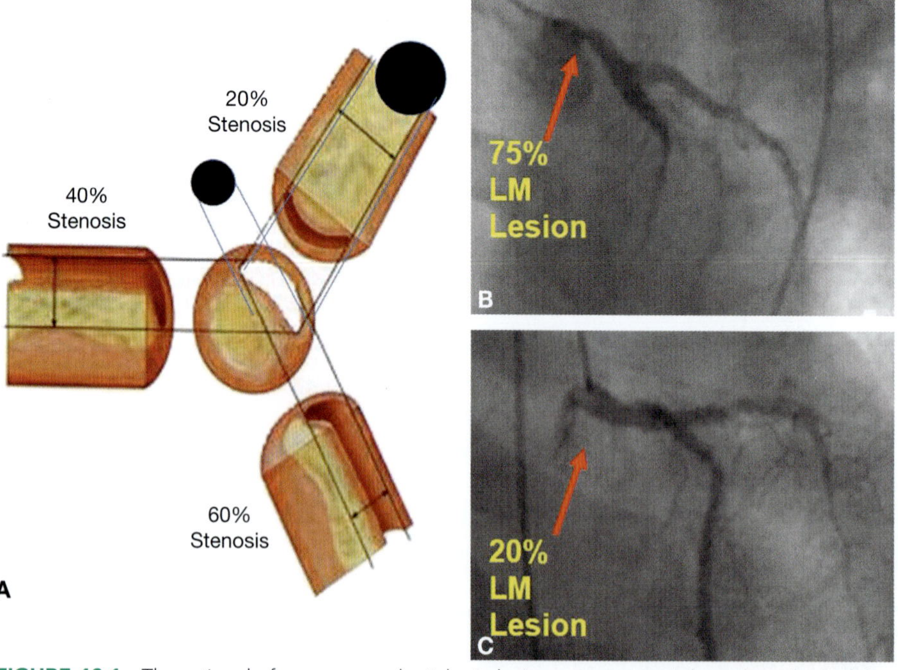

FIGURE 12.1 The rationale for coronary physiologic lesion assessment is based on the inability of the angiogram to accurately estimate stenosis severity. A true 3D depiction of any angiographic lumen requires multiple views. 2D stenosis measurements poor predictors of translesional pressure loss and ischemia. Viewed from different radiographic projections, an eccentric lumen produces an image with a high degree of uncertainty related to true lumen size. The same lesion may appear significantly different in one radiographic view compared to an orthogonal view. (B, left main [LM] in left anterior oblique cranial view. C, right anterior oblique caudal view).

TABLE 12.1 Indices of Coronary Pressure and Flow Measurements

BSR	$(P_{aorta} - P_{distal})$/APV (basal condition)
HSR	$(P_{aorta} - P_{distal})$/APV (during hyperemia)
P_d/P_a, distal coronary/aortic pressure ratio	mean P_{distal}/mean P_{aorta} (basal condition)
FFR	mean P_{distal}/mean P_{aorta} (during hyperemia)
NHPRs, iFR, dPR, dFR, RFR, Pd/Pa	mean P_{distal}/mean P_{aorta} (during diastole)
CFR	$APV_{hyperemia}/APV_{basal}$
HM	$P_d/APV_{hyperemia}$
IMR	$P_d \times T_{mn\ hyperemia}$

APV, average peak flow velocity; BSR, basal stenosis resistance index; CFR, coronary flow reserve; FFR, fractional flow reserve; HSR, hyperemic stenosis resistance index; HMR, hyperemic myocardial resistance; iFR, instantaneous wave-free ratio; IMR, index of microcirculatory resistance; NHPR, , nonhyperemic pressure ratio; P_{aorta}, aortic pressure; P_{distal}, distal coronary pressure; T_{mn}, mean transit time.

arterioles autoregulate the perfusion pressure at their origin within a finite pressure range.

The microcirculatory resistance (R3) consists of a dense network of capillaries (<100 mc) perfusing each myocyte adjacent to a capillary. Several conditions, such as left-ventricular (LV) hypertrophy, myocardial ischemia, or diabetes, can impair the microcirculatory resistance (R3) and blunt the normal increases in coronary flow in response to demand or pharmacologic agents. Increased R3 resistance may increase resting blood flow, resulting in reduced coronary flow reserve (CFR, the hyperemic/basal flow ratio).[2]

The invasive physiologic metrics used to measure the functions include fractional flow reserve (FFR) and nonhyperemic pressure ratio (NHPR) for the macrocirculatory responses and the index of microvascular resistance (IMR) and CFR (coronary vasodilator reserve [CVR]) spanning both macrocirculation and microcirculation.[2]

Pressure Loss Across a Stenosis

As blood traverses a diseased arterial segment, turbulence, friction, and separation of laminar flow cause energy loss, resulting in

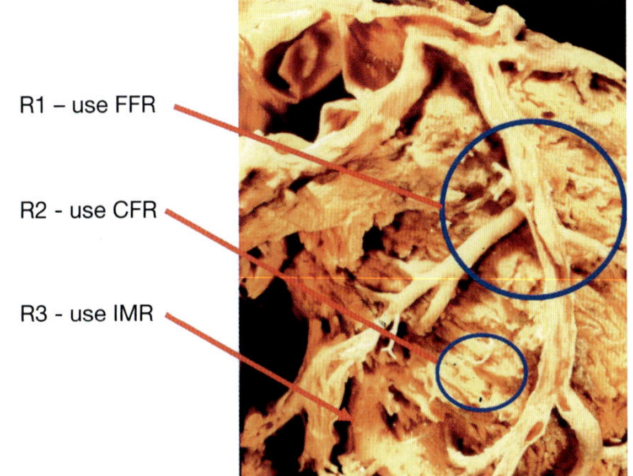

FIGURE 12.2 Specimen of the epicardial coronary artery showing severe luminal plaque and irregular surfaces of atherosclerotic disease. There are 3 sites of resistance to flow: R1 = epicardial; R2 = precapillary arterioles; and R3 = myocardial (microcirculation).

a pressure gradient (ΔP) across the stenosis. Resistance to flow is due to the morphologic features of the stenosis. Using a simplified Bernoulli formula for fluid dynamics, pressure loss across a stenosis can be estimated from blood flow as follows:

$$\Delta P = fQ + sQ^2$$

where ΔP is the pressure drop across a stenosis (mm Hg) and Q is the flow across the stenosis (mL/s). ΔP rises exponentially with reduced lumen cross-sectional area (the most commonly used measure of severity) and linearly with lesion length (**Fig. 12.4**). Additional factors (eg, A_s = stenotic segment cross-sectional area, p = blood density, μ = blood viscosity, L = stenosis length, and A_n = normal artery cross-sectional area) contributing to stenosis resistance include the shape of the entrance and exit orifices.

The first term (f) is linearly related to flow and accounts for energy losses owing to viscous friction of laminar flow through the stenosis. The second term (s) is related to flow in a quadratic manner (ie, squared) and reflects energy loss when the accelerated high-velocity flow exits the stenosis creating turbulent poststenotic distal flow, which then recovers some pressure becoming laminar flow beyond the stenosis. Because of the second term, the increases in the pressure-flow relationship are curvilinear. As a consequence, for a given stenosis with potentially several variables (ie, area and size of reference normal vessel), there may be a family of pressure-flow relationships reflecting the ischemic potential of the stenosis (**Fig. 12.5**).

By using aortic pressure obtained through the guide catheter and distal coronary pressure from the pressure sensor guidewire, one can measure both NHPR and hyperemic pressure ratios (**Figs. 12.6** and **12.7**).

Fractional Flow Reserve

While CFR was failed to define an angiographic stenosis because of the unknown presence of microvascular disease in patients with epicardial narrowings, Pijls et al and de Bruyne et al[3,4] found a pressure-only method to an accurate estimate of the percentage of normal coronary blood flow expected to go through a stenotic artery using the ratio of the poststenotic pressure to aortic pressure ratio during minimal and fixed resistance (ie, maximal hyperemia), called the FFR (**Fig. 12.6**).

FFR can be subdivided into three components describing the flow contributions by the coronary artery (FFR_{cor}), the myocardium (FFR_{myo}), and the collateral supply. FFR of the coronary artery is thus: $FFR_{cor} = FFR_{myo} - FFR_{coll}$. The following equations are used to calculate the FFR of a coronary artery and its dependent myocardium:

$$(FFR_{myo}) = 1 - \Delta P/P_a - P_V = (P_d - P_V)/(P_a - P_V)$$
$$(FFR_{cor}) = 1 - \Delta P/(P_a - P_W) = (P_d - P_W)/(P_a - P_W)$$
$$(FFR_{coll}) = FFR_{myo} - FFR_{cor}$$

where P_a is mean aortic pressure; P_d is mean distal coronary pressure; ΔP is mean translesional pressure gradient; P_v is mean right atrial pressure; and P_w is mean coronary wedge pressure or distal coronary pressure during balloon occlusion.[4] Because FFR_{cor} uses P_w, it can be calculated only during balloon coronary angioplasty. For daily clinical practice, FFR can be easily calculated by a simplified ratio of pressures assuming P_v is negligible relative to P_a and expressed as:

$$FFR \approx P_d/P_a$$

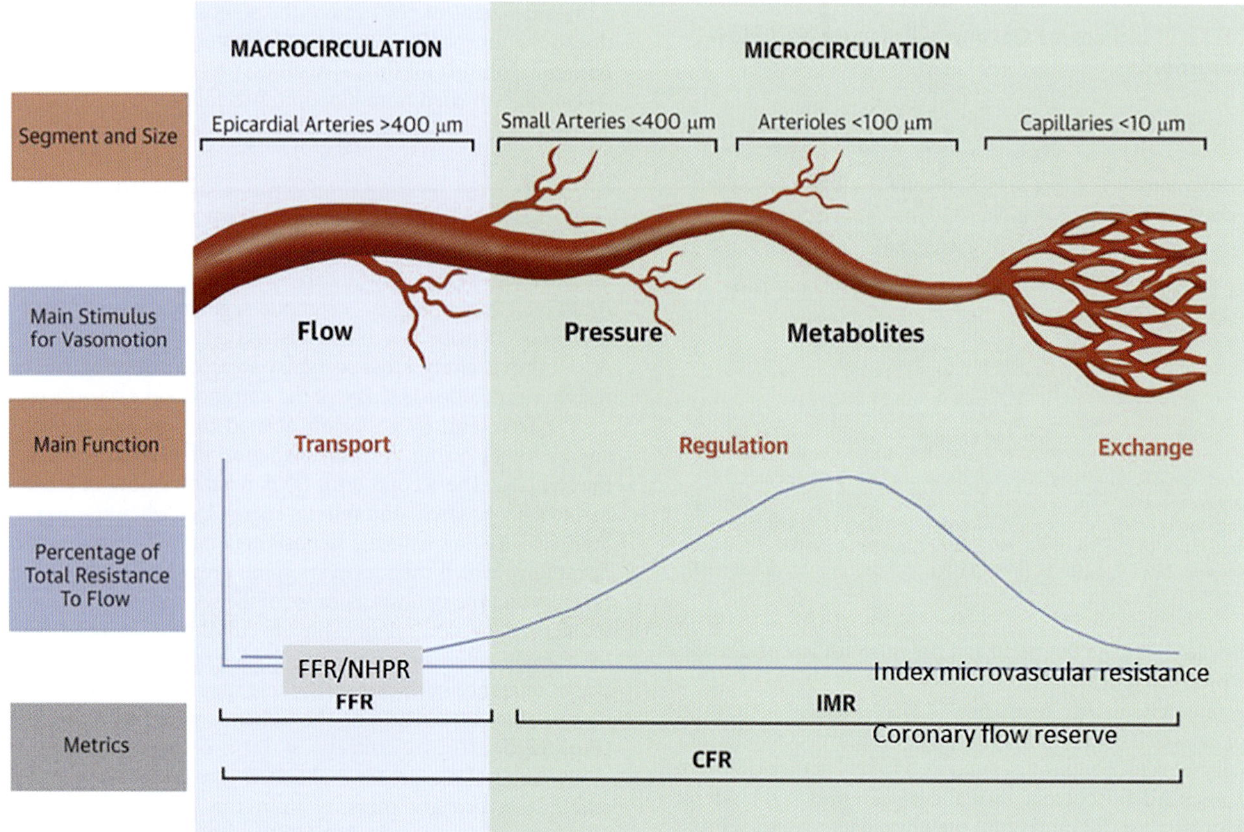

FIGURE 12.3 The macrovascular and microvascular coronary circulation are divided by size and function. Macrovascular disease involves epicardial arteries greater than 400 μm. The microcirculation is divided into small arteries 400 to 100 μm, arterioles of approximately 100 μm, and capillaries <10 μm. Each size artery is responsible for nutrient transport, flow regulation, and exchange oxygen and nutrients to the myocardium. Flow resistance increases dramatically across the arterial circuit to the capillaries. The invasive physiologic metrics used to measure the functions include FFR and nonhyperemic pressure ratio (NHPR) for the macrocirculatory responses and the index of microvascular resistance (IMR) and coronary flow reserve (CVR) spanning both macrocirculation and microcirculation. (From de Bruyne B, Oldroyd KG, Pijls NHJ. Microvascular (Dys)Function and clinical outcome in stable coronary disease. *J Am Coll Cardiol.* 2016;67(10):1170-1172. doi:10.1016/j.jacc.2015.11.066)

The normal value for FFR is unequivocally 1 for each patient, coronary artery, myocardial distribution, and microcirculatory status. An FFR value of <0.75 in patients with stable angina is strongly related to provocable myocardial ischemia using multiple stress testing methods. Because it is independent of hemodynamic and loading conditions, the FFR is a more epicardial lesion-specific measurement compared with CFR or resting trans-stenotic pressure gradients. FFR reflects both antegrade and collateral perfusion. Because it is calculated only at peak hyperemia, it excludes the microcirculatory resistance from the computation. FFR is largely independent of basal flow, driving pressure, heart rate, systemic blood pressure, or status of the microcirculation.

FFR is strongly related to provocable myocardial ischemia using different clinical stress testing modalities in patients with stable angina as the comparative standard. The nonischemic threshold value for FFR used in most recent clinical outcome studies is >0.80 for deferral of PCI. Even in patients with an abnormal microcirculation, a normal FFR indicates the epicardial conduit resistance (ie, a stenosis) is not a major contributing factor to perfusion impairment, and that stenting would not restore normal perfusion.

Nonhyperemic Pressure Ratios

Adenosine-free or nonhyperemic, resting pressure ratios were developed as alternative to hyperemic pressure ratios (FFR, contrast FFR) and are clinically noninferior to FFR in large multicenter trials. The first NHPR developed was the instantaneous wave-free ratio (iFR), a resting translesional pressure ratio taken during a specific diastolic interval in which the natural wave reflections in the cardiovascular system are quiescent. During this wave-free period, microvascular resistance is constant (but not minimal), and therefore, meeting one condition of FFR without inducing hyperemia (ie, need for adenosine).[5] All NHPRs use the ratio of distal coronary pressure and aortic pressure but differ in the portion of the diastolic period of the cardiac cycle that is measured (ie, dPR, DFR, relative CFR, Pd/Pa), and all have similar threshold values and are considered as a group with class action (**Figs. 12.8** and **12.9**).

In the Adenosine Vasodilator Independent Stenosis Evaluation (ADVISE) study, 157 stenoses were assessed with iFR and FFR to produce an 80% correspondence. The RESOLVE study[6] compared the diagnostic accuracy of the iFR and resting coronary artery pressure with the aortic pressure ratio Pd/Pa with respect to the FFR in a core laboratory. The iFR, Pd/Pa, and FFR were measured in 1768 patients from 15 clinical sites. The core lab analyzed the data, and thresholds corresponding to 90% accuracy in predicting ischemic versus nonischemic FFR were then identified. In 1974 lesions, the optimal iFR to predict an FFR <0.8 was 0.92 with an accuracy of 80%. For the resting Pd/Pa ratio, the cut point was 0.92 with an overall accuracy of 92% with no significant differences between iFR and Pd/Pa. Both measures have 90% accuracy to predict positive or negative FFR in 65% and 48% of lesions, respectively. These data suggest that resting indices of lesion severity demonstrated an

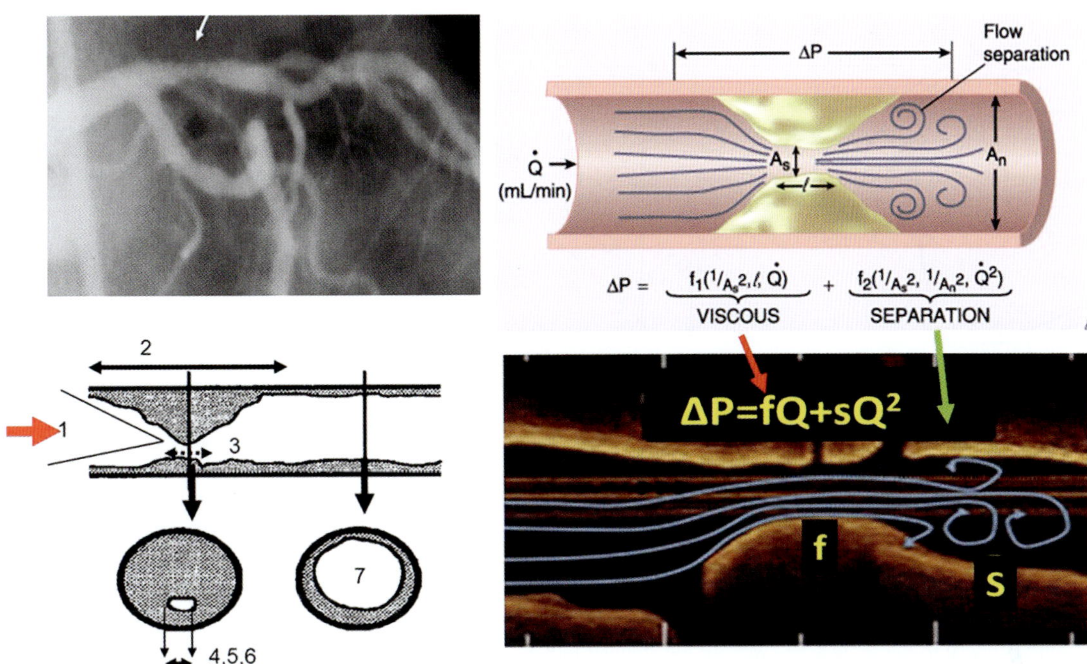

FIGURE 12.4 Determinants of pressure loss across a coronary stenosis. Top left, frame from the coronary angiogram. The 2D image cannot predict the pressure loss. Bottom left, there are at least 6 morphological factors that produce pressure loss across a stenosis, most of which cannot be measured from the angiogram. (1) Entrance angle, (2) length of disease, (3) length of lesion, (4-6) type of lesion (eccentric, concentric, irregular), and (7) reference vessel size. Top right, diagram of components responsible for the change in pressure across the stenosis. There are two major factors; the viscous friction coefficient and the separation coefficient, each of these are related to area stenosis, length of stenosis, but the separation coefficient also is impacted by the area of the normal reference vessel. Flow is linearly related to viscous friction and in an exponential fashion to the separation coefficient. Bottom right, an optical coherence tomography cross section showing the flow pattern of convergence and turbulence across the stenosis. The impact of the frictional coefficient occurs principally at the lesion, whereas separation coefficient results in energy loss principally in the poststenotic area.

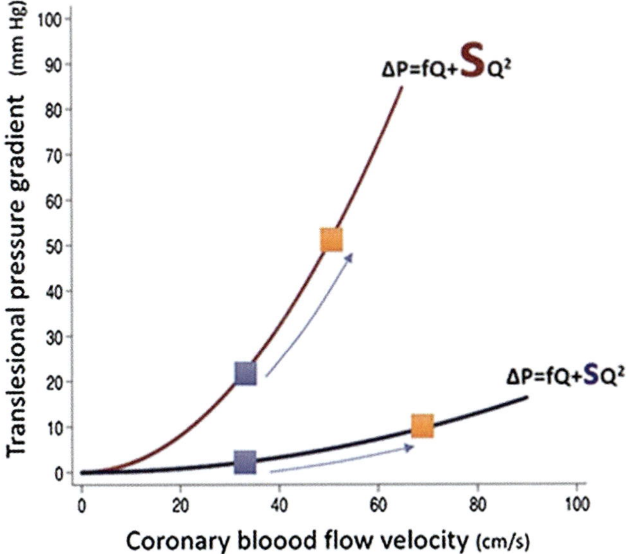

FIGURE 12.5 Based on the relationship between pressure and flow across a stenosis, the coronary pressure gradient versus flow velocity quadratic curves can be constructed. In this illustration, the top curve would be associated with ischemia having significant pressure loss for a small increase in flow compared to the lower curve with a small pressure loss for a substantial increase in flow. The coefficient of separation, S, in the top curve suggests an important focal stenosis compared to the bottom curve.

overall accuracy with FFR of about 80%, which can be improved to 90% in a subset of lesions.

The reproducibility of NHPRs depends on a stable resting coronary blood flow. Measurements obtained shortly after saline flushing, contrast, or nitroglycerin (NTG) administration may be artifactually lowered due to residual hyperemia. Other factors including drift, guide catheter dampening, and artifacts affect both NHPR and FFR. Advantages and limitations of hyperemic and NHPRs in the cath laboratory are summarized in **Table 12.2**.

Technique of Angioplasty Sensor-Guidewire Use

After diagnostic angiography, the sensor pressure guidewire is set to atmospheric pressure on the cath table. It is then passed through the guide catheter to the central aortic position, and the two pressure signals are matched. Heparin (60 U/kg) is given before inserting the guidewire. Intracoronary (IC) NTG (100-200 µg) is given to vasodilate and block vasoconstriction of the artery. NTG has no effect on hemodynamic measurements unless the stenosis is vasoconstricted.

After the sensor wire is passed beyond the lesion, baseline aortic and guidewire pressures are recorded, continuously recording both guide catheter and sensor-wire pressures. NHPR are acquired in duplicate at rest followed by FFR, measured during adenosine-induced hyperemia at the lowest Pd/Pa.

Coronary Hyperemia for FFR (Table 12.3)

Lesion assessment by FFR requires measurements during maximal hyperemia. At maximal hyperemia, autoregulation is abolished, and microvascular resistance is fixed and minimal. Under these conditions, coronary blood flow is directly related to coronary pressure.

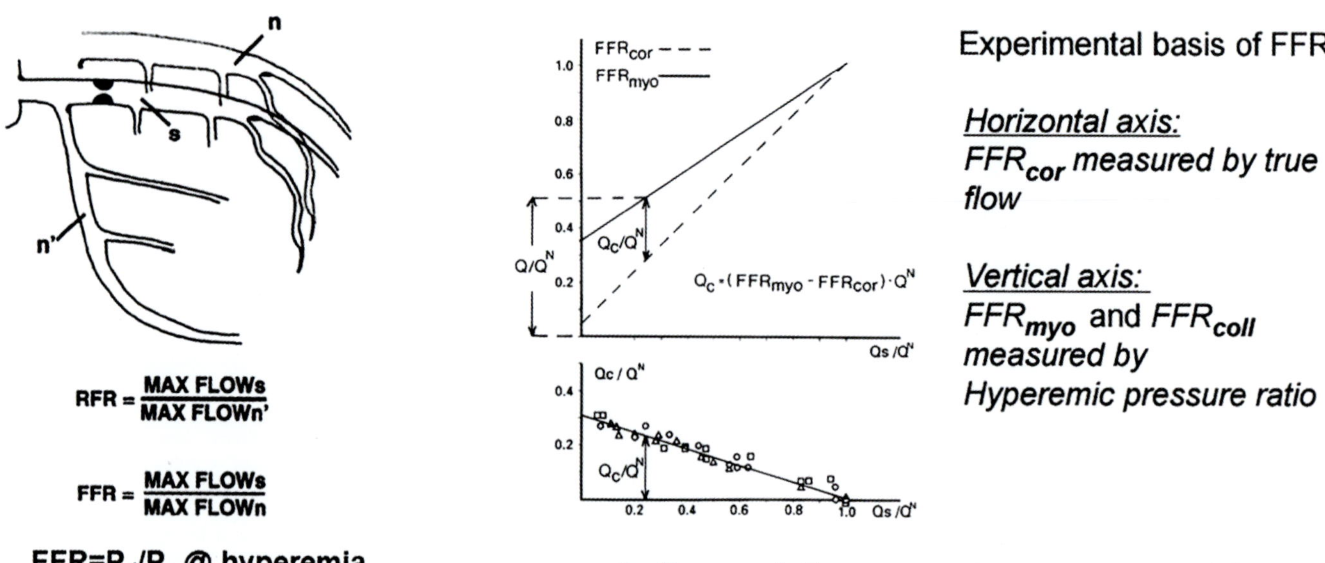

FIGURE 12.6 Concept behind fractional flow reserve (FFR). As depicted in the first human study of FFR from 1994, 67 FFR equals the ratio of maximal flow in a stenotic artery (s) to the same artery without the stenosis (n0). Relative coronary flow reserve (CFR) (RFR) equals the ratio of maximum flow in the stenotic artery to a neighboring normal artery (n). For isolated coronary artery stenosis, RFR equals FFR when normalized for distal myocardial mass. (From De Bruyne B, Baudhuin T, Melin JA, et al. Coronary flow reserve calculated from pressure measurements in humans. Validation with positron emission tomography. *Circulation*. 1994;89:1013-1022; with permission. From Johnson NP, Kirkeeide RL, Gould KL. History and development of coronary flow reserve and fractional flow reserve for clinical applications. *Intervent Cardiol Clin*. 2015;4:397-410, with permission from Elsevier.)

Adenosine, a potent short-acting hyperemic stimulus, is the most widely used hyperemic agent. Adenosine is benign in the appropriate dosages (50-100 µg in the right coronary artery (RCA) and 100-200 µg in the left coronary artery or infused intravenously at 140 µg/kg/min). Intravenous (IV) and IC adenosine produce equivalent hyperemia. **Table 12.4** lists the characteristics of pharmacologic hyperemia-inducing agents that can be used in coronary flow studies. IC nitroprusside (50 and 100-µg bolus) produces nearly identical results to IV and IC adenosine.

Pitfalls of measuring FFR and NHPR are listed in **Table 12.4**.

CORONARY FLOW RESERVE

CVR, also known as CFR, is the ratio of maximal hyperemic to resting coronary flow or flow velocity and describes the ability of the coronary vascular bed to increase flow in response to increased myocardial oxygen demand from mechanical (eg, exercise) or

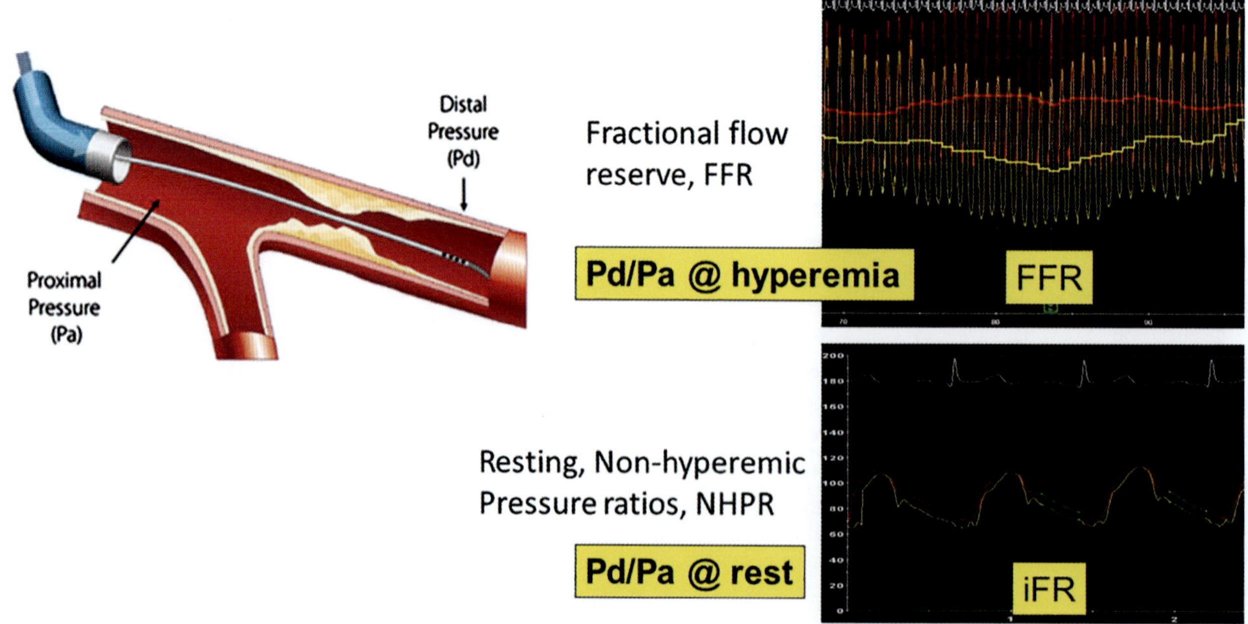

FIGURE 12.7 Invasive translesional pressure measurements obtained by fractional flow reserve (FFR) (top) and Pd/Pa (bottom). NHPR, nonhyperemic pressure ratio; Pa, aortic pressure is measured through the guide catheter. Pd, distal pressure in the coronary is measured by the pressure sensor guidewire.

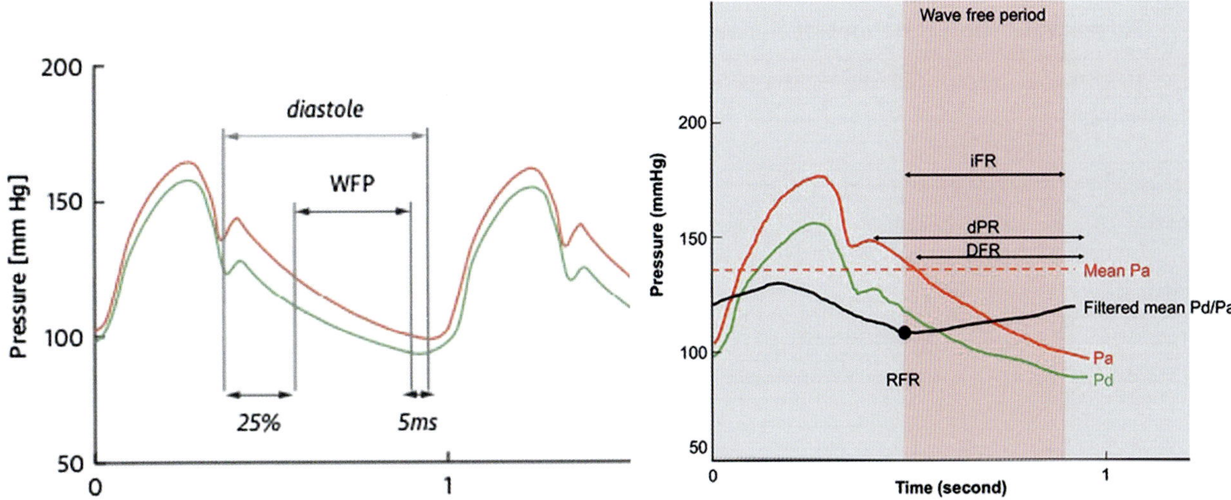

FIGURE 12.8 Calculations of nonhyperemic pressure ratios (NHPRs). (Left panel) Instantaneous wave-free ratio (iFR, Philips Medical) is defined as average Pd/Pa during the wave-free period (WFP). The WFP begins 25% of the way into diastole and ends 5 ms before the end of diastole. Right panel, There are several other NHPRs. The diastolic pressure ratio (dPR, Opsens, Inc) is defined as average P_d/P_a during entire diastole. The diastolic hyperemia-free ratio (DFR, Boston Scientific) is defined as average P_d/P_a during the diastolic period when the P_a is less than mean P_a with a negative slope. The resting full-cycle ratio (relative coronary flow reserve RFR], Abbott Vascular) is defined as the lowest filtered mean P_d/P_a during the entire cardiac cycle. (Modified from Kogame N, Ono M, Kawashima H, et al. The impact of coronary physiology on contemporary clinical decision making. *JACC Cardiovasc Interv*. 2020;13:1617-1638.)

pharmacologic (eg, adenosine) stimuli. CFR was initially thought to predict the ischemic potential of a stenosis. Gould et al[3] showed that increasing coronary stenosis severity was associated with a predictable decline in CFR, beginning to decline with a 60% diameter narrowing in dog experiments. It was thus initially thought that one could identify stenoses of physiologic importance by angiographic stenoses of >50%. Unfortunately, this observation does not extend consistently to human coronary angiography (**Fig. 12.10**).

Normal coronary flow at baseline and during hyperemia has a large range, from 2x to 5x resting flow in man.[3] At diameter stenoses >80% to 90%, all available coronary reserves have been exhausted, and resting flow begins to decline (**Fig. 12.10**). CFR can be reduced due to the angiographic epicardial stenoses as well as the presence of microvascular disease in patients. CFR may be abnormal if one or both are abnormal, and for this reason, an abnormal CFR cannot be determined to be solely due to a coronary stenosis. CFR is used to assess the presence of microvascular disease in the absence of epicardial obstructions. Factors responsible for reduced CFR in the absence of epicardial stenosis are shown in **Table 12.5**.

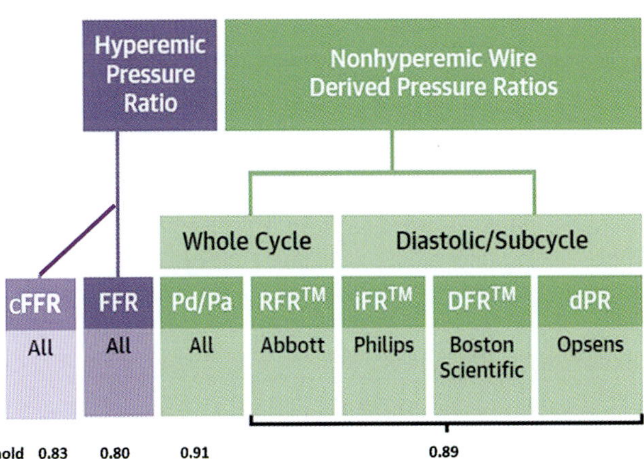

FIGURE 12.9 Translesional coronary hemodynamic indices. There are two hyperemic pressure ratios (using mean Pd/Pa at hyperemia): contrast fractional flow reserve (FFR) (cFFR is submaximal) and fractional flow reserve (FFR) (with adenosine and considered to be maximal hyperemic stimulus. There are five nonhyperemic pressure ratios; two whole cycle (Pd/Pa generic and relative coronary flow reserve [RFR] by Abbott), three diastolic subcycles (instantaneous wave-free ratio [Ifr] by Philips, DFR by Boston Scientific, and dPR by Opsens). Ischemic threshold values are displayed beneath each index. (Modified from Kogame N, Ono M, Kawashima H, et al. The impact of coronary physiology on contemporary clinical decision making. *JACC Cardiovasc Interv*. 2020;13:1617-1638.)

In adult patients with chest pain undergoing cardiac catheterization with angiographically normal vessels, the CFR averages 2.7 ± 0.64.[7] CFR values <2.0 have been associated with inducible myocardial ischemia on stress testing. Changes in heart rate, blood pressure, and contractility alter CFR by changing resting basal flow or maximal hyperemic flow or both.[4] **Fig. 12.11** demonstrates the differences among FFR, CFR, and NHPR.

Validation of FFR and NHPR

FFR values <0.75 are associated with ischemic stress testing with high sensitivity (88%), specificity (100%), positive predictive value (100%), and overall accuracy (93%). FFR values >0.80 are associated with negative ischemic results with a predictive accuracy of 95%. The initial FFR validation study[8,9] compared FFR to a panel of three different stress tests in the same patients both before and after PCI (**Fig. 12.12**.). Myocardial perfusion scintigraphy is a difficult standard for ischemia since it compares relative and not absolute myocardial flow in different coronary beds making the determination of the ischemic potential of individual lesions in patients with multivessel CAD challenging. Similarly, on stress echocardiography, severe ischemia in one region may mask the consequences of a less severe albeit hemodynamically significant lesion in another region. Single stress testing comparisons with variations in testing methods and patient cohorts have produced overlapping positive and negative FFR results (0.75-0.80). The interpretation of FFR values in this range requires clinical judgment. In contrast to noninvasive tests, FFR is a vessel- and lesion-specific index of ischemia.

TABLE 12.2 Advantages and Limitations of Hyperemic and NHPRs in the Catheterization Laboratory

FEATURE	NHPR	FFR	COMMENT
Established cutpoint	++	++	iFR compared to FFR
RCT data	++	+++	FFR has larger database in varied anatomy
Hyperemia required	-	+	Adenosine adds cost, time, reduces patient satisfaction
Signal variability	Varies with stimuli changing basal state	Varies with adenosine infusions, respiration	
Serial or tandem lesions	Less crosstalk	More crosstalk	Hyperemia magnifies interaction between individual lesions

RCT, randomized clinical trial.

TABLE 12.3 Characteristics of Pharmacologic Hyperemia-Inducing Agents for Coronary Flow Studies

DRUG	DOSE	PLATEAU (S)	HALF-LIFE (MIN)	SIDE EFFECTS	COMMENTS
Papaverine IC	15 mg LCA 10 mg RCA	30-60	2	Transient Q-T interval prolongation, torsades de pointes	Rarely used
Adenosine IV	140 µg/kg/min	60-120	1-2	Decreased blood pressure (10%-15%), chest burning	Avoid in patients with history of bronchospasm
Adenosine IC	100-200 µg LCA 50-100 µg RCA	10-15	0.5-1	Transient AV block when injected into the dominant artery	Must repeat with escalating doses to ensure that maximal hyperemia is reached
Dobutamine IV	20-40 µg/kg/min	60-120	3-5	Tachycardia, increase in blood pressure	May induce ischemia
Nitroprusside IC	0.3-0.9 µg/kg	20	1	Decreased blood pressure (20%)	
Regadenoson IV	0.4 mg	30	2-4[a]	Tachycardia	Exact length of hyperemia and ability to repeat bolus not studied in the cardiac catheterization lab for FFR

[a]Half-life is triphasic, with second phase lasting ~30 minutes and third phase lasting ~2 hours.
AV, atrioventricular; FFR, fractional flow reserve; IC, intracoronary; IV, intravenous; LCA, left coronary artery; RCA, right coronary artery.

TABLE 12.4 Pitfalls of FFR

1. **Equipment factors (FFR/NHPR):**
   - Erroneous zero, (tubing/connector leaks)
   - Faulty electric wire connection
   - Pressure signal drift, miscalibration, ECG
2. **Procedural factors**
   - Guide catheter damping
   - Incorrect sensor position
   - Inadequate hyperemia
   - Changing basal flow
3. **Physiological factors**
   - Serial lesion
   - LM/collateral myocardial bed size
   - STEMI
   - LVH?
     - LVEDP?
     - RA?

While FFR was validated against several different ischemic tests, iFR was validated against FFR and subsequently found to have a threshold value of 0.89, which correlated with FFR <0.80 and demonstrated a good diagnostic performance. iFR and FFR have similar diagnostic efficiency for detection of ischemia-inducing stenoses when tested against a third comparator[10] (**Fig. 12.13**). **Table 12.6** lists ischemic thresholds for IC physiologic measurements.

Discordance Between NHPR and Hyperemic Indices

iFR/FFR discordance occurs in 20% of cases. There are three common situations when one might expect FFR and NHPRs to be discordant: (1) conditions associated high flow (left anterior descending [LAD], large myocardial mass, and high CO) favors FFR+/NHPR−; (2) focal lesions favor FFR+/NHPR− because the separation coefficient (sQ^2) is larger in focal than in diffuse lesions; and (3) diffuse lesions favor FFR−/NHPR+ because of lower net CFR. In summary, most of the iFR−/FFR+ disparity is due to high translesional flow with high CFR, whereas the converse (iFR+/FFR−) has been seen more in diffuse coronary disease with lower CFR[11,12] (**Fig. 12.14**). The clinical significance of discordant FFR/NHPR remains under study. In the IRIS-FFR registry, Cook et al[13]

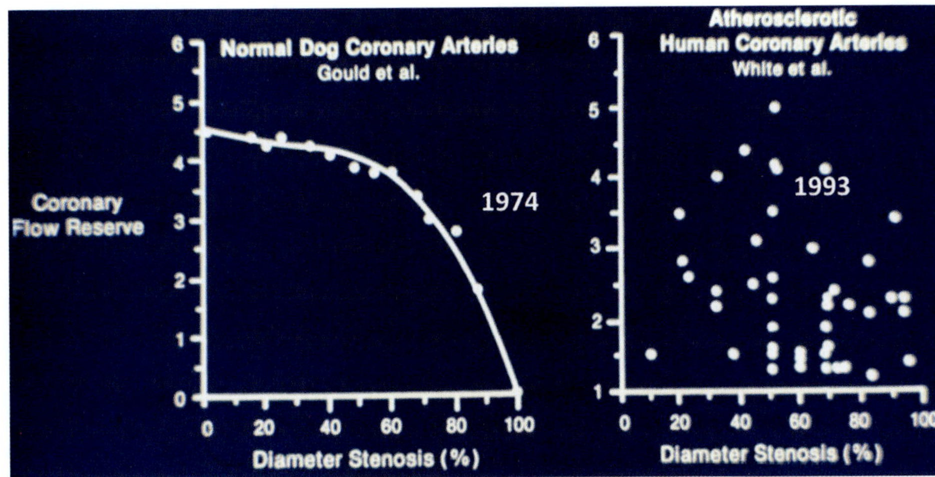

FIGURE 12.10 Left, Relationship of coronary flow reserve (CFR) to percent diameter narrowing from experimental dog model of Gould et al. CFR is preserved until percent narrowing exceeds 60%, and resting flow is not affected until narrowing exceeds 80%. Right panel, in patients, this relationship is not strong because the percent diameter stenosis is not accurate from the angiogram, and because patients have microvascular disease and thus can have an impaired CFR despite a normal coronary artery. (From Gould KL, Lipscomb K, Hamilton GW. Physiologic basis for assessing critical coronary stenosis: instantaneous flow response and regional distribution during coronary hyperemia as measures of coronary flow reserve. *Am J Cardiol.* 1974;33:87-94 and from Wilson R, White. *Am J Cardiol.* 1993;71:10D-16D.)

found that adverse clinical event rates are highest when both values are concordantly abnormal (iFR+/FFR+) with lower event rates for discordant iFR+/FFR−, iFR−/FFR+. Concordantly negative iFR−/FFR− are associated with the best outcomes for medical therapy. To provide more confidence in the decision in this setting, it is recommended to proceed in a step-wise fashion from the NHPR to cFFR and/or to adenosine FFR for a final decision on revascularization.

Clinical Outcomes of FFR and NHPR

Both FFR and NHPR can be used to determine the appropriateness of angioplasty. For example, the DEFER study randomized 325 patients scheduled for PCI into three groups and reported the 5-year outcomes.[14] If FFR was >0.75, patients were randomly assigned to the deferral group (n = 91, medical therapy for CAD) or the PCI performance group (n = 90, PCI with stents). If FFR was <0.75, PCI was performed as planned and patients were entered into the reference group (n = 144). The event-free survival was not different between the deferred and performed group (80% and 73%, respectively, P = .52), and both were significantly better than in the reference PCI group (63%, P = .03). The composite rate of cardiac death and acute myocardial infarction (MI) in the deferred, performed, and reference groups was 3.3%, 7.9%, and 15.7%, respectively (P = .21 for deferred vs performed and P = .003 for reference vs both the deferred and performed groups) (**Fig. 12.15**).

TABLE 12.5 Factors Responsible for Microvascular Disease and Reduction of Coronary Flow Reserve

Abnormal vascular reactivity
Abnormal myocardial metabolism
Abnormal sensitivity toward vasoactive substances
Coronary vasospasm
Myocardial infarction
Hypertrophy
Vasculitis syndromes
Hypertension
Diabetes
Recurrent ischemia

From Baumgart D, Haude M, Liu F, Ge J, Goerge G, Erbel R. Current concepts of coronary flow reserve for clinical decision making during cardiac catheterization. *Am Heart J.* 1998;136:136-149.

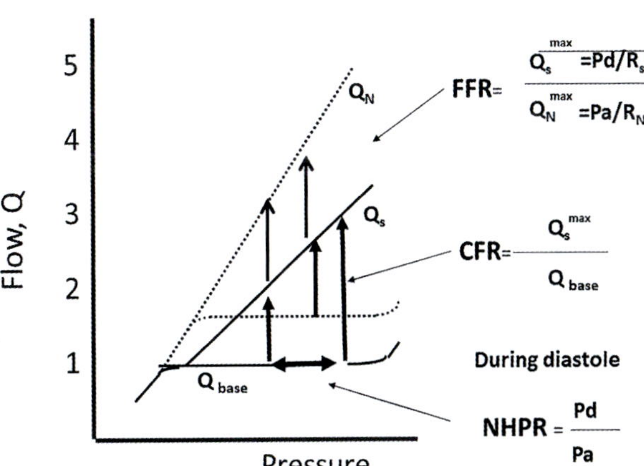

FIGURE 12.11 Comparison of fractional flow reserve (FFR), coronary flow reserve (CFR) and instantaneous wave-free ratio (iFR) nonhyperemic pressure ratio (NHPR). The Y-axis is the increase in flow from baseline value of 1. X-axis is the pressure during measurement. The diagonal line represents the line of maximal hyperemia. FFR is measured at hyperemia only and is unaffected by changes in basal flow. In contrast, CFR is the ratio of hyperemic to basal flow, and any change in either changes the CFR value. At constant basal flow, NHPR (eg, iFR, Pd/Pa) can be easily computed. Any change in basal flow will change the NHPR measurement.

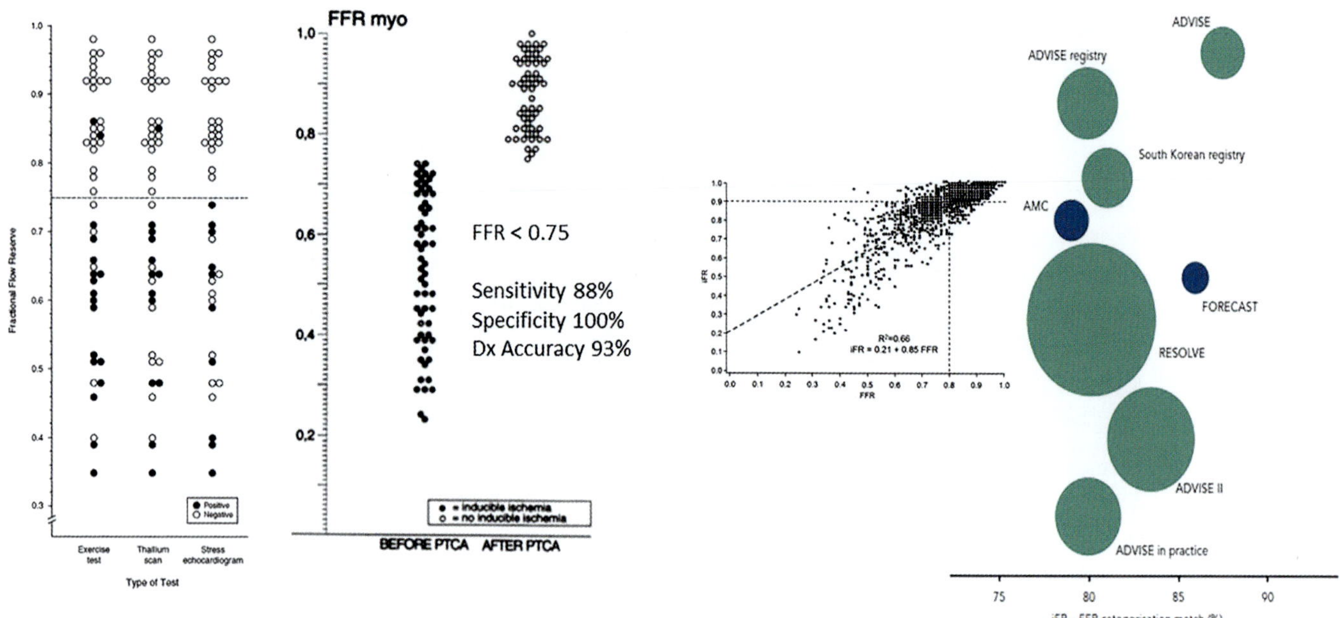

FIGURE 12.12 Left, Validation of fractional flow reserve (FFR) using three different stress tests in patients before and after percutaneous transluminal coronary angioplasty (PTCA). (Adapted with permission from Pijls NH, De Bruyne B, Peels K, et al. Measurement of fractional flow reserve to assess the functional severity of coronary-artery stenoses. *N Engl J Med.* 1996;334:1703-1708). The threshold of 0.75 was established by this study with subsequent studies using single stress tests of different kinds produced a range of the threshold value between 0.75 and 0.80. Clinical studies used 0.80 as their dichotomous cutpoint for clinical outcomes. Right, Comparisons of iFR to FFR from several studies. The size of circle represents the number of patients in the study. ADVISE, adenosine vasodilator independent stenosis evaluation; ADVISE II, adenosine vasodilator independent stenosis evaluation II; AMC, Academic Medical Center (Amsterdam); DEFINE-FLAIR, functional lesion assessment of indeterminant stenosis to guide revascularization; Dx, diagnostic; FFR, fractional flow reserve; FFR myo, myocardial fractional flow reserve; FORECAST, TCT-230 instantaneous wave-free ratio and gradient: new promising adenosine-independent alternative to fractional flow reserve; iFR, instantaneous wave-free ratio; iFR-SWEDEHEART, instantaneous wave-free ratio versus fractional flow reserve in patients with stable angina pectoris or acute coronary syndromes; PTCA, percutaneous transluminal coronary angioplasty; RESOLVE, multicenter core laboratory comparison of the instantaneous wave-free ratio and resting P d /P a with fractional flow reserve. (Adapted with permission from Jeremias A, Maehara A, Généreux P, et al. Multicenter core laboratory comparison of the instantaneous wave-free ratio and resting Pd/Pa with fractional flow reserve: the RESOLVE study. *J Am Coll Cardiol.* 2014;63:1253-1261.)

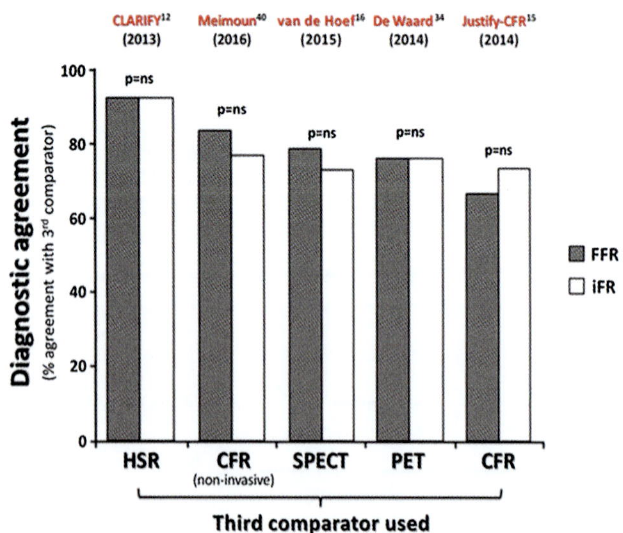

FIGURE 12.13 Comparison of the percent agreement of instantaneous wave-free ratio (iFR; white boxes) and fractional flow reserve (FFR; black boxes) to the third comparators used in single studies. CFR, coronary flow reserve; HFR, hyperemic stenosis resistance; PET, positron emission tomography; SPECT, single photon emission computerized tomography. Comparison with FFR. (From De Rosa S, Polimeni A, Petraco R, Davies JE, Indolfi C. Diagnostic performance of the instantaneous wave-free ratio: comparison with fractional flow reserve. *Circ Cardiovasc Interv.* 2018;11(1):e004613. doi:10.1161/CIRCINTERVENTIONS.116.004613)

TABLE 12.6 Ischemic Thresholds of Invasive Physiologic Indices

INDEX	NORMAL VALUE	ISCHEMIC THRESHOLD	FORMULA	COMMENTS
FFR	1.0	≤0.80	Pd/Pa, hyperemia	Standard for invasive physiologic indices
cFFR	1.0	0.83	Pd/Pa, contrast hyperemia	Avoids adenosine with use of contrast media
iFR (and NHPRs)	1.0	0.89	Pd/Pa during wave free and other diastolic cycle periods	Avoids adenosine. 80% accurate vs FFR
Resting Pd/Pa	1.0	0.92	Whole cycle Pd/Pa	Avoids adenosine. 80% accurate vs FFR

From Fearon W. Invasive coronary physiology for assessing intermediate lesions. *Circ Cardiovasc Interv.* 2015;8:e001942. doi:10.1161/CIRCINTERVENTIONS.114.001942

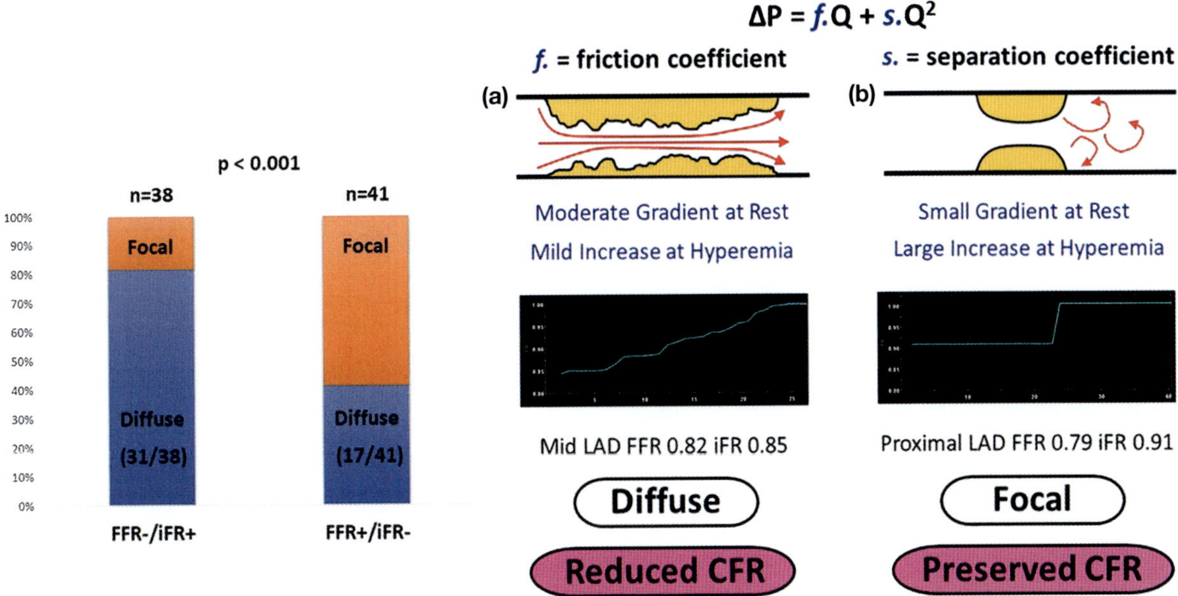

FIGURE 12.14 Disease patterns of instantaneous wave-free ratio (iFR)/fractional flow reserve (FFR) discordance. In patients with diffuse disease, the coefficient of friction contributes more to an FFR–/iFR+ discordance; however, in focal lesions, the separation coefficient plays a larger role and thus more FFR+/iFR– results. There is also an association of CFR to iFR/FFR discordance with reduced CFR more common with the FFR–/iFR+ and a preserved CFR seen more with FFR+/iFR–. (From Warisawa T, Cook CM, Howard JP, et al. Physiological pattern of disease assessed by pressure-wire pullback has an influence on fractional flow reserve/instantaneous wave-free ratio discordance. *Circ Cardiovasc Interv*. 2019;12(5):e007494.)

Multivessel Disease PCI

The foundational studies for use of FFR in multivessel disease patients are the FAME (FFR vs Angiography for Multivessel Evaluation) family of studies (**Fig. 12.16**). FAME 1 tested whether ischemia (FFR)-directed PCI was better than angiographically guided stenting of all angiographic lesions. FAME 1 found that compared to angiographically guided PCI, FFR-guided PCI demonstrated lower major adverse cardiac event (MACE) at 1, 2, and 5 years in the FAME trial. van Nunen et al[15] examined 1005 patients with multivessel CAD undergoing PCI with drug-eluting stents (DES). For the FFR-PCI group (n = 496), all lesions had FFR measurements and only those with an FFR <0.80 were stented. For the Angio-PCI group (n = 509), all lesions identified were stented. Clinical characteristics and angiographic findings were similar in both groups, with average SYNTAX score of 14.5 (indicating low-intermediate risk patients).

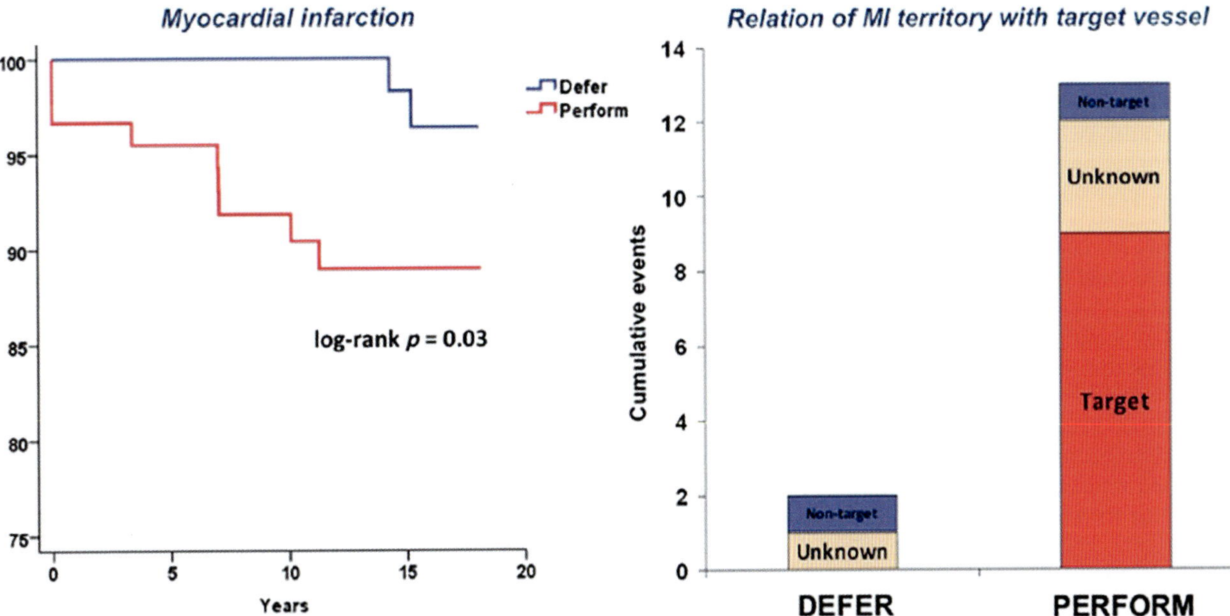

FIGURE 12.15 Results of the DEFER study at 15 years. Left, Kaplan-Meier survival curves for freedom from adverse cardiac events for 15 years follow-up for FFR+/treated, FFR–/treated, and FFR–/deferred. Right panel, Cardiac death and acute myocardial infarction rates at follow-up. (From Adjedj J, De Bruyne B, Floré V, et al. Significance of intermediate values of fractional flow reserve in patients with coronary artery disease. *Circulation*. 2016;133:502-508. doi:10.1161/CIRCULATIONAHA.115.018747)

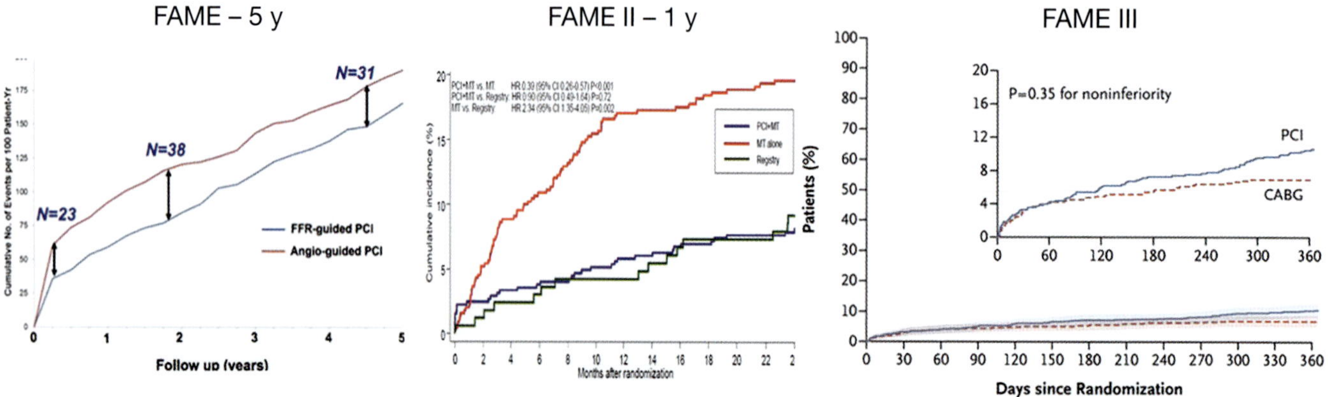

FIGURE 12.16 The three landmark studies of fractional flow reserve (FFR). Left, FAME (FFR Assessment in Multivessel coronary artery disease [CAD] Evaluation) study. The patients were randomized to the percutaneous coronary intervention (PCI) or angiographically guided treatment. The angiographic strategy had a significantly higher rate of death or myocardial infarction (MI) (12.7% vs 8.4%; *P* = .03) and a higher rate of needing or coronary artery bypass graft (CABG) or repeat PCI (9.5% vs 6.1mn%; *P* = .03). (From Zimmermann FM, Ferrara A, Johnson NP, et al. Deferral vs. performance of percutaneous coronary intervention of functionally non-significant coronary stenosis: 15-year follow-up of the DEFER trial. *Eur Heart J.* 2015;36(45):3182-3188, by permission of Oxford University Press.) Middle, The FAME II study compared optimal medical therapy (OMT) to OMT and PCI in patients with multivessel CAD and at least one lesion FFR+. The OMT group (red curve) had significantly more events than either the PCI (blue curve) or the control group (green curve, multivessel disease with FFR– and followed in the registry). FFR, fractional flow reserve. (Data from De Bruyne B, Pijls NH, Kalesan B, et al. Fractional flow reserve–guided PCI versus medical therapy in stable coronary disease. *N Engl J Med.* 2012;367:991-1001.) Right, FAME 3 study compared FFR-guided PCI versus CABG in patients with multivessel CAD. CABG had fewer events than FFR-guided PCI. In moderate and low syntax score patients, there was equipoise between PCI and CABG for outcomes. (From Fearon WF, Zimmermann FM, De Bruyne B, et al. Fractional flow reserve-guided PCI as compared with coronary bypass surgery. *N Engl J Med.* 2022;386:128-137.)

Compared to the Angio-PCI group, the FFR-PCI group used fewer stents per patient (1.9 ± 1.3 vs 2.7 ± 1.2; *P* < .001) and less contrast (272 vs 302 mL; *P* < .001) and had a lower procedure cost ($5332 vs $6007; *P* < .001) and shorter hospital stay (3.4 vs 3.7 days; *P* = .05). More importantly, the 2-year rates of mortality or MI were 13% in the Angio-PCI group compared with 8% in the FFR-PCI group (*P* = .02). Composite rates of death/nonfatal MI or revascularization were 22% and 18%, respectively (*P* = .08). For lesions deferred based on an FFR of >0.80, the rate of MI was only 0.2% and the rate of revascularization was 3.2% after 2 years.

The FFR-Guided PCI Versus Medical Therapy in Stable Coronary Disease (FAME 2) trial[16] addressed the question whether optimal medical therapy (OMT) for CAD was better than OMT with PCI in patients with multivessel CAD and who have proven ischemia by FFR.[17] A total of 1220 patients with angiographic disease in one, two, or three vessels that was suitable for PCI underwent FFR. All patients with lesions having an FFR of 0.80 or less were randomized to either PCI or medical therapy alone. A composite of all-cause mortality, nonfatal MI, or unplanned hospitalization leading to urgent revascularization during a 2-year follow-up was the primary end point. As in prior studies, patients whose lesions that had FFR values of >0.80 were entered into a registry and followed. The registry patients had a low rate of the primary end point of death (0), MI (1.8%), or urgent revascularization (2.4%) over the follow-up of 12 months, thus reproducing the findings of the pre-DES era DEFER trial. The FAME 1 and 2 trials demonstrate revascularization will not improve outcomes in patients with stenoses with nonischemic FFR.

The FAME 3 (FFR Versus Angiography for Multivessel Evaluation 3) study tested whether FFR-guided PCI would be noninferior to CABG for patients with multivessel CAD.[18] In this multicenter international trial, 1500 patients with three-vessel CAD were randomly assigned to undergo CABG or FFR-guided PCI. The 1-year incidence of the composite primary endpoint (death, MI, stroke, or repeat revascularization) was 10.6% compared with 6.9% for those having PCI compared with CABG (hazard ratio [HR], 1.5; 95% confidence interval, 1.1-2.2), not meeting the noninferiority boundaries for FFR-guided PCI (pnoninferiority = 0.35). However, the complexity of the CAD should be considered because, for the subset of patients with lower SYNTAX (Synergy Between Percutaneous Coronary Intervention with TAXUS and Cardiac Surgery) scores, FFR-guided PCI was better than CABG with respect to MACE.

Multiple large trials comparing FFR-guided PCI to angiographically guided PCI consistently demonstrate the superiority of an ischemia (FFR)-guided approach (**Fig. 12.17**).

NHPRs and Intermediate Lesion Assessment

The 2 largest randomized noninferiority trials of iFR and FFR were DEFINE-FLAIR[19] and IFR-SWEDEHEART[20] in which participants were randomized to iFR- or FFR-guided PCI or medical therapy. The DEFINE-FLAIR study was multinational trial that enrolled 2492 patients from 17 countries. IFR-SWEDEHEART enrolled 2037 patients at 15 centers in Sweden, Denmark, and Iceland. The dichotomous threshold of iFR <0.89 produced noninferior clinical outcomes when compared to FFR <0.80 (**Fig. 12.18**). At 1 year, there were no significant differences between iFR and FFR for the composite primary endpoint of all-cause mortality, MI, or revascularization. Both studies showed reduced chest discomfort and procedure times as would be expected by the administration of adenosine IV as the major methodologic difference between iFR and FFR. NHPRs are now in common use as they streamline the workflow for coronary lesion assessment by obviating the need for hyperemia.

Left Main Stenosis

Because angiographic assessment alone is often not reliable to determine the clinical importance of a left main (LM) artery narrowing, translesional physiology is a valuable tool for accurate decision making. For assessment by FFR, a number of large studies support the use of FFR >0.80 to safely defer revascularization in the LM intermediate stenosis. Modi et al summarized the LM FFR studies in **Fig. 12.19**.[21]

For iFR, Warisawa et al[22] examined 314 patients with intermediate LM stenosis. Based on an iFR threshold of 0.89, revascularization was deferred (n = 163) or instituted (n = 151). At the

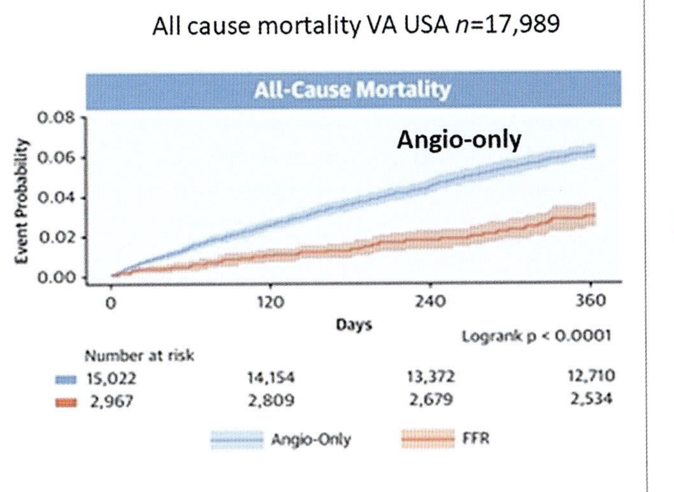

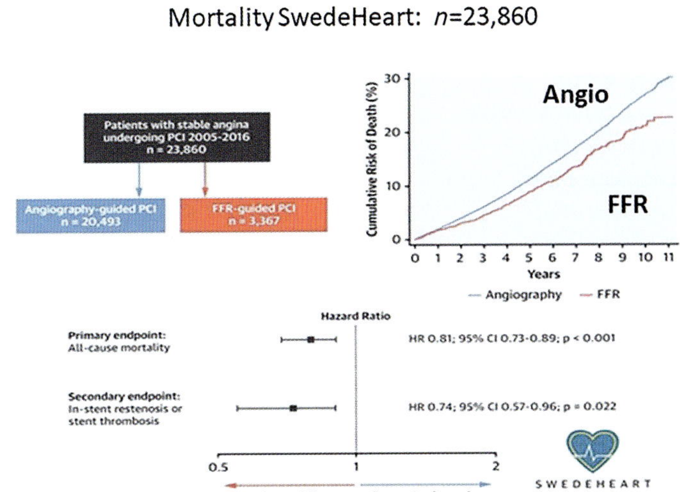

FIGURE 12.17 Fractional flow reserve (FFR)-guided percutaneous coronary intervention (PCI) compared to Angio-Guided PCI in stable ischemic heart disease. Left, the utilization of an FFR-guided revascularization strategy in patients with angiographically intermediate stenoses and stable ischemic heart disease increased from 2009 to 2017. An FFR-guided revascularization strategy is associated with significantly lower all-cause mortality at 1 year compared with an angiography (Angio)-only revascularization strategy. (From Parikh RV, Liu G, Plomondon ME, et al. Utilization and outcomes of measuring fractional flow reserve in patients with stable ischemic heart disease *J Am Coll Cardiol*. 2020;75:409-419.). Right, Data from the Swedish Coronary Angiography and Angioplasty Registry for 23,860 PCI patients with stable angina pectoris (2005 and March 2016) demonstrated that all-cause mortality and the secondary endpoints (stent thrombosis or restenosis and periprocedural complications) were reduced with the use of FFR. (From Völz S, Dworeck C, Redfors B, et al. Survival of patients with angina pectoris undergoing percutaneous coronary intervention with intracoronary pressure wire guidance. *J Am Coll Cardiol*. 2020;75:2785-2799.)

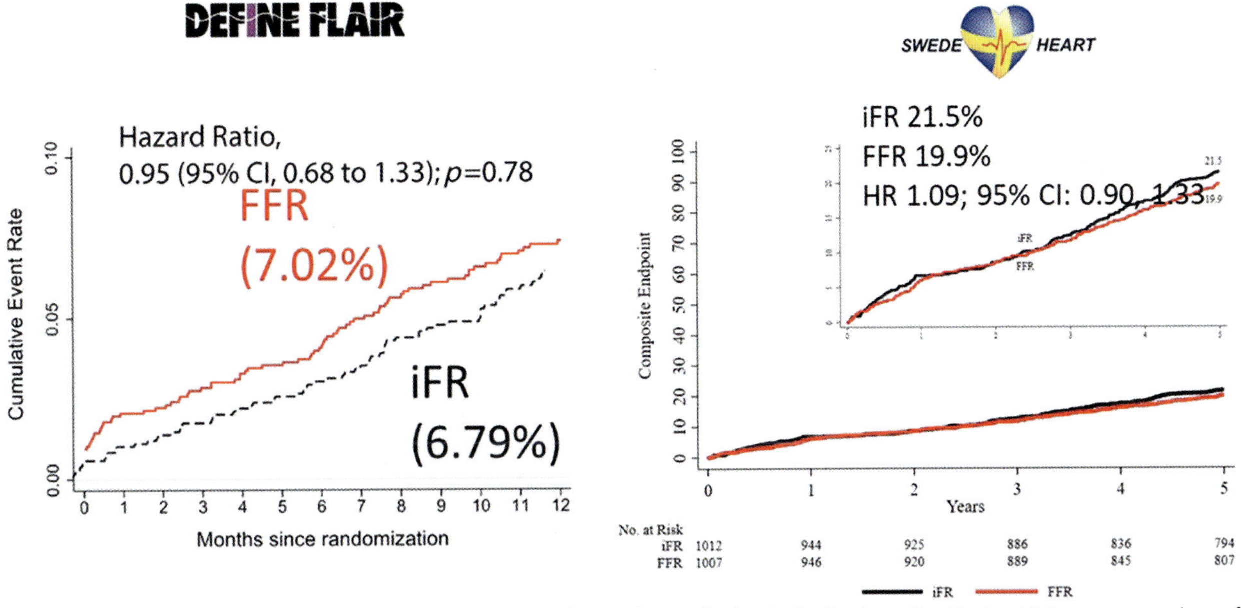

FIGURE 12.18 *Left*, DEFINE-FLAIR and *right*, SWEDEHEART randomized controlled trials. For both studies, Kaplan-Meier curves are shown for the cumulative risk of the composite of death from any cause, nonfatal myocardial infarction, or unplanned revascularization within 12 months after the index procedure. Both studies used a single cutoff of 0.89 for the threshold of treatment. (From Davies JE, Sen S, Dehbi HM, et al. Use of the instantaneous wave-free ratio or fractional flow reserve in PCI. *N Engl J Med*. 2017;376(19):1824-1834; Götberg M, Christiansen EH, Gudmundsdottir IJ, et al. Instantaneous wave-free ratio versus fractional flow reserve to guide PCI. *N Engl J Med*. 2017;376(19):1813-1823.)

30 months of follow-up, MACE occurred in 15 patients (9.2%) in the deferred group compared to 22 patients (14.6%) in the revascularized group (P = .26). There was no difference between the medical or revascularized groups. Although the number of iFR-LM studies is limited, the deferral of revascularization of LM stenosis based on iFR appears to be safe, with similar long-term outcomes to those who were revascularized. **Fig. 12.20** shows FFR and iFR LM outcomes.

For assessment of the LM with downstream CAD, such as an additional significant LAD stenosis, it is necessary to understand the relationship of the myocardial bed size and the FFR. The LM FFR reflects flow to the entire left heart myocardial bed through both the LAD and the circumflex coronary artery (CFX). To compute LM FFR, maximal flow in the bed supplied by the target vessel is required. Thus, the myocardial bed for the LM is the summed territories of both the LAD and the CFX (**Fig. 12.21**). The LM bed

Study	FFR cut-off	Total number of patients: Total	Total number of patients: Deferred	Mean FU (months)	Odds ratio
Bech et al (2001)	<0.75	54 (100)	24 (44)	29±15	1.316
Jimenez-Navarro et al (2005)	<0.75	27 (100)	20 (74)	26±12	0.625
Legutko et al (2005)	<0.75	38 (100)	20 (53)	24±12	0.889
Lindstaedt et al (2006)	<0.75	51 (100)	24 (47)	29±16	0.952
Courtis et al (2009)	<0.75	142 (100)	82 (58)	14±11	3.394*
Hamilos et al (2009)	≤0.80	213 (100)	138 (65)	35±25	1.415
Overall		525 (100)	308 (59)		1.424

FIGURE 12.19 Summary of results from meta-analysis of combined long-term outcomes in fractional flow reserve (FFR)-guided management of left main coronary artery disease. *Denotes $P < .05$. (From Modi BN, van de Hoef TP, Piek J, Perera D. Physiological assessment of left main coronary artery disease. *EuroIntervention.* 2017;13:820-827, published online June 2017. Physiological assessment of left main coronary artery disease.)

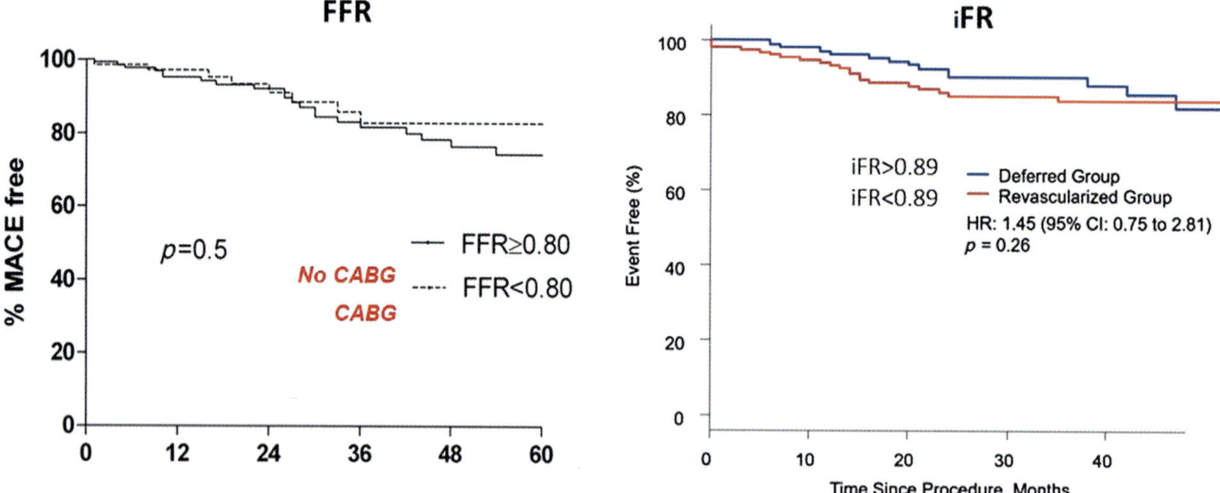

FIGURE 12.20 Coronary physiology and left main (LM) outcomes. Left, fractional flow reserve (FFR)-directed treatment outcomes (From Hamilos M, Muller O, Cuisset T, et al. Long-term clinical outcome after fractional flow reserve-guided treatment in patients with angiographically equivocal left main coronary artery stenosis. *Circulation.* 2009;120:1505-1512). Right, instantaneous wave-free ratio treatment-directed outcomes in LM. (From Warisawa T, Cook CM, Rajkumar C, et al. Safety of revascularization deferral of left main stenosis based on instantaneous wave-free ratio evaluation. *JACC Cardiovasc Interv.* 2020;13(14):1655-1664.)

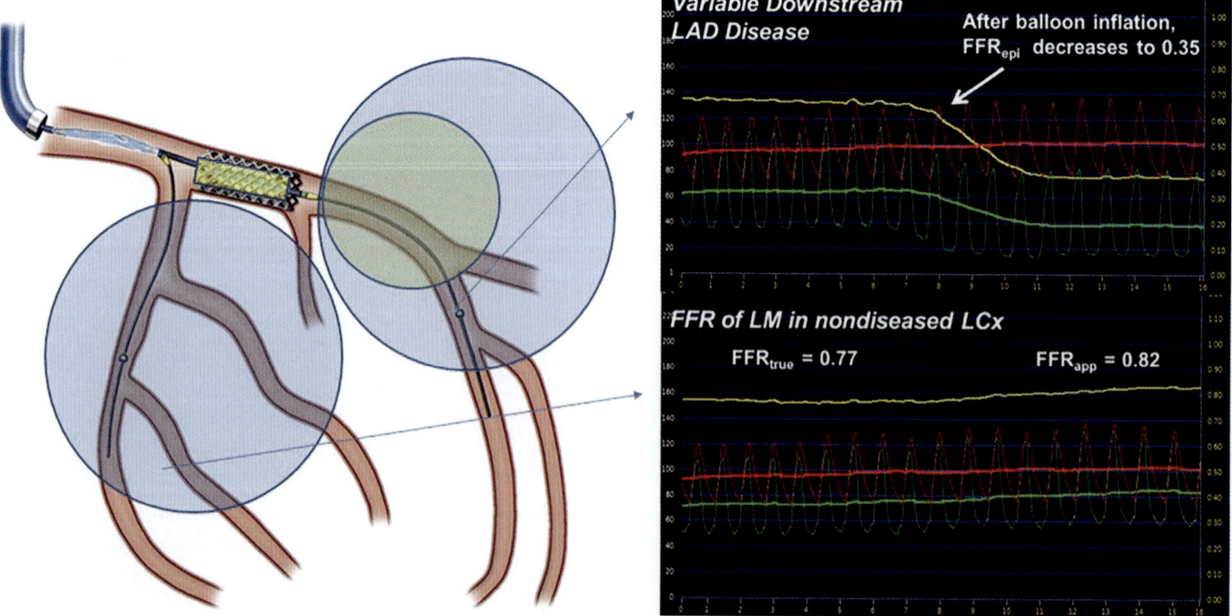

FIGURE 12.21 Impact of distal left anterior descending (LAD) stenosis on apparent fractional flow reserve (FFR) in the left main artery. The model in patients used those who had LAD stent placement with a second partially inflated balloon in the left main to simulate an intermediate left main (LM) lesion. Two pressure wires were used to measure simultaneous FFR in the LAD and circumflex zones (large blue circles, arrows connect the bed to their respective FFR tracing [yellow line on the right panel]). As the LAD balloon is inflated, the LAD territory diminishes (yellow circle) and the FFR in the circumflex as the apparent FFR of the left main rises indicating dependence on myocardial bed size to produce an accurate FFR of the left main. Only a very severe lesion (FFR <0.60) will raise the LM FFR apparent. (From Fearon W, et al. *JACC Cardiovasc Interv.* 2015;8(3):398-403.)

can be even larger if the RCA is occluded and if collateral is supplied from the left coronary system. In this case, the flow through the LM would involve supply to the inferior LV as well as the anterior LV. An LM narrowing without other disease (ie, no LAD, CFX, or RCA stenoses; top left, **Fig. 12.21**) reflects the physiologic significance of just the LM narrowing. An LM narrowing plus LAD stenosis (top right, **Fig. 12.21**) could produce a higher LM FFR; however, because the LM bed is decreased due to the LAD stenosis. The same considerations would apply in the setting of a CFX narrowing. The LM FFR alone cannot be accurately measured just when there are serial lesions. Fearon et al[23] demonstrated the impact of downstream disease on FFR measurement of LM in 25 patients by creating intermediate left main coronary artery stenosis, and LAD or CFX stenosis with deflated balloon catheters after PCI of the LAD/CFX, or both. FFR across the LM and LAD altered the FFR LM measured in the CFX only when the net LM/LAD FFR was <0.60.

Serial Lesions and Diffuse CAD

For lesions in series, FFR cannot identify an accurate individual lesion value. This limitation occurs because the first lesion blunts the hyperemia of the second and vice versa. The extent of this interaction, or crosstalk, between lesions is unpredictable. The individual FFR of each stenosis separately can be predicted by a different FFR equation from Pijls et al[24] using P_a, pressure between the two stenoses (P_m), P_d, and coronary occlusion wedge pressure (P_w) during maximum hyperemia:

$$FFR_{predicted} = \left(P_d - \left[\left(P_m/P_a\right) * P_w\right]\right) / \left(\left(P_a - P_m\right) + \left(P_d - P_w\right)\right)$$

This calculation requires the use of the P_w during balloon inflation, an impractical method for routine diagnostic measurements.

The use of pullback pressure tracings from distal to proximal at rest or during hyperemia provides more information and a more accurate method to determine the hemodynamic significance of multiple lesions in series or in the setting of diffuse disease. Using iFR to assess serial lesions is easier than FFR and may prove to be the preferred clinical approach. Kikuta et al[25] presented the value of iFR pullback measurements before angioplasty assessing how often the treatment strategy based on angiography alone was changed and predicting the post-PCI hemodynamic result. In 168 lesions, the iFR pullback procedure identified the relative ischemic contribution of each stenosed segment to the iFR value of the entire vessel. This information changed the revascularization plan 31% of the time with a reduction in the average number and length of stents implanted. At the same time, the pre-PCI iFR pullback was used to predict the post-PCI iFR measurement in 134 vessels (128 patients). Following PCI, the mean difference between predicted and actual post-PCI iFR was small at 0.011 ± 0.004 with a strong correlation (r = 0.73, P < .001). The angiographic coregistration of NHPR (eg, iFR) will improve the way PCI is performed and improve outcomes by reducing the residual and unsuspected ischemia. An example of iFR coregistration identifying lesions appropriate for revascularization is presented in **Fig. 12.22**.

The pressure pullback recording can identify the location of focal lesions in the setting of diffuse disease. An abnormal FFR can be seen in the absence of focal epicardial stenoses and is often best treated medically or with surgical revascularization. Diffuse disease is characterized by a continuous and gradual pressure recovery during pullback, without any abrupt increase in pressure related to a focal region.

Acute Coronary Syndromes

The acute phase of an ST-segment elevated myocardial infarction (STEMI) and non-ST-segment elevated myocardial infarction (NSTEMI) is associated with dynamic changes in both the target stenosis and the myocardial bed beyond the lesion. The territory remote from the infarct zone is impacted to a variable degree (**Fig. 12.23**). Resting flow, hyperemic flow, and microvascular function may be altered in the nonculprit artery, particularly when the nonculprit vessel is in proximity to the infarct zone. Changes in coronary flow related to the acute myocardial injury affects both NHPR and FFR. An increase in sympathetic tone may increase resting coronary flow, reducing iFR. In addition, microvascular dysfunction may extend into the infarct border zone potentially decreasing hyperemic flow in the nonculprit arteries producing a false negative FFR. This involvement would imply that FFR would underestimate stenosis severity in nonculprit vessels.

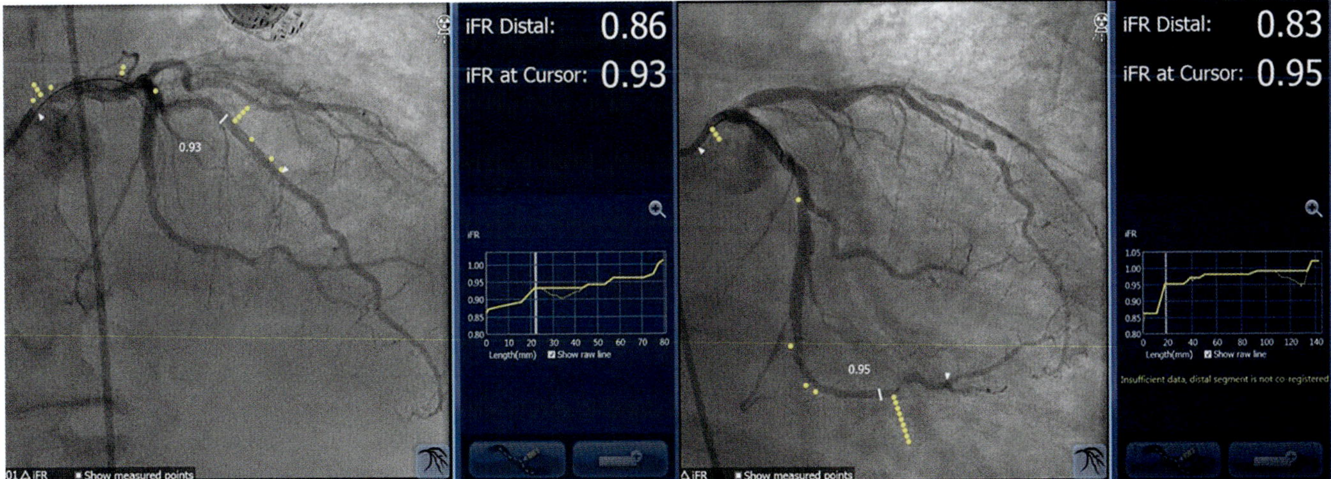

FIGURE 12.22 Instantaneous wave-free ratio (iFR) coregistration in left anterior descending (LAD) (left) and circumflex coronary artery (CFX) (right) coronary arteries. This elderly patient had angina and dyspnea 4 years after CFX stent placement. A recent exercise tolerance test (ETT) was negative, but angina persisted. Pull back pressures in the LAD were consistent with diffuse disease without a focal lesion, while pullback pressure recordings from the CFX showed a distal severe and focal lesion with large pressure drop but no pressure loss across the prior stent or left main percutaneous coronary intervention of the distal CFX eliminated the angina.

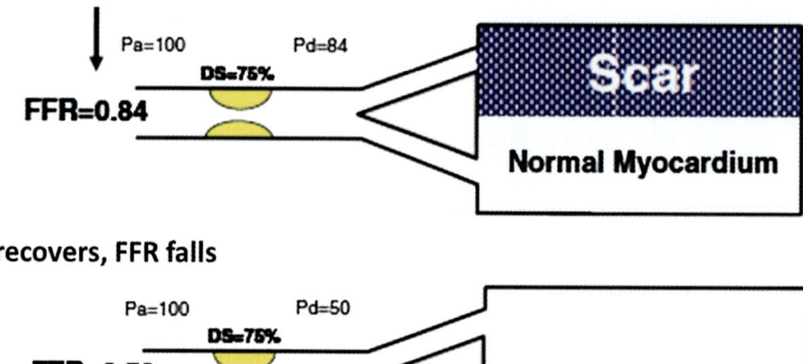

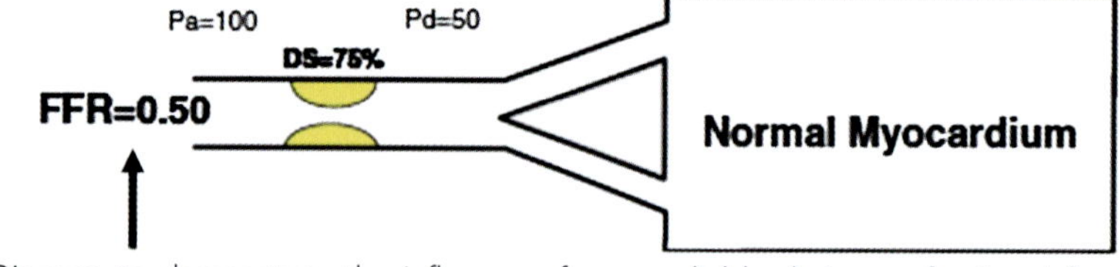

FIGURE 12.23 Diagram to demonstrate the influence of myocardial bed size on fractional flow reserve (FFR). Top: A mild lesion of 50% supplying a large territory of myocardium can have a low FFR of 0.75. Bottom: In contrast, a severe angiographic narrowing of 85% supplying a small myocardial territory can have a high FFR of 0.83. In an ST-segment elevated myocardial infarction (STEMI) patient, the lower panel might represent the acute phase, and the upper panel the recuperation phase, with changing FFR values influencing the decision making at the time of STEMI. Similar conditions may exist for the noninfarct-related artery assessments.

In sum, the predictive ability of FFR in acute coronary syndrome (ACS) is limited because (1) the microvascular bed in the infarct zone may not have uniform, constant, or minimal resistance; (2) the severity of stenosis may evolve as thrombus and vasoconstriction abate; and (3) FFR measurements are not meaningful when normal perfusion (ie, maximal hyperemia) cannot be achieved. In nonculprit lesions and target lesion assessment during the recovery phase of MI, FFR retains its value for clinically decision making.

Because of a changing myocardial bed during recuperation after an acute infarction, FFR is not used in the STEMI culprit artery until 4 to 6 days after the event, when myocardial function is believed to stabilize. For the non-IRA in STEMI/NSTEMI patients, the zone of myocardial injury of the culprit vessel is unknown but may extend close to the region supplied by the non-IRA. In a subset of the FAME study, 101 patients undergoing PCI for both STEMI and NSTEMI had 112 non-IRA lesions assessed by FFR at the index procedure and again 35 ± 4 days later. The non-IRA FFR was 0.77 ± 0.13 at baseline and identical at follow-up remeasurement, concluding that in ACS, FFR was unchanged over 3 months following the presentation.

Post PCI Physiology

Post-PCI functional assessment predicts long-term patient outcomes and provides insights into the residual ischemic potential of the treated vessel. Suboptimal functional results should be examined and if possible, treated.

Agarwal and Uretsky[26] demonstrated that the higher the final FFR/NHPR the fewer the adverse events (**Fig. 12.24**). Mechanisms for suboptimal post-PCI physiology are not always evident. The DEFINE-PCI study[27] showed that 25% of angiographically adequate interventions have residual hemodynamic impairment due to diffuse CAD, unsuspected new narrowing, edge stent dissection, proximal vessel narrowing, or vasospasm (**Fig. 12.25**). A significant association was observed between ΔFFR and symptomatic relief ($P = .02$). Thus, the larger the improvement in FFR, the larger the symptomatic relief and the lower the event rate. Measuring FFR before and after PCI provides clinically useful prognostic data (**Fig. 12.26**).

CFR TECHNIQUES

The invasive assessment of the coronary circulation involves macrovascular or epicardial (R1) testing and microvascular testing. Epicardial disease is characterized by NHPR or FFR while the microcirculation can be assessed by CFR or IMR, measured with either Doppler flow velocity or with thermodilution techniques (**Figs. 12.27** and **12.28**). IC Doppler flow velocity is measured at baseline and then continuously during bolus injection of IC adenosine (**Fig. 12.29**).

As the Doppler wire is not widely available, the most common method of measuring CFR is the coronary thermodilution technique, which uses thermistors on a pressure-sensor angioplasty guidewire. The shaft of the angioplasty pressure-guide wire (Abbott Medical) has a temperature-dependent electrical resistance and acts as a proximal thermistor, which allows for the detection of the start of the indicator (saline) injection (**Fig. 12.30**). Bolus saline is injected, and temperature arrival times are surrogates of coronary flow velocity. Measurements at rest and again during adenosine hyperemia are then used to compute CFR. Thermodilution CFR (CFR_{thermo}) is defined as:

CFRthermo = (1/Tmn rest)/1/Tmn hyper), where Tmn is the mean transit time arrival in seconds.

Simultaneous measurements of CFR and FFR are currently obtained for both clinical and research studies on coronary and myocardial resistance. When combined with pressure measurements, CFR measurements can provide a complete description of the pressure-flow relationship and the response of the microcirculation.

As mentioned previously, CFR differs from FFR in several significant ways. Because it uses basal flow as well as the specific hyperemic flow, CFR varies with any change in basal flow from changes in heart rate, blood pressure, and contractility (**Fig. 12.11**). Changes in the slope of maximal hyperemia will also alter the CFR. In contrast, FFR is largely independent of basal flow levels as it is computed only at maximal flow. FFR is unaffected by changing hemodynamics or the status of the microcirculation. For these

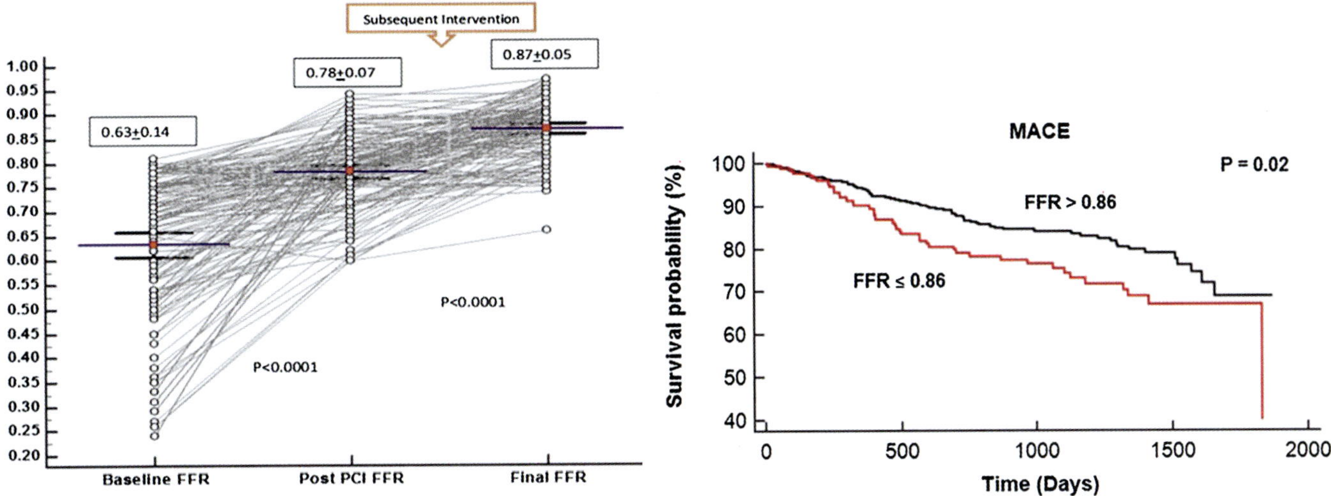

FIGURE 12.24 Impact of subsequent interventions on post-percutaneous coronary intervention (PCI) fractional flow reserve (FFR). Left panel, Serial interventions undertaken to address suboptimal post-PCI FFR. The FFR prior to reintervention was 0.63, which increased to 0.78 ± 0.07 after the initial intervention. Further interventions with IVUS assessment, additional stenting increased the FFR to 0.87 ± 0.05. Right panel, Kaplan-Meier curves of MACE for patients whose final FFR was >0.86 with significant reduction of adverse outcomes over 5 years. AS, additional stenting; IVUS, intravascular ultrasound; MACE, major adverse cardiac event; OCT, optical coherence tomography; PD, postdilation. (From Agarwal SK, Kasula S, Hacioglu Y, Ahmed Z, Uretsky BF, Hakeem A. Utilizing post-intervention fractional flow reserve to optimize acute results and the relationship to long-term outcomes. *JACC Cardiovasc Interv*. 2016;9(10):1022-1031. doi:10.1016/j.jcin.2016.01.046)

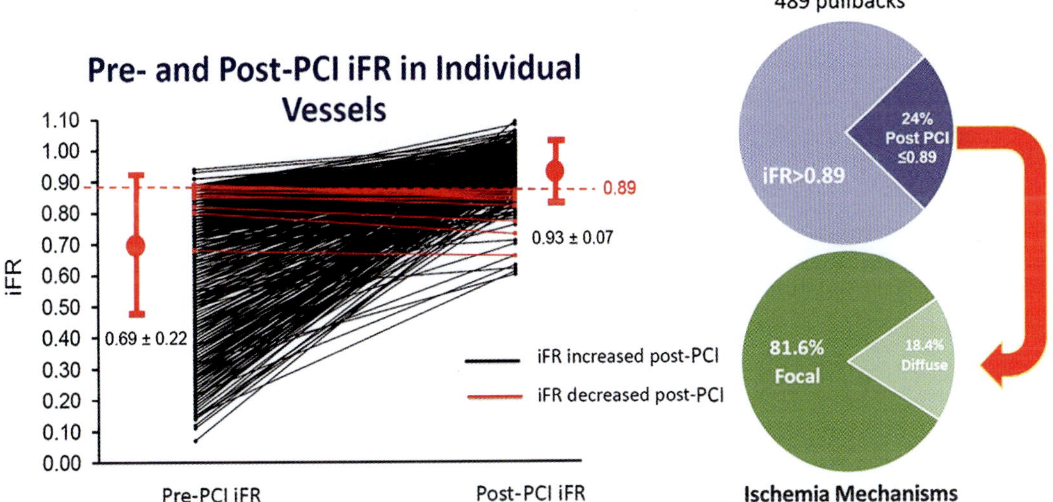

FIGURE 12.25 Significant residual ischemia after angiographically successful percutaneous coronary intervention (PCI) was not uncommon, occurring in 24% of patients. In a large majority of cases, residual pressure gradients were focal and thus potentially amenable to treatment with additional PCI. (From Jeremias A, Davies JE, Maehara A, et al. Blinded physiological assessment of residual ischemia after successful angiographic percutaneous coronary intervention: the DEFINE PCI study. *JACC Cardiovasc Interv*. 2019;12(20):1991-2001. doi:10.1016/j.jcin.2019.05.054)

reasons, FFR is preferred over CFR for in-lab lesion assessment. CFR is used for assessment of microvascular disease along with IMR.

Index of Microcirculatory Resistance

The IMR, defined as the ratio of distal coronary pressure to the inverse of the mean transit time during maximal hyperemia, provides prognostic information for STEMI patients. IMR is a quantitative index that is unique to the microcirculation and independent of epicardial CAD.[28,29] IMR is superior to CFR because it is not affected by resting hemodynamics, making it more reproducible, even after hemodynamic perturbations. After STEMI, IMR predicts the amount of myocardial damage and left ventricular recovery better than other indices and is an independent predictor of long-term clinical outcomes.

After primary angioplasty, Fearon et al[29] demonstrated the prognostic value of IMR compared with CFR, thrombolysis in MI perfusion grade, and clinical variables. Patients with an IMR >40 had a higher rate of death or rehospitalization at 1 year than those with an IMR ≤40 (17% vs 7%; *P* = .027). During follow-up (2.8 years), an IMR >40 was the only independent predictor of death alone (HR, 4.3; *P* = .02). IMR may potentially be used in selecting patients with relatively preserved postinfarct microvasculature that might most benefit from regional delivery of regenerative cell therapies.[30]

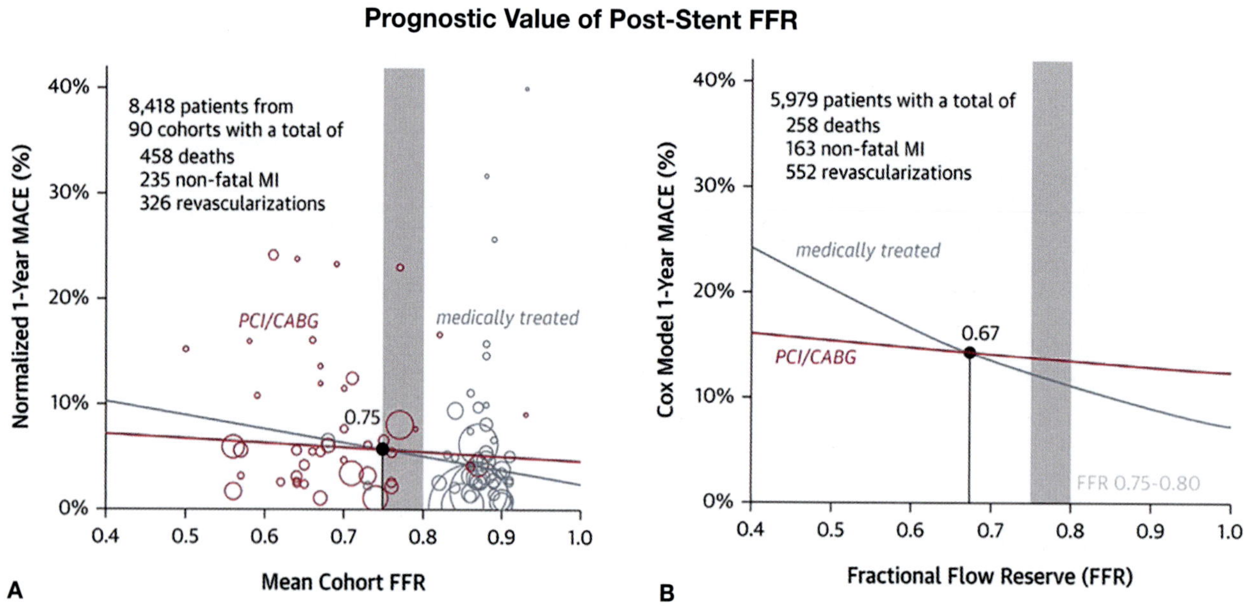

Prognostic Value of Post-Stent FFR

A

Normalized 1-Year MACE (%)

8,418 patients from
90 cohorts with a total of
458 deaths
235 non-fatal MI
326 revascularizations

PCI/CABG

medically treated

0.75

40%
30%
20%
10%
0%

0.4 0.5 0.6 0.7 0.8 0.9 1.0

Mean Cohort FFR

B

Cox Model 1-Year MACE (%)

5,979 patients with a total of
258 deaths
163 non-fatal MI
552 revascularizations

medically treated

0.67

PCI/CABG

FFR 0.75-0.80

40%
30%
20%
10%
0%

0.4 0.5 0.6 0.7 0.8 0.9 1.0

Fractional Flow Reserve (FFR)

FIGURE 12.26 Prognostic value of poststent fractional flow reserve (FFR). A, Normalized 1-year major adverse cardiac event (MACE) rate for study-level analysis. Meta regression for the study-level data fits the normalized 1-year. MACE rate (circles whose size reflects the number of patients) for cohorts treated with either revascularization (red) or medical therapy (slate) as a function of mean lesion FFR. Colored lines depict the metaregression fit. These curves cross at the optimal FFR threshold, shown here for a univariate model with random effects. See **Table 12.2** for results from other models. B, Cox model 1-year MACE rate for patient-level analysis. Patient-level analysis fits the outcomes data to a Cox proportional hazards model of survival, shown here with the best-fit 1-year MACE rate as a function of individual lesion FFR. Colored lines depict the model fit for revascularization (red) or medical therapy (slate) treatment. These curves cross at the optimal FFR threshold, here shown for the unadjusted model. MI, myocardial infarction. (From Johnson N, et al. *JACC*. 2014;64(16):1641-1654.)

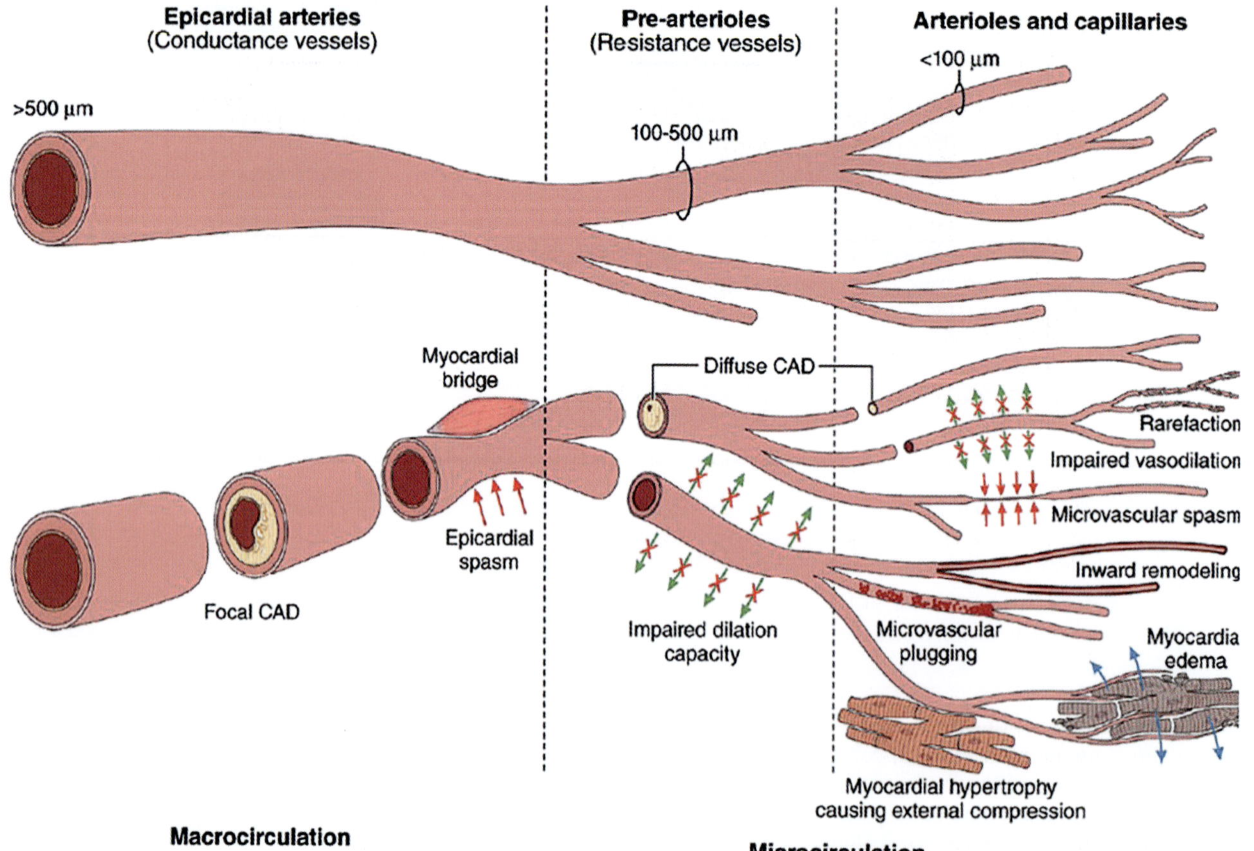

FIGURE 12.27 Proposed mechanisms of functional, structural, and compressive forces acting on the microcirculation. (From Smilowitz NR, Toleva O, Chieffo A, Perera D, Berry C. Coronary microvascular disease in contemporary clinical practice. *Circ Cardiovasc Interv*. 2023;16(6):e012568. Originally published June 1, 2023. doi:10.1161/CIRCINTERVENTIONS.122.012568)

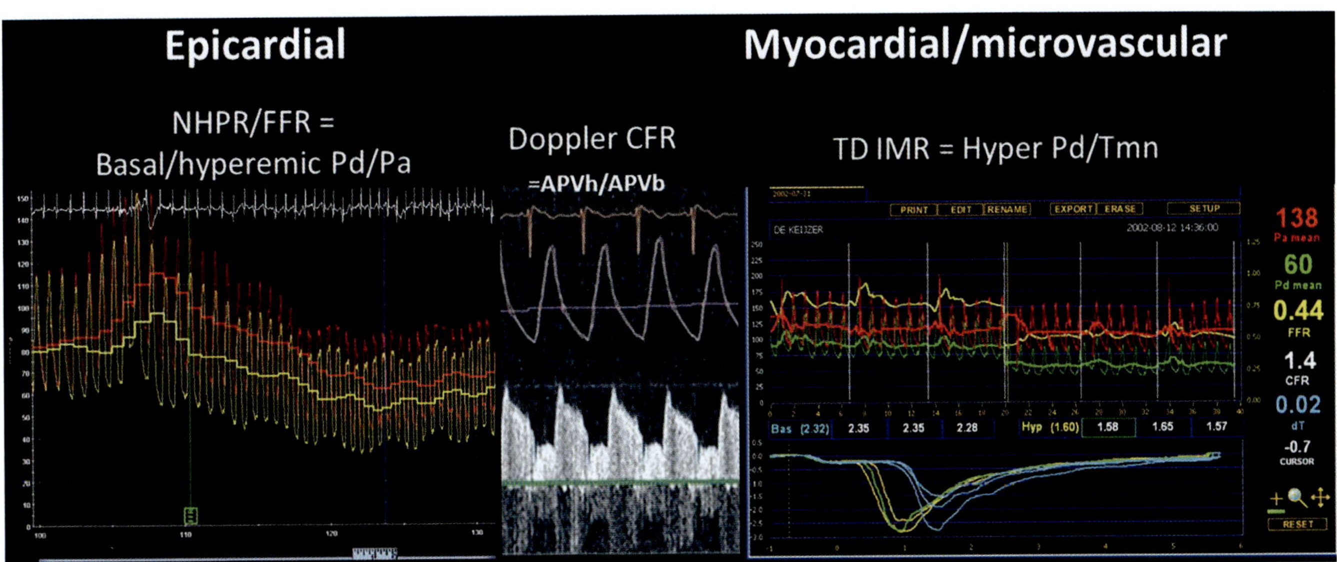

FIGURE 12.28 Tools for the invasive assessment of the coronary circulation. Epicardial or R1 resistances are measured with FFR or NHPR. The microvascular circulation can be assessed with coronary flow reserve, measured with Doppler flow velocity or with thermodilution techniques. FFR, fractional flow reserve; NHPR, nonhyperemic pressure ratio.

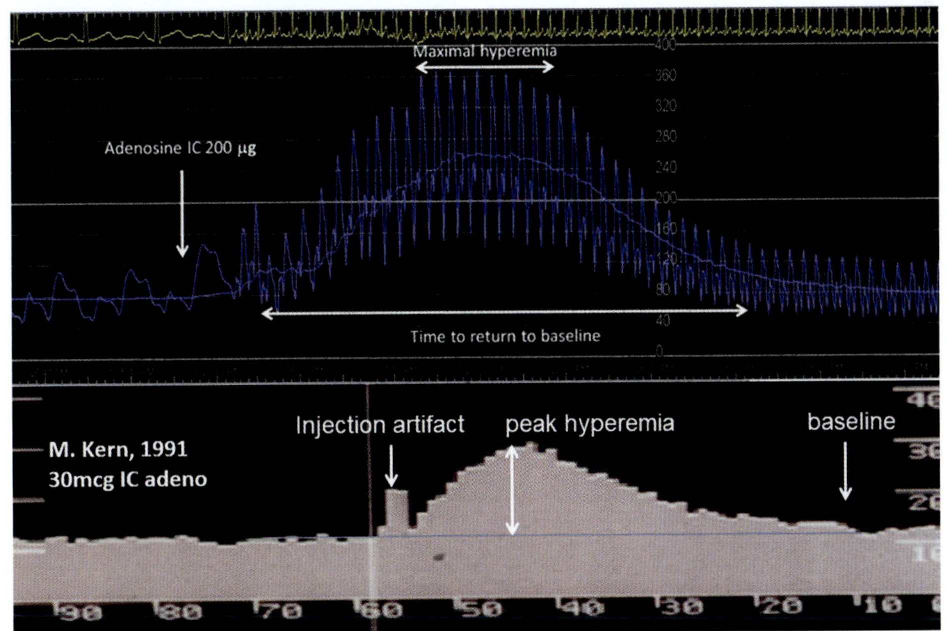

FIGURE 12.29 Intracoronary Doppler flow velocity used to measure coronary flow reserve (CFR) with intracoronary adenosine. Top panel depicts zero cross Doppler with the time course of hyperemia after a 200 μg bolus of intracoronary (IC) adenosine. Time to peak is about 30 to 45 seconds from injection (arrow) to return to baseline. Lower panel, spectral IC Doppler wire with adenosine bolus injection of 30 μg. Time on the x-axis is marked in 10 seconds divisions. (Top panel, adapted from Adjedj, et al. *JACC Cardiovasc Interv*. 2015;8(11):1422-1430. Lower panel, M. Kern 1993.)

Illustrative Cases

A 72-year-old man has typical angina. On angiography, there is a severe stenosis of the proximal circumflex artery (**Fig. 12.31**). Although FFR is not required, the PCI of the circumflex stenosis (left top, prestent, arrow) was performed with a 0.014 fiber optic pressure wire. (Right top) The significant initial gradient corresponded to an FFR prestent of 0.69). After stenting, the angiogram improved, and there was no residual gradient (bottom right, poststent FFR = 0.94).

A 56-year-old man had unstable angina. An electrocardiogram shows inferior lateral ST changes (**Fig. 12.32A**). Angiography showed a severe CFX lesion. While a pressure guidewire is not required, the FFR before stenting was 0.63 (**Fig. 12.32B**). After the stent, the angiogram was significantly improved and the final Pd/Pa = 1.0 (**Fig. 12.32B**). Attention was directed at the RCA. The RCA had a Pd/Pa = 0.97 and cFFR = 0.87 (**Fig. 12.32C**). No intervention was indicated.

- A practical approach to FFR/NHPR decisions is provided in **Fig. 12.33**, **Table 12.7**, and **Table 12.6**. Ischemic thresholds of invasive physiologic indices.

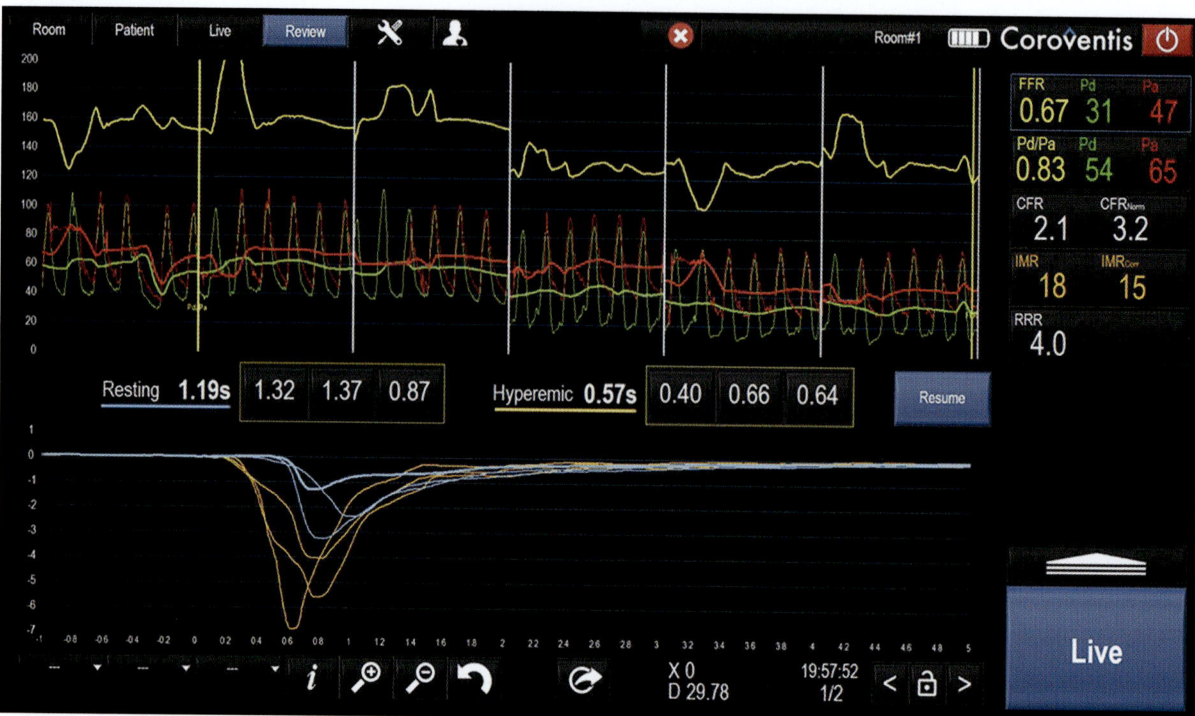

FIGURE 12.30 Determining coronary flow physiology (Pd/Pa, FFR, CFR, IMR, and RRR) use the thermodilution technique and software (CoroFlow) from Abbott Medical pressure-wire system. At the top of the figure, the *red* signals reflect the guide catheter pressure (P_a), the *green* signals reflect the coronary pressure (P_d), and the *yellow line* represents the calculated FFR. CFR is measured as the ratio of the averaged basal temperature arrival time divided by the average of the hyperemic arrival times. The blue and gold curves at the bottom represent the thermodilution temperature changes during rest and subsequently at maximal hyperemia, respectively. The numbers above the curves are the transit times in seconds. Hyperemic times are faster than basal times reflecting faster flow. Values for the calculations are shown on the right side of the figure. FFR, fractional flow reserve. CFR, coronary flow reserve; IMR, index of microvascular resistance.

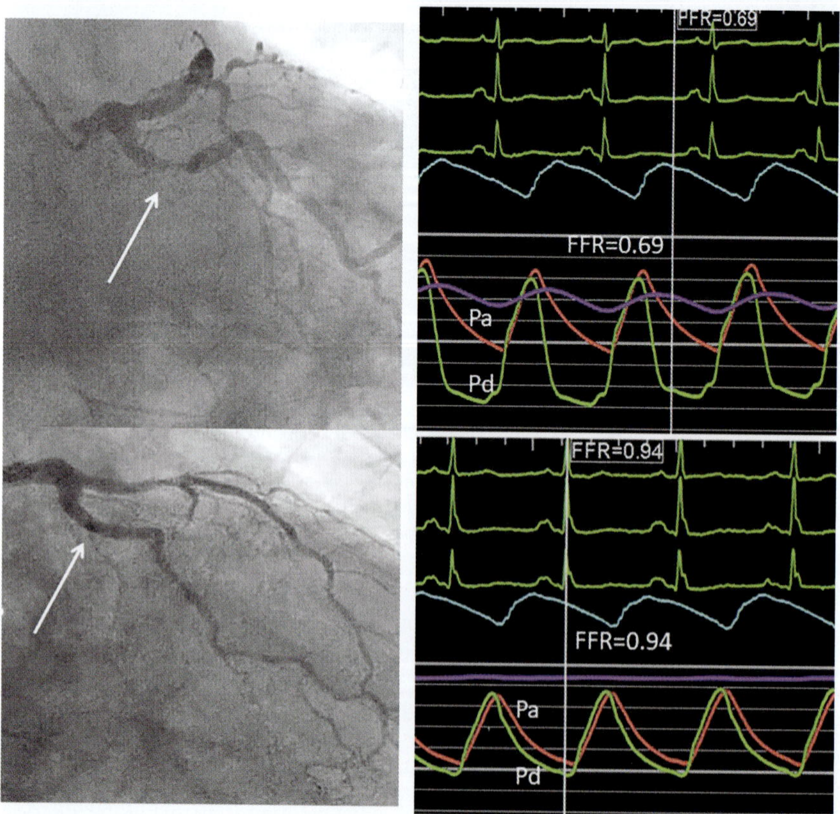

FIGURE 12.31 Case illustration. A 72-year-old man has typical angina. On angiography, there is a severe stenosis of the proximal circumflex artery. Although FFR is not required, the PCI of the circumflex stenosis (left top, prestent, arrow) was performed with a 0.014 fiber optic pressure wire. The significant initial gradient (right top corresponded to an FFR prestent of 0.69). After stenting, the angiogram improved and there was no residual gradient (bottom right, poststent FFR = 0.94). FFR, fractional flow reserve; PCI, percutaneous coronary intervention.

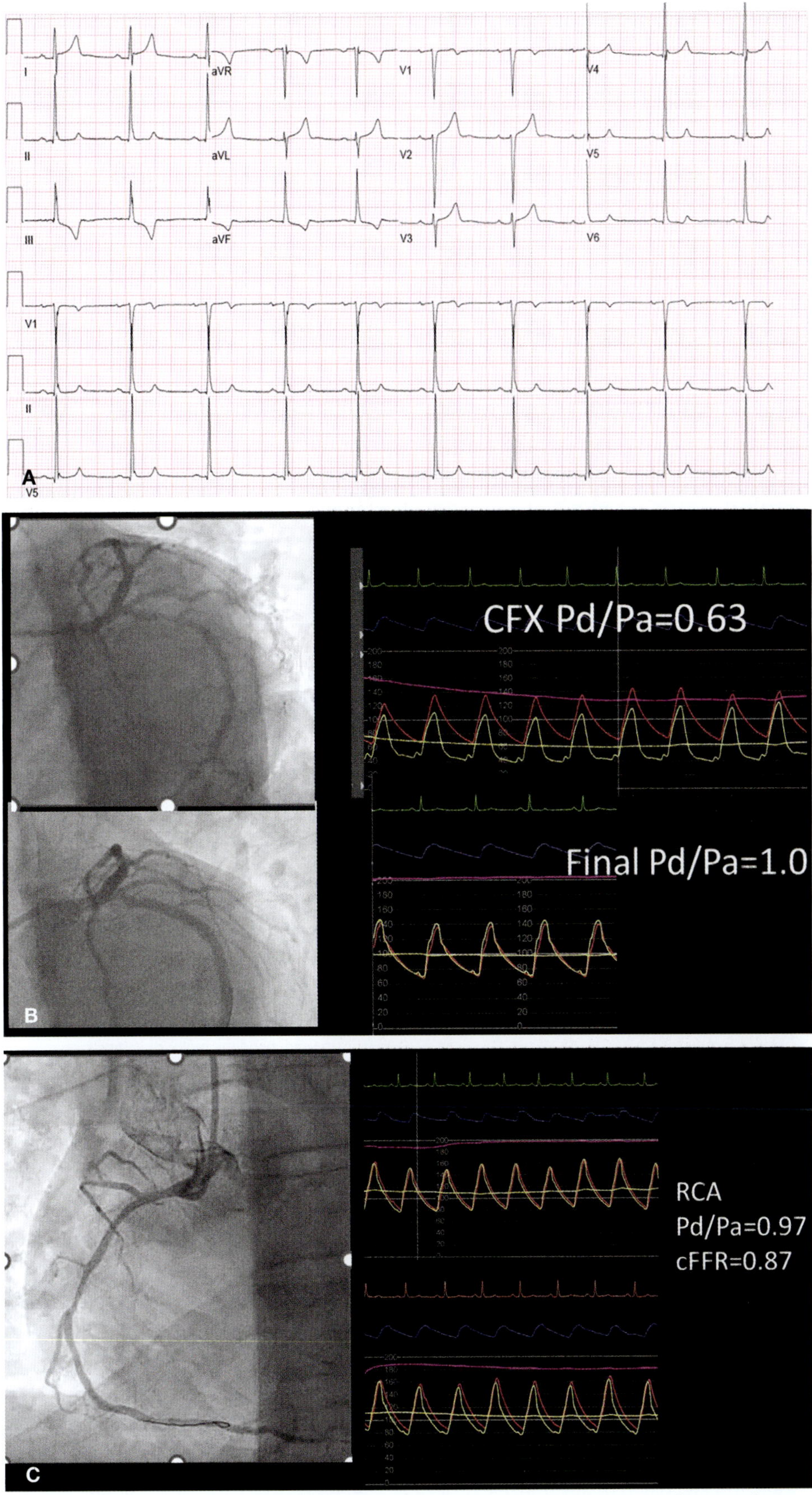

FIGURE 12.32 A, Case illustration. A 56-year-old man had unstable angina. An electrocardiogram shows inferior lateral ST changes. B, Top, angiography showed a severe CFX lesion. Right top, while a pressure guidewire is not required, the FFR before stenting was 0.63. Right bottom, after the stent, the angiogram was significantly improved and the final Pd/Pa = 1.0. C, Attention was directed at the right coronary artery (RCA). The RCA had a Pd/Pa = 0.97 and cFFR = 0.87. No intervention was indicated. CFX, circumflex coronary artery.

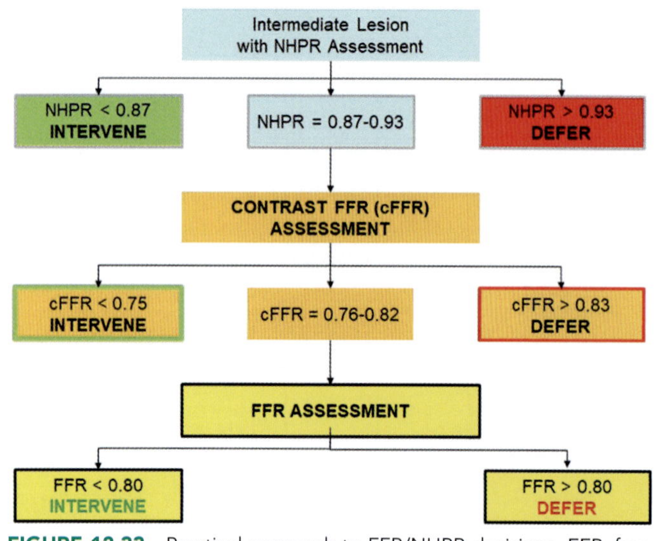

FIGURE 12.33 Practical approach to FFR/NHPR decisions. FFR, fractional flow reserve; NHPR, nonhyperemic pressure ratio.

TABLE 12.7 Uses of FFR and NHPR in Clinical Practice

CONDITION	BEST MODALITY	COMMENT
Stable ischemic HD	NHPR = FFR	If borderline, check cFFR, then FFR. Use pullback pressure recording
Acute coronary syndrome, nonculprit	FFR or NHPR	Little data on NHPR but FFR affected by proximity to infarct zone
Diffuse disease	NHPR > FFR	More iFR+/FFR− lesions. Use pullback pressure recording. See issues on disparity
Focal residual lesions	FFR = NHPR	Associated with more iFR−/FFR + results
Focal RCA lesions	FFR = NHPR but consider RFR > Ifr	Less impacted by systolic flow in RCA
TAVR	NHPR > FFR	Less flow change with NHPR

HD, heart disease; cFFR, contrast FFR; RFR, resting flow ratio; TAVR, transaortic valve replacement.

Key Points

- Angiography alone is insufficient to identify the physiologic impact of intermediate stenoses.
- While noninvasive stress testing has known limitations, translesional physiology (FFR and NHPR) provides an accurate reflection of lesion-specific ischemic potential.
- Treatment of stable CAD guided by FFR/NHPR demonstrates superiority over angiographically guided PCI with significant clinical and economic benefits. FFRs or NHPRs are reasonable to assess angiographic intermediate coronary lesions (50%-70% diameter stenosis) and can be useful for guiding revascularization decisions in patients with stable ischemic heart disease (SIHD). (Class IIa, level of evidence: A)
- According to the expert SCAI consensus paper, FFR is definitely beneficial in SIHD when noninvasive stress imaging is contraindicated, discordant, nondiagnostic, or unavailable. FFR should be used to assess the functional significance of intermediate coronary stenoses (50%-70%) and more severe stenoses (<90%).
- In patients with multivessel coronary disease, PCI guided by FFR measurement improves outcomes and saves resources when compared with PCI guided by angiography alone.
- In patients with three-vessel coronary disease, measuring FFR could allow reclassification of the number of vessels diseased and/or the SYNTAX score, thereby guiding decisions regarding revascularization by CABG or PCI.
- In SIHD, PCI of lesions with FFR <0.80 improves symptom control and decreases the need for hospitalization requiring urgent revascularization when compared with medical therapy alone.
- FFR is of no proven benefit for measurement of the culprit vessel in a patient with an acute STEMI or any unstable ACS presentation and should not be performed.
- NHPR outcomes are noninferior to FFR in SIHD studies.

References

1. Johnson NP, Kirkeeide RL, Gould KL. History and development of coronary flow reserve and fractional flow reserve for clinical applications. *Interv Cardiol Clin*. 2015;4:397-410.
2. de Bruyne B, Oldroyd KG, Pijls NHJ. Microvascular (Dys)Function and clinical outcome in stable coronary disease. *J Am Coll Cardiol*. 2016;67(10):1170-1172. doi:10.1016/j.jacc.2015.11.066
3. Pijls NH, Van Gelder B, Van der Voort P, et al. Fractional flow reserve. A useful index to evaluate the influence of an epicardial coronary stenosis on myocardial blood flow. *Circulation*. 1995;92(11):3183-3193.
4. de Bruyne B, Bartunek J, Sys SU, Pijls NH, Heyndrickx GR, Wijns W. Simultaneous coronary pressure and flow velocity measurements in humans. Feasibility, reproducibility, and hemodynamic dependence of coronary flow velocity reserve, hyperemic flow versus pressure slope index, and fractional flow reserve. *Circulation*. 1996;94(8):1842-1849.
5. Sen S, Escaned J, Malik IS, et al. Development and validation of a new adenosine-independent index of stenosis severity from coronary wave-intensity analysis: results of the ADVISE (ADenosine Vasodilator Independent Stenosis Evaluation) study. *J Am Coll Cardiol*. 2012;59(15):1392-1402.
6. Jeremias A, Maehara A, Généreux P, et al. Multicenter core laboratory comparison of the instantaneous wave-free ratio and resting Pd/Pa with fractional flow reserve: the RESOLVE study. *J Am Coll Cardiol*. 2014;63(13):1253-1261.
7. Kern MJ, Bach RG, Mechem CJ, et al. Variations in normal coronary vasodilatory reserve stratified by artery, gender, heart transplantation and coronary artery disease. *J Am Coll Cardiol*. 1996;28(5):1154-1160.
8. De Bruyne B, Bartunek J, Sys SU, Heyndrickx GR. Relation between myocardial fractional flow reserve calculated from coronary pressure measurements and exercise-induced myocardial ischemia. *Circulation*. 1995;92(1):39-46.
9. Pijls NH, De Bruyne B, Peels K, et al. Measurement of fractional flow reserve to assess the functional severity of coronary-artery stenoses. *N Engl J Med*. 1996;334(26):1703-1708.
10. De Rosa S, Polimeni A, Petraco R, Davies JE, Indolfi C. Diagnostic performance of the instantaneous wave-free ratio: comparison with fractional flow reserve. *Circ Cardiovasc Interv*. 2018;11(1):e004613. doi:10.1161/CIRCINTERVENTIONS.116.004613
11. Warisawa T, Cook CM, Howard JP, et al. Physiological pattern of disease assessed by pressure-wire pullback has an influence on fractional flow reserve/instantaneous wave-free ratio discordance. *Circ Cardiovasc Interv*. 2019;12(5):e007494.

12. Cook CM, Jeremias A, Petraco R, et al. Fractional flow reserve/instantaneous wave-free ratio discordance in angiographically intermediate coronary stenoses: an analysis using Doppler-derived coronary flow measurements. *JACC Cardiovasc Interv*. 2017;10(24):2514-2524.
13. Tonino PA, Fearon WF, De Bruyne B, et al. Angiographic versus functional severity of coronary artery stenoses in the FAME study fractional flow reserve versus angiography in multivessel evaluation. *J Am Coll Cardiol*. 2010;55(25):2816-2821.
14. Zimmermann FM, Ferrara A, Johnson NP, et al. Deferral vs. performance of percutaneous coronary intervention of functionally non-significant coronary stenosis: 15-year follow-up of the DEFER trial. *Eur Heart J*. 2015;36(45):3182-3188. PMID: 26400825. doi:10.1093/eurheartj/ehv452
15. van Nunen LX, Zimmermann FM, Tonino PA, et al, FAME Study Investigators. Fractional flow reserve versus angiography for guidance of PCI in patients with multivessel coronary artery disease (FAME): 5-year follow-up of a randomised controlled trial. *Lancet*. 2015;386(10006):1853-1860. PMID: 26333474. doi:10.1016/S0140-6736(15)00057-4
16. De Bruyne B, Pijls NH, Kalesan B, et al, FAME 2 Trial Investigators. Fractional flow reserve-guided PCI versus medical therapy in stable coronary disease. *N Engl J Med*. 2012;367(11):991-1001.
17. Xaplanteris P, Fournier S, Pijls NHJ, et al, FAME 2 Investigators. Five-year outcomes with PCI guided by fractional flow reserve. *N Engl J Med*. 2018;379(3):250-259. PMID: 29785878. doi: 10.1056/NEJMoa1803538
18. Fearon WF, Zimmermann FM, De Bruyne B, et al, FAME 3 Investigators. Fractional flow reserve-guided PCI as compared with coronary bypass surgery. *N Engl J Med*. 2022;386(2):128-137.
19. Davies JE, Sen S, Dehbi HM, et al. Use of the instantaneous wave-free ratio or fractional flow reserve in PCI. *N Engl J Med*. 2017;376(19):1824-1834.
20. Götberg M, Christiansen EH, Gudmundsdottir IJ, et al, iFR-SWEDEHEART Investigators. Instantaneous wave-free ratio versus fractional flow reserve to guide PCI. *N Engl J Med*. 2017;376(19):1813-1823.
21. Modi BN, van de Hoef TP, Piek J, Perera D. Physiological assessment of left main coronary artery disease. *EuroIntervention*. 2017;13(7):820-827.
22. Warisawa T, Cook CM, Rajkumar C, et al. Safety of revascularization deferral of left main stenosis based on instantaneous wave-free ratio evaluation. *JACC Cardiovasc Interv*. 2020;13(14):1655-1664.
23. Fearon WF, Yong AS, Lenders G, et al. The impact of downstream coronary stenosis on fractional flow reserve assessment of intermediate left main coronary artery disease: human validation. *JACC Cardiovasc Interv*. 2015;8(3):398-403.
24. Pijls NH, De Bruyne B, Bech GJ, et al. Coronary pressure measurement to assess the hemodynamic significance of serial stenoses within one coronary artery validation in humans. *Circulation*. 2000;102(19):2371-2377.
25. Kikuta Y, Cook CM, Sharp ASP, et al. Pre-angioplasty instantaneous wave-free ratio pullback predicts hemodynamic outcome in humans with coronary artery disease: primary results of the international multicenter iFR GRADIENT registry. *JACC Cardiovasc Interv*. 2018;11(8):757-767.
26. Agarwal SK, Kasula S, Hacioglu Y, Ahmed Z, Uretsky BF, Hakeem A. Utilizing post-intervention fractional flow reserve to optimize acute results and the relationship to long-term outcomes. *JACC Cardiovasc Interv*. 2016;9(10):1022-1031.
27. Jeremias A, Davies JE, Maehara A, et al. Blinded physiological assessment of residual ischemia after successful angiographic percutaneous coronary intervention: the DEFINE PCI study. *JACC Cardiovasc Interv*. 2019;12(20):1991-2001.
28. Fearon WF, Balsam LB, Farouque HMO, et al. Novel index for invasively assessing the coronary microcirculation. *Circulation*. 2003;107(25):3129-3132.
29. Fearon WF, Shah M, Ng M, et al. Predictive value of the index of microcirculatory resistance in patients with ST-segment elevation myocardial infarction. *J Am Coll Cardiol*. 2008;51(5):560-565.
30. Ng MK, Yong ASC, Ho M, et al. The index of microcirculatory resistance predicts myocardial infarction related to percutaneous coronary intervention. *Circ Cardiovasc Interv*. 2012;5(4):515-522.

Hemodynamics for Interventional Cardiologists

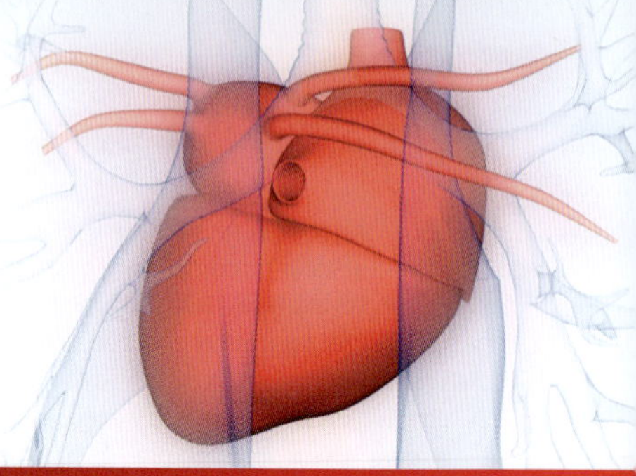

Morton J. Kern and Arnold H. Seto

Hemodynamics can confirm or establish the etiology of many surgically correctable cardiac diseases, but diagnoses can be inaccurate if the data are poorly collected or inaccurately obtained. Hemodynamics data play a critical role in teaching cardiovascular pathophysiology and should be a continued point of excellence for invasive cardiologists.

This chapter will review the essential hemodynamics applicable to coronary and structural interventions in the cardiac catheterization laboratory. Complete reviews of hemodynamics, both in general and those specifically applicable to complex conditions, can be found elsewhere.[1-6] An excellent summary of hemodynamics in the catheterization laboratory is presented by Nishimura and Carabello.[7]

THE CARDIAC CYCLE

All pressure waves of the cardiac cycle can be understood by reviewing the electrical and mechanical activity of the heart, as shown in the Wiggers diagram (**Fig. 13.1**). The timing of mechanical events, such as contraction and relaxation, and the generation of transvalvular and ventricular pressure gradients can be obtained from the electrocardiogram (ECG) matched to the corresponding pressure waveform. Each electrical event (eg, P wave, QRS, T wave) is followed normally by a mechanical function (either contraction or relaxation), resulting in a specific pressure wave.

While the ECG "P" wave correlates with the beginning of atrial contraction, the QRS with ventricular activation, and the "T" wave with ventricular relaxation, the normal sequence of contraction and relaxation of the heart muscle is disturbed by arrhythmias and conduction defects. Normal cardiac function may become inefficient or ineffective, as can be demonstrated with associated hemodynamic alterations.

NORMAL PRESSURE WAVE FORMS

Beginning the cardiac cycle, the P wave signals and initiates atrial contraction. Atrial systole and diastole are denoted as the "a" wave (**Fig. 13.1**, point a), followed by the "x" descent, respectively. The P wave, and the "A/x" pressures, is followed by the QRS, signaling depolarization of the ventricles (point b). The left ventricular (LV) pressure after the "a" wave is the end diastolic pressure, also known as LVEDP, and corresponds to the R wave (vertical line) intersection with the LV pressure (point b). About 15 to 30 ms after the QRS, the ventricles contract, the LV (and right ventricular [RV]) pressure increases rapidly during the isovolumetric contraction period (interval b-c). When LV pressure rises above aortic pressure, the aortic valve (AV) opens (point c). Systolic ejection continues until repolarization, signaled by the T wave (point d). After the T wave, the LV relaxation produces a fall in the LV and aortic pressure. When the LV pressure falls below the aortic pressures, the AV closes (point e). The ventricular pressure continues to fall, and when it falls below the left atrial (LA) pressure, the mitral valve (MV) opens and the LA empties into the LV (point f).

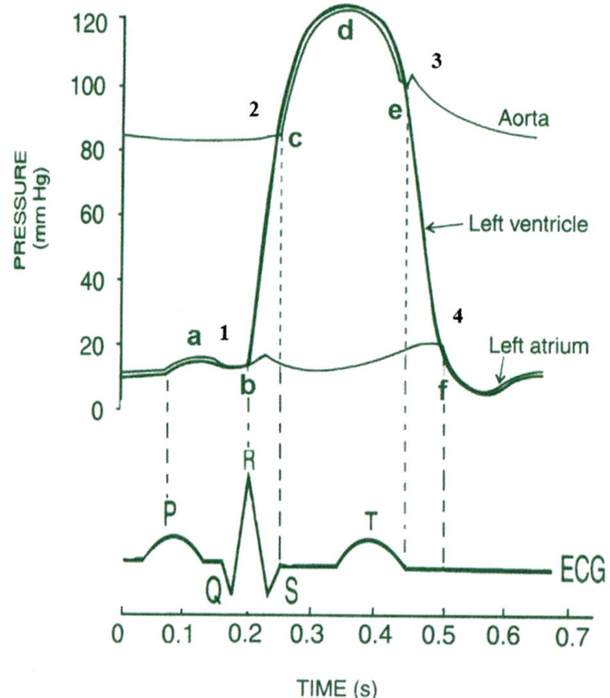

FIGURE 13.1 The Wiggers diagram. Pressure curves of the left atrium and left ventricle are superimposed with the corresponding portions of the electrocardiogram at the bottom. Points 1, 2, 3, and 4 represent the closure of the AV valves; 2 the opening of the semilunar valves (aortic in this case); 3 the closure of the aortic valve; 4 the opening of the AV (mitral valve). AV, aortic valve.

Returning to the atrial pressure wave across the cycle, after the "a" wave, atrial pressure slowly rises, with atrial filling during systole, continuing to increase until the end of systole when the pressure and volume of the LA are nearly maximal, producing a ventricular filling wave: the "v" wave. The "v" wave peak (point 4) is followed by a rapid fall, labeled "Y" descent, when the MV opens. The peaks and troughs of the atrial pressure waves are changed by pathologic conditions such as acute valvular regurgitation, heart failure, and infarction.

RIGHT HEMODYNAMICS

The normal right atrial (RA) and pulmonary capillary wedge (PCW) pressure wave forms are shown in **Fig. 13.2**. RA pressure normally decreases with intrathoracic pressure during spontaneous inspiration (**Fig. 13.3**, top). Nevertheless, in patients with congestive heart failure or other conditions impairing venous return to the right side of the heart (eg, pericardial constriction), RA pressure during

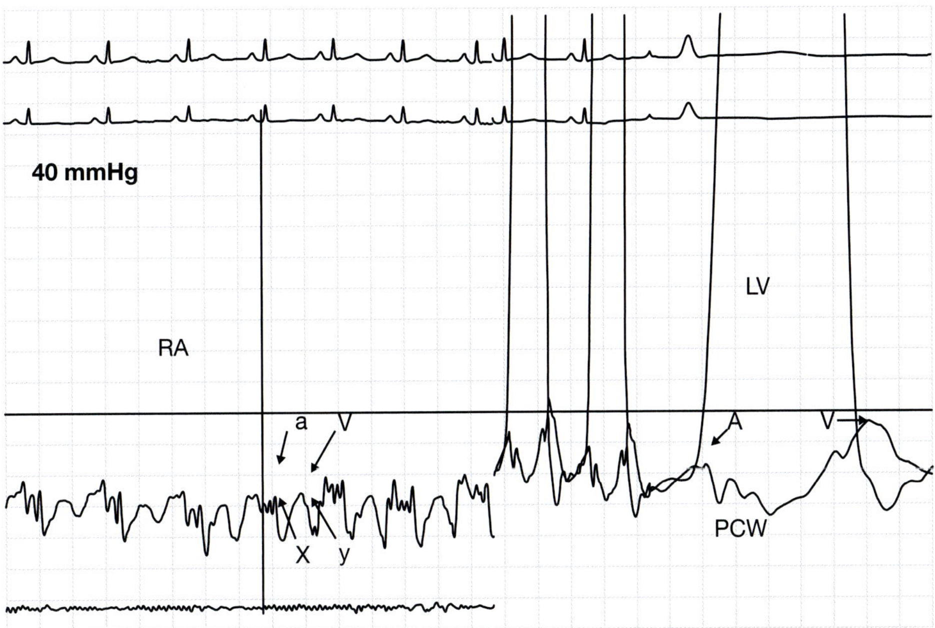

FIGURE 13.2 Normal RA (*left*) and PCW with LV pressure waveforms (*right*) demonstrate the "a" wave of LV pressure (a) and the "a" wave delayed of pulmonary capillary wedge (PCW) pressure ("a") and "v" wave of the PCW pressure (v) noted by large arrows. Normal RA pressures show typical "a" and "v" waves with corresponding "x" and "y" descents. LV, left ventricle, 0 to 40 mm Hg scale.

inspiration may fail to decrease, or might even increase during inspiration (**Fig. 13.3**, Kussmaul sign), reflecting impaired filling of the RV and elevated pressures. **Fig. 13.4** shows rapid "Y" descents during inspiration, with no change in mean RA pressure.

Pressure waves in the atria are a function of the pressure/flow relationship or compliance of the chamber. A poorly compliant chamber (ie, stiff) may demonstrate a large "v" wave despite normal flow, while a very compliant chamber may not register marked pressure wave changes despite torrential flow. A low-compliance LA can be seen by the pressure waves in a patient with mitral stenosis (MS). **Fig. 13.5** shows LA and RA pressures together. The high LA pressure is due to both MS and a stiff left atrium after rheumatic inflammation. The LA pressure waveform also has a marked "v" wave, which is due not to regurgitation but to the poor compliance of the atrium. In this example, atrial fibrillation is present, showing a lack of "a" waves and the presence of a "c" notch preceding the large "v" wave, demonstrating how arrhythmias may distort atrial and ventricular waveforms.

Normal RA waveforms have smaller "a" and "v" waves than the left atrium, but these become distorted in the setting of significant valve dysfunction. In patients with tricuspid regurgitation, the RA wave loses its characteristic "a" and "v" waves, which are replaced by a large and broad "s" (systolic) wave of blood reflux from the RV back into the LV. **Fig. 13.6** shows the RA waveform of a 67-year-old woman with dyspnea at rest, with systolic murmur, which varies with respiration. In **Fig. 13.7A**, note the corresponding pattern of RV and RA in a patient with severe tricuspid regurgitation. The RV angiogram of this patient is shown in **Fig. 13.7B**.

FUNDAMENTAL OBSERVATIONS OF PRESSURE-VOLUME LOOPS

Pressure-Volume Relationships

Cardiac ventricular hemodynamics can be represented by a pressure-volume (PV) loop, which plots the changes of these variables over a cardiac cycle.[6-8] The shape of the PV loop is specific for the ventricle/arterial circuit coupling. The PV loop (**Fig. 13.8**) for the left ventricle/aorta is different from the PV loop for the right ventricle/pulmonary artery (PA), but each represents one cardiac cycle. Beginning at end-diastole (point a), LV volume has received the atrial contribution and is maximal. Isovolemic contraction ("a"-"b") increases LV pressure, with no change in volume. At the end of isovolemic contraction, LV pressure exceeds aortic pressure, the AV opens, and blood is ejected from the LV into the aorta (point b). Over the systolic ejection phase, LV volume decreases, and as ventricular repolarization occurs, LV ejection ceases and relaxation begins. When LV pressure falls below aortic pressure, the AV closes, a point also known as the end-systolic pressure-volume point (ESPV) (point c). Isovolemic relaxation occurs until LV pressure decreases below the atrial pressure, opening the MV (point d).

The stroke volume (SV) is represented by the width of the PV loop, the difference between end-systolic and end-diastolic volumes. The area within the loop represents stroke work. Load-independent LV contractility, also known as E_{max}, is defined as the maximal slope of the ESPV points under various loading conditions; the line of these points is the ESPV relationship. Effective arterial elastance (E_a), a measure of LV afterload, is defined as the ratio of end-systolic pressure to SV. Under steady-state conditions, optimal LV contractile efficiency occurs when the ratio of E_a:E_{max} approaches 1.

The PV loop describes contractile function, relaxation properties, SV, cardiac work, and myocardial oxygen consumption. Hemodynamic alterations and interventions change the PV relationship in predictable ways, and comparisons of various hemodynamic interventions can be made more precisely by examining the PV loop (**Figs. 13.9** and **13.10**).

Acute changes in cardiac function, such as might occur with acute myocardial infarction, are also easily demonstrated (**Fig. 13.11**). In acute myocardial infarction, LV contractility (E_{max}) is reduced; LV pressure and SV and LV stroke work may be unchanged or reduced; and LVEDP is increased. In cardiogenic

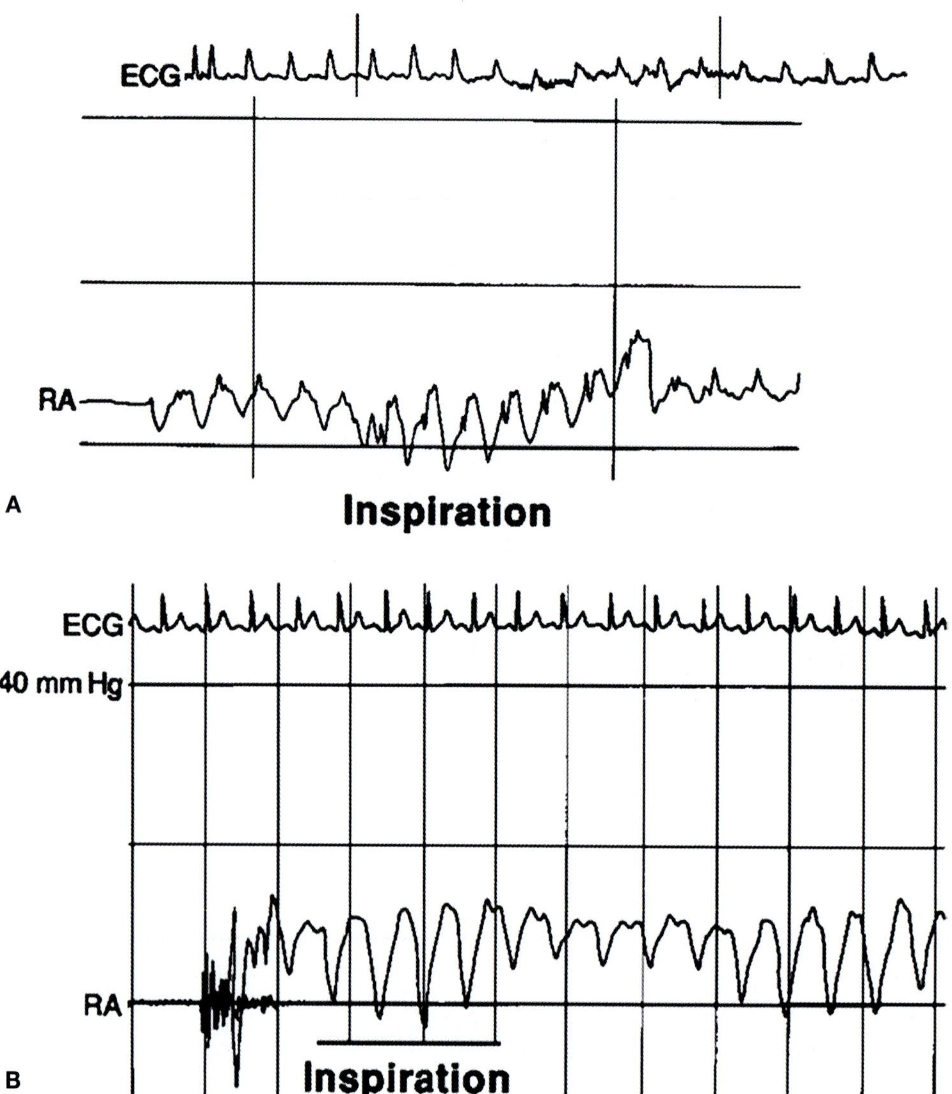

FIGURE 13.3 **A:** Right atrial (RA) pressure during inspiration. Note the fall in pressure as the negative intrathoracic pressure is transmitted to RA. **B:** RA pressure in patient with congestive heart failure showing failure to decrease with inspiration (Kussmaul sign).

shock, E_{max} is severely reduced, LV afterload (E_a) may be increased, LV end-diastolic volume (LVEDV) and LVEDP are increased, and SV is reduced, findings easily seen to display reduced LV contractile function, acute diastolic dysfunction, elevated LVEDV and LVEDP, and increased LV work (oxygen demand). In more severe cases of myocardial infarction that evolve into cardiogenic shock, LV contractile function is more severely reduced with associated significant increases in end-diastolic P and V. The LV impairment results in a markedly reduced SV, with an increased myocardial oxygen demand.

The most common applications of PV loops characterize only LV hemodynamics. For research into RV function or extracardiac problems, the standard PV loops become complex and affected by the unique factors altering the right-sided PV loop configuration. Interpretation of this is beyond the scope of this review.

Intracardiac Shunts

Blood moves across atrial, ventricular, and other anatomic communications due to differences in pressure over the cardiac cycle. For the most common shunt, the atrial septal defects (ASDs), the pressure changes across the atrial septum determine the flow across the shunt.

The LA pressure is typically lower than RA pressure until after birth when the lungs expand with air and the RV flow raises the LA pressure and closes the patent foramen ovale. Immediately after birth, the right atrium and right ventricle see the lower resistance of the pulmonary circuit, compared with the left atrium and ventricle, which receive more blood and also must pump across the higher resistance of the systemic circulation. This relationship is evident in a patient with aortic stenosis (AS) in whom transseptal LA to RA pressure pullback can be recorded showing large LA "v" waves compared with the lower RA pressure with much

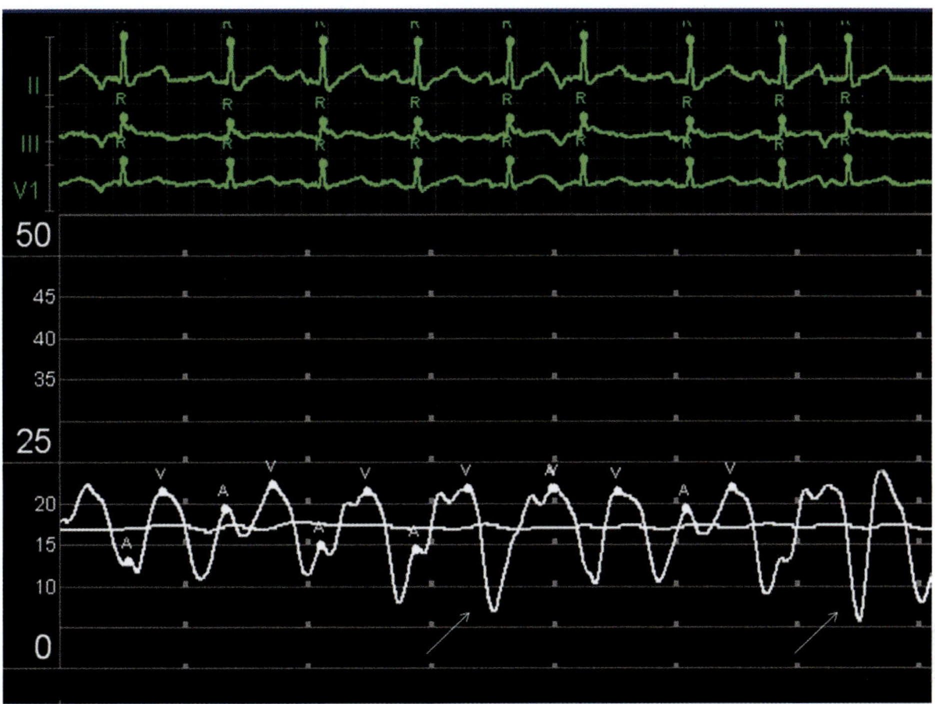

FIGURE 13.4 Right atrial (RA) pressure during inspiration in patient with CHF. The failure to decrease RA pressure during inspiration is Kussmaul sign. Note exaggeration of "v" waves during inspiration. CHF, congestive heart failure.

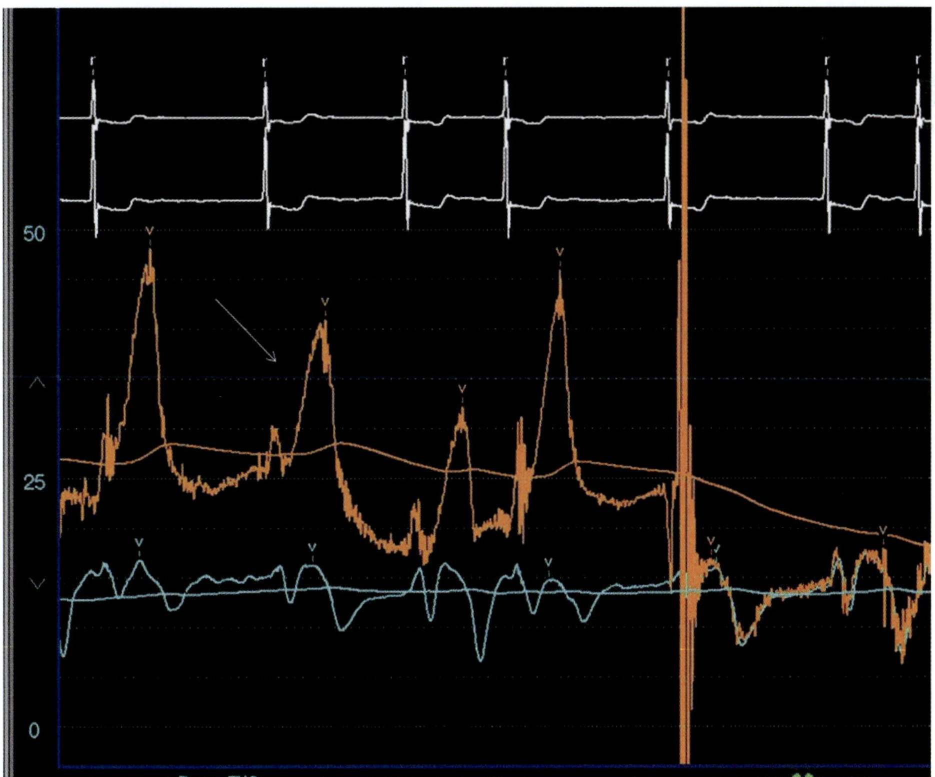

FIGURE 13.5 Left atrial (*orange*) and right atrial (*blue*) pressure tracings during pullback from the LA to the RA in a patient with mitral stenosis. Note the significantly higher LA pressure and large "v" waves (*arrow*). In the absence of mitral regurgitation, large "v" waves are a measure of LV compliance. After pulling back across the intra-atrial septum (vertical line artifact), the pressure wave from the LA matches the RA. Note the effect of the cardiac rhythm distorting the atrial waveforms. LA, left atrial; LV, left ventricular; RA, right atrial.

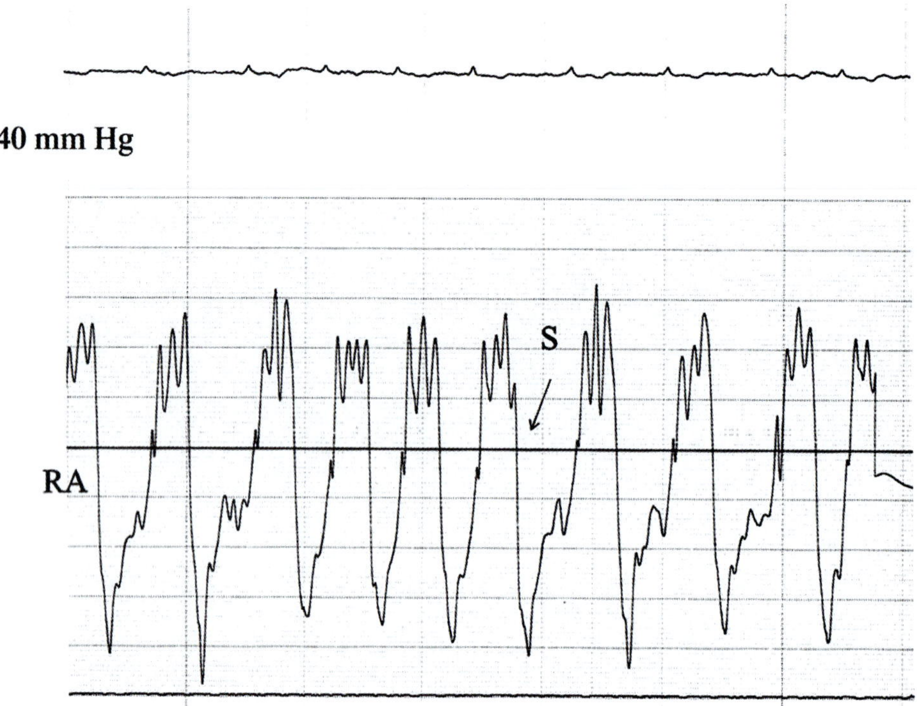

FIGURE 13.6 Right atrial (RA) waveform of a 67-year-old woman with dyspnea at rest and systolic murmur that varies with respiration. S, regurgitant wave.

reduced "a" and "v" waves (**Fig. 13.7**). Nevertheless, in certain situations, especially during the Valsalva maneuver, the RA pressure can transiently increase above the LA pressure, which in the presence of a patent foramen ovale (PFO) produces right-to-left shunting and possible transit of emboli-producing clinical sequelae.

Intracardiac Shunts: Atrial Septal Defects

Percutaneous closure of ASD and PFO are performed routinely in many laboratories by experienced operators. PFOs may be closed out of concern for paradoxical embolism, while ASDs are generally closed due to excessive volume loading of the right side of the heart. Measurement of atrial hemoglobin oxygen saturations enables precise quantification of the severity of interatrial shunting and is the gold standard for defining which ASDs require closure. Oxygen saturations from multiple locations are obtained during a diagnostic "saturation run" in a rapid but systematic manner. A standard balloon-tipped Swan-Ganz-type catheter is satisfactory, but a large-bore end-hole or side-hole (multipurpose) catheter performs better rapid sampling, particularly from left-sided structures. A left-to-right shunt is suggested when an oxygen step-up, or increase in oxygen content, in a chamber or vessel exceeds that of a proximal compartment. A step-up in oxygen saturation at the PA by more than 7% above the RA saturation is indicative of a significant left-to-right shunt at the atrial level. Similarly, the desaturation of arterial blood samples from the left-sided heart chambers and aorta suggests a right-to-left shunt. In determining the site of the right-to-left shunt, sequential samples from the pulmonary veins, LA, LV, and aorta can be easily obtained when an interatrial septal defect is present.

Mixed venous oxygen saturation can be assumed to be fully mixed PA blood in the absence of a shunt. If there is a left-to-right shunt, mixed venous blood is measured one chamber proximal to the step-up. In the case of an atrial septal defect, the mixed venous oxygen content is computed from the weighted average of vena caval blood (ie, as the sum of three times the superior vena cava plus one inferior vena the sum averaged divided by four). When pulmonary venous blood is not collected, PVO_2 (pulmonary vein) percentage saturation is assumed to be 95%.

Shunt Calculation

The Fick or left-sided indicator dilution methods of CO determination are employed to measure systemic flow. Using the Fick method, the following formulas apply:

1. Systemic flow

$$Q_s\,(L/\min) = \frac{O_2\ con\sup mtion\,(mL/\min)}{(arterial - mixed\ venous)\,O_2\ content}$$

2. Pulmonary flow

$$Q_P\,(L/\min) = \frac{O_2\ consumption\,(mL/\min)}{(pulmonary\ venous - pulmonary\ arterial)\,O_2\ content}$$

3. The effective pulmonary blood flow (EPB)

$$Q_{EPB} = \frac{Q_2\ consumption\,(mL/\min)}{(pulmonary\ venous - mixed\ venous)\,O_2\ content}$$

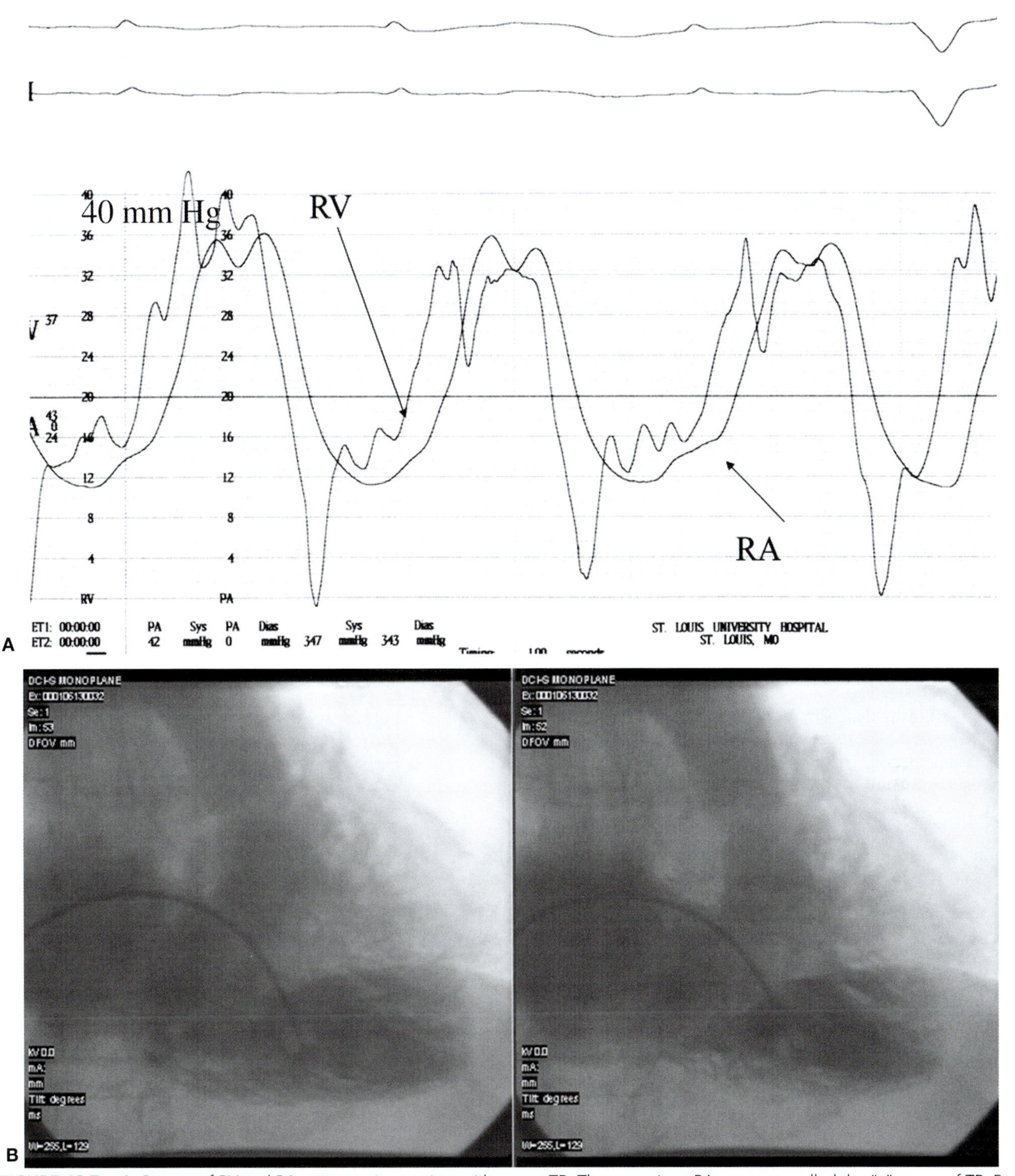

FIGURE 13.7 **A:** Pattern of RV and RA pressures in a patient with severe TR. The regurgitant RA waves are called the "s" waves of TR. Pressure scale 0 to 40 mm Hg. **B:** Cineangiographic frames from right ventriculography showing severe tricuspid regurgitation with reflux of contrast medium into the right atrium. RA, right atrial; RV, right ventricular; TR, tricuspid regurgitation.

Normally, the effective pulmonary blood flow is equal to the systemic blood flow. In a left-to-right shunt, the effective pulmonary blood flow is increased (by the amount of the shunt) as follows:

$$Q_{EPB} = \text{systemic flow} + \text{shunt flow}, (\text{left-toright}) \quad (13.1)$$

In a right-to-left shunt, the effective pulmonary blood flow is decreased (by the amount of the shunt):

$$Q_{EPB} = \text{systemic flow} - \text{shunt flow}, (\text{right-to-left}) \quad (13.2)$$

The shunt volume is determined by use of Equations (13.1) and (13.2). Intracardiac shunt calculations are summarized in **Figs. 13.12-13.14**. The ratio of pulmonary to systemic flow (called Q_p/Q_s) for a left-to-right shunt is called the shunt fraction. A $Q_p/Q_s > 1.5$ is considered the threshold shunt fraction that makes closure indicated.

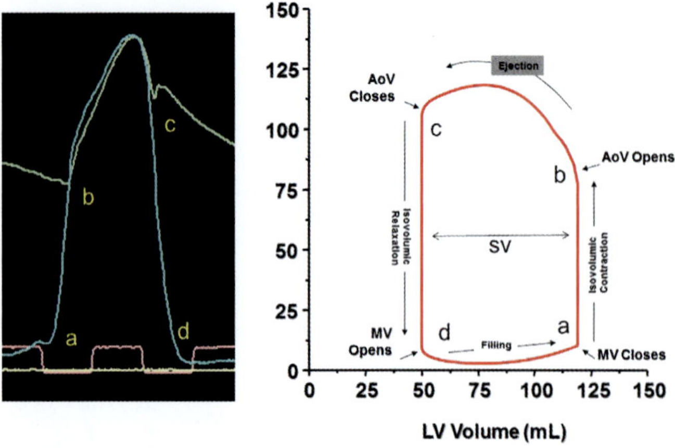

FIGURE 13.8 The pressure-volume (PV) loop characterizes the changes in pressure flow over the course of one cardiac cycle. *Left*, the left ventricular and aortic pressure as measured during cardiac catheterization. *Right*, the pressure-volume loop derived from the hemodynamics of LV pressure and volume. Point a, left ventricular end-diastolic pressure is followed by isovolumetric contraction ending at point b, the aortic valve opening. Ejection continues until the repolarization of the LV produces a fall in LV ejection. LV pressure falls past point c, aortic valve closure, and continues to fall along the line of isovolumetric relaxation to point d, mitral valve opening. Changes in the shape of the pressure-volume loop demonstrate changes in contractility, cardiac output. LV, left ventricular; SV, stroke volume.

Aortic Stenosis

Before reviewing hemodynamics of AS, examine the normal LV and aortic pressure obtained with a micromanometer dual transducer catheter shows nearly ideal waveforms of aortic and LV pressure (**Fig. 13.15**). As an aside, also note the normal LV filling pattern over the diastolic period. The normal LV pressure has an anachronism shoulder and a normal small impulse outflow tract gradient (red arrow). The pressure tracings most commonly used in clinical practice are acquired with electronic transducers and fluid-filled catheters such as the 5F pigtail catheter and 6F femoral artery (FA) sheath side arm (right side, **Fig. 13.15**). Note the resonant artifact (whip, fling, or ringing) compared with the high-fidelity tracings. It should be recalled that the FA pressure is not only higher due to resonant signal amplification but also delayed in time as the wave travels from the aortic location to the FA location. This is a normal finding of all peripheral pressures compared with central aortic pressures.

The hemodynamic assessment of AS and the subsequent success of valve therapies begin with accurate transvalvular gradient and cardiac output measurements. Many clinical catheterization laboratory measurements use the FA to represent aortic pressure. Owing to resonance and peripheral pressure amplification, the FA systolic pressure is higher and delayed relative to the central aortic pressure, which artefactually decreases the mean gradient relative to the LV. When using femoral pressure, precise pressure gradients cannot be obtained in patients with peripheral vascular disease at

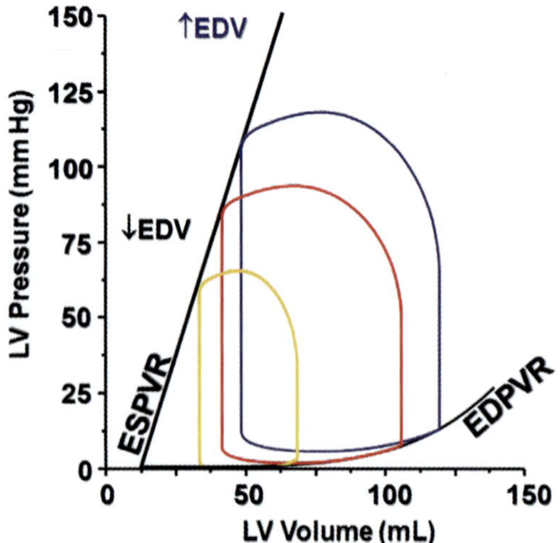

FIGURE 13.9 Effect of changes in left ventricular preload. Increasing the left ventricular end-diastolic pressure along the line of the end-diastolic pressure-volume relationship (EDPVR). As volume is increased, left ventricular end-diastole, stroke volume, and aortic pressure increase. EDV, end-diastolic volume; ESPVR, end-systolic pressure-volume relationship. (Courtesy of Dr. Dan Burkhoff, Columbia University, New York, NY.)

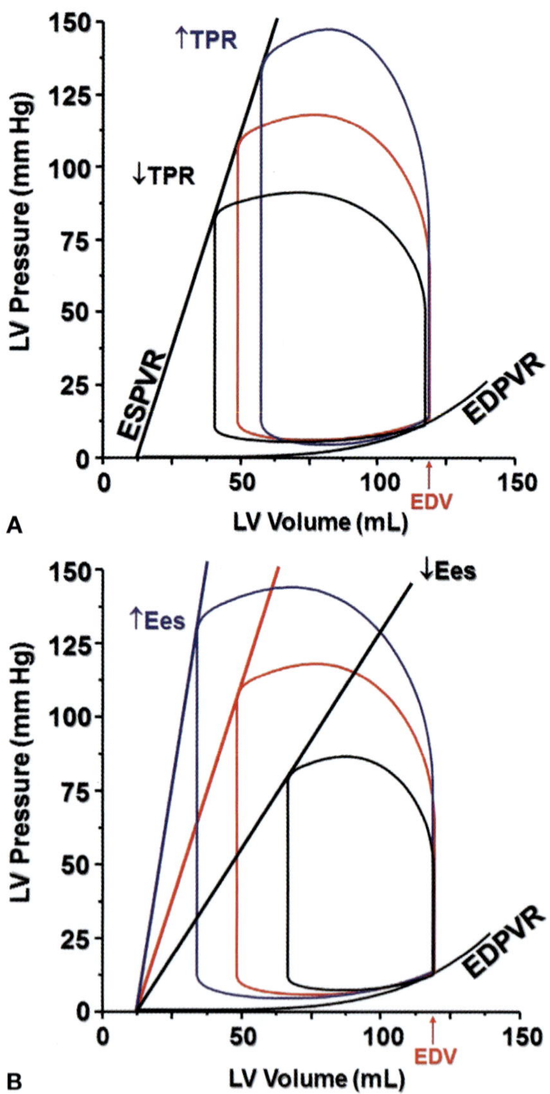

FIGURE 13.10 **A:** The effects of increasing afterload or total peripheral vascular resistance (TPR) decreases stroke volume (SV), increases aortic pressure, and minimally modifies LVEDP. **B:** The effect of increasing contractility. The increasing slope of the line of Ees increases SV, aortic pressure, with minimal effect on LVEDP. EDPVR, end-diastolic pressure-volume relationship; EDV, end-diastolic volume; Ees, end-systolic elastance; ESPVR, end-systolic pressure-volume relationship; LV, left ventricular; LVEDP, left ventricular end-diastolic pressure. (**A and B:** Courtesy of Dr. Dan Burkhoff, Columbia University, New York, NY.)

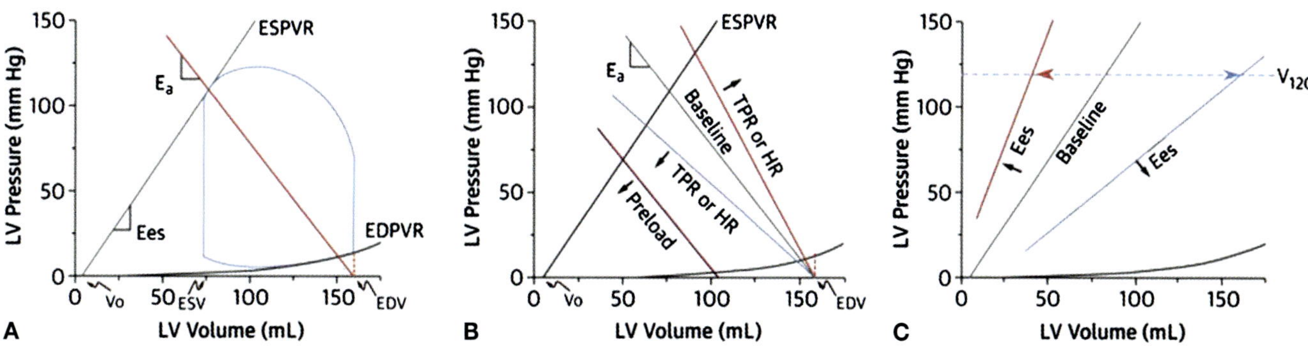

FIGURE 13.11 Overview of pressure-volume loops (PVLs) and relations.[9] **A:** Normal PVL, is bounded by the end-systolic pressure-volume relationship (ESPVR) and end-diastolic pressure-volume relationship (EDPVR). ESPVR is approximately linear with slope end-systolic elastance (Ees) and volume-axis intercept (Vo). Effective arterial elastance (E_a) is the slope of the line extending from the end-diastolic volume (EDV) point on the volume axis through the end-systolic pressure-volume point of the loop. **B:** Slope of the E_a line depends on total peripheral resistance (TPR) and heart rate (HR), and its position depends on EDV. **C:** The ESPVR shifts with changes in ventricular contractility, which can be a combination of changes in Ees and Vo. Changes in contractility can be indexed by V120, the volume at which the ESPVR intersects 120 mm Hg. Load-independent LV contractility also known as E_{max}, is defined as the maximal slope of the end-systolic pressure volume (ESPV) point under various loading conditions, known as the ESPV relationship (ESPVR). Effective arterial elastance (E_a) is a measure of LV afterload and is defined as the ratio of end-systolic pressure and stroke volume. ESV, end-systolic volume; LV, left ventricular. (From: Burkhoff D, Sayer G, Doshi D, Uriel N. Hemodynamics of mechanical circulatory support. *J Am Coll Cardiol*. 2015;66(23):2663.)

the level of the aortic bifurcation or lower. For improved accuracy in measuring the LV-Ao gradient, a double-lumen catheter or two arterial catheters are required.

There is considerable new information on the mechanisms of AS and its hemodynamic manifestations. Pibarot and Dumesnil[10] reviewed critical characteristics of blood flow and pressure across the AV (**Fig. 13.16**). The ejection of blood from the LV is forced through the fixed reduced aortic orifice area (ie, the anatomic orifice area). Energy is lost due to resistance (ie, a portion of the potential energy of the blood pressure), resulting in a pressure drop and acceleration of flow. After crossing the AV (ie, the effective orifice area), part of the kinetic energy is reconverted back to potential energy and the pressure increases (also called the "pressure recovery"). Doppler echocardiography measures the peak instantaneous gradient across the entire outflow tract and aorta and is thus able to capture this phenomenon of pressure recovery. Catheter-based measurements of aortic pressure are typically several centimeters distal in the aorta after pressure recovery has already occurred. There are several specialized measures of the relationship between hemodynamic load and arterial resistance or impedance to flow. The global hemodynamic load imposed on the left ventricle results from the summation of the valvular load and the arterial load. These subjects are addressed in detail elsewhere.[10-14]

In simple terms, AS is characterized by a delayed upslope of aortic pressure and a large LV-aortic pressure gradient (**Fig. 13.17**). The mean pressure gradient is the area between the aortic (Ao) and LV pressure tracings during systolic ejection. To quickly assess the significance of the LV-Ao pressure gradient, operators frequently use the peak-to-peak LV and aortic pressure difference.[15]

SVC/IVC to RA	*min 7%*	*ASD/PAPVR*
RA to RV	*min 5%*	*VSD*
RV to PA	*min 5%*	*PDA*
Any (SVC to PA)	*min 7%*	*Anywhere*

FIGURE 13.12 Intracardiac shunt calculations. ASD, atrial septal defect; IVC, inferior vena cava; PA, pulmonary artery; PDA, posterior descending artery; RA, right atrial; RV, right ventricular; SVC, superior vena cava; VSD, ventricular septal defect.

The peak-to-peak gradient is not equivalent to the mean gradient for mild and moderate stenosis but is often close to the mean gradient for severe stenosis. The peak-to-peak gradient should not be confused with the peak instantaneous gradient. Because of pressure recovery, catheter-based measurements of the peak instantaneous gradient are often lower than echocardiographic measurements.

When using the FA pressure, more accurate valve areas are obtained with unshifted LV-Ao pressure tracings (**Fig. 13.17**, right side), as the delay in FA pressure partially corrects for the effects of peripheral amplification. If the FA pressure is shifted back to match the upstroke of the LV, femoral pressure overshoot (amplification) reduces the true gradient. For the highest accuracy, pressures should be measured immediately above and below the AV with a dual-lumen catheter or two catheters, especially for patients with low cardiac output and a low transvalvular gradient.

Valve Area Calculations

Stenotic valve areas are calculated from pressure tracings and cardiac output.[16] Cardiac outputs are measured by thermodilution or from the Fick calculation. The Fick calculation uses either assumed oxygen consumption (3 mL/kg O_2 or 125 mL/min/m^2) or, for best accuracy, direct oxygen consumption with a metabolic oximeter.

The Gorlin formula (10) can be applied to both aortic and MVs:

$$\text{vlave area}\left(\text{cm}^2\right) = \frac{\text{value flow}\left(\text{mL/s}\right)}{\text{K}\times\text{C}\times\sqrt{\text{MVG}}},$$

where MVG is mean valvular gradient (mm Hg), K (44.3) is a derived constant by Gorlin and Gorlin, C is an empirical constant that is 1 for semilunar valves and tricuspid valves and 0.85 for MVs, and valve flow is measured in milliliters per second during the diastolic or systolic flow period. For MV flow, the diastolic filling period is used:

$$\frac{CO(mL/\text{min})}{(\textit{diastolic filling period})(HR)}$$

For AV flow, the systolic ejection period (SEP) is used:

$$\frac{CO(mL/\text{min})}{(\textit{systolic ejection period})(HR)}$$

Quick Method to Calculate Severity of Left-to-Right Shunt (Qp/Qs) Using Only Oxygen Saturation Values

$$\frac{PBF}{SBF} = \frac{\dfrac{O_2\ Consumption}{PV(\%)-PA(\%)}}{\dfrac{O_2\ Consumption}{AO(\%)-MV(\%)}} = \frac{AO-MV}{PV-PA}$$

Example:

MV=60%
PA=80%
PV=95%
AO=95%

$$\frac{95-60}{95-80} = \frac{35}{15} = 2.33$$

FIGURE 13.13 Left-to-right shunt calculations. AO, aorta; MV, mitral valve; PA, pulmonary artery; PBF, pulmonary blood flow; PV, pressure volume; SBF, systemic blood flow.

where SEP (s/min) = systolic period (s/beat) × HR. Computerized hemodynamic systems are generally used to perform these measurements and calculations.

A simplified formula (also known as the Hakke formula [10]) can provide a quick in-laboratory determination of AV area, estimated as:

Quick valve area = $CO/\sqrt{LV}$ ›aortic peak›to›peak pressure difference.

For example, peak-to-peak gradient = 65 mm Hg, CO = 5 L/min

$$\text{Quick valve area} = \frac{5L/min}{\sqrt{65}} = \frac{5L/min}{8} = 0.63cm^2$$

The quick formula differs from the Gorlin formula by 18% ± 13% in patients with bradycardia (<65 beats/min) or tachycardia (>100 beats/min). The Gorlin equation overestimates the severity of valve stenosis in low-flow states.

Hemodynamics of Transcatheter Aortic Valve Replacement

Hemodynamic measurements before and after transcatheter aortic valve replacement (TAVR) may demonstrate the effectiveness of the implant and also identify valvular regurgitation or LV dysfunction (see the section titled "Aortic Regurgitation" later in this chapter). An example of a patient's hemodynamics before and after TAVR is shown in **Fig. 13.18**. Features denoting successful implantation are the reduction of the LV-Ao gradient (80-0 mm Hg), an increase in aortic systolic pressure (105-122 mm Hg), and the absence of newly widened pulse pressure, which would suggest aortic insufficiency. In addition, after TAVR, there is restoration of a dicrotic notch (**Fig. 13.18**, point d) and anachrotic shoulder (**Fig. 13.18**, point a). The rapidly rising LV diastolic pressure may represent unmasked diastolic dysfunction (**Fig. 13.18**, point dd). The aortic pulse pressure suggests minimal or no aortic insufficiency.

Bidirectional Shunts

- Effective Blood flow:
- $Q_{eff} = O_2$ consumption/(PVO_2-MV O_2)
- Left-to-right shunt: Q_p- Q_{eff}
- Right-to-left shunt: Q_s- Q_{eff}

FIGURE 13.14 Bidirectional shunt calculations.

Aortic Regurgitation

Aortic regurgitation occurs when there is inadequate closure or malcoaptation of the AV leaflets, allowing blood to enter the LV cavity from the aorta during diastole (**Fig. 13.19**). The typical hemodynamics findings of aortic insufficiency include an elevated LV end-diastolic pressure (EDP) (**Fig. 13.19**, arrow), widened aortic pulse pressure (**Fig. 13.19**, arrowheads), and near equalization of LV and aortic EDP.[11] Depending on the extent of the valve leaflet and/or aortic root disruption, some patients may require urgent valve replacement. **Fig. 13.20** shows a patient with mixed aortic stenosis and regurgitation. Note the LV-Ao gradient, wide pulse pressure, and rapid LV diastolic filling slope up to the LVEDP and near equilibration of aortic diastolic pressure with LVEDP. **Fig. 13.21** illustrates the hemodynamics of a paravalvular leak following a TAVR procedure with an increase in LVEDP and the slope of diastolic pressure rise.

Evaluation of Aortic Stenosis in Patients With Low Gradient and Low Ejection Fraction

A continuing dilemma exists in patients with low cardiac output and small aortic-LV gradients (eg, the patient with dyspnea, poor LV function, and a 20-mm-Hg aortic-LV gradient with cardiac output of 3 L/min; AV area = 0.7 cm^2). Should this valve be replaced with a prosthetic valve that has an intrinsic gradient of 10 to 20 mm Hg? Because the Gorlin formula for AV area calculations uses an empiric constant (K) the true valve area may be variable under low-flow conditions.[12]

To assess whether low-gradient/low-flow AS is due to cardiomyopathy or true fixed valve stenosis, a dobutamine challenge is necessary to increase cardiac output and reassess gradients and valve area. **Figs. 13.22** and **13.23** illustrate hemodynamic changes observed under low- and high-flow states. In this example, a

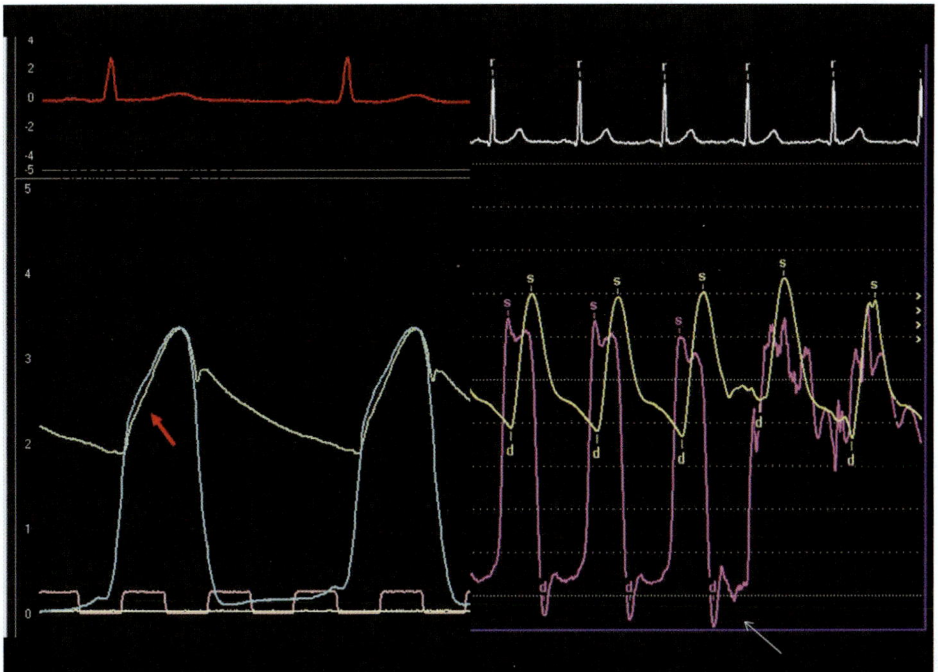

FIGURE 13.15 Normal left ventricular (LV) and aortic pressures. (*Left*) Micromanometer dual transducer pressure catheter with near-ideal wave forms of aortic and left ventricular pressure. *Red arrow* denotes anachrotic shoulder and small normal impulse LV outflow tract gradient. (*Right*) Pressures measured with fluid-filled transducer systems using 5F pigtail catheter through a 6F femoral artery sheath side arm. Note the resonant artifact (fling or ringing, *white arrow*).

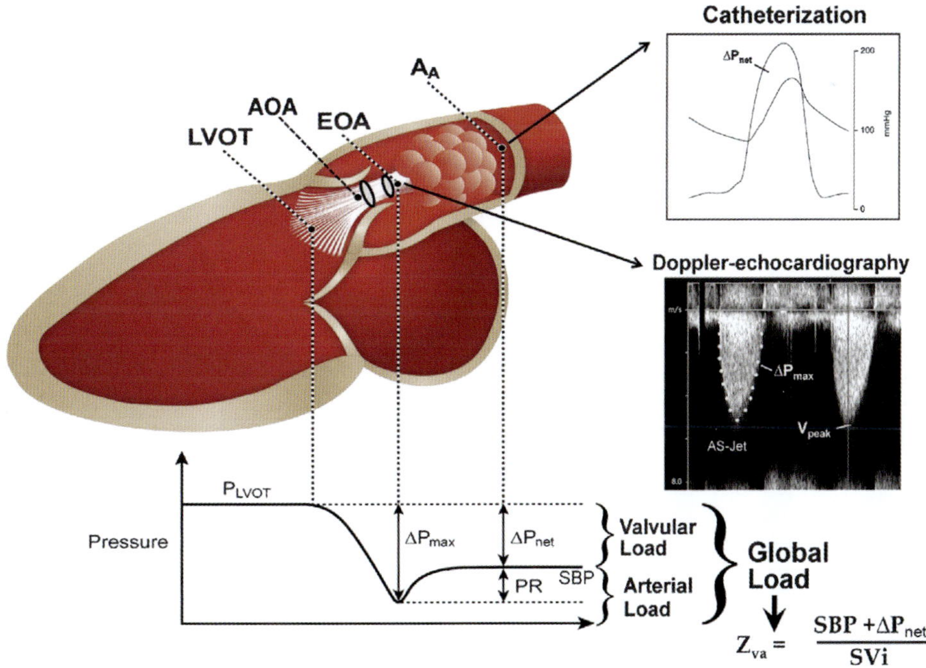

FIGURE 13.16 Pathophysiology of aortic stenosis (AS). Blood flow and pressure across LVOT, aortic valve, and ascending aorta during systole. When the blood flow contracts to pass through a stenotic orifice (ie, the anatomic orifice area [AOA]), a portion of the potential energy of the blood, namely, pressure, is converted into kinetic energy, namely, velocity, thus resulting in a pressure drop and acceleration of flow. Downstream of the vena contracta (ie, the effective orifice area [EOA]), a large part of the kinetic energy is irreversibly dissipated as heat because of flow turbulences. The remaining portion of the kinetic energy that is reconverted back to potential energy is called the "pressure recovery" (PR). The global hemodynamic load imposed on the left ventricle results from the summation of the valvular load and the arterial load. This global load can be estimated by calculating the valvuloarterial impedance. In patients with medium- or large-sized ascending aorta, the impedance can be calculated with the standard Doppler mean gradient in place of the net mean gradient. A_A, cross-sectional area of the aorta at the level of the sinotubular junction; ΔP_{max}, maximum transvalvular pressure gradient recorded at the level of vena contracta (ie, mean gradient measured by Doppler); ΔP_{net}, net transvalvular pressure gradient recorded after pressure recovery (ie, mean gradient measured by catheterization); LVOT, left ventricular outflow tract; P_{LVOT}, pressure in the LVOT; SBP, systolic blood pressure; SVi, stroke volume index; V_{peak}, peak aortic jet velocity; Z_{va}, valvuloarterial impedance. (From: Philippe Pibarot P, Dumesnil JG. Improving assessment of aortic stenosis. *J Am Coll Cardiol*. 2012;60(3):169-180.)

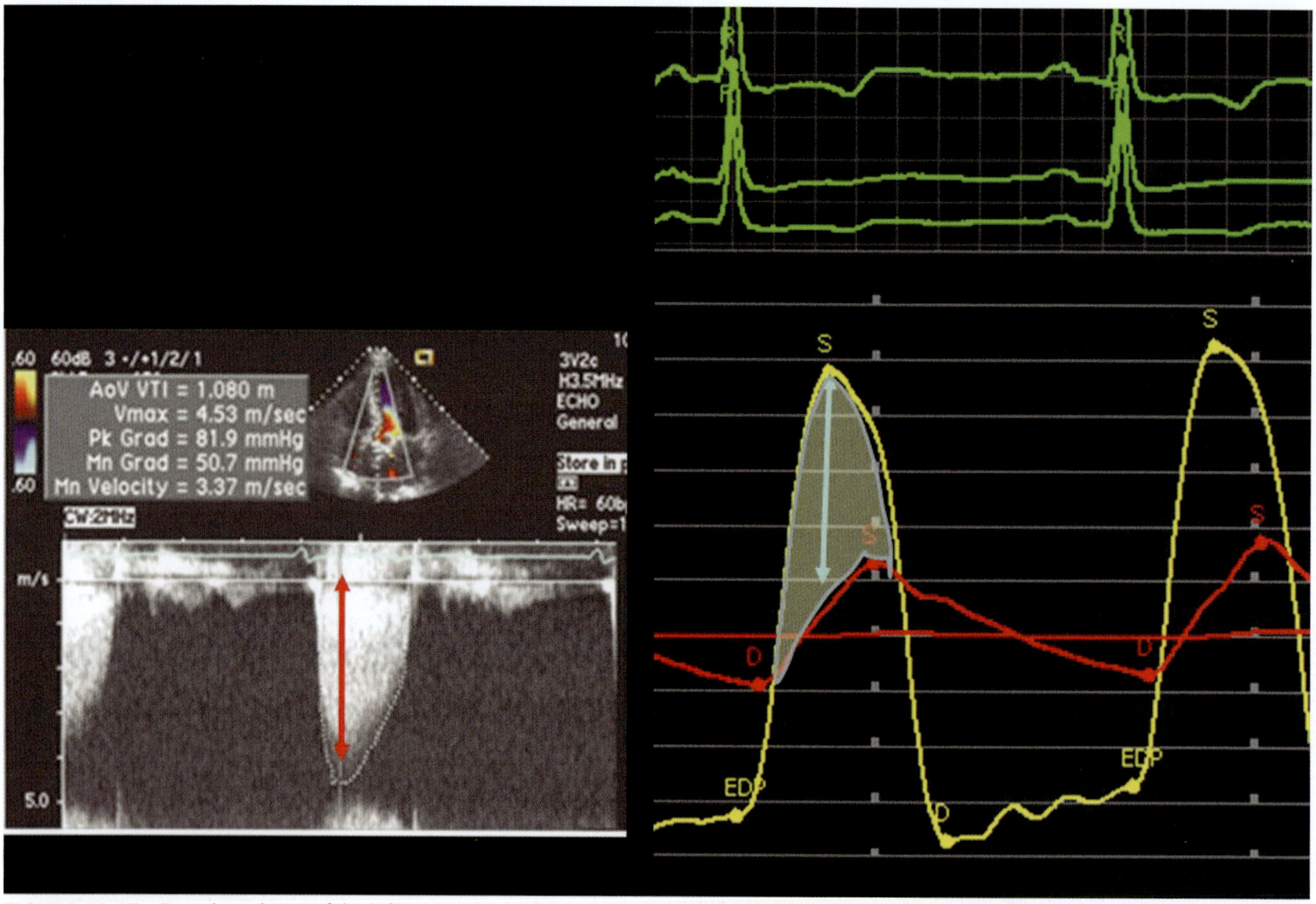

FIGURE 13.17 Doppler velocity of the left ventricular outflow tract in patient with aortic stenosis and corresponding hemodynamic LV-Ao pressure tracings. The peak instantaneous velocity (*red arrow*) is used to compute the transvalvular pressure gradient (4 V^2), which should correspond to the hemodynamic pressure gradient (*shaded area*) in moderate and severe stenosis. This relationship is weaker in some mild to minimal stenoses. EDP, end-diastolic pressure.

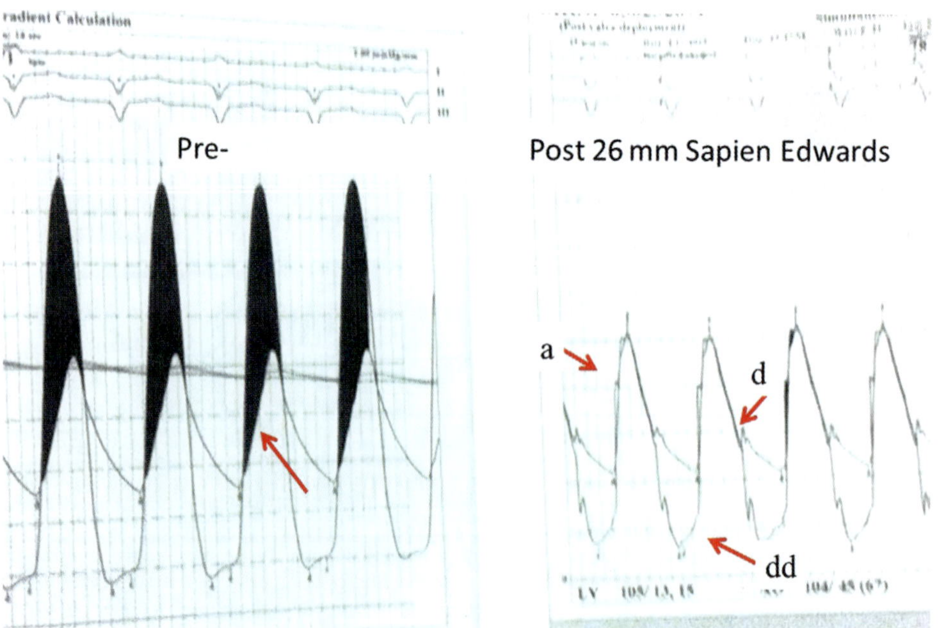

FIGURE 13.18 **Left:** LV-Ao pressure tracings before TAVR show classical delayed aortic pressure upstroke (*arrow*) and large pressure gradient (*black shaded area*), scale is 0 to 200 mm Hg. Aortic valve area was 0.6 cm^2. **Right:** Hemodynamics immediately after TAVR. Note the elimination of the pressure gradients, restoration of a dicrotic notch (d) and anachrotic shoulder (a). The rapidly rising LV diastolic pressure may represent unmasked diastolic dysfunction (dd) or mild aortic insufficiency. The aortic pulse pressure suggests minimal or no aortic insufficiency. LV-Ao, left ventricular and aortic; TAVR, transcatheter aortic valve replacement.

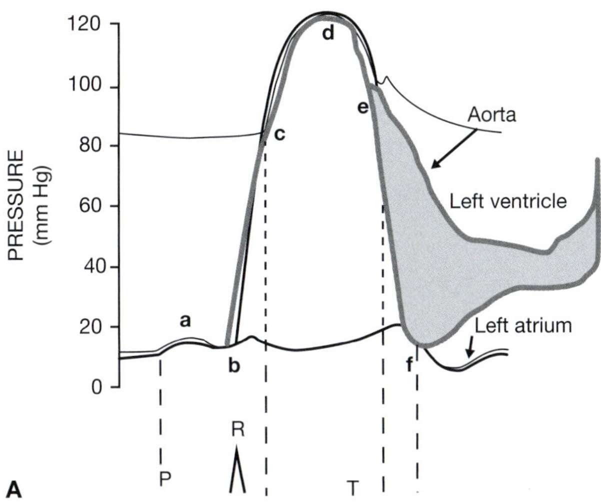

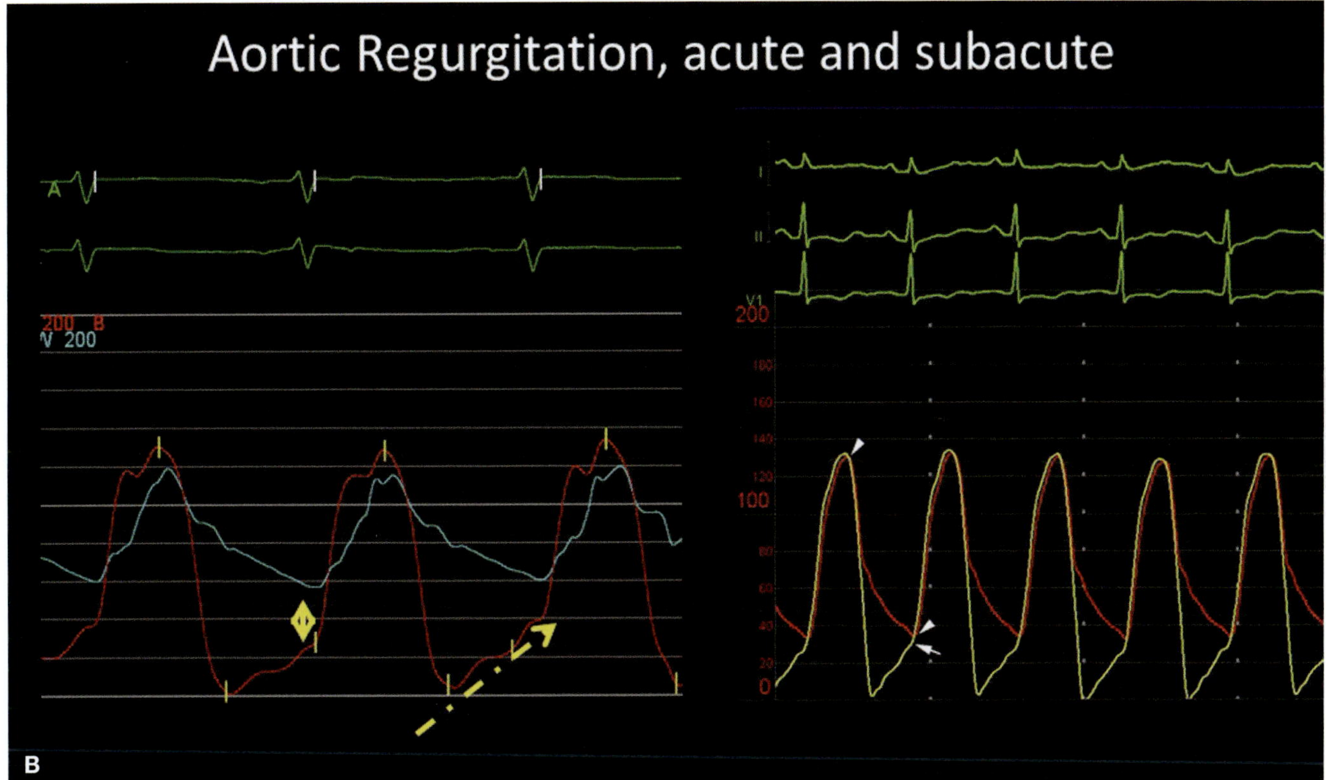

FIGURE 13.19 **A:** Hemodynamics of aortic insufficiency. Important findings include (1) the largest diastolic gradient occurs early; (2) left ventricular (LV) retrograde filling increases LV volume and pressure with rapid increase in LV pressure over diastole, left ventricular end-diastolic pressure (LVEDP) will have rapid upstroke until LV size compensates for increased volume; (3) there is wide aortic pulse pressure. **B:** Hemodynamic tracing showing elevated LV end-diastolic pressure (*arrow*), widened aortic pulse pressure (*arrowheads*), and near equalization of LV and aortic end-diastolic pressures. (From: Ren X, Banki NM. Classic hemodynamic findings of severe aortic regurgitation. *Circulation*. 2012;126:e28-e29.)

62-year-old man undergoes cardiac catheterization for AS. On examination of the hemodynamic tracings (**Fig. 13.22**), there is a LV-Ao gradient of 30 mm Hg with a cardiac output of 3.2 L/min and a calculated AV area of 0.7 mm^2. Dobutamine was then infused (**Fig. 13.22**) at 10 µg/min (with pacing), and then 20 µg/min, with an increased pacing rate of 95 beats/min. The LV-Ao gradient increased to 50 mm Hg, cardiac output of 4.2 L/min, and aortic valve area (AVA) remained fixed at 0.6 cm^2. **Fig. 13.23** shows a plot of the relationship between the mean gradient (y-axis) and the transvalvular flow (x-axis, bottom), according to the Gorlin formula for three different values of AVA (0.7, 1.0, and 1.5 cm^2). Cardiac output (x-axis, top) is also shown, assuming a heart rate of 75 beats/min and an SEP of 300 ms. At low transvalvular flows, the mean gradient is low at all three valve areas. Two different responses to the dobutamine challenge are illustrated for a hypothetical patient with a baseline flow of 150 mL/s, mean gradient of 23 mm Hg, and calculated AVA of 0.7 cm^2. In one scenario (dob 1), flow increases to 225 mL/s, mean gradient increases to 52 mm Hg, and AVA remains 0.7 cm^2, consistent with fixed AS. In the second scenario, flow increases to 275 mL/s, mean gradient increases to

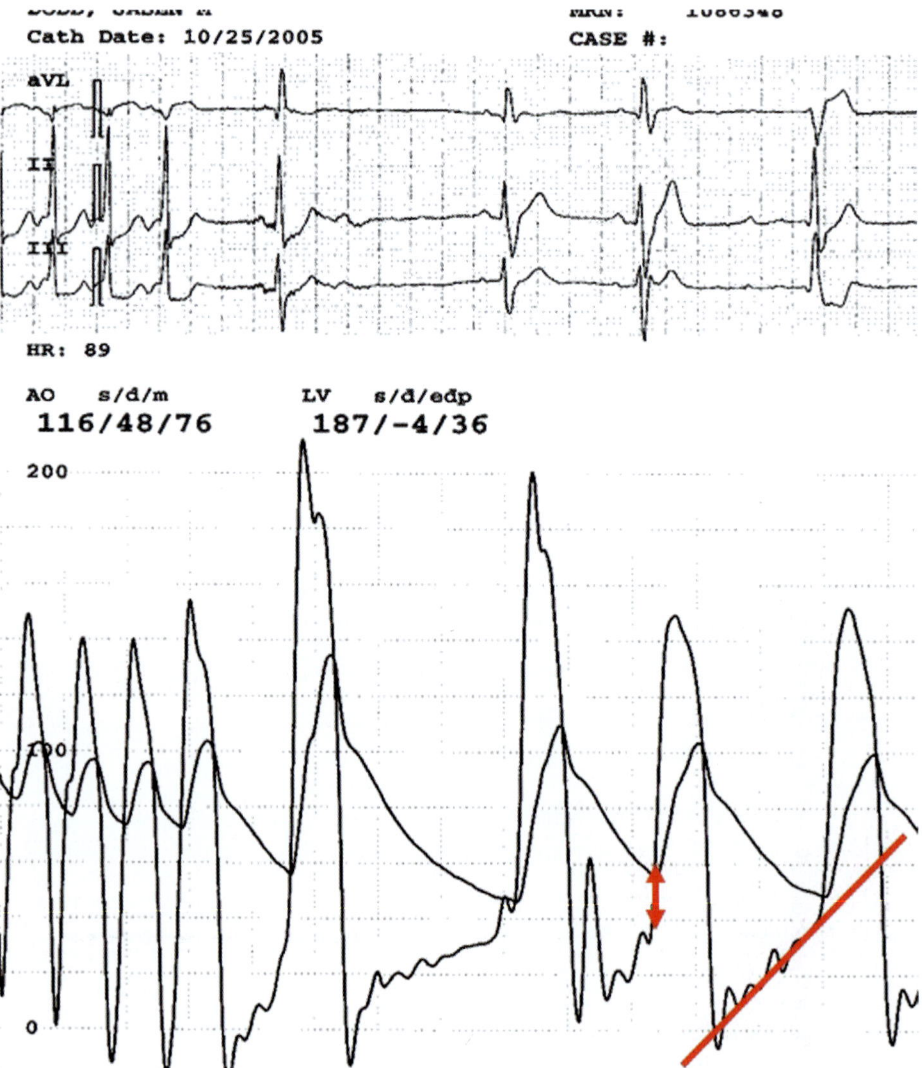

FIGURE 13.20 Hemodynamics of combined mixed AS and AI with LV-Ao systolic gradient and rapidly increasing diastolic LV filling pressure (*diagonal line*), wide pulse pressure, and close approximation of aortic diastolic pressure with LVEDP (*double arrow head*). AI, aortic insufficiency; AS, aortic stenosis; Top, hemodynamics before and after TAVR. LV-Ao, left ventricular and aortic; LVEDP, left ventricular end-diastolic pressure.

38 mm Hg, and AVA increases to 1.0 cm^2. This patient has changed to a different curve, consistent with relative or pseudo-AS. HR indicates heart rate; SEP, systolic ejection period.

Based on the response to dobutamine, aortic valve replacement is therefore appropriate for this patient, despite a low resting gradient and low ejection fraction.

Hypertrophic Obstructive Cardiomyopathy

The hemodynamic evaluation of hypertrophic obstructive cardiomyopathy (HOCM) centers on the degree of left ventricular outflow tract (LVOT) obstruction. LVOT obstruction in hypertrophic cardiomyopathy is dynamic and exquisitely sensitive to ventricular loading conditions and contractility, often producing disparate findings between echocardiographic and invasive measurements, and at different times and under different conditions. The LVOT gradient at rest should be compared with dynamic and provocable gradients (eg, variation with respiration, post–premature ventricular contraction [PVC] accentuation) before committing to alcohol septal ablation.

The assessment of the LVOT gradient is identical to that used for the assessment of AV stenosis. While acceptable in most circumstances, a pigtail catheter with shaft side holes should be replaced by an end hole or HALO (out of plane pigtail) catheter, because pigtail catheters have shaft side holes that may be positioned above the intracavitary obstruction, producing an erroneously low LVOT gradient. A HALO catheter with no shaft side holes is preferred. The most accurate hemodynamic assessment of LVOT obstruction uses a transseptal approach with a balloon-tipped catheter placed at the LV inflow region and a pigtail catheter in the ascending aorta for simultaneous measurement of the LVOT gradient. The transseptal approach helps to avoid catheter entrapment, which can be confused for LV pressure of LVOT obstruction. Use of an 8F Mullins sheath for transseptal access also enables the recording of LA pressure via the sidearm for assessment of concomitant diastolic dysfunction.

A typical HOCM pressure wave form at rest is shown in **Fig. 13.24**. The demonstration of LVOT obstruction, compared with intrinsic AV obstruction, is made by pullback of the LV catheter from apex to base. The large LV-aortic gradient disappears

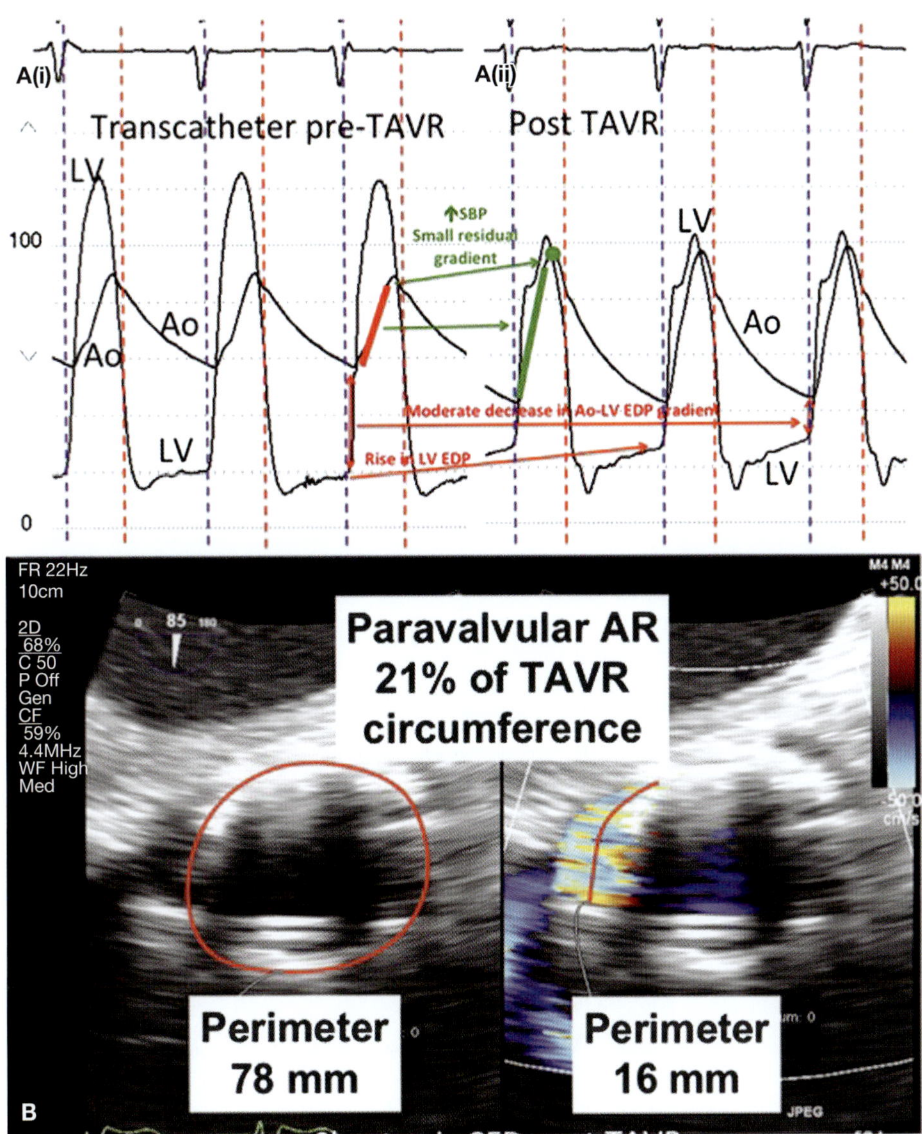

FIGURE 13.21 An illustration of the hemodynamics of a paravalvular leak following a TAVR procedure with an increase in LVEDP and the slope of a diastolic pressure rise. *Lower panel* shows echocardiographic images of Doppler paravalvular leakage. AR, paravalvular aortic regurgitation; LVEDP, left ventricular end-diastolic pressure; TAVR, transcatheter aortic valve replacement. (Courtesy of Dr. Raj Makkar.)

when the catheter is positioned just above the midcavity obstruction (**Fig. 13.24**).

Because of the dynamic nature of HOCM obstruction and its sensitivity to loading conditions, the hemodynamic recordings during a PVC can unmask the pathophysiology. The post-PVC hemodynamic tracings in a patient with HOCM (**Fig. 13.25**) is associated with three distinct features: (1) the rapid upstroke of aortic pressure, (2) a narrow aortic pulse pressure, and (3) a spike and dome configuration of early vigorous LV ejection, followed by delay in ejection of the remaining LV volume, with the resulting outflow gradient. Another method to demonstrate the severity of LVOT obstruction in patients with HOCM is to perform a Valsalva maneuver. At the beginning of the Valsalva strain phase, there is an increase in LVEDP and reduced arterial pulse pressure. The LVOT gradient begins to appear. It is most pronounced during the plateau phase and may be dramatic during a PVC in this setting.

Both AS and HOCM are associated with systolic outflow obstruction with systolic murmurs. AS can be easily differentiated from HOCM by examining the response to a PVC. A comparison of the post-PVC hemodynamic responses between HOCM and AS is shown in **Fig. 13.26**. In AS, the post-PVC hemodynamic tracings show a larger pulse pressure, a consistently slow aortic upstroke of fixed valve obstruction, and no change in the aortic waveform, all in contrast to the HOCM hemodynamics, which show a reduced pulse pressure, brisk aortic pressure upstroke (parallel to LV pressure), and deformation of the aortic waveform with a spike and dome of rapid early ejection with secondary outflow obstruction.

MV Stenosis

Rheumatic MS restricts LA outflow, increases LA pressure, and limits cardiac output. Characteristic changes include thickening of the

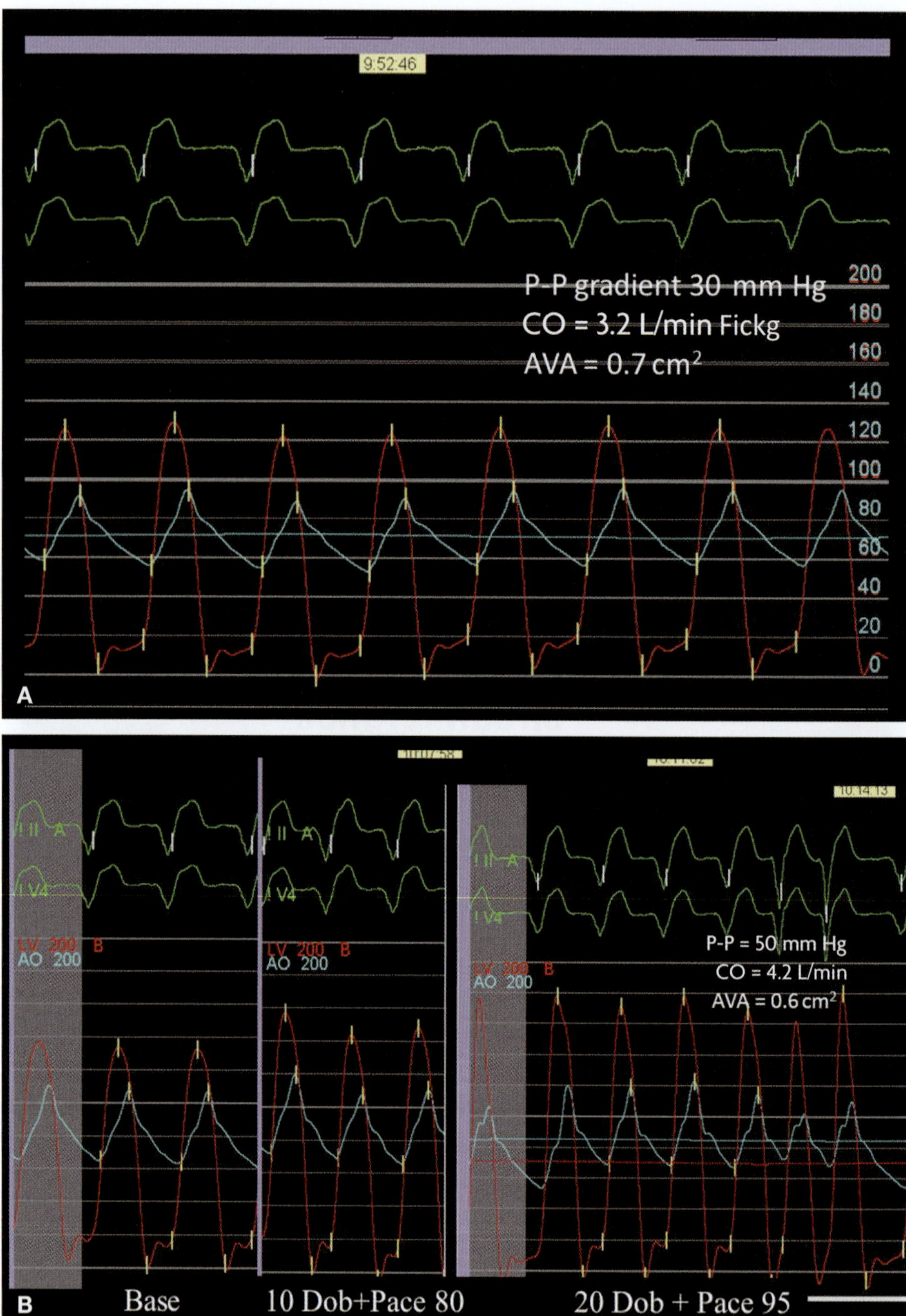

FIGURE 13.22 **A:** Patient with low-pressure-gradient AS and reduced LVEF (25%). There is no coronary artery disease. The peak-to-peak (P-P) gradient is 30 mm Hg with a cardiac output (CO) of 3.2 L/min Fick, resulting in aortic valve area (AVA) of 0.7 cm^2. Is this fixed AS or cardiomyopathy? **B:** Dobutamine challenge in patient with low-gradient/low-flow AS. After infusion of dobutamine 10 μg/min and 20 μg/min with ventricular pacing, the P-P gradient is now 50 mm Hg, CO is 4.2 L/min, and AVA is 0.6 cm^2. AS is fixed despite increased CO. Valve replacement is appropriate. AS, aortic stenosis; LVEF, left ventricular ejection fraction.

cusps and retraction of the subvalvular apparatus (**Fig. 13.27**). **Fig. 13.28** is a schematic representation of LV, aortic, and LA pressures, showing normal relationships and alterations with mild and severe MS. Corresponding classic auscultatory signs of MS are shown at the bottom. Compared with mild MS, with severe MS the higher LA "v" wave causes earlier pressure crossover and earlier MV opening, leading to a shorter time interval between AV closure and the opening snap. The higher LA EDP with severe MS also results in later closure of the MV. With severe MS, the diastolic rumble becomes longer and there is accentuation of the pulmonic component (P_2) of the second heart sound (S_2) in relation to the aortic component (A_2).

The hemodynamic assessment of the stenotic MV is performed initially with combined left and right heart hemodynamics, most often using a PCW pressure, compared with a simultaneous LV pressure at rest. In patients with borderline hemodynamic results, measurements

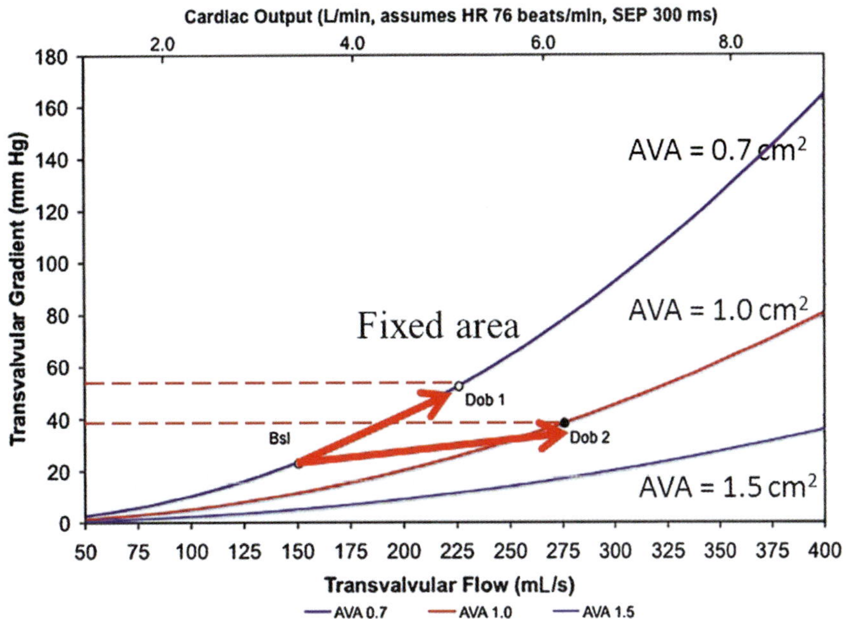

FIGURE 13.23 Plot of the relationship between mean gradient (y-axis) and transvalvular flow (x-axis, *bottom*) according to the Gorlin formula for three different values of AVA (0.7, 1.0, and 1.5 cm^2). Cardiac output (x-axis, *top*) is also shown, assuming a heart rate of 75 beats/min and a systolic ejection period of 300 ms. At low transvalvular flows, the mean gradient is low at all three valve areas. Two different responses to the dobutamine challenge are illustrated for a hypothetical patient (Bsl) with a baseline flow of 150 mL/s, mean gradient of 23 mm Hg, and calculated AVA 0.7 cm^2. In one scenario (dob 1), flow increases to 225 mL/s, mean gradient increases to 52 mm Hg, and AVA remains 0.7 cm^2, consistent with fixed AS. In the second scenario, flow increases to 275 mL/s, mean gradient increases to 38 mm Hg, and AVA increases to 1.0 cm^2. This patient has changed to a different curve, consistent with relative or pseudo-AS. AS, aortic stenosis; AVA, aortic valve area; HR, heart rate; SEP, systolic ejection period. (From: Grayburn PA. Assessment of low-gradient aortic stenosis with dobutamine. *Circulation.* 2006;113:604-606.)

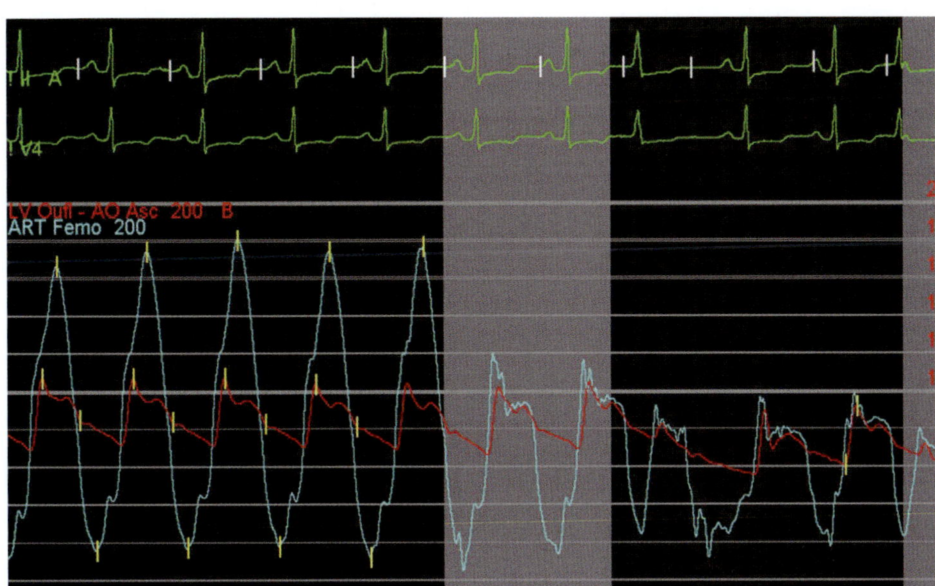

FIGURE 13.24 Hemodynamic left ventricular (*blue*) and aortic (*red*) pressure tracings in patient with hypertrophic cardiomyopathy. The LV catheter is pullback from distal LV (*left side*) to subaortic position (*right side*). Note the reduction in LV-Ao pressure gradient while still recording LV pressure. In addition, one can appreciate the configuration of the aortic pressure with a typical "spike and dome" appearance. LV, left ventricular.

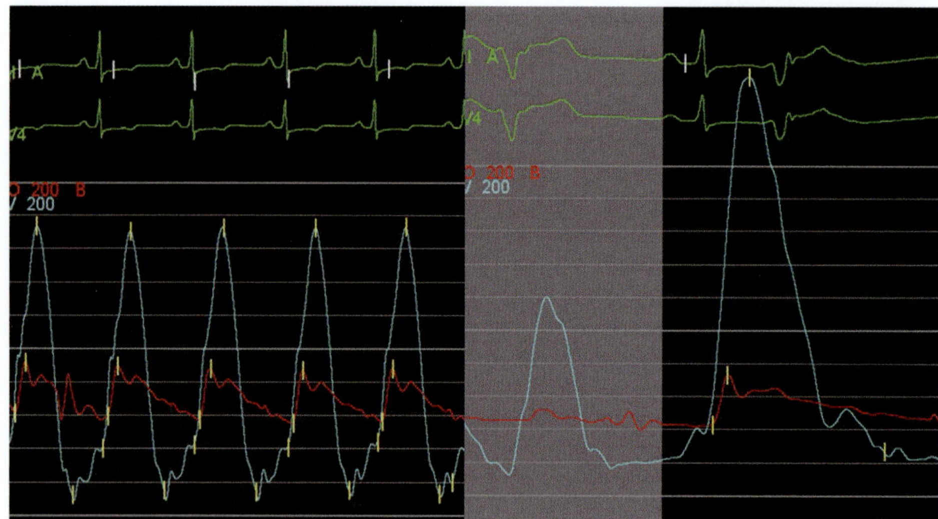

FIGURE 13.25 Hemodynamics in a patient with hypertrophic obstructive cardiomyopathy. LV (*blue*) and aortic (*red*) pressure tracings demonstrate the vertical upstroke of aortic pressure with a rapid early ejection and mid-systolic delay (*spike and dome pattern*). Following a PVC (*shaded bar*), the post-PVC reduction of the aortic pulse pressure is evident (called the Brockenbrough-Braunwald-Morrow sign) with a marked increase in the LVOT pressure gradient. LVOT, left ventricular outflow tract; PVC, premature ventricular contraction.

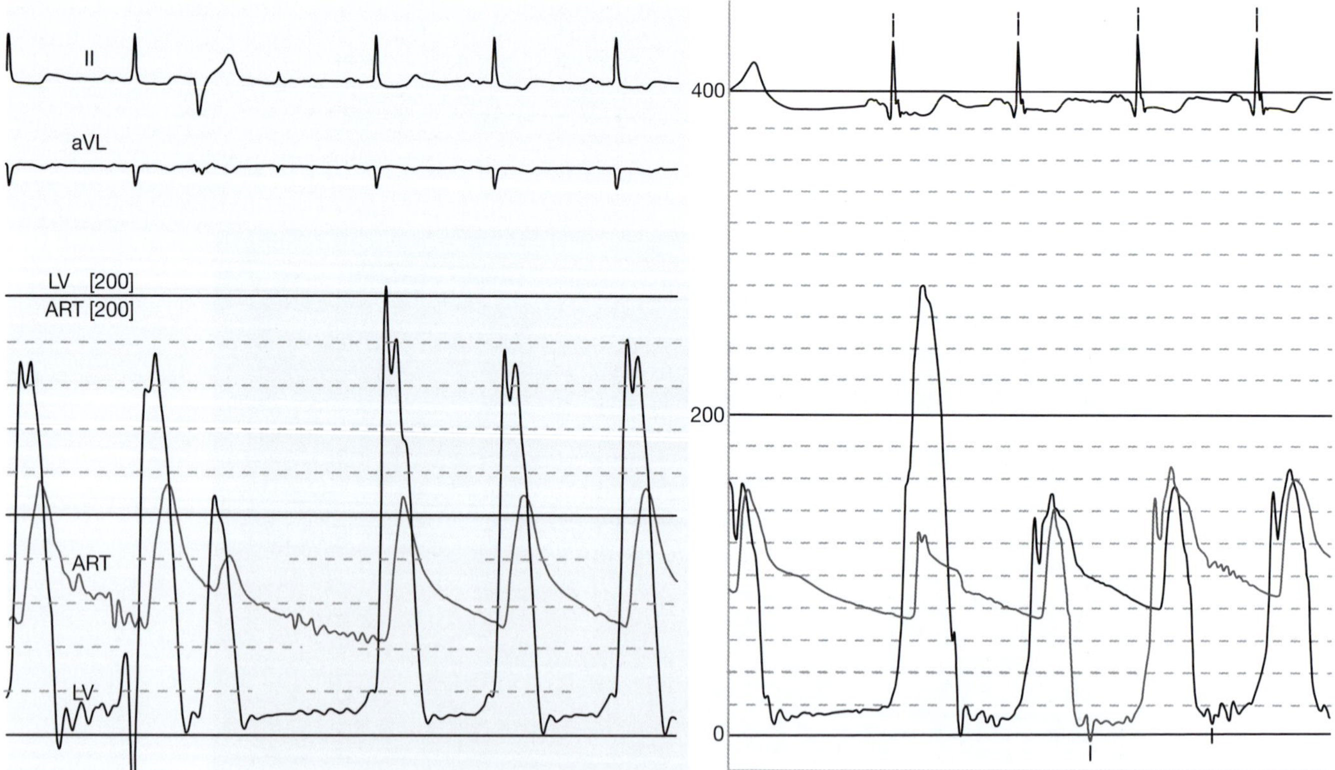

FIGURE 13.26 Hemodynamic tracings in a patient with AS (*left*) compared with one with HOCM (*right*). In AS, the post-PVC beat of the aortic pressure wave has a slow upstroke, wide pulse pressure, and the same waveform as normal beats. In HOCM, the post-PVC aortic pressure has a vertical upstroke, a narrow pulse pressure, and the typical alteration of the aortic pressure of obstruction with the spike and dome contour. AS, aortic stenosis; HOCM, hypertrophic obstructive cardiomyopathy; PVC, premature ventricular contraction.

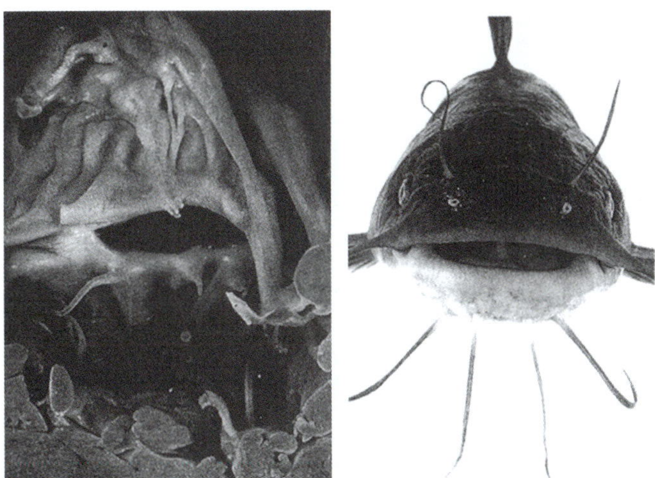

FIGURE 13.27 Rheumatic mitral stenosis with thickening of the cusps and retraction of the subvalvular apparatus. The right side is a fish-mouth shape similar to that of the mitral stenotic valve.

should be made during exercise (eg, arm lifting with weights). The PCW pressure often overestimates LA pressure in patients with MS or prosthetic MVs due to delayed and poor pressure transmission, making correct alignment of pressure tracings difficult.

For patients with elevated PCW pressure and suspected MV abnormalities, use of direct LA pressure by transseptal puncture is the most accurate method and should be used prior to MV surgery or valvuloplasty. **Fig. 13.29** shows a PCW pressure (red) and LA pressure (orange) demonstrating different timing of "v" waves and a higher mean for PCW, which would falsely increase MV gradient measurement. Nevertheless, if the PCW/LV pressure tracings show no significant gradients, transseptal catheterization is often unnecessary.

If the medical treatment of MS is ineffective, then percutaneous balloon mitral valvuloplasty (PBMV) is indicated. **Fig. 13.30**

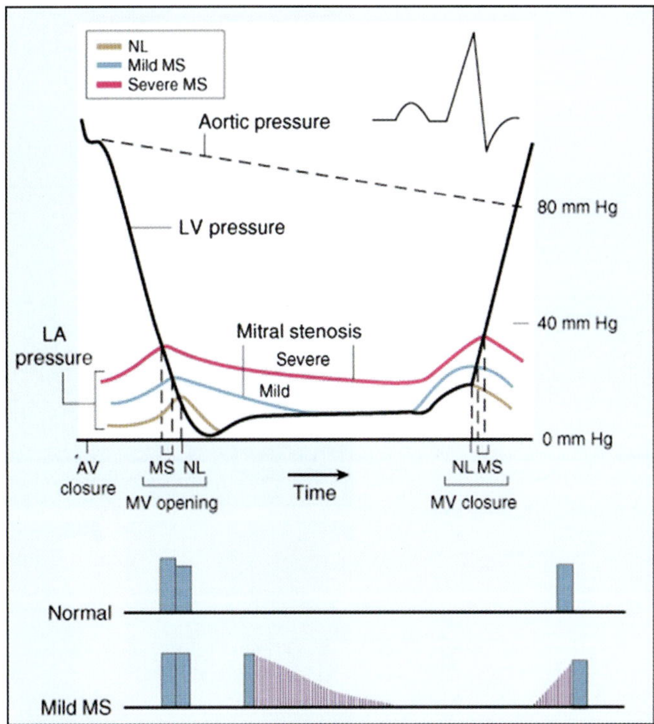

FIGURE 13.28 Schematic representation of the left ventricular (LV), aortic, and left atrial (LA) pressures, showing normal relationships and alterations with mild and severe mitral stenosis (MS). Corresponding classic auscultatory signs of MS are shown at the bottom. Compared with mild MS, severe MS has a higher left atrial "v" wave, causing earlier pressure crossover and an earlier mitral valve (MV) opening, leading to a shorter time interval between aortic valve (AV) closure and the opening snap (OS). The higher left atrial end-diastolic pressure with severe MS also results in later closure of the mitral valve. With severe MS, the diastolic rumble becomes longer and there is accentuation of the pulmonic component (P_2) of the second heart sound (S_2) in relation to the aortic component (A_2).

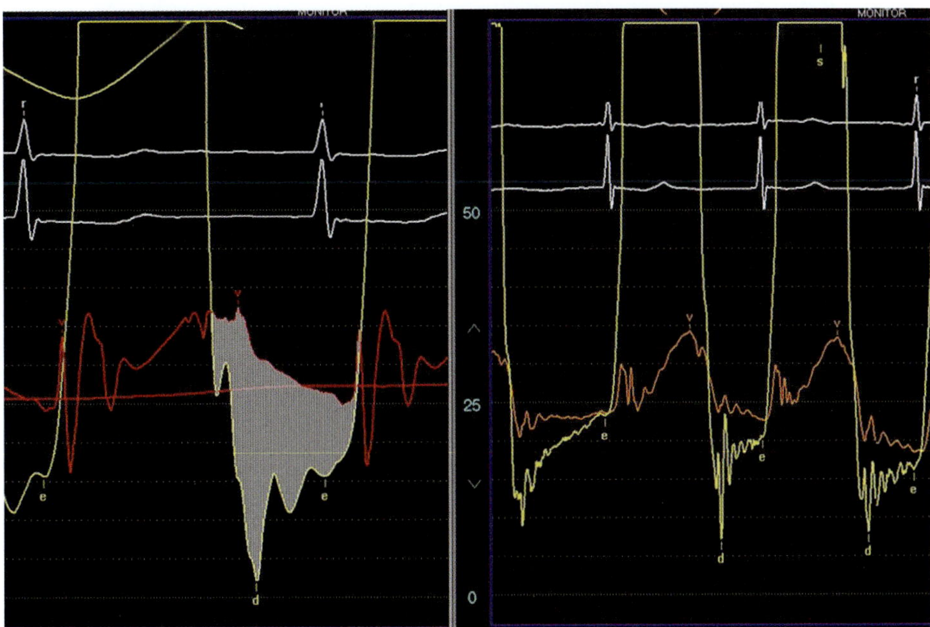

FIGURE 13.29 Hemodynamic tracings in a patient with mitral stenosis. The LV and PCW (*left*) tracings show a large mitral valve gradient of approximately 20 mm Hg (pressure scale is 0-50 mm Hg). On the *right*, LV and directly measured LA pressures (via transseptal approach) show higher fidelity pressure wave forms and marked reduction in the mitral pressure gradient (6 mm Hg). Note the "c" notch and "v" wave are distinct compared with the wave forms on the PCW. PCW does not always equal LA. LA, left atrial; LV, left ventricular; PCW, pulmonary capillary wedge.

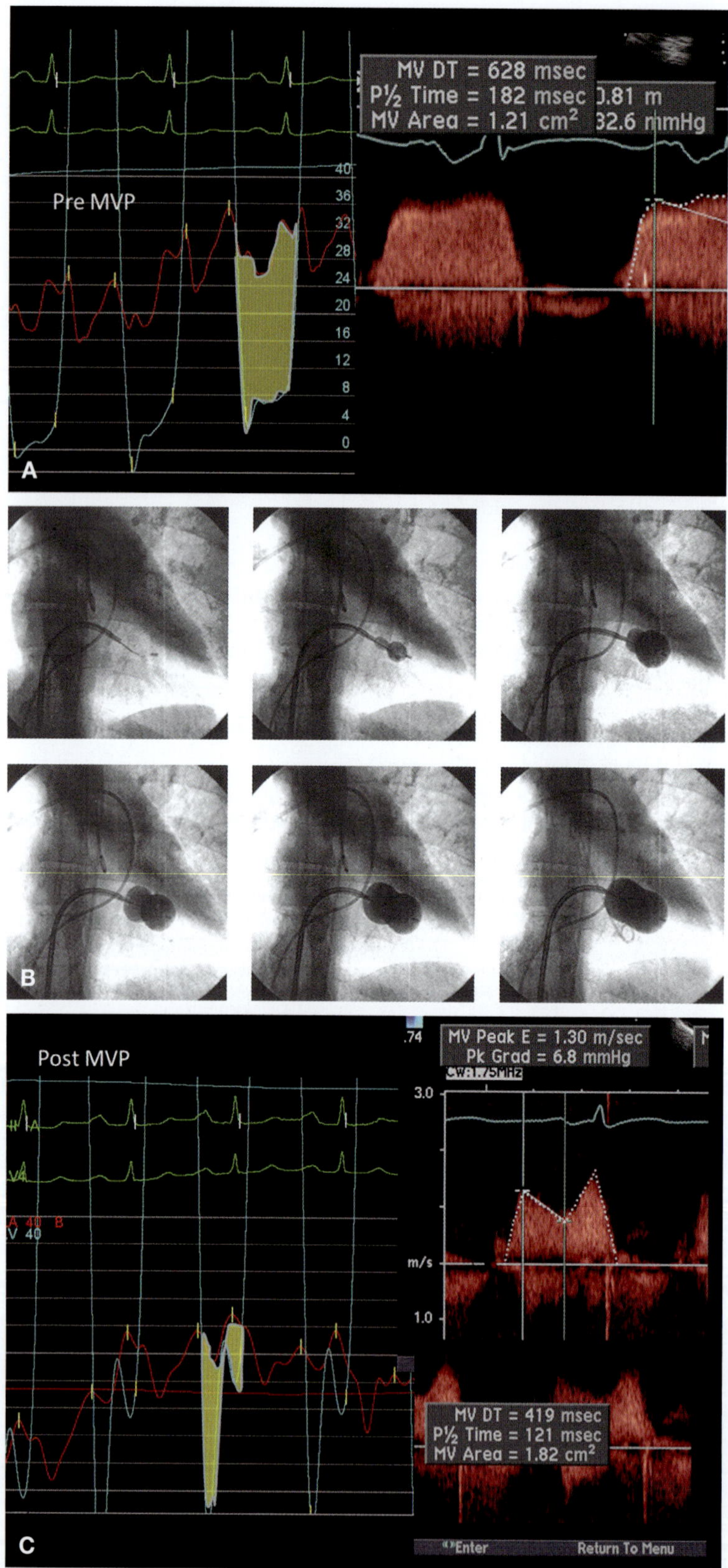

FIGURE 13.30 **A:** Hemodynamics and Doppler echo findings before mitral valve balloon valvuloplasty (PMBV). **Left:** LV (*blue tracing*) and LA (*red tracing*) demonstrate a large diastolic mitral valve gradient (*yellow*). **Right:** The Doppler velocity across the mitral valve shows a mitral valve area of 1.21 cm^2 with a 32-mm-Hg gradient. After evaluation by 2D echo and TEE, the results were a low Wilken score (<8) and no LA thrombus; mitral balloon valvuloplasty was performed. **B:** Cine frames of Inoue balloon expansion during Inoue mitral balloon valvuloplasty. Hemodynamics after PMBV are shown in **C**. **C:** Hemodynamic and Doppler echo findings after PMBV. **Left:** LV and LA pressures show marked reduction of diastolic mitral gradient. Right: Doppler flow after the procedure likewise shows reduced peak transvalvular velocities, an improved pressure half-time, and an increased mitral valve area of 1.82 cm^2. LA, left atrial; LV, left ventricular; PBMV, percutaneous balloon mitral valvuloplasty; TEE, transesophageal echocardiograms.

illustrates a case of MS treated with PBMV. Successful procedures produce an average decrease in MV gradient of approximately 50% to 75% of the baseline gradient and a doubling of the MV area: on average, about 2 cm^2.

Mitral Regurgitation

Mitral regurgitation (MR) is the result of the inability to maintain leaflet coaptation during systole. The mitral apparatus consists of the annulus, the anterior and posterior leaflets, and their tethers of the thin chordae tendinae attached to the papillary muscles. Failure of any of these structures can result in malcoaptation of the mitral leaflets and valvular regurgitation.

Acute MR produced by stretching or tearing of leaflets is characterized by a new and large "v" wave (**Fig. 13.31**). A new large "v" wave after PBMV is MR until proven otherwise. Nevertheless, the quality of "v" waves depends upon the compliance of the chamber, and large "v" waves can be seen in the absence of MR (**Fig. 13.32**). The PCW "v" wave is thus of limited value in the accurate identification of true MR. **Fig. 13.33** shows LA hemodynamics, with a large "v" wave due to a paravalvular mitral prosthetic valve leak.

Constrictive and Restrictive Cardiac Hemodynamics

Dyspnea, elevated neck veins, ascites, and pedal edema suggest right-sided heart failure with a potential differential diagnosis that includes both restrictive and constrictive pathophysiologic

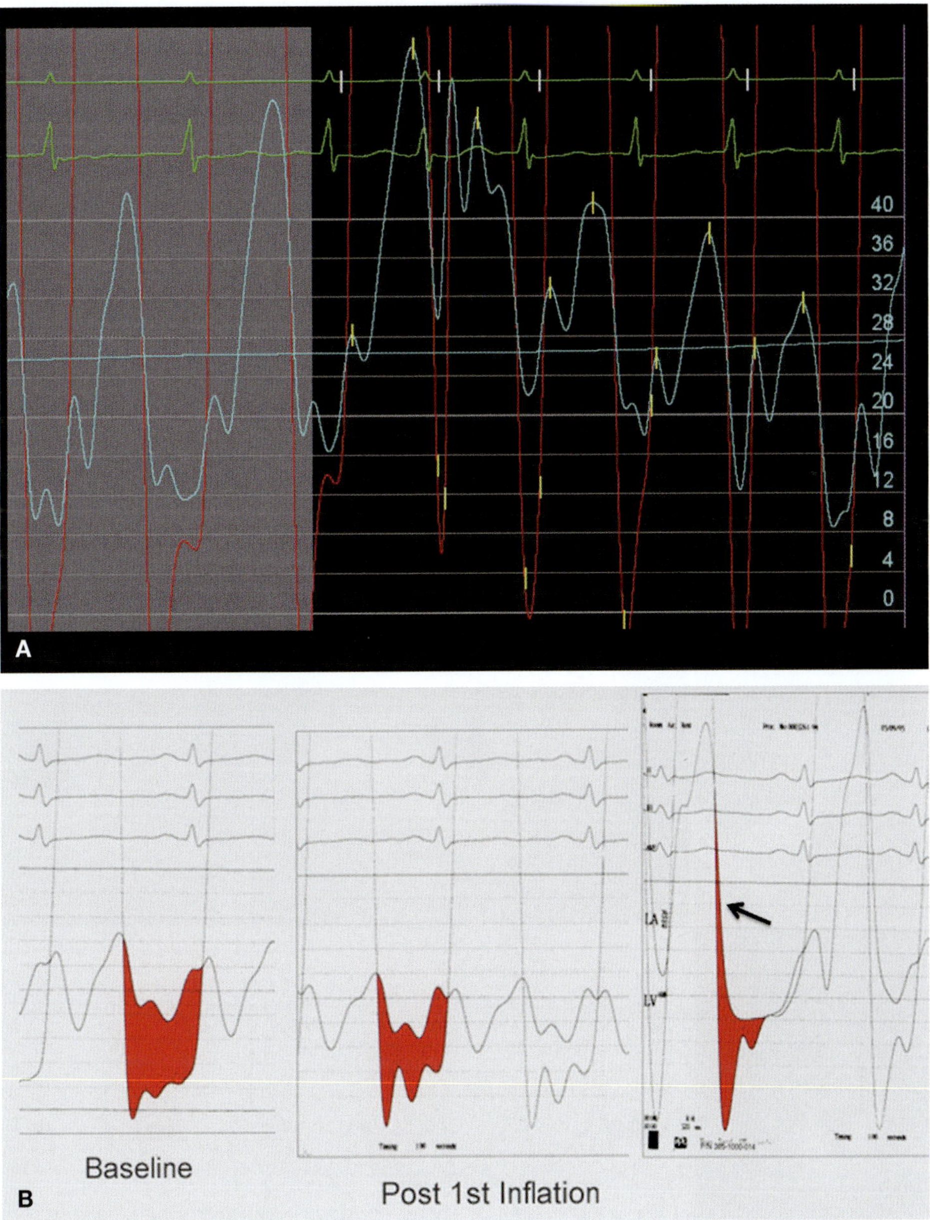

FIGURE 13.31 Hemodynamics of a case of MS treated with PBMV which resulted in mitral regurgitation (MR). **A:** Top tracing show acute MR produced by stretching or tearing of leaflets is characterized by a new and large "v" wave. A new large "v" wave after PBMV is MR until proven otherwise. **B:** Bottom tracings show mitral gradient t baseline, middle, post first inflation, right final inflation with minimal gradient but large V wave of acute MR. AO, aorta; LA, left atrium; LAA, left atrial appendage; LV, left ventricle. (Courtesy of Vuyisile T. Nkomo, Sorin V. Pislaru, Paul Sorajja, and Allison K. Cabalka, citation is unchange.)

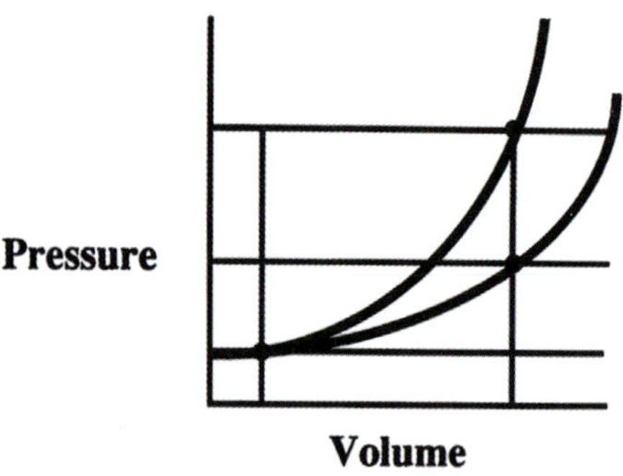

FIGURE 13.32 Pressure-volume relationship can produce different compliance curves. This graph illustrates the effect of high and lower compliance on a "v" wave. A highly compliant system (*bottom curve*) produces little pressure change as volume increases, whereas a low compliant or "stiff" (*top curve*) system produces large pressure increases during similar volume infusion.

diseases. The traditional hemodynamic criteria for the diagnosis of constrictive pericardial disease have been based largely on diastolic equalization of ventricular pressures, with a characteristic abrupt cessation of ventricular filling early in diastole and restriction of further filling demonstrated by a plateau of diastolic left and RV pressures (**Fig. 13.34**). Dynamic respiratory changes in right and left ventricular pressures in patients with constrictive pericarditis, as proposed by Hurrell et al,[13] have the highest sensitivity and specificity for true constrictive pericardial disease (**Table 13.1**).

With constrictive physiology, upon inspiration there is a decrease in the early transmitral gradient, demonstrating a dissociation of the intrathoracic and intracardiac pressures. The right and left ventricular systolic pressures move *discordantly* due to ventricular interdependence (ie, when the RV fills, the LV volume decreases, and vice versa). With inspiration, the LV systolic pressure decreases and the RV systolic pressure increases. **Fig. 13.35** shows an example of normal RV/LV dynamic pressure responses in a normal patient (left) and the discordant systolic pressure during respiration in a patient with constrictive pericardial disease (right).

In restrictive cardiomyopathy, the RV/LV systolic pressures move together during respiration because ventricular volumes can expand together[13] (**Fig. 13.36**).

Cardiac Tamponade

Cardiac tamponade is the most severe form of diastolic dysfunction and is associated with compression of the heart and an inability to fill due to pericardial pressure exceeding intracardiac pressure. Tamponade may occur during or after structural, coronary, or electrophysiologic interventions. A high index of suspicion is critical to rapidly detect and treat this life-threatening condition with pericardiocentesis. Fluid accumulating in the pericardial space produces an elevation of pericardial pressure. The magnitude of pericardial pressure increase depends on the rate of fluid accumulation and the compliance of the pericardium. Compression of the heart, as well as prevention of adequate ventricular filling, reduces SV, cardiac output, and arterial pressure and may rapidly progress to cardiogenic shock and death without intervention. Both tamponade and constriction may be associated with a paradoxical pulse (>10 mm Hg reduction in arterial pressure during inspiration [**Fig. 13.37**]), low cardiac output, tachycardia, and hypotension. Cardiac tamponade and constrictive pericarditis have important pathophysiologic differences. In constriction, early diastolic filling is very rapid, as the ventricle rapidly recoils after ejection. This results in the characteristic brisk "Y" descent that is almost universally observed. In contrast, elevated pericardial pressure in cardiac tamponade limits filling throughout all of diastole and the "Y" descent is characteristically blunted. **Fig. 13.38** illustrates the hemodynamics of cardiac tamponade and its relief after pericardiocentesis.

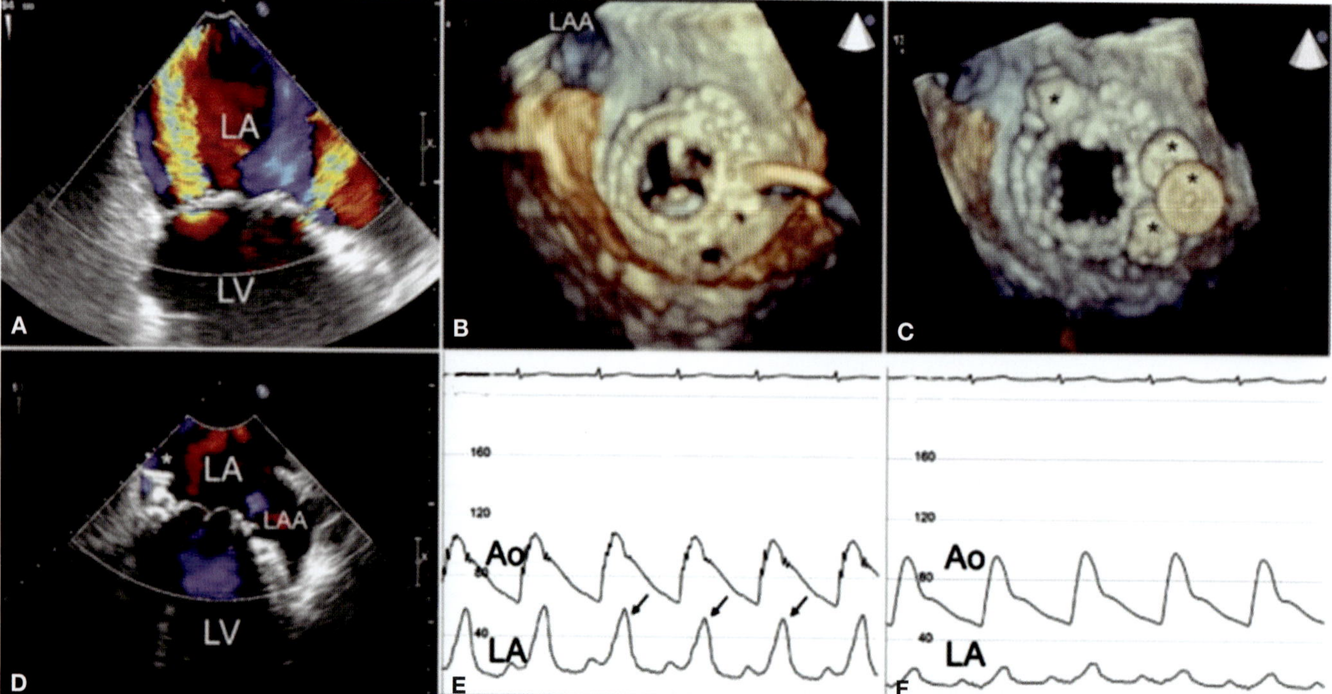

FIGURE 13.33 Transesophageal echocardiogram showed 1 small anterolateral and a larger posteromedial leak **(A)**. Under 3-dimensional echocardiographic guidance **(B)**, 3 Amplatzer vascular plugs (Plymouth, MN, USA) were deployed to close the posteromedial leak, and 1 additional device was placed in the anterolateral leak **(C)**. The procedure was uncomplicated, with marked reduction in paravalvular prosthetic mitral regurgitation **(D)**. There was significant hemodynamic **(E and F)** and clinical improvement post-procedure. Ao, aortic; LAA, left atrial appendage; LV, left ventricular. (From: Nkomo VT, Pislaru SV, Sorajja P, Cabalka AK. Plugged! *J Am Coll Cardiol*. 2013;61(3):356.)

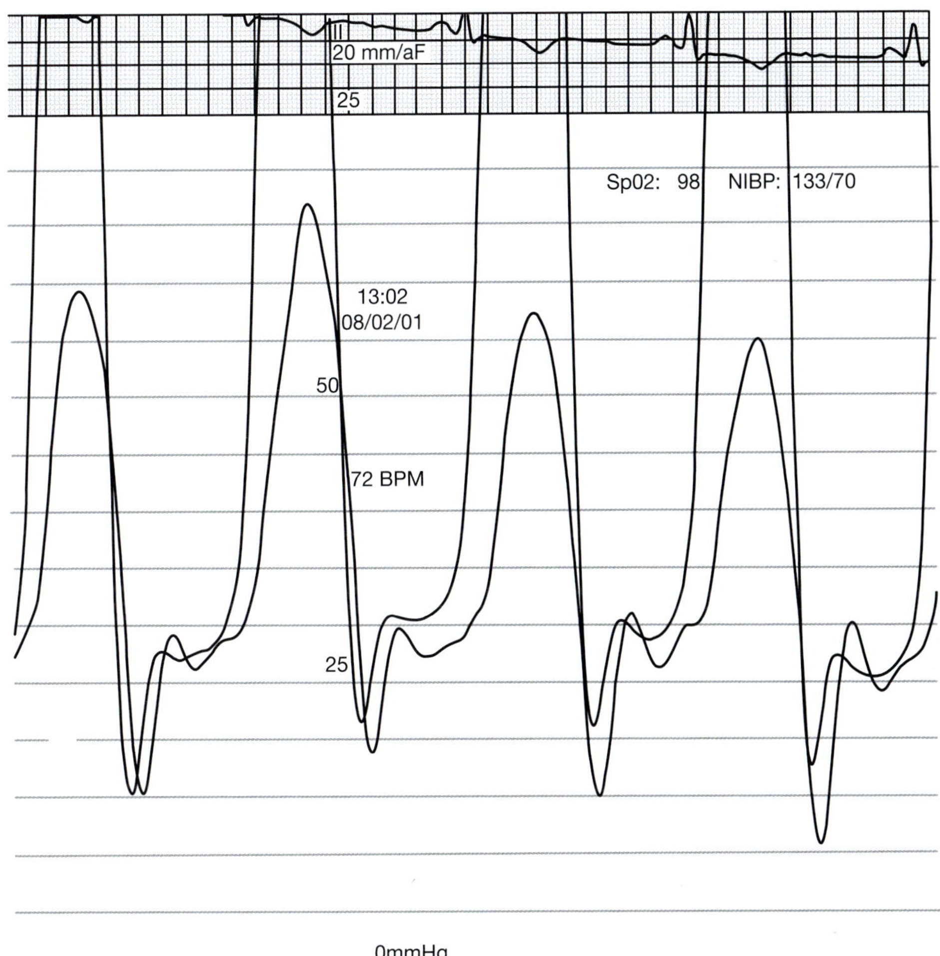

FIGURE 13.34 Hemodynamics of constrictive/restrictive physiology. LV and RV tracings (0-40 mm Hg scale) show an abrupt cessation of diastolic filling, with a dip and plateau configuration. This pattern is common but not diagnostic for constrictive pericarditis. LV, left ventricular; RV, right ventricular.

TABLE 13.1 Comparison of Traditional and Dynamic Respiratory Criteria for Diagnostic Constrictive Pericarditis

	CRITERIA	SENSITIVITY (%)	SPECIFICITY (%)	PPV	NPV
Traditional	LVEDP vs RVEDP <5	60	38	4	57
	RVEDP vs RVSP >1/3	93	38	52	89
	PASP <55	93	24	47	25
	Right ventricular free wall >7 mm	93	57	61	92
	Respiratory: Change of right atrial pressure <3 mm Hg	93	48	58	92
Dynamic respiratory factors	Pulmonary capillary wedge vs LV >5 mm Hg	93	81	78	94
	LV/RV interdependence	100	95	94	100

LV, left ventricular; LVEDP, left ventricular end-diastolic pressure; NPV, negative predictive value; PASP, pulmonary artery systolic pressure; PPV, positive predictive value; RV, right ventricular; RVEDP, right ventricular end-diastolic pressure; RVSP, right ventricular systolic pressure.

From Hurrell DG, Nishimura RA, Higano ST, et al. Value of dynamic respiratory changes in left and right ventricular pressures for the diagnosis of constrictive pericarditis. *Circulation.* 1996;93:2007-2013.

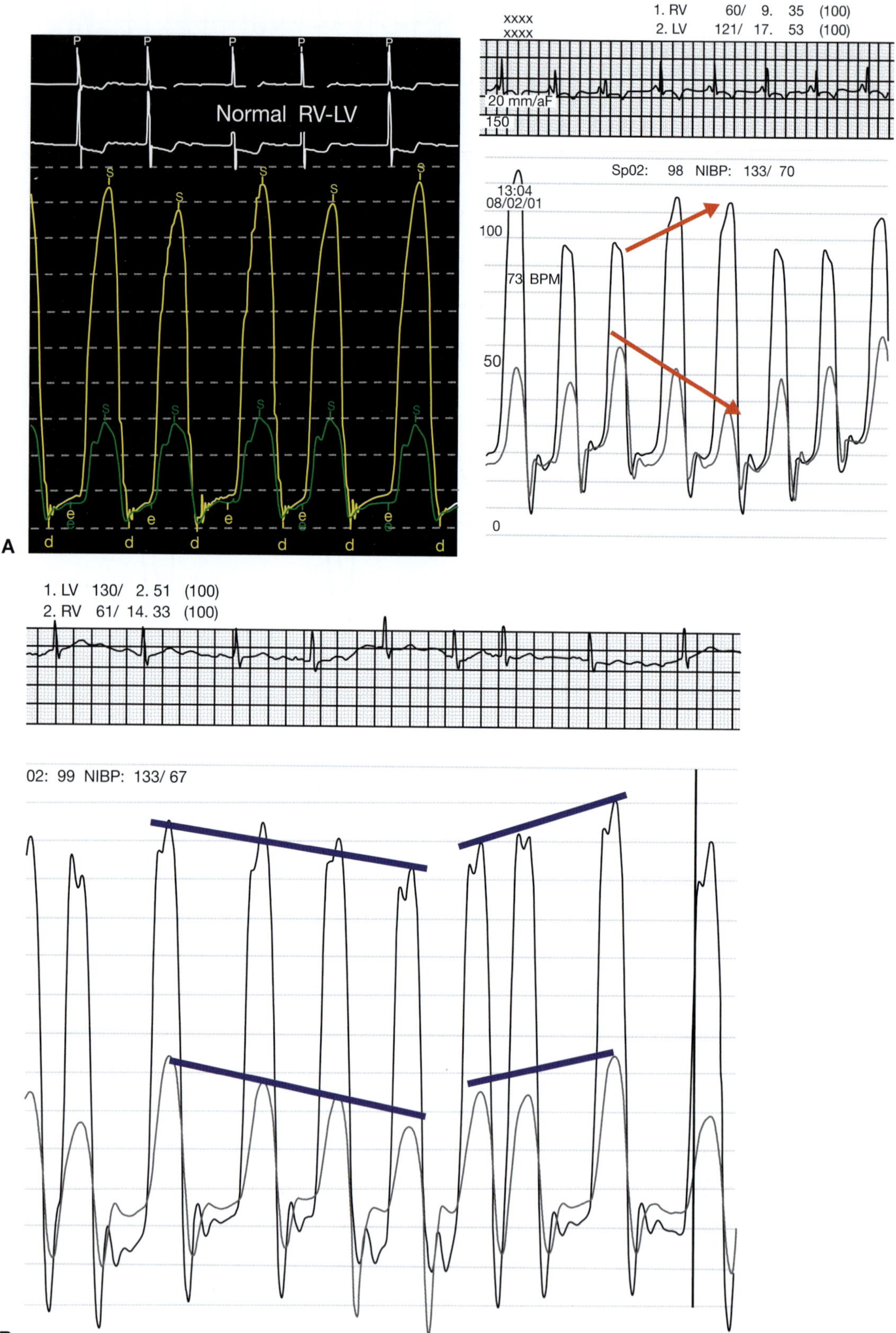

FIGURE 13.35 **A:** *Left*, normal LV/RV relationship over the respiratory cycle. *Right*, Dynamic respiratory variation of systolic RV and LV pressures demonstrates discordant respiratory motion. The discordant respiratory variation of pressures shown here is diagnostic for constrictive pericardial physiology. **B:** Dynamic respiratory variation of systolic RV and LV pressures demonstrates concordant respiratory motion. The concordant respiratory variation of pressures shown here is diagnostic for restrictive cardiomyopathy. LV, left ventricular; RV, right ventricular.

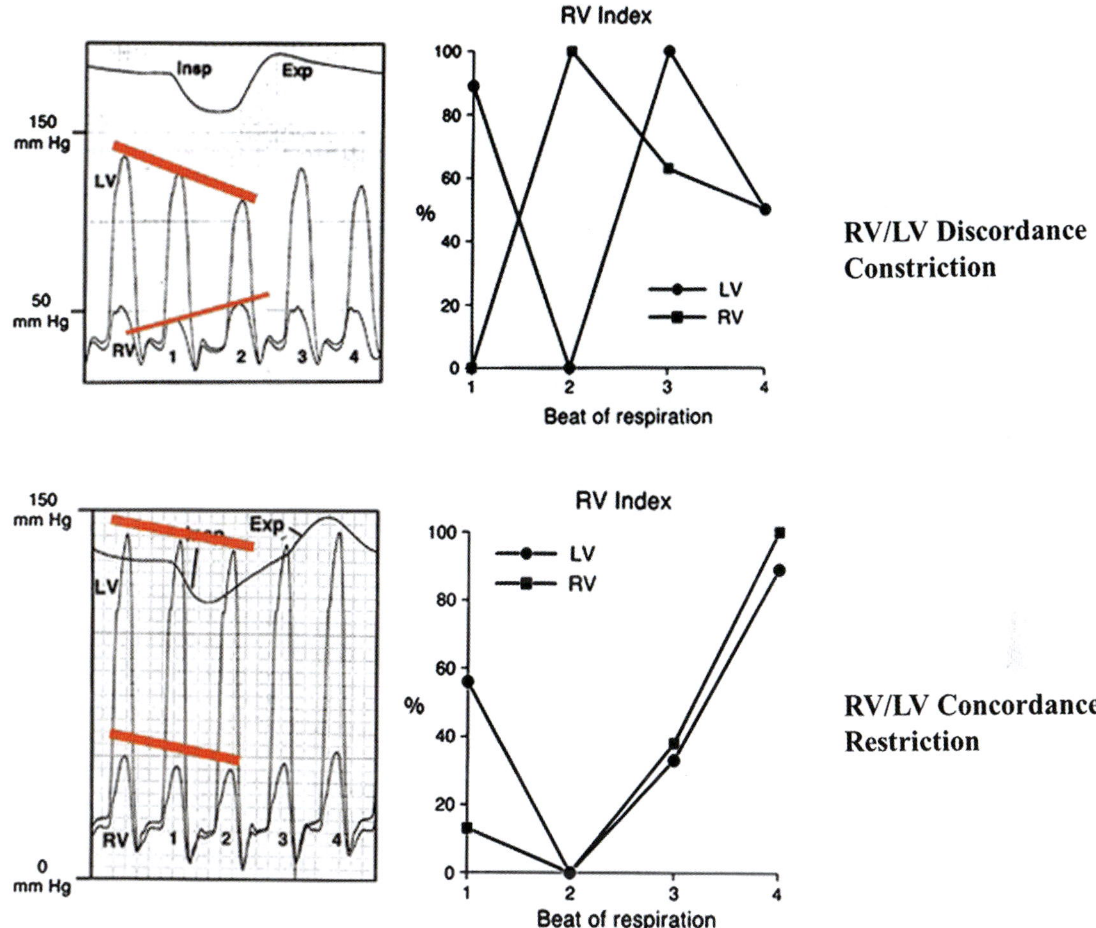

FIGURE 13.36 Dynamic respiratory variation of LV and RV systolic pressures differentiates constrictive from restrictive physiology. **Top:** RV/LV Discordance = Constriction. **Bottom:** RV/LV Concordance = Restriction. LV, left ventricular; RV, right ventricular. (From: Hurrell DG, Nishimura RA, Higano ST, et al. Value of dynamic respiratory changes in left and right ventricular pressures for the diagnosis of constrictive pericarditis. *Circulation.* 1996;93:2007-2013.)

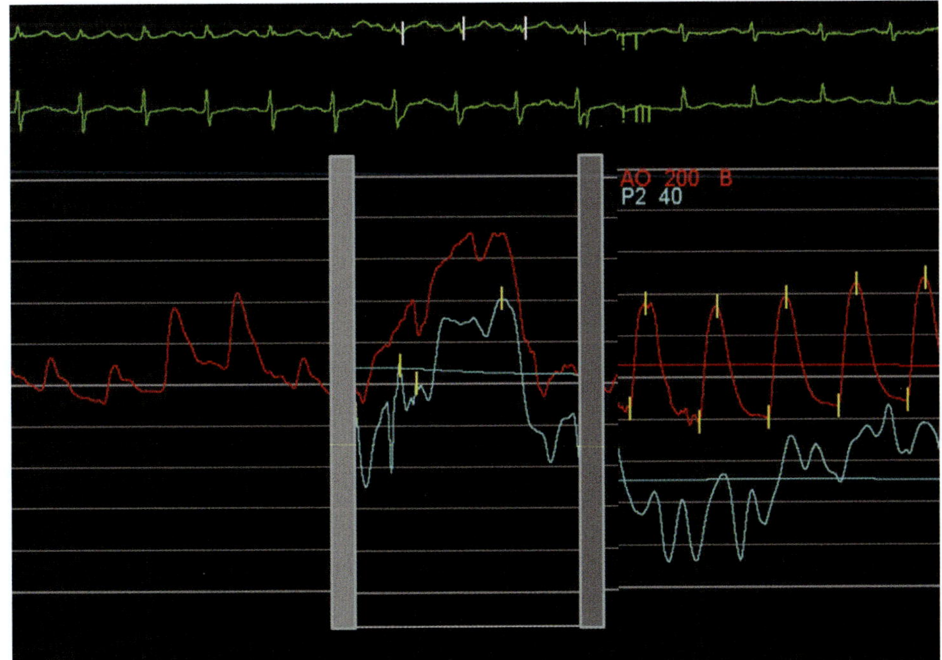

FIGURE 13.37 Hemodynamic findings in cardiac tamponade. **Left:** Aortic pressure (0-200 mm Hg scale) before pericardiocentesis in patient with clinical and echocardiographic findings of tamponade. **Middle:** RA and pericardial pressures (0-40 mm Hg scale) before pericardiocentesis. **Right:** Aortic pressure (0-200 mm Hg scale) and pericardial pressure (0-40 mm Hg scale) after pericardiocentesis. Note restoration of arterial pulse with loss of marked respiratory variance (pulsus paradoxus) and reduction of pericardial pressure from 22 to 12 mm Hg. RA, right atrial.

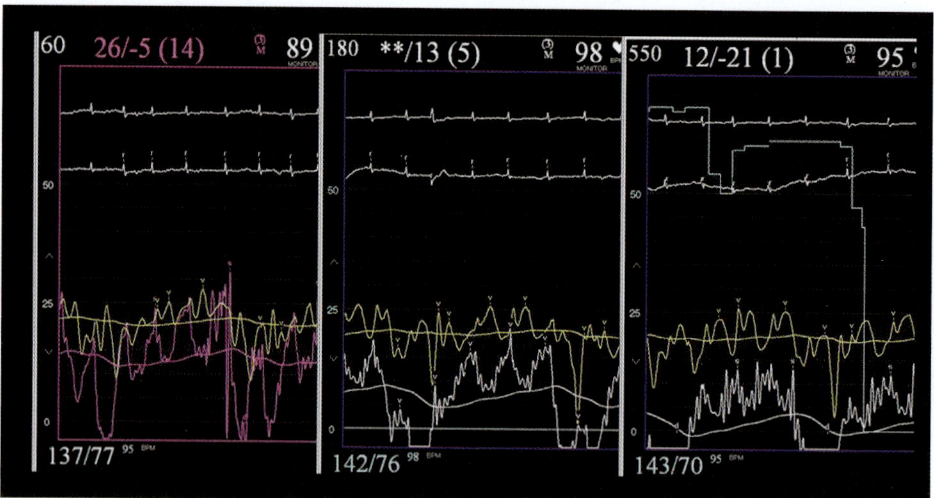

FIGURE 13.38 Hemodynamic tracings during pericardiocentesis in a patient with shortness of breath and pericardial effusion. The presumed cause of dyspnea was tamponade. *Left*, baseline hemodynamics. RA pressure is yellow tracing. *Middle*, RA and pericardial pressure after 180 mL was removed. *Right*, pressures after 550 mL fluid was removed from pericardium. Nevertheless, the relief of pericardial pressure by pericardiocentesis demonstrated no change in RA pressure. No cardiac tamponade is present. The diagnosis is effusive constrictive pericardial disease with LV dysfunction. LV, left ventricular; RA, right atrial.

Key Points

- The cardiac cycle and PV loops can be used to assess the effects of interventions on cardiac output (SV) and filling pressures.
- Right hemodynamics and shunt calculations are important to placement of closure devices.
- Left-sided heart hemodynamics are used to identify ventricular function, relaxation, and outflow obstruction due to valvular, subvalvular, or supravalvular lesions.
- Hypertrophic obstructive cardiomyopathy may be confused with AS in some patients.
- MV hemodynamics are critical to understand applications of balloon valvuloplasty and mitral clip for regurgitation.
- Pericardial hemodynamics must differentiate among constrictive, restrictive, and tamponade physiology.
- Basic hemodynamics and pressure wave interpretation can be appreciated from review of the Wiggers diagram.
- Valvular heart disease: Pressure waveforms demonstrate transvalvular gradients and identify mechanisms of valve function. HOCM versus AS has unique post-PVC hemodynamic configuration.
- Diastolic dysfunctional hemodynamics: constriction versus restriction.
- Diastolic "dip and plateau" configuration is present in several types of diastolic dysfunction whether due to pericardium or myocardium. The most specific differentiating features of the two disease states involve the dynamic respiratory interaction of left and right ventricular systolic pressures. Concordant respiratory systolic pressure changes are associated with restrictive cardiomyopathy, whereas discordant respiratory pressure changes are associated with constrictive pericardial disease.

References

1. Kern MJ, Lim MJ, Goldstein JA, eds. *Hemodynamic Rounds: Interpretation of Cardiac Pathophysiology from Pressure Waveform Analysis*. 4th ed. Wiley-Blackwell; 2017.
2. Sorajja PS, Lim MJ, Kern MJ, eds. *Kern's Cardiac Catheterization Handbook*. 7th ed. Elsevier; 2020:495.
3. Kern M, Seto AH. *Right and left heart hemodynamics*. In: *Cardiac Catheterization & Interventional Cardiology Self-Assessment Program (CathSAP)*. American College of Cardiology Foundation; 2020. Available at: www.acc.org/cathsap
4. Kern M, Seto AH, Herrmann J. Invasive hemodynamic diagnosis of cardiac disease. In: Libby P, Mann DL, Bonow RO, Tomeselli GF, Bhatt DL, eds. *Braunwald's Heart Disease*. 12th ed. Elseivier; 2021:38-409.
5. Lim MJ, Sorajja P, Kern MJ, eds. *The Interventional Cardiac Catheterization Handbook*. 5th ed. Elsevier; 2023:458.
6. Grossman MM. *Baim's Cardiac Catheterization, Angiography, and Intervention*. 8th ed. Wolters Kluwer/Lippincott Williams & Wilkins; 2013:223-272.
7. Nishimura RA, Carabello BA. Hemodynamics in the cardiac catheterization laboratory of the 21st century. *Circulation*. 2012;125(17):2138-2150.
8. Borlaug BA, Kass DA. Invasive hemodynamic assessment in heart failure. *Heart Fail Clin*. 2009;5(2):217-228.
9. Burkhoff D, Mirsky I, Suga H. Assessment of systolic and diastolic ventricular properties via pressure-volume analysis: a guide for clinical, translational, and basic researchers. *Am J Physiol Heart Circ Physiol*. 2005;289(2):H501-H512.
10. Pibarot P, Dumesnil JG. Improving assessment of aortic stenosis. *J Am Coll Cardiol*. 2012;60(3):169-180.
11. Ren X, Banki NM. Classic hemodynamic findings of severe aortic regurgitation. *Circulation*. 2012;126(3):e28-e29.
12. Grayburn PA. Assessment of low-gradient aortic stenosis with dobutamine. *Circulation*. 2006;113(5):604-606.
13. Hurrell DG, Nishimura RA, Higano ST, et al. Value of dynamic respiratory changes in left and right ventricular pressures for the diagnosis of constrictive pericarditis. *Circulation*. 1996;93(11):2007-2013.
14. Hakki AH, Iskandrian AS, Bemis CE, et al. A simplified valve formula for the calculation of stenotic cardiac valve areas. *Circulation*. 1981;63(5):1050-1055.
15. Remmelink M, Sjauw KD, Henriques JPS, et al. Acute left ventricular dynamic effects of primary percutaneous coronary intervention from occlusion to reperfusion. *J Am Coll Cardiol*. 2009;53(17):1498-1502.
16. Gorlin R, Gorlin SG. Hydraulic formula for calculation of the area of the stenotic mitral valve, other cardiac valves, and central circulatory shunts. I. *Am Heart J*. 1951;41:1-29.

Percutaneous Coronary Equipment Guide

Marvin Eng and Kathleen E. Kearney

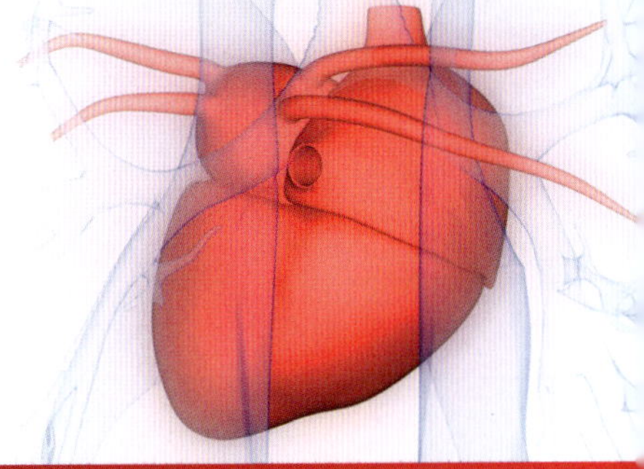

INTRODUCTION

The key to successful percutaneous coronary intervention (PCI) is proper selection of coronary equipment to provide stable, coaxial access for device delivery and safe, successful treatment of the target lesion. The goal of this chapter is to provide a framework for equipment selection for PCI.

CORONARY GUIDE CATHETERS

Guiding catheters must be able to accommodate PCI equipment, enable coaxial engagement, and support the delivery of equipment in the face of an obstructed pathway that may be tortuous or calcified. Size and shape of coronary guiding catheters selection is impacted by access site, aorta size, coronary vessel, disease complexity, intended PCI devices, bleeding risk, and contrast limit.

Coronary guide catheters are constructed in a manner to optimize lumen size for equipment delivery. Using three layers, an outer lubricious coating, embedded stainless steel mesh, and inner hydrophilic lining, guiding catheter design optimizes inner diameter to be larger than corresponding diagnostic catheters (**Fig. 14.1**). As PCI has evolved, iterative improvements in angioplasty catheters and adjunctive devices have enabled various combinations of devices to deliver simultaneously, depending on the guide catheter diameter. Provided is a table of several pragmatic permutations of PCI equipment based on guide catheter size (**Table 14.1**).[1]

Guide Curvature Selection

Considerable variability across coronary anatomy and operators exists; however, a small sample of commonly used shapes (**Fig. 14.2**) and a table of common curves is shown for right and left coronary cannulation (**Tables 14.2** and **14.3**). Certain guide catheter shapes are classified based on their backup support for equipment delivery (**Fig. 14.3**).[2]

Coaxial support for equipment delivery: Passive support is derived from a combination of the inherent material stiffness, guide curve coaxial alignment, contralateral aortic wall contact, catheter size, and angle of contact (**Fig. 14.4**). Larger catheters are inherently more stiffer and offer greater support than smaller guiding catheters.[2]

On the contrary, active support is achieved by guide manipulation to conform to the aortic root or deep engagement of the catheter (**Fig. 14.3**). Caveats to active guide support include vessel size and proximal disease as deep intubation may cause pressure dampening, flow obstruction, and/or vessel dissection especially if the proximal lumen is the same size or smaller than the guide.

Guide catheter size not only impacts the type and amount of equipment that can be delivered, but also larger guide catheters are stiffer and improve backup force for equipment delivery. However, these benefits can be offset by higher contrast volume utilization and higher rates of vascular complications. Body habitus and access route limit guiding catheter size, especially in radial access and if sheath/catheter size approaches the maximal diameter or stretches the vessel.[3] Sheathless guiding catheters allow for a step-up in guide size typically accommodated by the access site, such as 8F for radial access, but compromises in torque control, and the guides may be more prone to kinking in this configuration.

Sidehole guiding catheters are designed to engage vessels with ostial vessel disease that would normally cause pressure dampening. They prevent excessive pressurization of the coronary vessel, reducing the chance for hydraulic vessel dissection and enables reliable aortic pressure monitoring at the cost of higher contrast utilization. It is important to note that coronary flow is reduced during guide engagement despite the normalization of pressure waveform, so the monitoring for ischemia via other signals remains important in patent vessels.

Guide catheter length (90-125 cm) selection varies according to vessel distance from access site and according to equipment length used. For instance, some very tall patients or significant vessel tortuosity may require additional catheter length for coaxial coronary engagement, especially from radial access. Alternatively, shorter guide lengths facilitate cases in bypass grafts and complex chronic total occlusion (CTO) cases for retrograde gear delivery. Guide catheters may be manually shortened as well by trimming a distal section and reconnecting with an interposed cut sheath one size smaller than the guide catheter, at the expense of some stability and torque control.

Coronary Wire Selection

Lesion traversal using a guidewire is the first interventional step to performing PCI. The spectrum of available guidewires continues to grow as PCI becomes increasingly complex (**Table 14.4**). The fundamental construction of a coronary guidewire is composed of four main components (**Fig. 14.5**):

Core: The inner structure of the wire that extends from the proximal to distal end, but not all of cores reach the distal wire tip. Proximally, the core can be made of stainless steel, nitinol, or a composite of the two metals. The composition of the core determines tip load, flexibility, steerability, trackability and support for performing PCI. Core thickness is proportional to wire support. Some cores taper, and the length of the taper is inversely proportional to the propensity for the distal wire tip to prolapse.

Tip: The tip is the distal end of the wire. If the core extends to the entire length of the wire, it is a "core-to-tip" design that lends to increased tactile feedback and near 1:1 torque control. Wires where the cores do not reach the distal end have a small metal ribbon that provides shape retention, softness,

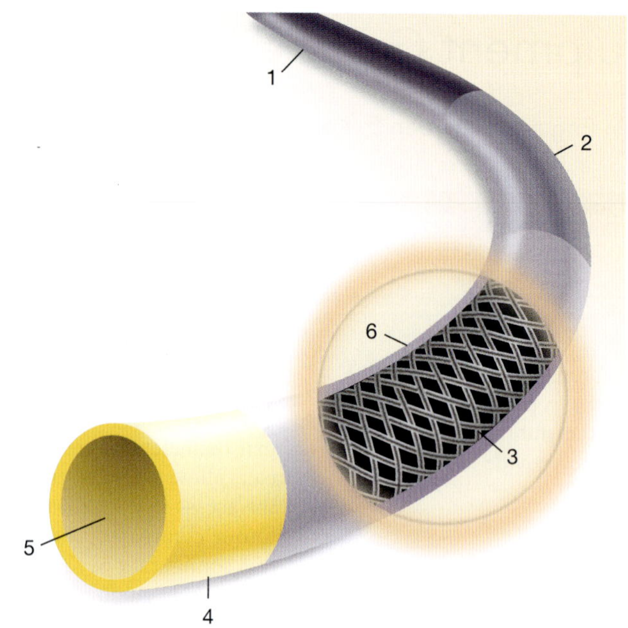

FIGURE 14.1 Guide catheter anatomy: (1) secondary curve; (2) primary curve; (3) stainless steel mesh; (4) atraumatic tip; (5) inner hydrophilic lining; (6) outer lubricious coating. (Image provided courtesy of Boston Scientific. ©2024 Boston Scientific Corporation or its affiliates. All rights reserved.)

TABLE 14.1 Compatibility of Various Combinations of Coronary Equipment With Differing Guiding Catheter Sizes

	5 FR	6 FR	7 FR	8 FR
Internal diameter (inches)	0.56-0.58	0.70-0.71	0.78-0.81	0.88-0.90
External diameter (mm)	2.3	2.52-2.6	2.85-3.1	3.2-3.5
Balloons ≥5 mm	N	Y	Y	Y
Stents ≥4.5 mm	N	Y	Y	Y
2 monorail balloons	N	Y	Y	Y
1 monorail balloon + 1 monorail stent	N	Y	Y	Y
Wire + 1 microcatheter	Y	Y	Y	Y
2 microcatheters	N	Y	Y	Y
1 microcatheter + 1 OTW balloon	N	N	Y	Y
2 OTW balloons	N	N	N	Y
2 monorail stents	N	N	Y	Y
1 monorail balloon + 1 microcatheter	N	Y	Y	Y
1 monorail balloon + OTW balloon	N	Y	Y	Y
IVUS + 2nd wire	Y	Y	Y	Y
IVUS + microcatheter	N	N	Y	Y
Rotablator	N	Y	Y	Y
Laser 0.9-1.4 mm	N	Y	Y	Y
3 monorail balloons	N	N	Y	Y

N, no; Y, yes.

Adapted from Ybarra L, Rinfret S. Access selection for chronic total occlusion percutaneous coronary intervention and complication management. *Interv Cardiol Clin.* 2021;10(1):109-120.

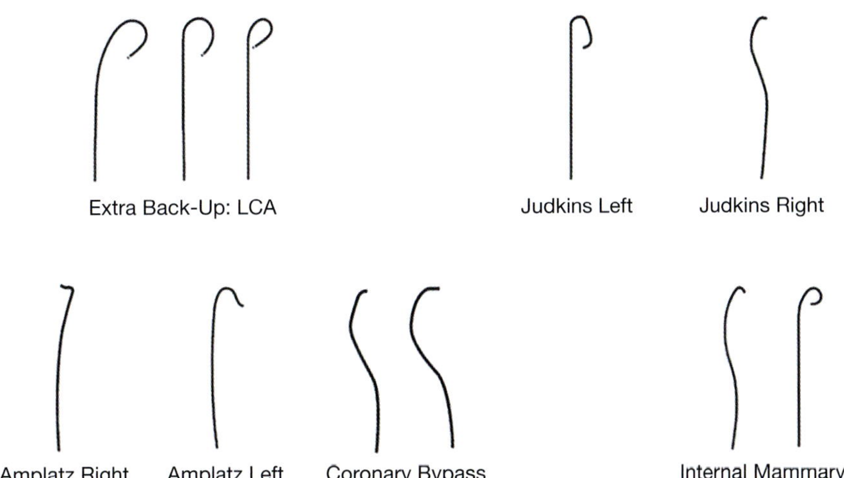

FIGURE 14.2 Commonly used guiding catheter shapes. There is an extensive list of guiding catheters from each manufacturer, some with specific curves for radial PCI that are not listed here.

TABLE 14.2 Some Suggestions for Guide Catheter Selection With Commonly Used Catheters for Differing Situations When Approaching the Coronary Vessels With Femoral Access

	LEFT CORONARY	RIGHT CORONARY
Normal root	JL4, AL-1, EBU 3.75, XB 3.5, VL4	JR4, AL-1, AR-1, AR-mod, HS
Dilated root	JL4.5, JL5, AL ≥ 2, EBU/XB ≥4, VL 5	JR ≥ 5, AL ≥ 2
	JL3.0-3.5, AL-0.75, EBU 3.5, XB 3, VL 3	JR 3, AL 0.75

AL, amplatz left; AR, amplatz right; EBU, extra back-up; HS, hockey stick; JL, judkins left; JR, judkins right; VL, voda left, XB, xtra back up.

TABLE 14.3 Suggestions for Guide Catheter Selection With Commonly Used Catheters for Differing Aortic Diameters When Using Radial Access. In General, When Using Left-Sided Radial Guides, Similar Shapes Will Work for Femoral Access But the Curve Must be Decreased, Often Approximately ½ Size to Achieve Coaxial Engagement

	LEFT CORONARY	RIGHT CORONARY
Normal root	JL3.5, AL-1, EBU 3.0-3.5, XB 3.0, VL3, IL 4.0	JR4, AL-1, AR-1, AR-mod, Ikari R or Ikari L 4.0, HS
Dilated root	JL ≥ 4, AL ≥ 2, EBU ≥ 3.75, XB ≥3.5, VL ≥ 4	JR ≥ 5, AL ≥ 2
Narrow root	JL3.0-3.5, AL-0.75, EBU 3.0, XB 3, VL 3	JR 3, AL 0.75, AR-1, AR mod

AL, amplatz left; AR, amplatz right; EBU, extra back-up; HS, hockey stick; JL, judkins left; JR, judkins right; VL, voda left; XB, xtra back up.

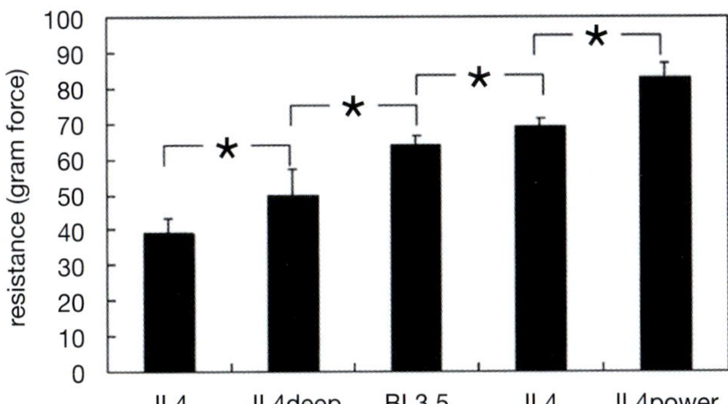

FIGURE 14.3 Comparative backup force of various 6 French (Fr) guiding catheters with automated balloon advancement in an ex vivo transradial dry model. Engagement with a JL4 guide (far left column) offers less backup support than deep engagement using the JL4 or an extra-backup left guide (center column). An Ikari left (IL4) and IL4 (far right column) with power position using deep engagement offered the highest degree of backup support in this model.[2] JL, Judkins Left. (Used with permission of H M P COMMUNICATIONS, from Ikari Y, Nagaoka M, Kim JY, Morino Y, Tanabe T. The physics of guiding catheters for the left coronary artery in transfemoral and transradial interventions. *J Invasive Cardiol.* 2005;17:636-641; permission conveyed through Copyright Clearance Center, Inc.)

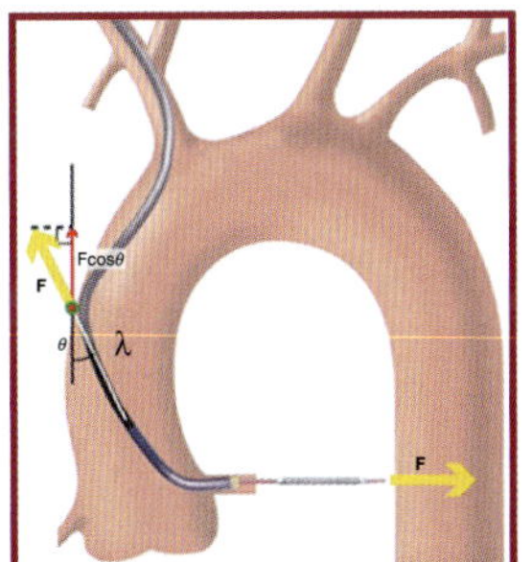

FIGURE 14.4 If *theta* is large and close to 90°, the backup force is greater. If FcosΘ ≤ λ, the guiding catheter should be stable. If FcosΘ ≥ λ, the system is vulnerable to collapse.[4] (Used with permission of H M P COMMUNICATIONS, from Ikari Y, Masuda N, Matsukage T et al. Backup force of guiding catheters for the right coronary artery in transfemoral and transradial interventions. *J Invasive Cardiol.* 2009;21:570-574; permission conveyed through Copyright Clearance Center, Inc.)

TABLE 14.4 A Nonexhaustive List of Coronary Guidewires With Differing Characteristics to Illustrate the Differentiation Between Classes of Wires

WIRE FUNCTION	WIRE CHARACTERISTICS	WIRES	TIP STIFFNESS (G)	MANUFACTURER
Workhorse	Steerable, trackable, good tactile feedback	Balanced middle weight Runthrough Sion Blue Prowater Choice PT		Abbott Terumo Asahi Intecc Terumo Boston Scientific
Navigating tortuosity and calcification	Polymer jacketed Tapered tip	Pilot 50 Fielder FC Sion Black Whisper		Abbott Terumo Asahi Intecc Abbott
Penetration	Polymer jacketed Non–polymer jacketed	Pilot 200 Gladius Confianza Pro 12 Gaia 1, 2, 3	4.1 3.0 12.4 1.7, 3.5, 4.5	Asahi Intecc Asahi Intecc Asahi Intecc Asahi Intecc

and tip flexibility at the expense of torque control. Wires are generally 0.014″ (0.36-mm) wires and have 0.014″ tips, but some have tapered tips (0.10″) (eg, Fielder XT [Asahi Intecc, Irvine, CA]).

Body: (coils, covers, sleeves): The wire body around the core is composed of coils or polymers. Hybrid wires may have polymer for the body, known as a sleeve, and the distal tip is left uncovered. The uncovered tip, better known as spring coils, provides good tactile feedback, shapeability, and shape retention. Some wire may have polymer coating that extends to the tip coils that improves deliverability across calcified or tortuous anatomy at the expense of tactile feedback (eg, Pilot 50 [Abbott Vascular, Santa Clara, CA]).

Coating: The wire body can be coated with an overlay that is hydrophilic or hydrophobic. These materials can reduce friction, improve guidewire tracking, and device delivery. Hydrophilic coatings make wires lubricious, thus decreasing tactile feedback but improving navigation through tortuosity and calcium. Hydrophobic coatings improve tactile feedback but are less slippery and decrease trackability. Again, hybrid designs exist that combine hydrophobic tip coils with hydrophilic intermediate coils to provide tactile feedback with trackability.

Guidewire selection for the gamut of coronary anatomies extends beyond this chapter, but there are several characteristics to differentiate wires:

Torquability: The translation of torque at the proximal end to the distal end for improved steering. The ultimate goal is 1:1 torque control from proximal shaft to distal tip.

Trackability, deliverability, or crossing: Once the distal tip crosses, the ability for the rest of the wire to follow and be advanced across stenoses or tortuosity is termed trackability.

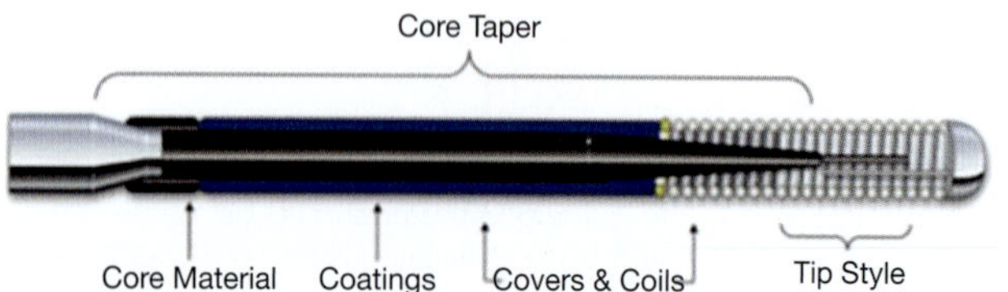

FIGURE 14.5 Anatomy of a guidewire. Guidewires are composed of the core, the tip, coatings, and covers.

Tactile feedback: Transmission of resistance to wire manipulation from distal tip to proximal body.

Tip load: The load is measured by force required to buckle the tip when applied orthogonally to a standard surface. Soft wires have low tip loads and are frequently used for their atraumatic nature and safety profile. Higher tip loads are specifically utilized for resistant plaque, frequently CTOs. Combining higher tip loads with tapered designs will increase the penetration power of a wire. Tip loads may vary from 0.5 to 25 g.

Support: Characterized as guidewire resistance to bending. Wires with more support assist with device delivery and vessel straightening. At times supportive wires are used as a "buddy," a second wire placed in parallel to straighten a vessel and assist with supporting device delivery. Less supportive wires navigate tortuosity better.

Length: Wires generally come in the short (180-190 cm) or long (300 cm) variety. There are some short wires that are compatible with wire extensions (eg, Asahi Extension [Asahi Intecc] or Doc wire [Abbott Vascular]) that convert a shorter wire to one appropriate for exchanging longer over-the-wire devices (~135-150 cm) out of the body. Longer wires sacrifice torque control and are more difficult to manage, so trapping techniques are usually preferable if guide size is sufficient, but not always feasible (for example, when using peripheral equipment off-label.) There are some specialty extra-long wires (eg, RG3, R350) specifically designed for externalization during CTO PCI, with extended coating to reduce friction and for greater ease of tracking.

ANGIOPLASTY BALLOON

In general, there are two types of commercially available balloons: over-the-wire (OTW) and monorail/rapid exchange balloons. OTW balloons have a central lumen throughout the balloon for the wire and a separate lumen (hypotube) for balloon inflation. Use of OTW balloons for wire support has largely been replaced by microcatheters due to improved performance. Monorail balloons only have a short segment of the catheter with a lumen for both the balloon and the wire allowing for lower-profile delivery and enables operators to fit more equipment into a guide. Furthermore, the short segment for the wire enables operators to perform single-operator PCI using 180-cm wires with monorail balloons. Lower-profile balloons facilitate bifurcation and multivessel PCI allowing more equipment to fit within guiding catheters.

There are specialty balloons that have different purpose such as cutting angioplasty (eg, Wolverine [Boston Scientific, Natick, MA]) and have adjunctive technology to improve angioplasty results such as lithotripsy (eg, Shockwave Medical, Santa Clara, CA). For instance, there are specialty balloons for dilation of ostial stents (Ostial Flash, Campbell, CA).

CORONARY MICROCATHETER SELECTION

Architecture: Microcatheters are supportive catheters that typically have a hydrophilic coating, and as compared with OTW balloons, the lumen is larger to minimize friction of torquing. Many catheters have a braided design to resist kinking when dealing with tortuous or calcified vessels.

Microcatheters support wire traversal by providing backup support and facilitate wire exchanges. Furthermore, they can dilate channels, allow distal drug delivery, and perform contrast injections. Commercially available microcatheters have variable crossing profiles, torquability, deliverability, and lengths (**Table 14.5**). One notable theme is that as catheter crossing profiles become smaller, pushabililty and torque transmission are sacrificed. For instance, the Caravel (Asahi Intecc), Finecross (Terumo, Shibuya, Japan), and micro-14 (Roxwood Medical, Redwood City, CA) microcatheters are good for navigating small channels but have difficulty traversing calcified channels. Corsair (Asahi Intecc) and Turnpike (Teleflex, Wayne, PA) catheters are more supportive, have better torque transmission, and cross calcified channels more easily. Turnpike LP (Teleflex), Mamba Flex (Boston Scientific, Marlborough, MA), and Corsair Pro XS (Asahi Intecc) are lower profile and specifically designed for retrograde collateral crossing.

There are two specialty coronary double-lumen microcatheters (Twin Pass [Teleflex] and Sasuke [Asahi Intecc]) specially designed for either delivery of a buddy wire or distal delivery of intracoronary medications. Specific wire techniques include bifurcation wiring, reverse wiring, parallel wiring to cross complex lesions, and of course distal delivery of buddy wires after crossing difficult lesions.

CORONARY GUIDE EXTENSION

Guide extenders increase the active support for coaxial delivery of coronary devices in crossing challenging lesions. The "mother and child" technique enables deep vessel engagement with the advantages of intubating with a softer, more flexible tubular device as compared with stiff guides that have primary curves. There are four guide extensions available in the United States: Guideliner (Teleflex), Guidezilla (Boston Scientific, Marlborough, MA), Telescope (Medtronic, St. Paul, MN), and the Trapliner (Teleflex) (**Table 14.6**). Other than improving active support for device delivery in tortuous and calcified coronary vessels, it can be used for thrombectomy, focusing contrast injections, and, in extreme cases, assisting with removal of trapped equipment such as atherectomy burrs.

Complications of using guide extensions include vessel dissection, stent deformation or dislodgement, and air embolism. With the most common complication of coronary dissection, best practices include using catheters to introduce the guide extension into a vessel. If the vessel is particularly tortuous, then balloon-assisted tracking is done by inflating a small balloon to cover the edges of the guide extension and either advancing the guide extension as a unit or advancing the balloon ahead of the guide extension then

TABLE 14.5 Coronary Microcatheters and Specific Characteristics

MICROCATHETER	LENGTH (CM)	DISTAL CROSSING DIAMETER (FR)	MANUFACTURER	SPECIAL CHARACTERISTICS
Micro-14	155	1.6	Roxwood Medical	Lowest profile, good trackability
Finecross	130, 150	1.8	Terumo	Low profile, supportive catheter, less pushability
Caravel	135, 150	1.9	Asahi Intecc	Good crossability and trackability
Corsair Pro XS	135, 150	2.1	Asahi Intecc	Good crossability and trackability
Mamba Flex	135, 150	2.1	Boston Scientific	Excellent trackability
Turnpike LP	135, 150	2.2	Teleflex	Enhanced crossability and trackability
Corsair	135, 150	2.6	Asahi Intecc	Excellent crossability and trackability
Turnpike	135, 150	2.6	Teleflex	Supportive catheter
Turnpike Spiral	130, 150	2.9	Teleflex	Supportive catheter for crossing calcified lesions
Turnpike Gold	135	2.9	Teleflex	Supportive catheter for crossing calcified lesions
Twinpass	135	2	Teleflex	Dual lumen catheter
Sasuke	135	2	Asahi Intecc	Dual lumen catheter
Supercross	130, 150	1.8	Teleflex	Flexible, angled-tip catheter provides directional support

Adapted from Dawson K, Cheney A, Hira RS. Toolbox for chronic total occlusion percutaneous coronary intervention. *Intervent Cardiol Clin.* 2021;10:25-31.

TABLE 14.6 Various Guide Extensions Available in the United States

CATHETER	MANUFACTURER	SIZE RANGE	OD (6 FR)	ID (6 FR)	RX LENGTH
Guideliner V3	Teleflex	5, 5.5-8 Fr	1.7 mm/0.067″	1.42 mm/0.056″	25 cm
Trapliner	Teleflex	6-8 Fr	1.7 mm/0.067″	1.42 mm/0.056″	13 cm
Guidezilla II	Boston Scientific	6-8 Fr (6 Fr Long [L])	1.71 mm/0.067″	1.45 mm/0.057″	25/40 cm (6Fr L)
Telescope	Medtronic	5.5-7 Fr	1.7 mm/0.067″	1.42 mm/0.056″	25 cm

ID, inner diameter; OD, outer diameter.

inflating the balloon followed by advancing the guide extension while the balloon is deflating.

The Trapliner (Teleflex) is a niche guide extension that has a balloon within its lumen for trapping coronary wires and enabling exchange of OTW microcatheters and balloons during cases.

ATHERECTOMY DEVICES

Rotablator: The Rotablator (Boston Scientific, Marlborough, MA) is a rotational atherectomy device composed of an egg-shaped diamond-coated burr, except the 1.25 mm size, which is bullet shaped (**Table 14.7**). It is available in many different sizes (1.25-2.5 mm) and is powered by compressed gas to spin a burr at speeds as high as 200K revolutions/minute. A lubricant (Rotaglide, Boston Scientific, Marlborough, MA) is mixed and infused through the shaft of the device to prevent the device from jamming or overheating during use. There are two modes, the normal mode and a lower spin mode. Dynaglide is typically used to minimize friction while traversing guide catheters or vessel tortuosity. The Rotablator ablates calcium antegrade to the burr path. The wire used is 0.010″ and the tip is 0.012″ designed to prevent the Rotaburr (Boston Scientific, Marlborough, MA) from traveling off the wire. There are two versions, the Rotafloppy and Rotasupport (Boston Scientific, Marlborough, MA) wires. The latter may be used preferentially to take advantage of wire bias in cases of eccentric calcium or ostial lesions but is associated with an increased risk of perforation, so its use remains selective.

CSI: The Diamondback 360 (Cardiovascular Systems Inc, St. Paul, MN) is an orbital atherectomy device that changes the diameter of the crown rotation based on the spin speed. There are two speeds, 80,000 and 120,000 revolutions per minute (rpm). The diameter of the ablation is contingent on not only the spin speed but also the speed of crown advancement and the duration of ablation. Longer spins and slower crown advancement are conducive to larger spin diameters. Unlike Rotablator, the CSI ablates calcium radial to the crown and does not treat calcium antegrade to the burr.

Laser: Excimer coronary laser atherectomy (ECLA) (Philips, Cambridge, MA) utilizes a xenon-chloride monochromatic exciter laser to produce ultraviolet light bursts at 308 nm with a pulse frequency of 25 to 80 Hz. The laser ablates calcium by breaking molecular bonds (photochemical), by thermal energy (photothermal), and with microbubble formation (photomechanical). The photochemical energy can be titrated, better known as fluency. For coronary interventions, operators generally choose between the 0.9 and 1.4 mm catheter sizes.

INTRAVASCULAR IMAGING

Recent data have reaffirmed the value of intravascular imaging to optimizing PCI outcomes.[5-9] There are currently two types of intravascular imaging, intravascular ultrasound (IVUS) and optical coherence tomography (OCT). Both provide cross-sectional intravascular anatomy that can provide detailed tissue composition and coronary dimensions. With use of automated pullback, intravascular imaging can provide lesion length and plaque volume as well as vessel diameter.

There are two main types of IVUS, rotational IVUS using a single rotating element to image the vessel and a nonrotating phased array of multiple elements (**Table 14.8**). Rotational IVUS all have higher imaging resolution at the expense of potential nonuniform

TABLE 14.7 Atherectomy Devices for Coronary PCI

DEVICE	MANUFACTURER	SIZE (MM)	MINIMUM GUIDE	ROTATIONAL SPEED
Rotablator	Boston Scientific	1.25	6 Fr (0.060″)	160,000-180,000 rpm
		1.5	6 Fr (0.063″)	160,000-180,000 rpm
		1.75	7 Fr (0.073″)	160,000-180,000 rpm
		2.0	8 Fr (0.083″)	160,000-180,000 rpm
		2.15	8 Fr (0.089″)	140,000-160,000 rpm
		2.25	9 Fr (0.093″)	140,000-160,000 rpm
CSI	CSI	1.25	6 Fr (0.066″)	80,000 rpm 120,000 rpm
ECLA laser	Philips	0.9-1.4	6 Fr (0.049-0.062″)	NA

NA, not applicable.

TABLE 14.8 Intravascular Ultrasound Devices and Specifications Available in the United States

CATHETER	MANUFACTURER	SIZE (F)	MINIMUM GUIDE (FR)	TRANSDUCER	MHZ	RANGE (MM)	LENGTH (CM)
OptiCross	Boston Scientific	3.0	5	Rotational	40	18	135
OptiCross HD	Boston Scientific	3.0	5	Rotational	60	18	135
OptiCross 6HD	Boston Scientific	3.6	6	Rotational	60	18	135
Eagle Eye and Eagle Eye Short Tip (ST)	Philips	3.5	5	Phased Array	20	20	150
Revolution	Philips	3.2	6	Rotational	45	14	135
Refinity Short Tip (ST)	Philips	3.0	5	Rotational	45	14	135
DualPro	Nipro	3.2	5	Rotational	35-65	16	135

rotational disturbance (NURD). Recent updates in catheter technology have decreased the incidence of NURD.

OCT uses near-infrared light to produce high-definition cross-sectional anatomy. The technique offers improved resolution compared with IVUS but with less tissue penetration. Therefore, viscous media such as contrast must be injected during interrogation to displace blood cells and prevent from obstructing the infrared light from the vessel wall. There are two catheters on the market that perform OCT, the Dragonfly (Philips) and Vis-Rx (Nipro, Bridgewater, NJ).

SUMMARY

With the aforementioned equipment, countless permutations can perform complex PCI for bifurcations, CTOs, or simple angioplasty. Use of thrombectomy devices, coronary filters, stent selection, and stent optimization extend beyond the scope of this chapter. Most importantly, with the above-mentioned fundamental tools, PCI equipment delivery and successful procedural completion is possible with even some of the most challenging scenarios.

Disclosures

Marvin H. Eng, MD is a clinical proctor for Edwards Lifesciences and Medtronic.

Kathleen Kearney reports consulting fees/honoraria from Abbott Vascular, Abiomed, Asahi, Inc, Boston Scientific, CSI, Medtronic, Teleflex, and Philips.

References

1. Ybarra LF, Rinfret S. Access selection for chronic total occlusion percutaneous coronary intervention and complication management. *Interv Cardiol Clin*. 2021;10(1):109-120.
2. Ikari Y, Nagaoka M, Kim JY, Morino Y, Tanabe T. The physics of guiding catheters for the left coronary artery in transfemoral and transradial interventions. *J Invasive Cardiol*. 2005;17(12):636-641.
3. Kotowycz MA, Johnston KW, Ivanov J, et al. Predictors of radial artery size in patients undergoing cardiac catheterization: insights from the Good Radial Artery Size Prediction (GRASP) study. *Can J Cardiol*. 2014;30(2):211-216.
4. Ikari Y, Masuda N, Matsukage T, et al. Backup force of guiding catheters for the right coronary artery in transfemoral and transradial interventions. *J Invasive Cardiol*. 2009;21(11):570-574.
5. Gao XF, Ge Z, Kong XQ, et al. 3-Year outcomes of the ULTIMATE trial comparing intravascular ultrasound versus angiography-guided drug-eluting stent implantation. *JACC Cardiovasc Interv*. 2021;14(3):247-257.
6. Hong SJ, Mintz GS, Ahn CM, et al. Effect of intravascular ultrasound-guided drug-eluting stent implantation: 5-year follow-up of the IVUS-XPL randomized trial. *JACC Cardiovasc Interv*. 2020;13(1):62-71.
7. Kinnaird T, Johnson T, Anderson R, et al. Intravascular imaging and 12-month mortality after unprotected left main stem PCI: an analysis from the British cardiovascular intervention society database. *JACC Cardiovasc Interv*. 2020;13(3):346-357.
8. Räber L, Mintz GS, Koskinas KC, et al. Clinical use of intracoronary imaging. Part 1: guidance and optimization of coronary interventions. An expert consensus document of the European Association of Percutaneous Cardiovascular Interventions. *Eur Heart J*. 2018;39(35):3281-3300.
9. Johnson TW, Räber L, di Mario C, et al. Clinical use of intracoronary imaging. Part 2: acute coronary syndromes, ambiguous coronary angiography findings, and guiding interventional decision-making—an expert consensus document of the European Association of Percutaneous Cardiovascular Interventions. *Eur Heart J*. 2019;40(31):2566-2584.

Calcified Lesion Management—Atherectomy, Specialty Balloons, Laser, and Intravascular Lithotripsy

Ahmed E. Kazem and Karim M. Al-Azizi

ROTATIONAL ATHERECTOMY

Device

The Rotablator and Rotapro (Boston Scientific; Marlboro, MA) are over-the-wire (OTW) systems that consist of a nickel-plated, diamond-coated brass burr attached to a drive shaft that can achieve speeds up to 200,000 rpm driven by compressed gas (**Fig. 15.1**). The 20- to 30-µm-sized diamond chips are located only on the front half of the olive-shaped burr. Much like a high-speed sander, the burr ablates and creates microparticulate debris when the burr comes into contact with relatively inelastic tissue. The turbine unit is cooled using a saline flush solution that also helps irrigate the vessel during activation of the burr, helping disperse the microparticulate debris through the vasculature. The reusable console can be adjusted to achieve burr speeds up to 200,000 rpm in the fully activated mode and speeds of 80,000 rpm when used in the Dynaglide mode (used almost solely for the purpose of removing the burr from the guide catheter). Each burr and drive shaft come as a separate unit and are attached to a disposable advancer using a locking mechanism. The advancer has a control knob that allows the operator to advance or retract the spinning burr and has a range of 10 cm before the burr position needs to be moved if additional atherectomy is desired. The burr and drive shaft accommodate a 0.09-inch guide wire with a floppy tip of 30 cm that has a 0.21 olive at the joint between the flexible tip and the shaft of the guide wire to prevent the burr from advancing to the flexible tip of the guide wire. A special wire clip is attached at the end of the guide wire as it exits the advancer and helps prevent the wire from spinning during the high-speed rotation. The advancer also has an internal brake that prevents the wire from spinning or advancing, which can be manually overridden by a "brake defeat" button at the back end of the device.

Principles of Atherectomy

The atheroablative effect of rotational atherectomy (RA) is based on the concept of differential cutting that is selective ablation of relatively inelastic materials such as calcified or heavily fibrotic atheromatous plaque with sparing of elastic nondiseased vessel segments. The analogy of rotablation is shaving with the razor preferentially cutting hair (inelastic tissue) and not skin (elastic tissue). The microparticulate debris generated during atherectomy range from 5 to 12 µm depending on the atherectomy speed and composition of the plaque. The debris passes through the coronary microcirculation and is ultimately taken up by the reticuloendothelial system of the spleen and liver. The rate and volume of microparticulate debris in relation to coronary flow will ultimately determine whether or not microvascular obstruction occurs, overwhelming the capacity of the capillary system. The rotablator device also takes advantage

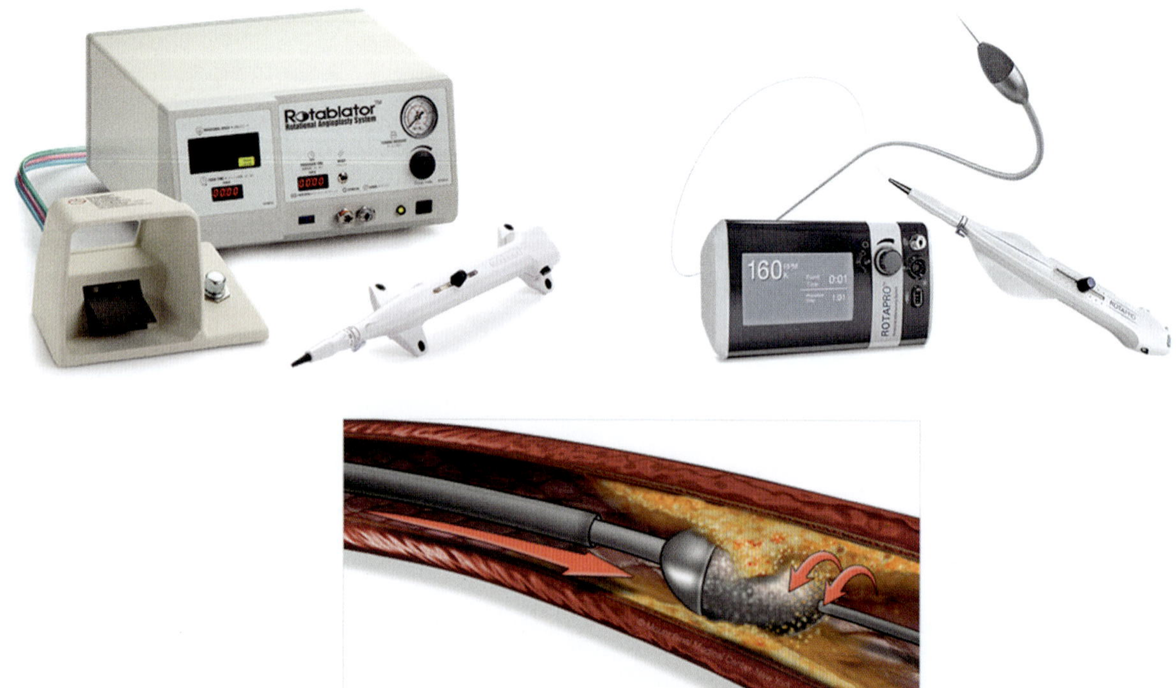

FIGURE 15.1 Composite images of the components (console and foot pedal, and advancer and catheter) of the Rotablator system on the left and the updated Rotapro system on the right. A cartoon illustration of the burr within a lesion is shown at the bottom.

of orthogonal displacement of friction as a result of the high rotational speeds, which essentially eliminates the longitudinal friction component of resistance. This characteristic distinguishes it from the passive movement of simple balloon and stent catheters within the coronary arterial system and guide catheter.

The optimal speed during an atherectomy procedure has undergone extensive evaluation.[1] Extremely low speeds potentially generate larger microparticulate debris and are inefficient in ablation, while very high speeds are associated with significant local rises in temperature and potentially thermal-mediated vascular changes, including a propensity for flow reduction. Rates of 140,000 to 160,000 RPM appear to provide an optimal compromise between the efficiency and extent of atherectomy in relation to local thermal effects and are the currently recommended range of speed for most atherectomy procedures.

Procedure

Burr Selection

Burr selection has undergone a substantial evolution since the introduction of RA. Initially, the device was used to debulk arteries, followed by balloon angioplasty. With the advent and success of intracoronary stents, and lack of data demonstrating that RA reduced restenosis rates, RA has been used almost exclusively for lesion preparation, prior to stenting, when a lesion is undilatable or extensive calcification is present. In contemporary use, burr sizes of 1.25 to 1.75 mm generally provide appropriate lesion preparation prior to stenting and it would only be under unusual circumstances that burr sizes beyond this would be chosen. In general, the greater the vessel angulation and/or extent of calcification, the smaller the burr sizes that would be chosen. The operator's comfort level will also help dictate whether the procedure will start with a 1.25- or 1.5-mm burr. One technical note that bears mentioning is that the 1.25-mm burr has a more tubular shape than the larger, more olive-shaped burrs, with many experts believing that the smallest burr is more prone to "jump forward" and potentially gets lodged in the vessel.

Guide Catheter Selection

Guide catheter selection for RA requires coaxial alignment, appropriate sizing to allow advancement and retraction of the burrs, and some measure of coronary flow during the procedure to help move microparticulate debris through the coronary microvasculature. The internal diameter of the guide catheter should be 0.04 inch larger than the burr to minimize difficulty during advancement and retraction of the burr. In addition, guide shapes require gentle transition from the shaft of the burr to the tip because acute angles, such as may be seen with a typical Judkins catheter, can impede the advancement and/or retraction of the burrs at the primary and secondary curves of the catheter. Finally, side holes may be useful so that continued flow occurs around the drive shaft of the rotablator device even during activation and advancement.

Procedural Technique

Atherectomy is begun approximately 1 cm proximal to the target lesion with constant flush through the drive shaft, controlled in an on-and-off fashion by either the foot pedal, if using the Rotablator system, or directly from the advancer, on the Rotapro system (**Table 15.1**). Expert consensus opinion is that optimal RA involves slow advancement of the burr with contact with the stenotic plaque for approximately 10 to 15 seconds and then withdrawal of the burr from the lesion allowing coronary flow to occur, followed by resumption of 10 seconds of atherectomy. Total atherectomy runs are recommended to last no more than 30 to 45 seconds to minimize the potential of overwhelming the microvasculature with the microparticulate debris. Atherectomy is continued with multiple runs until the lesion has been successfully crossed, the full extent of the 10-cm range of the advancer has been exhausted, or it appears that continued efforts would be futile with the burr chosen.

Adjunctive Techniques

The composition of the fluid used to cool the turbine of the advancer is often augmented to include nitroglycerin as a vasodilator, as well

TABLE 15.1 Procedural Approaches for Rotational Atherectomy

	TRADITIONAL	CONTEMPORARY
Arterial access	Femoral 8 Fr	Radial (6-7.5 Fr) or femoral (6-8 Fr), depending upon burr size requirement and operator experience.
Guiding catheter	Judkins catheters	Single curve with strong support. Operator preference but stable catheter position required.
Guide wire	Floppy rotawire or extra support rotawire for aorto-ostial lesions	Rotawire placement not always straightforward. Use of regular wire placement, with exchange using microcatheter placement is often required.
Burr size	Debulking up to 0.7 vessel ratio	Plaque modification with small burrs (1.25-1.5 mm) as initial strategy is default position. A step-up approach is encouraged to limit debris size and complications.
Ablation speed	180,000-200,000 rpm	Plaque modification usually achieved at low speeds (135,000-180,000 rpm) to reduce risk of complications.
Temporary pacemaker	Always for dominant RCA and left main PCI	Smaller burrs at lower speeds have led to lower incidence of transient heart block. Many operators use atropine to treat, avoiding any complications of temporary pacemaker placement.
Rotablation flush	Rotablation cocktail with verapamil, nitrates, and heparin in saline recommended	Rotablation cocktail with verapamil, nitrates, and heparin in saline recommended.

RCA, right coronary artery; PCI, percutaneous coronary intervention.

TABLE 15.2 Indications and Contraindications for Rotational Atherectomy

INDICATIONS	CONTRAINDICATIONS
Single-vessel atherosclerotic CAD[a]	Lesion cannot be crossed with guide wire[a]
Multivessel atherosclerotic CAD[a]	Last remaining vessel with compromised LV function[a]
Restenotic lesions[a]	Saphenous vein grafts[a]
Native vessel CAD with lesion length <25 mm[a]	Angiographic evidence of thrombus[a]
Heavily calcified lesions	Angiographic evidence of dissection at lesion site[a]
Undilatable lesions	

[a]Per instructions for use.
CAD, coronary artery disease; LV, left ventricular.

as Roto-glide (Boston Scientific) as a coronary lubricant. The latter consists of a sterile egg white and olive oil emulsion, which in animal testing appeared to minimize heat generation, permitting a higher rate of rotation of the burr if needed. General expert consensus also recommends liberal use of vasopressors to maintain an adequate perfusion pressure during RA. Practically, this is most easily performed with 100-μg bolus injections of Neo-Synephrine (phenylephrine). Additionally, liberal use of nitroglycerin throughout the procedure is recommended to enhance coronary flow and minimize microparticulate obstruction of the microvasculature. Prophylactic pacemakers have traditionally been used by some to counteract the bradycardia, which can be severe at times, that may accompany rotablation. Nevertheless, some operators use aminophylline and/or atropine to minimize atherectomy-associated bradycardia without use of temporary pacemakers.

Indications and Contraindications for Use

The manufacturers' and generally accepted clinical indications and contraindications for use of RA are shown in **Table 15.2**. Operator experience will dictate comfort levels with these parameters. Accepted indications are heavily calcified lesions able to be crossed with the rotablator guide wire, as well as undilatable lesions. In contemporary practice, RA has shown a resurgence in use due to a more elderly population enriched with more calcific disease, as well as use in more complex percutaneous coronary intervention (PCI) and chronic total occlusions (CTOs). Accepted contraindications include severe lesion entry or exit angulation and angiographically visible thrombus or dissection.

Outcomes

The studies evaluating the clinical efficacy and safety of RA were performed in the late 1990s.[2-4] As a result of these studies, RA was shown to be at most noninferior to percutaneous transluminal coronary angioplasty (PTCA) with respect to restenosis and associated with higher rates of adverse cardiac events. More recently, Arora and colleagues[5] published the results of PCI with and without RA from a nationwide patient sample from 107,131 cases in 2012 and showed higher overall complication rates with RA (12.7%) compared with without RA (9.1%), $P < .01$ (**Table 15.3**). With the advent of the stent era, continued interest in debulking prior to stent placement led to the evaluation of atherectomy as an adjunct to stenting. In the SPORT trial, patients with moderate to heavily

TABLE 15.3 Incidence of Periprocedural Complications of Percutaneous Coronary Intervention

	ATHERECTOMY		OVERALL	*P*-VALUE
	NO	YES		
Overall (unweighted)	103,759 (96.85)	3372 (3.15)	107,131	
Overall (weighted)	518,795 (96.85)	16,860 (3.15)	535,655	
Any complication[a]	9.05%	12.66%	9.16%	<0.001
Any complication or death	9.73%	13.5%	9.85%	<0.001
Any vascular complication	1.06%	1.57%	1.08%	<0.001
Postoperative hemorrhage requiring transfusion	0.4%	0.3%	0.4%	<0.001
Vascular injury	0.7%	1.28%	0.71%	<0.001
Cardiac complications	2.07%	4.06%	2.14%	<0.001
Iatrogenic cardiac complications	1.83%	3.56%	1.88%	<0.001
Pericardial complications	0.13%	0.3%	0.13%	<0.001
Open heart surgery	0.16%	0.24%	0.16%	0.01
Respiratory complications (postoperative respiratory failure)	5.46%	7.12%	5.51%	<0.001
Postoperative stroke/TIA	0.14%	0.12%	0.14%	0.507
Acute renal failure requiring dialysis	0.18%	0.24%	0.18%	0.107
Postoperative DVT/PE	0.52%	0.71%	0.53%	0.001
Postoperative infectious complications	1.44%	1.66%	1.45%	0.019

[a]Any periprocedural complication listed in supplemental **Table 15.1**.
DVT, deep venous thrombosis; PE, pulmonary embolism; TIA, transient ischemic attack.
Adapted from Arora S, Panaich SS, Patel N, et al. Coronary atherectomy in the United States (from a nationwide inpatient sample). *Am J Cardiol*. 2016;117:555-562.

calcified lesions were randomized to either RA, followed by stenting, or PTCA followed by stenting.[6] The trial was stopped early, but available data were presented that showed the primary endpoint of restenosis at 9 months was similar between the two groups, while major adverse cardiac events were higher with RA. More recently, outcomes after Taxus stent placement, with or without RA, were evaluated in 240 patients in the ROTAXUS trial.[7] They also did not observe a decrease in late lumen loss after RA, compared with balloon angioplasty.

More recently, following the production of the updated Rotapro RA system, the Rotapro study was conducted to evaluate the safety and feasibility of this system for lesion preparation in calcified coronary artery stenosis.[8] The study consisted of 597 patients treated with RA (246 Rotapro vs 351 Rotablator). Procedural outcomes were compared according to the applied system. The primary endpoint of in-hospital major adverse cardiac events (MACE) was comparable between the Rotapro and the Rotablator groups; however, Rotapro was associated with less fluoroscopy time, radiation dose, as well as contrast use.

As a result of these clinical trials, in the 2021 American College of Cardiology (ACC)/American Heart Association (AHA)/Society for Cardiovascular Angiography and Interventions (SCAI) update of coronary artery revascularization guidelines (**Table 15.4**), RA remains a class IIa recommendation for plaque modification in fibrotic or heavily calcified lesions that might not be crossed by a balloon catheter or adequately dilated prior to stent implantation, to improve procedural success (level of evidence: B-R).[9]

TABLE 15.4 2021 ACC/AHA/SCAI Coronary Artery Revascularization Guidelines

ROTATIONAL ATHERECTOMY: RECOMMENDATIONS
• Class IIa • In patients with fibrotic or heavily calcified lesions, plaque modification with rotational atherectomy can be useful to improve procedural success (*level of evidence: B-R*).

Complications

The operator should be aware of several procedural complications that are relatively common with the use of RA (**Table 15.5**). Bradycardia can accompany RA and can be severe. It is most commonly associated with treatment of the right coronary artery (RCA) but can be seen with treatment of both the left anterior descending and circumflex coronary arteries as well. Although some operators favor preprocedural placement of a temporary pacemaker, this is often not required with the use of aminophylline and/or atropine, as mentioned earlier. Coronary slow flow or no flow is a well-recognized complication of RA. Multiple preventive strategies have been outlined. Factors that have been implicated in slow flow include excessive burr speeds, prolonged atherectomy, as well as burr "deceleration" during atherectomy. The latter is defined as a decrease in more than 5000 rpm below the average working atherectomy speed and is signaled in the change in the frequency generated by the device during atherectomy. Although very uncommon, burr entrapment can occur as the burr deeply engages the vessel and plaque, causing stalling or complete cessation of rotation of the device. Once this occurs, coronary ischemia will develop due to flow obstruction. Because the device performs atherectomy in a clockwise fashion, it has been suggested that detachment of the burr from the advancer, and counterclockwise manual rotation of the burr, can help facilitate removal of the device. In extreme circumstances, it may be necessary to perform emergency surgery to remove the device.

Finally, coronary perforation remains one of the feared complications of coronary RA. In the largest cohort study to date of perforations associated with RA use, the incidence of coronary perforations was 1.3% (103/8047) and in multivariate analysis had an odds ratio of 2.37 (95% confidence interval 1.80-3.11; $P < .001$) for predicting a perforation.[10] In spite of differential cutting, the position of the guide wire across an angulated segment of the vessel may still result in ablation and ultimately perforation. The propensity for the guide wire to lie within the coronary vessel in the straightest path has been termed "wire bias" and may bring the burr into contact with nondiseased elements of the vessel wall.[1] Type I and type II perforations can often be managed with adjunct balloon angioplasty. Free-flowing type III perforations are much more difficult to treat and may often necessitate pericardiocentesis and/or emergency surgery. Although a covered stent would be attractive in these situations, these perforations often occur at severe angulations of vessels, in heavily calcified vessels, and in more distal locations of the coronary circulation, making placement of the bulky covered stents difficult at best. It should be noted that direct thrombin inhibitors were not used at the time of the initial experience with RA. In today's practice, direct thrombin inhibitors are frequently used and are potentially problematic with use of RA because their effect cannot be reversed in the setting of a perforation, and unfractionated heparin is the consensus recommendation of experts regarding use of this device.

TABLE 15.5 Complication Management—Avoid With Good Technique

	TECHNIQUE TO AVOID	STRATEGY FOR RESOLUTION
Slow flow	Small burrs and lower speeds	Optimize BP if low
	Be patient between ablation runs	Use of intracoronary nitrates/verapamil/adenosine/nitroprusside all described
		Use of flush cocktail
Dissection	Careful case selection to avoid excessive tortuosity	Avoid further rotablation if dissection identified
		Dissection management as for any PCI
Burr entrapment	Rare complication usually avoided with careful case selection and good technique	Controlled push and pull of rotablation shaft
		Position second wire to allow balloon placement
		Cautious deep intubation with mother-in-child catheter for more support
		Cardiothoracic surgical resolution occasionally required
Perforation	Commonly related to poor technique (oversizing of burr, too angulated, inappropriate speed)	Standard techniques to resolve any perforation, including emergency pericardiocentesis and use of covered stents

BP, blood pressure; PCI, percutaneous coronary intervention.

ORBITAL ATHERECTOMY

Device

The orbital atherectomy (OA) system (Cardiovascular Systems, Inc., St. Paul, MN) is an OTW system that has similarities to RA, but with notable differences in the mechanism of atherectomy and technique (**Fig. 15.2**). The OA device, the Diamondback 360, is a single, eccentrically mounted diamond-coated crown that orbits on the wire rather than spins, utilizing the mechanism of centrifugal force, which presses the crown against the lesion, resulting in differential sanding. An advantage of the system is its ability to exert sanding motions with both forward and backward advancement of the burr. The subsequent microparticulate debris is smaller than with RA (<2 vs 5-10 μm). The entire system consists of four components: the device (OAD, orbital atherectomy device), which is an OTW sheath-covered drive shaft and crown; a dedicated guide wire; a reusable external pump system; and a lubricant solution. The OAD has a single crown size that can be used for all cases. It is 6-Fr guide compatible, but can be used with a 7-Fr guide for more robust support. The radius of atherectomy is altered using the speed of orbit: 80,000 and 120,000 rpm. An advancer unit allows the operator to advance or retract the burr at a target travel rate of between 1 and 10 mm per second. Akin to RA, an infusion of mixture is used to cool and lubricate the mechanism, reducing friction between the drive shaft and the glide wire. The specified glide wire, the ViperWire Advance, is a stainless steel 0.012-inch wire with a silicon coating and spring tip, which measures 0.014 inch, in contrast to the body of the 0.009-inch rotablator wire. This tip must angiographically be at least 10 cm distal to the target lesion.

Principles of Orbital Atherectomy

The underlying mechanism of differential sanding is similar to that of RA (see earlier) in that there is selective ablation of inelastic materials, including heavily calcified or fibrotic plaque versus normal vessel. The notable differences involve the single crown size and orbit compared with the potentially larger burr sizes with RA.

Procedure

Burr Selection

In contrast to RA where burr size is a complex choice and has been well studied, in OA this is far more straightforward of a choice. Most cases are accomplished with one crown size (fixed "classic crown" of 1.25 mm), but the orbital path and speed allow for varied depth of orbital cutting.

Guide Catheter Selection

Guide catheter selection requires significant coaxial guide support and appropriate sizing. Extra backup guides for the left coronary system, and a MAC 3.0 (Medtronic) or the Amplatz Left curve guides, work well for the right coronary system. This can be accomplished through a 6- or 7-Fr system.

Procedural Technique

OA is begun by positioning the crown over the wire 1 cm proximal to the target lesion, visualizing that the tip is not within the lesion when the crown and drive shaft begin to spin. The advancement begins after ensuring that 5 mm exists between the

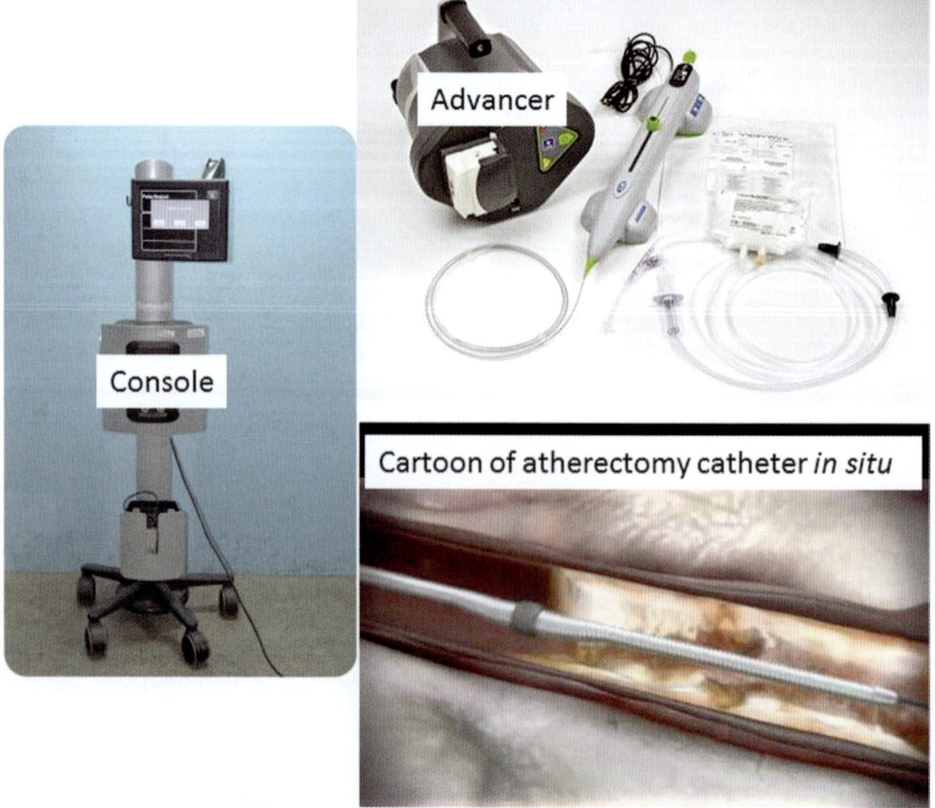

FIGURE 15.2 Composite images of the components (console, and advancer and catheter) of the orbital atherectomy system. The guide wire used to deliver the burr to the lesion site is not shown. A cartoon illustration of the crown within a lesion is shown on the bottom.

proximal end of the guide wire spring tip and the OAD drive shaft at the distal end of the lesion. The break lever is engaged and the control knob and button is used to turn on the device and control the forward advancement of the burr. A slow rate of travel through the lesion, between 1 and 10 mm per second, is desired in a slow forward-and-backward motion for a total of no more than 30 seconds—with a maximal treatment time of 5 minutes. An equal period of rest between runs is recommended, and the system provides an audible alarm at 25 seconds. Unlike RA, additional runs or passes with the device will provide further gain in luminal area due to the different mechanism of action and the contribution of increasing centrifugal force on the lesion. Longer lesions will require additional passes, not just longer-duration passes.

Adjunctive Techniques

The system includes ViperSlide (Cardiovascular Systems, Inc.), which is an emulsion comprising soybean oil, egg yolk phospholipids, glycerin, sodium hydroxide, and water. This decreases heat and friction between the OAD and the guide wire. Similar to RA, prophylactic pacemaker placement can be considered in RCA lesions or in left dominant circumflex lesions.

Indications and Contraindications for Use

The manufacturer's generally accepted clinical indication is to facilitate stent delivery in patients with coronary artery disease who are acceptable candidates for PTCA or stenting due to, de novo, severely calcified coronary artery lesions (**Table 15.6**). The accepted contraindications include an inability to pass the wire, a target in a bypass graft, a stent or last remaining conduit, and an angiographically visible dissection or thrombus. A strong relative contraindication would be that of severe tortuosity, with a particular focus on lesion entry or exit angles.

Outcomes

The data evaluating the clinical safety and efficacy of OA are derived from the ORBIT I and ORBIT II studies. There is no randomized controlled trial directly comparing RA with OA. The ORBIT I trial was a two-center, prospective, nonrandomized feasibility study in 50 patients.[11] Device success was 98%, and procedural success was 94%. Major adverse events occurred in 4% in-hospital; in 6% at 30 days; and in 8% at 6 months. The ORBIT II trial (Chambers) was a prospective multicenter nonblinded single-arm trial in 443 patients with severely calcified lesions. Successful stent delivery after OA occurred in 97.7% of patients. The rates of slow flow and no reflow were very low, occurring in less than 1% of patients. In-hospital myocardial infarction (MI) occurred in 0.7% of patients, target vessel revascularization in 0.7%, and cardiac death in 0.2%. The 2021 AHA/ACC/SCAI guidelines for coronary artery revascularization included a IIb recommendation given for OA to be considered to improve procedural success in patients with fibrotic or heavily calcified lesions (**Table 15.7**).[9]

Complications

The overall mix of complications with OA is similar to that of RA, including bradycardia, particularly in patients with culprit RCA or left-dominant large circumflex lesions; dissection; slow flow or no reflow; and, most alarmingly, coronary perforation. In the ORBIT II trial, the rate of any of these complications was low: 0.9% post OA and 1.8% overall (8/443).

TABLE 15.6 Indications and Contraindications for Orbital Atherectomy

INDICATIONS	CONTRAINDICATIONS
To facilitate stent delivery in patients with coronary artery disease who are acceptable candidates for PTCA or stenting due to de novo, severely calcified coronary artery lesions[a]	Inability to pass wire[a]
	Target in a bypass graft, stent, or last remaining conduit[a]
	Angiographically visible thrombus[a]

[a]Per instructions for use.
PTCA, percutaneous transluminal coronary angioplasty.

CUTTING BALLOON ANGIOPLASTY

Device

Cutting balloon angioplasty utilizes specialty balloons with microsurgical blades (atherotomes) that are aligned longitudinally causing localized atherosclerotic incisions during balloon inflation. The Flextome cutting balloon (Boston Scientific) was first introduced in the early 1990s and has since been upgraded to a newer, lower-profile Wolverine cutting balloon, which was designed for improved flexibility and deliverability. The Wolverine balloon is an OTW system that features a balloon with either three or four longitudinally aligned and fixed atherotomes (**Fig. 15.3**). The balloons are available in 6, 10, and 15 mm lengths, with diameters available from 2 to 3.25 mm, with three atherotomes, and 3.50 to 4 mm, which contain four atherotomes. These atherotomes are folded within the balloon material along its long axis in the deflated position and are slowly deployed over approximately 1 minute. This process creates controlled longitudinal incisions as a result of the deployment process. When the balloon is deflated, the atherotomes are folded within the balloon material to minimize the risk of trauma as the balloon is withdrawn from the coronary circulation. It should be noted that, because of the addition of the atherotomes, the balloons have a crossing profile that is larger than either compliant or noncompliant conventional balloons.

Procedure

The general preparation for the cutting balloon procedure is similar to that for a simple balloon angioplasty.[12] The one caveat may be that guides with additional backup support might be necessary to cross some lesions because of the bulkier nature of the cutting balloon compared with a conventional balloon. Similar to simple balloon angioplasty, the lesion is initially crossed with a coronary guide wire and the cutting balloon is advanced to the lesion site.

TABLE 15.7 2021 ACC/AHA/SCAI Coronary Artery Revascularization Guidelines

ORBITAL ATHERECTOMY: RECOMMENDATIONS
• Class IIb   • In patients with fibrotic or heavily calcified lesions, plaque modification with orbital atherectomy may be considered to improve procedural success (*level of evidence: B-NR*).

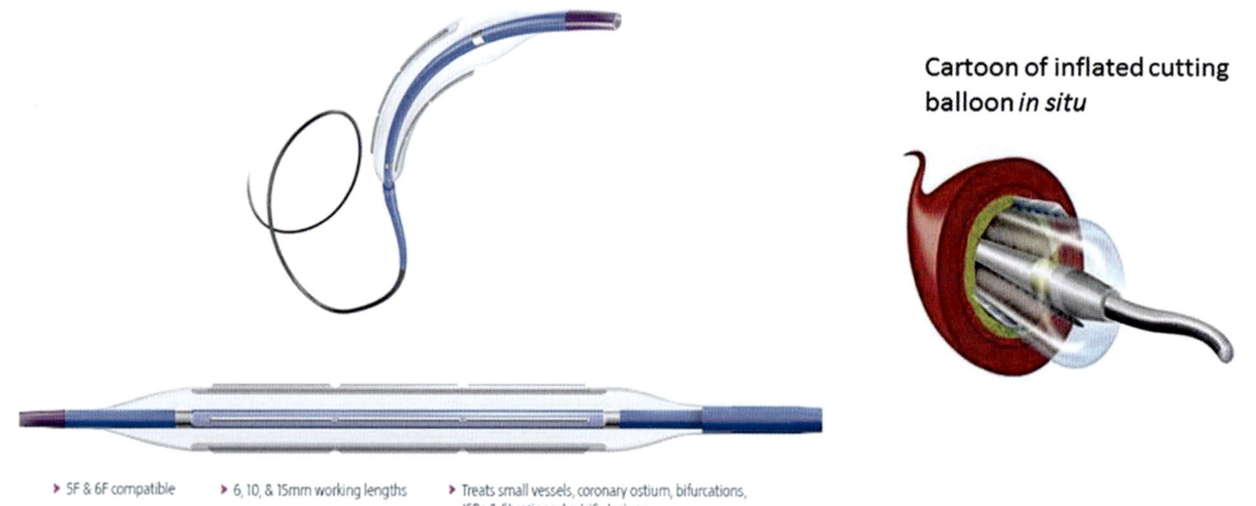

FIGURE 15.3 A magnified image of an inflated cutting balloon showing the exposed atherotomes fixed to the long axis of the balloon is shown on the left. A cartoon illustration of an inflated cutting balloon in a vessel is shown on the right.

As can be recognized by the short working lengths, the device is designed to treat short lesions. Once the lesion is crossed, the balloon is slowly inflated at 1 atm per 5 seconds, until nominal pressure (6 atm) is achieved. Deflation is performed similar to balloon angioplasty and the device withdrawn into the guide catheter. In some circumstances when the result is suboptimal, upsizing an additional half size may be necessary to achieve optimal enlargement of the vessel at the lesions site.

Indications for Use

The manufacturer's and generally accepted clinical indications and contraindications for use of cutting balloon angioplasty are shown in **Table 15.8**. Generally accepted indications are for focal-resistant lesions, in-stent restenosis, and ostial and bifurcation lesions. Contraindications are angiographically visible thrombus and concentric severe calcification. The manufacturer warns about using the cutting balloon distal to a stent, or through a stent strut, because the device may become entangled in the stent and be difficult to remove and/or disrupt the stent architecture.

Outcomes

The cutting balloon was introduced in the mid-1990s and underwent evaluation in comparison with simple balloon angioplasty for de novo coronary artery lesions.[13] In the CAPAS[14] trial, angiographic restenosis was lower than with balloon angioplasty, but in the much larger global restenosis trial (GST)[15] and REDUCE I[16] trial, angiographic restenosis at 9 months was similar for both devices. Overall cumulative rates of major adverse clinical events were similar for both devices, although there was a trend in favor of the cutting balloon.

In the RESCUT trial, the cutting balloon was compared with balloon angioplasty for treatment of in-stent restenosis, with binary restenosis as a primary endpoint again.[17] In this trial, 9-month angiographic restenosis rates were similar for the two devices, as was cumulative major adverse cardiac events at 1 year.

More recently, the COPS trial was a randomized study that compared the use of cutting balloon versus noncompliant balloon (NCB) use in 100 patients with severe de novo calcified coronary lesions.[18] The study concluded that treatment of calcified lesions with high-pressure cutting balloon results in a larger minimal stent area and more symmetric stent expansion at the level of the calcified segment compared with NCB.

Based on the results of these clinical trials, the 2021 update of the coronary artery revascularization guidelines gave balloon atherotomy (cutting or scoring balloons) a class IIb recommendation in patients with fibrotic or heavily calcified lesions, to improve procedural success (**Table 15.9**).[9]

TABLE 15.8 Indications and Contraindications for Cutting Balloon Angioplasty

INDICATIONS	CONTRAINDICATIONS
High-pressure, balloon-resistant lesion[a]	Angiographic evidence of thrombus[a]
Discrete (<15 mm) or tubular (<10-20 mm) lesions[a]	Vessel angulation >45°[a]
Reference vessel diameter 2-4 mm[a]	Use through stent struts or a lesion distal to a recently implanted stent[a]
In-stent restenosis	Presence of coronary spasm[a]
Bifurcation lesions	
Ostial lesions	

[a]Per instructions for use.

Complications

The complications associated with cutting balloon angioplasty are in general similar to those of simple balloon angioplasty. Although the device is intended to create controlled dissections, extensive dissections nonetheless have been observed. Additionally, perforations and other ischemic complications have been observed similar to simple balloon angioplasty.

SCORING BALLOON ANGIOPLASTY

Device

The AngioSculpt RX scoring balloon (Philips; San Diego, CA) is a novel balloon catheter consisting of a semicompliant balloon catheter, around which three rectangular nitinol scoring wires are

TABLE 15.9 2021 ACC/AHA/SCAI Coronary Artery Revascularization Guidelines

CUTTING/SCORING BALLOON ANGIOPLASTY: RECOMMENDATIONS
Class IIb
• In patients with fibrotic or heavily calcified lesions, plaque modification with balloon atherotomy may be considered to improve procedural success (*level of evidence: B-NR*).

wrapped in a helical fashion (**Fig. 15.4**). The balloon catheter can be expanded to 20 atm of pressure, allowing greater force to be applied focally compared with standard balloon angioplasty. The device is 0.014-inch guide wire and 6-Fr guide catheter compatible. It is available in diameters of 2, 2.5, 3, and 3.5 mm and lengths of 6, 10, and 15 mm.

The Scoreflex NC scoring balloon (Cardiovascular Systems, Inc.) is an NCB with dual wires on opposite sides of the balloon surface, which creates a focal stress pattern to facilitate safe and controlled plaque modification. The catheter features a short rapid exchange tip that enables the combined effect of the built-in nitinol wire and the conventional guide wire on the opposite side to score lesions (**Fig. 15.4**). It is available in diameters of 1.75 mm up to 4.0 mm and lengths of 10, 15, and 20 mm.

Procedure

The general preparation for the scoring balloon procedure is similar to that for a simple balloon angioplasty.[12] Similar to simple balloon angioplasty, the lesion is initially crossed with a coronary guide wire and the scoring balloon is advanced to the lesion site. Once the lesion is crossed, the balloon is inflated at 2-atm increments, over 10 to 20 seconds, until a final deployment pressure is achieved. The scoring balloon has the potential advantage over conventional balloons in restenotic lesions where slippage with conventional balloons occurs frequently. The AngioSculpt features a helical cage design and square, rather than round, wire shape, which provides circumferential scoring and helps minimize slippage, locking the device within the lesion (**Fig. 15.4**). Deflation is performed similar to balloon angioplasty, and the device is withdrawn into the guide catheter. In some circumstances when the result is suboptimal, upsizing an additional half size may be necessary to achieve optimal enlargement of the vessel at the lesion's site.

Indications for Use

The AngioSculpt as well as the Scoreflex scoring balloon catheters are indicated for use in the treatment of hemodynamically significant coronary artery stenosis, including in-stent restenosis and complex type C lesions, for the purposes of improving myocardial perfusion (**Table 15.10**).

Outcomes

The results of a US multicenter trial evaluating the safety and efficacy of the AngioSculpt scoring balloon indicated a high success rate and low incidence of coronary dissections (13.7%).[19] In an observational trial of 299 patients, ultrasound imaging was used to assess drug-eluting stent placement (Cypher or Taxus) after direct stenting, predilatation with a conventional balloon, and after scoring balloon pretreatment. Use of the scoring balloon resulted in greater luminal gain and a higher percentage of lesions achieving a final stent diameter >5.0 mm^2, compared with either direct stenting or predilation with a conventional balloon.[20] Outcomes after use of a drug-coated balloon in in-stent restenosis, with or without pretreatment with a scoring balloon, were evaluated in the ISAR-DESIRE 4 trial and showed that scoring balloon use significantly improved the angiographic antirestenotic efficacy of paclitaxel-coated balloon angioplasty.[21] Finally, the scoring balloon was used to treat the side branch of bifurcation lesions treated with a drug-eluting stent in 93 patients in the AGILITY trial.[22] The postscoring balloon dissection rate was 6.0% (2.1% after stenting), and the 9-month MACE rate was 5.4%.

As previously mentioned, the 2021 update of the coronary artery revascularization guidelines has given balloon atherotomy (cutting or scoring balloons) a class IIb recommendation in patients with fibrotic or heavily calcified lesions, to improve procedural success (**Table 15.9**).[9]

Complications

The complications associated with scoring balloon angioplasty are in general similar to those of simple balloon angioplasty and cutting

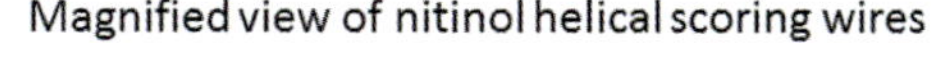

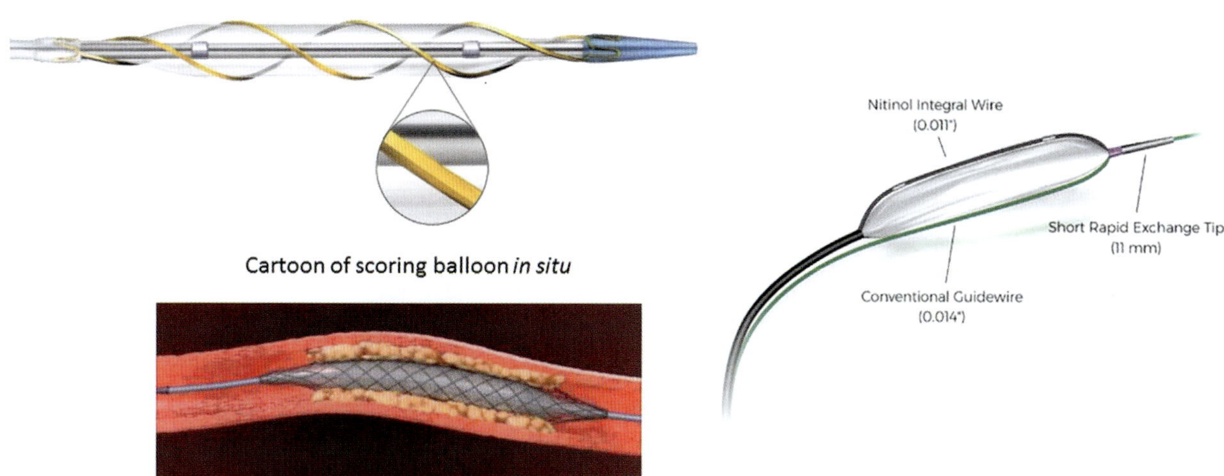

FIGURE 15.4 Magnified view of the nitinol helical scoring wires, with a blowup of the wire itself. An illustration of a scoring balloon within a lesion is shown at the bottom. On the right is a magnified image of the Scoreflex NC scoring balloon.

TABLE 15.10 Indication and Contraindications for Scoring Balloon Angioplasty

INDICATIONS	CONTRAINDICATIONS
Use in the treatment of hemodynamically significant coronary artery stenosis, including in-stent restenosis, and complex type C lesions for the purpose of improving myocardial perfusion[a]	Use through stent struts or a lesion distal to a recently implanted stent[a]
Bifurcation lesions	Presence of coronary spasm[a]
Ostial lesions	Excessive vessel angulation
Lesion preparation in conjunction with bioresorbable stents	Angiographic evidence of thrombus

[a]Per instructions for use.

balloon angioplasty. Although the device is intended to create controlled dissections, extensive dissections nonetheless have been observed. Additionally, perforations and other ischemic complications have been observed similar to simple balloon angioplasty.

LASERS

Device

The excimer laser coronary atherectomy (ELCA) system (Spectranetics, Colorado Springs, CO) consists of a multifiber catheter and a CVX-300 console, which emits light at ultraviolet wavelengths of 308 nm (**Fig. 15.5**). It is 0.014-inch guide wire–compatible and is available in either Rx or OTW configurations. Catheters are available in sizes ranging from 0.9 to 2.0 mm for the Rx configuration and 0.9 mm in the OTW configuration. The catheters are 6- to 8-Fr compatible, depending on the catheter size. Fluence of 30 to 60 mJ/mm^2 is available for all catheters, while the 0.9-mm X-80 has the unique quality of delivering fluence up to 80 mJ/mm^2.

Principles of Laser Angioplasty

Laser-mediated coronary angioplasty was developed and offered for clinical application in order to approach lesions that were challenging for routine balloon angioplasty, such as nondilatable lesions, as well as CTOs. Most interventionalists are familiar with the general concept of laser performance because it is used in multiple medical applications, including lead extraction for pacemaker lead removal. Lasers produce intense electromagnetic energy delivered through coaxial optical fibers bundled inside a coronary delivery catheter. The optimal lasing technique involves delivery of the tip of the laser catheter to the area of interest. Activation of the device produces a cone of laser energy that extends no more than 50 µm beyond the tip of the catheter and leads to vaporization of plaque. The vaporization of organic material such as plaque is achieved by photochemical effects, in which the pulses destroy carbon bonds; photothermal effects where intracellular water is heated causing cellular destruction; and photomechanical effects where bubbles burst and alter obstructive material.[23] The laser beam does not interact with inorganic material, such as calcium or steel; thus, it can be used safely near a guide wire or stent. Not surprisingly, the tremendous energy generated by the laser beam can also lead to gas bubbles and acoustic effects, which have the untoward effect of possible dissection and perforation, but which can be minimized by good technique and continuous saline irrigation of the vessel.

Laser Technique

Optimal lasing requires guide wire positioning across a lesion, as well as coaxial movement within the coronary circulation. Lasing also generates a tremendous amount of heat, which is dissipated a number of ways: via control of the energy intensity used to deliver the energy, limiting the length of each of the lasing sequences, and the liberal use of a heparin flush throughout the procedure. The lasing technique currently used is similar to that reported in the LEONARDO trial, a prospective registry evaluating the safety and efficacy of fluence rates up to 80 mJ/mm^2 in patients with complex coronary lesions using the X-80 laser catheter.[20] Initial lasing was initiated at 60 mJ/mm^2 (40 Hz) and increased to 80 mJ/mm^2 (80 Hz) for resistant lesions.

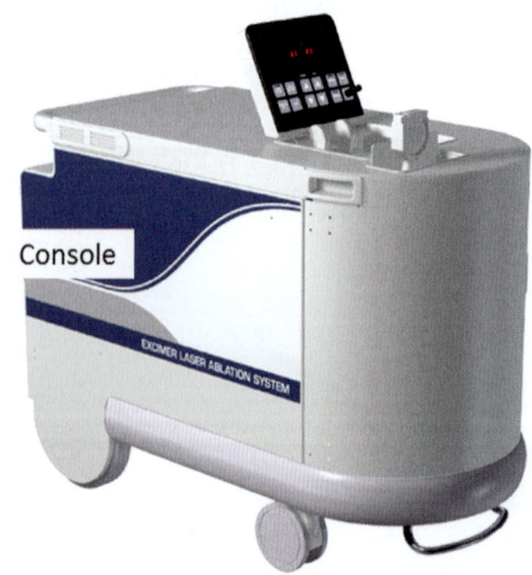

Cartoon of laser *in situ*

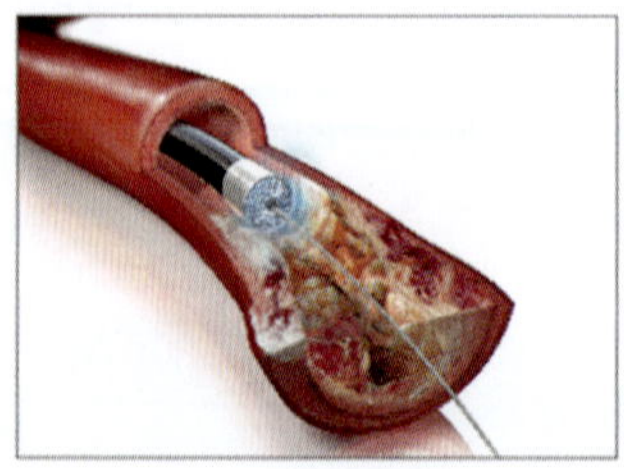

FIGURE 15.5 The excimer laser ablation system console is shown on the left. An illustration of the laser within a lesion is shown on the right.

The laser pulse length is 185 nanoseconds, with cycles of 5 seconds on and 10 seconds off (except for the X-80 catheter, which uses a 10 seconds on and 5 seconds off cycle). Successful coronary laser angioplasty is followed by stenting.

Indications for Use

The manufacturer's and generally accepted clinical indications and relative contraindications for use of laser angioplasty are shown in **Table 15.11**. Current indications are for occluded saphenous vein bypass grafts, ostial lesions, long lesions, moderately calcified lesions, CTOs, lesions that previously failed balloon angioplasty, and restenosis in 316L stainless steel stents. Contraindications include inability to cross the lesion with a guide wire, lesion located within a bifurcation, excessive lesion entry and exit angulation of the lesion and vessel, and lesion is located in an unprotected left main artery.

Outcomes

Use in De Novo Coronary Artery Lesions

In the AMRO[6] and LAVA[24] trials, laser and balloon angioplasty were evaluated with a primary endpoint of 6-month clinical outcomes. Rates of revascularization were higher with laser versus balloon angioplasty and were also associated with a significant increase in rates of coronary complication compared with simple balloon angioplasty alone. Based on these studies, routine use of laser angioplasty is not recommended for de novo coronary lesions.

Use in In-stent Restenosis, Chronic Total Occlusions, Thrombus-Rich Lesions, and Undilatable Stents

Prior to the advent of drug-eluting stents, restenosis after simple balloon angioplasty and after bare-metal stenting remained a clinical challenge. Because of the physical characteristics of the restenotic material, use of simple balloon angioplasty was challenging because of the propensity of the balloon to slip (watermelon seed) within the stenotic region. A number of devices, such as the rotablator and cutting balloon, were developed specifically to address this limitation of balloon angioplasty. Laser angioplasty, similarly, was also added to the devices attempting to treat this specific lesion subset. Successful treatment of in-stent restenosis has been reported in single-center registries, but no trial has been conducted to determine its efficacy and safety compared with other modalities. Optimal use of the laser angioplasty is performed in an OTW fashion. Nevertheless, some lesions are not amenable to wire crossing, such as CTOs, and so present a unique clinical challenge. A laser-tipped wire was developed to facilitate passage through an occluded vessel. In the TOTAL randomized trial, laser-assisted angiography and stenting was successful in 91% of cases.[25] Six-month angiographic restenosis rates were similar and high for both groups, including a 20% reocclusion rate. MACE was similar for both groups.

Recent experience in patients with stents inadequately expanded using high-pressure NCBs indicates that ELCA can be useful to facilitate full stent expansion, presumably by ablating organic elements within the vessel wall, thus constraining calcium within the vessel wall.[26] Additionally, interest in use of ELCA for thrombotic lesions, especially in degenerated vein grafts and in patients with acute MI, has grown as the safety and feasibility of ELCA in these settings has been described.[27,28]

Based on the data obtained, although limited, the ACC/AHA/SCAI has issued the following recommendations: There is a class IIb recommendation for laser angioplasty for use in patients with heavily calcified lesions to improve procedural success (level of evidence: B-NR) (**Table 15.12**).[9]

TABLE 15.11 Indications and Contraindications for Coronary Laser Angioplasty

INDICATIONS	CONTRAINDICATIONS
Occluded SVGs[a]	Unprotected LM lesion[a]
Ostial lesions[a]	Lesion is beyond acute bends or is in a location where the catheter cannot traverse[a]
Long lesions >20 mm[a]	Lesion cannot be reached by catheter[a]
Moderately calcified stenoses[a]	Bifurcation lesion[a]
CTOs crossable by guide wire[a]	Patient is not a CABG candidate[a]
Lesion that previously failed PTCA[a]	
In-stent Restenosis in 316L stainless steel stents, prior to the administration of intravascular brachytherapy[a]	

[a]Per instructions for use.

CABG, coronary artery bypass grafting; CTO, chronic total occlusion; LM, left main; PTCA, percutaneous transluminal coronary angioplasty; SVG, saphenous vein graft.

Complications

Similar to most other coronary interventional devices, the use of laser angioplasty is associated with potential dissection, perforation, and acute closure. The use of saline flushes in conjunction with compulsive attention to technique and a methodical approach to laser angioplasty has minimized the potential for these complications, but given the intense energy at the tip of the catheter, the potential for serious coronary complications persists. The treatment of these complications is similar to that for complications arising from other interventional devices. Similar to the potential concern for coronary perforation during coronary RA, general expert consensus is that anticoagulation accompanying the use of laser angioplasty should be unfractionated heparin because it can be readily reversed with protamine.

INTRAVASCULAR LITHOTRIPSY

Device

Intravascular lithotripsy (IVL) (Shockwave Medical Inc., Santa Clara, CA) is a rapid exchange system that consists of three main

TABLE 15.12 2021 ACC/AHA/SCAI Coronary Revascularization Guidelines

LASER ANGIOPLASTY: RECOMMENDATIONS
• Class IIb   • In patients with fibrotic or heavily calcified lesions, plaque modification with laser angioplasty may be considered to improve procedural success (*level of evidence: B-NR*).

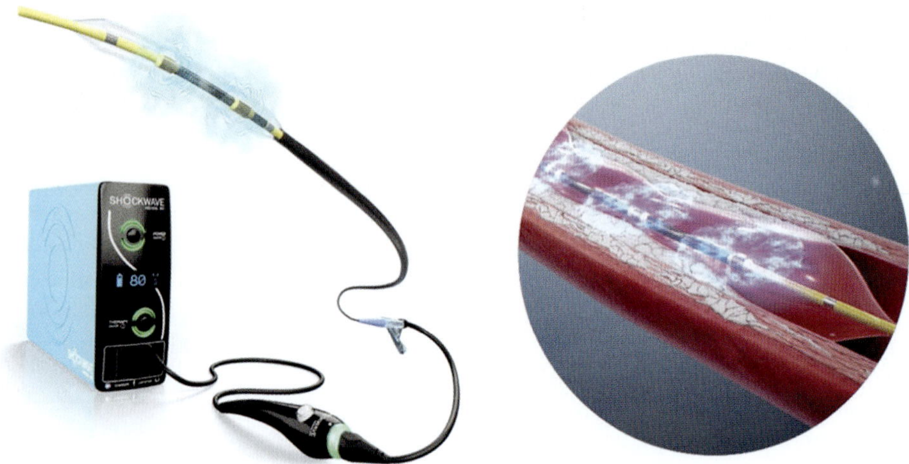

FIGURE 15.6 Illustration of the intravascular lithotripsy system, with the components including the IVL generator, connector cable, and IVL catheter, which operates using a conventional balloon containing several emitters positioned within the affixed balloon. An illustration of the IVL balloon within a lesion is shown on the right.

components: an IVL catheter, IVL connector cables, and the IVL generator (**Fig. 15.6**). The coronary IVL catheter consists of a 0.014-inch guide wire–compatible, fluid-filled balloon angioplasty catheter with lithotripsy emitters incorporated into the shaft of the 12-mm-long balloon segment. The rapid exchange catheter facilitates the delivery of the coronary IVL system, which comes in diameters of 2.5, 3, 3.5, and 4 mm. The system can be delivered via a 6-Fr or greater coronary guide catheter.

IVL represents an innovative technique for treatment of calcified arterial disease, rooted in a well-established treatment approach initially devised for renal calculi. IVL utilizes a conventional balloon catheter containing several emitters positioned within the affixed balloon segment. These emitters generate rapid sonic pressure waves, traversing the length and breadth of the mounted balloon. As these waves propagate through soft tissue, they induce shear stress, causing the fracture of intimal and medial calcium within the vessel wall. The use of IVL was first described in the treatment of calcified peripheral artery lesions. Successively, as the safety and efficacy of this technology was shown in peripheral arteries, the use of IVL expanded to the treatment of calcified coronary artery disease. IVL received US Food and Drug Administration approval for use within calcified peripheral arteries in 2017 and for coronary artery use in 2021.

Principles of Lithotripsy

IVL has emerged as an instinctive and captivating approach for managing extensively calcified lesions within coronary arteries. It combines the calcium-disrupting proficiency of lithotripsy with the well-known nature of balloon catheters, presenting an appealing therapeutic modality. The IVL semicompliant balloon involves two radiopaque lithotripsy emitters 6 mm apart and two conventional markers at the proximal and distal edges of the balloon. These emitters receive electrical pulses from the generator, vaporizing the fluid (a standard mixture of 50% NaCl 0.9% and 50% radiopaque contrast) within the balloon and creating a rapidly expanding and collapsing bubble. This bubble has the ability to transmit circumferential pulsatile mechanical energy into the vessel wall, in the form of sonic pressure waves equivalent to approximately 50 atmospheres (atm).[29] Crucially, it is the acoustic wave and not the balloon that generates the disruptive force, allowing for low-pressure balloon inflation, and hence mitigating the risk of barotrauma, vascular dissection, and perforation.

The technology of IVL does not rely on direct vascular tissue injury for plaque modification but rather on sonic waves with the purpose of breaking both superficial and deep calcium deposits with minimal soft tissue impairment. Several mechanisms have been shown to play a role in calcific fragmentation by IVL, including axial splitting by compressive circumferential forces; generation and violent collapse of cavitation bubbles by shock waves inside the saline-contrast-filled balloon that impact the surface of the calcific plaque, as well as the fatigue mechanism involving progressive expansion of microfractures into macrofractures by the cumulative impact of the repetitive multiple shock wave pulses.[30] In contrast to debulking techniques of atherectomy, the calcium fragments resulting from the IVL therapy remain unmoved, reducing the likelihood of distal embolization.

Procedure

Similar to coronary balloon angioplasty, a 0.014″ coronary guide wire is passed distal to the calcified coronary lesion. The IVL catheter is equipped by connecting a balloon indeflator, filled with a 1:1 mix of saline and contrast, to the inflation port. The IVL catheter balloon should then be prepared and deaired like conventional coronary balloons. Particular attention should be applied to the deairing procedure since air in the balloon reduces the effectiveness of the IVL therapy. The connector cable is placed within a sterile sleeve and attached to the catheter emitter cable, connected to the generator. The IVL catheter is then introduced over the wire, with use of the rapid exchange system and advanced over the guide wire to the coronary artery. Radiopaque markers are present on the catheter, which are used under fluoroscopy to position the catheter within the calcified coronary lesion. In the rare event that the IVL catheter is not able to initially cross a calcified lesion, predilation with low-profile angioplasty balloons could be performed or even RA may be used to facilitate IVL catheter delivery.

The IVL catheter balloon is then gently expanded at a pressure slightly below nominal (approximately 4 atm) and placed against the vessel wall. This positioning establishes a proficient interface between the fluid and tissue, which have comparable acoustic impedances. As a result, the transmission of shock wave energy to the vessel wall becomes notably efficient. The control button on the connector cable is pressed to activate a treatment cycle, which consists of a total 10 pulses, with 1 pulse per second. Each IVL catheter has the ability to deliver a maximum of either 8 treatment cycles (a total of 80 pulses), with use of the Shockwave C2 catheter, or 12 treatment cycles (a total of 120 pulses), with use of the newer rendition of the IVL catheter, the Shockwave C^{2+}, which is designed to treat longer lesions and more challenging eccentric and nodular calcium.

Following every cycle, the balloon can optionally be inflated to 6 atm, in order to compress the fractured calcium prior to a new treatment cycle. In lesions requiring more than the allowed treatment cycles, a second IVL catheter would need to be used. After performing IVL therapy, a standard PCI approach is taken.

Indications for Use

The Shockwave IVL system is indicated for severely calcified, stenotic de novo coronary arteries prior to stenting. While the literature presents numerous clinical cases demonstrating the utilization and effectiveness of IVL in managing in-stent restenosis linked to insufficiently expanded coronary stents, there is currently a lack of substantial data to firmly validate this off-label application for IVL.[31] According to the manufacturers, the Shockwave coronary IVL system is contraindicated and not intended for use for stent delivery, nor is it intended for application within carotid or cerebrovascular arteries.

Outcomes

There have been three major trials that have assessed the use of IVL within the coronary artery realm (**Table 15.13**). The initial study to evaluate the use of IVL in the coronary field was DISRUPT CAD I.[32] This single-arm, premarket study enrolled 60 patients with severely calcified lesions. Device success was 98%, with stenting performed in 86.7% of cases. Clinical success (residual stenosis <50% without in-hospital MACE) was 95%. At 30 days, the cumulative MACE rate was 5%, with no cardiac deaths, Q-wave MIs, or target vessel revascularizations. Procedural safety was achieved with no complications such as coronary dissections, perforations abrupt vessel closure, slow flow, or no reflow.

The DISRUPT CAD II was a postmarket study to again assess the safety and performance of the IVL system.[33] This single-arm trial enrolled 120 patients with severe calcified coronary artery disease to be treated with IVL and stenting. Device success was achieved in all patients. The composite primary endpoint of in-hospital MACE (cardiac death, MI, and target vessel revascularization) occurred in 5.8% of patients. There was no procedural abrupt closure, slow or no reflow, or perforations following IVL.

Then, the Disrupt CAD III study was a prospective, single-arm multicenter study designed for regulatory approval of coronary IVL.[34] With the largest patient population, this study enrolled 431 patients with severe coronary calcification who underwent IVL and stenting. The primary safety endpoint of freedom from MACE at 30 days occurred in 92.2% with a procedural success rate of 92.4%.

Based on the data obtained, the ACC/AHA/SCAI guidelines on coronary revascularization have issued a class IIb recommendation for plaque modification with IVL use in patients with fibrotic or heavily calcified lesions, similar to the recommendations given to laser atherectomy, OA, and balloon atherotomy (**Table 15.14**).[9]

Complications

Potential complications are consistent with standard catheter-based cardiac interventions and include dissection, perforation, and acute closure. Coronary artery perforation may occur due to barotrauma from either low-pressure balloon inflation or high-energy acoustic wave emission, although rates have remained low in clinical trials.

Moreover, IVL therapy has been shown to cause atrial and/or ventricular capture, particularly in patients with bradycardia. While there is no electric current that leaves the IVL catheter, the small amount of transformed mechanical energy is theorized to couple with the cardiac conduction system, producing ectopic captures, termed "shocktopics." The Disrupt CAD III trial assessed the frequency and clinical consequences of this phenomenon.[34] IVL-induced capture was noted during IVL in 41.1% of cases, and intraprocedural hypotension was more common in patients with IVL-induced capture than those without (40.5% vs 24.5%, P = .0007). In none of the patients did IVL-induced capture result in sustained ventricular arrhythmias during or immediately after the procedure, nor were they associated with any adverse events. However, in the event of clinically significant hemodynamic effects from IVL-induced capture, you may have to temporarily interrupt IVL therapy.

TABLE 15.13 Studies Evaluating Coronary Artery IVL Use

	DISRUPT CAD I	DISRUPT CAD II	DISRUPT CAD III
Design	Multicenter, single arm	Multicenter, single arm	Multicenter, single arm
Number of patients	60	120	431
Number of sites	7	15	47
Inclusion criteria	• De novo moderate/severe calcific coronary lesions • Stenosis ≥50% • Reference vessel diameter = 2.5-4.0 mm • Lesion length ≤32 mm	• Single de novo severe calcific lesion • Stenosis ≥50% • Reference vessel diameter = 2.5-4.0 mm • Lesion length ≤32 mm	• Single de novo severe calcific lesion • Stenosis ≥70% but <100%, OR ≥50% and <70% with evidence of ischemia[a] • Reference vessel diameter = 2.5-4.0 mm • Lesion length ≤40 mm
Acute gain	1.7 mm	1.6 mm	1.7 mm
30-d MACE	5.0%	7.6%	7.8%
6-mo MACE	8.3%	-	-
1-y MACE	-	-	13.8%

[a]Via positive stress test, or fractional flow reserve value ≤ 0.80, or iFR <0.90, or IVUS or OCT minimum lumen area ≤4.0 mm^2.

TABLE 15.14 2021 ACC/AHA/SCAI Coronary Revascularization Guidelines

INTRAVASCULAR LITHOTRIPSY: RECOMMENDATIONS
• Class IIb • In patients with fibrotic or heavily calcified lesions, plaque modification with intravascular lithotripsy may be considered to improve procedural success (*level of evidence: B-NR*).

Key Points

- Rotational atherectomy
  - RA achieves atheroablation with an OTW diamond-tipped burr spinning at >140,000 rpm based on the concept of differential cutting; ie, selective ablation of relatively inelastic materials such as calcified or heavily fibrotic atheromatous plaque with sparing of elastic nondiseased vessel segments.
  - RA was not superior to PTCA or laser atherectomy in reducing restenosis in multiple clinical trials in de novo or restenotic lesions.
  - The 2021 ACC/AHA/SCAI guidelines for coronary revascularization have issued a class IIa recommendation for preparation of fibrotic or heavily calcified lesions that might not be crossed by a balloon catheter or adequately dilated prior to stent implantation (level of evidence: B-R)
  - Contemporary practice uses RA for lesion preparation prior to stenting, particularly in calcified vessels.
- Orbital atherectomy
  - The mechanism of differential sanding occurring during OA is similar to that of RA with selective ablation of inelastic materials, including heavily calcified or fibrotic plaque, and sparing of elastic tissue.
  - The safety and efficacy of OA was evaluated in ORBIT I and ORBIT II trials, both prospective registries of patients undergoing PCI of heavily calcified vessels. Procedural success was high, and complication rates were similar to, or lower than, historical studies of RA.
  - Similar to RA, OA is used for lesion preparation prior to stenting, particularly in moderate to severely calcified lesions.
  - The 2021 ACC/AHA/SCAI guidelines for coronary revascularization have issued a class IIb recommendation for plaque modification with use of OA in patients with fibrotic or heavily calcified lesions
- Scoring balloon angioplasty
  - The AngioSculpt scoring balloon is composed of three rectangular nitinol wires wrapped in a helical fashion about a semicompliant balloon. On inflation, there is circumferential scoring of the vessel while minimizing slippage, which is ideal for treating restenotic lesions.
  - The scoring balloon angioplasty is indicated for treatment of in-stent restenosis and complex type C lesions.
- Cutting balloon angioplasty
  - Cutting balloon atherectomy achieves vessel dilation with three or four atherotomes attached to the surface of a conventional angioplasty balloon by controlled longitudinal incision of the vessel wall.
  - The cutting balloon is used in contemporary practice for lesion preparation in restenotic or ostial main or branch vessel disease.
  - In the 2021 update of the coronary artery revascularization guidelines, cutting or scoring balloon angioplasty received a class IIb indication for fibrotic or heavily calcified lesions to improve procedural success (level of evidence: B-NR).
- Laser atherectomy
  - Lasers produce intense electromagnetic energy at ultraviolet wavelengths of 308 nm delivered through coaxial optical fibers bundled inside a coronary delivery catheter. Vaporization of plaque is achieved by photochemical, photomechanical, and photothermal effects.
  - Based on limited clinical data, the 2021 update of the coronary revascularization guidelines has issued the following recommendations: There is a class IIb recommendation for laser angioplasty that might be considered for fibrotic or moderately calcified lesions that cannot be crossed or dilated with conventional balloon angioplasty (level of evidence: B-NR).
  - Contemporary practice with a laser is useful for lesion preparation in lesions that have failed PTCA. Lasers can also be useful in mild to moderately calcified lesions, or long lesions, and in CTOs, including occluded vein grafts.
- Intravascular lithotripsy
  - IVL has emerged as an instinctive and captivating approach for managing extensively calcified lesions within coronary arteries as it combines the calcium-disrupting proficiency of lithotripsy with the well-known nature of balloon catheters.
  - The IVL balloon contains emitters that receive electrical pulses, which then vaporize the fluid within the balloon, creating a rapidly expanding and collapsing bubble. This bubble can transmit circumferential pulsatile mechanical energy into the vessel wall, in the form of sonic pressure waves.
  - Based on the Disrupt CAD studies, the ACC/AHA/SCAI guidelines for coronary revascularization have issued a class IIb recommendation for plaque modification with IVL use in patients with fibrotic or heavily calcified lesions.

References

1. Reisman M, Shuman BJ, Harms V. Analysis of heat generation during high-speed rotational ablation: technical implications. *J Am Coll Cardiol*. 1996;27:292A.
2. Whitlow PL, Bass TA, Kipperman RM, et al. Results of the study to determine rotablator and transluminal angioplasty strategy (STRATAS). *Am J Cardiol*. 2001;87(6):699-705.
3. Dill T, Dietz U, Hamm CW, et al. A randomized comparison of balloon angioplasty versus rotational atherectomy in complex coronary lesions (COBRA study). *Eur Heart J*. 2000;21:1759-1766.
4. Reifart N, Vandormael M, Krajcar M, et al. Randomized comparison of angioplasty of complex coronary lesions at a single center: excimer laser, rotational atherectomy, and balloon angioplasty comparison (ERBAC) study. *Circulation*. 1997;96(1):91-98.
5. Arora S, Panaich SS, Patel N, et al. Coronary atherectomy in the United States (from a nationwide inpatient sample). *Am J Cardiol*. 2016;117(4):555-562.
6. Buchbinder M,Fortuna R, Sharma SK, Bass T, Kipperman R, Greenberg J. Debulking prior to stenting improves acute outcomes: early results from the SPORT trial. *J Am Coll Cardiol*. 2000;35:8A.

7. Abdel-Wahab M, Richardt G, Joachim Büttner H, et al. High-speed rotational atherectomy before paclitaxel-eluting stent implantation in complex calcified coronary lesions: the randomized ROTAXUS (rotational atherectomy prior to Taxus stent treatment for complex native coronary artery disease) trial. *JACC Cardiovasc Interv*. 2013;6(1):10-19.
8. Ayoub M, Tajti P, Ferenc M, et al. Feasibility and outcome of the Rotapro system in treating severely calcified coronary lesions: the Rotapro study. *Cardiol J*. 2021. doi:10.5603/CJ.a2021.0128
9. Lawton JS, Tamis-Holland JE, Bangalore S, et al. 2021 ACC/AHA/SCAI guideline for coronary artery revascularization. Executive summary: a report of the American College of Cardiology/American Heart Association Joint Committee on clinical practice guidelines. *Circulation*. 2022;145(3):e4-e17. Erratum in: *Circulation*. 2022;145(11):e771. doi:10.1161/CIR.0000000000001039
10. Kinnaird T, Kwok CS, Kontopantelis E, et al. Incidence, determinants, and outcomes of coronary perforation during percutaneous coronary intervention in the United Kingdom between 2006 and 2013: an analysis of 527,121 cases from the British Cardiovascular Intervention Society database. *Circ Cardiovasc Interv*. 2016;9(8):e003449. doi:10.1161/CIRCINTERVENTIONS.115.003449
11. Parikh K, Chandra P, Choksi N, Khanna P, Chambers J. Safety and feasibility of orbital atherectomy for the treatment of calcified coronary lesions: the ORBIT I trial. *Catheter Cardiovasc Interv*. 2013;81(7):1134-1139.
12. Lee MS, Singh V, Nero TJ, Wilentz JR. Cutting balloon angioplasty. *J Invasive Cardiol*. 2002;14(9):552-556.
13. Barath P, Fishbein MC, Vari S, Forrester JS. Cutting balloon: a novel approach to percutaneous angioplasty. *Am J Cardiol*. 1991;68(11):1249-1252.
14. Izumi M, Tsuchikane E, Funamoto M, et al. Final results of the CAPAS trial. *Am Heart J*. 2001;142(5):782-789.
15. Mauri L, Bonan R, Weiner BH, et al. Cutting balloon angioplasty for the prevention of restenosis: results of the cutting balloon global randomized trial. *Am J Cardiol*. 2002;90(10):1079-1083.
16. Bittl JA, Chew DP, Topol EJ, Kong DF, Califf RM. Meta-analysis of randomized trials of percutaneous transluminal coronary angioplasty versus atherectomy, cutting balloon atherotomy, or laser angioplasty. *J Am Coll Cardiol*. 2004;43(6):936-942.
17. Albiero R, Silber S, Di Mario C, et al. Cutting balloon versus conventional balloon angioplasty for the treatment of in-stent restenosis: results of the restenosis cutting balloon evaluation trial (RESCUT). *J Am Coll Cardiol*. 2004;43(6):943-949.
18. Mangieri A, Nerla R, Castriota F, et al. Cutting balloon to optimize predilation for stent implantation: the COPS randomized trial. *Catheter Cardiovasc Interv*. 2023;101(4):798-805. doi:10.1002/ccd.30603
19. Mooney MR, Teirstein P, Carlier S. Final results from the U.S. multi-center trial of the AngioSculpt scoring balloon catheter for the treatment of complex coronary artery lesions. *Am J Cardiol*. 2006;98:121.
20. de Ribamar Costa J Jr, Mintz GS, Carlier SG, et al. Nonrandomized comparison of coronary stenting under intravascular ultrasound guidance of direct stenting without predilation versus conventional predilation with a semi-compliant balloon versus predilation with a new scoring balloon. *Am J Cardiol*. 2007;100(5):812-817.
21. Kufner S, Joner M, Schneider S, et al, ISAR-DESIRE 4 Investigators. Neointimal modification with scoring balloon and efficacy of drug-coated balloon therapy in patients with restenosis in drug-eluting coronary stents: a randomized controlled trial. *JACC Cardiovasc Interv*. 2017;10(13):1332-1340. PMID: 28683939. doi:10.1016/j.jcin.2017.04.024
22. Weisz G, Metzger DC, Liberman HA, et al. A provisional strategy for treating true bifurcation lesions employing a scoring balloon for the side branch: final results of the AGILITY trial. *Catheter Cardiovasc Interv*. 2013;82(3):352-359.
23. Ambrosini V, Sorropago G, Laurenzano E, et al. Early outcome of high energy Laser (Excimer) facilitated coronary angioplasty ON hARD and complex calcified and balloOn-resistant coronary lesions: LEONARDO study. *Cardiovasc Revasc Med*. 2015;16(3):141-146.
24. Stone GW, de Marchena E, Dageforde D, et al. Prospective, randomized, multicenter comparison of laser-facilitated balloon angioplasty versus stand-alone balloon angioplasty in patients with obstructive coronary artery disease. The Laser Angioplasty versus Angioplasty (LAVA) trial investigators. *J Am Coll Cardiol*. 1997;30(7):1714-1721.
25. Serruys PW, Hamburger JN, Koolen JJ, et al. Total occlusion trial with angioplasty by using laser guidewire. The TOTAL trial. *Eur Heart J*. 2000;21:1797-1805.
26. Badr S, Ben-Dor I, Dvir D, et al. The state of the excimer laser for coronary intervention in the drug-eluting stent era. *Cardiovasc Revasc Med*. 2013;14(2):93-98.
27. Nishino M, Mori N, Takiuchi S, et al. Indications and outcomes of excimer laser coronary atherectomy: efficacy and safety for thrombotic lesions-The ULTRAMAN registry. *J Cardiol*. 2017;69(1):314-319.
28. Giugliano GR, Falcone MW, Mego D, et al. A prospective multicenter registry of laser therapy for degenerated saphenous vein graft stenosis: the COronary graft Results following Atherectomy with Laser (CORAL) trial. *Cardiovasc Revasc Med*. 2012;13(2):84-89.
29. Kereiakes D, Virmani R, Hokama J, et al. Principles of intravascular lithotripsy for calcific plaque modification. *JACC Cardiovasc Interv*. 2021;14(12):1275-1292. DOI: 10.1016/j.jcin.2021.03.036
30. Dini CS, Tomberli B, Mattesini A, et al. Intravascular lithotripsy for calcific coronary and peripheral artery stenoses. *EuroIntervention*. 2019;15(8):714-721.
31. Tovar Forero MN, Wilschut J, Van Mieghem NM, Daemen J. Coronary lithoplasty: a novel treatment for stent underexpansion. *Eur Heart J*. 2019;40(2):221. PMID: 30289452. doi:10.1093/eurheartj/ehy593
32. Brinton TJ, Ali ZA, Hill JM, et al. Feasibility of Shockwave coronary intravascular lithotripsy for the treatment of calcified coronary stenoses. *Circulation*. 2019;139(6):834-836. PMID: 30715944. doi:10.1161/CIRCULATIONAHA.118.036531
33. Ali ZA, Nef H, Escaned J, et al. Safety and effectiveness of coronary intravascular lithotripsy for treatment of severely calcified coronary stenoses: the disrupt CAD II study. *Circ Cardiovasc Interv*. 2019;12(10):e008434. PMID: 31553205. doi:10.1161/CIRCINTERVENTIONS.119.008434
34. Hill JM, Kereiakes DJ, Shlofmitz RA, et al, Disrupt CAD III Investigators. Intravascular lithotripsy for treatment of severely calcified coronary artery disease. *J Am Coll Cardiol*. 2020;76(22):2635-2646. PMID: 33069849. doi:10.1016/j.jacc.2020.09.603

Coronary Stents

David W. Louis and J. Dawn Abbott

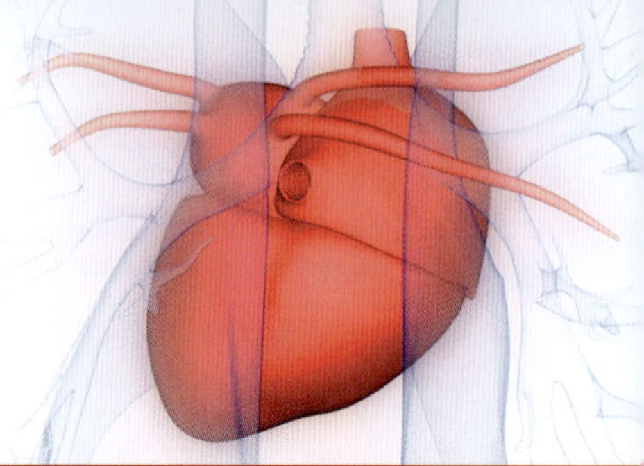

Numerous technologic and procedural advances have occurred in interventional cardiology since the first successful balloon angioplasty in 1977 by Andreas Gruentzig. This chapter will discuss coronary stents, from their initial development through contemporary platforms, and their usage in various clinical indications.

MEASURES OF DEVICE AND PROCEDURAL SUCCESS

Quantitative coronary angiography is used to assess and compare the efficacy of balloon and stent-based angioplasty (**Fig. 16.1**). A basic understanding of these terms is required to evaluate the mechanisms and clinical outcomes of percutaneous coronary intervention (PCI).

Angiographic Outcomes

- *Acute gain* = post minimal luminal diameter (MLD) - pre MLD (often measured in millimeters)
- *Late loss* = post MLD - late MLD (usually measured 6-9 months after initial procedure)

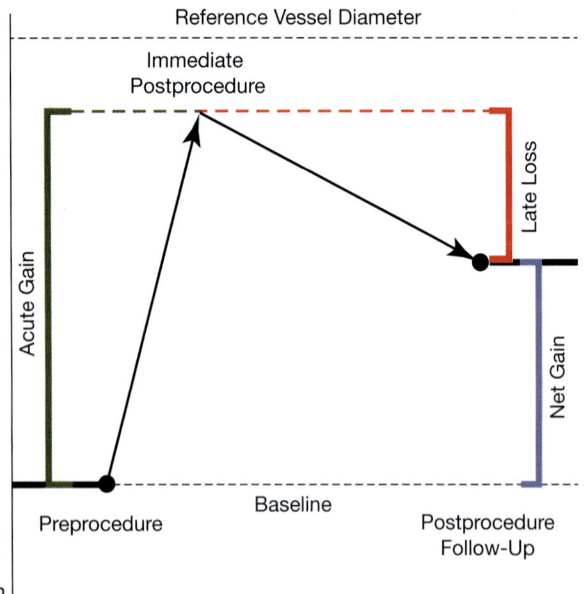

FIGURE 16.1 Acute gain, late loss, and net gain. Prior to coronary intervention, a stenotic segment has a minimal lumen diameter. The intervention results in an *acute gain*, illustrated by the upward arrow showing improvement in minimal lumen diameter. In subsequent angiographic follow-up, the minimal lumen diameter decreases due to neointimal hyperplasia and neoatherosclerosis, a phenomenon referred to as *late loss*. The resultant overall improvement in minimal lumen diameter is referred to as *net gain*.

- *Late loss index* = late loss/acute gain
- *Net gain* = late MLD – pre MLD
- *Angiographic (binary) restenosis* is typically defined as a late lesion diameter stenosis >50%.

Clinical Outcomes

- *Target lesion revascularization (TLR)*: Any repeat revascularization of the original lesion, which includes the stented segment and 5 mm proximal and/or distal to the stent, usually measured 6 to 12 months after the procedure.
- *Target vessel revascularization (TVR)*: Any repeat revascularization involving the previously treated vessel.
- *Major adverse cardiac events (MACE)*: Although component definitions vary, endpoints commonly reported include death, nonfatal myocardial infarction (MI), nonfatal stroke, and TLR/TVR.
- *Target vessel failure (TVF)*: Composite of TVR, target vessel MI, or cardiac death.

OVERVIEW OF STENT DESIGN

Coronary stents are classified by mode of implantation, material composition, scaffold configuration, and stent coatings.

- *Mode of implantation*—self-expanding or balloon expandable. While the initial coronary stent (Gianturco-Roubin stent) was self-expanding, contemporary coronary stents are balloon expandable.
- *Material composition*—specific stent material used to construct the scaffold. Historically, the most widely used material was 316L stainless steel. The introduction of cobalt or a cobalt-chromium or platinum-chromium alloy into the stent composition offered the ability to create thin (75-82 μm) and ultrathin (<75 μm) struts without sacrificing radiologic visibility or radial strength. Additional stent compositions include nitinol, a nickel/titanium alloy (often used in self-expanding stents), and biodegradable polymers (used in bioabsorbable scaffolds).
- *Scaffold configuration*—refers to the shape and construction of the stent design. Stents can be assigned to one of three subgroups: (1) coiled wire, (2) slotted tube/multicellular (most commonly used), and (3) modular ring. The coiled-wire configuration was used in early coronary stents (Gianturco-Roubin-1) and utilized a single strand of stainless steel wire forming a cylinder of interdigitating loops. The Palmaz-Schatz stent was the first slotted-tube balloon-expandable stent and provided improved scaffolding, but it was limited by a high delivery profile, inflexibility, and the requirement of a protective delivery sheath to maintain the stent on the balloon. Modifications to the slotted-tube design to improve trackability, flexibility, and deliverability were implemented in the development of second- and third-generation stents used in the contemporary

TABLE 16.1 Stent Coatings Designed to Reduce Stent Thrombosis

Carbon
Ionic oxygen
Gold
Nitric oxide scavengers
Heparin
IIb/IIIa inhibitors
Activated protein C
Hirudin and bivalirudin
Prostacyclin
CD34 antibody
Phosphorylcholine
Fluorinated copolymer
BioLinx polymer
Trifluoroethanol (Polyzene-F)
Protein coating
PET fiber mesh

PCI era. Multicellular stents can be subclassified as open-cell or closed-cell stents. Open-cell designs are made of parallel wire loops with few connections, resulting in varied side strut size, which improves flexibility, deliverability, and side-branch access while maintaining radial strength. Closed-cell designs employ a repeating unicellular element with a higher number of crossing and connecting struts, which reduces the area per cell and increases the total area of stent contact with vessel intima, thereby improving scaffolding. Modular ring design stents are constructed from a series of sinusoidal rings in series, allowing for greater stent flexibility, but there is potential for greater plaque prolapse. Stents currently in use have open-cell designs.

- *Stent coatings*—Stents may be uncoated (bare metal), contain passive coatings such as polytetrafluoroethylene (PTFE), or contain polymers to reduce thrombogenicity and/or allow for controlled delivery of antiproliferative drug therapy. A multitude of stent coatings have been designed and studied in an attempt to promote vascular healing and prevent complications (**Table 16.1**). These polymers may be further classified as durable or bioresorbable and have varying degrees of biocompatibility and vascular responses.

In summation, stent design is critical. An ideal stent (**Table 16.2**) affords trackability, flexibility, and visibility; allows for accurate placement; provides scaffolding; and remains patent without significant risk of stent thrombosis and in-stent restenosis (ISR). However, a trade-off is often required as flexibility and conformability are inversely related to scaffolding and radial strength.

Bare-Metal Stent Overview

The initial invasive therapy for coronary artery disease (CAD) was percutaneous transluminal balloon coronary angioplasty (PTCA), which resulted in plaque fracture, expansion of the external elastic media, and axial plaque redistribution. While many vessels treated with PTCA demonstrated procedural success and reduction in stenosis severity, resultant vascular inflammation with platelet and clotting activation and smooth muscle proliferation commonly led to acute vessel closure (5%-8% of cases) and restenosis (30%-40% of cases).[1] As a result, coronary stents were developed to scaffold balloon-induced coronary dissection, increase acute gain, and prevent elastic recoil.

TABLE 16.2 Factors Associated With In-Stent Restenosis or Target Lesion Revascularization After Drug-Eluting Stent Implantation

Patient	Age
	Female
	Comorbidities including diabetes mellitus
	Multivessel coronary artery disease
Lesion	In-stent restenosis
	Bypass graft
	Chronic total occlusion
	Small vessels
	Calcified lesion
	Ostial lesion
	Left anterior descending lesion
	Long lesions
	Thrombotic lesion
Procedure	Treatment of multiple lesions
	Type of drug-eluting stents
	Final diameter stenosis
	Minimal stent area
	Stent edge dissection
	Stent inflow or outflow disease
	Lack of intracoronary imaging use

The first balloon-expandable bare-metal stent (BMS) was developed in 1988 by Cesare Gianturco and Gary Roubin and gained US Food and Drug Administration (FDA) approval in 1993 for the reversal of postangioplasty acute or threatened vessel closure.[2] Subsequently, the stainless steel, slotted tube, Palmaz-Schatz stent (Johnson and Johnson, Interventional Systems, Warren, NJ) became the dominant coronary stent design after the STRESS and BENESTENT trials showed superiority of stenting compared with PTCA, driven largely by significantly lower rates of angiographic restenosis and TLR.[2,3] Long-term follow-up of these stents have demonstrated few late clinical or angiographic recurrences from years 1 to 5 after implantation, with progressive decrements in luminal diameter beyond 10 years.[4] The utilization of dual antiplatelet therapy (DAPT) and routine high-pressure dilation with noncompliant balloons has further lowered the risk of stent thrombosis.[5]

While coronary stents increase acute gain more than PTCA, an exaggerated poststent implantation response of neointimal hyperplasia ultimately results in greater late loss compared with PTCA alone. Despite this, the net gain with stents remains favorable compared with balloon angioplasty with less overall restenosis. Nevertheless, TLR and stent thrombosis remained problematic[6] and were attributed to intrinsic stent properties including strut thickness and cell design.[7,8] Two randomized controlled trials, ISAR-STEREO (Intracoronary Stenting and Angiographic Results: Strut Thickness Effect on Restenosis Outcomes Trial) and ISAR-STEREO-2, found significantly lower rates of angiographic and clinical restenosis with a thin strut and open-cell design compared with thick strut and closed-cell design.[9,10]

Drug-Eluting Stents Overview

Despite serial advancements in BMS design including the use of cobalt and platinum-chromium alloys, lower-profile stent struts, improved flexibility/deliverability, and enhancements to radial/longitudinal strength, restenosis rates remain high, often approaching

20% to 40% at 6 to 12 months.[11] First-generation drug-eluting stents (DESs) were successful in reducing TLR and stent thrombosis compared with BMS,[12] but subacute and late stent thrombosis as well as challenges with deliverability remained problematic.[13-15] Newer generations of stents employing polymer coatings to prolong drug delivery are most commonly used today, with biocompatible polymers, biodegradable polymers, and polymer-free DES platforms all under investigation.[16] At present, DESs are considered the gold standard for percutaneous intervention of coronary artery stenoses,[17] and the 2021 ACC/AHA/SCAI Guideline for Coronary Revascularization gives a class I indication for DES use in preference to BMS to reduce the risk of restenosis, MI, and acute stent thrombosis.[18] A limited summary of BMS and DES is shown in **Table 16.3** (**Fig. 16.2**).

TABLE 16.3 Summary of Bare-Metal Stents and Drug-Eluting Stents

GENERATION	DRUG	POLYMER	STENT	STRUT THICKNESS (μm)
Past Bare-Metal Stents (BMSs)				
Wall Stent	n/a	n/a	Self-expanding	80-100
Gianturco-Roubin	n/a	n/a	Wire coil	127
Palmaz-Schatz	n/a	n/a	Slotted tube with articulating bridge	70
Newer BMSs				
Integrity	n/a	n/a	Cobalt-chromium	90
Vision	n/a	n/a	Cobalt-chromium	81
REBEL	n/a	n/a	Platinum-chromium	81
Polymer-Coated BMS				
COBRA	n/a	Poly(bis[trifluoroethoxy] phosphazene)	Cobalt-chromium	71
First-Generation Drug-Eluting Stents (DESs)				
Cypher	Sirolimus	Biostable mix of poly-*n*-butyl methacrylate (PBMA) and polyethylene-vinyl acetate	Bx Velocity	140
Taxus Express	Paclitaxel	Styrene-isobutylene-styrene (SIBS)	Express	132
Taxus Liberté	Paclitaxel	SIBS	Liberté	97
Taxus Element	Paclitaxel	SIBS	Element (platinum-chromium)	81
Second/Third-Generation DESs				
Endeavor	Zotarolimus	Phosphorylcholine	Driver (cobalt alloy)	91
Xience	Everolimus	PBMA and PVDF-HF	Multi-Link Vision/8 (cobalt-chromium)	81
Promus	Everolimus	PBMA and PVDF-HFP	Platinum-chromium	81
Resolute	Zotarolimus	BioLinx polymer	Integrity (cobalt alloy)	91
Bioabsorbable Polymer or Polymer-Free DESs				
Synergy	Everolimus	Abluminal poly- (d, l-lactide-co-glycolide) (bioabsorbable)	Platinum-chromium	74
Orsiro	Sirolimus	Abluminal poly-l-lactic acid (bioabsorbable)	PK Papyrus (cobalt-chromium)	60 (2.25-3.0 mm); 80 (3.5-4.0 mm)
Biomatrix[a]	Biolimus A9	Abluminal poly-l-lactic acid (bioabsorbable)	Juno (stainless steel)	120
Nobori[a]	Biolimus A9	Abluminal poly-l-lactic acid (bioabsorbable)	S-stent	120
BioFreedom[a]	Biolimus A9	n/a	Gazelle (stainless steel)	120
Ultimaster[a]	Sirolimus	Poly (d, l-lactide-co-caprolactone) (bioabsorbable)	Cobalt-chromium	80

n/a, none; PVDF-HF, polyvinylidene fluoride-hydrogen fluoride; PVDF-HFP, poly vinylidene fluoride-co-hexafluoropropylene.
[a]Not FDA approved.

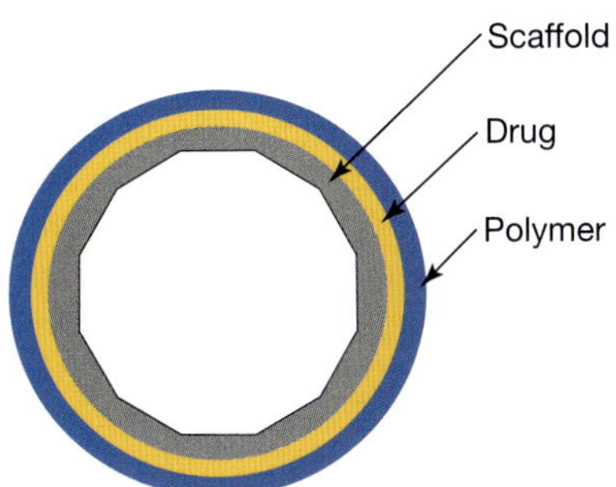

FIGURE 16.2 Components of drug-eluting stents. Modern drug-eluting stents are composed of three key components: the stent, the antiproliferative agent, and the polymer/carrier.

FIRST-GENERATION DRUG-ELUTING STENTS

Sirolimus-Eluting Stents

The Cordis CYPHER sirolimus-eluting stent (SES) was the first FDA-approved DES for patients with symptomatic ischemic disease due to discrete de novo lesions of length ≤30 mm in native coronary arteries with a reference diameter of ≥2.5 to ≤3.5 mm. The device consisted of a stainless steel (316L) stent in a sinusoidal pattern, coated with a nonerodible polymer and sirolimus mixture. This design allowed for a "slow release" of sirolimus, whereby approximately 80% of the sirolimus was released within the first month after stent implantation. The RAVEL trial and SIRIUS trial were two prospective randomized trials that evaluated adverse outcomes after CYPHER stent implantation. The RAVEL trial found significantly lower rates of late luminal loss, suggesting reductions in neointimal hyperplasia in the sirolimus-stent group compared with the standard-stent group.[19] Furthermore, the total number of cardiac adverse events was notably lower with the sirolimus stent (5.8% vs 28.8%, $P < .001$), driven by TLR (0 vs 27 patients), and cumulative event-free survival was higher in those with the sirolimus stent (94.1% vs 70.9%, $P < .001$).[19] The SIRIUS trial compared an SES with an analogous BMS and found a significant reduction in the primary endpoint of TVF among SES patients (8.6% vs 21.0%, $P < .001$).[20] Similar to the RAVEL trial, results were largely driven by reduction in TVR attributable to decreased rates of neointimal hyperplasia and late loss.[20] Long-term follow-up analyses have demonstrated sustained reductions in clinical restenosis endpoints with similar rates of death, MI, and stent thrombosis compared with BMS.[21,22] This stent is no longer commercially available due to the availability of newer stent platforms and designs.

Paclitaxel-Eluting Stents

The TAXUS paclitaxel-eluting coronary stent (PES) system was approved in 2008 shortly after the CYPHER stent and was indicated for improving luminal diameter for the treatment of de novo lesions ≤28 mm in length in native coronary arteries ≥2.5 to ≤3.75 mm in diameter. The TAXUS stent was made of stainless steel (316L) and coated with a nonerodible polymer carrier loaded with paclitaxel in a slow-release (SR) formulation. By adjusting the ratio of paclitaxel to polymer, drug-release kinetics could be altered to allow for slower drug elution, of which the SR formulation resulted in approximately 8% paclitaxel elution in 30 days. While the majority of early clinical trial data was based on the Express open-cell, slotted-tube, stainless steel stent platform (PES[E]), serial iterations of TAXUS stent design have varied, including the Liberte stent (a thinner-strut open-cell stainless steel design) and the Element stent (a platinum-chromium-based stent). The PES(E) has been studied in multiple randomized trials and observational analyses, with consistent findings of improved angiographic and clinical restenosis endpoints compared with BMS.[23] This platinum-chromium alloy stent platform is no longer in use.

Comparison Among First-Generation Drug-Eluting Stents

A series of comparisons between the SES and PES have been conducted to assess superiority of one stent over the other. Evidence from these trials shows similar clinical performance with a decreased rate of neointimal hyperplasia in the SES-treated patients. In a meta-analysis of 16 randomized trials (n = 8695) comparing SES with PES, SES was found to significantly reduce TLR (hazard ratio [HR] 0.74; 95% confidence interval [CI] 0.63-0.87; $P < .001$) and stent thrombosis (HR 0.66; 95% CI 0.46-0.94; $P = .02$) without a statistical difference in the risk for death or MI.[24] In two randomized clinical trials with 10 years of long-term follow-up data, the rate of definite stent thrombosis was similar between groups. **Table 16.4** lists the Academic Research Consortium Classification of Stent Thrombosis.

SECOND-GENERATION DRUG-ELUTING STENTS

Despite the demonstrated efficacy of the SES and PES platforms, adverse vessel responses to these first-generation stents were observed, which included delayed re-endothelialization, hypersensitivity, and eosinophilic inflammatory reactions, and, importantly, late stent thrombosis. Two studies reported an increase in mortality with the first-generation DES compared with the BMS,[13,25] resulting in a significant decrease in the clinical use of DES.[26] While many potential mechanisms may contribute to stent thrombosis, summarized in **Table 16.5**, these findings led to additional modifications in stent design. As a result, serial refinements to the stent platform, polymer composition, pharmacologic agent, and its elution kinetics have been implemented in order to address the safety issues while maintaining efficacy.

TABLE 16.4 Academic Research Consortium Classification and Definition of Stent Thrombosis Summarized

Definite stent thrombosis
Angiographic or pathologic evidence of thrombus that originates within or 5 mm adjacent to the stent, and clinical evidence of an acute coronary syndrome within a 48-h time window
Probable stent thrombosis
Unexplained death within the first 30 d after stent implantation Target vessel infarction without angiographic confirmation
Possible stent thrombosis
Unexplained death beyond 30 d after the procedure
Stent thrombosis timing
Acute stent thrombosis: 0-24 h after stent implantation Subacute stent thrombosis: >24 h to 30 d after stent implantation Late stent thrombosis: >30 d to 1 y after stent implantation Very late stent thrombosis: >1 y after stent implantation.

TABLE 16.5 Potential Mechanisms of Stent Thrombosis

Patient	Premature discontinuation of dual antiplatelet therapy Smoking Diabetes Chronic kidney disease Acute coronary syndrome presentation High posttreatment platelet reactivity CYP2C19 genetic polymorphism Early postimplantation surgical procedures
Lesion	Diffuse coronary artery disease with long-stented segment Small vessel disease Bifurcation disease Thrombus-containing lesions Significant inflow or outflow lesions proximal or distal to the stented segment
Stent	Stent underexpansion Edge dissection Poor endothelialization Thick stent struts Strut fracture Hypersensitivity/inflammatory reactions to DES components (eg, some polymers) Late malapposition Neoatherosclerosis with plaque rupture

DES, drug-eluting stent.

Zotarolimus-Eluting Stents

The Endeavor Zotarolimus-Eluting Coronary Stent System was the first zotarolimus-eluting stent (ZES) and was indicated for improving coronary luminal diameter in patients with ischemic heart disease due to de novo lesions of length ≤27 mm in native coronary arteries with reference vessel diameters of ≥2.5 to ≤3.5 mm. This device comprises a cobalt-chromium alloy stent and a formulation of zotarolimus contained in a biocompatible polymer. This stent was limited by a rapid release rate of zotarolimus (90% within 7 days, 100% within 30 days), which resulted in more neointimal proliferation and greater late loss than observed with the first-generation DESs.[27,28] Although angiographic efficacy was lower with the Endeavor stent, it had very low rates of late adverse events, including very late stent thrombosis, cardiac death, or MI.[29,30]

The Resolute Onyx ZES (Medtronic) is manufactured by coating a metallic stent substrate (a cobalt-based alloy shell and a platinum-iridium alloy core) with zotarolimus and Medtronic's proprietary biocompatible polymer (BioLinx). This tripolymer is designed to slow the elution of zotarolimus (60% elution by 30 days, 100% by 180 days). In a single-arm trial, these modifications resulted in reduced rates of restenosis compared with those seen with the prior ZES(E) or BMS.[31]

The new Onyx Frontier was approved by the FDA in 2022 and comes with improved catheter flexibility and deliverability via a lower crossing profile when compared with the Resolute Onyx DES, according to unpublished bench test data. This stent shares recent approval for patients who are at high risk of bleeding who may benefit from short-term DAPT of 1 month.[32]

Everolimus-Eluting Stents

Everolimus-eluting stent (EES) systems (Xience, Abbott Vascular, Santa Clara, CA; Promus, Boston Scientific, Natick, MA) incorporate the sirolimus derivative, everolimus, combined with a durable biocompatible polymer coated onto a low-profile cobalt-chromium (Xience) or platinum-chromium (Promus Element/Premier) stent. The release kinetics of EES are similar to that seen with SES (approximately 80% release of the drug at 30 days, 100% after 120 days). The EES polymer has been demonstrated to be noninflammatory in porcine experiments, with the additional property of resisting platelet and thrombus deposition in blood-contact applications.[15] Furthermore, EESs demonstrate more rapid functional re-endothelialization compared with SESs, PESs, or ZESs.[33] The EES has been studied in multiple randomized clinical trials comparing the device with BMS, PES, SES, and ZES platforms. Randomized comparisons of EES with PES demonstrated marked differences, with significant reductions in TLR, stent thrombosis, and MI with EES.[34,35] These benefits were sustained at 3 years.[36] Furthermore, both all-cause mortality (3.2% vs 5.1%, P = .02) and death or MI (5.9% vs 9.1%, P = .001) were reduced with EES compared with PES. On the other hand, when EES was compared with SES, smaller differences have been observed. Lastly, very low rates of stent thrombosis have been observed with EES in both clinical trials and observational studies.[37-39]

Additional modifications of stent technology continue to develop. As an example, the Synergy stent (Boston Scientific) incorporates a thin-strut platinum-chromium EES with a bioresorbable polymer, which enables complete polymer absorption to occur by 4 months after implantation. In a 5-year follow-up of the EVOLVE trial, these modifications resulted in no probable/definite stent thrombosis events and a low rate of target lesion failure (TLF) at 5.5%.[40]

Biolimus A9–Eluting Stents

Biolimus A9, a semisynthetic sirolimus analogue with enhanced lipophilicity, has been incorporated into two clinically available stent platforms that utilize a fully biodegradable abluminal polymer (poly-l-lactic acid [PLLA]), which is coreleased with Biolimus A9 and converted to carbon dioxide and water via the Krebs cycle over a 6- to 9-month period.[41] The BioMatrix (Biosensors International, Switzerland) stent and Nobori DES (Terumo Medical Corporation, Japan) utilize a stainless steel platform. While initial results comparing the Biolimus A9–eluting stent (BES) with SES demonstrate similar results of primary endpoints, longer-term follow-up out to 5 years suggests decreased rates of very late stent thrombosis.[42] The noninferiority trial NEXT compared the biodegradable polymer BES with the durable polymer EES and demonstrated similar safety and efficacy outcomes 3 years after stent implantation.[43]

As an alternative stent design utilizing Biolimus A9, the BioFreedom drug-coated stent is a polymer- and carrier-free stent. In a randomized trial comparing this platform with BMS in a population of high-bleeding-risk patients utilizing 30 days of DAPT, the BioFreedom BES outperformed its comparable BMS platform with regard to both safety (composite of cardiac death, MI, and stent thrombosis) and efficacy (clinically driven TLR) at 1 year, with findings preserved at 2-year follow-up.[44] These findings further support the use of modern DES in high-bleeding-risk patients.

Hybrid Sirolimus-Eluting Stents

Additional novel stent designs have incorporated drug delivery with a bioresorbable polymer coupled with a durable protective stent coating. One such stent platform is the Orsiro (Biotronik) stent, which uses a hybrid of active (sirolimus with bioabsorbable polymer matrix PLLA) and passive coatings (silicon carbide sealant) on a 60-µm or 80-µm strut for the 2.25- to 3.00-mm or the 3.50- to 4-mm stent platform, respectively. Conceptually, this allows for controlled drug release, followed by bioabsorption of the polymer, leaving a sealed stent to reduce interaction with the tissue or blood with the metallic surface of the stent. Initial studies of this platform compared with the durable polymer EES demonstrated comparable safety and efficacy at 2 years.[45] There have been at least nine randomized trials comparing the Orsiro to second-generation durable polymer DES. A systematic review and meta-analysis including 11,302 patients, TLF, favored the bioresorbable SES (odds ratio [OR], 0.82; 95% CI, 0.69-0.98; P = .03) at a mean follow-up of 2.8 years, driven primarily by a reduction in target vessel myocardial infarction without significant differences in cardiac death, TLR, and stent thrombosis.[46]

Late Outcomes of Drug-Eluting Stents

The use of polymer coatings has been associated with mid- and long-term adverse events after DES implantation. The development of polymer-free DES and newer-generation durable polymer-coated DES has helped mitigate these adverse outcomes. Ultimately, however, little data exist on late and very late outcomes after stenting. In the RESOLUTE All-Comers trial, an inferiority randomized controlled trial that assigned 2292 patients with either stable CAD or acute MI to ZES (n = 1140) or EES (n = 1152), both stents were found to have similar composite and individual efficacy and safety outcomes at 5 years.[47] ISAR-TEST-5 randomized 3002 patients with ischemic symptoms or evidence of myocardial ischemia to either a sirolimus- and probucol-eluting stent or a ZES. At 12 months, the polymer-free stent was noninferior to the newer-generation ZES with respect to the primary endpoint of cardiac death, TVR, or target vessel–related, as well as definite/probable stent thrombosis, or binary angiographic restenosis out to 12 months.[48] In an extended 10-year follow-up, no differences were observed in either device-oriented outcomes (cardiac death, MI related to target vessel, TLR) or patient-oriented outcomes (all-cause death, any MI, or any revascularization).[49] Additionally, rates of stent thrombosis were very low in both groups out to 10 years (<1% in both groups). It should be noted, however, that, while outcomes were similar, adverse outcomes occurred at high rates (cardiac death 26%, cardiac death or MI related to target vessel 29%, any revascularization [46%-47%]), illustrating the need for close outpatient follow-up and optimization of medications and comorbid conditions.

Drug-Eluting Stents in Patients at High Bleeding Risk

The management of patients with ischemic heart disease and high bleeding risk is challenging. Strategies to mitigate bleeding risk have included the use of BMS with 1 month of DAPT; however, higher rates of ISR and resultant TLR have been observed. Although current guidelines recommend 12 months of DAPT in patients with acute coronary syndrome and 6 months of DAPT in patients with stable CAD, shorter DAPT durations in combination with newer-generation DES and polymer-free stents have shown promise. In the LEADERS FREE trial, a polymer-free and carrier-free drug-coated stent (BioFreedom stent, Biosensors, Europe) was found to be superior in terms of safety and effectiveness compared with BMS in patients who received 1 month of DAPT.[50] The ONYX ONE trial compared ZES with polymer-free Biolimus A9–coated stents in patients at high bleeding risk subjected to 1 month of DAPT and found similar safety and effectiveness outcomes.[51] The SENIOR trial studied 1 month of DAPT in stable elderly patients (>75 years old) and 6 months of DAPT in unstable elderly patients undergoing PCI with the SYNERGY BP-DES (Boston Scientific) or REBEL BMS (Boston Scientific). At 1 year, there was a significant reduction in the composite primary endpoint of all-cause mortality, MI, stroke, or ischemia-driven TLR in patients who received DES compared with BMS, driven primarily by the need for TLR at 180 days to 1 year. No significant difference in stent thrombosis was noted between groups.[52]

Bioabsorbable Drug-Eluting Stents

Current-generation DESs have become the standard upon which novel PCI technologies are compared. Based on the contention that the ability to scaffold the vessel without requirement of a permanent scaffold would be superior for vascular remodeling, vasomotor function, limiting chronic inflammation, and preserving side branch access, bioresorbable scaffolds (BRSs) were developed. The first FDA-approved bioabsorbable stent, the Absorb BRS System (BVS-EES, Abbott Vascular, Santa Clara, CA) became commercially available in 2016. This device was a polymeric bioabsorbable scaffold constructed of PLLA, with a thin mixture of poly-d, l-lactic acid that serves as the drug carrier for everolimus. Similar to EES and SES, everolimus is 80% eluted at 30 days. While initial data regarding safety and efficacy were promising, as demonstrated by a low MACE rate, longer follow-up revealed a significantly higher rate of very late scaffold thrombosis compared with DES.[53-55] This risk resulted in withdrawal from the market in 2017. Currently, there are no FDA-approved BRSs. While there are BRSs that have CE mark in Europe, the current recommendations are to limit use to clinical trials. Factors that may have resulted in the increased thrombosis risk include thickness of struts, delayed resorption kinetics, implantation techniques with inaccurate sizing, and scaffold fracture.[56]

Covered Stents

Coronary perforations are a rare complication of PCI, but tamponade, cardiogenic shock, and death can occur if not rapidly identified and managed. Covered coronary stents are approved for use in the United States under a Humanitarian Device Exemption and all uses are reported. The JOSTENT GRAFTMASTER (Abbott Laboratories, Abbott Park, IL) covered stent has been used to treat vessels 2.75 to 5 mm in diameter and consisted of a "sandwich" stent design in which two coaxially aligned stainless steel stents are wrapped around an expandable nonbiodegradable (PTFE) membrane. The first-generation device was physician mounted, but this was replaced with a rapid exchange platform. While the device had high success at treating perforations, the limitations included difficult deliverability and high rates of restenosis. More recently, the PK Papyrus Covered Coronary Stent System (Biotronik, Berlin, Germany) was FDA approved. This stent graft is a balloon-expandable, ultrathin, single-stent design made from cobalt-chromium with a proBIO (amorphous silicon carbide) coating. This covered stent is compatible with a 5F guide catheter (up to stent size 4.0) and 6F guide catheter (for 4.5 and 5 stents) and available in 17 sizes ranging from 2.5 to 5 mm in diameter and 15, 20, and 26 mm in length. Compared with the JOSTENT GRAFTMASTER, the Papyrus covered stent has a lower crossing profile, is more flexible, and has a shorter delivery time. In a large series of over 1000 patients with perforation, PK Papyrus delivery was successful in 97.7% of cases and perforation sealing in 92.1%. Rates of pericardiocentesis and in-hospital death occurred in 30.2% and 12.4% of cases, respectively.[57] Given the only indication for covered stents is emergency use for perforations, there are no prospective clinical trials of the device.

CONCLUSIONS

Considerable improvements in coronary intervention over the past three decades have led to remarkable progress in the treatment of coronary disease. While balloon angioplasty enabled coronary interventions to become possible, abrupt vessel closure and restenosis remained problematic. The development of the BMS largely addressed acute vessel closure, but restenosis rates, albeit improved, were still clinically significant. The development of first-generation DES dramatically reduced the rates of restenosis and subsequent revascularization, but challenges with stent deliverability and adverse vessel reactions leading to stent thrombosis have led to serial improvements involving the pharmacologic agent, drug polymer, and stent design. These changes have further improved the safety, efficacy, and clinical utility of these newer stent platforms, becoming the preferred modality for most lesion and patient subsets. Recent stent upgrades have focused on improvements in drug platforms and polymers to include the development of bioresorbable polymers, BRSs, and polymer-free DESs. Among current-generation DESs, there are minimal differences in outcomes. The ultrathin-strut bioresorbable polymer sirolimus EES appears to have lower risk of target vessel MI compared with durable polymer DES. The data, however, are not compelling enough to recommend one current-generation DES platform over another or a durable versus bioresorbable polymer DES. Despite the theoretical advantages of bioresorbable polymers and polymer-free DESs, there is no evidence that these devices have improved safety or efficacy profiles in the short or long term. First-generation BRS had increased rates of late scaffold thrombosis, and thinner-strut PLLA devices and other bioresorbable materials are under study.

Key Points

- Compared with PTCA, BMSs result in a larger acute gain and larger late loss but maintain a larger net gain.
- Compared with PTCA, BMSs reduce the rates of acute vessel closure. Restenosis rates remain problematic, occurring in 10% to 20% of cases.
- DESs are composed of three key components: the stent, the antiproliferative agent, and the drug carrier (polymer), all of which can impact clinical and angiographic results.
- Compared with the BMS, first-generation DESs demonstrate a 55% reduction in TVR, largely attributable to reduced rates of in-stent late loss, resulting in reduced angiographic and clinical restenosis.
- Compared with the BMS, first-generation DESs have similar mortality or MI rates.
- Concerns regarding late/very late stent thrombosis resulted in prolonged duration of DAPT and development of newer stent platforms.
- In comparing first-generation DESs, the SES is superior to the PES in terms of TVR and stent thrombosis without differences in death or MI rates.
- Second-generation DESs, including durable polymer ZES and EES, are safer and more effective than first-generation DESs.
- Second-generation DESs demonstrate similar MACE compared with BMSs but with lower rates of definite/probable stent thrombosis.
- Second-generation DESs are superior to BMSs in various complex lesion subsets, including chronic total occlusions, saphenous vein grafts, diabetic patients, and acute MI.
- Most clinically available second-generation DESs demonstrate similar safety and efficacy.
- The improved safety profile of second-generation DESs has allowed for progressive reductions in recommended duration of DAPT, best demonstrated in patients with elevated bleeding risks.
- Lesion, patient, and procedural factors influence restenosis and TLR following DES implantation.
- First-generation biodegradable vascular scaffolds showed similar MACE to DES in the first year; however, increased risk of very late scaffold thrombosis resulted in removal from the US market.
- Rapid exchange covered stents are available for the treatment of free coronary perforations of vessels 2.5 to 5 mm in diameter. The Papyrus covered stent has a single stent layer and lower crossing profile compared with the earlier-generation covered stent platform.

For further review and interactivities, please see the chapter-based multiple choice questions and videos accessible in the complimentary eBook bundled with this text. Access instructions are located in the inside front cover.

References

1. Gruentzig AR, King SB III, Schlumpf M, Siegenthaler W. Long-term follow-up after percutaneous transluminal coronary angioplasty. The early Zurich experience. *N Engl J Med.* 1987;316(18):1127-1132.
2. George BS, Voorhees WD III, Roubin GS, et al. Multicenter investigation of coronary stenting to treat acute or threatened closure after percutaneous transluminal coronary angioplasty: clinical and angiographic outcomes. *J Am Coll Cardiol.* 1993;22(1):135-143.
3. Fischman DL, Leon MB, Baim DS, et al. A randomized comparison of coronary-stent placement and balloon angioplasty in the treatment of coronary artery disease. Stent Restenosis Study Investigators. *N Engl J Med.* 1994;331(8):496-501.
4. Yamaji K, Kimura T, Morimoto T, et al. Very long-term (15 to 20 years) clinical and angiographic outcome after coronary bare metal stent implantation. *Circ Cardiovasc Interv.* 2010;3(5):468-475.
5. Leon MB, Baim DS, Popma JJ, et al. A clinical trial comparing three antithrombotic-drug regimens after coronary-artery stenting. Stent Anticoagulation Restenosis Study Investigators. *N Engl J Med.* 1998;339(23):1665-1671.
6. Cutlip DE, Chhabra AG, Baim DS, et al. Beyond restenosis: five-year clinical outcomes from second-generation coronary stent trials. *Circulation.* 2004;110(10):1226-1230.
7. Garasic JM, Edelman ER, Squire JC, Seifert P, Williams MS, Rogers C. Stent and artery geometry determine intimal thickening independent of arterial injury. *Circulation.* 2000;101(7):812-818.
8. Rogers C, Edelman ER. Endovascular stent design dictates experimental restenosis and thrombosis. *Circulation.* 1995;91(12):2995-3001.

9. Kastrati A, Mehilli J, Dirschinger J, et al. Intracoronary stenting and angiographic results strut thickness effect on restenosis outcome (ISAR-STEREO) trial. *Vestn Rentgenol Radiol*. 2012;2012(2):52-60.
10. Pache J, Kastrati A, Mehilli J, et al. Intracoronary stenting and angiographic results: strut thickness effect on restenosis outcome (ISAR-STEREO-2) trial. *J Am Coll Cardiol*. 2003;41:1283-1288.
11. Cutlip DE, Chauhan MS, Baim DS, et al. Clinical restenosis after coronary stenting: perspectives from multicenter clinical trials. *J Am Coll Cardiol*. 2002;40(12):2082-2089.
12. Kirtane AJ, Gupta A, Iyengar S, et al. Safety and efficacy of drug-eluting and bare metal stents: comprehensive meta-analysis of randomized trials and observational studies. *Circulation*. 2009;119(25):3198-3206.
13. Pfisterer M, Brunner-La Rocca HP, Buser PT, et al. Late clinical events after clopidogrel discontinuation may limit the benefit of drug-eluting stents: an observational study of drug-eluting versus bare-metal stents. *J Am Coll Cardiol*. 2006;48(12):2584-2591.
14. Palmerini T, Biondi-Zoccai G, Della Riva D, et al. Stent thrombosis with drug-eluting and bare-metal stents: evidence from a comprehensive network meta-analysis. *Lancet*. 2012;379(9824):1393-1402.
15. Kolandaivelu K, Swaminathan R, Gibson WJ, et al. Stent thrombogenicity early in high-risk interventional settings is driven by stent design and deployment and protected by polymer-drug coatings. *Circulation*. 2011;123(13):1400-1409.
16. Garg S, Serruys PW. Coronary stents: looking forward. *J Am Coll Cardiol*. 2010;56(10 suppl):S43-S78.
17. Piccolo R, Bonaa KH, Efthimiou O, et al. Drug-eluting or bare-metal stents for percutaneous coronary intervention: a systematic review and individual patient data meta-analysis of randomised clinical trials. *Lancet*. 2019;393(10190):2503-2510.
18. Writing Committee Members; Lawton JS, Tamis-Holland JE, Bangalore S, et al. 2021 ACC/AHA/SCAI guideline for coronary artery revascularization: a report of the American College of Cardiology/American Heart Association Joint Committee on clinical practice guidelines. *J Am Coll Cardiol*. 2022;79:e21-e129.
19. Morice MC, Serruys PW, Sousa JE, et al. A randomized comparison of a sirolimus-eluting stent with a standard stent for coronary revascularization. *N Engl J Med*. 2002;346(23):1773-1780.
20. Moses JW, Leon MB, Popma JJ, et al. Sirolimus-eluting stents versus standard stents in patients with stenosis in a native coronary artery. *N Engl J Med*. 2003;349(14):1315-1323.
21. Caixeta A, Leon MB, Lansky AJ, et al. 5-year clinical outcomes after sirolimus-eluting stent implantation insights from a patient-level pooled analysis of 4 randomized trials comparing sirolimus-eluting stents with bare-metal stents. *J Am Coll Cardiol*. 2009;54(10):894-902.
22. Weisz G, Leon MB, Holmes SR Jr, et al. Five-year follow-up after sirolimus-eluting stent implantation results of the SIRIUS (Sirolimus-Eluting stent in de-novo native coronary lesions) trial. *J Am Coll Cardiol*. 2009;53(17):1488-1497.
23. Stone GW, Ellis SG, Cox DA, et al. A polymer-based, paclitaxel-eluting stent in patients with coronary artery disease. *N Engl J Med*. 2004;350(3):221-231.
24. Schomig A, Dibra A, Windecker S, et al. A meta-analysis of 16 randomized trials of sirolimus-eluting stents versus paclitaxel-eluting stents in patients with coronary artery disease. *J Am Coll Cardiol*. 2007;50(14):1373-1380.
25. Camenzind E, Steg PG, Wijns W. Stent thrombosis late after implantation of first-generation drug-eluting stents: a cause for concern. *Circulation*. 2007;115(11):1440-1455. discussion 1455.
26. Krone RJ, Rao SV, Dai D, et al. Acceptance, panic, and partial recovery the pattern of usage of drug-eluting stents after introduction in the U.S. (a report from the American College of Cardiology/National Cardiovascular Data Registry). *JACC Cardiovasc Interv*. 2010;3(9):902-910.
27. Burke SE, Kuntz RE, Schwartz LB. Zotarolimus (ABT-578) eluting stents. *Adv Drug Deliv Rev*. 2006;58(3):437-446.
28. Kandzari DE, Leon MB, Popma JJ, et al. Comparison of zotarolimus-eluting and sirolimus-eluting stents in patients with native coronary artery disease: a randomized controlled trial. *J Am Coll Cardiol*. 2006;48(12):2440-2447.
29. Kandzari DE, Leon MB, Meredith I, Fajadet J, Wijns W, Mauri L. Final 5-year outcomes from the Endeavor zotarolimus-eluting stent clinical trial program: comparison of safety and efficacy with first-generation drug-eluting and bare-metal stents. *JACC Cardiovasc Interv*. 2013;6(5):504-512.
30. Wijns W, Steg PG, Mauri L, et al. Endeavour zotarolimus-eluting stent reduces stent thrombosis and improves clinical outcomes compared with cypher sirolimus-eluting stent: 4-year results of the PROTECT randomized trial. *Eur Heart J*. 2014;35(40):2812-2820.
31. Meredith IT, Worthley SG, Whitbourn R, et al. Long-term clinical outcomes with the next-generation resolute stent system: a report of the two-year follow-up from the RESOLUTE clinical trial. *EuroIntervention*. 2010;5(6):692-697.
32. Kandzari DE, Kirtane AJ, Windecker S, et al. One-month dual antiplatelet therapy following percutaneous coronary intervention with zotarolimus-eluting stents in high-bleeding-risk patients. *Circ Cardiovasc Interv*. 2020;13(11):e009565.
33. Joner M, Nakazawa G, Finn AV, et al. Endothelial cell recovery between comparator polymer-based drug-eluting stents. *J Am Coll Cardiol*. 2008;52(5):333-342.
34. Smits PC, Vlachojannis GJ, McFadden EP, et al. Final 5-year follow-up of a randomized controlled trial of everolimus- and paclitaxel-eluting stents for coronary revascularization in daily practice: the COMPARE trial (A trial of everolimus-eluting stents and paclitaxel stents for coronary revascularization in daily practice). *JACC Cardiovasc Interv*. 2015;8(9):1157-1165.
35. Stone GW, Rizvi A, Newman W, et al. Everolimus-eluting versus paclitaxel-eluting stents in coronary artery disease. *N Engl J Med*. 2010;362(18):1663-1674.
36. Brener SJ, Kereiakes DJ, Simonton CA, et al. Everolimus-eluting stents in patients undergoing percutaneous coronary intervention: final 3-year results of the Clinical Evaluation of the XIENCE V Everolimus Eluting Coronary Stent System in the Treatment of Subjects With de Novo Native Coronary Artery Lesions trial. *Am Heart J*. 2013;166(6):1035-1042.
37. Bønaa KH, Mannsverk J, Wiseth R, et al. Drug-eluting or bare-metal stents for coronary artery disease. *N Engl J Med*. 2016;375(13):1242-1252.
38. Palmerini T, Benedetto U, Biondi-Zoccai G, et al. Long-term safety of drug-eluting and bare-metal stents: evidence from a comprehensive network meta-analysis. *J Am Coll Cardiol*. 2015;65(23):2496-2507.
39. Sabate M, Brugaletta S, Cequier A, et al. Clinical outcomes in patients with ST-segment elevation myocardial infarction treated with everolimus-eluting stents versus bare-metal stents (EXAMINATION): 5-year results of a randomised trial. *Lancet*. 2016;387(10016):357-366.
40. Kereiakes DJ, Meredith IT, Windecker S, et al. Efficacy and safety of a novel bioabsorbable polymer-coated, everolimus-eluting coronary stent: the EVOLVE II Randomized Trial. *Circ Cardiovasc Interv*. 2015;8(4):e002372.
41. Grube E, Buellesfeld L. BioMatrix Biolimus A9-eluting coronary stent: a next-generation drug-eluting stent for coronary artery disease. *Expert Rev Med Devices*. 2006;3(6):731-741.
42. Ghione M, Wykrzykowska JJ, Windecker S, et al. Five-year outcomes of chronic total occlusion treatment with a biolimus A9-eluting biodegradable polymer stent versus a sirolimus-eluting permanent polymer stent in the LEADERS all-comers trial. *Cardiol J*. 2016;23(6):626-636.
43. Natsuaki M, Kozuma K, Morimoto T, et al. Final 3-year outcome of a randomized trial comparing second-generation drug-eluting stents using either biodegradable polymer or durable polymer: NOBORI biolimus-eluting versus XIENCE/PROMUS everolimus-eluting stent trial. *Circ Cardiovasc Interv*. 2015;8(10):e002817.
44. Garot P, Morice MC, Tresukosol D, et al. 2-Year outcomes of high bleeding risk patients after polymer-free drug-coated stents. *J Am Coll Cardiol*. 2017;69(2):162-171.
45. Zbinden R, Piccolo R, Heg D, et al. Ultrathin strut biodegradable polymer sirolimus-eluting stent versus durable-polymer everolimus-eluting stent for percutaneous coronary revascularization: 2-year results of the BIOSCIENCE trial. *J Am Heart Assoc*. 2016;5(3):e003255.
46. Monjur MR, Said CF, Bamford P, Parkinson M, Szirt R, Ford T. Ultrathin-strut biodegradable polymer versus durable polymer drug-eluting stents: a meta-analysis. *Open Heart*. 2020;7(2):e001394.
47. Iqbal J, Serruys PW, Silber S, et al. Comparison of zotarolimus- and everolimus-eluting coronary stents: final 5-year report of the RESOLUTE all-comers trial. *Circ Cardiovasc Interv*. 2015;8(6):e002230.

48. Massberg S, Byrne RA, Kastrati A, et al. Polymer-free sirolimus- and probucol-eluting versus new generation zotarolimus-eluting stents in coronary artery disease: the intracoronary stenting and angiographic results—test efficacy of sirolimus- and probucol-eluting versus zotarolimus-eluting stents (ISAR-TEST 5) trial. *Circulation*. 2011;124(5):624-632.
49. Kufner S, Ernst M, Cassese S, et al. 10-Year outcomes from a randomized trial of polymer-free versus durable polymer drug-eluting coronary stents. *J Am Coll Cardiol*. 2020;76(2):146-158.
50. Urban P, Meredith IT, Abizaid A, et al. Polymer-free drug-coated coronary stents in patients at high bleeding risk. *N Engl J Med*. 2015;373(21):2038-2047.
51. Windecker S, Latib A, Kedhi E, et al. Polymer-based or polymer-free stents in patients at high bleeding risk. *N Engl J Med*. 2020;382(13):1208-1218.
52. Varenne O, Cook S, Sideris G, et al. Drug-eluting stents in elderly patients with coronary artery disease (SENIOR): a randomised single-blind trial. *Lancet*. 2018;391(10115):41-50.
53. Chevalier B, Onuma Y, van Boven AJ, et al. Randomised comparison of a bioresorbable everolimus-eluting scaffold with a metallic everolimus-eluting stent for ischaemic heart disease caused by de novo native coronary artery lesions: the 2-year clinical outcomes of the ABSORB II trial. *EuroIntervention*. 2016;12(9):1102-1107.
54. Rizik DG, Hermiller JB, Simonton CA, Klassen KJ, Kereiakes DJ. Bioresorbable vascular scaffolds for the treatment of coronary artery disease: what have we learned from randomized-controlled clinical trials? *Coron Artery Dis*. 2017;28(1):77-89.
55. Toyota T, Morimoto T, Shiomi H, et al. Very late scaffold thrombosis of bioresorbable vascular scaffold: systematic review and a meta-analysis. *JACC Cardiovasc Interv*. 2017;10(1):27-37.
56. Sotomi Y, Suwannasom P, Serruys PW, Onuma Y. Possible mechanical causes of scaffold thrombosis: insights from case reports with intracoronary imaging. *EuroIntervention*. 2017;12(14):1747-1756.
57. Kandzari DE, Sarao RC, Waksman R. Clinical experience of the PK Papyrus covered stent in patients with coronary artery perforations: results from a multi-center humanitarian device exemption survey. *Cardiovasc Revasc Med*. 2022;43:97-101.

17 Elective Percutaneous Coronary Intervention for Chronic Coronary Disease

Dhaval Kolte and Douglas E. Drachman

DEFINITION AND EPIDEMIOLOGY OF CHRONIC CORONARY DISEASE

Chronic coronary disease (CCD) represents a heterogeneous group of conditions that include obstructive and nonobstructive coronary artery disease (CAD) with or without prior acute coronary syndrome (ACS) or revascularization, ischemic heart disease diagnosed only by noninvasive testing, and chronic anginal syndromes with varying underlying etiologies.[1,2] CCD or chronic coronary syndromes encompass (i) patients with stable angina symptoms (or angina equivalents such as dyspnea) with or without positive results of an imaging test; (ii) patients with new onset of heart failure (HF) or left ventricular (LV) systolic dysfunction and known or suspected CAD or patients with established cardiomyopathy deemed to be of ischemic origin; (iii) patients discharged after admission for an ACS event or after coronary revascularization and stabilization of all acute cardiovascular issues; (iv) patients with angina and evidence of vasospastic or microvascular disease; and (v) asymptomatic patients diagnosed with CCD based solely on the results of a screening study.[1,2]

It is estimated that 20.5 million persons in the United States (US) ≥20 years of age have CAD, and 10.8 million have chronic stable angina pectoris.[3] Both within the US and worldwide, the prevalence of CAD and chronic stable angina vary by age, sex, race/ethnicity, and geographic region.[3] Despite a 19.2% relative reduction in the annual death rate attributable to CAD over the past decade, it remains the leading cause of death in the US and worldwide, and is associated with substantial health care burden at the individual and societal levels.[3]

MANAGEMENT OF CCD

The goals of management of patients with CCD are three-fold: relief of anginal symptoms, prevention of nonfatal events such as myocardial infarction (MI), and improvement of long-term survival. Lifestyle modifications and optimal medical therapy (OMT) are the cornerstones of management of patients with CCD. However, in CCD patients with lifestyle-limiting angina despite OMT, revascularization is indicated to improve symptoms and quality of life (QOL).[1,2,4-6] Similarly, in selected CCD patients, particularly patients with multivessel CAD, revascularization with either Percutaneous coronary intervention (PCI) or Coronary artery bypass grafting (CABG) has been shown to lower the risk of cardiac death, MI, and urgent revascularization (**Fig. 17.1**).[7-9] However, the role of revascularization in improving long-term survival among patients with CCD remains a topic of debate. Numerous studies and meta-analyses comparing PCI versus OMT alone in CCD have found no difference in all-cause mortality.[6,8,9] However, in CCD patients with LV systolic dysfunction—particularly left ventricular ejection fraction (LVEF) ≤35%—and multivessel CAD, and in patients with left main disease, CABG has been shown to be superior to OMT alone for improving survival (**Fig. 17.1**).[10-12]

PCI VERSUS OMT

In 1977, Andreas Grüentzig performed the first PCI to treat anginal symptoms.[13] Over the past 4 decades, with the technical progress in PCI and evolution of OMT, multiple randomized controlled trials (RCTs) have compared PCI versus no PCI on the background of OMT in patients with stable CAD (**Table 17.1**).

In the Angioplasty Compared to Medicine (ACME) trial, 212 patients with stable angina, exercise-induced myocardial ischemia, and 70% to 99% stenosis of one epicardial coronary artery were randomized to percutaneous transluminal coronary angioplasty (PTCA) or OMT (aspirin and a combination of β blockers, nitrates, and calcium-channel blockers [CCBs] titrated to eliminate angina).[14] Primary end points included change in exercise tolerance, frequency of angina, and nitroglycerin use; and exercise stress nuclear testing was evaluated at the baseline and 6 months postrandomization. Compared with OMT, PTCA improved exercise duration and reduced time to onset of angina and frequency of angina episodes. Mortality or MI rates did not differ significantly between the two treatment groups.[14] In a pilot study (ACME 2), 101 patients with 2-vessel CAD were evaluated using the same inclusion criteria, outcomes, and study protocol.[15] No difference was identified between the PTCA and OMT groups with respect to any of the end points.

In the Medicine, Angioplasty, or Surgery Study (MASS), 214 patients with stable angina, normal left ventricular systolic function, and a proximal left anterior descending coronary artery stenosis of >80% were randomized to OMT, PTCA, or CABG using an internal mammary artery conduit.[16] The primary end point was a composite of cardiac death, MI, or refractory angina requiring revascularization. OMT consisted of aspirin, β blockers, CCBs, and nitrates. At an average follow-up period of 3 years, the primary end point occurred in 3% of patients in the CABG group compared with 24% in the PTCA group and 17% in the OMT group, with no statistically significant difference between the latter two.[16] The difference was driven mainly by lower rates of refractory angina requiring revascularization in the CABG group. There were no differences in mortality or MI rates in the three groups. Both the CABG and PTCA groups had significantly higher percentages of patients free of angina compared with OMT (CABG 98%, PTCA 82%, and OMT 32%).

In the RITA 2 (second Randomized Intervention Treatment of Angina) trial, 1018 patients with at least 1-vessel CAD were randomized to OMT or PTCA with a median follow-up of 2.7 years.[17] This trial did not exclude patients with low LVEF or totally occluded coronary arteries. The combined primary end point of death or nonfatal MI occurred in 3.3% of patients in the OMT group versus 6.3% in the PTCA group (P = .02). There was no difference in mortality between the two groups, although there were more nonfatal MIs in the PTCA group (4.2% vs 2.0%), primarily driven by periprocedural MI.[17] Symptom relief was greater following PTCA in patients with Canadian Cardiovascular Society (CCS) Class ≥2 angina, but this benefit was lost at 2-year follow-up.[17]

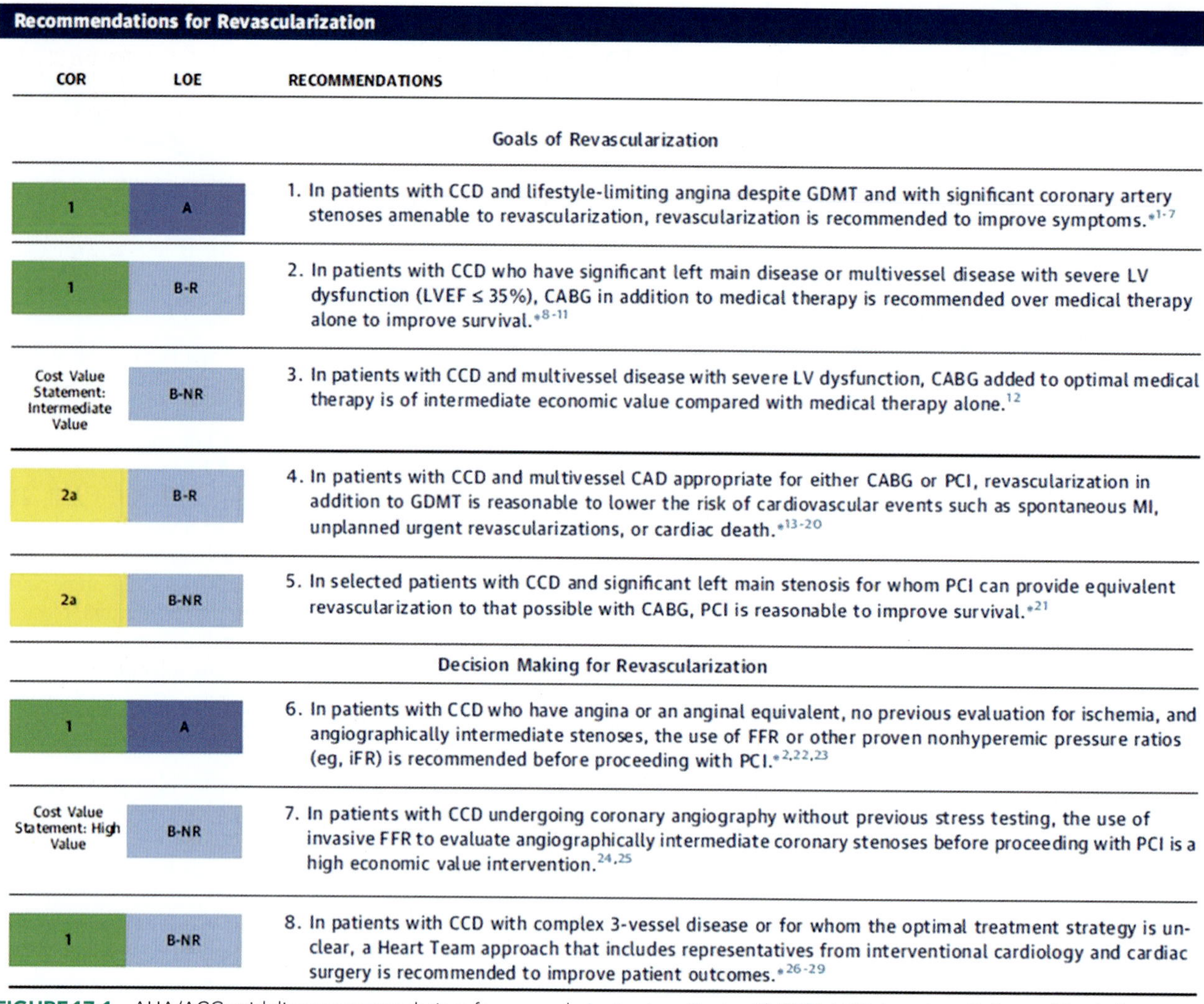

Recommendations for Revascularization

COR	LOE	RECOMMENDATIONS
		Goals of Revascularization
1	A	1. In patients with CCD and lifestyle-limiting angina despite GDMT and with significant coronary artery stenoses amenable to revascularization, revascularization is recommended to improve symptoms.*[1-7]
1	B-R	2. In patients with CCD who have significant left main disease or multivessel disease with severe LV dysfunction (LVEF ≤ 35%), CABG in addition to medical therapy is recommended over medical therapy alone to improve survival.*[8-11]
Cost Value Statement: Intermediate Value	B-NR	3. In patients with CCD and multivessel disease with severe LV dysfunction, CABG added to optimal medical therapy is of intermediate economic value compared with medical therapy alone.[12]
2a	B-R	4. In patients with CCD and multivessel CAD appropriate for either CABG or PCI, revascularization in addition to GDMT is reasonable to lower the risk of cardiovascular events such as spontaneous MI, unplanned urgent revascularizations, or cardiac death.*[13-20]
2a	B-NR	5. In selected patients with CCD and significant left main stenosis for whom PCI can provide equivalent revascularization to that possible with CABG, PCI is reasonable to improve survival.*[21]
		Decision Making for Revascularization
1	A	6. In patients with CCD who have angina or an anginal equivalent, no previous evaluation for ischemia, and angiographically intermediate stenoses, the use of FFR or other proven nonhyperemic pressure ratios (eg, iFR) is recommended before proceeding with PCI.*[2,22,23]
Cost Value Statement: High Value	B-NR	7. In patients with CCD undergoing coronary angiography without previous stress testing, the use of invasive FFR to evaluate angiographically intermediate coronary stenoses before proceeding with PCI is a high economic value intervention.[24,25]
1	B-NR	8. In patients with CCD with complex 3-vessel disease or for whom the optimal treatment strategy is unclear, a Heart Team approach that includes representatives from interventional cardiology and cardiac surgery is recommended to improve patient outcomes.*[26-29]

FIGURE 17.1 AHA/ACC guideline recommendations for revascularization in patients with CCD. ACC, American College of Cardiology; AHA, American Heart Association; CABG, coronary artery bypass grafting; CAD, coronary artery disease; CCD, chronic coronary disease; FFR, fractional flow reserve; GDMT, guideline-directed medical therapy; iFR, instantaneous wave-free ratio; LV, left ventricle; LVEF, left ventricular ejection fraction; PCI, percutaneous coronary intervention. (Adapted from Virani SS, Newby LK, Arnold SV, et al. 2023 AHA/ACC/ACCP/ASPC/NLA/PCNA guideline for the management of patients with chronic coronary disease: a report of the American Heart Association/American College of Cardiology Joint Committee on clinical practice guidelines. *J Am Coll Cardiol.* 2023;82(9):833-955.)

Because these trials recruited patients before the results of RCTs of the hydroxymethylglutaryl (HMG)-CoA inhibitors were published, statin use was not mandated, and lipid-lowering drugs were prescribed at the discretion of the supervising clinician. The Atorvastatin vs Revascularization Treatment (AVERT) trial randomized 341 patients with stable CAD, relatively normal LVEF, no symptoms or Canadian Cardiovascular Society (CCS) class I or II angina, and a serum level of low-density lipoprotein (LDL) cholesterol of at least 115 mg/dL who were referred for percutaneous revascularization to receive medical therapy with atorvastatin 80 mg/d or to undergo the recommended PTCA followed by usual care.[18] The primary end point was occurrence of a first ischemic event (cardiac death, cardiac arrest, nonfatal MI, stroke, CABG, PCI, or hospitalization for angina). Of patients in the medical therapy arm, 13% had an ischemic event compared with 21% in the PTCA group (P = .045). The authors concluded that in low-risk patients with stable CAD, aggressive lipid lowering therapy with a statin is at least as effective as PTCA and usual care.[18]

In the MASS-II trial, 611 patients with at least 2-vessel CAD were randomized to OMT, PCI, or CABG.[19] This was the first trial to require not only coronary stenosis but also ischemia (as detected by stress testing or presence of CCS class II or III angina), and to introduce the use of stents in the PCI arm. Statins were used in 68%, 73%, and 49% of patients assigned to the OMT, PCI, and CABG groups, respectively. There was no significant difference in the three groups with regard to cardiac death or acute MI during the 1-year follow-up. Freedom from angina at 1-year follow-up was more common in the CABG (88%) and PCI (79%) groups compared with that of the OMT group (46%); however, rates of angina requiring revascularization were higher in the PCI group (13.3% vs 8.3% in the OMT group and 0.5% in the CABG group).[19]

Improvement in Medical Therapy

A new chapter of revascularization trials began when it was recognized that the incremental effect of revascularization should be assessed in the setting of comprehensive guideline-directed medical therapy applied aggressively to patients in both arms of the trial.

The Clinical Outcomes Utilizing Revascularization and Aggressive Drug Evaluation (COURAGE) trial randomized 2287 patients with stable CAD (≥70% stenosis in at least 1 proximal epicardial coronary artery and objective evidence of myocardial

TABLE 17.1 RCTs of PCI + OMT Versus OMT Alone in Chronic Coronary Disease

TRIAL	KEY INCLUSION CRITERIA	N (PCI/OMT)	PCI	OMT	PRIMARY END POINT	FOLLOW-UP	RESULT
ACME, 1992	Clinical (stable angina pectoris, +ETT with STD ≥3 mm, or MI within past 3 mo); Angiographic (70%-99% diameter stenosis in proximal two-thirds of 1 epicardial coronary artery; ETT (≥1 mm STD)	105/107	PTCA	Isosorbide dinitrate with sublingual nitroglycerin, β blockers, CCBs, or a combination of these agents in a progressive stepped approach.	Change in exercise tolerance, frequency of angina attacks and use of nitroglycerin	6 mo	↑ exercise duration, ↓ time to onset of angina, and ↑ freedom from angina with PCI vs OMT
ACME-2, 1997	Same as ACME, except the presence of 2-vessel CAD	51/50	PTCA	Aspirin plus nitrates, β blockers, and CCBs in a progressive stepped approach.	Change in exercise duration, freedom from angina, QoL	6 mo	No difference
MASS, 1995	≥80% diameter stenosis in proximal LAD	72/72	PTCA	Aspirin, nitrates, β blockers, CCBs	Composite of cardiac death, MI, or refractory angina requiring revascularization	3 y	No difference
RITA-2, 1997	≥1-vessel CAD	504/514	BMS 9%	β blockers, CCBs, long-acting nitrates	Composite of all-cause death and nonfatal MI	2.7 y (median)	↑ nonfatal MI with PCI
AVERT, 1999	1- or 2-vessel CAD (≥50% stenosis), relatively normal LVEF, asymptomatic or mild-to-moderate angina, and LDL-C ≥115 mg/dL	177/164	BMS 30%	Atorvastatin 80 mg/d	Ischemic events	18 mo	↓ ischemic events (*P* = NS) and longer time to first ischemic event (*P* = .03) with OMT vs PCI
MASS-II, 2004	Proximal multivessel CAD >70%; ischemia (+ETT or CCS class II or III)	205/203	BMS 72%	Aspirin, statins, nitrates, β blockers, CCBs, ACEi	Cardiac death, Q-wave MI, or refractory angina requiring revascularization	1 y	No difference in cardiac death and Q-wave MI, but ↑ rates of refractory angina requiring revascularization with PCI
COURAGE, 2007	≥1-vessel CAD (≥70% stenosis and objective evidence of myocardial ischemia, or ≥80% stenosis and classic angina without provocative testing)	1149/1138	BMS 91%; DES 3%	Aspirin or clopidogrel; long-actine metoprolol, amlodipine, and isosorbide mononitrate alone or in combination; lisinopril or losartan; simvastatin ± ezetimibe; extended-release niacin and/or fibrates.	Composite of all-cause death and nonfatal MI	4.6 y (median)	No difference

(continued)

TABLE 17.1 RCTs of PCI + OMT Versus OMT Alone in Chronic Coronary Disease (*Continued*)

TRIAL	KEY INCLUSION CRITERIA	N (PCI/ OMT)	PCI	OMT	PRIMARY END POINT	FOLLOW-UP	RESULT
BARI 2D, 2009	DM2 (treatment with insulin or oral hypoglycemic drugs, or a confirmed elevated blood glucose level) and CAD (≥50% stenosis with a positive stress test, or ≥70% stenosis and classic angina)	798/807 (in the PCI stratum)	BMS 56%; DES 34.7%	Guideline-directed medical therapy with a target level of HbA1c <7%, LDL-C <100 mg/dL, BP < 130/80 mm Hg	All-cause death and MACE (composite of all-cause death, MI, stroke)	5 y	No difference
SWISSI II, 2007	MI within the preceding 3 mo, myocardial ischemia detected by bicycle exercise test and verified by stress imaging, and 1- or 2-vessel CAD	96/105	PTCA	Aspirin, statin; bisoprolol 5-10 mg/d, amlodipine 5-10 mg/d, molsidomine 4-12 mg twice daily, or combinations thereof	MACE (composite of cardiac death, nonfatal MI, and/or symptom-driven revascularization)	10.2 y (median)	↓ MACE with PCI vs OMT
DEFER, 2007	1-vessel CAD (>50% stenosis in a native coronary artery with a reference diameter of >2.5 mm), no evidence of reversible ischemia by noninvasive testing within the prior 2 mo, and FFR >0.75	90/91	BMS	Aspirin, statins, β blockers, CCBs, nitrates	Adverse cardiac events	5 y	No difference
FAME 2, 2012	1-, 2-, or 3-vessel CAD (>50% stenosis) and at least 1 stenosis with FFR ≤0.80	447/441	DES	Aspirin, β blockers, CCBs, ACEi or ARB, statin ± ezetimibe to reduce LDL-C to <70 mg/dL	Composite of all-cause death, MI, or urgent revascularization	213 d (mean)	↓ events (driven by lower rates of urgent revascularization) with PCI vs OMT
ISCHEMIA, 2020	Moderate or severe reversible ischemia on imaging tests or severe ischemia on exercise tests without imaging. (*Key exclusion criteria* were eGFR <30 mL/min/1.73 m^2, recent ACS, unprotected LM stenosis of ≥50% on CT, LVEF <35%, NYHA class III or IV heart failure, unacceptable angina despite maximal tolerated medical therapy)	2588/2591	Revascularization in 79% (PCI with DES in 74% and CABG in 26%)	Aspirin or clopidogrel; statins ± ezetimibe ± evolocumab for goal LDL-C <70 mg/dL; ACEi/ARB and β blockers according to guidelines	Composite of cardiovascular death, MI, or hospitalization for unstable angina, heart failure, or resuscitated cardiac arrest	3.2 y (median)	No difference in primary end point; ↑ improvement in angina-related health status (SAQ summary scores) with invasive vs conservative strategy

TABLE 17.1 RCTs of PCI + OMT Versus OMT Alone in Chronic Coronary Disease *(Continued)*

TRIAL	KEY INCLUSION CRITERIA	N (PCI/ OMT)	PCI	OMT	PRIMARY END POINT	FOLLOW-UP	RESULT
ISCHEMIA-CKD, 2020	Same as ISCHEMIA, and eGFR <30 mL/ min/1.73 m^2 or dialysis)	388/389	Revascularization in 50.2% (PCI with DES in 85% and CABG in 15%)	Same as ISCHEMIA	Composite of cardiovascular death, MI, or hospitalization for unstable angina, heart failure, or resuscitated cardiac arrest	2.2 y (median)	No difference in primary end point; ↑ stroke with invasive vs conservative strategy
ORBITA, 2018	1-vessel CAD (≥70% stenosis)	105/95 (PCI/ placebo procedure)	DES	Guideline-directed antianginal therapy with a prespecified target of ≥2 antianginals; DAPT; statins	Difference in exercise time increment	6 wk	No difference

ACEi, angiotensin converting enzyme inhibitor; ACME, Angioplasty Compared to Medicine; ARB, angiotensin II receptor blocker; AVERT, Atorvastatin versus Revascularization Treatment; BARI-2D, Bypass Angioplasty Revascularization Investigation 2 Diabetes; BMS, bare metal stent; BP, blood pressure; CABG, coronary artery bypass grafting; CAD, coronary artery disease; CCBs, calcium channel blockers; CCS, Canadian Classification System; CKD, chronic kidney disease; COURAGE, Clinical Outcomes Utilizing Revascularization and Aggressive Drug Evaluation; CT, computed tomography; DAPT, dual antiplatelet therapy; DEFER, ; DES, drug-eluting stent; DM2, type 2 diabetes mellitus; eGFR, estimated glomerular filtration rate; ETT, exercise treadmill test; FAME 2, Fractional Flow Reserve versus Angiography for Multivessel Evaluation 2; FFR, fractional flow reserve; HbA1c, hemoglobin A1c; ISCHEMIA, International Study of Comparative Health Effectiveness with Medical and Invasive Approaches; LAD, left anterior descending coronary artery; LDL-C, low-density lipoprotein cholesterol; LM, left main coronary artery; LVEF, left ventricular ejection fraction; MACE, major adverse cardiovascular events; MASS, Medicine, Angioplasty or Surgery Study; MI, myocardial infarction; NS, nonsignificant; NYHA, New York Heart Association; OMT, optimal medical therapy; ORBITA, Objective Randomized Blinded Investigation with optimal medical Therapy of Angioplasty in stable angina; PCI, percutaneous coronary intervention; PTCA, percutaneous transluminal coronary angioplasty; QoL, quality of life; RITA-2, second Randomized Intervention Treatment of Angina; SAQ, Seattle Angina Questionnaire; STD, ST-segment depression; SWISSI II, Swiss Interventional Study on Silent Ischemia Type II.

ischemia or at least one coronary stenosis of ≥80% and classic angina without provocative testing) to PCI + OMT or OMT alone.[20] More than 90% of patients in each arm received aspirin and statins, >80% received β blockers, and >60% received angiotensin-converting enzyme inhibitor (ACEi) or angiotensin receptor blocker (ARB) therapy. The primary outcome was a composite of all-cause death or nonfatal MI. After a median follow-up of 4.6 years, the cumulative primary event rates were 19.0% in the PCI group and 18.5% in the OMT group (P = .62).[20] There were no significant differences between the two groups in the composite of death, MI, and stroke (20.0% vs 19.5%, P = .62); hospitalization for ACS (12.4% vs 11.8%, P = .56); or MI (13.2% vs 12.3%, P = .33). In an extended survival analysis up to 15 years, there was no difference in survival between the initial strategy of PCI + OMT and OMT alone (25% vs 24, P = .76).[21] Nevertheless, this analysis was limited by a large percentage of patients who were lost to follow-up (47%), an unknown amount of crossover to PCI, and unknown causes of death.

In the Bypass Angioplasty Revascularization Investigation 2 Diabetes (BARI 2D) trial, 2368 patients with type 2 diabetes and stable CAD (≥50% stenosis of a major epicardial coronary artery associated with a positive stress test or ≥70% stenosis of a major epicardial coronary artery and classic angina) were randomized in a 2 × 2 factorial design to OMT or prompt revascularization and to insulin sensitization therapy or insulin-provision therapy to achieve a target glycated hemoglobin level of less than 7.0%.[22] Randomization was stratified according to the method of revascularization (PCI or CABG). More than 90% of patients in each arm received aspirin, statin, and ACEi/ARB, and >80% received β blockers. Primary end points were the rate of death and a composite of death, myocardial infarction, or stroke (major cardiovascular events). At 5 years, rates of survival did not differ significantly between the revascularization and the medical therapy groups (88.3% vs 87.8%, P = .97). The rates of freedom from major cardiovascular events also did not differ significantly between the two groups (77.2% vs 75.9%, P = .70).[22] In the PCI stratum, there was no significant difference in primary end points between the revascularization and the medical-therapy groups. In the CABG stratum, the rate of major cardiovascular events was significantly lower in the revascularization group (22.4%) than in the medical-therapy group (22.4% vs 30.5%, P = .01; interaction P-value = .002).[22]

Role of Ischemia Evaluation

In the Swiss Interventional Study on Silent Ischemia Type II SWISSI II) trial, 201 patients with a recent MI, myocardial ischemia detected by bicycle exercise test and verified by stress imaging, and 1- or 2-vessel CAD were randomized to PCI or intensive anti-ischemic medical therapy (β blockers, CCBs, nitrates).[23] During a mean follow-up of 10.2 years, the PCI group versus the anti-ischemic medical therapy group had lower rates of major adverse cardiac events defined as cardiac death, nonfatal MI, and/or symptom-driven revascularization (adjusted hazard ratio 0.33; 95% confidence interval 0.20-0.55; P < .001), lower rates of ischemia (11.6% vs 28.9%, P = .03), and improved LVEF.[23] Similarly, in the COURAGE Trial Nuclear Substudy of 314 patients who underwent serial rest/stress SPECT MPI before treatment and 6 to 18 months after randomization, the reduction in ischemic myocardium was greater with PCI + OMT versus OMT alone (−2.7% vs −0.5%, P < .0001).[24] The primary end point of ≥5% ischemia reduction occurred in 33% of patients in the PCI + OMT group versus 19% of those in the OMT group (P = .0004). Patients with ischemia reduction had lower unadjusted risk for death or MI (P = .037 [risk-adjusted P = .26]), particularly if baseline ischemia was moderate to severe (P = .001 [risk-adjusted P = .08]). Death or MI rates ranged from 0% to 39% for patients with no residual ischemia to ≥10% residual ischemia on follow-up (P = .002 [risk-adjusted P = .09]).[24] These data were consistent with a prior observational study of 10,627 patients demonstrating a survival advantage of revascularization over OMT in patients with moderate to severe ischemia (≥10% ischemia) detected by SPECT MPI.[25] On the contrary, in a post hoc substudy of the COURAGE trial including 1381 randomized patients (OMT n = 699, PCI + OMT n = 682) who underwent baseline stress myocardial perfusion imaging (MPI) with single-photon emission computed tomography (SPECT), the extent of ischemia (none to mild [<3 ischemic segments] vs moderate to severe [≥3 ischemic segments]) neither predicted adverse events and nor altered treatment effectiveness (rates of death or MI in OMT vs PCI + OMT groups were 18% vs 19% [P = .92] in patients with none to mild ischemia, and 19% vs 22% [P = .053] in patients with moderate to severe ischemia, respectively; interaction P-value = .65).[26] Furthermore, in a follow-up COURAGE core laboratory study in 621 patients, the extent of baseline ischemia did not correlate with the rate of death, MI, or ACS after mean follow-up of 4.7 years.[27]

Noninvasive testing often indicates the presence of ischemia in patients with multivessel CAD, but may fail to distinguish the specific territory or stenosis responsible. Moreover, in the case of balanced ischemia, noninvasive testing may not identify a perfusion abnormality, and may provide a false sense of security. The use of intracoronary pressure wire technology, permitting the evaluation of coronary fractional flow reserve (FFR), has emerged as an accurate and lesion-specific index that indicates whether a particular stenosis is responsible for downstream myocardial ischemia.[28] Several recent clinical trials have shown that FFR-guided intervention may provide a sound basis for decision making in the catheterization laboratory, permitting selective intervention only on lesions responsible for ischemia.[29,30]

In the DEFER trial, 325 patients with a >50% coronary stenosis and a negative perfusion study within 2 months underwent coronary angiography with measurement of FFR.[29] If FFR was ≥0.75, patients were randomly assigned to deferral (defer group; n = 91) or performance of PCI (perform group; n = 90). If FFR was <0.75, PCI was performed as planned (reference group; n = 144). At 5 years of clinical follow-up, the risk of death or MI from a nonischemic (FFR ≥ 0.75) lesion was very low, and not altered by PCI. In contrast, ischemia-causing lesions (FFR < 0.75) were the most important predictor of death or MI in follow-up.[29] The DEFER trial established the safety of not performing PCI in a nonsignificant stenosis as identified by FFR. Building on the findings of the DEFER trial, the use of FFR in the evaluation of patients with multivessel disease was examined in the Fractional Flow Reserve versus Angiography for Multivessel Evaluation trial (FAME).[30] In FAME, 1005 patients with ≥50% stenosis in at least two of the three major epicardial coronary vessels were randomized to undergo FFR-guided revascularization of only ischemia-causing lesions versus angiographically guided PCI of all angiographically significant stenoses.[30] The primary endpoint was a composite of death, MI, and revascularization at 2-year follow-up. The FFR-guided PCI had significantly fewer primary end-point events, 17.9% overall versus 22.4% for the angiographically guided PCI group. The FAME study demonstrated that routine FFR assessment in patients with multivessel disease results in lower rates of stent use, and significantly reduces the composite endpoint of death, MI, and revascularization. In the lesions with FFR >0.80, deferral of PCI appeared safe, resulting in a 2-year rate of MI of 0.2% and revascularization of 3.2%.[30]

The FAME 2 trial examined whether FFR-guided PCI in addition to OMT would be superior to OMT alone in patients with 1-, 2-, or 3-vessel CAD (>50% stenosis) and at least one stenosis in a major coronary artery with FFR ≤0.80.[7] Patients in whom all stenoses had an FFR of >0.80 were entered into a registry and received the best available medical therapy. The primary end point included a composite of death, MI, or urgent revascularization. The trial was halted prematurely by the data safety monitoring board after the enrollment of 1220 patients in light of a substantial between-group difference in the primary end-point event rate: 4.3% in the PCI group and 12.7% in the medical therapy group (hazard ratio, 0.32; 95% confidence interval 0.19-0.53; P < .001).[7] The difference was driven by a lower rate of urgent revascularization in the PCI group compared to the medical therapy group (1.6% vs 11.1%; hazard ratio, 0.13; 95% CI, 0.06-0.30; P < .001). In particular, in the PCI group, fewer urgent revascularizations were triggered by an MI or evidence of ischemia on electrocardiography (hazard ratio, 0.13; 95% CI, 0.04-0.43; P < .001). The FAME 2 trial demonstrated that in patients with stable CAD and functionally significant stenoses, FFR-guided PCI plus the best available medical therapy, as compared with the best available medical therapy alone, decreased the need for urgent revascularization.[7]

The International Study of Comparative Health Effectiveness with Medical and Invasive Approaches (ISCHEMIA) trial was designed to overcome two potential caveats of all prior RCTs comparing PCI + OMT versus OMT alone in patients with stable CAD.[31] First, in trials requiring angiographic evidence of obstructive CAD, it is possible that patients with high-risk anatomical features may have been excluded, and knowledge of the anatomy may have led to revascularization in patients who were randomly assigned to a conservative strategy. Second, previous studies allowed the enrollment of patients with any level of ischemia, which resulted in a minority of patients with moderate or severe ischemia for whom an invasive strategy might be most beneficial. In the ISCHEMIA trial, 5179 patients with stable CAD were enrolled after clinically indicated stress testing showed moderate or severe reversible ischemia on imaging tests or severe ischemia on exercise tests without imaging.[32] Most enrolled trial patients (73%) underwent coronary computed tomographic (CT) angiography to rule out left main coronary disease and nonobstructive coronary disease. Patients were randomized in 1:1 ratio to an initial invasive strategy of medical therapy, angiography, and revascularization when feasible or to an initial conservative strategy of medical therapy alone, with angiography reserved for failure of medical therapy. Patients who were assigned to the invasive strategy were to undergo angiography within 30 days after randomization and complete revascularization of all ischemic territories if feasible. Decisions about the type of revascularization (PCI or CABG) were deferred to the local heart team. Among patients in the invasive-strategy group, 96% underwent angiography and 79% underwent revascularization (PCI in 74% and CABG in 26%). The primary outcome was the composite of death from cardiovascular causes, MI, or hospitalization for unstable angina, HF, or resuscitated cardiac arrest. The key secondary outcomes were the composite of death from cardiovascular causes or MI and angina-related QOL. Over a median follow-up of 3.2 years, there were no significant differences in the rates of the primary outcome between the two groups.[32] The cumulative event rates in the invasive-strategy group versus the conservative-strategy group were 5.3% versus 3.4% (difference, 1.9 percentage points; 95% confidence interval [CI], 0.8-3.0) at 6 months, and 16.4% versus 18.2% (difference, −1.8 percentage points; 95% CI, −4.7-1.0) at 5 years.[32] Results were similar with respect to the key secondary outcome of death from cardiovascular causes or MI. However, patients randomly assigned to the invasive strategy had greater improvement in angina-related health status than those assigned to the conservative strategy (4.1 points, 4.2 points, and 2.9 points higher increases in the Seattle Angina Questionnaire [SAQ] summary scores at 3, 12, and 36 months with the invasive strategy than with the conservative strategy).[33] Differences were larger among participants who had more frequent angina at the baseline (8.5 vs 0.1 points at 3 months and 5.3 vs 1.2 points at 36 months among participants with daily or weekly angina as compared with no angina).[33] Similarly, in the ISCHEMIA Comprehensive QOL Substudy of 1819 participants (901 invasive strategy, 912 conservative strategy), patients with more frequent baseline angina had greater improvements in the symptom, physical functioning, and psychological well-being dimensions of QOL when treated with an invasive strategy, whereas patients who had rare/absent angina at the baseline reported no consistent treatment-related QOL differences.[5]

In the ISCHEMIA-CKD trial, 777 patients with advanced kidney disease (defined as an estimated glomerular filtration rate [eGFR] of <30 mL/min/1.73 m^2 of body-surface area or the receipt of dialysis) and moderate or severe myocardial ischemia were randomized to an initial invasive strategy of medical therapy, angiography, and revascularization when feasible or to an initial conservative strategy of medical therapy alone, with angiography reserved for failure of medical therapy.[34] The primary outcome was a composite of death or nonfatal MI. A key secondary outcome was a composite of death, nonfatal MI, or hospitalization for unstable angina, HF, or resuscitated cardiac arrest. At a median follow-up of 2.2 years, there were no significant differences in the rates of the primary outcome in the invasive-strategy group versus the conservative-strategy group (estimated 3-year event rate, 36.4% vs 36.7%; adjusted hazard ratio, 1.01; 95% confidence interval [CI], 0.79-1.29; P = .95).[34] Results for the key secondary outcome were similar (38.5% vs 39.7%; hazard ratio, 1.01; 95% CI, 0.79-1.29). Importantly, the invasive strategy was associated with a higher incidence of stroke and death or initiation of dialysis than the conservative strategy.

A pooled analysis of the ISCHEMIA and ISCHEMIA-CKD trials demonstrated no significant difference in death or death or MI with an initial invasive strategy versus an initial conservative strategy in patients with or without diabetes.[35] In contrast, another analysis of ISCHEMIA comparing outcomes by treatment strategy in participants with versus without history of HF or LV systolic dysfunction found that in the high-risk subgroup of patients with HF and LVEF 35% to 45%, an initial invasive strategy was associated with lower rates of the trial primary outcome, all-cause mortality, and cardiovascular mortality.[36]

Although ISCHEMIA selected participants primarily on the basis of the presence of moderate or severe ischemia on stress testing, ~15% had less than moderate ischemia according to core laboratory review.[37] In a post-hoc analysis of the ISCHEMIA trial, ischemia severity was not associated with increased risk of adverse outcomes, whereas more severe CAD was associated with increased risk of death and nonfatal MI, consistent with findings from a similar analysis of the COURAGE trial.[27,37] Ischemia severity did not identify a subgroup with treatment benefit on mortality, MI, the trial primary end point, or cardiovascular death or MI.[37] In the most severe CAD subgroup (n = 659), the 4-year rate of cardiovascular death or MI was lower in the invasive strategy group (difference, 6.3% [95% CI, 0.2%-12.4%]), but 4-year all-cause mortality was similar.[37]

Recently, Hochman et al[38] reported the interim 7-year all-cause, cardiovascular, and non-cardiovascular mortality rates for the ongoing ISCHEMIA-EXTEND (ISCHEMIA Extended Follow-up) study. During a median follow-up of 5.7 years, there was no difference in all-cause mortality with an initial invasive strategy compared with an initial conservative strategy (7-year rate, 12.7% vs 13.4%; adjusted hazard ratio, 1; 95% CI, 0.85-1.18), but there was lower risk of cardiovascular mortality (7-year rate, 6.4% vs 8.6%; adjusted hazard ratio, 0.78; 95% CI, 0.63-0.96) and higher risk of non-cardiovascular mortality (7-year rate, 5.6% vs 4.4%; adjusted hazard ratio, 1.44; 95% CI, 1.08-1.91) with an initial invasive strategy.[38]

Placebo Effect in Angina Relief After PCI

The ORBITA (Objective Randomied Blinded Investigation with optimal medical Therapy of Angioplasty in stable angina) trial was designed to assess the effect of PCI versus a placebo procedure for angina relief in patients with severe (≥70% stenosis) single-vessel CAD.[39] After enrollment, patients underwent 6 weeks of medical optimization, which focused on the initiation and up-titration of guideline directed antianginal therapy (97.5% reached the prespecified target of ≥2 antianginals). Patients then had prerandomization assessments with cardiopulmonary exercise testing, symptom questionnaires, and dobutamine stress echocardiography (DSE). All patients were pretreated with dual antiplatelet therapy. In both groups, the duration of dual antiplatelet therapy was the same and continued until the final (unblinding) visit. Coronary angiography was done via a radial or femoral arterial approach with auditory isolation achieved by placing over-the-ear headphones playing music on the patient throughout the procedure. In all patients, a research invasive physiological assessment of FFR and instantaneous wave-free ratio (iFR) was done. The clinical operator was blinded to the physiology values and therefore did not use them to guide treatment. After physiological assessment, sedation was established, auditory isolation was continued, and the patients were randomized 1:1 to undergo PCI (n = 105) or a placebo procedure (n = 95). For patients allocated to PCI, DESs were used for treating all lesions that were deemed to be angiographically significant, with a mandate to achieve angiographic complete revascularization. In the placebo group, patients were kept sedated for at least 15 minutes on the catheterization laboratory table, and the coronary catheters were withdrawn with no intervention performed. No information about the nature of the procedure (whether PCI or placebo) was transferred from the catheterization laboratory staff to the recovery staff. The study physicians present during the procedure had no further contact with the patient during the study. After 6 weeks of follow-up, the assessments done before randomization were repeated. The ORBITA trial found no significant difference in the primary endpoint of exercise time increment between groups (PCI minus placebo 16.6 s, 95% CI −8.9-42.0, P = .200).[39] However, subsequent physiology-stratified and stress echocardiography score-stratified analyses of the ORBITA trial showed that PCI improved stress echocardiography score more than the placebo (1.07 segment units; 95% CI, 0.70-1.44; P < .00001), and the placebo-controlled effect of PCI on stress echocardiography score increased progressively with decreasing FFR ($p_{interaction}$ < .00001) and decreasing iFR ($p_{interaction}$ < .00001).[40] Furthermore, there was a significant interaction between prerandomization stress echocardiography score and the effect of PCI on angina frequency score with a larger placebo-controlled effect in patients with the highest stress echocardiography score ($p_{interaction}$ = .031).[41] Limitations of the ORBITA trial include the small sample size (n = 230), limited generalizability due to inclusion of patients with single-vessel CAD and normal LVEF, and the choice of primary end point. Some of these limitations will be addressed by ORBITA-2, a double-blind, randomized, placebo-controlled trial that will compare the effect of PCI versus placebo procedure on angina frequency in patients with single- or multivessel disease, at 12 weeks, without background antianginal therapy.[42]

Meta-Analysis of RCTs

Several meta-analyses performed have consolidated the disparate trial designs and patient populations to determine the effect of PCI + OMT versus OMT alone in patients with stable CAD. In a meta-analysis of 14 RCTs that enrolled 14,877 patients with a weighted mean follow-up of 4.5 years, revascularization compared with medical therapy alone was not associated with improved survival but was associated with a lower risk of non-procedural MI and unstable angina with greater freedom from angina at the expense of higher rates of procedural MI.[6] Two other meta-analyses focused on "hard" clinical end points demonstrated that revascularization compared with medical therapy alone was associated with lower rates of cardiac mortality and spontaneous MI with no difference in all-cause mortality and stroke.[8,9] By meta-regression, Navarese et al.[8] showed that the cardiac mortality risk reduction after revascularization, compared with medical therapy alone, was linearly associated with follow-up duration, spontaneous MI absolute difference, and percentage of multivessel disease at the baseline.

CONCLUSION

CAD remains the leading cause of death in the United States and worldwide. Lifestyle modifications and OMT (aspirin, statins, ACEi/ARB, and antianginals [β blockers, CCBs, nitrates, ranolazine]) comprise the cornerstone of management of patients with CCD. Numerous RCTs and meta-analyses have shown that in patients with stable CAD and anginal symptoms with or without objective evidence of ischemia, PCI compared with OMT alone does not confer an overall survival benefit. However, in patients with multivessel CAD appropriate for either PCI or CABG, revascularization in addition to OMT is reasonable to lower the risk of cardiovascular events such as cardiac death, spontaneous MI, and unplanned urgent revascularization. In patients with lifestyle-limiting angina despite OMT, revascularization is indicated to improve symptoms and QOL; however, the perceived benefit of PCI in improving symptoms and QOL needs to be further investigated in large sham-controlled randomized trials.

Key Points

- The key objectives in the management of chronic coronary disease are relief of angina and reduction of major adverse cardiovascular events (MACE).
- Lifestyle modification and guideline-directed medical therapy comprise the cornerstones of management.
- In select individuals, particularly patients with multivessel coronary artery disease, revascularization may reduce the risk of cardiac death, myocardial infarction, and urgent revascularization, but the effect on long-term survival remains a topic of debate.

Disclosures

Dhaval Kolte, MD, PhD, FACC, FSCAI: Research grant from the National Heart, Lung, and Blood Institute outside the submitted work.

Douglas E. Drachman, MD, FACC, FSCAI: Boston Scientific (consulting), Broadview Ventures (consulting), Cardiovascular Systems Inc. (consulting), Cordis (consulting).

References

1. Knuuti J, Wijns W, Saraste A, et al. 2019 ESC guidelines for the diagnosis and management of chronic coronary syndromes. *Eur Heart J*. 2020;41(3):407-477.
2. Virani SS, Newby LK, Arnold SV, et al. 2023 AHA/ACC/ACCP/ASPC/NLA/PCNA guideline for the management of patients with chronic coronary disease: a report of the American Heart Association/American College of Cardiology Joint Committee on clinical practice guidelines. *J Am Coll Cardiol*. 2023;82(9):833-955.
3. Tsao CW, Aday AW, Almarzooq ZI, et al. Heart disease and stroke statistics-2023 update: a report from the American Heart Association. *Circulation*. 2023;147(8):e93-e621.
4. Writing Committee Members; Lawton JS, Tamis-Holland JE, et al. 2021 ACC/AHA/SCAI guideline for coronary artery revascularization: a report of the American College of Cardiology/American Heart Association Joint Committee on clinical practice guidelines. *J Am Coll Cardiol*. 2022;79:e21-e129.
5. Mark DB, Spertus JA, Bigelow R, et al. Comprehensive quality-of-life outcomes with invasive versus conservative management of chronic coronary disease in ISCHEMIA. *Circulation*. 2022;145(17):1294-1307.
6. Bangalore S, Maron DJ, Stone GW, Hochman JS. Routine revascularization versus initial medical therapy for stable ischemic heart disease: a systematic review and meta-analysis of randomized trials. *Circulation*. 2020;142(9):841-857.
7. De Bruyne B, Pijls NH, Kalesan B, et al. Fractional flow reserve-guided PCI versus medical therapy in stable coronary disease. *N Engl J Med*. 2012;367(11):991-1001.
8. Navarese EP, Lansky AJ, Kereiakes DJ, et al. Cardiac mortality in patients randomised to elective coronary revascularisation plus medical therapy or medical therapy alone: a systematic review and meta-analysis. *Eur Heart J*. 2021;42(45):4638-4651.
9. Vij A, Kassab K, Chawla H, et al. Invasive therapy versus conservative therapy for patients with stable coronary artery disease: an updated meta-analysis. *Clin Cardiol*. 2021;44(5):675-682.
10. Velazquez EJ, Lee KL, Deja MA, et al. Coronary-artery bypass surgery in patients with left ventricular dysfunction. *N Engl J Med*. 2011;364(17):1607-1616.
11. Velazquez EJ, Lee KL, Jones RH, et al. Coronary-artery bypass surgery in patients with ischemic cardiomyopathy. *N Engl J Med*. 2016;374(16):1511-1520.
12. Chaitman BR, Fisher LD, Bourassa MG, et al. Effect of coronary bypass surgery on survival patterns in subsets of patients with left main coronary artery disease. Report of the Collaborative Study in Coronary Artery Surgery (CASS). *Am J Cardiol*. 1981;48(4):765-777.
13. Gruntzig A. Transluminal dilatation of coronary-artery stenosis. *Lancet*. 1978;1(8058):263.
14. Parisi AF, Folland ED, Hartigan P. A comparison of angioplasty with medical therapy in the treatment of single-vessel coronary artery disease. Veterans Affairs ACME Investigators. *N Engl J Med*. 1992;326(1):10-16.
15. Folland ED, Hartigan PM, Parisi AF. Percutaneous transluminal coronary angioplasty versus medical therapy for stable angina pectoris: outcomes for patients with double-vessel versus single-vessel coronary artery disease in a Veterans Affairs Cooperative randomized trial. Veterans Affairs ACME InvestigatorS. *J Am Coll Cardiol*. 1997;29(7):1505-1511.
16. Hueb WA, Bellotti G, de Oliveira SA, et al. The Medicine, Angioplasty or Surgery Study (MASS): a prospective, randomized trial of medical therapy, balloon angioplasty or bypass surgery for single proximal left anterior descending artery stenoses. *J Am Coll Cardiol*. 1995;26(7):1600-1605.

17. Coronary angioplasty versus medical therapy for angina: the second Randomised Intervention Treatment of Angina (RITA-2) trial. RITA-2 trial participants. *Lancet*. 1997;350:461-468.
18. Pitt B, Waters D, Brown WV, et al. Aggressive lipid-lowering therapy compared with angioplasty in stable coronary artery disease. Atorvastatin versus Revascularization Treatment Investigators. *N Engl J Med*. 1999;341(2):70-76.
19. Hueb W, Soares PR, Gersh BJ, et al. The medicine, angioplasty, or surgery study (MASS-II): a randomized, controlled clinical trial of three therapeutic strategies for multivessel coronary artery disease—one-year results. *J Am Coll Cardiol*. 2004;43(10):1743-1751.
20. Boden WE, O'Rourke RA, Teo KK, et al. Optimal medical therapy with or without PCI for stable coronary disease. *N Engl J Med*. 2007;356(15):1503-1516.
21. Sedlis SP, Hartigan PM, Teo KK, et al. Effect of PCI on long-term survival in patients with stable ischemic heart disease. *N Engl J Med*. 2015;373(20):1937-1946.
22. BARI 2D Study Group; Frye RL, August P, et al. A randomized trial of therapies for type 2 diabetes and coronary artery disease. *N Engl J Med*. 2009;360:2503-2515.
23. Erne P, Schoenenberger AW, Burckhardt D, et al. Effects of percutaneous coronary interventions in silent ischemia after myocardial infarction: the SWISSI II randomized controlled trial. *JAMA*. 2007;297(18):1985-1991.
24. Shaw LJ, Berman DS, Maron DJ, et al. Optimal medical therapy with or without percutaneous coronary intervention to reduce ischemic burden: results from the Clinical Outcomes Utilizing Revascularization and Aggressive Drug Evaluation (COURAGE) trial nuclear substudy. *Circulation*. 2008;117(10):1283-1291.
25. Hachamovitch R, Hayes SW, Friedman JD, Cohen I, Berman DS. Comparison of the short-term survival benefit associated with revascularization compared with medical therapy in patients with no prior coronary artery disease undergoing stress myocardial perfusion single photon emission computed tomography. *Circulation*. 2003;107(23):2900-2907.
26. Shaw LJ, Weintraub WS, Maron DJ, et al. Baseline stress myocardial perfusion imaging results and outcomes in patients with stable ischemic heart disease randomized to optimal medical therapy with or without percutaneous coronary intervention. *Am Heart J*. 2012;164(2):243-250.
27. Mancini GBJ, Hartigan PM, Shaw LJ, et al. Predicting outcome in the COURAGE trial (clinical outcomes utilizing revascularization and aggressive drug evaluation): coronary anatomy versus ischemia. *JACC Cardiovasc Interv*. 2014;7(2):195-201.
28. Pijls NH, Sels JW. Functional measurement of coronary stenosis. *J Am Coll Cardiol*. 2012;59(12):1045-1057.
29. Pijls NH, van Schaardenburgh P, Manoharan G, et al. Percutaneous coronary intervention of functionally nonsignificant stenosis: 5-year follow-up of the DEFER study. *J Am Coll Cardiol*. 2007;49(21):2105-2111.
30. Tonino PA, De Bruyne B, Pijls NH, et al. Fractional flow reserve versus angiography for guiding percutaneous coronary intervention. *N Engl J Med*. 2009;360(3):213-224.
31. ISCHEMIA Trial Research Group; Maron DJ, Hochman JS, et al. International study of comparative health effectiveness with medical and invasive approaches (ISCHEMIA) trial: rationale and design. *Am Heart J*. 2018;201:124-135.
32. Maron DJ, Hochman JS. Invasive or conservative strategy for stable coronary disease. Reply. *N Engl J Med*. 2020;383(10):e66.
33. Spertus JA, Jones PG, Maron DJ, et al. Health-status outcomes with invasive or conservative care in coronary disease. *N Engl J Med*. 2020;382(15):1408-1419.
34. Bangalore S, Maron DJ, O'Brien SM, et al. Management of coronary disease in patients with advanced kidney disease. *N Engl J Med*. 2020;382(17):1608-1618.
35. Newman JD, Anthopolos R, Mancini GBJ, et al. Outcomes of participants with diabetes in the ISCHEMIA trials. *Circulation*. 2021;144(17):1380-1395.
36. Lopes RD, Alexander KP, Stevens SR, et al. Initial invasive versus conservative management of stable ischemic heart disease in patients with a history of heart failure or left ventricular dysfunction: insights from the ISCHEMIA trial. *Circulation*. 2020;142(18):1725-1735.
37. Reynolds HR, Shaw LJ, Min JK, et al. Outcomes in the ISCHEMIA trial based on coronary artery disease and ischemia severity. *Circulation*. 2021;144(13):1024-1038.
38. Hochman JS, Anthopolos R, Reynolds HR, et al. Survival after invasive or conservative management of stable coronary disease. *Circulation*. 2023;147(1):8-19.
39. Al-Lamee R, Thompson D, Dehbi HM, et al. Percutaneous coronary intervention in stable angina (ORBITA): a double-blind, randomised controlled trial. *Lancet*. 2018;391(10115):31-40.
40. Al-Lamee R, Howard JP, Shun-Shin MJ, et al. Fractional flow reserve and instantaneous wave-free ratio as predictors of the placebo-controlled response to percutaneous coronary intervention in stable single-vessel coronary artery disease. *Circulation*. 2018;138(17):1780-1792.
41. Al-Lamee RK, Shun-Shin MJ, Howard JP, et al. Dobutamine stress echocardiography ischemia as a predictor of the placebo-controlled efficacy of percutaneous coronary intervention in stable coronary artery disease: the stress echocardiography-stratified analysis of ORBITA. *Circulation*. 2019;140(24):1971-1980.
42. Nowbar AN, Rajkumar C, Foley M, et al. A double-blind randomised placebo-controlled trial of percutaneous coronary intervention for the relief of stable angina without antianginal medications: design and rationale of the ORBITA-2 trial. *EuroIntervention*. 2022;17(18):1490-1497.

Acute Coronary Syndromes

Arnold H. Seto and Kaushik Darbha

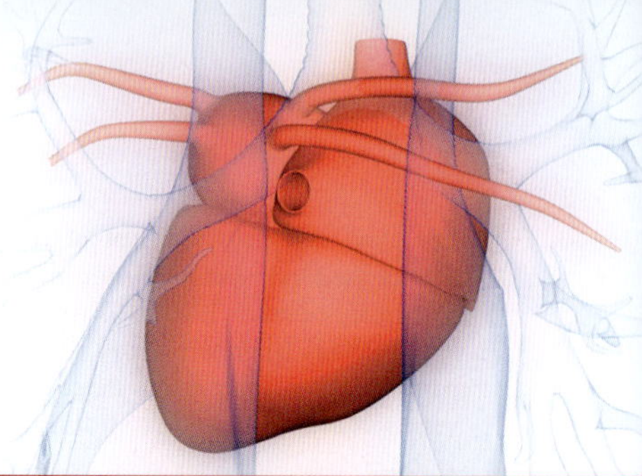

Acute coronary syndromes (ACS) include unstable angina (UA), non-ST segment elevation myocardial infarction (NSTEMI), and ST-segment elevation myocardial infarction (STEMI) (**Fig. 18.1**). Patients presenting with chest pain without persistent ST-elevation are typically admitted to the hospital with the diagnosis of non–ST-elevation ACS (NSTE-ACS), and are later classified into UA or NSTEMI on the basis of cardiac biomarkers.

Patients with ACS constitute the vast majority of patients (>80%) who require percutaneous coronary intervention (PCI). With the publication of the COURAGE trial and increasing scrutiny from payers, the use of PCI for stable angina is increasingly reserved for medically refractory symptoms.[1]

EPIDEMIOLOGY

The estimated annual incidence of myocardial infarction (MI) is ~805,000 according to the 2005 to 2014 ARIC study. Compared to men, women were less likely to undergo coronary angiography or percutaneous coronary intervention and were at higher risk of mortality from MI, with overall MI prevalence being 4.5% in males and 2.1% for females. Females experienced longer door-to-balloon time along with lower rates of guideline-directed medical therapy compared to males.[2] Extremely young patients (<35 years of age) were found more likely to be white, obese, a smoker, or with a family history of CAD, and were more likely to have a late presentation of STEMI and cardiogenic shock compared to older individuals.[2]

The acute in-hospital mortality of STEMI (7%) is higher than that for NSTE-ACS (3%-5%), but equalizes by 6 months. Longer-term follow-up demonstrates that NSTE-ACS has a higher mortality than STEMI. This is explained by different patient profiles: NSTE-ACS patients, on average, tend to be older and have more comorbidities, such as diabetes and renal failure, whereas STEMI patients tend to be younger smokers. Rates of STE-ACS are declining in North America due to reduced rates of smoking along with improved medical therapy.

PATHOLOGY

ACSs result from coronary artery obstruction causing myocardial ischemia and subsequent myocardial necrosis. Acute coronary artery obstruction typically results from thrombosis of a ruptured coronary plaque, with or without concomitant vasoconstriction. In contrast to the previous conception that coronary artery disease (CAD) is a slowly progressive disease, the current understanding is that of a stuttering inflammatory process of repeated plaque rupture and healing on top of a lipid core.

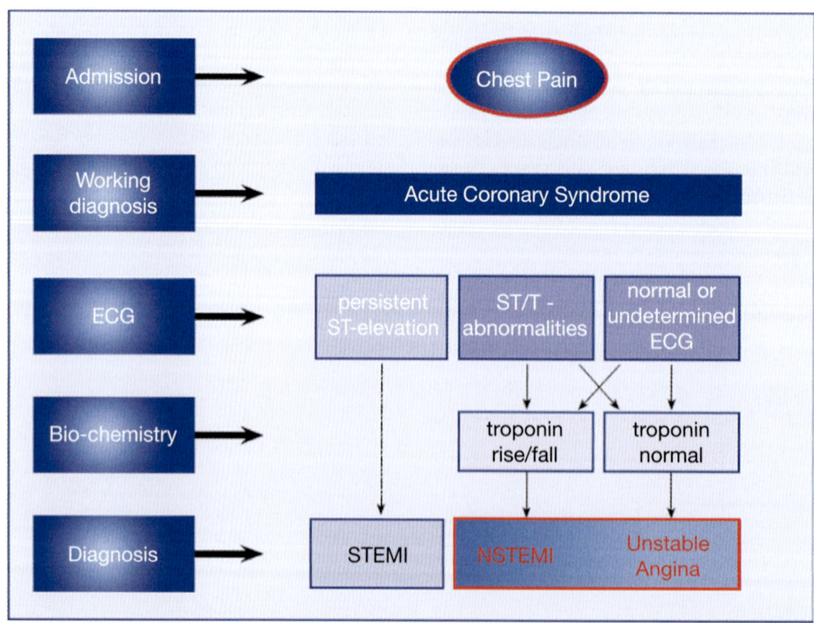

FIGURE 18.1 Spectrum of ACS. ACS, acute coronary syndrome. (From: Hamm CW, Bassand JP, Agewall S, et al. ESC guidelines for the management of acute coronary syndromes in patients presenting without persistent ST-segment elevation: the task force for the management of acute coronary syndromes (ACS) in patients presenting without persistent ST-segment elevation of the European Society of Cardiology (ESC). *Eur Heart J*. 2011;32:2999-3054.)

Abrupt thrombotic occlusion can thus occur with plaques that are not obstructive at baseline, although plaques that are already obstructive are more likely to be metabolically active and lead to clinical syndromes.

Coronary thrombosis involves endothelial dysfunction and disruption, platelet activation, and circulating coagulation proteins. The platelet is a central actor and regulates the process of thrombosis. When endothelial cells are injured, thrombosis begins with rapid adhesion of platelets to the site of injury. Within seconds, the platelets are activated, degranulated, and recruit additional platelets to the developing thrombus. The secretory granules release adenosine diphosphate (ADP), which stimulates further platelet activation, and thrombin, which initiates the coagulation system. Thromboxane is generated from the platelet phospholipase A2, and has an additional effect on platelet activation. Ultimately, glycoprotein IIb/IIIa receptors on the platelet are activated. Glycoprotein IIb/IIIa receptors bind to fibrinogen, cross-linking platelets together. Repetitive platelet activation and fibrinogen cross-linking brings about platelet aggregation, which can then lead to occlusive thrombus formation. Although there are multiple pathways to platelet activation, the platelet GP IIb/IIIa receptor is the final common pathway in platelet aggregation that would lead to NSTEMI.

When plaque rupture results in complete (100%) thrombotic occlusion and is sustained, the MI that results is typically transmural and associated with ST-segment elevation. Without reperfusion, a transmural infarction classically results in a Q-wave on ECG. With subtotal (99% or less) or temporary occlusion, the presentation may be either UA or NSTEMI, depending on the degree and duration of ischemia. When ischemia is sufficient to cause myonecrosis detectable by serum biomarkers, NSTEMI is diagnosed. With the use of high-sensitivity troponin (hsTn) assays, patients who would have formerly been categorized as UA (based on negative creatine kinase) are increasingly diagnosed as NSTEMI.

Other less common causes of ACS include spontaneous coronary dissection, spasm (Prinzmetal angina, cocaine), inflammatory arteritis, trauma, and thromboembolism. These rare causes should be considered in patients lacking CAD risk factors. For instance, a younger peripartum woman with chest pain and ECG changes may be more likely to have spasm or coronary dissection than atherosclerotic disease.

Intracoronary imaging studies have demonstrated that separately from plaque rupture, plaque erosion and calcific nodules can cause ACS (both STE and NSTE). The presence of clinically diagnosed MI with no obstructed coronary arteries seen on angiography (MINOCA), and spontaneous coronary artery dissection (SCAD) have been of particular interest, but are discussed elsewhere.[3]

CLINICAL PRESENTATION

The clinical presentation of ACS classically includes substernal chest discomfort associated with diaphoresis and dyspnea. This sensation may variably be described as pressure or sharp pain depending on the patient. The chest discomfort may radiate to the left arm, but also to the shoulder, neck, or jaw. Relief of chest pain with nitroglycerin, and exacerbation of the chest pain with manual pressure, may point toward a **cardiac** cause for chest pain, but these signs are insufficiently reliable for clinical diagnosis.

Atypical presentations occur frequently, particularly among diabetics and women. Dyspnea, epigastric pain, nausea, syncope, or unexplained tachycardia may be the only symptoms to suggest a cardiac pathology.

Physical examination of the ACS patients is often unremarkable. Signs of left ventricular dysfunction (rales, third heart sound, hypotension, jugular venous distention) or cardiogenic shock (cold clammy extremities, tachycardia) may be present in patients with extensive MI or prior injury.

INITIAL DIAGNOSIS

Patients with chest pain require prompt triage and risk assessment in an emergency room. An electrocardiography (ECG) should be immediately performed on presentation. Serial ECGs are recommended for patients with nondiagnostic ECGs or those who continue to be symptomatic. Comparison with prior ECGs can be extremely valuable, particularly in patients with baseline abnormalities such as hypertrophy or early repolarization. ECGs should be reviewed for ST-segment elevation (>1 mm in two contiguous leads) or new left bundle branch block, which may indicate acute STEMI. Isolated ST-segment depression in right precordial leads (V1-V3) with tall R-waves may indicate a true posterior infarction, which should also be treated as a STEMI. NSTE-ACS may present as ST-segment depression, T-wave inversions, or be electrically silent. Dynamic ST-segment or T-wave changes increase the specificity of the ECG for ACS.

The history, physical, and ECG are sufficient to diagnose ACS in less than half of cases. Cardiac biomarkers should thus be drawn on all patients with suspected ACS. Biomarkers may not be elevated in the first 4 hours after the onset of symptoms, thus serial biomarkers should be drawn at 6- or 8-hour intervals. The preferred cardiac biomarker is the troponin assay (cTnI or cTnT), which has a very high (>95%) sensitivity for myocardial injury. Ultrahigh–sensitivity (>99%) troponin assays are increasingly becoming available and may reduce the time to diagnosis of ACS.[4] Abnormal troponin levels connote an increased risk for major adverse cardiac events and death, with higher concentrations indicating progressively elevated risk.[5] The specificity of the cardiac troponin for ACS is reported to be very high (>95%) when used in patients with chest pain. Nevertheless, when used in a broader patient population than that of clinical trials, the test is frequently abnormal for reasons besides ACS, and there may still be a role for less-sensitive (but more specific) markers such as creatine kinase-MB (CK-MB). For instance, following PCI, troponin assays are overly sensitive to clinically silent periprocedural necrosis, and do not carry the same prognostic value as elevations in CK-MB.[6]

B-type natriuretic peptide (BNP) is increasingly used as a cardiac biomarker. Elevated levels may reflect either acquired or preexisting left ventricular dysfunction and are associated with an increased risk of complications.[5]

IS IT ACS?

Although not typically the subject of board examination questions, the diagnosis of ACS is commonly misapplied clinically. With the use of hsTn assays as the preferred cardiac marker, one of the most common consultations received by the interventional cardiologist is for the positive troponin, which in the absence of chest pain or ECG changes is often due to demand ischemia, heart failure, or renal failure rather than ACS.[7] The **fourth** universal definition of MI (**Table 18.1**) includes patients with positive biomarkers with either ischemic symptoms, ECG changes of ischemia or infarction,

TABLE 18.1 Classification of Different Types of Myocardial Infarction

Type 1: Spontaneous Myocardial Infarction (MI)
Spontaneous MI related to atherosclerotic plaque rupture, ulceration, assuring, erosion, or dissection with resulting intraluminal thrombus in one or more of the coronary arteries leading to decreased myocardial blood flow or distal platelet emboli with ensuing myocyte necrosis. The patient may have underlying severe CAD but on occasion nonobstructive or no CAD. hsTn values with at least 1 value above the 99th percentile URL and with at least 1 of the following: • Symptoms of acute myocardial ischemia; • New ischemic ECG changes; • Development of pathological Q waves; • Imaging evidence of new loss of viable myocardium or new regional wall motion abnormality in a pattern consistent with an ischemic etiology; • Identification of a coronary thrombus by angiography including intracoronary imaging or by autopsy.
Type 2: MI Secondary to an Ischemic Imbalance
In instances of myocardial injury with necrosis where a condition other than CAD contributes to an imbalance between myocardial oxygen supply and/or demand—e.g., coronary endothelial dysfunction, coronary artery spasm, coronary embolism, tachy-/brady-arrhythmias, anemia, respiratory failure, hypotension, and hypertension with or without LVH. hsTn values with at least one value above the 99th percentile URL, and **evidence of an imbalance between myocardial oxygen supply and demand unrelated to acute coronary atherothrombosis,** requiring at least one of the following: • Symptoms of acute myocardial ischemia; • New ischemic ECG changes; • Development of pathological Q waves; • Imaging evidence of new loss of viable myocardium or new regional wall motion abnormality in a pattern consistent with an ischemic etiology
Type 3: MI Resulting in Death when Biomarker Values are Unavailable
Patients who suffer cardiac death, with symptoms suggestive of myocardial ischemia accompanied by presumed new ischemic ECG changes or ventricular fibrillation, but die before blood samples for biomarkers can be obtained, or before increases in cardiac biomarkers can be identified, or MI is detected by autopsy examination.
Type 4a: MI Related to Percutaneous Coronary Intervention (PCI)
MI associated with PCI is arbitrarily defined by elevation of cTn values >5 × 99th percentile URL in patients with normal baseline values (<99th percentile URL) or a rise of cTn values >20% if the baseline values are elevated and are stable or falling. In addition, either (i) symptoms suggestive of myocardial ischemia, or (ii) new ischemic ECG changes or new LBBB, or (iii) angiographic loss of patency of a major coronary artery or a side branch or persistent slow- or no-flow or embolization, or (iv) imaging demonstration of new loss of viable myocardium or new regional wall motion abnormality are required.
Type 4b: MI Related to Stent Thrombosis
MI associated with stent thrombosis is detected by coronary angiography or autopsy in the setting of myocardial ischemia and with a rise and/or fall of cardiac biomarkers values with at least one value above the 99th percentile URL.
Type 4c: MI Related to Stent restenosis
MI occurring after PCI caused by focal or diffuse in-stent restenosis, or restenosis following balloon angioplasty in the infarct territory. This is often the only explanation when no other culprit lesion or thrombus can be identified, with a rise and/or fall of cTn values above the 99th percentile URL applying, the same criteria utilized for type 1 MI.
Type 5: MI Related to Coronary Artery Bypass Grafting (CABG)
MI associated with CABG is arbitrarily defined by elevation cardiac biomarker values >10 × 99th percentile URL in patients with normal baseline cTn values (<99th percentile URL). In addition, either (i) new pathological Q waves or new LBBB, or (ii) angiographic documented new graft or new native coronary artery occlusion, or (iii) imaging evidence of new loss of viable myocardium or new regional wall motion abnormality.

CAD, coronary artery disease; ECG, electrocardiography; LBBB, left bundle branch block; LVH, left ventricular hypertrophy; URL, upper reference limit.
Adapted from: Thygesen K, Alpert JS, Jaffe AS, et al. Fourth universal definition of myocardial infarction. *Circulation.* 2018;138(20):e618-e651.

echocardiographic evidence of infarction or angiographic evidence of coronary thrombus. This definition includes infarctions due to ACS, supply/demand imbalance, sudden cardiac death, PCI complications, or post-CABG.[3] The terminology is thus muddled, in that a patient may have an MI without having an ACS, particularly when nondiagnostic symptoms (esp. dyspnea, hypotension) and ECG (T-wave inversions) are present. Changes in the concentration of troponin may be helpful in differentiating acute from chronic causes of myocardial damage, with a rise of 20% typically being used as a criterion for an acute injury, especially in patients with renal failure, heart failure, or left ventricular hypertrophy.[8]

Antithrombotic therapies and PCI are beneficial only for patients with primary acute thrombotic coronary events. An incorrect diagnosis will be, at best, a distraction from the underlying illness, and at worst will be a therapeutic misadventure that will result in hemorrhagic or vascular complications. Caution is advisable when symptoms or ECG evidence of ACS are absent, or when clear alternative causes of troponin elevation are present.

TABLE 18.2 Recommended Anti-ischemic Therapies

Class Ia
1. Bed rest with continuous ECG monitoring
2. Supplemental oxygen in patients with respiratory distress or hypoxemia
3. Nitroglycerin for ischemic symptoms, heart failure, or hypertension
4. Oral β-blockers for patients without shock, heart failure, or heart block
5. ACE-inhibitors or angiotensin receptor blockers within 24 h in patients with left ventricular dysfunction
Class IIa
1. Morphine for chest discomfort refractory to nitroglycerin
2. Intravenous β-blockers for patients without contraindications

ACE, angiotensin converting enzyme; ECG, electrocardiography.

INITIAL MEDICAL MANAGEMENT

ACC/AHA Guidelines for the management of UA/NSTEMI were updated in complete form in 2014.[9] A thorough review of these guidelines is suggested for board preparation.

Anti-ischemic Therapies

Anti-ischemic therapies reduce myocardial oxygen demand or increase myocardial oxygen supply. Recommended anti-ischemic therapies are listed in **Table 18.2**. Nonpharmacologic therapies include bed rest and supplemental oxygen. Nitroglycerin can cause coronary vasodilatation and increase myocardial blood flow. β-blockers and calcium-channel blockers reduce myocardial demand by reducing heart rate, contractility, and afterload.

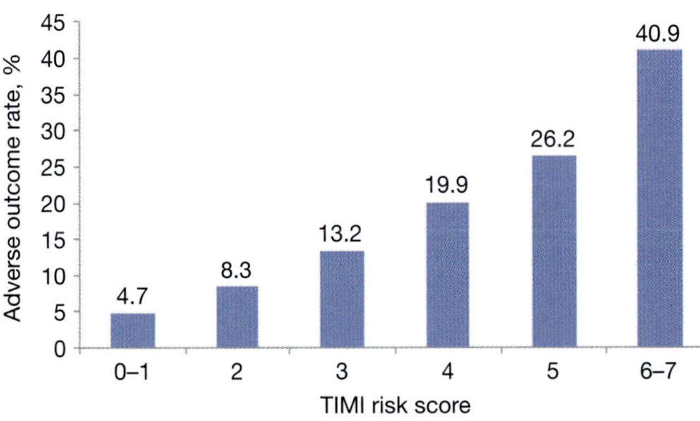

FIGURE 18.2 TIMI risk score in UA/NSTEMI. Adverse outcome: all-cause mortality, new or recurrent MI, or severe recurrent ischemia requiring urgent revascularization through 14 days after randomization (%). TIMI, thrombolysis in myocardial infarction. (Reprinted from: Anderson JL, Adams CD, Antman EM, et al. ACC/AHA 2007 guidelines for the management of patients with unstable angina/non-ST-elevation myocardial infarction: a report of the American College of Cardiology/American Heart Association Task Force on Practice Guidelines (Writing Committee to revise the 2002 guidelines for the management of patients with unstable angina/non-ST-elevation myocardial infarction) developed in collaboration with the American College of Emergency Physicians, the Society for Cardiovascular Angiography and Interventions, and the Society of Thoracic Surgeons endorsed by the American Association of Cardiovascular and Pulmonary Rehabilitation and the Society for Academic Emergency Medicine. *J Am Coll Cardiol*. 2007;50(7):e1-e157, with permission.)

β-blockers should not be administered for patients with shock, heart failure, or heart block. Morphine is reserved for angina refractory to nitroglycerin, but by relieving pain and anxiety, this also reduces myocardial oxygen demand.

Risk Stratification

Early risk stratification for ischemic complications is critical to form a management strategy for the heterogeneous NSTE-ACS population. A focused history and physical, a prompt EKG, and cardiac biomarkers (as described previously) helps distinguish UA and NSTEMI from noncardiac chest pain. Patients with a normal EKG and cardiac biomarkers can be safely sent for noninvasive stress testing for further risk assessment.

For those with UA/NSTEMI, risk-stratification models such as the thrombolysis in myocardial infarction (TIMI) or Global Registry of Acute Coronary Events (GRACE) risk score should be used for further identifying those patients at high risk for cardiovascular death, recurrent MI, or urgent revascularization (**Fig. 18.2**; **Table 18.3**). The TIMI risk score is simpler to remember, but has a less discriminating power. Patients at low risk for cardiac events (TIMI score <3, GRACE score <108) are candidates for a

TABLE 18.3 TIMI and GRACE Risk Score Components

TIMI RISK SCORE	
RISK SCORE COMPONENTS	
Age >65	Two anginal events in prior 24 h
>3 CAD risk factors	Use of aspirin in prior 7 d
Prior coronary stenosis of >50% ST-segment deviation on presentation	Elevated serum biomarkers
Risk Score	**Risk of Death, MI, or Urgent Revascularization**
0-1	4.7%
2	8.3%
3	13.2%
4	19.9%
5	26.2%
6-7	40.9%
Variable	**Odds Ratio**
Older age	1.7/10 y
Killip class	2.0/class
Systolic BP	1.4/20 mm Hg ↑
ST-segment deviation	2.4
Cardiac arrest during presentation	4.3
Serum creatinine level	1.2/1-mg/dL ↑
Positive initial cardiac biomarkers	1.6
Heart rate	1.3/30-beat/min ↑

BP, blood pressure; CAD, coronary artery disease; MI, myocardial infarction; TIMI, thrombolysis in myocardial ischemia.

Adapted from: Eagle KA, Lim MJ, Dabbous OH, et al. A validated prediction model for all forms of acute coronary syndrome: estimating the risk of 6-month postdischarge death in an international registry. *JAMA*. 2004;291:2727-2733.

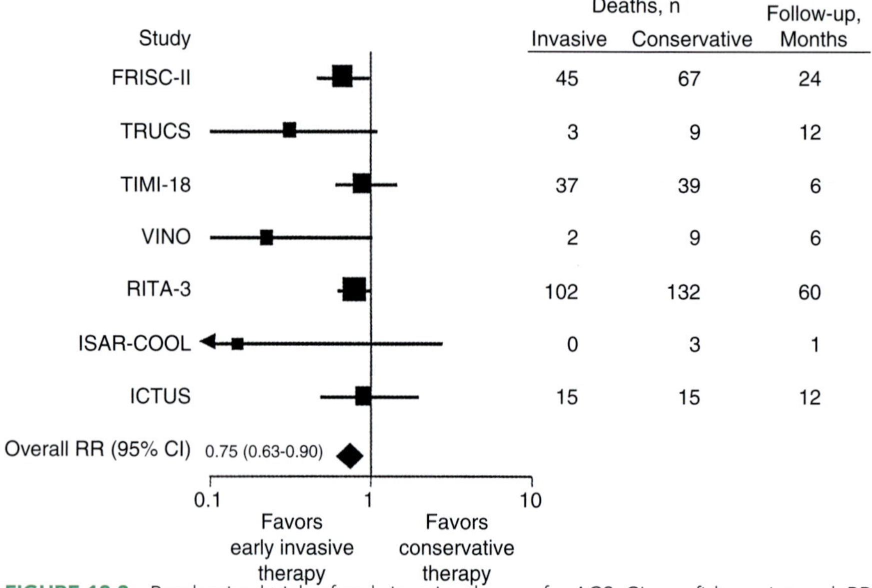

FIGURE 18.3 Randomized trials of early invasive therapy for ACS. CL, confidence interval; RR, relative risk. (From: Bavry AA, Kumbhani DJ, Rassi AN, et al. Benefit of early invasive therapy in acute coronary syndromes: a meta-analysis of contemporary randomized clinical trials. *J Am Coll Cardiol*. 2006;48:1319-1325, reprinted with permission from Elsevier.)

conservative approach, whereas patients with a moderate or high score are best treated with an invasive approach (see below).[10,11]

Risk stratification of bleeding risks is recommended to guide the choice of pharmacology, strategy, and access site. Bleeding, especially major bleeding requiring blood transfusion, has been strongly correlated with adverse outcomes in ACS including mortality. The cause of this correlation is yet to be determined, but likely includes the need to discontinue beneficial antithrombotic medications when bleeding occurs, along with an overlap of the risks of bleeding with risks of overall mortality. Blood transfusions may themselves exhibit an immunosuppressant effect that leads to complications.

A patient at high risk of bleeding might be more likely to benefit from a strategy of bivalirudin or radial access, or a conservative approach with fondaparinux. Another patient with a large NSTEMI and low bleeding risk might benefit from a triple antiplatelet strategy of aspirin, clopidogrel, and glycoprotein inhibitors (GPI).

Multiple scoring systems have been developed, with common risk factors including female gender, advanced age, renal insufficiency, diabetes, shock, baseline anemia, and extremes of weight.[12] Most of these have been primarily validated when using femoral access, with potentially less validity when a radial access approach is chosen. All the risk stratification tools are now readily available online or using portable electronic applications.

EARLY INVASIVE VERSUS CONSERVATIVE APPROACH

Multiple randomized controlled trials have compared a strategy of a routine invasive approach (angiography and revascularization) to a conservative approach (medical management with angiography only for recurrent angina, high-risk stress test findings, or hemodynamic compromise). The preponderance of the evidence favors the routine invasive approach for patients at moderate-to-high risk of cardiac complications from ACS, with low-risk patients having less benefit. The most definitive trials have included the FRISC2, TACTICS-TIMI 18, and RITA-3 trials. A meta-analysis of seven trials demonstrated a reduction in all-cause mortality (RR 0.75, 95% CI 0.63-0.90), recurrent MI (RR 0.83, 95% CI 0.72-0.96), and recurrent unstable angina (RR 0.69, 95% CI 0.65-0.74) (**Fig. 18.3**) with a routine invasive approach compared with a conservative approach.[13]

An early invasive approach within the first 24 hours of presentation is indicated if the hsTn levels are elevated, GRACE score is >140, or if there are new dynamic ST segment changes, with urgent invasive treatment being indicated for the presence of significant ischemia and/or hemodynamic instability. This strategy has shown a reduction in complications and potential improvement in overall outcomes.[14]

The TIMI and GRACE scores generally stratify patients adequately; nevertheless, other conditions not included in the model place patients at higher risk for cardiac events. Renal insufficiency, diabetes, and left ventricular dysfunction are conditions that would generally lead to favoring routine revascularization over conservative management. Low-risk patients (especially women with negative biomarkers) and those with comorbidities that make them high risk for bleeding complications may be among the few patients where a conservative strategy is superior.

TIMING OF PCI

The optimal timing of angiography and PCI has been extensively studied. Patients at high risk—including those with heart failure, refractory angina, and hemodynamic instability—should be taken emergently to the catheterization laboratory for evaluation. Previously, it was suggested that a short period of medical management or "cooling off" of an acute infarction could lead to increased safety for PCI, but no benefit was seen from delaying PCI in the ISAR-COOL trial.[15] The large TIMACS[16] trial demonstrated that an early invasive strategy (within the first 24 hours of presentation) compared with a delayed invasive strategy (>36 hours) was associated with a significant reduction in refractory ischemia, and a trend toward MACE reduction (9.6% vs 11.6%, P = .15), particularly in the highest-risk patients. Unlike in acute STEMI, there may be little demonstrable benefit in NSTEMI of immediate revascularization (<2 hours) compared with deferral until the next working day (<24 hours), although one trial (RIDDLE-NSTEMI[17]) suggested that immediate revascularization effectively reduced reinfarction during the precatheterization period.

CORONARY ARTERY BYPASS SURGERY (CABG)

There have been no randomized trials comparing PCI and CABG specifically in patients with ACS. In general, the preferred revascularization technique is made in a similar fashion as in stable CAD. Nevertheless, where there is a clear thrombotic culprit lesion, PCI may be preferable even in the presence of multivessel CAD. A staged PCI or CABG can subsequently be performed when the patient stabilizes. Alternatively, calculation of the angiographic SYNTAX score can guide whether CABG would be advantageous for the patient. $P2Y_{12}$ inhibitors should be discontinued for 5 days prior to urgent CABG.

The proportion of ACS patients requiring CABG sometime during their initial hospitalization is approximately 10%, with only less than 2% requiring emergency surgery. Although guidelines recommend preloading of clopidogrel or ticagrelor before PCI for ACS, the benefit of preloading remains debatable and may be limited to clopidogrel due to its slower onset of action. In current clinical practice, only 40% of ACS patients are preloaded, primarily due to concerns of delaying bypass surgery when needed.[18]

ANTIPLATELET THERAPIES

Aspirin

Aspirin (acetylsalicylic acid) irreversibly binds and inhibits platelet cyclo-oxygenase type 1 (COX-1), inhibiting thromboxane A2 formation for the lifetime of the platelet (7 days). Because it provides relatively weak platelet inhibition, it is considered safe for nearly every patient with potential ACS, often in conjunction with other agents. It should be administered as soon as possible after presentation, and continued indefinitely (Class I recommendation, LOE A), although evolving data suggest P2Y12 monotherapy may be a more effective alternative. For more rapid absorption, a loading dose of 162 to 325 mg of plain (not enteric-coated) aspirin is recommended to be chewed and swallowed. A subsequent daily dose of 75 to 100 mg was recently shown to be as effective as 325 mg with fewer gastrointestinal reactions (CURRENT-OASIS 7).[19] Nonsteroidal anti-inflammatory drugs such as ibuprofen interfere with the antiplatelet effects of aspirin, have been associated with increased cardiovascular risk, and should be discontinued on hospital admission.

ADP Receptor Antagonists

The oral $P2Y_{12}$ inhibitors ticlopidine, clopidogrel, prasugrel, and ticagrelor inhibit ADP-induced amplification of platelet aggregation. Dual antiplatelet therapy with aspirin and either an ADP-receptor antagonist or a GPI IIb/IIIa is recommended for all patients with ACS at medium to high risk or in whom an invasive strategy is planned.

Ticlopidine was the first agent in this class tested in ACS, but was associated with serious hematologic reactions, including agranulocytosis and thrombotic thrombocytopenic purpura (TTP). Although used until recently for patients with allergic reactions to clopidogrel, ticlopidine has no remaining role with the availability of the newer agents, prasugrel and ticagrelor.

Clopidogrel

Clopidogrel is a thienopyridine prodrug whose active metabolite irreversibly binds and inhibits the ADP receptor $P2Y_{12}$. It has an onset of action of 2 to 4 hours, with a 600-mg loading dose having more rapid onset than the 300-mg dose and generally preferred. A 75-mg maintenance dose is recommended for 12 months after PCI for ACS.

Clopidogrel is indicated for patients allergic to aspirin, and for most patients as a second antiplatelet agent. Due to its prolonged effect on platelet activity, it should be discontinued for 5 days prior to major surgery, especially cardiac surgery.

The landmark CURE trial demonstrated that a 300-mg dose of clopidogrel, followed by a daily 75-mg dose added to aspirin, reduced the risk of cardiovascular death, MI, or stroke from 11.4% to 9.3% (RR 0.80, P < .001) in patients with NSTE-ACS. Within the CURE trial, only 20% of patients received PCI (PCI-CURE), but the benefits of clopidogrel were more pronounced in this group (RR 0.70, P = .03).[20] Due to its delayed onset of action, clopidogrel should be administered on presentation to obtain maximal platelet inhibition at the time of PCI, although this is a subject of debate (as noted earlier).

Clopidogrel requires a two-step hepatic conversion to its active metabolite. Its clinical effect on platelet aggregation is highly variable among individual patients, due in part to variations in the cytochrome P450 system, especially CYP2C19. Patients who are poor metabolizers of clopidogrel are at increased risk for ischemic events, however, and the use of genetic testing to identify and treat such patients has not yet been found to be effective in reducing thrombotic risk.

Clopidogrel and aspirin increase the risk of gastrointestinal bleeding. Although in vivo studies have demonstrated an inhibition of clopidogrel metabolism with omeprazole, this has not been shown to have a clinical effect in the COGENT[21] study, and has not been shown with other agents. Due to the risk of bleeding, patients with prior gastrointestinal bleeding should be treated with a non-omeprazole proton-pump inhibitor.

Prasugrel

Prasugrel is a thienopyridine prodrug the metabolite of which irreversibly inhibits the ADP receptor. Similar to clopidogrel, it requires a two-step metabolism, but one step is rapidly mediated by serum esterases. As a result, prasugrel exhibits a high degree of platelet inhibition regardless of CYP inhibitors or variants. Its onset of action is rapid at 30 minutes, perhaps explaining why the ACCOAST trial demonstrated no benefit to up-front or preloaded prasugrel compared with prasugrel administered following PCI.[22] The duration of effect of prasugrel is longer than that of clopidogrel at 5 to 10 days, and thus should be discontinued 7 days prior to a major surgery.

The TRITON-TIMI 38 trial randomized 13,608 patients with ACS (74% NSTE-ACS) to either prasugrel (60-mg loading dose and 10-mg maintenance dose) or clopidogrel (300-mg loading and 75-mg daily). Among patients with NSTE-ACS undergoing PCI, prasugrel was administered only after diagnostic angiography.

The primary efficacy endpoint of cardiovascular death, MI, or stroke occurred in 9.9% of patients on prasugrel versus 12.1% of patients taking clopidogrel (HR 0.81, $P < .001$), mainly driven by recurrent MI. Nevertheless, the rate of major bleeding was increased with prasugrel from 1.8% to 2.4% (HR 1.32, $P = .03$), including fatal bleeding and CABG-related bleeding. Patients with a history of stroke or transient ischemic attack, patients older than 75 years of age, and patients with low body weight (<60 kg) had a higher risk of bleeding and no net benefit with prasugrel over clopidogrel.[23]

Ticagrelor

Ticagrelor is a newer ADP-receptor antagonist called a cyclopentyl-triazolo-pyrimidine. It binds reversibly to the $P2Y_{12}$ receptor and has a half-life of 12 hours. Ticagrelor requires no metabolism for activity, exhibits a rapid onset of action, and high levels of platelet inhibition. Based on its shorter half-life and reversible inhibition, ticagrelor may be held for as little as 1 to 3 days prior to CABG, although 5 days is preferred. Given its short half-life, ticagrelor must be administered twice daily. There is up to a 15% rate of dyspnea and an increase in bradycardia with ticagrelor, which may be confusing and complicating symptoms following MI.

The PLATO trial randomized 18,624 patients with ACS (11,067 NSTE-ACS) to clopidogrel (300 mg/75 mg) or ticagrelor (180-mg loading with 90-mg twice daily maintenance). Patients receiving PCI were given an additional 300-mg load of clopidogrel, or 90-mg ticagrelor if PCI occurred >24 hours after the initial loading dose. Major adverse cardiovascular events were reduced from 11.7% in the clopidogrel group to 9.8% in the ticagrelor group (HR 0.84, $P < .001$). This benefit to ticagrelor appeared to result without any difference in the rates of major bleeding from clopidogrel (11.2% vs 11.6%, $P = .43$). Finally, ticagrelor was found to have an overall mortality benefit compared with clopidogrel (4.7% vs 9.7% $P < .01$), which was driven by reductions in cardiovascular death.[24] As a result, ticagrelor has become the oral antiplatelet agent of choice in many laboratories, with the caveat of a higher cost and higher rates of intolerance in some patients.

GLYCOPROTEIN IIB/IIIA INHIBITORS

The intravenous GPI IIb/IIIa abciximab, eptifibatide, and tirofiban all inhibit the final pathway of platelet aggregation: the binding of the platelet to fibrinogen. These agents exhibit high levels (>90%) of platelet inhibition, causing reduced ischemic complications (~9% relative risk reduction) but also increased risks of bleeding in patients with ACS.[25]

The majority of the trials of these agents (EPIC, EPILOG, PURSUIT, PRISM) were conducted prior to the availability of clopidogrel, putting their ischemic benefits in the current era of dual-antiplatelet therapy with aspirin and clopidogrel in question.

The administration and pharmacology of the GPIs are reviewed. Key points include the risk of thrombocytopenia (0.5%-5.6%) with their use, which may be especially profound with repeated use of the monoclonal antibody abciximab. Eptifibatide and tirofiban have a relatively short half-life of ~2 hours, making CABG safe 6 hours after administration. Abciximab has a prolonged effect of 48 hours, requiring platelet transfusion in the case of excessive bleeding.

GPI have primarily demonstrated a benefit in patients treated with an invasive approach; patients managed conservatively with a dual-antiplatelet regimen of aspirin and clopidogrel may not benefit from the approach. The benefits of GP IIb/IIIa inhibition is highest in patients with elevated TIMI-risk scores (>4), especially those with positive troponin assays. It is reasonable to delay the administration of GP IIb/IIIa agents until the time of PCI, because the benefit of "upstream" treatment is nearly balanced by an increased risk of bleeding.

The use of GPIs has decreased with the availability of bivalirudin and more potent oral antiplatelet agents. Nevertheless, in patients who do not receive a loading dose of clopidogrel prior to PCI, there may be inadequate platelet inhibition during stenting, and GP IIb/IIIa inhibition has a Class IIa recommendation. ACS, especially STEMI, is associated with high levels of platelet activation and a delayed onset of action of all the oral $P2Y_{12}$ inhibitors. This increases the risk of acute stent thrombosis, especially when bivalirudin is used. Intravenous GPIs may effectively "bridge" the patient with dual antiplatelet inhibition until the oral agents take effect, a strategy that has demonstrated benefit with cangrelor.

Cangrelor

Cangrelor is an intravenous (IV), direct-acting ADP inhibitor that is both rapidly acting and rapidly reversible. The plasma half-life of cangrelor is 3 to 5 minutes, and platelet function normalizes within 1 to 2 hours of discontinuation of the drug, which may be useful when coronary anatomy is unknown and pretreatment with dual antiplatelet therapy has not occurred. Cangrelor was compared against a 600-mg loading dose of clopidogrel administered immediately before or after PCI in the recent CHAMPION-PHOENIX trial.[26] This demonstrated a reduction in the primary ischemic endpoint (4.7% vs 5.9%, $P = .005$) with an increase in minor bleeding such as small hematomas.

Cangrelor inhibits binding of clopidogrel and prasugrel metabolites to the $P2Y_{12}$ receptor. The package insert recommends that cangrelor be discontinued prior to the administration of clopidogrel or prasugrel, making cangrelor less helpful in bridging to these oral antiplatelet agents. The binding of ticagrelor is unaffected by cangrelor.

Cangrelor was not compared against a strategy of pretreatment with clopidogrel, or against prasugrel, ticagrelor, or GPIs. With its unique pharmacokinetic properties and safety profile, cangrelor may have a niche role for bridging off of other oral antiplatelet agents or as a safer alternative to GPIs.

ANTITHROMBOTIC THERAPIES

Unfractionated Heparin

Unfractionated heparin (UFH) is a mixture of polysaccharide molecules, one-third of which contain the key pentasaccharide sequence that binds to antithrombin. Antithrombin is then activated to inhibit factor Xa and thrombin. Due to variability in various heparin preparations, and protein binding, monitoring of the anticoagulant effect is necessary, with a goal of an activated partial thromboplastin time (aPTT) of 50 to 75 seconds, or 1.5 to 2.5 the upper limit of normal. For PCI, anticoagulation is measured using the whole blood activated clotting time (ACT), with a goal of 250 to 350 seconds, or 200 to 250 seconds if using a GPI. Typical bolus intravenous (IV) UFH doses in the catheterization laboratory are 70 to 100 IU/kg, or 50 to 60 IU/kg with GPIs. Repeated ACT measurements should be made with prolonged procedures. Continued anticoagulation following a successful PCI procedure has been associated with an increased risk of bleeding without ischemic benefits, and is not recommended.

Low-Molecular-Weight Heparins

The low-molecular-weight heparins (LMWH) (enoxaparin, tinzaparin, dalteparin) are heparin derivatives with a more consistent dose-response relationship than UFH. Similar to UFH, LMWH binds to antithrombin, causing inhibition of factor Xa and thrombin. Due to improved subcutaneous absorption, LMWH can be administered either subcutaneously (SQ) or by IV. Monitoring LMWH effects is considered unnecessary except for extremely obese patients, or those with renal insufficiency (CrCl < 30 mL/min). The ACT assay does not reliably measure LMWH effect; the anti-factor Xa assay is preferred but is not routinely available on a rapid basis.

Enoxaparin is the best studied among the LMWH for ACS. The therapeutic dose is 1 mg/kg SQ every 12 hours, or 0.75 to 1 mg/kg IV for elective PCI where no other anticoagulant has been administered. To optimize anti-Xa activity for PCI, an additional IV booster dose of 0.3 mg/kg is administeredif PCI is performed 8 to 12 hours after the prior SQ dose, particularly if fewer than three previous SQ doses have been received by the patient. Switching from one anticoagulant strategy to another (ie, LMWH to UFH) is associated with increased bleeding risk and is discouraged.

Early studies comparing LMWH to UFH in ACS have demonstrated a reduction of MI (10.1% vs 11%) without increases in bleeding. Nevertheless, many of these trials were performed without an invasive approach, putting the benefit in question. The more recent large SYNERGY trial of 9978 patients undergoing PCI for NSTE-ACS demonstrated equivalent efficacy between enoxaparin and UFH (14% vs 14.5%, *P* = NS) with more TIMI-major bleeding events (9.1% vs 7.6%, *P* = .008), possibly due to switching of anticoagulation strategies.[27]

Overall, LMWH is considered equivalent to UFH for ACS and PCI. Its advantages include the lack of monitoring, ease of administration, and lower risk of heparin-induced thrombocytopenia. The lack of monitoring can be a double-edged sword, because the inability to assess the adequacy of anticoagulation at the time of PCI may be perceived as a risk. LMWH has primarily been used in ACS in Europe and Canada, with a much lower market share than in the United States.

Fondaparinux

The heparinoid fondaparinux is a synthetic pentasaccharide derived from the binding regions of UFH and LWH. It inhibits factor Xa with antithrombin at high potency, with an SQ dose of 2.5 mg daily. Compared with LMWH, the use of fondaparinux demonstrated noninferiority for ischemic complications in the OASIS-5 trial, but decreased major bleeding from 4.1% to 2.2% (HR 0.52, *P* < .001). Major bleeding was associated with mortality, which was reduced with fondaparinux (2.9% vs 3.5%, *P* = .02).[28] Unexpected episodes of catheter thrombosis were noted with fondaparinux (0.9% vs 0.4%), but can be avoided with a standard bolus (85 IU/kg, or 60 IU/kg with GPI) of UFH at the time of PCI.

Fondaparinux carries a Class I recommendation for anticoagulation for ACS, but with a lower level of evidence than UFH, LMWH, and bivalirudin. Despite its mortality benefit in the OASIS-5 trial, fondaparinux has not been widely accepted by practicing interventionalists due to the small risk of catheter thrombosis. Nevertheless, it is the preferred agent for patients when a conservative, noninvasive approach is selected.

Bivalirudin

Bivalirudin is a direct thrombin inhibitor that does not require antithrombin as a cofactor. It inhibits both free thrombin and fibrin-bound thrombin, which may increase its efficacy in ACS. The drug generates a predictable anticoagulant effect that can be measured with the aPTT and ACT, but wherein repeated measurement is not required. Bivalirudin is given as an IV bolus of 0.75 mg/kg, with an infusion of 1.75 mg/kg/h. It is excreted by the kidney, and the infusion must be dose-adjusted in renal insufficiency.

The ACUITY trial was a randomized, open-label trial of 13,819 patients with ACS planned for an invasive strategy. Patients were randomized to heparin with GPI, bivalirudin with GPI, or bivalirudin alone strategies, in a background of aspirin and clopidogrel loading. There was no significant difference among any of the groups with respect to a composite ischemia endpoint. Nevertheless, the bivalirudin alone strategy demonstrated a reduction in ACUITY-defined major bleeding (3.0% vs 5.7%, RR 0.53, *P* < .001). The net clinical outcome (ie, the risk of major adverse cardiac events added to the risk of major bleeding) was thus reduced from 11.7% to 10.1% with bivalirudin when compared to heparin with GPI. Crossover from heparin to bivalirudin did not result in excess bleeding, and may have had a beneficial effect on ischemia.[29]

Because 40% of patients in the ACUITY did not end up having positive biomarkers and receiving PCI, the ISAR-REACT 4 trial tested 1721 patients with NSTEMI receiving PCI, to either UFH with GPI, or bivalirudin alone. The trial also used a more rigorous definition of major bleeding than the ACUITY trial. Nevertheless, the ISAR-REACT 4 trial demonstrated similar results: equivalent ischemic efficacy of bivalirudin compared with UFH + GPI, but with decreased major bleeding (2.6% vs 4.6%, *P* = .02).[30]

In the MATRIX trial, 7213 ACS patients were randomized to bivalirudin (with or without an extended infusion) or heparin with selective GPI. There were no significant differences between the two groups in terms of MACE or net adverse clinical events, including bleeding. The risk of stent thrombosis was higher with bivalirudin. Continuation of the bivalirudin infusion after PCI did not change the results.[31]

Finally, in the recent BRIGHT-4 trial, bivalirudin with a bolus and high-dose 2- to 4-hour infusion was shown to reduce major bleeding and mortality in STEMI patients compared with heparin monotherapy.[32]

Overall, and as described in several meta-analyses, bivalirudin is equivalent to heparin in terms of ischemic MACE, with a reduction in bleeding risk due in part to differential GPI use, but at the cost of an increased risk of acute stent thrombosis.

Postprocedure Care

Optimal care following revascularization should include referral for cardiac rehabilitation, smoking cessation assistance, and medical management of heart failure, arrhythmias, and risk factors. Dual antiplatelet therapy should be continued for 12 months after ACS, with the more potent $P2Y_{12}$ antagonists prasugrel or ticagrelor preferred. Antithrombotic treatment beyond dual antiplatelet therapy (DAPT) is available for selected patients at high risk for recurrent events, with some benefit demonstrated for low-dose rivaroxaban and the new PAR-1 antagonist vorapaxar, but at the cost of increased bleeding.

CONCLUSIONS

PCI is a highly proven revascularization strategy for ACSs. The benefit of PCI is greatest for patients at moderate to high risk for cardiac complications, and for patients who receive PCI early (<24 hours). Early risk stratification, preferably with a quantitative scoring system such as the TIMI or GRACE score, is the key guide to selecting a management strategy. An expanding array of antithrombotic agents—such as bivalirudin, prasugrel, and ticagrelor—give the informed interventionist the ability to adjust each patient's regimen in accordance with their clinical presentation, ischemic risk, and bleeding profile.

Key Points

- History, physical exam, and ECG are essential for rapid diagnosis of ACS.
- Elevated cardiac biomarkers are highly sensitive for myocardial damage.
- Noncoronary causes for troponin elevation should be considered when the history and ECG are not consistent with ACS.
- Early risk stratification of ischemic and bleeding risks is critical to subsequent management decisions.
- Moderate- and high-risk patients benefit from an early invasive approach, preferably with revascularization within the first 24 hours.
- Aspirin should be administered to all ACS patients without an allergy.
- Dual antiplatelet inhibition with an ADP-receptor antagonist is indicated for all patients with ACS.
- Prasugrel and ticagrelor have superior and more consistent platelet inhibition than clopidogrel.
- GPI benefit patients with an early invasive approach but increase bleeding.
- UFH with a goal ACT of 250 to 300 seconds provides adequate anticoagulation for PCI.
- Low-molecular-weight heparin is an alternative to heparin, but is associated with increased bleeding if switching to UFH occurs.
- Fondaparinux reduces bleeding and mortality in ACS, and may be preferable for conservatively managed patients.
- Bivalirudin reduces bleeding compared with unfractionated heparin + glycoprotein inhibitors, without increased ischemic complications when used with a dual antiplatelet regimen.

References

1. Ahmed B, Dauerman HL, Piper WD, et al. Recent changes in practice of elective percutaneous coronary intervention for stable angina. *Circ Cardiovasc Qual Outcomes*. 2011;4(3):300-305.
2. Tsao CW, Aday AW, Almarzooq ZI, et al. Heart disease and stroke statistics—2023 update: a report from the American Heart Association. *Circulation*. 2023;147(8):e93-e621.
3. Thygesen K, Alpert JS, Jaffe AS, et al. Fourth universal definition of myocardial infarction 2018. *Circulation*. 2018;138(20):e618-e651.
4. Reichlin T, Hochholzer W, Bassetti S, et al. Early diagnosis of myocardial infarction with sensitive cardiac troponin assays. *N Engl J Med*. 2009;361(9):858-867.
5. Eggers KM, Lagerqvist B, Venge P, Wallentin L, Lindahl B. Prognostic value of biomarkers during and after non-ST-segment elevation acute coronary syndrome. *J Am Coll Cardiol*. 2009;54(4):357-364.
6. Moussa ID, Klein LW, Shah B, et al. Consideration of a new definition of clinically relevant myocardial infarction after coronary revascularization: an expert consensus document from the Society for Cardiovascular Angiography and Interventions (SCAI). *J Am Coll Cardiol*. 2013;62(17):1563-1570.
7. Newby LK, Jesse RL, Babb JD, et al. ACCF 2012 expert consensus document on practical clinical considerations in the interpretation of troponin elevations: a report of the American College of Cardiology Foundation task force on Clinical Expert Consensus Documents. *J Am Coll Cardiol*. 2012;60(23):2427-2463.
8. NACB Writing Group; Wu AHB, Jaffe AS, et al. National Academy of Clinical Biochemistry laboratory medicine practice guidelines: use of cardiac troponin and B-type natriuretic peptide or N-terminal proB-type natriuretic peptide for etiologies other than acute coronary syndromes and heart failure. *Clin Chem*. 2007;53(12):2086-2096.
9. Amsterdam EA, Wenger NK, Brindis RG, et al. 2014 AHA/ACC guideline for the management of patients with non-ST-elevation acute coronary syndromes: a report of the American College of Cardiology/American Heart Association Task Force on practice guidelines. *J Am Coll Cardiol*. 2014;64(24):e139-e228.
10. Antman EM, Cohen M, Bernink PJ, et al. The TIMI risk score for unstable angina/non-ST elevation MI: a method for prognostication and therapeutic decision making. *JAMA*. 2000;284(7):835-842.
11. Fox KA, Dabbous OH, Goldberg RJ, et al. Prediction of risk of death and myocardial infarction in the six months after presentation with acute coronary syndrome: prospective multinational observational study (GRACE). *BMJ*. 2006;333(7578):1091.
12. Rao SV, McCoy LA, Spertus JA, et al. An updated bleeding model to predict the risk of post-procedure bleeding among patients undergoing percutaneous coronary intervention: a report using an expanded bleeding definition from the National Cardiovascular Data Registry CathPCI Registry. *JACC Cardiovasc Interv*. 2013;6(9):897-904.
13. Bavry AA, Kumbhani DJ, Rassi AN, Bhatt DL, Askari AT. Benefit of early invasive therapy in acute coronary syndromes: a meta-analysis of contemporary randomized clinical trials. *J Am Coll Cardiol*. 2006;48(7):1319-1325.
14. Collet JP, Thiele H, Barbato E, et al. 2020 ESC Guidelines for the management of acute coronary syndromes in patients presenting without persistent ST-segment elevation: the Task Force for the management of acute coronary syndromes in patients presenting without persistent ST-segment elevation of the European Society of Cardiology (ESC). *Eur Heart J*. 2021;42(14):1289-1367.
15. Neumann FJ, Kastrati A, Pogatsa-Murray G, et al. Evaluation of prolonged antithrombotic pretreatment ('cooling-off' strategy) before intervention in patients with unstable coronary syndromes: a randomized controlled trial. *JAMA*. 2003;290(12):1593-1599.
16. Mehta SR, Granger CB, Boden WE, et al. Early versus delayed invasive intervention in acute coronary syndromes. *N Engl J Med*. 2009;360(21):2165-2175.
17. Milosevic A, Vasiljevic-Pokrajcic Z, Milasinovic D, et al. Immediate versus delayed invasive intervention for non-STEMI patients: the RIDDLE-NSTEMI study. *JACC Cardiovasc Interv*. 2016;9(6):541-549.
18. Fan W, Plent S, Prats J, Deliargyris EN. Trends in P2Y12 inhibitor use in patients referred for invasive evaluation of coronary artery disease in contemporary US practice. *Am J Cardiol*. 2016;117(9):1439-1443.
19. Mehta SR, Tanguay JF, Eikelboom JW, et al. Double-dose versus standard-dose clopidogrel and high-dose versus low-dose aspirin in individuals undergoing percutaneous coronary intervention for acute coronary syndromes (CURRENT-OASIS 7): a randomised factorial trial. *Lancet*. 2010;376(9748):1233-1243.
20. Yusuf S, Zhao F, Mehta SR, et al. Effects of clopidogrel in addition to aspirin in patients with acute coronary syndromes without ST-segment elevation. *N Engl J Med*. 2001;345(7):494-502.
21. Bhatt DL, Cryer BL, Contant CF, et al. Clopidogrel with or without omeprazole in coronary artery disease. *N Engl J Med*. 2010;363(20):1909-1917.
22. Montalescot G, Bolognese L, Dudek D, et al. Pretreatment with prasugrel in non-ST-segment elevation acute coronary syndromes. *N Engl J Med*. 2013;369(11):999-1010.

23. Wiviott SD, Braunwald E, McCabe CH, et al. Prasugrel versus clopidogrel in patients with acute coronary syndromes. *N Engl J Med*. 2007;357(20):2001-2015.
24. Wallentin L, Becker RC, Budaj A, et al. Ticagrelor versus clopidogrel in patients with acute coronary syndromes. *N Engl J Med*. 2009;361(11):1045-1057.
25. Roffi M, Chew DP, Mukherjee D, et al. Platelet glycoprotein IIb/IIIa inhibition in acute coronary syndromes. Gradient of benefit related to the revascularization strategy. *Eur Heart J*. 2002;23(18):1441-1448.
26. Bhatt DL, Stone GW, Mahaffey KW, et al. Effect of platelet inhibition with cangrelor during PCI on ischemic events. *N Engl J Med*. 2013;368(14):1303-1313.
27. Ferguson JJ, Califf RM, Antman EM, et al. Enoxaparin vs unfractionated heparin in high-risk patients with non-ST-segment elevation acute coronary syndromes managed with an intended early invasive strategy: primary results of the SYNERGY randomized trial. *JAMA*. 2004;292(1):45-54.
28. Fifth Organization to Assess Strategies in Acute Ischemic Syndromes Investigators; Yusuf S, Mehta SR, et al. Comparison of fondaparinux and enoxaparin in acute coronary syndromes. *N Engl J Med*. 2006;354(14):1464-1476.
29. Stone GW, McLaurin BT, Cox DA, et al. Bivalirudin for patients with acute coronary syndromes. *N Engl J Med*. 2006;355(21):2203-2216.
30. Kastrati A, Neumann FJ, Schulz S, et al. Abciximab and heparin versus bivalirudin for non-ST-elevation myocardial infarction. *N Engl J Med*. 2011;365(21):1980-1989.
31. Valgimigli M, Frigoli E, Leonardi S, et al. Bivalirudin or unfractionated heparin in acute coronary syndromes. *N Engl J Med*. 2015;373(11):997-1009.
32. Li Y, Liang Z, Qin L, et al. Bivalirudin plus a high-dose infusion versus heparin monotherapy in patients with ST-segment elevation myocardial infarction undergoing primary percutaneous coronary intervention: a randomised trial. *Lancet*. 2022;400(10366):1847-1857.

STEMI Intervention: Emphasis on Guidelines

Mohamad B. Moumneh and Abdulla A. Damluji

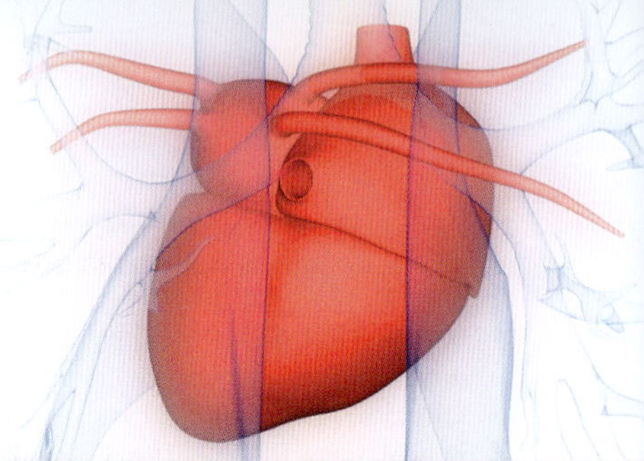

In 1990, specific and separate guidelines pertaining to ST-elevation myocardial infarction (STEMI) treatment and management were first introduced in the United States (US). Over the years, the clinical practice guidelines evolved substantially, covering various aspects and changes involved in the management and care of these complex patients, including the ability to understand and integrate both STEMI and percutaneous coronary intervention (PCI) guidelines, systems-of-care issues, reperfusion choices (pharmacologic and/or mechanical), risk stratification, adjunctive medical therapies, technical issues related to PCI, and postreperfusion management. This chapter focuses on acute intervention for STEMI, as well as related adjunctive medical therapies, with a focus on guidelines. A detailed review of adjunctive medical therapies (including anticoagulants, thrombolytics, and platelet-inhibitor agents) is covered elsewhere.

PRIMARY INTERVENTIONS

PCI Versus Fibrinolytic Therapy

Patients presenting for STEMI must undergo rapid evaluation for reperfusion therapy and have a reperfusion strategy implemented promptly when required. Among the interventions for immediate revascularization in such patients are primary PCI, fibrinolytic therapy, and acute surgical reperfusion, with the latter being rarely utilized in practice. No one intervention is superior in all settings. The choice of the revascularization approach is influenced by the availability of resources, such as PCI capability; systems of care; time to treatment; risks associated with the therapy, both medical and procedural; patient characteristics like symptom onset, ischemic time, presentation status, and comorbidities; and the expected benefits of the reperfusion strategy.[1]

While the fibrinolytic therapy can achieve reperfusion, re-occlusion of the artery can occur in approximately 20% of cases. Thus, the utilization of PCI offers lower rates of reinfarction, recurrent ischemia, and intracranial hemorrhage. While fibrinolytic therapy reduced the mortality rate of patients with STEMI by half, PCI further reduces these rates and generally has even lower mortality rates.[2] Other factors that limit the use of the fibrinolytic therapy include the failure to reperfuse the infarct-related artery (IRA) in nearly one-fifth of cases. However, PCI can achieve higher rates of thrombolysis in myocardial infarction (TIMI) grade 3 flow and infarct artery patency with reperfusion.

The utilization of PCI might sometimes be limited due to logistical and geographic barriers that necessitates the use of the widely available and easily accessible fibrinolytic therapy.[1,3,4] The 2013 American College of Cardiology Foundation (ACCF)/American Heart Association (AHA) STEMI guidelines emphasize that fibrinolysis should generally be limited to hospitals without on-site PCI capability and when there is an anticipated delay to performing primary PCI beyond 120 minutes of first medical contact[5,6] (**Table 19.1**). In these cases, the following recommendations to use fibrinolytic therapy in practice apply:

1. STEMI (ST-elevation >0.1 mV in at least two contiguous precordial leads or at least two adjacent limb leads), onset of ischemic symptoms <12 hours (Class I).
2. STEMI, PCI not available, clinical and/or electrocardiographic (ECG) evidence of ongoing ischemia within 12 to 24 hours of symptom onset and large area of myocardium at risk or hemodynamic instability (Class IIa).

In such instances, improved outcomes including survival and prevention of major adverse cardiovascular outcomes (MACE) are achieved compared to delayed PCI.[7] The 2013 STREAM (Strategic Reperfusion Early After Myocardial Infarction) trial randomized 1892 patients with symptom onset within 3 hours of medical contact, who could not undergo primary PCI within 1 hour, to primary PCI or fibrinolysis, and who were then transferred to a PCI-capable hospital. The trial noted that despite increased intracranial hemorrhage in the fibrinolysis group, no significant difference in the primary endpoint of death from any cause, including congestive heart failure (CHF), shock, or reinfarction at 30 days, was observed.[8] This trial further supports the notion that prompt fibrinolysis should be administered when primary PCI is not available to be performed in a timely fashion.

While fibrinolytic therapy remains a valid revascularization strategy when PCI is not available, the efficacy of fibrinolysis to achieve reperfusion diminishes as the duration from symptom onset to presentation lengthens. The optimal benefits are seen in patient presenting within the first 3 hours of the onset of symptoms. A moderate benefit persists up to 12 hours, but beyond 12 to 24 hours after symptom onset, the advantages are either minimal or undetermined.[4] There are a number of absolute and relative contraindications to fibrinolytic therapy (**Table 19.2**).

TABLE 19.1 Indications for Fibrinolytic Therapy When There Is a >120-min Delay From First Medical Contact to Primary PCI

	COR	LOE
Ischemic symptoms <12 h	I	A
Evidence of ongoing ischemia 12-24 h after symptom onset and a large area of myocardium at risk or hemodynamic instability	IIa	C
ST depression, except if true posterior (inferobasal) MI is suspected or when associated with ST elevation in lead AVR	III: harm	B

AVR, augmented vector right; COR, class of recommendation; LOE, level of evidence; MI, myocardial infarction; PCI, percutaneous coronary intervention.
Modified from O'Gara PT, Kushner FG, Ascheim DD, et al. 2013 ACCF/AHA guideline for the management of ST-elevation myocardial infarction. *Circulation*. 2013;127(4):e362-e425, with permission.

TABLE 19.2 Contraindications to Fibrinolytic Therapy in Patients Presenting With STEMI[a]

Absolute Contraindications
• Any prior ICH • Known structural cerebral vascular lesions (eg, AVM) • Known malignant intracranial neoplasm (primary or metastatic) • Ischemic stroke within 3 mo EXCEPT acute ischemic stroke within 3 h • Suspected aortic dissection • Active bleeding or bleeding diathesis (excluding menses) • Significant closed head or facial trauma within 3 mo • Intracranial or intraspinal surgery within 2 mo • Severe uncontrolled hypertension (unresponsive to emergency therapy) • For streptokinase, prior treatment within the previous 6 mo
Relative Contraindications
• History of chronic, severe, poorly controlled hypertension • Severe uncontrolled hypertension or presentation (SBP > 180 mm Hg or DBP > 110 mm Hg) • History of ischemic stroke prior to 3 mo, dementia, or known intracranial pathology not covered in contraindications • Traumatic or prolonged (>10 min) CPR • Major surgery (<3 wk) • Recent (within 2-4 wk) internal bleeding • Noncompressible vascular punctures • For streptokinase/anistreplase: prior exposure (more than 5 d ago) or prior allergic reaction to these agents • Pregnancy • Active peptic ulcer • Current use of anticoagulants: the higher the INR, the higher the risk of bleeding

AVM, arteriovenous malformation; CPR, cardiopulmonary resuscitation; DBP, diastolic blood pressure; ICH, intracranial hemorrhage; INR, International Normalized Ratio; SBP, systolic blood pressure.

Modified from O'Gara PT, Kushner FG, Ascheim DD, et al. 2013 ACCF/AHA guideline for the management of ST-elevation myocardial infarction. *Circulation*. 2013;127(4):e362-e425, with permission.

[a]Viewed as advisory for clinical decision-making and may not be all-inclusive or definitive.

Points Helpful to Clinical Practice

1. Various revascularization strategies for patients presenting with STEMI exist, and these include PCI, fibrinolytic therapy, and acute surgical reperfusion.
2. PCI is preferred to fibrinolytic therapy because it offers reduced mortality, reinfarction, recurrent ischemia, and intracranial hemorrhage risks, while achieving higher rates of TIMI grade 3 flow reperfusion.
3. Given its easy accessibility and broad availability, fibrinolytic therapy serves as an alternative when PCI is unavailable or delayed by more than 120 minutes.
4. Delay in the time to reperfusion diminishes the efficacy of fibrinolytic therapy to achieve successful revascularization.

RELATIONSHIP BETWEEN TIME OF ISCHEMIA, MYOCARDIAL SALVAGE, AND SURVIVAL

Benefits of reperfusion therapy are time-dependent. The longer the interval from symptom onset (coronary artery occlusion) to reperfusion, the less myocardium there is to rescue or salvage, which increases the risk of mortality. Reperfusion therapy offers the maximum benefits of myocardial salvage and improvement in survival within the first few hours of therapy[9] (**Fig. 19.1**). Several factors including the presence of collateral circulation, intermittent occlusion, myocardial oxygen consumption, ischemic preconditioning, persistence of residual blood flow, and hibernation can influence the precise time window of successful myocardial salvage. Time-independent benefits of opening the artery have also been suggested to exist and include improving infarct healing and electrical stability and reducing reinfarction.[1,10]

Current clinical practice guidelines recommend a systems goal of 90 minutes or less from the first medical contact to balloon angioplasty for hospitals that perform primary PCI.[11] A number of variables may influence the total time of reperfusion with primary PCI including patient and prehospital variables (eg, symptom onset to first medical contact, prehospital transport and arrival to a PCI-capable hospital, prehospital notification, and emergency medical services (EMS)-administered medical therapies) or in-hospital factors (eg, time of diagnosis, catheterization laboratory staffing, and procedure-related factors). Symptom onset to balloon time and door-to-balloon time are significantly associated with mortality following primary PCI. Earlier reperfusion reduces mortality risks, particularly in those patients presenting early after symptom onset (<2 hours). Delays in therapy affect mortality benefit to a greater extent in patients who are considered to be in the high risk groups (eg, large territory of myocardium at risk, anterior infarcts, CHF, advanced age or pathologic aging, and renal insufficiency).[12] Data from the National Cardiovascular Data Registry (NCDR) reveal a direction association between door-to-balloon time and in-hospital mortality. This relationship persists both below and above the 90-minute cutoff, suggesting any delay even when below 90 minutes can potentially carry an increased risk of mortality risk (**Fig. 19.2**).[13] System-related delays to achieve door-to-balloon time including prehospital, transfer, and in-hospital delays have also been shown to be independently associated with worse long-term mortality; each hour of delay was associated with an increase in the risk of death.[14] Hospitals without PCI capabilities also affect the relationship between time of ischemia,

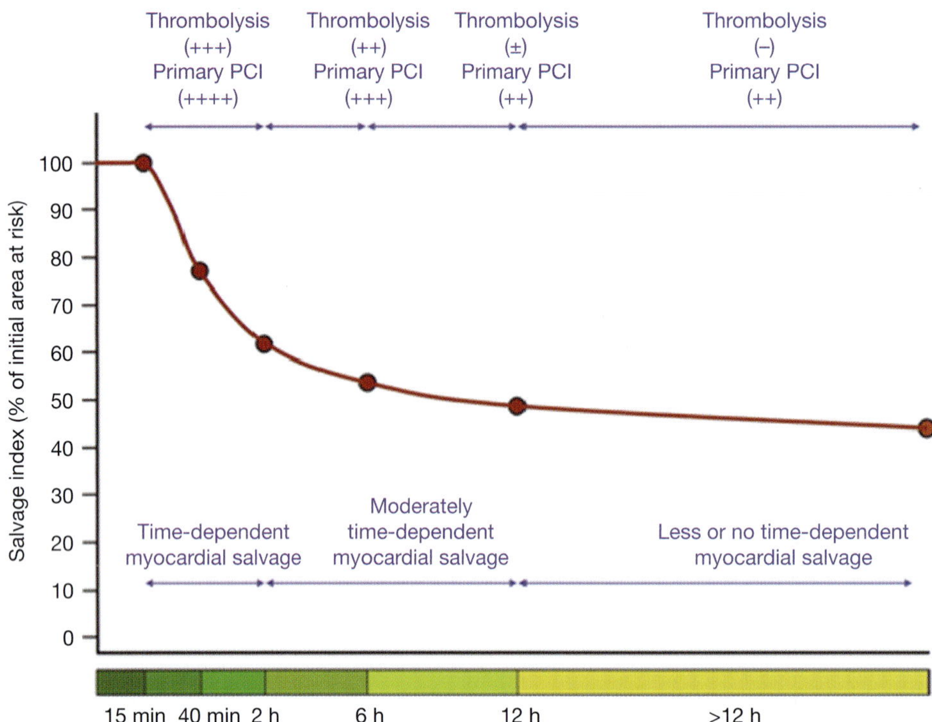

FIGURE 19.1 Time dependency of myocardial salvage expressed as percentage of initial area at risk. The initial parts of the curve up to 2 hours were reconstructed based on the experimental studies. For the first 15 minutes after coronary occlusion, myocardial necrosis is not observed. At 40 minutes after coronary occlusion, myocardial cell death develops rapidly, and the myocardial necrosis is confluent. After this point, progression to necrosis is slowed considerably. The other parts of the curve showing myocardial salvage from 2 to >12 hours from the symptom onset are reconstructed according to the data of scintigraphic studies in patients with acute myocardial infarction. Efficacy of reperfusion is expressed as follows: ++++, very effective; +++, effective; ++, moderately effective; ±, uncertainly effective; –, not effective. PCI, percutaneous coronary intervention. (From Schömig A, Ndrepepa G, Kastrati A. Late myocardial salvage: time to recognize its reality in the reperfusion therapy of acute myocardial infarction. *Eur Heart J.* 2006;27:1900-1907, with permission.)

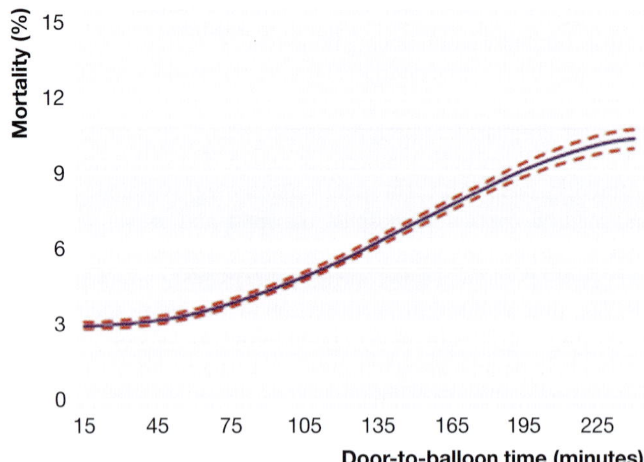

FIGURE 19.2 Adjusted in-hospital mortality as a function of door-to-balloon time. Median D2B time was 83 minutes, with 4.6% mortality. Longer door-to-balloon times were associated with a higher adjusted risk of mortality in hospital in a continuous nonlinear fashion (30 minutes = 3.0%, 60 minutes = 3.5%, 90 minutes = 4.3%, 120 minutes = 5.6%, 150 minutes = 7.0%, 180 minutes = 8.4%, $P < .001$). A reduction in door-to-balloon time from 90 to 60 minutes was associated with 0.8% lower mortality, and a reduction from 60 to 30 minutes with a 0.5% lower mortality. Data were from 43,801 STEMI patients undergoing primary PCI in NCDR (2005-2006). NCDR, national cardiovascular data registry; PCI, percutaneous coronary intervention; STEMI, ST-elevation myocardial infarction. (Modified from Rathore SS, Curtis JP, Chen J, et al. Association of door-to-balloon time and mortality in patients admitted to hospital with ST elevation myocardial infarction: national cohort study. *BMJ.* 2009;338:b1807, with permission from BMJ Publishing Group Ltd.)

myocardial salvage, and survival. Less than half of the US hospitals are capable of performing primary PCI, but 79% of the population lives within 1 hour of a PCI-capable hospital.[15]

In the US, efforts were made to improve the quality of care, reduce hospital treatment delays, and maximize access to primary PCI. These include the continuum of care from EMS activation to transfer to PCI-capable facilities, in addition to the AHA Mission Lifeline and Door-to-Balloon Alliance.[16] These hospitals should have an established treatment plans and algorithms designating how to approach patients with STEMI. The selection of the initial treatment strategy should be based on a predetermined institution-specific plan tailored to the available healthcare system of the community. For patients with STEMI presenting to hospitals without primary PCI capability, the decision should be made whether EMS can safely transfer the patient in a timely fashion to hospital systems equipped with primary PCI capability. If the referring hospital and the receiving PCI hospital have established a protocol that can minimize transfer delays, then transfer for primary PCI is generally recommended. For hospitals without such a plan or if the timeframe cannot be achieved, a decision to initiate fibrinolytic therapy must be made by the treating clinician. Immediate transfer of patients from hospitals without PCI capabilities to PCI-capable facilities following fibrinolysis is recommended as part of a "pharmaco-invasive" approach in high-risk patients. If these patients are not candidates for thrombolytic therapy, or if such treatments fail, a new program focused on interhospital transfers could offer significant benefit, eg, the Mission LifeLine 9-1-1 STAT TRANSFER Program.[17] **Figure 19.3** and **Table 19.3** summarize current recommendations regarding the triage, treatment, and transfer of patients presenting with STEMI.

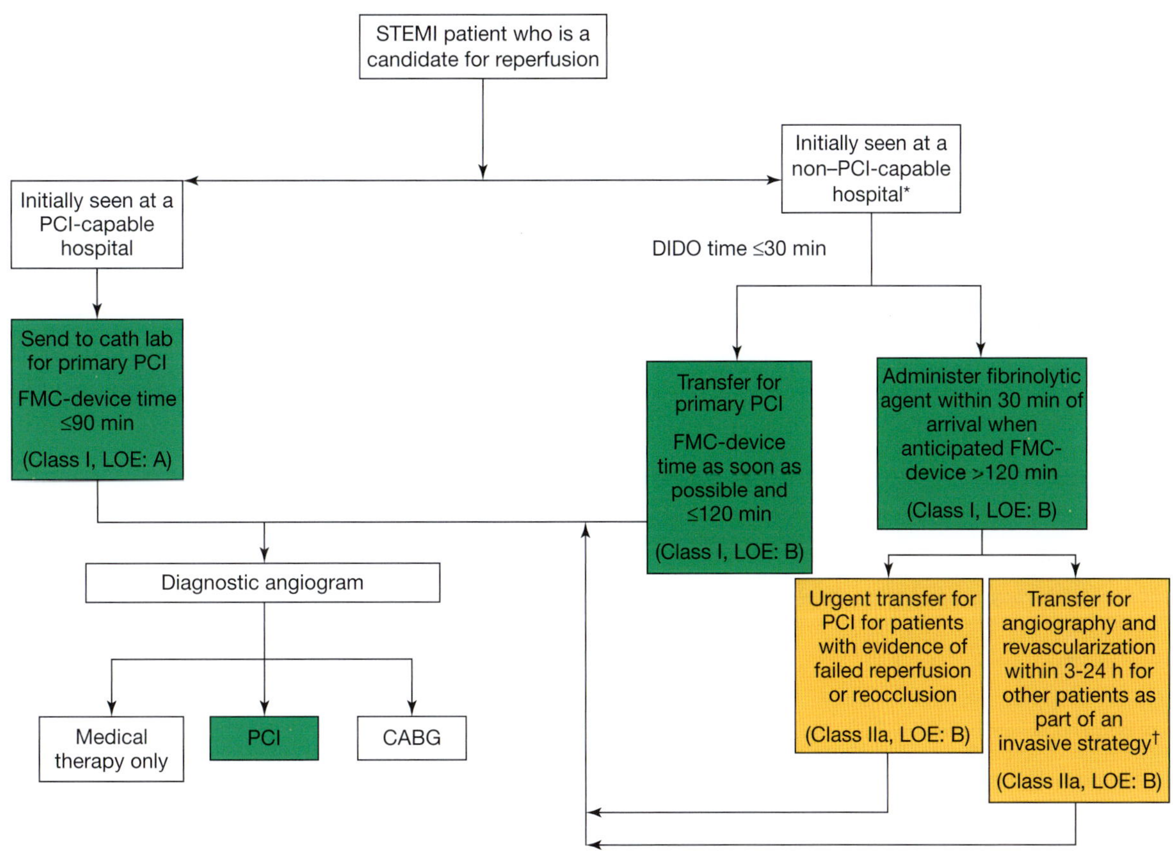

FIGURE 19.3 Guideline recommendations for triage and transfer for PCI in STEMI. Reperfusion therapy for patients with STEMI. The bold arrows and boxes are the preferred strategies. Performance of PCI is dictated by an anatomically appropriate culprit stenosis. *Patients with cardiogenic shock or severe heart failure initially seen at a non-PCI-capable hospital should be transferred for cardiac catheterization and revascularization as soon as possible, irrespective of time delay from MI onset (Class I, LOE: B). †Angiography and revascularization should not be performed within the first 2 to 3 hours after administration of fibrinolytic therapy. CABG, coronary artery bypass graft; DIDO, door-in–door-out; FMC, first medical contact; LOE, level of evidence; MI, myocardial infarction; PCI, percutaneous coronary intervention; and STEMI, ST-elevation myocardial infarction. (From O'Gara PT, Kushner FG, Ascheim DD, et al. 2013 ACCF/AHA guideline for the management of ST-elevation myocardial infarction. *Circulation*. 2013;127(4):e362–e425, with permission.)

Points Helpful to Clinical Practice

1. Delays in time to reperfusion therapies associated with increased mortality rates and MACE are affected by patient, prehospital, and in-hospital factors.
2. Guidelines recommend a time of 90 minutes or less from the first medical contact to balloon angioplasty to perform primary PCI and achieve revascularization.
3. Non–PCI-capable hospitals must have an established treatment plan when approaching patients presenting with STEMI.
4. A decision should be made whether enough time is available for interhospital transfer or if patients should be started on fibrinolytic therapy. When PCI is not available or fibrinolysis fails to achieve successful perfusion, the STAT TRANSFER Program to PCI-capable hospital may provide benefit.

INDICATIONS FOR PRIMARY PCI OF THE INFARCT ARTERY

Nearly all patients with STEMI presenting within 12 hours of symptom onset (with either clinical or ECG evidence of ongoing ischemia (Class I) or with ongoing symptoms of hemodynamic instability or cardiogenic shock (CS) (Class I)) are candidates for primary PCI (including those with true posterior infarcts or other equivocal ECG findings and with a newly occluded artery in a clinical setting consistent with STEMI). Other indications for PCI in patients with STEMI include failed reperfusion after the fibrinolytic therapy (Class I), stability, presenting 12 to 24 hours after symptom onset (Class IIa), or if complications of ischemia, heart failure (HF), or life-threatening arrhythmia (Class IIa) are present.[1]

Only in patients in whom the risk of revascularization outweighs benefit, or when the patient or designee does not agree to the procedure, would PCI be considered inappropriate. The greatest mortality benefit of primary PCI is in patients who present early or are at the highest risk. For example, over the last 20 years, patients with CS complicating their acute myocardial infarction (AMI) have reduced mortality rates following invasive intervention as reported by the SHOCK trial.[18]

Prior clinical practice guidelines recognized that there is an indication for primary PCI in asymptomatic patients presenting between 12 and 24 hours after symptom onset and who are at higher risk (Class IIb). The BRAVE-2 trial and the Prospective National Observational study support this observation. In the BRAVE-2 trial, PCI reduced infarct size in asymptomatic patients with STEMI and symptom onset between 12 and 48 hours before presentation and recorded a reduction in the 4-year mortality rate

TABLE 19.3 Triage and Transfer Decisions for Reperfusion: Recommendations for STEMI Systems of Care

Class I

1. All communities should create and maintain a regional system of STEMI care that includes assessment and continuous quality improvement of EMS and hospital-based activities.[a] Performance can be facilitated by participating in programs such as Mission: Lifeline and the D2B Alliance (LOE B).
   - Destination protocols to STEMI Receiving center
   - Transfer protocols for patients who arrive at STEMI Referral center and are primary PCI candidates, and/or are fibrinolytic ineligible and/or in cardiogenic shock (STEMI Referral Centers)
2. Performance of a 12-lead ECG by EMS personnel at the site of first medical contact (FMC) is recommended in patients with symptoms consistent with STEMI (LOE: B).
3. Reperfusion therapy should be administered to all eligible patients with STEMI with symptom onset within the prior 12 h (LOE: A).
4. Primary PCI is the recommended method of reperfusion when it can be performed in a timely fashion by experienced operators (LOE: A).
5. EMS transport directly to a PCI-capable hospital for primary PCI is the recommended triage strategy for patients with STEMI, with an ideal FMC-to-device time system goal of 90 min or less[b] (LOE: B).
6. Immediate transfer to a PCI-capable hospital for primary PCI is the recommended triage strategy for patients with STEMI who initially arrive at or are transported to a non–PCI-capable hospital, with an FMC-to-device time system goal of 120 min or less[b] (LOE: B).
7. In the absence of contraindications, fibrinolytic therapy should be administered to patients with STEMI at non–PCI-capable hospitals when the anticipated FMC-to-device time at a PCI-capable hospital exceeds 120 min because of unavoidable delays (LOE: B).
8. When fibrinolytic therapy is indicated or chosen as the primary reperfusion strategy, it should be administered within 30 min of hospital arrival[b] (LOE: B).

Class IIa

1. Reperfusion therapy is reasonable for patients with STEMI and symptom onset within the prior 12-24 h who have clinical and/or ECG evidence of ongoing ischemia. Primary PCI is the preferred strategy in this population (LOE: B).

ECG, electrocardiography; EMS, emergency medical services; LOE, level of evidence; PCI, percutaneous coronary intervention; STEMI, ST-elevation myocardial infarction.

Modified from O'Gara PT, Kushner FG, Ascheim DD, et al. 2013 ACCF/AHA guideline for the management of ST-elevation myocardial infarction. *Circulation.* 2013;127(4):e362-e425.

[a]Ensure streamlined care paths that focus on primary PCI as the first-choice treatment for STEMI. Protocols for triage, diagnosis, and cardiac catheterization lab activation should be established within the primary PCI-capable hospitals (STEMI Receiving Centers), process for prehospital identification and activation.

[b]The proposed time windows are system goals. For any individual patient, every effort should be made to provide reperfusion therapy as rapidly as possible.

when compared with conservative strategies.[19] The Prospective National Observational study also reported lower mortality rates in patients with STEMI and symptom onset 12 to 24 hours before presentation.[20] Current revascularization guidelines indicate a Class III (no benefit) for asymptomatic stable patients with STEMI who have a totally occluded infarct artery after symptom onset and have no ischemia.[1] **Table 19.4** summarizes the current guidelines for angiography and primary PCI in patients with STEMI.

Points Helpful to Clinical Practice

1. Patients with STEMI presenting within 12 hours of symptom onset are unstable and suffering from CS or HF, have a failed reperfusion following fibrinolytic therapy, or are stable, and those presenting between 12 and 24 hours after symptom onset are candidates for PCI.
2. Asymptomatic stable patients with a totally occluded infarct artery after symptom onset and no ischemia are not candidates.

TABLE 19.4 Indications for Primary PCI and Angiography in Patients With STEMI

INDICATIONS	COR	LOE
Primary PCI		
STEMI and ischemic symptoms within 12 h	I	A
Hemodynamic instability or cardiogenic shock irrespective of time delay from MI onset	I	B-R
Failed reperfusion after fibrinolytic therapy	I	C-LD
Treated with fibrinolytic therapy, angiography is performed within 3-24 h with the intent to perform PCI	IIa	B-R
Stable, presenting 12-24 h after symptom onset	IIa	B-NR
Complicated by ongoing ischemia, acute severe heart failure, or life-threatening arrhythmia irrespective of time delay from MI onset	IIa	C-EO
Asymptomatic stable patients with a totally occluded infarct artery after symptom onset and no ischemia, PCI should not be performed	III: no benefit	B-R

Updated recommendation from the 2021 ACC/AHA/SCAI guideline for coronary artery revascularization.

COR, class of recommendation; LOE, level of evidence; MI, myocardial infarction; PCI, percutaneous coronary intervention; STEMI, ST-segment elevation.

Modified from Members WC, Lawton JS, Tamis-Holland JE, et al. 2021 ACC/AHA/SCAI guideline for coronary artery revascularization: a report of the American College of Cardiology/American Heart Association Joint Committee on Clinical Practice Guidelines. *J Am Coll Cardiol.* 2022;79(2):e21-e129.

INDICATIONS FOR PRIMARY PCI: NON-INFARCT ARTERY AND IN MULTIVESSEL DISEASE

A substantial number of patients (40%-60%) presenting with STEMI have multivessel disease with significant stenosis in at least one non-IRA. These patients present the operator with several PCI options, including (1) primary PCI of the culprit vessel only, with

PCI of nonculprit arteries only for high-risk features; (2) multivessel PCI at the time of primary PCI; (3) or primary PCI followed by staged PCI of the nonculprit vessels. The previous STEMI guidelines did not recommend PCI of nonculprit vessels at the time of primary PCI in the setting of STEMI and gave a Class III (harmful) recommendation.[21] For a high-risk cohort with CS, the CULPRIT SHOCK trial showed that patients with culprit-only PCI had lower rates of mortality and renal dysfunction after a 30-day follow-up. Recent clinical trials and sub-studies, however, argue for an attempt to achieve complete revascularization because obstructive nonculprit vessel lesions may eventually lead to incident MACE.

The Preventive Angioplasty in Acute Myocardial Infarction (PRAMI) trial (n = 465) showed that patients undergoing multivessel PCI had a lower composite endpoint of cardiac death, nonfatal myocardial infarction (MI), or refractory angina than those undergoing culprit PCI only (**Fig. 19.4**). Similarly, the Complete vs Lesion-Only Primary PCI Trial (CvLPRIT) trial (n = 296) demonstrated a lower composite outcome of death, reinfarction, HF, and ischemia-driven revascularization at 12 months in multivessel PCI during index hospitalization than during culprit-only PCI. The Third Danish Trial in Acute Myocardial Infarction–Primary PCI in Patients With ST-Elevation Myocardial Infarction and Multivessel Disease (DANAMI-3-PRIMULTI) trial (n = 627) compared multivessel PCI guided by angiography and fractional flow reserve (FFR) occurring before discharge versus culprit-artery-only PCI and found the composite primary outcome of all-cause mortality, nonfatal MI, or ischemia-driven revascularization of nonculprit artery occurred in 13% of multivessel PCI versus 22% of culprit-artery-only PCI.[22] The Compare-Acute trial[23] (n = 885) showed that patients had a lower composite endpoint of death, nonfatal MI, revascularization, and stroke, while the Complete vs Culprit-Only Revascularization Strategies to Treat Multivessel Disease after Early PCI for STEMI (COMPLETE) trial (n = 4041) showed that patients had lower composite endpoints of cardiovascular death and nonfatal MI.[24] Finally, the Flow Evaluation to Guide Revascularization in Multivessel ST-Elevation Myocardial Infarction (FLOWER-AMI) trial (n = 1171) showed lower composite endpoints of death, nonfatal MI, and urgent revascularization.[25] **Table 19.5** illustrates additional details on these clinical trials. Taken together, the data on multivessel PCI during STEMI are mixed, but recent randomized controlled trials (RCTs) have suggested benefits either at the time of primary PCI or staged during the index hospitalization.

According to the 2021 AHA/ACC/Society for Cardiovascular Angiography and Interventions (SCAI) revascularization guidelines, patients with STEMI, who have multivessel disease, are hemodynamically stable, and those who have underwent primary PCI are candidates for staged PCI of significant non-IRA stenosis (Class I). Patients who are hemodynamically stable with low-complexity multivessel disease are candidates for PCI of the non-IRA (Class IIb), while patients who have complications like CS are not candidates for PCI of the non-IRA at the same time as the primary PCI (Class III: harm;[1] **Table 19.6**).

Points Helpful to Clinical Practice

1. On various occasions, patients with STEMI present with multivessel disease, creating a debate whether PCI of nonculprit vessels should be performed.
2. Based on results from the CULPRIT SHOCK, only culprit vessel PCI should be performed for patients with STEMI complicated by CS.
3. Based on results from trials such as PRAMI, DANAMI-3-PRIMULTI, COMPARE-ACUTE, COMPLETE, and FLOWER-AMI, patients with multivessel disease, who are hemodynamically stable and have underwent primary PCI, are candidates for staged PCI of significant non-IRA stenosis.
4. Factors that influence the decision to perform complete revascularization include symptoms, clinical stability, and presence of mechanical complications or CS.

SURGICAL AND NONSURGICAL HOSPITALS FOR PRIMARY PCI

Nearly all regions of the US allow PCI (either primary and/or elective) at hospitals without on-site surgery (SOS).[26] Such procedures take place at either office-based laboratories (OBLs) or ambulatory

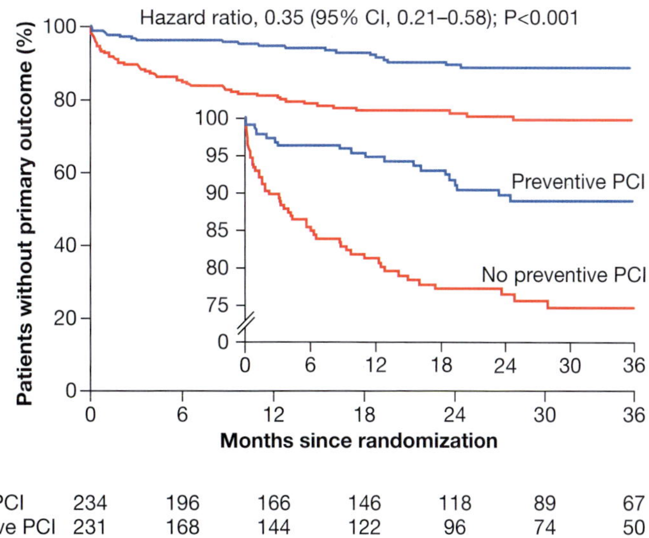

FIGURE 19.4 The primary outcome was a composite of death from cardiac causes, nonfatal myocardial infarction, or refractory angina. The inset graph shows the same data on a larger scale. All patients in the trial underwent infarct-artery PCI immediately before randomization. PCI, percutaneous coronary intervention. (From Wald DS, Morris JK, Wald NJ, et al. Randomized trial of preventive angioplasty in myocardial infarction. *N Engl J Med.* 2013;369(12):1115-1123, with permission.)

TABLE 19.5 Summary of Multivessel PCI Trials

	CVLPRIT			PRIMULTI			PRAMI			COMPARE-ACUTE			COMPLETE			FLOWER AMI			CULPRIT SHOCK		
Non-IRA lesion criteria	>70% DS or >50% DS in two views			>50% DS and FFR <0.80 or >90% DS			>50% DS			>50% DS and FFR = or <0.8			>70% DS or DS 50%-69% and FFR = or <0.8			>50% DS			>70% DS		
Randomization for non-IRA lesions	Immediate or staged complete revascularization (angio-guided) within index admission vs culprit only			Staged complete revascularization (FFR-guided) within index admission vs culprit only			Immediate complete revascularization (angio-guided) vs culprit only			Complete revascularization (FFR-guided) vs culprit only			Complete revascularization (angio-guided) vs culprit only			Complete revascularization (FFR-guided) vs culprit only			Immediate or staged revascularization (angio-guided)		
1° endpoint	D, MI, HF, ischemia-driven revascularization at 1 y			D, MI, ischemia-driven revascularization at 1 y			D, MI or refractory angina			D, MI, Revascularization, Stroke			D, nonfatal MI			D, nonfatal MI, urgent revascularization			D, renal replacement therapy at 30 d		
Results	MV PCI	Culprit-only	*P*	MV PCI	Culprit-only	*P*	MV PCI	Culprit-only	*P*	MV PCI	Culprit-only	*P*	MV PCI	Culprit-only	*P*	MV PCI	Culprit-only	*P*	MV PCI	Culprit-only	*P*
1° endpoint	10%	21.2%	0.009	13%	22%	0.004	9%	23%	<0.001	8%	21%	<0.001	7.8%	10.5%	0.004	5.5%	4.2%	0.31	55.4%	45.9%	0.01
Death	1%	4%	0.14	5%	4%	0.43	1.7%	4.3%	0.07	1.4%	1.7%	0.7	4.8%	5.2%	-	1.5%	1.7%	-	51.6%	43.3%	0.03
Reinfarction	1%	3%	0.39	5%	5%	0.87	3%	8.6%	0.009	-	-	-	-	-		5.5%	3.3%	-	-	-	-
Heart failure	3%	6%	0.14	-	-	-	-	-	-	-	-	-	2.9%	1.0%	-	1.5%	1.9%	-	-	-	-
Revascularization	5%	8%	0.20	5%	17%	17%	6.8%	19.9	<0.001	6.1%	17.5%	<0.001	1.4%	0.5%	-	2.6%	1.9%	-	3.8%	21.5%	<0/001
Renal replacement	-	-	-	-	-	-	-	-	-	-	-	-	-	-	-	-	-	-	16.4%	11.6%	0.07

D, death; DS, diameter stenosis; FFR, fractional flow reserve; HF, heart failure; IRA, infarct-related artery; MI, myocardial infarction; MV PCI, multi-vessel percutaneous coronary intervention.
Derived from Alasnag MA, Al-Shaibi KF. *PCI for Multivessel Disease in STEMI*. American College of Cardiology.

TABLE 19.6 Indications for PCI of the Non-Infarct-Related Artery and in Multivessel Disease in Patients With STEMI

COR	LOE	RECOMMENDATION
I	A	Patients with STEMI and multivessel disease who are hemodynamically stable and who have underwent primary PCI are candidates for staged PCI of significant non-IRA stenosis
IIB	B-R	Patients who are hemodynamically stable with low-complexity multivessel disease are candidates for PCI of the non-IRA
III: Harm	B-R	Patients who have complications like CS are not candidates for PCI of the non-IRA at the same time as the primary PCI

Updated recommendation from the 2021 ACC/AHA/SCAI guideline for coronary artery revascularization.
COR, class of recommendation; CS, cardiogenic shock; IRA, infarct-related artery; LOE, level of evidence; PCI, percutaneous coronary intervention; STEMI, ST-segment elevation.
Modified from Members WC, Lawton JS, Tamis-Holland JE, et al. 2021 ACC/AHA/SCAI guideline for coronary artery revascularization: a report of the American College of Cardiology/American Heart Association Joint Committee on Clinical Practice Guidelines. *J Am Coll Cardiol*. 2022;79(2):e21-e129.

surgery centers (ASCs).[27] The 2014 SCAI guidelines refer to primary PCI without SOS as Class IIa. These guidelines dictate that primary PCI without surgical backup should not be performed at institutions without a proven plan for rapid transport to a cardiac surgery hospital or without appropriate hemodynamic support capability for transfer (Class III: harm).[28] They also focus on volume-outcome relationships: (a) Volume threshold of 50 PCIs for an individual operator is needed, (b) optimal threshold for institutional volume of PCI should be >400 annually (Class I), (c) volumes of 200 to 400 PCIs/year are acceptable (Class IIa), (d) primary PCI is not recommended (Class III: no benefit) at low-volume hospitals (<200/y) by low-volume operators (<50/y), and (e) hospitals performing <36 PCIs/y are classified as not having PCI capabilities.[29]

However, recent advancements in the operators' experience, procedural techniques, equipment, and pharmacotherapeutics resulted in a change in consensus on best practices for PCI in hospital without surgical backup. In 2023, SCAI published an updated consensus document that incorporates factors such as patients' clinical and lesion risks, the rescue capability of the site for select cases, and the experience of the operator.[26] These updated recommendations are summarized in **Tables 19.7** and **19.8**. Recent studies have shown noninferiority of PCI in non-SOS hospitals compared to centers equipped for cardiac surgeries. For example, the mortality rates observed with PCI were either similar or lower in the non-SOS hospitals than those in hospitals quipped for cardiac surgeries.[30-32] To conclude, advancements in PCI techniques, operator expertise, and improvement in devices allow PCI in hospitals without an on-sight cardiac surgery setting if certain safety measures are in place within the system.

Points Helpful to Clinical Practice

1. Almost all regions in the US allow PCI to be performed at SOS.
2. The 2014 SCAI guidelines Class II recommendations refer to PCI in the absence of SOS, while Class III refers to PCI being performed in institutions that lack the ability to

TABLE 19.7 PCI Without On-Site Surgery: Recommendations for Patient Selection Based on SCAI Consensus Document on PCI Without On-Site Surgical Backup

	OBL/ASC	LEVEL 1 NON-SOS	LEVEL 2 NON-SOS	CARDIAC SURGERY FACILITY
Facility characteristics	Lacking ICU, blood bank, and code team	Low volume (<200 PCIs/year)	ICU, radiology, anesthesia, OR, multiple catheterization labs, experienced interventional cardiologists, well-staffed team (>4/room)	Multiple ORs, catheterization labs, structural heart procedures experienced interventional cardiologists, well-staffed team, and on-call cardiac surgeon and perfusionist Shock team
Rescue and support capabilities	IABP	IABP	IABP, pVAD, ECMO, vascular and/or thoracic surgery	IABP, pVAD, cardiopulmonary bypass, with or without ECMO, RVAD, LVAD, and transplantation
Plaque modification devices	Cutting balloon or IVL	Cutting balloon or IVL	Cutting balloon, IVL, rotational atherectomy, and orbital atherectomy	Cutting balloon, IVL, rotational atherectomy, and orbital atherectomy
Avoid intervention	High transfusion risk, calcified lesions atherectomy, low EF, CTO, unprotected left main, and degenerated vein grafts	Calcified lesion atherectomy, low EF, CTO, unprotected left main, and degenerated vein grafts	Epicardial retrograde CTO or last remaining vessel	

ASC, ambulatory surgery centers; CTO, chronic total occlusion; ECMO, extracorporeal membrane oxygenation; EF, ejection fraction; IABP, intra-aortic balloon pump; ICU, intensive care unit; IVL, intravascular lithotripsy; LVAD, left ventricular assist device; OBL, office-based laboratories; OR, operating room; PCI, percutaneous coronary intervention; pVAD, percutaneous ventricular assist device; RVAD, right ventricular assist device; SCAI, Society for Cardiovascular Angiography and Interventions; SOS, on-site surgery.
Modified from Grines CL, Box LC, Mamas MA, et al. SCAI expert consensus statement on percutaneous coronary intervention without on-site surgical backup. *Cardiovasc Interv*. 2023;16(7):847-860.

TABLE 19.8 Operator Experience to Perform PCI in Patient Presenting With ST-Elevation Myocardial Infarction Based on SCAI Consensus Document on PCI Without On-Site Surgical Backup

NEW (<3 Y)	EXPERIENCED (3-10 Y)	VERY EXPERIENCED (>10 Y)
Limited in judgment, guidelines, STEMI/shock experience, and use of atherectomy devices	Good judgment, familiar with guidelines, intermediate STEMI/shock experience, adequate use of atherectomy devices	Good judgment, familiar with guidelines, significant STEMI/shock experience, extensive use of atherectomy devices
Should avoid ASCs and independent atherectomy cases, ask colleague for case selection review	Performs procedures independently	Performs procedures independently

ASC, ambulatory surgery centers; PCI, percutaneous coronary intervention; SCAI, Society for Cardiovascular Angiography and Interventions; STEMI, ST-segment elevation myocardial infarction.

Modified from Grines CL, Box LC, Mamas MA, et al. SCAI expert consensus statement on percutaneous coronary intervention without on-site surgical backup. *Cardiovasc Interv.* 2023;16(7):847-860.

transport patients to a cardiac surgery hospital or to maintain hemodynamic stability prior to transfer.

3. The same guidelines discuss volume-outcome relations, with Class I referring to >400 PCIs/y, Class IIa referring to 200 to 400 PCIs/y, and Class III referring to <200 PCIs/y. Hospitals performing <36 PCIs/y do not have PCI capabilities.
4. A more recent SCAI consensus document provided guidance on performing elective PCI in hospitals with no SOS and focused on factors that influence patient selection including clinical lesion risk characteristics, operators' experience, and rescue treatment plan at the performing facility.

PCI FOLLOWING FIBRINOLYSIS

PCI can be performed in a number of different scenarios following fibrinolysis. Changes in PCI availability, evolution of triage and transfer capabilities, and research in pharmacologic therapy have allowed the evolution of a number of terms in parallel, including "rescue PCI," "facilitated PCI," and "pharmacoinvasive PCI." These strategies are summarized in **Table 19.9**. Failed fibrinolysis can be recognized by ongoing symptoms or failure of ECG evidence of reperfusion. ECG evidence of failed reperfusion is most easily made by <50% resolution of ST-segment elevation in the anterior leads or <70% in the inferior leads. Chest pain is not a requirement of failed reperfusion.[8] Immediate PCI, referred to as rescue PCI or rescue angioplasty, is used when fibrinolytic therapies fail. When compared to conservative treatments, reduced cardiovascular events such as recurrent MIs and repeat revascularization, improved event-free survival, but increased bleeding and stroke rates are recorded in rescue PCI.[11]

Facilitated PCI is a strategy for patients with STEMI that combines fibrinolytic therapy followed by PCI at hospitals without PCI capabilities, with the ideal interval between these approaches being <2 hours. The "facilitated PCI" term is no longer used in current guidelines.[3] Multiple regimens have been studied in clinical trials. Pharmacologic regimens have included full-dose or reduced-dose fibrinolytic therapy and the combination of a glycoprotein (GP) IIb/IIIa inhibitor with a reduced-dose fibrinolytic agent (eg, a fibrinolytic dose typically reduced 50%) and GP IIb/IIIa inhibitors alone. Facilitated PCI is inferior when compared to primary PCI according to a number of studies. In fact, this approach has the potential to introduce harm by increasing the risk of MACE. The Assessment of the Safety and Efficacy of a New Treatment Strategy with Percutaneous Coronary Intervention 4 (ASSENT-4) study compared up-front full-dose tenecteplase followed by PCI with primary PCI. The study was prematurely terminated because of increased in-hospital mortality, CHF, and shock within a 3-month period. On the basis of these outcomes, facilitated PCI is no longer recommended by clinical practice guidelines.[33]

A safer and more effective approach to revascularization is the pharmacoinvasive, also known as the delayed PCI. Unlike the facilitated approach where the ideal time between thrombolytic therapy and PCI at hospitals without PCI capabilities is <2 hours, the time for the pharmacoinvasive approach is between 2 and 24 hours. Current guidelines (Class IIa) recommend the transfer of high-risk patients who receive fibrinolytic therapy as primary reperfusion therapy at a facility without PCI capabilities to a PCI-capable

TABLE 19.9 Definitions of PCI for Patient Presenting With ST-Elevation Myocardial Infarction

Primary PCI
PCI used as the primary reperfusion method in patients with STEMI.
Rescue Angioplasty
PCI following the use of fibrinolysis for STEMI, when based on evidence of failed reperfusion by fibrinolysis. Generally, this requires time for fibrinolysis (60-90 min) to allow time for reperfusion and assessment of reperfusion to determine the need for PCI.
Facilitated Angioplasty
A strategy of planned immediate PCI after administration of an initial pharmacologic regimen intended to improve coronary patency before the emergency PCI procedure. A strategy upstream use of a pharmacologic therapy to "facilitate" primary PCI.
Early Routine Angioplasty/Pharmacoinvasive Approach
Immediate referral for PCI (following initial fibrinolytic therapy). Performed within several hours after fibrinolytic administration, regardless of whether or not clinical or electrocardiographic evidence of ongoing myocardial injury is present. Generally applies to patients presenting to hospitals without primary PCI who cannot undergo timely primary PCI. Sometimes referred to as "delayed" PCI, or as "immediate" PCI after administration of fibrinolysis at non–PCI-capable facilities.
Delayed Angioplasty in STEMI
The angioplasty is delayed, either due to delays from transport to a PCI facility or the choice of initial fibrinolysis for reperfusion.

PCI, percutaneous coronary intervention; STEMI, ST-segment elevation myocardial infarction.

facility as soon as possible, where PCI can be performed either when needed or as a pharmacoinvasive strategy. Transfer of all patients, regardless of risk, who receive fibrinolytic therapy as primary reperfusion therapy at facilities without PCI capabilities may also be considered (Class IIb) for transfer as soon as possible to a PCI-capable facility, where PCI can be performed when needed or as part of a pharmacoinvasive strategy.[34] Recommendations are primarily based on the two largest studies, CARESS and TRANSFER-AMI[3] (**Figs. 19.5** and **19.6**). Bleeding risk is an obvious concern when performing PCI after fibrinolysis; nevertheless, radial access, improvements in equipment, and adjunctive pharmacotherapies have improved success rates, while keeping bleeding risks low. TRANSFER-AMI and a large meta-analysis have not observed a significantly increased risk of TIMI major bleeding, although minor bleeding increased.[35]

Points Helpful to Clinical Practice

1. PCI can be performed following fibrinolysis through either rescue PCI or pharmacoinvasive PCI.
2. Rescue PCI is performed when fibrinolysis fails; pharmacoinvasive PCI is performed when the time between fibrinolysis and PCI is between 2 and 24 hours, and this approach generally carries favorable outcomes.
3. Facilitated PCI is no longer recommended due its adverse events when PCI is performed in hospitals without PCI capabilities and the time between fibrinolysis and PCI is less than 2 hours.

PCI FOR LATE-ARRIVING STEMI PATIENTS

The Occluded Artery Trial (OAT) trial tested the hypothesis that routine PCI for total occlusion 3 to 28 days after MI would reduce the composite of death, reinfarction, or Class IV HF in otherwise stable patients. The minimal time from symptom onset to angiography in patients with a total occlusion of the IRA (TIMI grade 0 or 1) was just over 24 hours. Important exclusion criteria were New York Heart Association (NYHA) Class III or IV HF, resting angina, renal impairment, left main or three-vessel disease, clinical instability, or severe inducible ischemia on stress testing. The 4-year cumulative endpoint was 17% in the PCI group and 16% in the medical therapy group (hazard ratio (HR) 1.16; 95% confidence interval (CI) 0.92-1.45; P = .2). Reinfarction rates tended to be higher in the PCI group, which may have attenuated any benefit in left ventricular (LV) remodeling.[36] Total Occlusion Study of Canada (TOSCA-2), an angiographic sub-study of OAT, demonstrated high success rates of IRA reperfusion but no significant benefit. These two studies demonstrate that elective PCI of an occluded infarct artery 1 to 28 days after MI in stable patients with single- or double-vessel disease had no incremental benefit beyond optimal medical therapy (aspirin, β-blockers, angiotensin-converting enzyme (ACE) inhibitors, and statins) in preserving LV function and preventing subsequent cardiovascular events.[37] It should be noted that delayed PCI of the IRA is indicated in patients who become unstable because of the development of CS, acute severe HF, or unstable postinfarction angina. Delayed PCI can also be performed in patients who did not receive reperfusion therapy but who did demonstrate significant residual ischemia during hospitalization. The DANAMI trial[38] evaluated the benefit of angioplasty in patients with residual ischemia following fibrinolysis. A total of 1008 patients, with inducible ischemia after fibrinolytic therapy for a first AMI, were randomized to

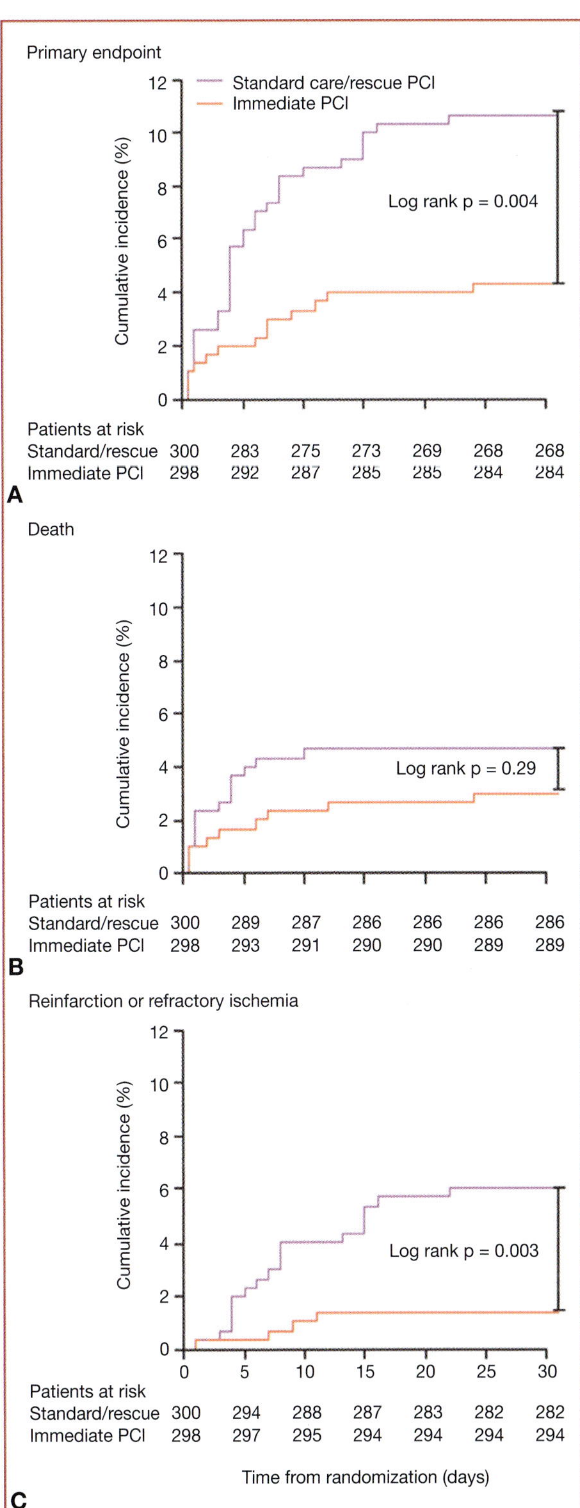

FIGURE 19.5 Results from the CARESS-in-AMI study: immediate transfer for PCI versus standard medical therapy with transfer as needed for rescue PCI, following fibrinolysis in STEMI patients presenting to hospitals without PCI capability. Shown are Kaplan–Meier event curves for the primary outcome (with 95% CI) **(A)**, for death **(B)**, and for reinfarction, refractory ischemia, or both **(C)**. Primary outcome was a composite of death, reinfarction, or refractory ischemia at 30 days. PCI, percutaneous coronary intervention; STEMI, ST-elevation myocardial infarction. (From Di Mario C, Dudek D, Piscione F, et al. Immediate angioplasty vs standard therapy with rescue angioplasty after thrombolysis in the Combined Abciximab REteplase Stent Study in Acute Myocardial Infarction (CARESS-in-AMI): an open, prospective, randomised, multicentre trial. *Lancet.* 2008;371:559-568, with permission.)

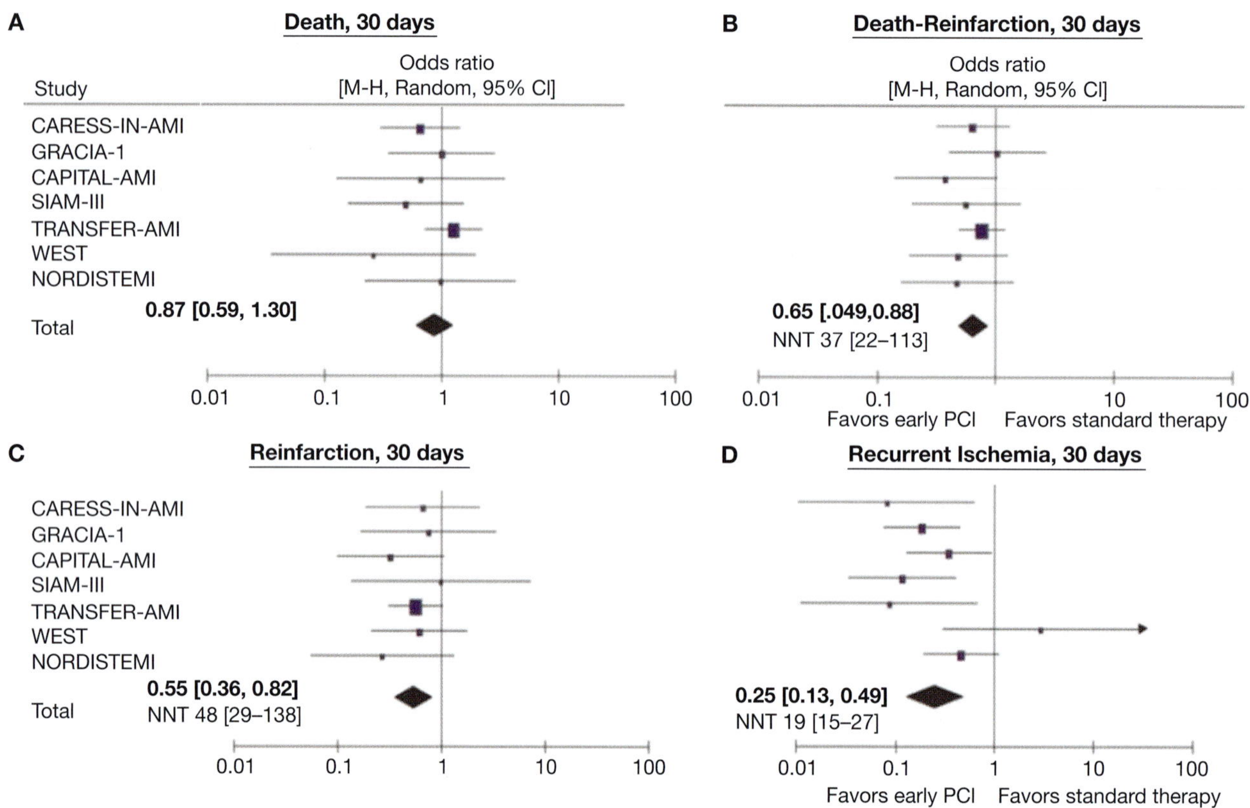

FIGURE 19.6 Meta-analysis of rescue PCI versus conservative therapy. Efficacy endpoints for rescue PCI versus conservative therapy. Clinical end points at 30 days for **(A)** death, **(B)** death and reinfarction, **(C)** reinfarction, and **(D)** recurrent ischemia. AMI, acute myocardial infarction; CARESS, Clopidogrel and Aspirin for Reduction of Emboli in Symptomatic Carotid Stenosis; CI, confidence interval; NNT, number needed to treat; PCI, percutaneous coronary intervention. (From Borgia F, Goodman SG, Halvorsen S, et al. Early routine percutaneous coronary intervention after fibrinolysis vs. standard therapy in ST-segment elevation myocardial infarction: a meta-analysis. *Eur Heart J.* 2010;31(17):2156-2169.)

conservative care or to catheterization followed by revascularization with balloon angioplasty or coronary artery bypass grafting (CABG) surgery. At 2.4 years of follow-up (median), mortality was 4% in the invasive treatment group and 4% in the conservative treatment group (P = NS). Invasive treatment was associated with a lower incidence of reinfarction (5.6% vs 10.5%; $P = .0038$) and a lower incidence of admission for unstable angina (17.9% vs 29.5%; $P < .001$). The primary endpoint (composite endpoint of death, reinfarction, or readmission for unstable angina) was 15.4% and 29.5% at 1 year, 23.5% and 36.6% at 2 years, and 31.7% and 44.0% at 4 years ($P \leq .001$) in the invasive and conservative treatment groups, respectively. The study supports the use of delayed or elective PCI in patients, following fibrinolysis with inducible ischemia (Class IIa). Patients with objective evidence of recurrent MI or spontaneous or provocable ischemia during recovery from STEMI are also suitable candidates (Class I). PCI can be beneficial when performed hours, days, or weeks after successful fibrinolytic therapy, by reducing unstable angina, reinfarction, and long-term mortality. PCI of a hemodynamically significant stenosis >24 hours after STEMI in a patent infarct artery, as part of a revascularization strategy, has been shown to improve contemporary outcomes.[39] In a large Danish registry of over 20,000 STEMI patients, early revascularization (within 14 days) in individuals with AMI was associated with a substantial reduction in 1-year mortality.[40] A summary of indications for PCI in patients who were managed with fibrinolytics or who did not receive reperfusion therapy is listed in **Table 19.10**.

TABLE 19.10 Indications for PCI of an Infarct Artery in Patients Who Were Managed With Fibrinolytic Therapy or Who Did Not Receive Reperfusion Therapy

	COR	LOE
Cardiogenic shock or acute severe HF	I	B
Intermediate- or high-risk findings on predischarge noninvasive ischemia testing	I	C
Spontaneous or easily provoked myocardial ischemia	I	C
Patients with evidence of failed reperfusion or re-occlusion after fibrinolytic therapy (as soon as possible)	IIa	B
Stable[a] patients after successful fibrinolysis, ideally between 3 and 24 h	IIa	B
Stable[a] patients >24 h after successful fibrinolysis	IIb	B
Delayed PCI of a totally occluded infarct artery >24 h after STEMI in stable patients	III: no benefit	B

COR, class of recommendation; HF, heart failure; LOE, level of evidence; PCI, percutaneous coronary intervention; STEMI, ST-elevation myocardial infarction.
From O'Gara PT, Kushner FG, Ascheim DD, et al. 2013 ACCF/AHA guideline for the management of ST-elevation myocardial infarction. *Circulation.* 2013;127(4):e362-e425.
[a]Although individual circumstances will vary, clinical stability is defined by the absence of low output, hypotension, persistent tachycardia, apparent shock, high-grade ventricular or symptomatic supraventricular tachyarrhythmias, and spontaneous recurrent ischemia.

Points Helpful to Clinical Practice

1. PCI of an occluded infarct artery 1 to 28 days after MI in stable patients with single- or double-vessel disease has no incremental benefit beyond optimal medical therapy in preserving LV function and preventing subsequent cardiovascular events.
2. Delayed PCI of the IRA is indicated in unstable patients due to the development of CS, acute severe HF, or unstable postinfarction angina or in patients who did not receive reperfusion therapy but demonstrated significant residual ischemia during hospitalization.

PCI VS CABG REVASCULARIZATION AND CABG IN STEMI

Not infrequently, a patient is brought to the catheterization lab, and diagnostic angiography demonstrates a reperfused vessel with adequate flow (TIMI 3 flow).[41] If the patient is asymptomatic and there is no evidence of ongoing ischemia, CHF, or instability, then there is a window for careful decision utilizing the heart team regarding the optimal approach to revascularization. Based on the 2021 ACC/AHA/SCAI guidelines, CABG is preferred over PCI in patients with coronary artery disease (CAD) who require revascularization for significant left main involvement associated with high-complexity (Class I) or revascularization for multivessel CAD with complex and diffuse CAD (SYNTAX score ≥33) (Class IIa).[42]

For patients with STEMI, emergency CABG surgery can either be a primary reperfusion strategy or can follow primary PCI. CABG is performed in patients with STEMI who are hemodynamically unstable or suffering from CS, when PCI is not feasible (Class I), in patients with STEMI who have certain mechanical complications (eg, ventricular septal rupture, mitral valve insufficiency due to papillary muscle rupture or infarction, or free-wall rupture; Class I), or when a large area of the myocardium is at risk and PCI is not feasible (Class IIa).[43] CABG should not be performed in patients with STEMI, when (1) primary PCI has failed and there is absence of ischemia or a large area of myocardium at risk; (2) surgical revascularization is not feasible due to poor distal targets; or (3) if there is no reflow (Class III: harm).[1] **Table 19.11** summarizes the recommendations for CABG surgery utilization in patients presenting with STEMI.

Points Helpful to Clinical Practice

1. While PCI remains the standard approach to revascularization in patients with STEMI, certain conditions may favor the use of CABG instead.
2. Such conditions include hemodynamic instability, CS, or large areas of myocardial at risk when PCI is not being feasible and mechanical complications of MI.

BALLOON ANGIOPLASTY VERSUS STENTING IN PRIMARY PCI

In the last two decades, randomized clinical trials and numerous comprehensive meta-analyses demonstrated superior outcomes associated with primary PCI using stenting compared to plain old balloon angioplasty. Such outcomes focused on reduced reinfarction risks and mortality rates, where stenting recorded 5% reocclusion rates compared to 15% in percutaneous transluminal coronary angioplasty (PTCA). Similarly, stenting reduced the incidence of overall major adverse cardiac events (MACEs; OR 0.49 [0.40-0.59]), primarily driven by a significant reduction in target vessel revascularization (TVR; OR 0.44 [0.36-0.54]) with a nonsignificant trend toward a decrease in reinfarction[44,45] (**Fig. 19.7**). However, primary PCI with stenting still carries long-term risk of thrombosis due to the presence of a permanent implant and risk of bleeding due to dual antiplatelet therapy (DAPT).

TABLE 19.11 Recommendations for CABG as a Primary Revascularization Strategy in Patient Presenting With STEMI

COR	LOE	RECOMMENDATION
I	B-R	Patients who are hemodynamically unstable or suffering from CS, when PCI is not feasible
I	B-NR	Patients who have certain mechanical complications (eg, ventricular septal rupture, mitral valve insufficiency due to papillary muscle rupture or infarction, or free wall rupture)
IIa	B-NR	Patients with a large area of the myocardium is at risk and PCI is not feasible
III: Harm	C-EO	Patients for whom primary PCI failed, in the absence of ischemia or large area of myocardium being at risk, or if surgical revascularization is not feasible due to poor distal targets or if there is no reflow

Updated recommendation from the 2021 ACC/AHA/SCAI guideline for coronary artery revascularization.
CABG, coronary artery bypass graft; COR, class of recommendation; CS, cardiogenic shock; LOE, level of evidence; PCI, percutaneous coronary intervention; STEMI, ST-segment elevation.
Modified from Members WC, Lawton JS, Tamis-Holland JE, et al. 2021 ACC/AHA/SCAI guideline for coronary artery revascularization: a report of the American College of Cardiology/American Heart Association Joint Committee on Clinical Practice Guidelines. *J Am Coll Cardiol*. 2022;79(2):e21-e129.

Recent trials have focused on a possible alternative for stenting with reduced long-term effects and need for DAPT. The REVELATION randomized trial explored the safety and efficacy of paclitaxel-coated balloon angioplasties. Its findings identified the drug-coated balloon angioplasty (DCB) to be safe and efficient, as well as noninferior to drug-eluted stents (DES) in terms of FFR at 9 months following PCI.[46] Such findings indicate that while additional research is needed for the use of DCB, an alternative to permanent implants with similar results might come into play.

Points Helpful to Clinical Practice

1. In the past *two* decades, multiple studies have shown that primary PCI using stenting is superior to plain old balloon angioplasty during STEMI.
2. Long-term thrombotic due to permanent implants and bleeding risk due to DAPT during primary PCI with stenting are small but not insignificant.
3. Recent trials have showed noninferiority of DCB when compared to DES, shedding the light on future alternative therapies for select patients presenting with STEMI.

COMPARISON BETWEEN DES AND BARE-METAL STENTS IN PRIMARY PCI

As previously discussed, stent placement in a highly thrombogenic milieu of the IRA may predispose to acute or late-stent thrombosis. The higher risk of stent thrombosis with both bare-metal stents (BMSs) and DESs is seen in patients with STEMI compared to

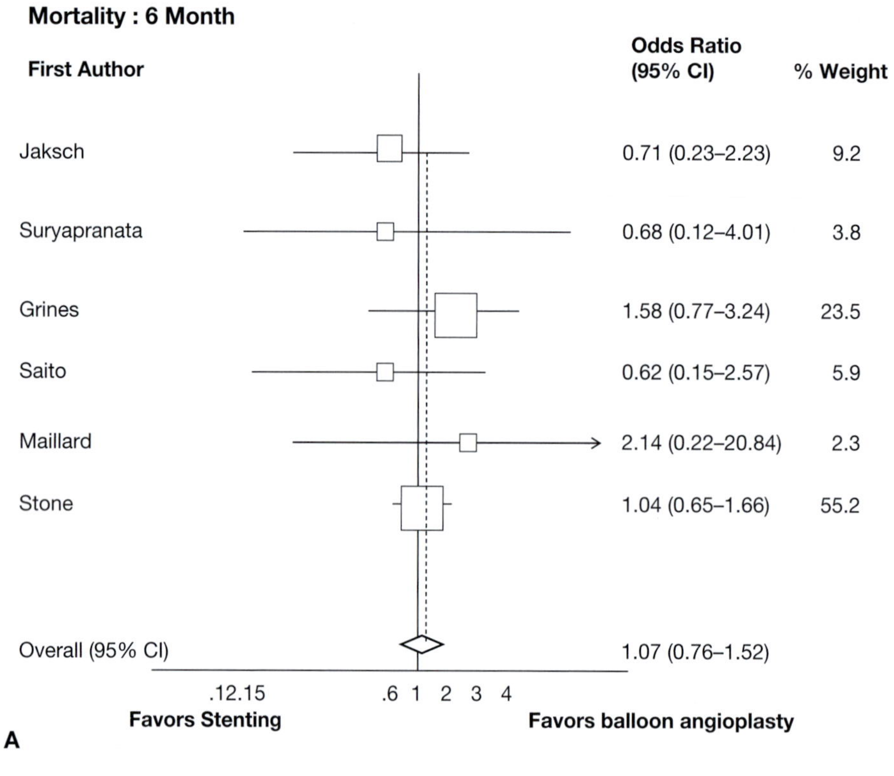

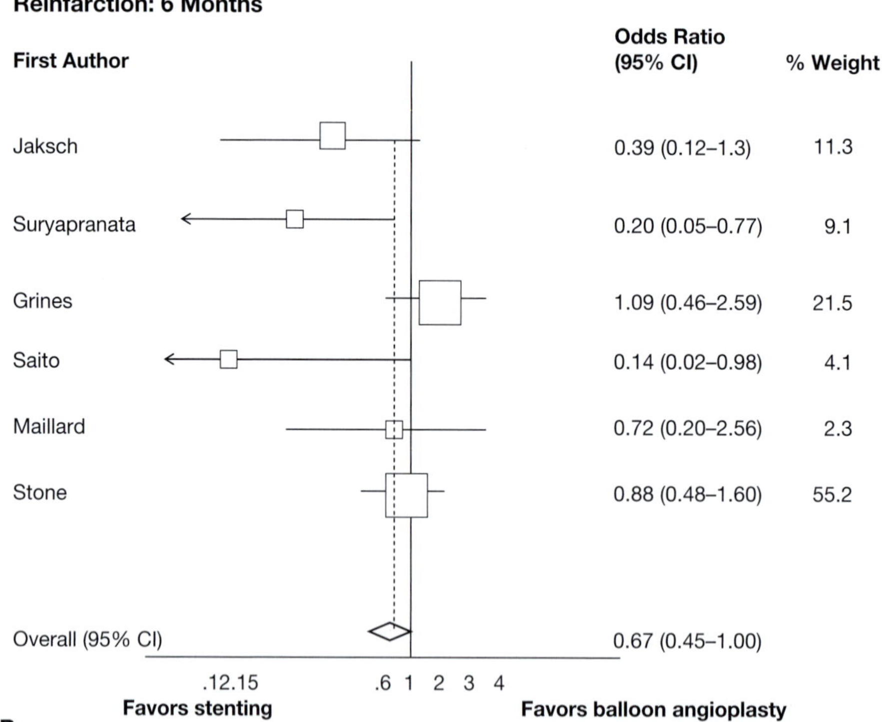

FIGURE 19.7 Bare-metal stenting versus balloon angioplasty for STEMI. Meta-analysis results (6 months) comparing patients with myocardial infarction who were treated with primary stenting versus balloon angioplasty. **A.** Odds ratios for mortality. **B.** Odds ratio for reinfarction.

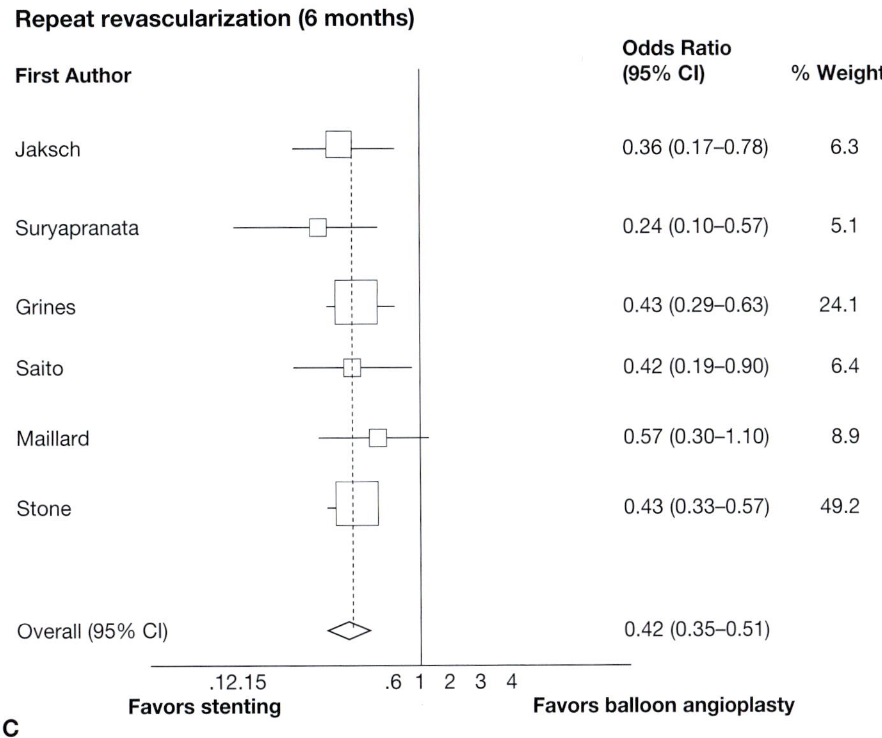

FIGURE 19.7 (*continued*) **C.** Odds ratios for repeat revascularization. CI, confidence interval; STEMI, ST-elevation myocardial infarction. (From Nordmann AJ, Hengstler P, Harr T, Young J, Bucher HC. Clinical outcomes of primary stenting vs balloon angioplasty in patients with myocardial infarction: a meta-analysis of randomized controlled trials. *Am J Med.* 2004;116:253-262, with permission.)

elective PCI. Other lesion and patient subsets also have higher rates of thrombosis: smaller arteries (<2.5 mm diameter), longer lesions, bifurcations, and diabetic vessels. These risk factors predict both stent thrombosis and restenosis. The greatest risk of stent thrombosis is within the first 30 days with BMS and within the first year with DES. Because the risk of stent thrombosis caused by BMSs is greatest within the first 30 days after implantation, the use of thienopyridine (in addition to aspirin) is necessary for a minimum of 30 days. When BMS are placed in the setting of STEMI, 1 year of DAPT is recommended (Class I), and aspirin should be continued indefinitely. As for DES, the greatest risk of thrombosis is due to early discontinuation of DAPT, associated with stent thrombosis rehospitalization and death.[47,48] In the Premier Registry, a surprisingly high number of DES-treated MI patients (13.6%) stopped their thienopyridine within 30 days. Patients who stopped this therapy by 30 days were more likely to die during the next year (7.5% vs 0.7%; $P < .0001$; adjusted HR 9.0; 95% CI 1.3-60.6) or to be re-hospitalized (23% vs 14%; $P = .08$; adjusted HR > 1.5; 95% CI 0.78-3.0).[49]

When comparing DESs and BMSs, DESs significantly reduce intimal proliferation, restenosis, and the need for TVR more than BMSs.[18] In the acute setting of STEMI, a constant debate exists in practice on the safety of the route used of DES placement. The safety and efficacy of DES in STEMI has been evaluated through prospective registries, RCT, and meta-analysis. The prevailing consensus is that while DES did not mark reduce mortality risk compared with BMS, they do mitigate the risk of restenosis, as evidenced by target lesion revascularization (TLR) and TVR. However, stent thrombosis remains a small but significant concern. As a result, second-generation DESs were developed with novel biodegradable polymers in an attempt to reduce such risks; however, long-term clinical outcomes are yet to address these concerns.[50] Findings pertaining to DES and BMS readmission and mortality in patients with STEMI remain limited. In terms of readmission, DES has lower rates than BMS (15.3% compared to 24.3%) based on nonrandomized data collected in 47,334 patients from the Nationwide Readmission Database in 2016. The same sample indicated that the mortality rates were 5.5% after 6 months in DES patients compared to 10.3% in BMS patients.[51] Data from other studies record conflicting findings in terms of mortality. The GRACE registry on 5093 patients with STEMI showed propensity and risk-adjusted mortality that were similar between BMS and DES up to 6 months, but late postdischarge mortality was higher in DES patients from 6 months to 2 years (HR 4.90; $P = .01$) or from 1 to 2 years (HR: 7.06; $P = .02$).[45] In contrast, a registry for Massachusetts State data, including 7217 patients with STEMI, described in a matched-paired analysis that the 2-year risk-adjusted mortality was lower for patients who received a DES than for those who received a BMS among patients with STEMI (8.5% vs 11.6%; $P = .008$).[44] The HORIZONS-AMI study randomized (in a 3:1 ratio) 3006 patients presenting with ST-segment elevation MI to receive paclitaxel-eluting stents or otherwise identical BMSs. The trial showed that placement of a paclitaxel-eluting stent rather than a BMS reduced the 1-year rates of ischemia-driven repeat-target lesion (4.5% vs 7.5%; HR 0.59; 95% CI 0.43-0.83; $P = .002$) and TVR (5.8% vs 8.7%; HR 0.65; 95% CI 0.48-0.89; $P = .006$), with no significant difference in rates of the composite safety endpoint (stent thrombosis, reinfarction, stroke, or death). Patients had similar 12-month rates of death and stent thrombosis. The rate of 13-month angiographic binary restenosis was significantly decreased by DES compared with BMS (10.0% vs 22.9%; HR 0.44; 95% CI 0.33-0.57; $P < .001$; **Table 19.12**). Results at 3 years demonstrated that the use of paclitaxel-eluting stents significantly reduced the 3-year rates of ischemia-driven TLR from 15.1% to 9.4% (40% relative reduction;

TABLE 19.12 Drug-Eluting Stents Compared With Bare-Metal Stents: 1- and 3-Year Results From the HORIZONS-AMI Study

	DES PACLITAXEL-ELUTING STENTS (%)	BMS	*P*	HAZARD RATIO (95% CI)
Ischemia-Driven Target Lesion Revascularization				
1 y	4.5	7.5	0.002	0.59 (0.43-0.83)
3 y	9.4	15.1	<0.0001	0.60 (0.48-0.76)
Ischemia-Driven Target Vessel Revascularization				
1 y	5.8	8.7	0.006	0.65 (0.48-0.89)
3 y	12.4	17	0.0003	
Death				
1 y	3.5	3.5	0.98	
3 y	5.6	6.6	0.31	
Reinfarction				
1 y	3.7	4.5	0.31	
3 y	7.0	6.6	0.77	
Death or Reinfarction				
1 y	6.8	7.0	0.83	
3 y	11.8	11.5	0.88	
Stroke				
1 y	1.0	0.7	0.39	
3 y	1.6	1.4	0.70	
Stent Thrombosis (Definite or Probable)				
1 y	3.2	3.4	0.77	
3 y	4.8	4.3	0.63	1.10 (0.74-1.65)
Safety MACE (Death, Reinfarction, Stroke, and Stent Thrombosis)				
1 y	8.1	8.0	0.92	1.02 (0.76-1.36)
3 y	13.6	12.9	0.66	

BMS, bare-metal stent; CI, confidence interval; DES, drug-eluting stent; MACE, major adverse cardiac events; TLR, target lesion revascularization.

Data taken from Stone GW, Lansky AJ, Pocock SJ, et al. Paclitaxel-eluting stents versus bare-metal stents in acute myocardial infarction. *N Engl J Med.* 2009;360:1946-1959; Stone GW, Witzenbichler B, Guagliumi G, et al. Heparin plus a glycoprotein IIb/IIIa inhibitor versus bivalirudin monotherapy and paclitaxel-eluting stents versus bare-metal stents in acute myocardial infarction (HORIZONS-AMI): final 3-year results from a multicentre, randomised controlled trial. *Lancet.* 2011;377(9784):2193-2204, with permission.

Fig. 19.8 and **Table 19.13**). The HORIZONS-AMI study also showed that patients who had a combination of risk factors associated with restenosis—insulin-dependent diabetes, small vessel size (<3.0 mm), and long lesion length (>30 mm)—benefited from DES rather than BMS for reducing TVR and angiographic restenosis. Patients without these risk factors had no benefit in terms of 1-year TLR with the use of DESs compared with BMSs[52] (**Fig. 19.9**).

In summary, the benefit of DESs compared to BMSs in STEMI cases is reducing restenosis and the need for repeat revascularization (target vessel and target lesion). DESs do not reduce the incidence of death or recurrent MI when compared to BMS. Stent thrombosis does not appear to be increased with DESs over BMSs in randomized trials, although it remains a concern in the real-world setting.

Points Helpful to Clinical Practice

1. In STEMI patients, higher risk of stent thrombosis with both BMSs and DESs is seen compared to elective PCI. DESs reduce intimal proliferation, restenosis, and the need for TVR more than BMSs, but the risk of stent thrombosis remains a concern in practice. Studies have conflicting results in terms of mortality, but data from randomized trials showed no mortality benefit with DES over BMS.
2. Discontinuation of DAPT is considered to lead to the greatest risk of DES thrombosis that may ultimately increase the risk of mortality and hospitalization.
3. Findings from the HORIZONS-AMI study indicate lower rates of ischemia-driven repeat target lesion and TVR after 1 and 3 years in DESs compared to BMSs but no difference in the rates of thrombosis, reinfarction, stroke, or death. Patients at increased risks benefited from DESs more than BMSs.

ADJUNCTIVE THERAPIES FOR PRIMARY PCI IN PATIENTS WITH STEMI

Management of Thrombus Formation

Previously, there was great enthusiasm for the use of routine manual aspiration thrombectomy in the setting of STEMI, especially after the results of the TAPAS study came out in 2008. TAPAS was a large single-center study that randomized 1071 patients with STEMI to aspiration thrombectomy prior to primary PCI versus primary PCI only and demonstrated that aspiration thrombectomy provided improved TVR with improved myocardial blush and ST-segment resolution, as well as lower mortality in those with better myocardial blush grade and ST-segment resolution.[53,54] In the prior 2013 clinical practice guidelines on STEMI, aspiration thrombectomy had a Class IIa recommendation. However, larger and more recent studies showed that aspiration thrombectomy in STEMI patients before primary PCI is of no benefit and does not improve cardiovascular outcomes, leading to a change in this recommendation. Based on the 2021 ACC/AHA/SCAI revascularization guidelines, routine aspiration thrombectomy received a Class III recommendation (**Table 19.14**).[1]

The TASTE trial (n = 7244), a large RCT published in 2013 comparing routine aspiration thrombectomy before primary PCI to primary PCI only, showed no difference in 30-day, as well as 1-year outcomes including death, hospitalization for recurrent MI, stent thrombosis, TVR, or MACE between the two groups (**Fig. 19.10**).[55,56] Another large RCT comparing manual thrombectomy versus PCI alone in STEMI was evaluated in the TOTAL trial (*n* = 10,732). Published in 2015, it showed similar results to TASTE, with no difference in the primary outcome of death from cardiovascular causes, recurrent MI, CS, or NYHA Class IV HF within 180 days. TOTAL also showed an increased risk of stroke within 30 days in patients receiving manual thrombectomy (0.7% vs 0.3%, HR 2.06; 95% CI 1.13-3.75; *P* = .02).[57] Finally, an updated meta-analysis was performed, which included the trials mentioned earlier and found no significant reduction in death, reinfarction, or stent thrombosis with routine aspiration thrombectomy prior to primary PCI. In addition, the study showed a small but nonsignificant increase in the risk of stroke in patients

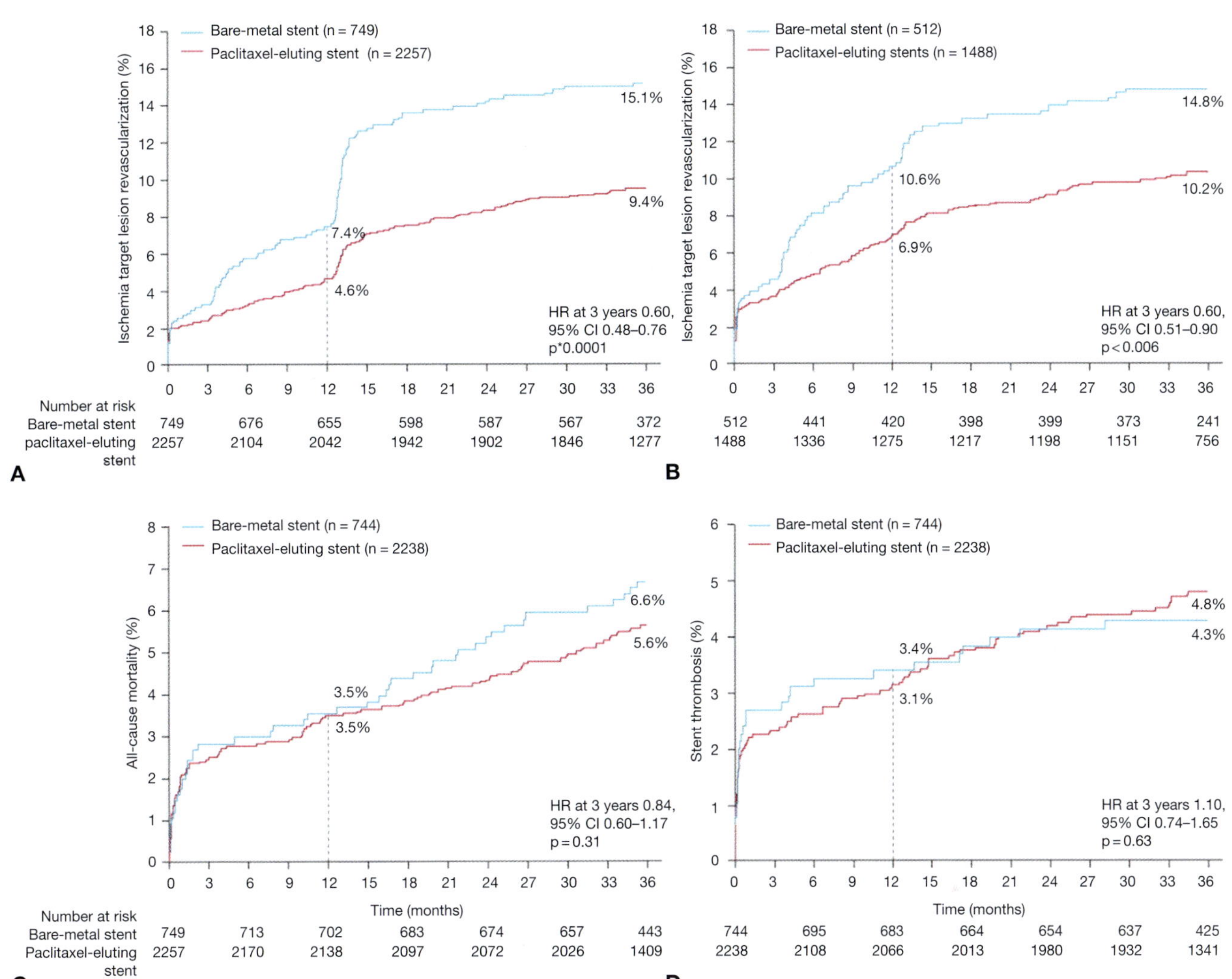

FIGURE 19.8 Bare-metal compared with drug-eluting stenting during primary PCI for STEMI in the HORIZONS-AMI study. Shown are the time-to-event curves for 3 years for major bleeding not related to coronary artery bypass graft surgery **(A)**, cardiac mortality **(B)**, reinfarction **(C)**, and definite or probable stent thrombosis **(D)** in patients randomized to heparin plus a GPI or bivalirudin monotherapy. GPI, glycoprotein IIb/IIIa inhibitor; HR, hazard ratio; PCI, percutaneous coronary intervention; STEMI, ST-elevation myocardial infarction. The vertical dotted line shows the 1-year event rate. One-year rates are also displayed. (From Stone GW, Witzenbichler B, Guagliumi G, et al. Heparin plus a glycoprotein IIb/IIIa inhibitor versus bivalirudin monotherapy and paclitaxel-eluting stents versus bare-metal stents in acute myocardial infarction (HORIZONS-AMI): final 3-year results from a multicentre, randomised controlled trial. *Lancet.* 2011;377(9784):2193-2204, with permission.)

TABLE 19.13 Meta-Analysis of DES Compared With BMS During Primary PCI: Long-Term (>3 y) Follow-Up of Major Randomized Clinical Trials

TRIAL	DEATH OR (95% CI)	TVR OR (95% CI)	STENT THROMBOSIS[a]
Dedication	1.73 (0.97-3.08)	0.40 (0.25-0.64)	0.90 (0.36-2.24)
Paseo	0.65 (0.29-1.49)	0.24 (0.11-0.54)	0.49 (0.07-3.57)
Strategy	1.19 (0.54-2.62)	0.33 (0.14-0.75)	0.86 (0.28-2.66)
Sesami	0.61 (0.20-1.92)	0.46 (0.23-0.92)	1.00 (0.37-2.73)
Mission	0.69 (0.25-1.85)	0.54 (0.27-1.09)	1.69 (0.40-7.20)
Typhoon	0.61 (0.27-1.36)	0.49 (0.30-0.80)	0.92 (0.42-2.00)
Passion	0.75 (0.45-1.27)	0.73 (0.42-1.26)	1.19 (0.52-2.69)
Meta-analysis	0.89 (0.64-1.24)	0.46 (0.36-0.58)	0.99 (0.68-1.45)

BMS, bare-metal stent; CI, confidence interval; DES, drug-eluting stent; PCI, percutaneous coronary intervention; TVR, target vessel revascularization.
Modified from Ziada KM, Charnigo R, Moliterno DJ. Long-term follow-up of drug-eluting stents placed in the setting of ST-segment elevation myocardial infarction. *JACC Cardiovasc Interv.* 2011;4(1):39-41, with permission.
[a]Definition of stent thrombosis differed among studies.

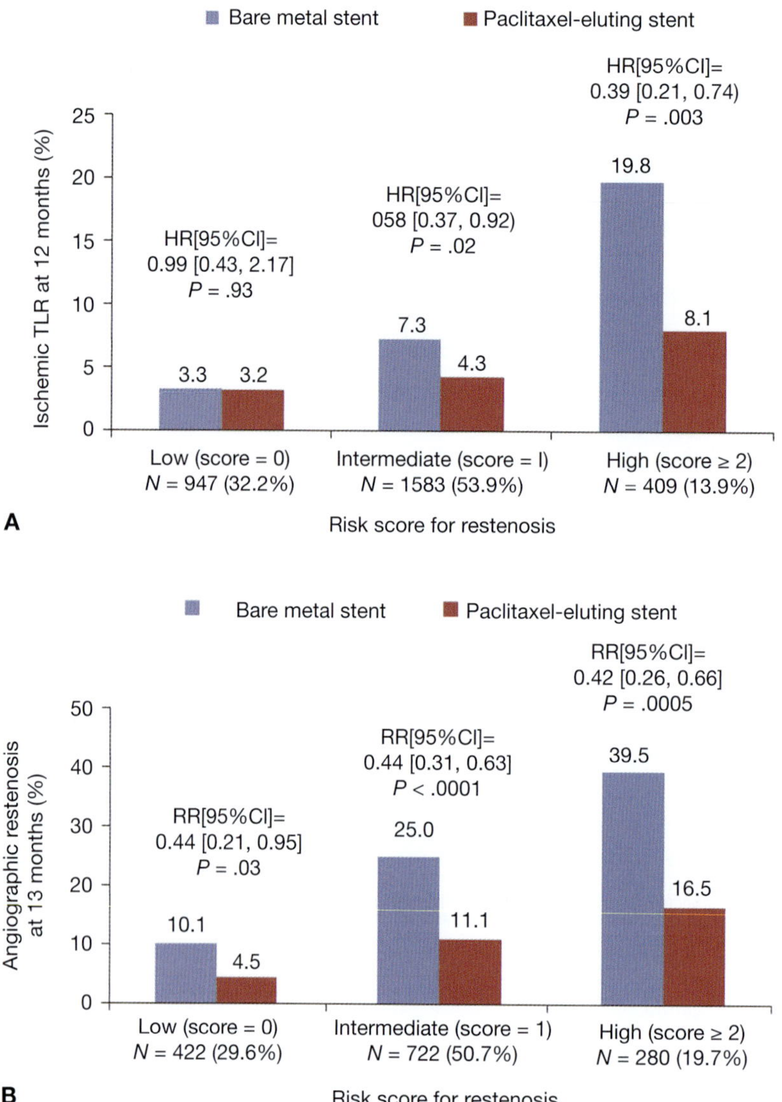

FIGURE 19.9 Risk for restenosis comparing DESs and BMSs in the HORIZONS-AMI study. Rates of 12-month target-lesion revascularization (TLR) and 13-month angiographic restenosis. **(A)** Rates of 12-month ischemic TLR and **(B)** 13-month angiographic restenosis in patients randomly allocated to paclitaxel-eluting stents (red bars) or to bare-metal stents (blue bars), according to the risk strata for restenosis. BMSs, bare-metal stents; CI, confidence interval; DESs, drug-eluting stents; HR, hazard ratio; RR, relative risk. Low-, intermediate-, and high-risk groups for restenosis were created using three variables (one point each): (a) RVD < 3.0 mm, (b) lesion length >30 mm, and (c) insulin-treated diabetes. Patients with 0, 1, and >2 of these three risk factors were defined as being at low, intermediate, or high risk for TLR and restenosis, respectively. (From Stone GW, Parise H, Witzenbichler B, et al. Selection criteria for drug-eluting vs bare-metal stents and the impact of routine angiographic follow-up: 2-year insights from the HORIZONS-AMI (Harmonizing Outcomes With Revascularization and Stents in Acute Myocardial Infarction) trial. *J Am Coll Cardiol.* 2010;56:1597-1604, with permission.)

TABLE 19.14 Recommendation for Routine Aspiration Thrombectomy in STEMI

COR	LOE	RECOMMENDATION
III: No Benefit	A	Aspiration thrombectomy in STEMI patients before primary PCI is of no benefit

Updated recommendation from 2021 ACC/AHA/SCAI Guideline for Coronary Artery Revascularization.

COR, class of recommendation; LOE, level of evidence; PCI; percutaneous coronary intervention; STEMI, ST-segment elevation.

Modified from Members WC, Lawton JS, Tamis-Holland JE, et al. 2021 ACC/AHA/SCAI guideline for coronary artery revascularization: a report of the American College of Cardiology/American Heart Association Joint Committee on Clinical Practice Guidelines. *J Am Coll Cardiol.* 2022;79(2):e21-e129.

receiving aspiration thrombectomy.[58] Selective or bailout thrombectomy has a Class IIb recommendation based on the 2015 ACC/AHA guidelines and can be considered, but its usefulness is not well established (**Table 19.15**).[59]

Rheolytic thrombectomy is a technique to remove the thrombus by using high-velocity saline jets around the catheter tip that entrain thrombus toward the inflow windows. In all cases (AngioJet device; Boston Scientific, Marlborough MA), routine rheolytic thrombectomy for AMI has not consistently shown any clinical benefit, and its use is not recommended in current guidelines. The JETSTENT trial (n = 501) compared rheolytic thrombectomy with stenting to stenting alone and showed improvement in reperfusion but not in infarct size in

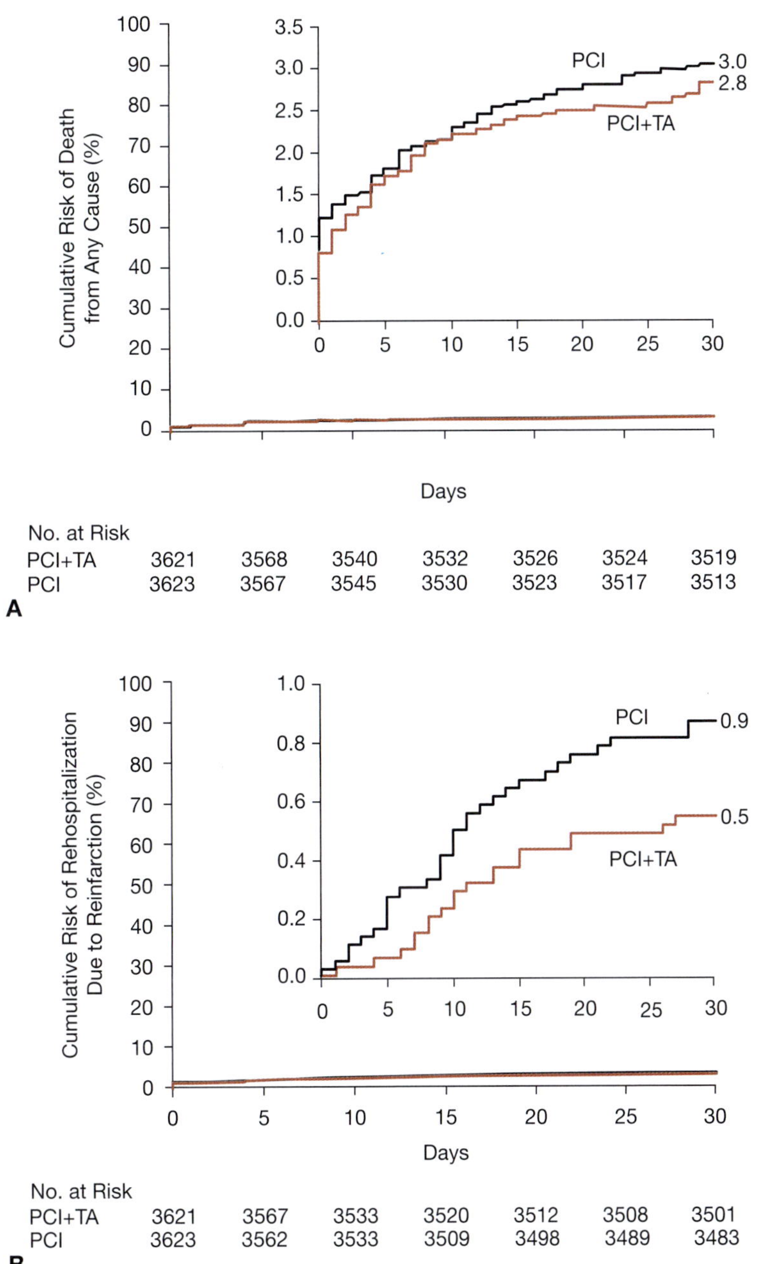

FIGURE 19.10 Kaplan–Meier curves are shown for the cumulative probability of death from any cause **(A)** and of hospitalization due to reinfarction **(B)** up to 30 d after PCI only (PCI) or after PCI with thrombus aspiration (PCI + TA). The insets show the same data on an enlarged y-axis. PCI, percutaneous coronary interventions. (From Fröbert O, Lagerqvist B, Olivecrona GK, et al. Thrombus aspiration during ST-segment elevation myocardial infarction. *N Engl J Med.* 2013;369(17):1587-1597. Copyright © 2013 Massachusetts Medical Society. Reprinted with permission from Massachusetts Medical Society.)

TABLE 19.15 Recommendation for Selective or Bailout Aspiration Thrombectomy for Select Patient Presenting With ST-Elevation Myocardial Infarction

COR	LOE	RECOMMENDATION
IIb	C-LD	Use of selective or bailout aspiration thrombectomy in STEMI patients undergoing primary PCI is not well established

From Levine GN, Bates ER, Blankenship JC, et al. 2015 ACC/AHA/SCAI focused update on primary percutaneous coronary intervention for patients with ST-elevation myocardial infarction: an update of the 2011 ACCF/AHA/SCAI guideline for percutaneous coronary intervention and the 2013 ACCF/AHA guideline for the management of ST-elevation myocardial infarction. *J Am Coll Cardiol.* 2016;67:1235-1250.
COR, class of recommendation; LOE, level of evidence; PCI; percutaneous coronary intervention; and STEMI, ST-segment elevation.

the rheolytic thrombectomy group, suggesting that aspiration thrombectomy remains the preferential choice.[60] In a meta-analysis of rheolytic therapy involving small studies and one larger study (AIMI study), rheolytic thrombectomy was associated with increased mortality risk.[61] Selective use by experienced operators in cases of large thrombus may provide some benefit in select cases.

Three principal categories of embolic protection devices (EPDs) exist: proximal occlusive devices, distal occlusive devices, and filter-based systems. EPDs have been clearly demonstrated to be advantageous during saphenous vein graft (SVG) interventions (Class I). Nevertheless, their effectiveness during primary PCI in native coronary arteries has not been shown in randomized clinical trials (neutral effect).[1,62]

Points Helpful to Clinical Practice

1. Early trials such as the TAPAS, encouraged the use of aspiration thrombectomy prior to PCI due to improved TVR, myocardial blush, and ST-segment resolution, as well as lower mortality rates. However, more recent studies such as the TASTE and TOTAL trials showed no improvement in cardiovascular outcomes with aspiration thrombectomy prior to PCI, leading to a change in classification (Class III according to 2021 guidelines).
2. The use of rheolytic thrombectomy and EPD during STEMI in native coronary circulation are not associated with improved outcomes, and routine use is not recommended.

Pharmacotherapies: Parenteral Anticoagulants

This group includes unfractionated heparin (UFH), the mainstay treatment (Class I), bivalirudin, enoxaparin, and argatroban.[63] Treatment with anticoagulation in patients with STEMI undergoing PCI is needed to prevent thrombotic complications. A number of trials have evaluated the safety and efficacy of parenteral anticoagulants in the setting of primary PCI for STEMI.[63]

Previous trials reported superiority of bivalirudin compared to heparin when used in patients with STEMI. The HERO-1[64] and HERO-2 trials,[65] comparing bivalirudin with heparin among STEMI patients receiving aspirin and streptokinase, showed higher coronary patency rates at 90 to 120 minutes and had sustained coronary patency at 3 days among bivalirudin recipients. In order to further investigate the efficacy of bivalirudin in the setting of STEMI, the HORIZONS-AMI trial was performed in 2008.[52] This pivotal trial prospectively compared UFH in combination with a GP IIb/IIIa inhibitor with bivalirudin (primarily as monotherapy although with provisional abciximab or double-bolus eptifibatide), among 3600 patients. The primary endpoint of composite major bleeding plus MACE (death, reinfarction, TVR for ischemia, and stroke) within 30 days was lower among bivalirudin recipients (9% vs 12%), largely because of lower rates of major bleeding both at 30 days (5% vs 8.4%) and at 1 year (6% vs 9%; **Fig. 19.11**). There was no significant difference in MACE alone (5.5% vs 5.5%). There was a significant absolute 1% increased rate of stent thrombosis within the first 24 hours with the use of bivalirudin (1.3% vs 0.3%, $P < .001$), but there was no significant difference between the two groups beyond this period. Finally, cardiac mortality (1.8% vs

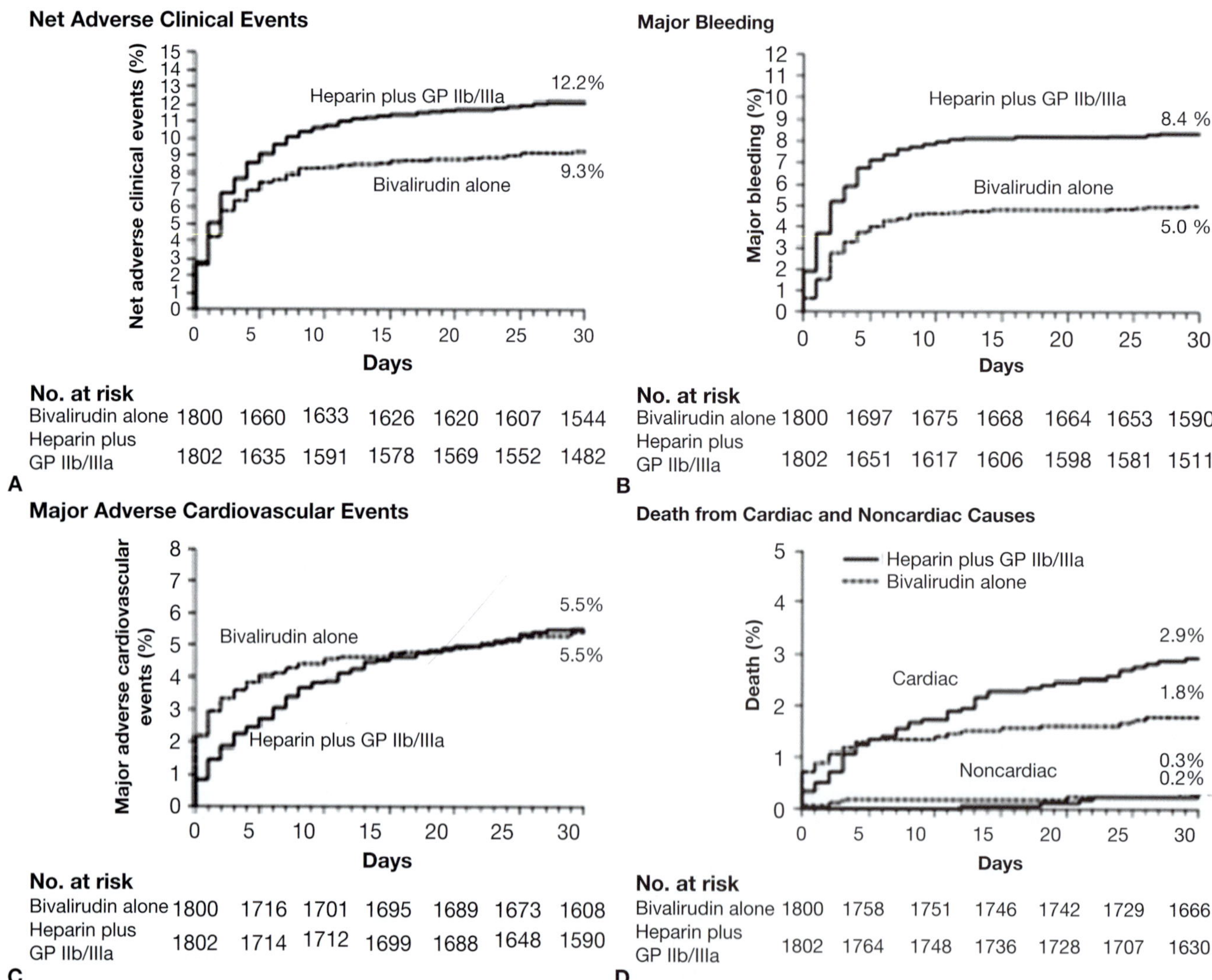

FIGURE 19.11 Time-to-event through 30 d for net adverse clinical events, $P = .006$ **(A)**, major bleeding, $P < .0001$ **(B)**, MACE, $P =$ NS **(C)**, and death from cardiac causes, $P = .03$ **(D)**. GP, glycoprotein; MACE, major adverse cardiac events. (From Stone GW, Witzenbichler B, Guagliumi G, et al. Bivalirudin during primary PCI in acute myocardial infarction. *N Engl J Med.* 2008;358(21):2218-2230. Copyright © 2008 Massachusetts Medical Society. Reprinted with permission from Massachusetts Medical Society.)

TABLE 19.16 Dosing of Parenteral Anticoagulants During PCI

ANTICOAGULANT	PREVIOUS ANTICOAGULANT THERAPY	NO PREVIOUS ANTICOAGULANT THERAPY
UFH	Add as needed to achieve therapeutic ACT (250-300 s)	70-100 U/kg bolus to achieve therapeutic ACT (250-300 s)
Bivalirudin	Repeat ACT if UFH was administered If ACT therapeutic range not achieved, give 0.75 mg/kg IV bolus, then 1.75 mg/kg/h IV infusion	0.75 mg/kg bolus, 1.75 mg/kg/h IV infusion
Enoxaparin	If one SC dose was administered or if the last SC dose was between the last 8 and 12 h, give 0.3 mg/kg IV dose Nothing is given if last SC dose was given within the last 8 h	0.5-0.75 mg/kg IV bolus
Argatroban	200 μg/kg IV bolus, followed by 15 μg/kg/min IV infusion	350 μg/kg, followed by 15 μg/kg/min IV infusion

Updated recommendation from 2021 ACC/AHA/SCAI Guideline for Coronary Artery Revascularization.
ACT, activated clotting time; IV, intravenous; PCI, percutaneous coronary intervention; SC, subcutaneous; UFH, unfractionated heparin.
Modified from Members WC, Lawton JS, Tamis-Holland JE, et al. 2021 ACC/AHA/SCAI guideline for coronary artery revascularization: a report of the American College of Cardiology/American Heart Association Joint Committee on Clinical Practice Guidelines. *J Am Coll Cardiol*. 2022;79(2):e21-e129.

2.9%) and all-cause mortality (2.1% vs 3.1%) rates were both significantly lower in the bivalirudin group. At 3 years, bivalirudin had lower rates of all-cause mortality (5.9% vs 7.7%, HR 0.75 [0.58-0.97]; *P* = .03), cardiac mortality (2.9% vs 5.1%, HR 0.56 [0.40-0.80]; *P* = .001), reinfarction, and major bleeding (not related to bypass graft surgery), with no significant differences in ischemia-driven TVR, stent thrombosis, or composite adverse events (MACE 21.9% vs 21.8%, *P* = .95).[66] The HEAT-PPCI trial was a randomized, single-center study comparing heparin to bivalirudin (with similar utilization of GP IIb/IIIa inhibitors in both arms: 13% and 15%). The primary efficacy outcome (composite of all-cause mortality, cerebrovascular accident, reinfarction, or unplanned TLR at 28 days) occurred in 8.7% in the bivalirudin group and 5.7% in the heparin group (absolute risk difference 3.0%; RR 1.52, 95% CI 1.09-2.13, *P* = .01). Notably, the rates of acute stent thrombosis were 3.4% versus 0.9% (*P* = .001), and reinfarction 2.7% versus 0.9% (*P* = .004), favoring the use of heparin. There was no difference in major bleeding (BARC 3-5; 3.5% vs 3.1% *P* = .59).[67]

The MATRIX trial also demonstrated no significant difference in outcomes or net adverse clinical events with heparin (and discretionary use of GP IIb/IIIa inhibitors) versus bivalirudin in 7213 acute coronary syndrome (ACS) patients (over one-half were STEMI). Neither MACE (10.3% and 10.9%, respectively, *P* = .44) nor net adverse clinical events (NACE; composite of major bleeding or MACE) were different (NACE 11.2% and 12.4%; *P* = .12). The rate of definite stent thrombosis was significantly higher in the bivalirudin group than in the heparin group. Post-PCI bivalirudin infusion, as compared with no infusion, did not significantly decrease the rate of urgent TVR, definite stent thrombosis, or NACE (11.0% and 11.9%, respectively; RR, 0.91; 95% CI, 0.74-1.11; *P* = .34). Nevertheless, bivalirudin was associated with lower rates of death from any cause (1.7% vs 2.3%; rate ratio, 0.71; 95% CI 0.51-0.99; *P* = .04), cardiac death (1.5% vs 2.2%; *P* = .03), and major bleeding (BARC 3 or 5; 1.4% vs 2.5%; *P* < .001), but the absolute differences were small.[68] Similarly, the VALIDATE-SWEDEHEAR, an RCT on 3005 patients with STEMI receiving either heparin or bivalirudin, showed no significant difference in outcome (death from any cause in bivalirudin vs heparin: 1.9% vs 1.7%, respectively, *P* = .21; MI 0.8% vs 1.1%, *P* = .18; major bleeding 5.1% vs 5.6%, *P* = .32; and stroke 0.7% vs 0.8%, *P* = 1.00).[69] Bivalirudin and argatroban, another direct thrombin inhibitor, can be used in the place of UFH due to their mechanism of not binding platelet factor 4 and thus causing heparin-induced thrombocytopenia (HIT; Class I).

As for enoxaparin, it can also be used in the place of UFH, as trials have showed no difference in terms of adverse events.[63] The SYNERGY trial showed similar rates between enoxaparin and UFH in terms of abrupt closure (1.3% vs 1.7%), threatened abrupt closure (1.1% vs 1.0%), unsuccessful PCI (3.6% vs 3.4%), and emergency CABG (0.3% vs 0.3%).[70] Current guidelines recommended to avoid the use of UFH if enoxaparin was administered in the last 12 hours, as stacking of both medications increases the risk of bleeding[1] (Class III: harm). **Table 19.16** shows current recommendations regarding parenteral anticoagulation therapy dosing during PCI, while **Table 19.17** shows current recommendations regarding parenteral anticoagulation therapy during PCI.

Pharmacotherapies: Antiplatelet Agents

Oral and parenteral antiplatelet agents play a critical role as adjunctive therapies in primary PCI for STEMI. The basic mechanisms of the various agents are summarized in **Fig. 19.12**. The following agents will be discussed in this section: GP IIb/IIIa inhibitors

TABLE 19.17 Recommendations of Parenteral Anticoagulants During PCI for Patient Presenting With ST-Elevation Myocardial Infarction

COR	LOE	RECOMMENDATION
I	C-EO	UFH administration in patients undergoing PCI is useful in reducing ischemic events
I	C-LD	Bivalirudin and argatroban can be used in the place of UFH in patients with HIT undergoing PCI
IIb	A	Bivalirudin can replace UFH in patients undergoing PCI to reduce bleeding risk
III: harm	B-R	Avoid the use of UFH if enoxaparin was administered in the last 12 h, as stacking of both medications increases the risk of bleeding

Updated recommendation from 2021 ACC/AHA/SCAI Guideline for Coronary Artery Revascularization.
COR, class of recommendation; HIT, heparin-induced thrombocytopenia; LOE, level of evidence; PCI, percutaneous coronary intervention; UFH, unfractionated heparin.
Modified from Members WC, Lawton JS, Tamis-Holland JE, et al. 2021 ACC/AHA/SCAI guideline for coronary artery revascularization: a report of the American College of Cardiology/American Heart Association Joint Committee on Clinical Practice Guidelines. *J Am Coll Cardiol*. 2022;79(2):e21-e129.

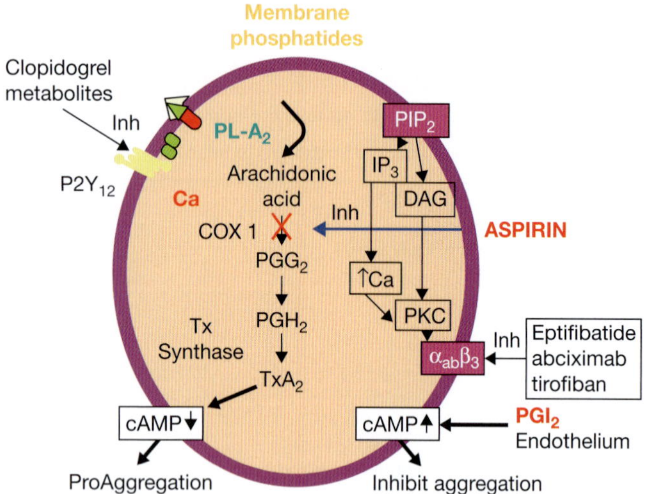

FIGURE 19.12 Activation of phospholipase A2 liberates arachidonic acid (AA) from the cell membrane. AA then metabolizes to thromboxane A2 (TxA2) by cyclooxygenase (COX), which is inhibited by aspirin (AS). TxA2 is a potent platelet agonist and vasoconstrictor. When ADP is released from activated platelets, it binds to the P2Y12 receptor of circulating platelets, which initiates platelet aggregation and amplification. Clopidogrel, prasugrel, and ticlopidine all irreversibly bind the P2Y12 receptor, thereby preventing ADP. Ticagrelor, in contrast, is a reversible P2Y12 receptor inhibitor. Inosine diphosphate (IP2) is released after the activation of the P2Y12 receptor. IP2 is phosphorylated to IP3. The release of both IP3 and diacylglycerol leads to activation of protein kinase C (PKC) and to the eventual activation of GP IIb/IIIa, which permits its binding to fibrinogen, the final step in platelet activation and aggregation. ADP, adenosine diphosphate; cAMP, cyclic adenosine monophosphate; GP, glycoprotein; P2Y12, platelet adenosine diphosphate receptor. (Redrawn from Dupont AG, Gabriel DA, Cohen MG. Antiplatelet therapies and the role of antiplatelet resistance in acute coronary syndrome. *Thromb Res.* 2009;124(1):6-13, with permission.)

(eptifibatide, abciximab, tirofiban), thienopyridines (clopidogrel, prasugrel), aspirin, cangrelor, and ticagrelor.

Only a few trials have studied GP IIb/IIIa inhibitors in conjunction with oral antiplatelet therapies. The BRAVE-3 trial studied 800 patients pretreated with 600 mg of clopidogrel randomly assigned to either abciximab or placebo prior to PCI. At 30 days, the composite of death, recurrent MI, stroke, or urgent revascularization of the IRA was not significantly different. There was also no difference in infarct size or major bleeding.[71] The On-TIME 2 study randomized 491 patients to tirofiban versus placebo prior to primary PCI. All patients received IV heparin bolus, aspirin, and 600-mg clopidogrel prior to randomization. Tirofiban recipients had improved ST-segment resolution before and after PCI; nevertheless, there were no significant differences in TIMI grade 3 coronary flow, major or minor bleeding rates, or in death, recurrent MI, or urgent TVR.[72] A meta-analysis by Gurm et al compared abciximab with small-molecule GP IIb/IIIa inhibitors (eptifibatide or tirofiban). There were no differences in 30-day mortality (1.9% small molecule vs 2.3% abciximab, P = NS) or in reinfarction rates (1.3% vs 1.2%, P = NS). Rates of TVR were identical (1.7%) for both groups. Both major and minor bleeding rates were similar for both groups.[73] Finally, one study, FINESSE, investigated the issue of timing of a GP IIb/IIIa antagonist administration. This double-blind, placebo-controlled study randomized 2453 patients to pre-PCI treatment with half-dose fibrinolysis plus abciximab, pre-PCI abciximab alone, and abciximab during the time of PCI. The primary endpoint was a composite of all-cause death, ventricular function >48 hours after randomization, CS, and CHF during the first 90 days of randomization. The trial showed no benefit (including mortality) with pre-PCI abciximab compared with abciximab at the time of PCI. Based on the preceding studies, among others, the guideline-writing committee concluded that the various GP IIb/IIIa antagonists have similar efficacy and that in the setting of DAPT, it is reasonable to start treatment with GP IIb/IIIa antagonists at the time of primary PCI (with or without stenting) in selected patients such as those with a large thrombus burden, no reflow, or slow flow (Class IIa).[1,74]

The TRITON-TIMI 38 trial evaluated the safety and efficacy of the most-recent member of the thienopyridine family, prasugrel. This double-blinded study randomized 13,600 ACS patients to prasugrel (loading dose 60 mg followed by 10 mg daily) versus clopidogrel (loading dose 300 mg followed by 75 mg daily) for 6 to 15 months. Twenty-six percent of patients in the TRITON-TIMI 38 trial presented with STEMI. In the overall cohort, the primary efficacy endpoint of death from cardiovascular causes, nonfatal MI, or nonfatal stroke was seen in 12.1% of clopidogrel patients and in 9.9% of prasugrel patients ($P < .001$); there was a significant benefit of prasugrel seen in the STEMI subset as well. The benefit of prasugrel in the primary efficacy endpoint was seen within the first 24 hours of randomization and persisted through 15 months of follow-up (**Fig. 19.13**). The difference in the primary endpoint was largely due to the reduction in MI among prasugrel recipients (7.4% vs 9.7%, $P < .001$). Subgroups of patients also had a significant benefit with prasugrel, and this included diabetics and patients receiving GP IIb/IIIa inhibitors. Rates of stent thrombosis (definite or probable) were also reduced in the prasugrel group (1.1% vs 2.4%, $P < .001$). These improved efficacy outcomes but did come at a price with respect to safety endpoints. Major bleeding was seen in 2.4% of prasugrel patients compared with 1.8% seen in the clopidogrel group, and life-threatening bleeding, including both fatal and nonfatal bleeding rates, was also higher among prasugrel recipients. Three groups in particular were found not to have a net clinical benefit from prasugrel: patients with a prior transient ischemic attack (TIA) or stroke, patients weighing <60 kg, and patients aged >75 years. Patients with prior TIA or stroke were in fact found to have net adverse events from prasugrel.[75] Based on these data, the US Food and Drug Administration (FDA) declared prasugrel to be contraindicated in these patients,[76] while the current ACC/AHA/SCAI guidelines recommended against using prasugrel in patients who have a history of TIA or stroke (Class III: harm).[1]

The use of ticagrelor was evaluated in the PLATO trial, which randomized 18,600 patients with ACS to either clopidogrel (300-mg or 600-mg loading dose, followed by 75 mg daily) or ticagrelor (180-mg loading dose, followed by 90 mg twice daily). A total of 38% of patients presented with STEMI. The primary endpoint of death from vascular causes or cerebrovascular causes, or death from an unknown cause, was seen in 9.8% in the ticagrelor group versus 11.7% in the clopidogrel group ($P < .001$), with the difference in treatment effect being apparent within the first 30 days of therapy. Furthermore, the composite of all-cause death, MI, or stroke was also reduced in the ticagrelor group (10.2% vs 12.3%, $P < .001$). Rates of stent thrombosis were also lower among those who received ticagrelor (1.3% vs 1.9%, $P = .009$), although the absolute difference is still small. The rates of major bleeding and TIMI major bleeding were also similar between the two groups. Although intracranial bleeding episodes were more common among ticagrelor recipients, there were no significant differences in the rates of stroke, including hemorrhagic stroke.[77] Based on the PLATO trial, ticagrelor was FDA-approved for patients with ACS as of July 2011. Current guidelines recommend the use of

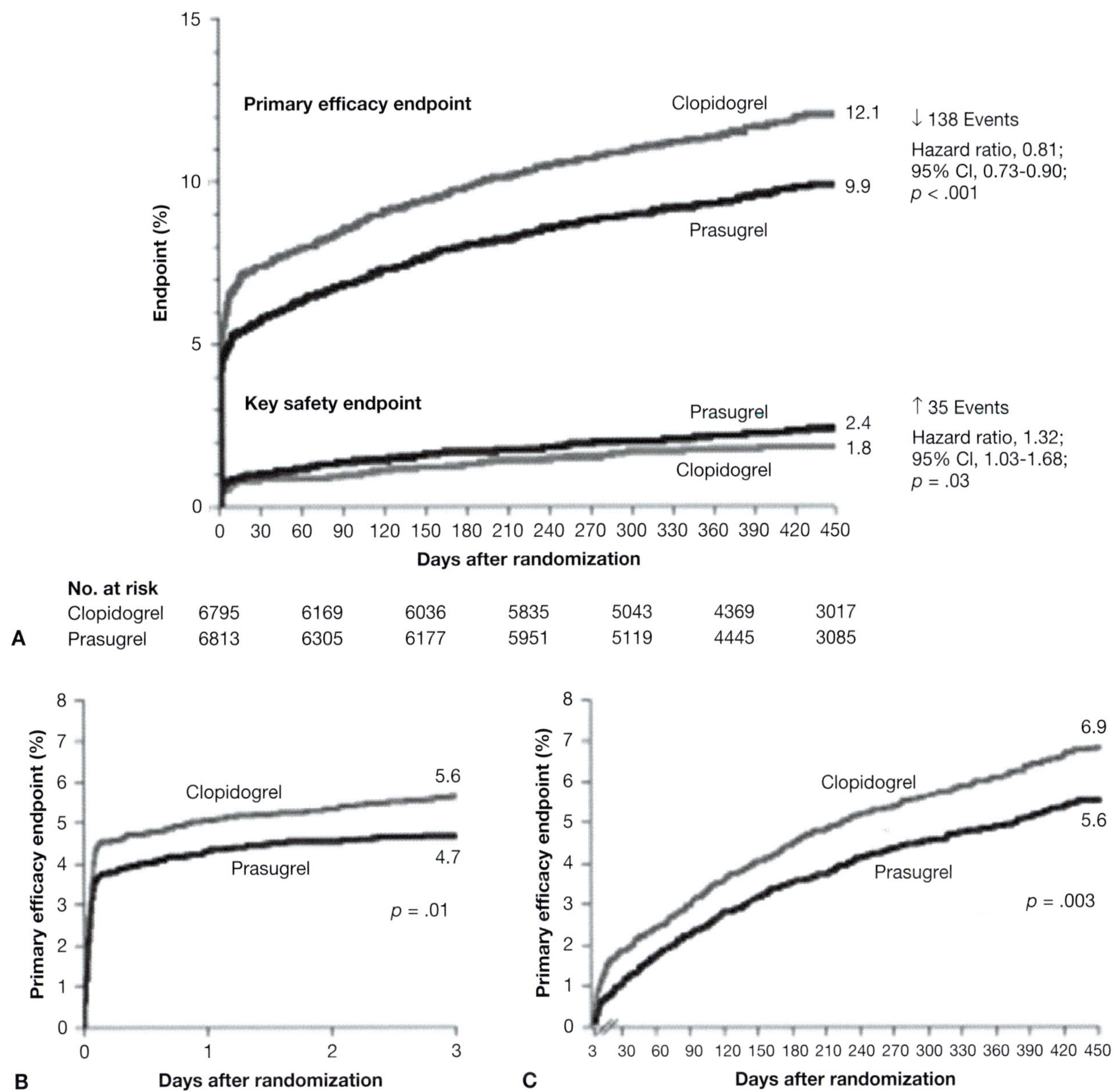

FIGURE 19.13 Kaplan–Meier survival curves comparing clopidogrel and prasugrel. **A.** Data for the primary efficacy end point (death from cardiovascular causes, nonfatal myocardial infarction [MI], or nonfatal stroke) (top) and for the key safety end point (Thrombolysis in Myocardial Infarction [TIMI] major bleeding not related to coronary-artery bypass grafting) (bottom) during the full follow-up period. The hazard ratio for prasugrel, as compared with clopidogrel, for the primary efficacy end point at 30 days was 0.77 (95% confidence interval [CI], 0.67-0.88; $P > .001$), and that at 90 days was 0.80 (95% CI, 0.71-0.90; $P < .001$). Data for the primary efficacy end point are also shown from the time of randomization to day 3 **(B)** and from 3 days to 15 months, with all end points occurring before day 3 censored **(C)**. **C.** The number at risk includes all patients who were alive (regardless of whether a nonfatal event had occurred during the first 3 days after randomization) and had not withdrawn consent for follow-up. The *P* values in **(A)** for the primary efficacy end point were calculated with the use of the Gehan–Wilcoxon test; all other *P* values were calculated with the use of the log-rank test. (From Wiviott SD, Braunwald E, McCabe CH, et al. Prasugrel vs clopidogrel in patients with acute coronary syndromes. *N Engl J Med.* 2007;357(20):2001-2015. Copyright © 2007 Massachusetts Medical Society. Reprinted with permission from Massachusetts Medical Society.)

ticagrelor or prasugrel in preference to clopidogrel in patients who have ACS and are undergoing PCI to avoid ischemia and stent thrombosis (Class IIa), and also the use of ticagrelor as an alternative to clopidogrel in patients who are younger than 75 years undergoing PCI to also reduce the risk of ischemic events (Class IIb).[1] For patients older than 75 years, the use of clopidogrel is preferred over newer P2Y12 inhibitors because of the increased risk of bleeding.[78] The PLATO trial also showed that low doses of aspirin (usually <100 mg) should be used in patients receiving ticagrelor, while current guidelines recommend a loading dose of aspirin, followed by a daily dose in patients undergoing PCI to reduce risks of ischemia (Class I).[1]

Before prasugrel and ticagrelor, clopidogrel was the main thienopyridine used in practice. The CREDO trial is an RCT that assigned patients to receive either 300 mg of clopidogrel ($n = 1053$) or a placebo ($n = 1063$). The group receiving clopidogrel recorded a 26.9% reduction in the combined risk of death, MI, and stroke a year following PCI.[79] Clopidogrel is also still the only P2Y12 inhibitor studied in patients immediately after fibrinolytic therapy. In the CLARITY-TIMI 28 ($n = 1863$) trial, in patients aged <75 years undergoing PCI after mandatory angiography to either clopidogrel (300-mg oral loading dose followed by 75 mg daily) or placebo, the primary efficacy endpoint was a composite of an occluded IRA (defined TIMI flow grade of 0 or 1) on angiography or death or recurrent MI before angiography. This totaled 21.7% in the placebo group and 15.0% in the clopidogrel group, representing a 36% reduction in the odds of the endpoint with clopidogrel. The primary 30-day outcome of the composite of cardiovascular death, recurrent MI, or stroke from PCI to 30 days after randomization was seen in 3.6% in the clopidogrel group versus 6.2% in the placebo group (P = .008). Pretreatment with clopidogrel additionally reduced the incidence of MI or stroke prior to PCI (4.0% vs 6.2%, P = .03), with no significant difference in both major and minor bleeding risks.[80] Current dosing recommendations are a maintenance dose of 75 mg/d, a loading dose of 600 mg, or a loading dose of 300 mg after fibrinolytic therapy (Class I). As for the recent clinical practice guidelines, the use of clopidogrel followed by daily dosing is recommended in patients undergoing PCI (Class I).[1] The evidence in favor of the use of thienopyridines in addition to aspirin in the setting of STEMI treated with fibrinolysis is also compelling. The COMMIT-CCS-2 study randomized 45,852 patients in China to clopidogrel, 75 mg daily (treatment was to continue until discharge or up to 4 weeks in hospital), with no loading dose versus placebo in addition to aspirin (162 mg/d). The use of clopidogrel produced a highly significant 9% (CI 3-14) reduction in death, reinfarction, or stroke (2121 [9.2%] clopidogrel vs 2310 [10.1%] placebo; P = .002) and a significant 7% reduction in any death (1726 [7.5%] vs 1845 [8.1%]; P = .03). There was no significant increase in the risk of major bleeding.[81]

No studies comparing cangrelor to prasugrel or ticagrelor exist to date, but 3 clinical trials that compared cangrelor to clopidogrel have been reported. A meta-analysis on the CHAMPIONS trials reported lower rates of mortality, AMI, ischemia-driven revascularization, and stent thrombosis with the cangrelor group than with the clopidogrel group.[82] Current revascularization guidelines recommend the use of cangrelor in patients undergoing PCI when they are P2Y12 inhibitor naïve.[1] **Table 19.18** includes the latest ACC/AHA/SCAI guideline recommendations for antiplatelet therapy dosing during PCI, while **Table 19.19** includes the latest guideline recommendations for antiplatelet therapy during PCI.

In 2016, the ACC/AHA released a focused guideline update on duration of DAPT in patients with CAD.[47] The recommendations are summarized in **Table 19.20**. However, a newer supplementary update on DAPT duration was published, with recommendations focused on a shorter duration of DAPT followed by P2Y12 monotherapy. The 2021 ACC/AHA/SCAI revascularization guidelines recommend at least a duration of 1 to 3 months of DAPT in patients undergoing PCI before transitioning to the P2Y12 monotherapy for patients with high bleeding risk (**Fig. 19.14**).[1]

Pharmacotherapies: Antiplatelet Agents

1. For patients undergoing primary PCI for STEMI, anticoagulation with either UFH or bivalirudin must be given in order to reach a therapeutic activating clotting time. Both anticoagulants have proven beneficial in the setting of STEMI.
2. Compared with clopidogrel, prasugrel has been found to have reduced rates of death from cardiovascular causes, nonfatal MI, or nonfatal stroke; nevertheless, current guidelines recommend against using prasugrel in patients who have a history of TIA or stroke, low body mass, or are above the age of 75 years. Similarly, ticagrelor has lower all-cause death, MI, and stroke rates than clopidogrel during percutaneous revascularization for patients presenting with STEMI.
3. Studies published after the 2016 update on guidelines on the use of DAPT in patients with STEMI encourage a shorter duration (1-3 months) before transitioning to the P2Y12 monotherapy for high-bleeding-risk patients.

ADJUNCTIVE ANTITHROMBOTICS TO SUPPORT REPERFUSION WITH FIBRINOLYTIC THERAPY

Fibrinolytic therapy (fibrin-specific agents preferred) requires the concurrent use of adjunctive antiplatelet and/or anticoagulant therapies to optimize the effectiveness of reperfusion and prevent re-occlusion. Further details regarding anticoagulation, fibrinolysis, and antiplatelet therapy can be found in other Chapters.

TABLE 19.18 Dosing of Antiplatelet Agents During PCI Among Patient Presenting With ST-Elevation Myocardial Infarction

ANTIPLATELET	LOADING DOSE	MAINTENANCE DOSE
Aspirin (oral agent)	162-325 mg	75-100 mg daily
Clopidogrel (oral agent)	600 mg, after fibrinolytic therapy a lower dose of 300 mg	75 mg daily
Prasugrel (oral agent)	60 mg	10 mg daily, 5 mg in patients with body weight less than 60 kg and in adults aged more than 75 (if deemed necessary)
Ticagrelor (oral agent)	180 mg	90 mg daily BID
Abciximab (intravenous agent)	0.25 mg/kg bolus	0.125 μg/kg/min (maximum 10 μg/min) for 12 h
Eptifibatide (intravenous agent)	double bolus: 180 μg/kg (10-min interval)	2.0 μg/kg/min up to 18 h
Tirofiban (intravenous agent)	high dose bolus: 25 μg/kg over 3 min	0.15 μg/kg/min up to 18 h
Cangrelor (intravenous agent)	0.25 mg/kg	4.0 μg/kg/min for duration of procedure or for 2 h

Updated recommendation from 2021 ACC/AHA/SCAI Guideline for Coronary Artery Revascularization.
BID, twice a day; PCI, percutaneous coronary intervention.
Modified from Members WC, Lawton JS, Tamis-Holland JE, et al. 2021 ACC/AHA/SCAI guideline for coronary artery revascularization: a report of the American College of Cardiology/American Heart Association Joint Committee on Clinical Practice Guidelines. *J Am Coll Cardiol.* 2022;79(2):e21-e129.

TABLE 19.19 Recommendations of Antiplatelets During PCI

COR	LOE	RECOMMENDATION
I	B-R	A loading dose of aspirin, followed by a daily dose in patients undergoing PCI is recommended
I	B-R	A loading dose of P2Y12, followed by a daily dose in patients with ACS undergoing PCI is recommended
I	C-LD	A loading dose of clopidogrel, followed by a daily dose in patients with SIHD undergoing PCI is recommended
I	C-LD	A loading dose of 300 mg clopidogrel after fibrinolytic therapy, followed by a daily dose in patients undergoing PCI is recommended
IIa	A	A shorter duration (1-3 mo) of DAPT in patients undergoing PCI is recommended, with transition to P2Y12 monotherapy following
IIa	B-R	Ticagrelor or prasugrel can be used instead of clopidogrel in patients with ACS undergoing PCI
IIa	C-LD	Glycoprotein IIb/IIIa can be used in patients with ACS undergoing PCI who have large thrombus burden, no re-flow, or slow flow
IIb	B-R	Ticagrelor can be used as an alternative to clopidogrel in patients who are younger than 75 years undergoing PCI
IIb	B-R	Cangrelor can be used in patients undergoing PCI who are P2Y12 naïve
III: No benefit	B-R	Glycoprotein IIb/IIIa in patients with SIHD undergoing PCI is not recommended
III: Harm	B-R	Prasugrel is not recommended in patients with a history of TIA or stroke undergoing PCI

Updated recommendation from 2021 ACC/AHA/SCAI Guideline for Coronary Artery Revascularization.
ASC, acute coronary syndrome; COR, class of recommendation; DAPT, dual antiplatelet therapy; LOE, level of evidence; PCI; percutaneous coronary intervention; SIHD, stable ischemic heart disease; TIA, transient ischemic attack.
Modified from Members WC, Lawton JS, Tamis-Holland JE, et al. 2021 ACC/AHA/SCAI guideline for coronary artery revascularization: a report of the American College of Cardiology/American Heart Association Joint Committee on Clinical Practice Guidelines. *J Am Coll Cardiol*. 2022;79(2):e21-e129.

TABLE 19.20 Recommendations for DAPT in ACS Patients From the 2016 ACC/AHA Focused Update on DAPT Duration in ACS Patients

RECOMMENDATIONS FOR DURATION OF DAPT IN PATIENTS WITH ACS TREATED WITH FIBRINOLYTIC THERAPY		
RECOMMENDATION	**COR**	**LOE**
In patients with STEMI treated with DAPT in conjunction with fibrinolytic therapy, $P2Y_{12}$ inhibitor therapy (clopidogrel) should be continued for a minimum of 14 d (level of evidence: A) and ideally at least 12 mo (level of evidence: C).	I	A C
In patients treated with DAPT, a daily aspirin dose of 81 mg (range, 75-100 mg) is recommended.	I	B
In patients with STEMI treated with fibrinolytic therapy who have tolerated DAPT without bleeding complications and who are not at high bleeding risk (eg, prior bleeding on DAPT, coagulopathy, oral anticoagulant use), continuation of DAPT for longer than 12 mo may be reasonable	IIb	A
Recommendations for Duration of DAPT in Patients With ACS Treated With PCI		
In patients with ACS treated with DAPT after BMS or DES implantation, $P2Y_{12}$ inhibitor therapy (clopidogrel, prasugrel, or ticagrelor) should be given for at least 12 mo.	I	B
In patients treated with DAPT, a daily aspirin dose of 81 mg (range, 75-100 mg) is recommended.	I	B
In patients with ACS treated with DAPT after coronary stent implantation, it is reasonable to use ticagrelor in preference to clopidogrel for maintenance $P2Y_{12}$ inhibitor therapy.	IIa	B
In patients with ACS treated with DAPT after coronary stent implantation, who are not at high risk for bleeding complications and who do not have a history of stroke or TIA, it is reasonable to choose prasugrel over clopidogrel for maintenance P2Y12 inhibitor therapy.	IIa	B
In patients with ACS treated with coronary stent implantation who have tolerated DAPT without bleeding complications and who are not at high bleeding risk (eg, prior bleeding on DAPT, coagulopathy, oral anticoagulant use), continuation of DAPT for longer than 12 mo may be reasonable.	IIb	A
In patients with ACS treated with DAPT after DES implantation who develop a high risk of bleeding (eg, treatment with oral anticoagulant therapy), are at high risk of severe bleeding complications (eg, major intracranial surgery), or develop significant overt bleeding, discontinuation of $P2Y_{12}$ therapy after 6 mo may be reasonable.	IIb	C
Prasugrel should not be administered to patients with a prior history of stroke or TIA.	III: harm	B

ACS, acute coronary syndrome; BMS, bare-metal stent; COR, class of recommendation; DAPT, dual antiplatelet therapy; DESs, drug-eluting stents; LOE, level of evidence; PCI, percutaneous coronary intervention; STEMI, ST-elevation myocardial infarction; TIA, transient ischemic attack.
Modified from Levine GN, Bates ER, Bittl JA, et al. 2016 ACC/AHA guideline focused update on duration of dual antiplatelet therapy in patients with coronary artery disease. *J Am Coll Cardiol*. 2016;68(10):1082.

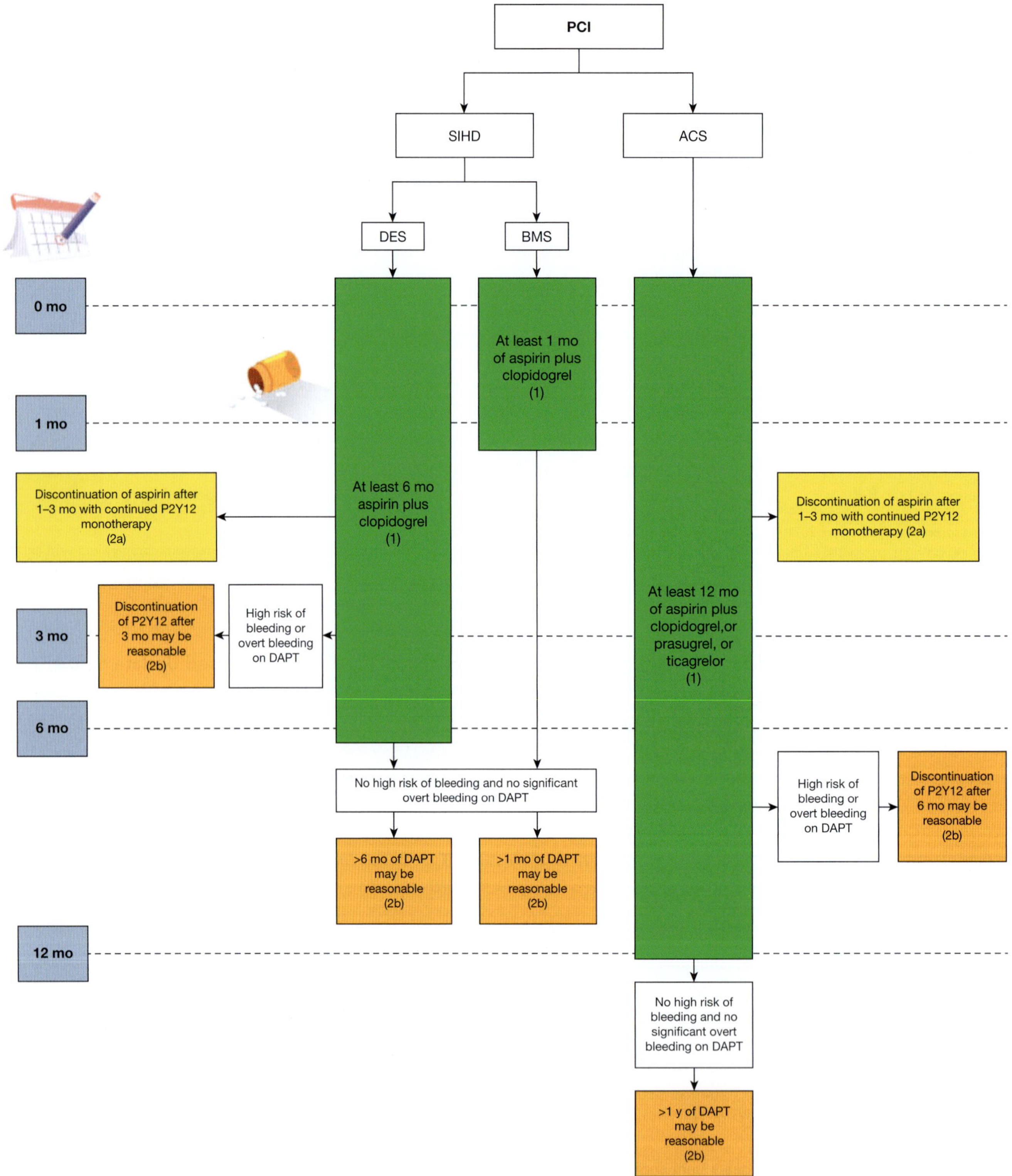

FIGURE 19.14 The use of DAPT for patients after PCI based on the 2016 DAPT guidelines with new recommendations from 2021 ACC/AHA/SCAI guidelines. ACS, acute coronary syndrome; BMS, bare metal stent; DAPT, dual antiplatelet therapy; DES, drug-eluting stent; P2Y12, platelet adenosine diphosphate receptor; PCI, percutaneous coronary intervention; SIHD, stable ischemic heart disease. It is not meant to encompass every patient scenario or situation, and clinicians are encouraged to use a Heart Team approach when care decisions are unclear and to see the accompanying supportive text for each recommendation. (Figure from Members WC, Lawton JS, Tamis-Holland JE, et al. 2021 ACC/AHA/SCAI guideline for coronary artery revascularization: a report of the American College of Cardiology/American Heart Association Joint Committee on Clinical Practice Guidelines. *J Am Coll Cardiol.* 2022;79:e21-e129.)

References

1. Members WC, Lawton JS, Tamis-Holland JE, et al. 2021 ACC/AHA/SCAI guideline for coronary artery revascularization: a report of the American College of Cardiology/American Heart Association Joint Committee on Clinical Practice Guidelines. *J Am Coll Cardiol*. 2022;79:e21-e129.
2. Chacko L, P Howard J, Rajkumar C, et al. Effects of percutaneous coronary intervention on death and myocardial infarction stratified by stable and unstable coronary artery disease: a meta-analysis of randomized controlled trials. *Circ Cardiovasc Qual Outcomes*. 2020;13(2):e006363.
3. Fazel R, Joseph TI, Sankardas MA, et al. Comparison of reperfusion strategies for STsegment–elevation myocardial infarction: a multivariate network meta-analysis. *J Am Heart Assoc*. 2020;9(12):e015186.
4. Kastrati A, Coughlan J, Ndrepepa G. *Primary PCI, Late Presenting STEMI, and the Limits of Time*. American College of Cardiology Foundation; 2021:1306-1308.
5. Jneid H, Addison D, Bhatt DL, et al. 2017 AHA/ACC clinical performance and quality measures for adults with ST-elevation and non–ST-elevation myocardial infarction: a report of the American College of Cardiology/ American Heart Association Task Force on Performance Measures. *Circ Cardiovasc Qual Outcomes*. 2017;10:e000032.
6. Sim DS, Jeong MH, Ahn Y, et al; Korea Acute Myocardial Infarction Registry KAMIR Investigators. Pharmacoinvasive strategy versus primary percutaneous coronary intervention in patients with ST-segment–elevation myocardial infarction: a propensity score–matched analysis. *Circ Cardiovasc Interv*. 2016;9:e003508.
7. Jamal J, Idris H, Faour A, et al. Late outcomes of ST-elevation myocardial infarction treated by pharmaco-invasive or primary percutaneous coronary intervention. *Eur Heart J*. 2023;44(6):516-528.
8. Engel Gonzalez P, Omar W, Patel KV, et al. Fibrinolytic strategy for ST-segment–elevation myocardial infarction: a contemporary review in context of the COVID-19 pandemic. *Circ Cardiovasc Interv*. 2020;13(9):e009622.
9. Dauerman HL, Ibanez B. *The edge of time in acute myocardial infarction*. American College of Cardiology Foundation; 2021:1871-1874.
10. Kloner RA. Stunned and hibernating myocardium: where are we nearly 4 decades later? *J Am Heart Assoc*. 2020;9(3):e015502.
11. Vetrovec GW. *Important Trial Results for Interventional Cardiology From TCT 2017 and AHA 2017*. American College of Cardiology. 2018.
12. Park J, Choi KH, Lee JM, et al; KAMIR-NIH Korea Acute Myocardial Infarction Registry–National Institutes of Health Investigators. Prognostic implications of door-to-balloon time and onset-to-door time on mortality in patients with ST-segment–elevation myocardial infarction treated with primary percutaneous coronary intervention. *J Am Heart Assoc*. 2019;8(9):e012188.
13. Nathan AS, Raman S, Yang N, et al. Association between 90-minute door-to-balloon time, selective exclusion of myocardial infarction cases, and access site choice: insights from the cardiac care outcomes assessment program (COAP) in Washington State. *Circ Cardiovasc Interv*. 2020;13(9):e009179.
14. Koul S, Andell P, Martinsson A, et al. Delay from first medical contact to primary PCI and all-cause mortality: a nationwide study of patients with ST-elevation myocardial infarction. *J Am Heart Assoc*. 2014;3(2):e000486.
15. Nallamothu BK, Bates ER, Wang Y, Bradley EH, Krumholz HM. Driving times and distances to hospitals with percutaneous coronary intervention in the United States: implications for prehospital triage of patients with ST-elevation myocardial infarction. *Circulation*. 2006;113(9):1189-1195.
16. Jollis JG, Al-Khalidi HR, Roettig ML, et al; Mission: Lifeline STEMI Systems Accelerator Project. Regional systems of care demonstration project: American Heart Association Mission—lifeline STEMI systems accelerator. *Circulation*. 2016;134(5):365-374.
17. French WJ, Gunderson M, Travis D, et al. Emergency interhospital transfer of patients with ST-segment–elevation myocardial infarction: call 9-1-1—the American Heart Association mission—lifeline program. *Am Heart Assoc*. 2022;11(22):e026700.
18. Henry TD, Tomey MI, Tamis-Holland JE, et al; American Heart Association Interventional Cardiovascular Care Committee of the Council on Clinical Cardiology; Council on Arteriosclerosis, Thrombosis and Vascular Biology; and Council on Cardiovascular and Stroke Nursing. Invasive management of acute myocardial infarction complicated by cardiogenic shock: a scientific statement from the American Heart Association. *Circulation*. 2021;143(15):e815-e829.
19. Schömig A, Mehilli J, Antoniucci D, et al; Beyond 12 hours Reperfusion AlternatiVe Evaluation BRAVE-2 Trial Investigators. Mechanical reperfusion in patients with acute myocardial infarction presenting more than 12 hours from symptom OnsetA randomized controlled trial. *JAMA*. 2005;293(23):2865-2872. doi:10.1001/jama.293.23.2865
20. Ndrepepa G, Kastrati A, Mehilli J, Antoniucci D, Schömig A. Mechanical reperfusion and long-term mortality in patients with acute myocardial infarction presenting 12 to 48 hours from onset of symptoms. *JAMA*. 2009;301(5):487-488. doi:10.1001/jama.2009.32
21. O'gara PT, Kushner FG, Ascheim DD, et al. 2013 ACCF/AHA guideline for the management of ST-elevation myocardial infarction: a report of the American College of Cardiology Foundation/American Heart Association Task Force on Practice Guidelines. *J Am Coll Cardiol*. 2013;61(4):e78-e140.
22. Engstrøm T, Kelbæk H, Helqvist S, et al; DANAMI-3—PRIMULTI Investigators. Complete revascularisation versus treatment of the culprit lesion only in patients with ST-segment elevation myocardial infarction and multivessel disease (DANAMI-3—PRIMULTI): an open-label, randomised controlled trial. *Lancet*. 2015;386(9994):665-671. doi:10.1016/s0140-6736(15)60648-1
23. Smits PC, Abdel-Wahab M, Neumann FJ, et al; Compare-Acute Investigators. Fractional flow reserve–guided multivessel angioplasty in myocardial infarction. *N Engl J Med*. 2017;376(13):1234-1244. doi:10.1056/NEJMoa1701067
24. Mehta SR, Wood DA, Storey RF, et al; COMPLETE Trial Steering Committee and Investigators. Complete revascularization with multivessel PCI for myocardial infarction. *N Engl J Med*. 2019;381(15):1411-1421. doi:10.1056/NEJMoa1907775
25. Alasnag MA, Al-Shaibi KF, *PCI for Multivessel Disease in STEMI*. American College of Cardiology.
26. Grines CL, Box LC, Mamas MA, et al. SCAI Expert consensus statement on percutaneous coronary intervention without on-site surgical backup. *JACC Cardiovasc Interv*. 2023;16(7):847-860.
27. Grines CL, Box LC, Mamas MA, et al. SCAI Expert consensus statement on percutaneous coronary intervention without on-site surgical backup. *Journal of the Society for Cardiovascular Angiography & Interventions*. 2023;2:100560. doi:10.1016/j.jscai.2022.100560
28. Affronti A, Ruel M. Emergency surgery for iatrogenic injuries attributable to percutaneous coronary interventions: when planning and time matter. *Am Heart Assoc*. 2019;8(1):e011525.
29. Aikawa T, Yamaji K, Nagai T, et al. Procedural volume and outcomes after percutaneous coronary intervention for unprotected left main coronary artery disease—report from the National Clinical Data (J-PCI Registry). *J Am Heart Assoc*. 2020;9:e015404.
30. Waldo SW, Hebbe A, Grunwald GK, Doll JA, Schofield R. Clinical and anatomic complexity of patients undergoing coronary intervention with and without on-site surgical capabilities: insights from the Veterans Affairs Clinical Assessment, Reporting and Tracking (CART) Program. *Circ Cardiovasc Interv*. 2021;14(1):e009697.
31. Hannan EL, Zhong Y, Wu Y, et al. Treatment of coronary artery disease and acute myocardial infarction in hospitals with and without on-site coronary artery bypass graft surgery. *Circ Cardiovasc Interv*. 2019;12(1):e007097.
32. Dziewierz A, Brener SJ, Siudak Z, et al. Impact of on-site surgical backup on periprocedural outcomes of primary percutaneous interventions in patients presenting with ST-segment elevation myocardial infarction (from the ORPKI polish national registry). *Am J Cardiol*. 2018;122(6):929-935. doi:10.1016/j.amjcard.2018.05.047
33. McCartney PJ, Eteiba H, Maznyczka AM, et al; T-TIME Group. Effect of low-dose intracoronary alteplase during primary percutaneous coronary intervention on microvascular obstruction in patients with acute myocardial infarction: a randomized clinical trial. *JAMA*. 2019;321(1):56-68.
34. Walters D, Mahmud E. Thrombolytic therapy for st-elevation myocardial infarction presenting to non-percutaneous coronary intervention centers during the COVID-19 crisis. *Curr Cardiol Rep*. 2021;23(10):152-158.
35. Arbel Y, Ko DT, Yan AT, et al; TRANSFER-AMI Trial Investigators. Long-term follow-up of the trial of routine angioplasty and stenting after fibrinolysis to

enhance reperfusion in acute myocardial infarction (TRANSFER-AMI). *Can J Cardiol*. 2018;34(6):736-743. doi:10.1016/j.cjca.2018.02.005

36. Hochman JS, Lamas GA, Buller CE, et al; Occluded Artery Trial Investigators. Coronary intervention for persistent occlusion after myocardial infarction. *N Engl J Med*. 2006;355(23):2395-2407.
37. Džavík V., Buller CE, Lamas GA, et al; TOSCA-2 Investigators. Randomized trial of percutaneous coronary intervention for subacute infarct-related coronary artery occlusion to achieve long-term patency and improve ventricular function: the Total Occlusion Study of Canada (TOSCA)–2 Trial. *Circulation*. 2006;114(23):2449-2457.
38. Madsen JK, Grande P, Saunamäki K, et al. Danish multicenter randomized study of invasive versus conservative treatment in patients with inducible ischemia after thrombolysis in acute myocardial infarction (DANAMI). DANish trial in Acute Myocardial Infarction. *Circulation*. 1997;96(3):748-755.
39. Zeymer U, Uebis R, Vogt A, et al; ALKK-Study Group. Randomized comparison of percutaneous transluminal coronary angioplasty and medical therapy in stable survivors of acute myocardial infarction with single vessel disease: a study of the Arbeitsgemeinschaft Leitende Kardiologische Krankenhausarzte. *Circulation*. 2003;108(11):1324-1328.
40. Stenestrand U, Wallentin L. Early revascularisation and 1-year survival in 14-day survivors of acute myocardial infarction: a prospective cohort study. *Lancet*. 2002;359(9320):1805-1811. doi:10.1016/s0140-6736(02)08710-x
41. Liu T, Howarth AG, Chen Y, et al. Intramyocardial hemorrhage and the "Wave front" of reperfusion injury compromising myocardial salvage. *J Am Coll Cardiol*. 2022;79(1):35-48. doi:10.1016/j.jacc.2021.10.034
42. Virani SS, Newby LK, Arnold SV, et al; Peer Review Committee Members. 2023 AHA/ACC/ACCP/ASPC/NLA/PCNA guideline for the management of patients with chronic coronary disease: a report of the American Heart Association/American College of Cardiology Joint committee on clinical practice guidelines. *Circulation*. 2023;148(9):e9-e119. doi:10.1161/cir.0000000000001168
43. Damluji AA, van Diepen S, Katz JN, et al; American Heart Association Council on Clinical Cardiology; Council on Arteriosclerosis, Thrombosis and Vascular Biology; Council on Cardiovascular Surgery and Anesthesia; and Council on Cardiovascular and Stroke Nursing. Mechanical complications of acute myocardial infarction: a scientific statement from the American Heart Association. *Circulation*. 2021;144(2):e16-e35. doi:10.1161/cir.0000000000000985
44. Nordmann AJ, Hengstler P, Harr T, Young J, Bucher HC. Clinical outcomes of primary stenting versus balloon angioplasty in patients with myocardial infarction: a meta-analysis of randomized controlled trials. *Am J Med*. 2004;116(4):253-262. doi:10.1016/j.amjmed.2003.08.035
45. Zhu MM, Feit A, Chadow H, Alam M, Kwan T, Clark LT. Primary stent implantation compared with primary balloon angioplasty for acute myocardial infarction: a meta-analysis of randomized clinical trials. *Am J Cardiol*. 2001;88(3):297-301. doi:10.1016/s0002-9149(01)01645-9
46. Vos NS, Fagel ND, Amoroso G, et al. Paclitaxel-coated balloon angioplasty versus drug-eluting stent in acute myocardial infarction: the REVELATION randomized trial. *JACC Cardiovasc Interv*. 2019;12(17):1691-1699. doi:10.1016/j.jcin.2019.04.016
47. Levine GN, Bates ER, Bittl JA, et al. 2016 ACC/AHA guideline focused update on duration of dual antiplatelet therapy in patients with coronary artery disease: a report of the American College of Cardiology/American Heart Association Task Force on clinical practice guidelines—an update of the 2011 ACCF/AHA/SCAI guideline for percutaneous coronary intervention, 2011 ACCF/AHA guideline for coronary artery bypass graft surgery, 2012 ACC/AHA/ACP/AATS/PCNA/SCAI/STS guideline for the diagnosis and management of patients with stable ischemic heart disease, 2013 ACCF/AHA guideline for the management of ST-elevation myocardial infarction, 2014 AHA/ACC guideline for the management of patients with non-ST-elevation acute coronary syndromes, and 2014 ACC/AHA guideline on perioperative cardiovascular evaluation and management of patients undergoing noncardiac surgery. *Circulation*. 2016;134(10):e123-e155. doi:10.1161/cir.0000000000000404
48. Kereiakes DJ, Yeh RW, Massaro JM, et al; Dual Antiplatelet Therapy DAPT Study Investigators. Antiplatelet therapy duration following bare metal or drug-eluting coronary stents—the dual antiplatelet therapy randomized clinical trial. *JAMA*. 2015;313(11):1113-1121. doi:10.1001/jama.2015.1671
49. Grines CL, Bonow RO, Casey DE, Jr, et al, American Heart Association, American College of Cardiology, Society for Cardiovascular Angiography and Interventions, American College of Surgeons, American Dental Association, American College of Physicians. Prevention of premature discontinuation of dual antiplatelet therapy in patients with coronary artery stents: a science advisory from the American Heart Association, American College of Cardiology, Society for cardiovascular angiography and interventions, American College of Surgeons, and American Dental Association, with representation from the American College of Physicians. *Catheter Cardiovasc Interv*. 2007;69(3):334-340. doi:10.1002/ccd.21124
50. Kuramitsu S, Ohya M, Shinozaki T, et al. Risk factors and long-term clinical outcomes of second-generation drug-eluting Stent thrombosis: insights from the REAL-ST registry. *Circ Cardiovasc Interv*. 2019;12(6):e007822.
51. Malik AH, Shetty S, Yandrapalli S, et al. 6-month readmission and mortality differences in DES vs. BMS for STEMI in the contemporary era-A nationwide analysis. *Circulation*. 2019;140:A9514.
52. Hamirani YS, Jibrin I, Abraham D, Merriman B, Wenz C, Bahr RD. Paclitaxel-eluting versus bare-metal stents in acute ST elevation myocardial infarction (STEMI). *Crit Pathw Cardiol*. 2008;7(4):232-238. doi:10.1097/HPC.0b013e3181805e0b
53. Vlaar PJ, Svilaas T, van der Horst IC, et al. Cardiac death and reinfarction after 1 year in the Thrombus Aspiration during Percutaneous coronary intervention in Acute myocardial infarction Study (TAPAS): a 1-year follow-up study. *Lancet*. 2008;371(9628):1915-1920. doi:10.1016/s0140-6736(08)60833-8
54. Svilaas T, Vlaar PJ, van der Horst IC, et al. Thrombus aspiration during primary percutaneous coronary intervention. *N Engl J Med*. 2008;358(6):557-567. doi:10.1056/NEJMoa0706416
55. Lagerqvist B, Fröbert O, Olivecrona GK, et al. Outcomes 1 year after thrombus aspiration for myocardial infarction. *N Engl J Med*. 2014;371(12):1111-1120. doi:10.1056/NEJMoa1405707
56. Fröbert O, Lagerqvist B, Olivecrona GK, et al; TASTE Trial. Thrombus aspiration during ST-segment elevation myocardial infarction. *N Engl J Med*. 2013;369(17):1587-1597. doi:10.1056/NEJMoa1308789
57. Jolly SS, Cairns JA, Yusuf S, et al; TOTAL Investigators. Randomized trial of primary PCI with or without routine manual thrombectomy. *N Engl J Med*. 2015;372(15):1389-1398. doi:10.1056/NEJMoa1415098
58. Elgendy IY, Huo T, Bhatt DL, Bavry AA. Is aspiration thrombectomy beneficial in patients undergoing primary percutaneous coronary intervention? Meta-analysis of randomized trials. *Circ Cardiovasc Interv*. 2015;8(7):e002258. doi:10.1161/circinterventions.114.002258
59. Pruthi S, Bangalore S. The state of coronary thrombus aspiration. *J Am Heart Assoc*. 2022;11(16):e026849. doi:10.1161/jaha.122.026849
60. Migliorini A, Stabile A, Rodriguez AE, et al; JETSTENT Trial Investigators. Comparison of AngioJet rheolytic thrombectomy before direct infarct artery stenting with direct stenting alone in patients with acute myocardial infarction. The JETSTENT trial. *J Am Coll Cardiol*. 2010;56(16):1298-1306. doi:10.1016/j.jacc.2010.06.011
61. Ali A, Cox D, Dib N, et al; AIMI Investigators. Rheolytic thrombectomy with percutaneous coronary intervention for infarct size reduction in acute myocardial infarction: 30-day results from a multicenter randomized study. *J Am Coll Cardiol*. 2006;48(2):244-252. doi:10.1016/j.jacc.2006.03.044
62. Sharma S, Lardizabal JA. Embolic protection devices in saphenous vein graft intervention: a stitch in time saves nine. *Circ Cardiovasc Interv*. 2017;10(12):e006124. doi:10.1161/circinterventions.117.006124
63. Damluji AA, Otalvaro L, Cohen MG. Anticoagulation for percutaneous coronary intervention: a contemporary review. *Curr Opin Cardiol*. 2015;30(4):311-318. doi:10.1097/hco.0000000000000182
64. White HD, Aylward PE, Frey MJ, et al. Randomized, double-blind comparison of hirulog versus heparin in patients receiving streptokinase and aspirin for acute myocardial infarction (HERO). Hirulog Early Reperfusion/Occlusion (HERO) Trial Investigators. *Circulation*. 1997;96(7):2155-2161. doi:10.1161/01.cir.96.7.2155
65. White H; Hirulog and Early Reperfusion or Occlusion HERO-2 Trial Investigators. Thrombin-specific anticoagulation with bivalirudin versus heparin in patients receiving fibrinolytic therapy for acute myocardial

infarction: the HERO-2 randomised trial. *Lancet*. 2001;358(9296):1855-1863. doi:10.1016/s0140-6736(01)06887-8

66. Stone GW, Witzenbichler B, Guagliumi G, et al; HORIZONS-AMI Trial Investigators. Heparin plus a glycoprotein IIb/IIIa inhibitor versus bivalirudin monotherapy and paclitaxel-eluting stents versus bare-metal stents in acute myocardial infarction (HORIZONS-AMI): final 3-year results from a multicentre, randomised controlled trial. *Lancet*. 2011;377(9784):2193-2204. doi:10.1016/s0140-6736(11)60764-2
67. Shahzad A, Kemp I, Mars C, et al; HEAT-PPCI trial investigators. Unfractionated heparin versus bivalirudin in primary percutaneous coronary intervention (HEAT-PPCI): an open-label, single centre, randomised controlled trial. *Lancet*. 2014;384(9957):1849-1858. doi:10.1016/s0140-6736(14)60924-7
68. Valgimigli M, Frigoli E, Leonardi S, et al; MATRIX Investigators. Bivalirudin or unfractionated heparin in acute coronary syndromes. *N Engl J Med*. 2015;373(11):997-1009. doi:10.1056/NEJMoa1507854
69. James S, Koul S, Andersson J, et al. Bivalirudin versus heparin monotherapy in ST-segment-elevation myocardial infarction. *Circ Cardiovasc Interv*. 2021;14(12):e008969. doi:10.1161/circinterventions.120.008969
70. Ferguson JJ, Califf RM, Antman EM, et al; SYNERGY Trial Investigators. Enoxaparin vs unfractionated heparin in high-risk patients with non-ST-segment elevation acute coronary syndromes managed with an intended early invasive strategy: primary results of the SYNERGY randomized trial. *JAMA*. 2004;292(1):45-54. doi:10.1001/jama.292.1.45
71. Mehilli J, Kastrati A, Schulz S, et al; Bavarian Reperfusion Alternatives Evaluation-3 BRAVE-3 Study Investigators. Abciximab in patients with acute ST-segment-elevation myocardial infarction undergoing primary percutaneous coronary intervention after clopidogrel loading: a randomized double-blind trial. *Circulation*. 2009;119(14):1933-1940. doi:10.1161/circulationaha.108.818617
72. Kushner FG, Hand M, Smith SC Jr, et al; American College of Cardiology Foundation, American Heart Association Task Force on Practice Guidelines. 2009 focused updates: ACC/AHA guidelines for the management of patients with ST-elevation myocardial infarction (updating the 2004 guideline and 2007 focused update) and ACC/AHA/SCAI guidelines on percutaneous coronary intervention (updating the 2005 guideline and 2007 focused update)—a report of the American College of Cardiology Foundation/American Heart Association Task Force on Practice Guidelines. *Catheter Cardiovasc Interv*. 2009;74(7):E25-E68. doi:10.1002/ccd.22351
73. Gurm HS, Tamhane U, Meier P, Grossman PM, Chetcuti S, Bates ER. A comparison of abciximab and small-molecule glycoprotein IIb/IIIa inhibitors in patients undergoing primary percutaneous coronary intervention: a meta-analysis of contemporary randomized controlled trials. *Circ Cardiovasc Interv*. 2009;2(3):230-236. doi:10.1161/circinterventions.108.847996
74. Ellis SG, Tendera M, de Belder MA, et al; FINESSE Investigators. Facilitated PCI in patients with ST-elevation myocardial infarction. *N Engl J Med*. 2008;358(21):2205-2217. doi:10.1056/NEJMoa0706816
75. Thomas A, Gitto M, Shah S, et al. Antiplatelet strategies following PCI: a review of trials informing current and future therapies. *J Soc Cardiovasc Angiogr Interv*. 2023:2:100607.
76. Jia M, Li Z, Chu H, Li L, Chen K. Novel oral P2Y12 inhibitor prasugrel vs. clopidogrel in patients with acute coronary syndrome: evidence based on 6 studies. *Med Sci Monit*. 2015;21:1131-1137. doi:10.12659/msm.893914
77. Wallentin L, Becker RC, Budaj A, , et al; PLATO Investigators. Ticagrelor versus clopidogrel in patients with acute coronary syndromes. *N Engl J Med*. 2009;361(11):1045-1057. doi:10.1056/NEJMoa0904327
78. Damluji AA, Forman DE, Wang TY, et al; American Heart Association Cardiovascular Disease in Older Populations Committee of the Council on Clinical Cardiology and Council on Cardiovascular and Stroke Nursing; Council on Cardiovascular Radiology and Intervention; and Council on Lifestyle and Cardiometabolic Health. Management of acute coronary syndrome in the older adult population: a scientific statement from the American Heart Association. *Circulation*. 2023;147(3):e32-e62. doi:10.1161/CIR.0000000000001112
79. Steinhubl SR, Berger PB, Mann JT III, et al, CREDO Investigators. Clopidogrel for the Reduction of Events During Observation. Early and sustained dual oral antiplatelet therapy following percutaneous coronary intervention: a randomized controlled trial. *JAMA*. 2002;288(19):2411-2420. doi:10.1001/jama.288.19.2411
80. Sabatine MS, Cannon CP, Gibson CM, et al; CLARITY-TIMI 28 Investigators. Addition of clopidogrel to aspirin and fibrinolytic therapy for myocardial infarction with ST-segment elevation. *N Engl J Med*. 2005;352(12):1179-1189. doi:10.1056/NEJMoa050522
81. Chen ZM, Jiang LX, Chen YP, et al; COMMIT ClOpidogrel and Metoprolol in Myocardial Infarction Trial Collaborative Group. Addition of clopidogrel to aspirin in 45,852 patients with acute myocardial infarction: randomised placebo-controlled trial. *Lancet*. 2005;366(9497):1607-1621. doi:10.1016/s0140-6736(05)67660-x
82. Steg PG, Bhatt DL, Hamm CW, et al; CHAMPION Investigators. Effect of cangrelor on periprocedural outcomes in percutaneous coronary interventions: a pooled analysis of patient-level data. *Lancet*. 2013;382(9909):1981-1992. doi:10.1016/s0140-6736(13)61615-3

Cardiogenic Shock and Mechanical Circulatory Support Devices

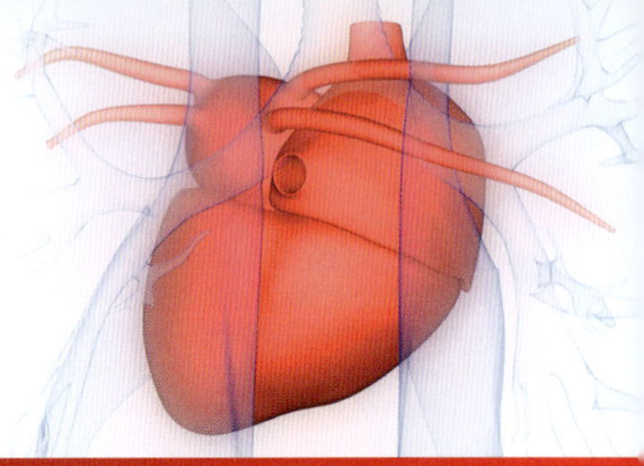

Modar Alom and Karim M. Al-Azizi

In the past 2 decades, the field of interventional cardiology has witnessed significant clinical and technological advancements, leading to a revolution in practice. The dividing lines between what could traditionally be accomplished only through surgery and what can now be described as the standard of care in the catheterization laboratory continue to blur. Accordingly, the risk profile of patients referred to percutaneous coronary intervention (PCI) has changed, with a heightened level of acuity. Furthermore, the treatment of cardiogenic shock (CS) has advanced with the introduction of percutaneously inserted hemodynamic support devices. PCI-related risk, the nature and hemodynamics of CS, and the relative merits of support in the management of both have become increasingly relevant and important over the past few years. This chapter serves to review high-risk PCI, CS, and outlines the role of mechanical circulatory support devices utilized in the catheterization laboratory.

HIGH-RISK PCI

While no PCI is truly free of procedural complications, the spectrum of patients and lesions treated by PCI is associated with a wide range of risks. Advances in technology and the advent of hemodynamic support have enhanced our ability to treat more complex and higher-risk patient subsets.

Understanding the clinical and anatomical features associated with elevated procedural risk is paramount to ensuring optimal case management and patient outcomes. With appropriate preparation and anticipation, adjunct procedural strategies can be employed to mitigate risks and optimize care.

DEFINING RISK

PCI-related risk is associated with both clinical and anatomical features. From the clinical perspective, patient presentation, along with baseline characteristics, such as age, gender, diabetes, prior myocardial infarction (MI), left ventricular (LV) dysfunction, peripheral artery disease, and renal insufficiency, have all been associated with increased risk of complications, including death, MI, stroke, and stent thrombosis.[1] Importantly, many of these factors are not modifiable and cannot be improved prior to the procedure. Conversely, some preprocedural characteristics such as renal function or volume status can be medically optimized prior to PCI, and an effort to mitigate risk should logically focus on optimization where possible.

Anatomically, numerous factors have been associated with an increased risk of procedural failure and/or complications. These factors include left main (LM) stenosis, bifurcation disease, trifurcation lesions, saphenous vein graft stenosis, ostial stenosis, heavily calcified lesions, and chronic total occlusions[2] (**Table 20.1**). Recognizing the inherent risk associated with each lesion, especially in the context of clinical risk factors, allows for appropriate planning of treatment strategy and adjunct equipment. Specific strategies to treat these types of lesions are covered elsewhere in this text.

TABLE 20.1 Angiographic Features Contributing to Increasing Complexity of CAD

Left main or proximal LAD artery lesion
Chronic total occlusion
Trifurcation lesion
Complex bifurcation lesion
Heavy calcification
Severe tortuosity
Aorto-ostial stenosis
Diffusely diseased and narrowed segments distal to the lesion
Thrombotic lesion
Lesion length >20 mm

CAD, coronary artery disease; LAD, left anterior descending.

Assessing Risk

Incorporating patient presentation, baseline characteristics, and relevant anatomy, a subjective assessment of risk is a basic component of any interventional procedure. To help objectify this process, multiple risk calculators have been developed and validated. Two of the best validated and commonly used calculators are the Mayo Clinic Risk Score and the New York State PCI Database. The Mayo Clinic Risk Score was originally derived from 7457 patients undergoing PCI at a single center.[3] It was reiterated in 2007 and validated with data collected by the NCDR Cath PCI Registry of over 300,000 patients undergoing PCI between 2004 and 2006 (**Fig. 20.1**).[4] The New York State PCI Database analyzed 45,000 PCI procedures in 2002 and identified nine factors associated with an increased risk of adverse events, assigning weighted integer scores to each variable.[5] Both the Mayo Clinic and NY State risk scores continue to accurately predict in-hospital mortality in the current era.[6]

Anatomic risk scores have also been developed. The *SYNTAX score* was developed as part of a trial comparing PCI to coronary artery bypass surgery in patients with LM or multivessel disease.[7] Based upon anatomic factors for each lesion, an overall score is derived to depict complexity of the interventional procedure. Divided by tertiles, the SYNTAX score has been shown to predict death, MI, stroke, and/or repeat revascularization at 1 year.[8] Importantly, the SYNTAX score does not predict in-hospital outcomes, and the score lacks any clinical modifiers of risk. The SYNTAX II score was developed to incorporate both the anatomic SYNTAX score and clinical predictors of risk, such as age, gender, ejection fraction, renal function, and the presence of peripheral or

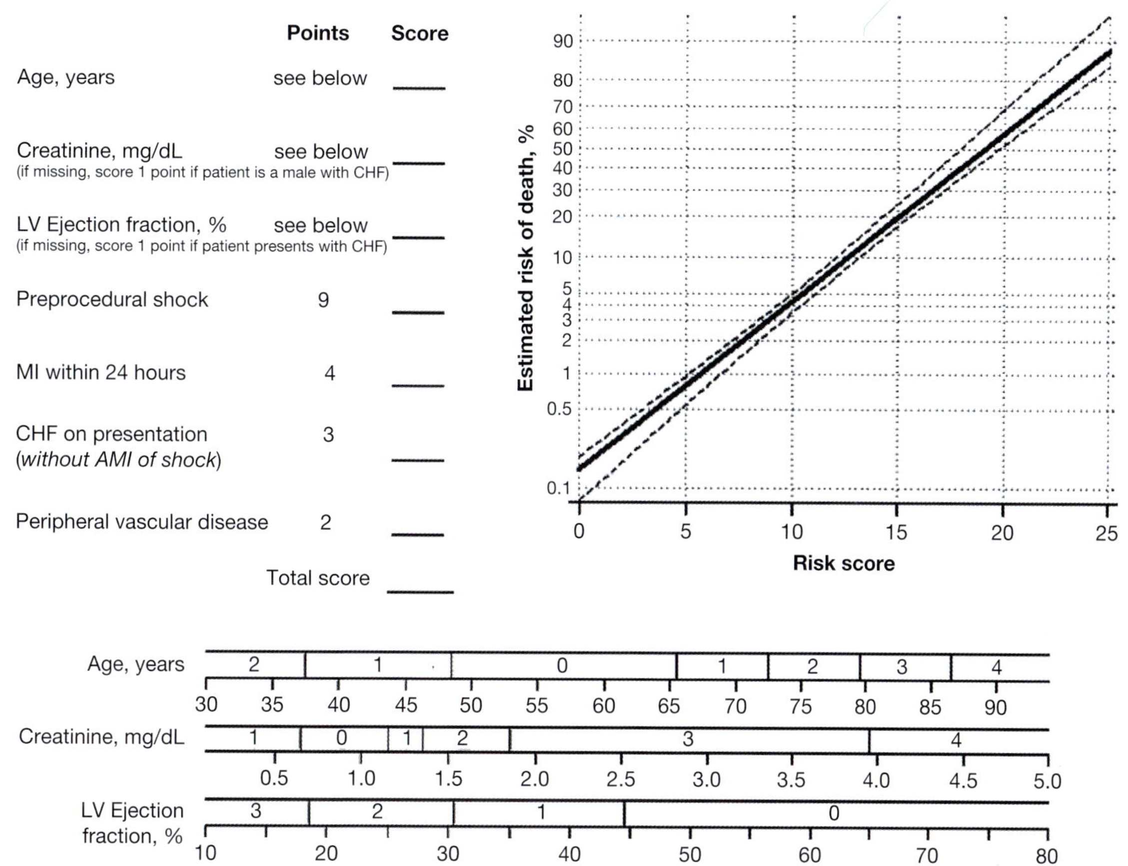

FIGURE 20.1 Mayo Clinic risk calculator. AMI, acute myocardial infarction; CHF, congestive heart failure; LV, left ventricular; MI, myocardial infarction.

chronic lung disease to predict in hospital and mortality for both PCI and coronary artery bypass grafting (CABG). The SYNTAX II score predictive accuracy on 4-year mortality was validated in an analysis of 1480 patients enrolled in two studies comparing PCI and CABG for multivessel or LM coronary disease.[9] While no single calculator will capture every variable, these calculators all serve to provide a conceptual framework upon which to gauge periprocedural risk.

While high-risk PCI applies to a wide spectrum of clinical and anatomic scenarios, an important subset relates to the potential for hemodynamic collapse and CS. Patients undergoing PCI targeting an unprotected LM coronary artery or a last remaining conduit, especially in the setting of complex disease and reduced ejection fraction, are at particularly high risk. The remainder of this chapter focuses on this subset of high-risk PCI and CS, including the use of circulatory support devices for the management of both.

CARDIOGENIC SHOCK

CS is a major cause of global morbidity and mortality. CS most commonly occurs after an acute myocardial infarction (AMI) or in patients with advanced heart failure (HF). Shock from any cause is characterized by tissue hypoperfusion leading to end-organ damage, and CS is defined as tissue hypoperfusion secondary to cardiac failure despite adequate circulatory volume and LV filling pressure. Hemodynamic criteria for CS include the following: a systolic blood pressure <90 mm Hg for >30 minutes or a fall in mean arterial blood pressure greater than 30 mm Hg below baseline with a cardiac index (CI) of <1.8 L/min/m^2 without hemodynamic support or <2.2 L/min/m^2 with support and a pulmonary capillary wedge pressure (PCWP) >15 mm Hg.[10-12]

The Society for Cardiac Angiography and Interventions (SCAI) shock stages classify CS into five stages (A-E). Stage A represents patients at risk, while stage E signifies severe shock with multiorgan failure. The classification assists in assessing severity and determining therapy, with each stage correlating to increased mortality risk. It provides a structured approach for clinicians treating patients with HF and shock (**Fig. 20.2**).

CAUSES OF CS

A wide range of conditions can lead to CS (**Table 20.2**). CS can develop in the setting of AMI and can occur after both ST-elevation myocardial infarction (STEMI) and non-ST-elevation myocardial infarction (NSTEMI), either as a manifestation of primary pump failure or as a mechanical complication. While thrombotic coronary artery occlusion is often well tolerated, approximately 5% to 8% of AMI patients develop clinical manifestations of hemodynamic collapse.[13] Early preclinical studies suggest that approximately 40% of the myocardium must be involved in an AMI to cause CS,[14] and risk factors include occlusion of the left anterior descending (LAD) artery, age over 65, hypertension, prior infarction, or multivessel disease.[15] Mortality associated with CS after AMI is high, with in-hospital mortality approaching 60% in multiple studies.[16]

Postmyocardial mechanical complications (acute mitral regurgitation, papillary muscle rupture, ventricular septal rupture, and free wall rupture) are important and clinically dramatic events that can lead to CS. In the revascularization era, these events are fortunately

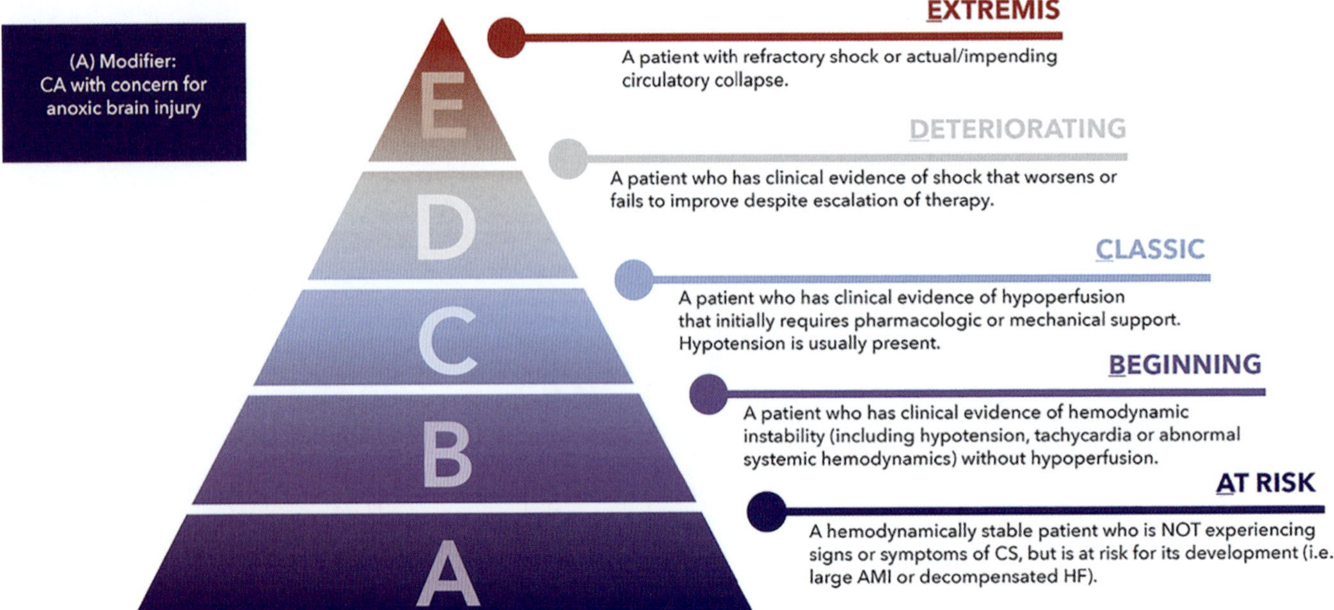

FIGURE 20.2 SCAI SHOCK classification pyramid. AMI, acute myocardial infarction; CS, cardiogenic shock; HF, heart failure; SCAI, Society for Cardiovascular Angiography and Interventions.

rare, with papillary muscle rupture and ventricular septal or free wall rupture collectively occurring in only about 1% of cases. Risk factors include female gender and the absence of coronary artery disease, suggesting the relevance of "at risk" myocardium and the importance of collateral circulation in chronic disease. When it does occur, papillary muscle rupture most commonly involves the posteromedial papillary muscle because it receives a singular blood supply from the dominant coronary vessel supplying the posterior descending artery.[17] It manifests as acute, severe mitral regurgitation, and HF. Septal rupture occurs within subtended territory from the infarcted related artery (anteroapical with LAD occlusion or posterobasal with right coronary artery [RCA] occlusion) and presents as acute HF from a left-right shunt.[18,19] Free wall rupture can occur anywhere within subtended territory and manifests most commonly as pulseless electrical activity and tamponade.[20,21]

While CS following AMI is typically related to left-sided HF, right ventricular (RV) myocardial infarction (RVMI) can also lead to CS, and it is associated with a high risk of morbidity and mortality, ventricular fibrillation, and high-grade AV-conduction block.[22,23] As the RV receives blood from acute marginal branches of the RCA and the posterior descending artery, RVMI occurs most commonly after acute proximal right coronary occlusion but can occur after occlusion of a dominant circumflex artery.[24,25] RV ischemia leads to RV systolic failure and reduced LV preload. As RV pressure and volume (PV) overload develop, the interventricular septum shifts toward the LV cavity, further reducing LV stroke volume. Hemodynamic indices of RV failure in AMI include measurements of RV stroke work, right atrial to PCWP (RA:PCWP) ratio of >0.8, and pulmonary artery pulse pressure.[26] In the SHOCK registry, isolated RV failure accounted for 49 (5.3%) of the 933 patients with myocardial dysfunction as the primary mechanism underlying CS.[27]

CS in the absence of AMI occurs most commonly in the presence of advanced HF. In 2017, there were 1.2 million HF hospitalizations in the United States among 924,000 patients with HF.[28] As a manifestation of acutely decompensated HF, CS is included among several HF classification systems (**Table 20.3**). The New York Heart Association (NYHA) classifies HF severity based on symptoms. CS is categorized as a manifestation of NYHA Class IV HF. For patients with advanced HF (NYHA class III or IV), the Interagency Registry

TABLE 20.2 Causes of Cardiogenic Shock

ISCHEMIC	NONISCHEMIC	NONCARDIAC
Acute myocardial infarction	Chronic systolic heart failure	Severe sepsis
Pump failure	Myocarditis	Subarachnoid hemorrhage
Right ventricular infarction	Hypertrophic cardiomyopathy	Hypothyroidism
Post-myocardial infarction complications	Valvular heart disease	
Arrhythmia	Myocardial contusion	
Papillary muscle rupture	Stress cardiomyopathy	
Ventricular septal rupture	Arrhythmia	
Free wall rupture/tamponade		

TABLE 20.3 Classifications of Heart Failure and Cardiogenic Shock

ACC/AHA STAGE	NYHA	INTERMACS	TERMINOLOGY
D	IV	I	"Crash and burn," emergent mechanical support
D	IV	II	Intravenous inotropes, may need mechanical support
D	IV	III	Stable, but inotrope-dependent
D	IV (ambulatory)	IV	Resting symptoms, oral therapy, peak VO_2 <12 L/min
D	IV (ambulatory)	V	ADL is severely limited, peak VO_2 <12 L/min
D	III	VI	ADL is possible but limited
D	III	VII	Advanced class III symptoms
C	I–III	–	Structural disease, current or past symptoms
B	I	–	Structural disease, no symptoms
A	I	–	At risk, no structural disease or symptoms

for Mechanically Assisted Circulatory Support (INTERMACS) has defined seven clinical profiles before implantation of an LV assist device (LVAD).[29] CS is identified by INTERMACS profiles 1 and 2, where patients may be "crashing" despite aggressive therapy or "sliding fast on inotropes," respectively. Both INTERMACS 1 and 2 subjects may be considered for temporary circulatory support as a bridge to recovery, surgical LVAD, or cardiac transplantation.

Primary valvular heart disease is another important cause of CS. Endocarditis, mitral valve prolapse, chordal rupture, or aortic dissection extending to the aortic annulus may cause CS secondary to valve failure.[30-34] Patients with chronic valve disease, including aortic/mitral stenosis, may also develop CS secondary to progressive LV failure or arrhythmias.[35]

HEMODYNAMICS OF CS

As defined earlier, CS is characterized by sustained hypotension, low cardiac output, and impaired tissue perfusion despite adequate intravascular volume. Cardiac function is best represented by the PV loop. Each PV loop represents one cardiac cycle (**Fig. 20.3A**).[36]

The PV loop can be modulated in various ways (**Fig. 20.3B-D**). Increasing preload will increase SV without changing E_{max} or E_a. Vasopressors designed to increase afterload will increase E_a, which may reduce stroke volume, without affecting E_{max}. Inotropes will primarily increase E_{max}, while decreasing E_a. These approaches increase cardiac stroke work and myocardial oxygen demand, which may propagate myocardial ischemia.

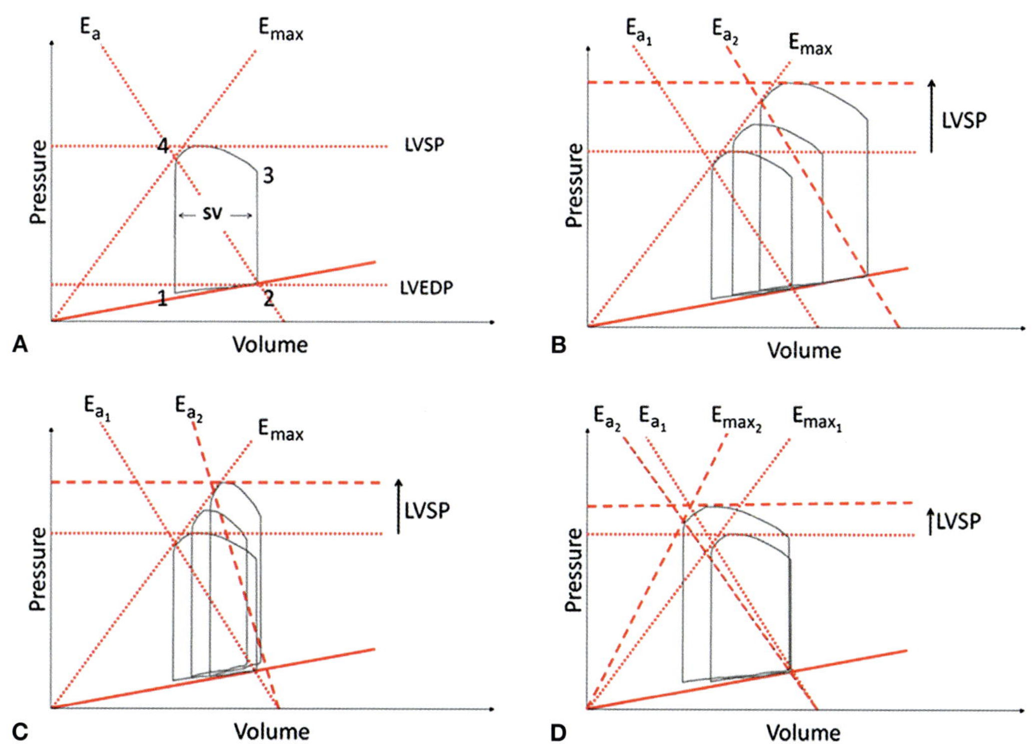

FIGURE 20.3 Pressure-volume (PV) loops. **A,** Normal PV loop. The impact of **(B)** increased LV preload (volume resuscitation), **(C)** increased LV afterload (vasopressors), and **(D)** increased LV contractility (inotropes). LV, left ventricular.

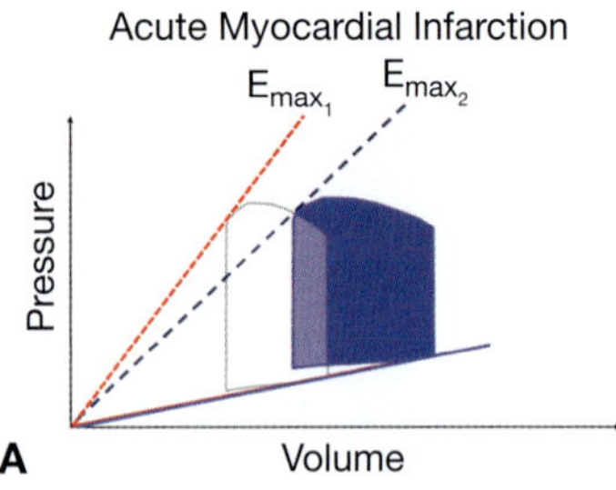

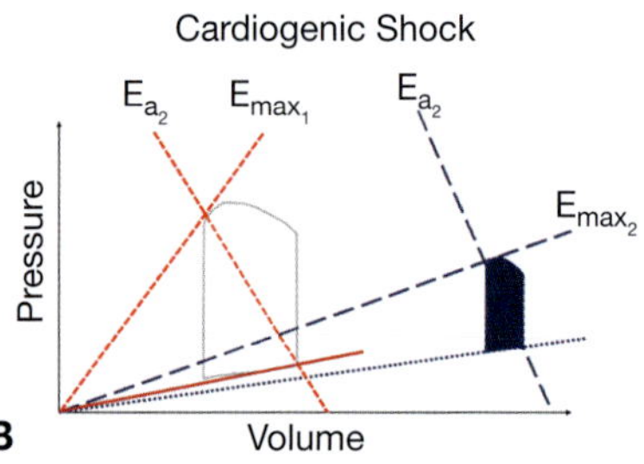

FIGURE 20.4 PV loops in AMI and cardiogenic shock. Cardiac hemodynamics in AMI **(A)** and cardiogenic shock **(B)**. AMI, acute myocardial infarction; PV, pressure–volume.

In the setting of an AMI, E_{max} and stroke volume may be reduced, while E_a increases to compensate for hypotension (**Fig. 20.4A**).[37,38] Without treatment, cardiac function worsens, and significant reductions in E_{max} and stroke volume are observed, which contribute to both systemic hypotension and progressively increasing LV end-diastolic volume. Increased systemic vascular resistance (SVR) is reflected as an increase in E_a. As CS progresses, the PV loop becomes smaller and shifts to the right of the PV plane (**Fig. 20.4B**). The goal of therapy in the setting of CS is to increase contractility, improve stroke volume, and reduce intracardiac volume overload while maintaining an adequate mean arterial pressure (MAP) to support end-organ tissue perfusion.

Changes in afterload are variable in CS. Reduced cardiac output activates the sympathetic nervous system, which increases SVR through adrenergic agonists, including norepinephrine and epinephrine. Nevertheless, measured SVR in the setting of CS can often be normal or low. In the SHOCK trial, nearly 20% of subjects with CS had signs of systemic inflammatory response syndrome, as defined by fever, leukocytosis, and low SVR.[39,40] A postulated mechanism for low SVR in these CS subjects was the activation of inducible nitric oxide synthase by inflammatory mediators, thereby leading to systemic vasodilatation.

MANAGEMENT OF CS

Diagnosis and Initial Stabilization

Early diagnosis is essential for successful management of CS. Rapid bedside assessment of signs and symptoms include hypotension, tachycardia, oliguria, change in mental status, hypoxia, cyanosis, and cold or clammy skin. Rales suggestive of pulmonary edema may not be consistently present in CS. Initial diagnostic testing includes electrocardiography to diagnose AMI or arrhythmia. Bedside echocardiography can rapidly define cardiac etiologies for CS, including primary systolic failure, tamponade, valvular insufficiency, valvular stenoses, or septal/free wall rupture. Pulmonary artery (PA) catheterization may help discriminate noncardiac from cardiac causes of shock and help define the underlying cause of cardiac failure, including LV failure, RV failure, cardiac tamponade, severe mitral regurgitation, and ventricular septal defects. PA catheterization provides critical information, including intracardiac filling pressures, screening oximetry, and quantification of cardiac output. PA catheterization is a IIB recommendation to define hemodynamic subsets and help develops appropriate management strategies patients with CS.[41]

The goal of initial treatment for CS includes maintenance of tissue perfusion, which includes both maintaining MAP and oxygenation. Early mechanical ventilation should be considered in patients with persistent hypoxemia despite supplemental oxygen. Volume resuscitation should be attempted to maintain MAP in subjects without evidence of overt volume overload (elevated jugular venous pressure or pulmonary congestion). In the setting of symptomatic bradycardia, transvenous pacing may be required to enhance cardiac output.

Pharmacologic Therapy

Pharmacologic support with inotropes or vasopressors is recommended for individuals not responsive to volume resuscitation or in the setting of decompensated HF. Each pharmacologic agent provides a unique profile of hemodynamic support (**Table 20.4**).[42] First-line agents for blood pressure support include escalating doses of dopamine, norepinephrine, or epinephrine. High-dose dopamine, norepinephrine, or epinephrine will stimulate both α- and β-adrenergic receptors, thereby providing primarily vasopressor and minimal inotropic support. Inotropes such as dobutamine and milrinone should be initiated in individuals with primary cardiac failure. Both agents will provide β-receptor agonism by stimulating the receptor directly or promoting accumulation of cyclic adenosine monophosphate, respectively.

Through inotropic and vasopressor support, these pharmacologic agents serve to increase cardiac output and maintain an MAP to sustain vital organ perfusion. Disadvantages of inotropes include increased risk for ventricular arrhythmia, increased myocardial oxygen demand, and increased stroke work. All these can lead to myocardial ischemia—especially in the setting of obstructive coronary artery disease.[43] Inotropes may also promote systemic hypotension and may require use of concomitant vasopressors to sustain blood pressure while enhancing cardiac output. While maintaining central MAP, vasopressor agents may lead to peripheral vasoconstriction and related complications. In cases of refractory shock despite pharmacologic support, mechanical assist devices may be considered.

Revascularization

In patients with STEMI and CS or hemodynamic instability, PCI or CABG (when PCI is not feasible) is indicated to improve survival, irrespective of the time delay from MI onset (2+).[44,45] Mechanical revascularization, or primary PCI, of the infarct artery is the preferred method of restoring coronary perfusion because of its superior efficacy and decreased risk of complications compared with fibrinolytic therapy.[46]

The SHOCK trial randomized 302 patients with STEMI complicated by CS to emergent revascularization (ER) within 6 hours via coronary angioplasty (64%), or CABG (36%), or intensive medical therapy (including thrombolytics) and delayed (≥54 hours) revascularization if clinically and angiographically appropriate.[47] While there was a difference in the primary endpoint of 30-day survival between ER and optimal medical therapy (OMT) (53% vs 44%), it did not reach statistical significance (95% confidence interval: 0.96-1.53; $P = .109$). Nevertheless, at 6 months, 1 year, and 6 years, absolute survival was significantly better after ER compared with

TABLE 20.4 Pharmacologic Agents in Cardiogenic Shock

AGENT	GENERAL MECHANISM	RECEPTORS				DOSE RANGE	OVERALL EFFECT	CAUTIONS
		α-1	β-1	β-2	DA			
Phenylephrine	Pure α	+++	0	0	0	Up to 180 μg/min	= to ↑ CO ↑ SVR	Caution with high SVR
Norepinephrine	α-1, some β-1	+++	++	0	0	Up to 350 μg/min	↑ CO ↑ SVR	Reflex bradycardia
Epinephrine	β-1 at low doses, increasing α-1 and β-2 with higher doses	+++	+++	++	0	Up to 0.5 μg/kg/min	↑ CO, ↓ SVR at low dose ↑ SVR at high dose	May induce vasospasm
Dopamine	Low dose—DA Mid doses—β-2 High doses—α-1	0 + ++	+ + ++	0 0 0	++ ++ ++	0.5–2 μg/kg/min 2–10 μg/kg/min 10–20 μg/kg/min	↑ CO at all doses ↑ SVR at higher doses	Arrhythmogenic
Dobutamine	β-1, β-2 at low doses, some α-1 with higher doses	+	+++	++	0	Up to 40 μg/kg/min	↑ CO ↓ SVR	Arrhythmogenic
Milrinone	Nonadrenergic PDE inhibitor, but similar effects as dobutamine	PDE inhibitor				Up to 0.5 μg/min	↑ CO ↓ SVR	Hypotension, thiocyanate poisoning

CO, cardiac output; PDE, phosphodiesterase; SVR, systemic vascular resistance.

OMT.[48] No significant survival difference was observed in subjects undergoing coronary angioplasty compared with CABG. Of note, although there was a suggestion of increased mortality in the 56 patients over age 75 who were enrolled in the SHOCK trial, several studies have since demonstrated improved survival with ER in elderly patients presenting with AMI and CS.[49,50]

Circulatory Support Devices

Mechanistically, the goals of hemodynamic support devices are to improve oxygen delivery to the vital organs, improve cardiac output, decrease LV oxygen demand, and increase coronary flow. Indications for mechanical cardiac support (MCS) can range from short-term protection during a PCI procedure to indefinite term support in fulminant CS. Currently available options for LV support include the intra-aortic balloon pump (IABP), Impella CP and 5.5 (Abiomed, Danvers, MA), TandemHeart (Cardiac Assist, Pittsburgh, PA), and extracorporeal membrane oxygenation (ECMO). Right-sided support devices include the Impella RP, Impella RP Flex, and ProtekDuo (Cardiac Assist, Pittsburgh, PA) (**Table 20.5**). Each device (**Fig. 20.5**) has a role in the management of high-risk PCI or CS, and their relative characteristics are discussed in the following text.

As noted earlier, a subset of high-risk PCI relates to the potential for hemodynamic collapse and CS, including unprotected LM and last remaining conduit in patients with reduced ejection fractions. In these patients, it is important to have hemodynamic support available. In fact, it can be argued that the prophylactic support may even be of benefit.

For those in CS related from any cause, mechanical support devices are often beneficial. These devices allow for adequate distal tissue perfusion while allowing the heart time to recover from a transient insult or serving as a bridge to more definitive therapy (revascularization, durable LV assist, or transplantation). In these cases, the underlying cause of shock, stability of the system, degree of support necessary, and expected time course to definitive outcome are important in choosing the appropriate device.

Intra-Aortic Balloon Pump

An IABP is a balloon catheter placed percutaneously, most commonly through the femoral artery (FA), into the descending aorta distal to the left subclavian artery. The IABP is connected to a pump console. Helium inflation and deflation is gated to the electrocardiogram or aortic pressure tracing and serves to enhance coronary perfusion during diastole by displacing blood volume within the descending aorta and augment cardiac output via pressure sink in the aorta during systole. The primary effects of IABP support are to (a) increase coronary perfusion, (b) reduce LV afterload, (c) increase LV SV, and (d) reduce LV end-diastolic pressure (**Fig. 20.6A**).[51] The degree of hemodynamic support afforded by an IABP is dictated by the size of the IABP, which ranges between 34 and 50 mL.

While intuitively attractive in high-risk PCI, the routine use of the IABP is not without controversy. The Balloon Pump Assisted Coronary Intervention Study (BCIS-1) evaluated routine IABP support versus no routine support in 301 patients undergoing HR-PCI.[52] While there was no difference in major adverse cardiovascular and cerebrovascular endpoints at 28 days (15.2% routine vs 16.0% no routine IABP), there were significantly fewer major procedural complications in those who received routine IABP. The Counterpulsation to Reduce Infarct Size Pre-PCI Acute MI (CRISP-AMI) trial was a multicenter, prospective, randomized to 337 patients with acute ST-segment elevation MI without shock undergoing planned primary PCI to either IABP support prior to PCI (n = 161) or primary PCI without IABP (n = 176). The

TABLE 20.5 Circulatory Support Devices

DEVICE	IABP	IMPELLA CP	IMPELLA 5.5	TANDEMHEART	VA ECMO	IMPELLA RB	PROTEKDUO
Pump mechanism	Pneumatic	Axial flow	Axial flow	Centrifugal	Centrifugal	Axial flow	Centrifugal
Canula size	8F	14F	23f	Inflow: 21F Outflow: 15-17F	Inflow: 15-22F Outflow: 18-21F	23F	29F-31F
Pump capacity	0.5-1 L/min	3.5 L/min	6.2 L/min	3.5 (15) and 5.0 (17) L/min	3-6 L	>4 L/min	>4.5 L/min
Hemodynamic support	LV	LV	LV	BiV	BiV	RV	RV
Effect on afterload	↓	↔	↔	↑	↑	↔	↔
Effect on LVEDP	↓	↓	↓	↓	↑	↔	↔
Effect on coronary perfusion	↑	Unknown possibly ↑	Unknown possibly ↑	Unknown possibly ↓	Unknown possibly ↓	↔	↔
Risk of limb ischemia	+	++	++	+++	+++	-	-
Risk of hemolysis	+	++	++	++	++	++	++
Anticoagulation	+	+	+	+++	+++	+	+++

BiV, biventricular; ECMO, extracorporeal membrane oxygenation; IABP, intra-aortic balloon pump; LV, left ventricular; LVEDP, LV end-diastolic pressure; RV, right ventricular.

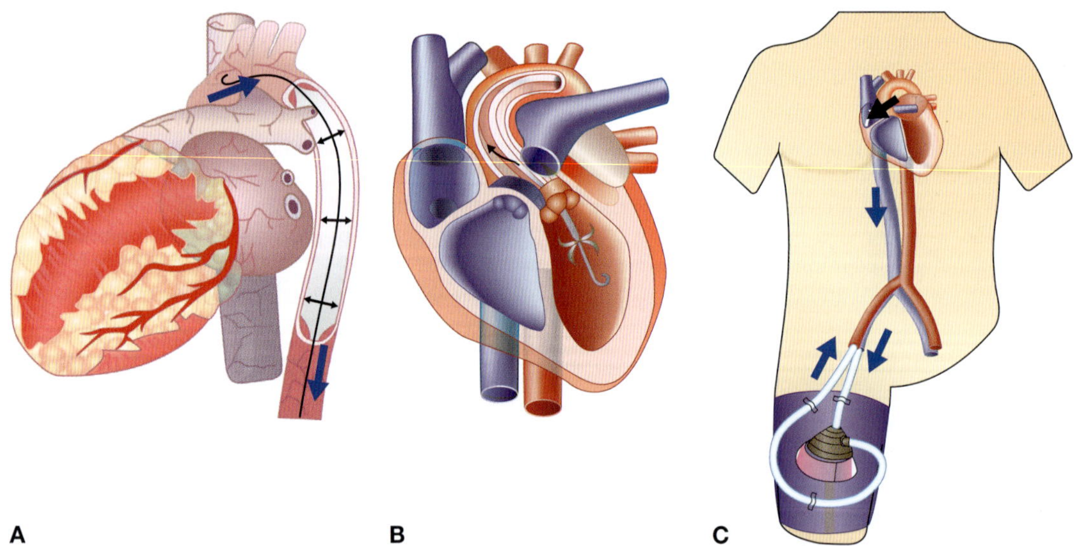

FIGURE 20.5 Percutaneous support devices. Percutaneous mechanical support devices **(A)** IABP, **(B)** Impella, **(C)** TandemHeart. IABP, intra-aortic balloon pumping.

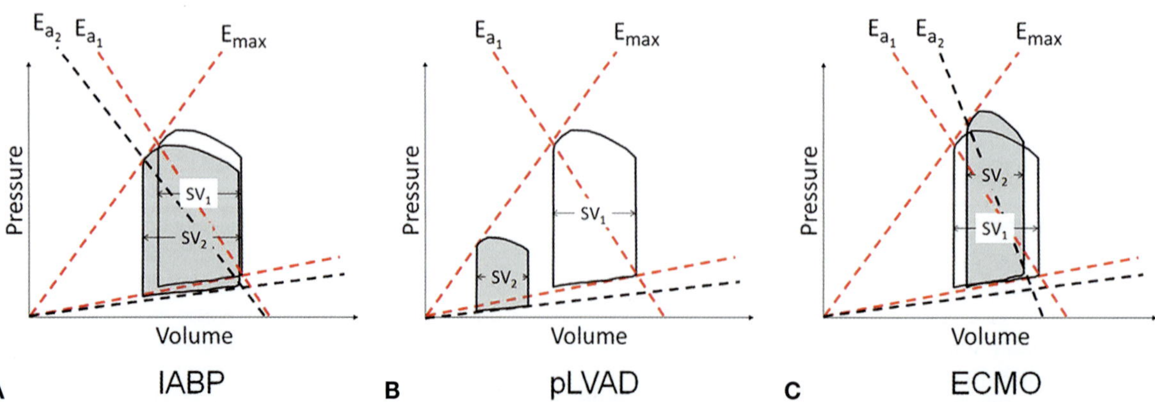

FIGURE 20.6 Hemodynamics of IABP, Impella/Tandem, and VA ECMO. Pressure-volume (PV) loops after treatment with **(A)** intra-aortic balloon counterpulsation, **(B)** percutaneous LV assist devices: Impella and TandemHeart, or **(C)** venoarterial ECMO. ECMO, extracorporeal membrane oxygenation; LV, left ventricular.

primary endpoint was infarct size, measured by cardiac magnetic resonance imaging. Mean infarct size was not significantly different between the groups (42.1% vs 37.5%); nevertheless, a trend toward reduced 6-month mortality was observed in the patients receiving up-front IABP.[53]

In patients with AMI and CS, IABP was associated with a significant reduction in mortality from 67% to 49% in the NRMI-2 database.[54] This survival benefit may relate to several factors, including improved delivery of drugs to the site of occlusion, improved penetration into the thrombus, or rapid reversal of hypotension.

Though an IABP can improve vital organ perfusion, the increase in cardiac output is modest and estimated at about 1 L/min. Additionally, the IABP depends on cardiac performance to function appropriately. For high-risk PCI and CS, this support may not prove adequate, and more aggressive mechanical support is necessary. The primary goal of a pLVAD is to reduce native LV SV, thereby reducing LV stroke work, while maintaining systemic perfusion.

Impella

The Impella is an axial flow device placed in retrograde fashion across the aortic valve that directly unloads the left ventricle and directs blood flow into the proximal aorta. The primary hemodynamic effect of the Impella is to reduce native LV SV and LV end-diastolic pressure (LVEDP).[55] The Impella is available in two forms: Impella Cardiac Power (CP) and Impella 5.5, providing an estimated 3.5 or 6.2 L/min of flow. Those are the newer generation that replaced 2.5 and 5. The Impella CP can be inserted percutaneously either as a standalone device or through a 14 French sheath, while the 5.5 is generally placed by surgical cutdown to the axillary artery.

For patients undergoing high-risk PCI, Impella may have some advantage over the IABP. The PROTECT II trial was a randomized trial comparing the Impella 2.5 to the IABP in 448 patients with LV ejections fraction <35% undergoing nonemergent PCI to either unprotected LM or a last patent coronary vessel (or ejection fraction <30% with three vessel coronary disease). Approximately two-thirds of patients had NYHA class III or IV systolic HF symptoms, with an average ejection fraction of less than 25% and similarly high PCI risk (New York, Mayo, and SYNTAX) scores. The Impella was associated with improved hemodynamic support measured by CP output. In the intention to treat population, the primary endpoint of 30-day major adverse cardiac events (MACEs) was similar between the two groups (35.1% Impella vs 40.1% IABP, $P = .227$), but a trend toward the reduction of MACE with Impella was noted at 90 days (40.6% Impella vs 49.3% IABP, $P = .066$).[56] A new study published in 2022 compared Impella and IABP support for high-risk PCI. The study involved 2156 patients undergoing nonemergent high-risk PCI. The use of Impella was associated with a higher survival rate in-hospital, showing 95.3% survival compared to 91.0% with IABP.[57]

The US-Pella registry analyzed 154 patients with AMI and CS who underwent revascularization with mechanical support via an Impella 2.5. In 38 patients, no hemodynamic support was provided during the PCI, and the Impella was placed following the procedure. In 53 patients, an IABP was placed prior to the PCI, and an Impella was placed following the procedure. In the remaining 63 patients, the Impella was placed prior to revascularization. Respective survival rates were 41% for the patients not receiving support, 42.3% for those under IABP support during PCI, and 62.1% for those with Impella support prior to the procedure.[58] These results imply utility of early Impella placement in patients with AMI and CS.

For patients with CS complicating AMI, nonrandomized trials have compared the Impella 2.5 to IABP with no significant survival benefit demonstrated. The lack of difference was largely attributed to the fact that 2.5 L/min of support was inadequate for CS. The IMPella versus IABP Reduces mortality in STEMI patients treated with primary PCI in Severe CS (IMPRESS in Severe Shock) trial compared Impella CP to IABP in 48 patients with a primary endpoint of 30-day mortality. All patients underwent primary PCI, and the two devices were associated with similar mortality rates at both 30 days (46% Impella vs 50% IABP, $P = .92$) and 6 months (50% vs 50%, $P = .92$).[59] There are no randomized controlled studies comparing IABP to Impella 5.5 or 5.0 in patients with AMI and CS.

For patients with isolated right-sided failure or biventricular failure, the Impella RP provides support via RA to PA configuration. The device is inserted through 23 French access in the right femoral vein, and it is generally guided to the left PA. With appropriate placement, it bypasses the RV by taking blood from the right atrial and pumping it through to the PA. It is capable of up to 5 L/min. The device has a humanitarian device exemption.

The RECOVER RIGHT study evaluated 30 patients with RV failure (the majority from postcardiotomy shock).[60] There was significant hemodynamic improvement (CO 1.8 ± 0.2-3.3 ± 0.2 L/min). The 30-day survival rate was 73.3% with 100% survival among discharged patients at 180 days.

A new RP Flex Impella has received Food and Drug Administration approval in 2022. It has 11F catheter and inserted via internal jugular vein. Although not widely used yet, it is expected to replace the RP impella eventually given it is advantage in facilitating patient mobility.

The ProtekDuo consists of a single cannula with two lumens designed for bidirectional flow. The cannula removes blood from the RA with the 29F outer lumen of the cannula and then returns it to the pulmonary artery through the 16F inner lumen. A larger 31F outer cannula with an 18.5F inner cannula is also available. The blood withdrawn from the outer cannula is circulated by a TandemHeart centrifugal pump, which can provide 4.5 to 5 L/min of RV support. If the patient is hypoxemic, an oxygenator can be added to provide VV ECMO.

TandemHeart

The TandemHeart is a centrifugal continuous flow pump that can generate between 3.5 and 5 L/min of flow. It is typically configured from the left atrium (LA)-to-FA, drawing oxygenated blood from the LA and circulating it back to the common FA, effectively bypassing the native LV. This original device requires a trans-septal puncture for LV support, and configurations now exist to provide pure ECMO through inferior vena cava inflow, oxygenation, and FA outflow, as well as RV support via cannula placement in the RA and PA with or without an oxygenation.

As with the Impella device, the primary hemodynamic effect of the TandemHeart device is to reduce native LV SV and LVEDP (**Fig. 20.6B**).[61] Compared to IABP in CS, these devices are associated with higher CI, MAP, and lower PCWP in a meta-analysis of three trials involving 100 patients, 40 of whom were treated with the TandemHeart device.[62] Nevertheless, despite improved hemodynamic profiles in CS, no difference in 30-day mortality was observed across the studies in this analysis, and patients treated with TandemHeart experienced an increase in bleeding complications. Future studies are required to determine the clinical utility of percutaneous ventricular assist devices in CS.

Potential complications associated with pMCS devices include peripheral vascular obstruction and ischemia, bleeding, infection, and stroke. IABP-specific complications include the following: malposition resulting in subclavian, mesenteric, or renal arterial obstruction; aortic dissection; and air or plaque embolism. Complications associated with the Impella CP device include ventricular arrhythmias and hemolysis, while complications specific to the TandemHeart device include the risk of left atrial perforation during trans-septal cannula insertion, cannula migration (antegrade or retrograde), and the potential for interatrial shunting after device removal.

Extracorporeal Membrane Oxygenation

For individuals with cardiorespiratory or biventricular failure, ECMO can be considered. Specifically, venoarterial ECMO is performed by pumping blood from the venous system into the arterial system using a centrifugal pump attached to an external oxygenator. Multiple ECMO pump devices are in commercial production, and ECMO can be rapidly initiated by percutaneous cannulation. While providing peripheral support by circulating oxygenated blood into the arterial system, ECMO effectively decreases LV SV by decreasing preload to the LV. As a result, increased afterload has been observed with ECMO due to retrograde flow through the arterial system (**Fig. 20.6C**).[63] For patients with severe LV dysfunction, "venting" the LV with an Impella may provide adequate decompression while maintaining sufficient systemic support through ECMO. This strategy may lead to improved survival compared to venoarterial ECMO alone. In a propensity matched study of 63 patients with CS, the 42 patients receiving venoarterial ECMO alone had a significantly lower in-hospital survival rate compared to the 21 patients receiving venoarterial ECMO and Impella support (20% vs 53%, $P < .01$). Further study is clearly required, but the results of this study suggest that LV decompression is an important component in the management of CS.[64]

CONCLUSIONS

The clinical and hemodynamic profiles of patients presenting to the catheterization laboratory have come to include increasingly complex, high-risk, and high-acuity situations. From high-risk PCI to CS, the various characteristics, physiology, and treatment modalities continue to develop and evolve. Over the coming decade, we can expect new advancements and emerging clinical evidence to further refine the approaches to high-risk PCI and CS.

Key Points

- Hemodynamic criteria for CS include a systolic blood pressure <90 mm Hg for >30 minutes or a fall in mean arterial blood pressure greater than 30 mm Hg below baseline with a CI of <1.8 L/min/m^2 without hemodynamic support or <2.2 L/min/m^2 with support and a PCWP > 15 mm Hg.
- Post-MI complications leading to CS include acute mitral regurgitation, ventricular septal rupture, ventricular free wall rupture, and RV failure.
- The goal of initial treatment for CS includes maintenance of tissue perfusion, which includes maintaining both MAP and oxygenation. CS refractory to volume resuscitation or that associated with decompensated HF may require escalating doses of dopamine, norepinephrine, or epinephrine. Hypotension and ventricular arrhythmias may occur with initiation of inotropes such as dobutamine and milrinone.
- ER was associated with a statistically significant difference in survival compared with OMT after 6 months, 1 year, and 6 years of follow-up in the SHOCK trial.
- Percutaneous mechanical support options for CS include IABP, Impella axial flow pumps, the TandemHeart centrifugal flow pump, or ECMO.
- The American College of Cardiology (ACC)/American Heart Association (AHA) definition of a "successful" PCI can be classified into three categories: angiographic, procedural, and clinical success. Each of these should be carefully considered when approaching a high-risk coronary intervention.
- Clinical variables of risk predict clinical outcomes, while anatomical lesion characteristics predict angiographic success.
- The ACC/AHA and SCAI lesion classification systems remain highly relevant in the modern era for grading the likelihood of technical success.
- The Mayo Clinic Clinical Scoring system demonstrates a high predictive value for identifying complications associated with PCI.
- The overall goals of percutaneous mechanical support devices are to (a) maintain vital organ perfusion, (b) improve native cardiac output by reducing intracardiac filling pressures, (c) reduce LV volumes, wall stress, and myocardial oxygen consumption, and (d) augment coronary perfusion during high-risk PCI.
- Based on emerging data and experience, the updated PCI guidelines have incorporated hemodynamic support devices as an adjunct to HR-PCI in select cases, as a class IIB recommendation.

References

1. Virani SS, Newby LK, Arnold SV, et al. 2023 AHA/ACC/ACCP/ASPC/NLA/PCNA guideline for the management of patients with chronic coronary disease: a report of the American heart association/American College of cardiology Joint Committee on clinical Practice guidelines. *Circulation*. 2023;148(9):e9-e119.
2. Lawton JS, Tamis-Holland JE, Bangalore S, et al. 2021 ACC/AHA/SCAI guideline for coronary artery revascularization: executive summary—a report of the American College of Cardiology/American Heart Association Joint Committee on clinical practice guidelines. *Circulation*. 2022;145(3):e4-e17.
3. Singh M, Rihal CS, Lennon RJ, Spertus J, Rumsfeld JS, Holmes DR Jr. Bedside estimation of risk from percutaneous coronary intervention: the new Mayo Clinic risk scores. *Mayo Clin Proc*. 2007;82(6):701-708.
4. Singh M, Peterson ED, Milford-Beland S, Rumsfeld JS, Spertus JA. Validation of the mayo clinic risk score for in-hospital mortality after percutaneous coronary interventions using the national cardiovascular data registry. *Circ Cardiovasc Interv*. 2008;1:36-44.
5. Wu C, Hannan EL, Walford G, et al. A risk score to predict in-hospital mortality for percutaneous coronary interventions. *J Am Coll Cardiol*. 2006;47(3):654-660.
6. Brener SJ, Colombo KD, Haq SA, Bose S, Sacchi TJ. Precision and accuracy of risk scores for in-hospital death after percutaneous coronary intervention in the current era. *Catheter Cardiovasc Interv*. 2010;75(2):153-157.
7. Sianos G, Morel MA, Kappetein AP, et al. The SYNTAX score: an angiographic tool grading the complexity of coronary artery disease. *EuroIntervention*. 2005;1(2):219-227.

8. Serruys PW, Morice MC, Kappetein AP, et al. Percutaneous coronary intervention versus coronary-artery bypass grafting for severe coronary artery disease. *N Engl J Med*. 2009;360(10):961-972.
9. Sotomi Y, Cavalcante R, van Klaveren D, et al. Individual long-term mortality prediction following either coronary stenting or bypass surgery in patients with multivessel and/or unprotected left main disease: an external validation of the SYNTAX Score II Model in the 1,480 patients of the BEST and PRECOMBAT randomized controlled trials. *JACC Cardiovasc Interv*. 2016;9(15):1564-1572.
10. Antonelli M, Levy M, Andrews PJD, et al. Hemodynamic monitoring in shock and implications for management. International Consensus Conference, Paris, France, 27-28 April 2006. *Intensive Care Med*. 2007;33(4):575-590.
11. Reynolds HR, Hochman JS. Cardiogenic shock: current concepts and improving outcomes. *Circulation*. 2008;117(5):686-697.
12. Topalian S, Ginsberg F, Parrillo JE. Cardiogenic shock. *Crit Care Med*. 2008;36(1 suppl):S66-S74.
13. Goldberg RJ, Samad NA, Yarzebski J, Gurwitz J, Bigelow C, Gore JM. Temporal trends in cardiogenic shock complicating acute myocardial infarction. *N Engl J Med*. 1999;340(15):1162-1168.
14. Alonso DR, Scheidt S, Post M, Killip T. Pathophysiology of cardiogenic shock. Quantification of myocardial necrosis, clinical, pathologic and electrocardiographic correlations. *Circulation*. 1973;48(3):588-596.
15. Lindholm MG, Køber L, Boesgaard S, Torp-Pedersen C, Aldershvile J; Trandolapril Cardiac Evaluation Study Group. Cardiogenic shock complicating acute myocardial infarction; prognostic impact of early and late shock development. *Eur Heart J*. 2003;24(3):258-265.
16. Babaev A, Frederick PD, Pasta DJ, et al. Trends in management and outcomes of patients with acute myocardial infarction complicated by cardiogenic shock. *JAMA*. 2005;294(4):448-454.
17. Barbour DJ, Roberts WC. Rupture of a left ventricular papillary muscle during acute myocardial infarction: analysis of 22 necropsy patients. *J Am Coll Cardiol*. 1986;8(3):558-565.
18. Radford MJ, Johnson RA, Daggett WM Jr, et al. Ventricular septal rupture: a review of clinical and physiologic features and an analysis of survival. *Circulation*. 1981;64(3):545-553.
19. Moore CA, Nygaard TW, Kaiser DL, Cooper AA, Gibson RS. Postinfarction ventricular septal rupture: the importance of location of infarction and right ventricular function in determining survival. *Circulation*. 1986;74(1):45-55.
20. Shapira I, Isakov A, Burke M, Almog C. Cardiac rupture in patients with acute myocardial infarction. *Chest*. 1987;92(2):219-223.
21. Mann JM, Roberts WC. Rupture of the left ventricular free wall during acute myocardial infarction: analysis of 138 necropsy patients and comparison with 50 necropsy patients with acute myocardial infarction without rupture. *Am J Cardiol*. 1988;62(13):847-859.
22. Chockalingam A, Gnanavelu G, Subramaniam T, Dorairajan S, Chockalingam V. Right ventricular myocardial infarction: presentation and acute outcomes. *Angiology*. 2005;56(4):371-376.
23. Engstrom AE, Vis MM, Bouma BJ, et al. Right ventricular dysfunction is an independent predictor for mortality in ST-elevation myocardial infarction patients presenting with cardiogenic shock on admission. *Eur J Heart Fail*. 2010;12(3):276-282.
24. Verani MS, Tortoledo FE, Batty JW, Raizner AE. Effect of coronary artery recanalization on right ventricular function in patients with acute myocardial infarction. *J Am Coll Cardiol*. 1985;5:1029-1035.
25. Andersen HR, Falk E, Nielsen D. Right ventricular infarction: frequency, size and topography in coronary heart disease—a prospective study comprising 107 consecutive autopsies from a coronary care unit. *J Am Coll Cardiol*. 1987;10(6):1223-1232.
26. Dell'Italia LJ, Starling MR, Crawford MH, Boros BL, Chaudhuri TK, O'Rourke RA. Right ventricular infarction: identification by hemodynamic measurements before and after volume loading and correlation with noninvasive techniques. *J Am Coll Cardiol*. 1984;4(5):931-939.
27. Jacobs AK, Leopold JA, Bates E, et al. Cardiogenic shock caused by right ventricular infarction: a report from the SHOCK registry. *J Am Coll Cardiol*. 2003;41(8):1273-1279.
28. Agarwal MA, Fonarow GC, Ziaeian B. National trends in heart failure hospitalizations and readmissions from 2010 to 2017. *JAMA Cardiol*. 2021;6(8):952-956. doi:10.1001/jamacardio.2020.7472
29. Stevenson LW, Pagani FD, Young JB, et al. INTERMACS profiles of advanced heart failure: the current picture. *J Heart Lung Transplant*. 2009;28(6):535-541.
30. Erbel R. Role of transesophageal echocardiography in dissection of the aorta and evaluation of degenerative aortic disease. *Cardiol Clin*. 1993;11(3):461-473.
31. Tiong IY, Novaro GM, Jefferson B, Monson M, Smedira N, Penn MS. Bacterial endocarditis and functional mitral stenosis: a report of two cases and brief literature review. *Chest*. 2002;122(6):2259-2262.
32. Brizzio ME, Zapolanski A. Acute mitral regurgitation requiring urgent surgery because of chordae ruptures after extreme physical exercise: case report. *Heart Surg Forum*. 2008;11(4):E255-E256.
33. Yuan SM. Clinical significance of mitral leaflet flail. *Cardiol J*. 2009;16(2):151-156.
34. Wang A. Recent progress in the understanding of infective endocarditis. *Curr Treat Options Cardiovasc Med*. 2011;13(6):586-594.
35. Otto CM, Nishimura RA, Bonow RO, et al. 2020 ACC/AHA guideline for the management of patients with valvular heart disease: executive summary—a report of the American College of Cardiology/American Heart Association Joint Committee on clinical practice guidelines. *Circulation*. 2021;143(5):e35-e71.
36. Burkhoff D, Mirsky I, Suga H. Assessment of systolic and diastolic ventricular properties via pressure-volume analysis: a guide for clinical, translational, and basic researchers. *Am J Physiol Heart Circ Physiol*. 2005;289(2):H501-H512.
37. Shioura KM, Geenen DL, Goldspink PH. Assessment of cardiac function with the pressure-volume conductance system following myocardial infarction in mice. *Am J Physiol Heart Circ Physiol*. 2007;293(5):H2870-H2877.
38. Remmelink M, Sjauw KD, Henriques JPS, et al. Acute left ventricular dynamic effects of primary percutaneous coronary intervention from occlusion to reperfusion. *J Am Coll Cardiol*. 2009;53(17):1498-1502.
39. Hochman JS. Cardiogenic shock complicating acute myocardial infarction: expanding the paradigm. *Circulation*. 2003;107(24):2998-3002.
40. Kohsaka S, Menon V, Lowe AM, et al. Systemic inflammatory response syndrome after acute myocardial infarction complicated by cardiogenic shock. *Arch Intern Med*. 2005;165(14):1643-1650.
41. Heidenreich PA, Bozkurt B, Aguilar D, et al. 2022 AHA/ACC/HFSA guideline for the management of heart failure: executive summary—a report of the American College of Cardiology/American Heart Association Joint Committee on clinical practice guidelines. *Circulation*. 2022;145(18):e876-e894.
42. Mann HJ, Nolan PE Jr. Update on the management of cardiogenic shock. *Curr Opin Crit Care*. 2006;12(5):431-436.
43. Petersen JW, Felker GM. Inotropes in the management of acute heart failure. *Crit Care Med*. 2008;36(1 suppl):S106-S111.
44. Fernandez AR, Sequeira RF, Chakko S, et al. ST segment tracking for rapid determination of patency of the infarct-related artery in acute myocardial infarction. *J Am Coll Cardiol*. 1995;26(3):675-683.
45. Mehta RH, Lopes RD, Ballotta A, et al. Percutaneous coronary intervention or coronary artery bypass surgery for cardiogenic shock and multivessel coronary artery disease? *Am Heart J*. 2010;159(1):141-147.
46. Keeley EC, Boura JA, Grines CL. Primary angioplasty versus intravenous thrombolytic therapy for acute myocardial infarction: a quantitative review of 23 randomised trials. *Lancet*. 2003;361(9351):13-20.
47. Hochman JS, Sleeper LA, Webb JG, et al. Early revascularization in acute myocardial infarction complicated by cardiogenic shock. SHOCK investigators. Should we emergently revascularize occluded coronaries for cardiogenic shock. *N Engl J Med*. 1999;341(9):625-634.
48. Hochman JS, Sleeper LA, White HD, et al. One-year survival following early revascularization for cardiogenic shock. *JAMA*. 2001;285(2):190-192.
49. Dauerman HL, Ryan TJ Jr, Piper WD, et al. Outcomes of percutaneous coronary intervention among elderly patients in cardiogenic shock: a multicenter, decade-long experience. *J Invasive Cardiol*. 2003;15(7):380-384.
50. Prasad A, Lennon RJ, Rihal CS, Berger PB, Holmes DR Jr. Outcomes of elderly patients with cardiogenic shock treated with early percutaneous revascularization. *Am Heart J*. 2004;147(6):1066-1070.
51. Kawaguchi O, Pae WE, Daily BB, Pierce WS. Ventriculoarterial coupling with intra-aortic balloon pump in acute ischemic heart failure. *J Thorac Cardiovasc Surg*. 1999;117(1):164-171.

52. Perera D, Stables R, Thomas M, et al. Elective intra-aortic balloon counterpulsation during high-risk percutaneous coronary intervention: a randomized controlled trial. *JAMA*. 2010;304(8):867-874.
53. Patel MR, Smalling RW, Thiele H, et al. Intra-aortic balloon counterpulsation and infarct size in patients with acute anterior myocardial infarction without shock: the CRISP AMI randomized trial. *JAMA*. 2011;306(12):1329-1337.
54. Goldberg RJ, Gore JM, Thompson CA, Gurwitz JH. Recent magnitude of and temporal trends (1994-1997) in the incidence and hospital death rates of cardiogenic shock complicating acute myocardial infarction: the second national registry of myocardial infarction. *Am Heart J*. 2001;141(1):65-72.
55. Valgimigli M, Steendijk P, Sianos G, Onderwater E, Serruys PW. Left ventricular unloading and concomitant total cardiac output increase by the use of percutaneous Impella Recover LP 2.5 assist device during high-risk coronary intervention. *Catheter Cardiovasc Interv*. 2005;65(2):263-267.
56. O'Neill WW, Kleiman NS, Moses J, et al. A prospective, randomized clinical trial of hemodynamic support with Impella 2.5 versus intra-aortic balloon pump in patients undergoing high-risk percutaneous coronary intervention: the PROTECT II study. *Circulation*. 2012;126(14):1717-1727.
57. Lansky AJ, Tirziu D, Moses JW, et al. Impella versus intra-aortic balloon pump for high-risk PCI: a propensity-adjusted large-scale claims dataset analysis. *Am J Cardiol*. 2022;185:29-36.
58. O'Neill WW, Schreiber T, Wohns DHW, et al. The current use of Impella 2.5 in acute myocardial infarction complicated by cardiogenic shock: results from the USpella Registry. *J Interv Cardiol*. 2014;27:1-11.
59. Ouweneel DM, Eriksen E, Sjauw KD, et al. Percutaneous mechanical circulatory support versus intra-aortic balloon pump in cardiogenic shock after acute myocardial infarction. *J Am Coll Cardiol*. 2017;69(3):278-287.
60. Anderson MB, Goldstein J, Milano C, et al. Benefits of a novel percutaneous ventricular assist device for right heart failure: the prospective RECOVER RIGHT study of the Impella RP device. *J Heart Lung Transplant*. 2015;34(12):1549-1560.
61. Goldstein AH, Pacella JJ, Clark RE. Predictable reduction in left ventricular stroke work and oxygen utilization with an implantable centrifugal pump. *Ann Thorac Surg*. 1994;58(4):1018-1024.
62. Cheng JM, den Uil CA, Hoeks SE, et al. Percutaneous left ventricular assist devices vs. intra-aortic balloon pump counterpulsation for treatment of cardiogenic shock: a meta-analysis of controlled trials. *Eur Heart J*. 2009;30(17):2102-2108.
63. Kawashima D, Gojo S, Nishimura T, et al. Left ventricular mechanical support with Impella provides more ventricular unloading in heart failure than extracorporeal membrane oxygenation. *ASAIO J*. 2011;57(3):169-176.
64. Pappalardo F, Schulte C, Pieri M, et al. Concomitant implantation of Impella® on top of veno-arterial extracorporeal membrane oxygenation may improve survival of patients with cardiogenic shock. *Eur J Heart Fail*. 2017;19(3):404-412.

Multivessel Percutaneous Coronary Intervention

Judit Karacsonyi and Yader Sandoval

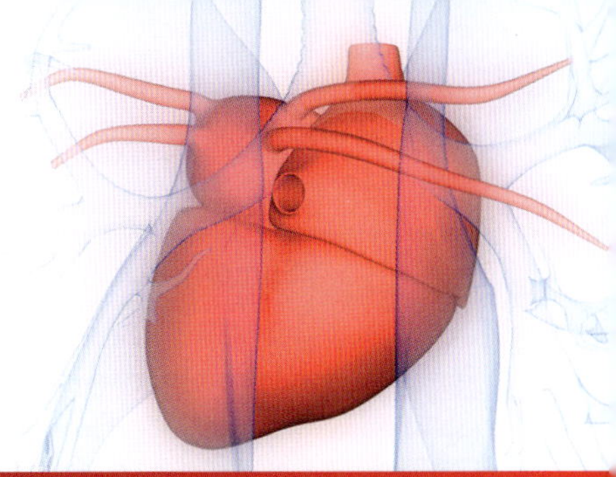

Approximately 40% to 60% of patients undergoing percutaneous coronary interventions (PCIs) have multivessel coronary artery disease (CAD).[1] Technical advancements in PCI and improvements in medical therapy have enabled multivessel PCI as a therapeutic option in patients with both acute and chronic CAD.[2,3] Multivessel PCI, particularly in nonemergent situations, benefits from a heart team-based approach that includes careful consideration of potential therapeutic options, including medical therapy, coronary artery bypass graft (CABG) surgery, and shared decision making that involves discussion of the risks and benefits of each modality. Likewise, it is important to consider patient factors, such as age, diabetes, renal dysfunction, and left ventricular (LV) dysfunction, that may influence decisions about revascularization, as well as anatomical factors such as the presence of left main (LM) disease, bifurcation lesions, coronary calcification, and coronary chronic total occlusions (CTOs), and the degree to which each revascularization modality can achieve complete revascularization.[4]

INDICATIONS AND EVIDENCE FOR MULTIVESSEL PCI

Clinical Practice Guidelines and Evidence

The American College of Cardiology (ACC)/American Heart Association (AHA) clinical practice guidelines for multivessel PCI are summarized in **Table 21.1**.[5] **Table 21.2** summarizes appropriateness use criteria for coronary revascularization addressing multivessel PCI.

ST-Elevation Myocardial Infarction

In ST-elevation myocardial infarction (STEMI) patients with multivessel CAD, following successful primary PCI, the 2021 ACC/AHA/Society for Cardiovascular Angiography and Interventions (ACC/AHA/SCAI) Guideline for Coronary Artery Revascularization recommend (class I, A) staged PCI of a significant noninfarct artery stenosis in selected *hemodynamically stable* patients to reduce the risk of death or myocardial infarction (MI).[5] In those with low-complexity multivessel CAD, PCI may be considered at the time of primary PCI (class 2b, B-R).

Previous guidelines[7] endorsed against (class III, harm) performing PCI in the noninfarct artery at the time of primary PCI in patients with STEMI that were hemodynamically stable. Following multiple randomized controlled trials (RCTs) and meta-analyses demonstrating the benefit of complete revascularization in STEMI patients with multivessel CAD, the 2021 guidelines recommend multivessel PCI in hemodynamically stable patients.

PRAMI (Preventive Angioplasty in Acute Myocardial Infarction) was the first trial (5 centers, 465 patients) addressing the role of PCI in noninfarct coronary arteries with major stenoses and showed a significant reduction in the risk of adverse cardiovascular events (death from cardiac causes, nonfatal MI, or refractory angina) as compared with PCI limited to the infarct artery only (9% vs 23%, hazard ratio [HR] in the preventive-PCI group, 0.35; 95% confidence interval [CI], 0.21-0.58; $P < .001$).[8]

In the DANAMI-3-PRIMULTI (The Third DANish Study of Optimal Acute Treatment of Patients With STEMI: PRImary PCI in MULTIvessel Disease) trial, 627 patients with STEMI were randomized, and a fractional flow reserve (FFR)-guided complete revascularization strategy was superior to treatment of the infarct-related artery (IRA) only (13% vs 22%; HR, 0.56; 95% CI, 0.38-0.83; $P = .004$) with respect to the composite primary endpoint of all-cause mortality, nonfatal reinfarction, and ischemia-driven revascularization of lesions in non-IRAs.[9] In the CvLPRIT (Complete vs Lesion-only Primary PCI) trial, 296 patients with STEMI and multivessel disease were enrolled across seven UK centers and randomized to complete revascularization or IRA revascularization. The results showed that 10.0% of patients in the complete revascularization group met the primary endpoint (all-cause death, recurrent MI, heart failure, and ischemia-driven revascularization within 12 months) as compared to 21.2% in the IRA-only revascularization group (HR, 0.45; 95% CI, 0.24-0.84; $P = .009$).[9] Similar findings were reported in the Compare-Acute trial that randomly assigned 885 patients with STEMI and multivessel disease to complete revascularization of non-infarct-related coronary arteries guided by FFR or no revascularization of non-infarct-related coronary arteries. The primary endpoint was met in 8% of the patients in the complete-revascularization group and 21% in IRA PCI-only group (HR, 0.35; 95% CI, 0.22-0.55; $P < .001$; composite of death from any cause, nonfatal MI, revascularization, and cerebrovascular events at 12 months).[10]

COMPLETE (Complete Vs Culprit-Only Revascularization Strategies to Treat Multivessel Disease after Early PCI for STEMI) trial was the largest RCT that enrolled 4041 patients and found that complete revascularization (performed within 45 days of STEMI) was superior to culprit-lesion-only PCI in reducing the risk of cardiovascular death or MI (7.8% vs 10.5%; HR, 0.74; 95% CI, 0.60-0.91; $P = .004$; **Fig. 21.1**), as well as the risk of cardiovascular death, MI, or ischemia-driven revascularization (8.9% vs 16.7%; HR, 0.51; 95% CI, 0.43-0.61; $P < .001$).[11]

The majority of these trials excluded patients with LM disease, CTO of the noninfarct artery, complex noninfarct disease, and only approximately one-third of the enrolled patients had triple-vessel disease. A heart team-based approach involving shared decision making therefore remains important, particularly in those with complex residual CAD.

Complete revascularization at the time of the primary PCI is reasonable in carefully selected patients with low-complexity noninfarct artery disease, normal LV filling pressures, and normal renal function. Clinical data, lesion complexity, hemodynamics, patient stability, radiation, and contrast dose should be carefully assessed before pursuing immediate complete revascularization.[5]

TABLE 21.1 Summary of ACC/AHA Clinical Practice Guidelines for Multivessel PCI[5]

CLINICAL SETTING	COR	LOE
STEMI and Non-Infarct-Related Artery		
In selected hemodynamically stable patients with STEMI and multivessel disease, after successful primary PCI, staged PCI of a significant noninfarct artery stenosis is recommended to reduce the risk of death or MI	1	A
In selected hemodynamically stable patients with STEMI and low-complexity multivessel disease, PCI of a noninfarct artery stenosis may be considered at the time of primary PCI to reduce cardiac event rates	2b	B-R
In patients with STEMI complicated by cardiogenic shock, routine PCI of a noninfarct artery at the time of primary PCI should not be performed because of the higher risk of death or renal failure	3: Harm	B-R
NSTEMI and Nonculprit Artery		
In patients with NSTE-ACS who present in cardiogenic shock, routine multivessel PCI of nonculprit lesions in the same setting should not be performed	3: Harm	B-R
SIHD		
Left ventricular dysfunction and multivessel CAD		
In patients with SIHD and multivessel CAD appropriate for CABG with severe LV systolic dysfunction (LVEF <35%), CABG is recommended to improve survival	1	B-R
In selected patients with SIHD and multivessel CAD appropriate for CABG and mild-to-moderate LV systolic dysfunction (EF 35%-50%), CABG (to include an LIMA graft to the LAD) is reasonable to improve survival	1	B-R
Left main CAD		
In patients with SIHD and significant left main stenosis, CABG is recommended to improve survival	1	B-R
In selected patients with SIHD and significant left main stenosis for whom PCI can provide equivalent revascularization to that possible with CABG, PCI is reasonable to improve survival	2a	B-NR
Multivessel CAD		
In patients with SIHD, normal ejection fraction, significant stenosis in three major coronary arteries (with or without proximal LAD), and anatomy suitable for CABG, CABG may be reasonable to improve survival	2b	B-R
In patients with SIHD, normal ejection fraction, significant stenosis in three major coronary arteries (with or without proximal LAD), and anatomy suitable for PCI, the usefulness of PCI to improve survival is uncertain	2b	B-R
Stenosis in the proximal LAD artery		
In patients with SIHD, normal LVEF, and significant stenosis in the proximal LAD, the usefulness of coronary revascularization to improve survival is uncertain	2b	B-R
Single- or double-vessel disease not involving the proximal LAD		
In patients with SIHD, normal LVEF, and 1- or 2-vessel CAD not involving the proximal LAD, coronary revascularization is not recommended to improve survival	3: No benefit	B-R
In patients with SIHD, who have >1 coronary arteries that are not anatomically or functionally significant (<70% diameter of non-left main coronary artery stenosis, FFR>0.80), coronary revascularization should not be performed with primary or sole intent to improve survival	3: Harm	B-NR
In patients with SIHD and multivessel CAD appropriate for either CABG or PCI, revascularization is reasonable to lower the risk of cardiovascular events, such as spontaneous MI, unplanned urgent revascularizations, or cardiac death	2a	B-R
In patients with refractory angina despite medical therapy and with significant coronary artery stenosis amendable to revascularization, revascularization is recommended to improve symptoms	1	A
In patients with angina but no anatomic or physiological criteria for revascularization, neither CABG nor PCI should be performed	3: Harm	C-LD
Patients With Complex Disease		
In patients who require revascularization for significant left main CAD with high-complexity CAD, it is recommended to choose CABG over PCI to improve survival	1	B-R
In patients who require revascularization for multivessel CAD with complex or diffuse CAD (eg, SYNTAX score >33), it is reasonable to choose CABG over PCI to confer a survival advantage	2a	B-R
Diabetes		
In patients with diabetes and multivessel CAD with the involvement of the LAD, who are appropriate candidates for CABG, CABG (with a LIMA to the LAD) is recommended in preference to PCI to reduce mortality and repeat revascularizations	1	A

TABLE 21.1 Summary of ACC/AHA Clinical Practice Guidelines for Multivessel PCI[5] (*Continued*)

CLINICAL SETTING	COR	LOE
In patients with diabetes and multivessel CAD amendable to PCI and an indication for revascularization and are poor candidates for surgery, PCI can be useful to reduce long-term ischemic outcomes	2a	B-NR
In patients with diabetes who have left main stenosis and low- or intermediate-complexity CAD in the rest of the coronary anatomy, PCI may be considered an alternative to CABG to reduce major adverse cardiovascular outcomes	2b	B-R
Patients With Previous CABG		
In patients with previous CABG with a patent LIMA to the LAD who need repeat revascularization, if PCI is feasible, it is reasonable to choose PCI over CABG	2a	B-NR
In patients with previous CABG and refractory angina on GDMT that is attributable to LAD disease, it is reasonable to choose CABG over PCI when an IMA can be used as a conduit to LAD	2a	C-LD
In patients with previous CABG and complex CAD, it may be reasonable to choose CABG over PCI when an IMA can be used as a conduit to LAD	2b	B-NR

B-NR, level B nonrandomized; B-R, level B randomized; CABG, coronary artery bypass graft; CAD, coronary artery disease; C-EO, level C expert opinion; C-LD, level C limited data; COR, Class of Recommendation; FFR, fractional flow reserve; GDMT, guideline-directed medical therapy; IMA, internal mammary artery; LAD, left anterior descending; LIMA, left internal mammary artery; LOE, level of evidence; LVEF, left ventricular ejection fraction; MACE, major adverse cardiovascular event; MI, myocardial infarction; NSTEMI, non-ST-segment-elevation myocardial infarction; PCI, percutaneous coronary intervention; SIHD, stable ischemic heart disease; STEMI, ST-segment-elevation myocardial infarction; SYNTAX, Synergy between PCI With TAXUS and Cardiac Surgery.

Derived from Lawton JS, Tamis-Holland JE, Bangalore S, et al. 2021 ACC/AHA/SCAI guideline for coronary artery revascularization: executive summary: a report of the American College of Cardiology/American Heart Association Joint Committee on Clinical Practice Guidelines. *Circulation.* 2021:CIR0000000000001039.

Whereas in hemodynamically stable patients, multivessel PCI is an option during primary PCI or as a staged procedure, in STEMI patients with cardiogenic shock culprit vessel-only, primary PCI is recommended. Routine PCI of noninfarct artery at the time of primary PCI in cardiogenic shock received a class 3 (Level of Evidence [LOE] B-R) in the 2021 ACC/AHA/SCAI Guideline for Coronary Artery Revascularization because of higher risk of death or renal failure.[5] This recommendation was largely based on the results of the CULPRIT-SHOCK (Culprit Lesion Only PCI Vs Multivessel PCI in Cardiogenic Shock) trial that randomized 706 patients with multivessel disease, acute MI, and cardiogenic shock to either PCI of the culprit lesion only, with the option of staged revascularization of nonculprit lesions, or immediate multivessel PCI. The study found that the primary endpoint at 30 days (composite of death or severe renal failure leading to renal-replacement therapy) occurred in 45.9% in the culprit-lesion-only PCI group and in 55.4% in the multivessel PCI group (relative risk [RR], 0.83; 95% CI, 0.71-0.96; P = .01; **Fig. 21.2**). Furthermore, death rate from any cause was significantly lower in the culprit-lesion-only PCI group compared with the multivessel PCI group (43.3% vs 51.6%; RR, 0.84; 95% CI, 0.72-0.98; P = .03).[13]

The risks associated with immediate multivessel PCI include contrast nephropathy, volume overload, and ischemic complications in the nonculprit artery that could enhance hemodynamic deterioration.[5] At 1-year follow-up of the CULPRIT-SHOCK trial, mortality was similar between the two groups; death from any cause had occurred in 50.0% in the culprit-lesion only PCI and 56.9% in the multivessel PCI group, respectively (RR, 0.88; 95% CI, 0.76-1.01). The incidence of rehospitalization for heart failure, however, was higher, and repeat revascularization was more frequent with culprit-lesion-only PCI compared with multivessel PCI.[14] In addition to the randomized trial, a meta-analysis including 5850 patients and 11 nonrandomized trials confirmed similar results and suggested no benefit with multivessel PCI in cardiogenic shock with STEMI compared with culprit-only PCI. It found no difference in short-term mortality between multivessel PCI versus culprit-only PCI (odds ratio [OR], 1.08; 95% CI, 0.81-1.43; P = .61) or long-term mortality (OR, 0.84; 95% CI, 0.54-1.30,

TABLE 21.2 Appropriate Use Criteria for Coronary Revascularization[6] (Patients With Ischemic Symptoms on ≥2 Antianginals)

	CABG	PCI
Two-vessel CAD with proximal LAD stenosis	Appropriate	Appropriate
Three-vessel CAD with low CAD complexity (focal stenoses, SYNTAX score ≤22)	Appropriate	Appropriate
Three-vessel CAD with intermediate to high CAD complexity (SYNTAX score >22)	Appropriate	May be appropriate
Isolated left main disease (ostial/midshaft)	Appropriate	Appropriate
Left main stenosis (ostial/midshaft) with low CAD burden (one to two additional vessels, SYNTAX score ≤22)	Appropriate	Appropriate
Left main stenosis (bifurcation) with low CAD burden (one to two additional vessels, SYNTAX score ≤22)	Appropriate	May be appropriate
Left main stenosis (bifurcation) and additional CAD with intermediate to high CAD burden (SYNTAX score >22)	Appropriate	Rarely appropriate
Nonculprit lesion in ACS for symptomatic ischemia, FFR <0.80, or positive stress test	Appropriate	Appropriate

ACS, acute coronary syndrome; CAD, coronary artery disease; FFR, fractional flow reserve; SYNTAX, Synergy between PCI With TAXUS and Cardiac Surgery.

From Patel MR, Calhoon JH, Dehmer GJ, et al. ACC/AATS/AHA/ASE/ASNC/SCAI/SCCT/STS 2017 appropriate use criteria for coronary revascularization in patients with stable ischemic heart disease: a report of the American College of Cardiology Appropriate Use Criteria Task Force, American Association for Thoracic Surgery, American Heart Association, American Society of Echocardiography, American Society of Nuclear Cardiology, Society for Cardiovascular Angiography and Interventions, Society of Cardiovascular Computed Tomography, and Society of Thoracic Surgeons. *J Am Coll Cardiol.* 2017;69(17):2212-2241.

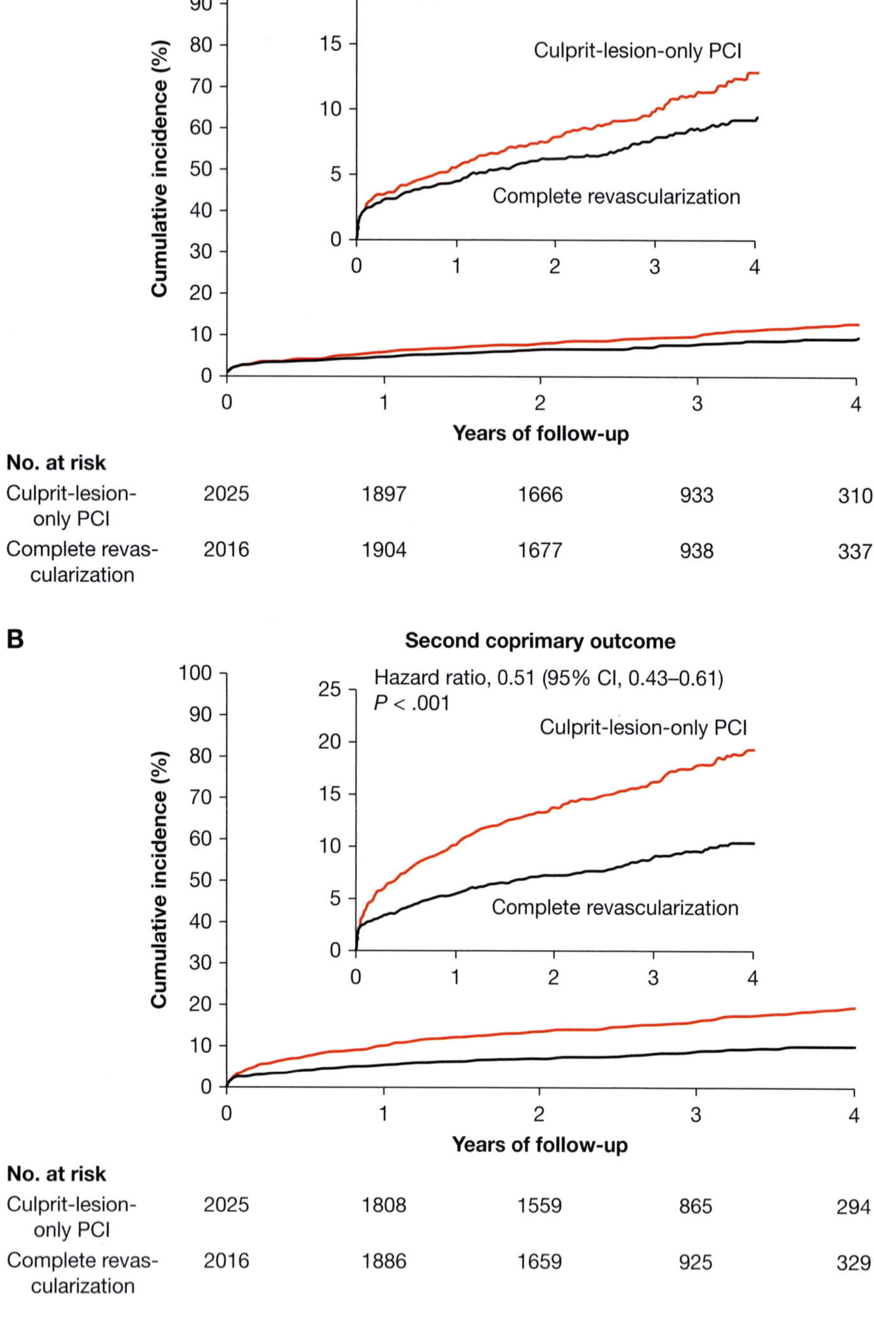

FIGURE 21.1 COMPLETE trial. Cumulative incidence of the first and second coprimary outcomes.[11] PCI, percutaneous coronary intervention. (From Mehta SR, Wood DA, Storey RF, et al. Complete revascularization with multivessel PCI for myocardial infarction. *N Engl J Med.* 2019;381(15):1411-1121. Figure 1. Copyright © 2019 Massachusetts Medical Society. Reprinted with permission from Massachusetts Medical Society.)

P = .54). There was no significant difference between the two groups regarding cardiovascular death (OR, 0.72; 95% CI, 0.42-1.23; *P* = .23), reinfarction (OR, 1.65; 95% CI, 0.84-3.26; *P* = .15), or repeat revascularization (OR, 1.13; 95% CI, 0.76-1.69; *P* = .54). There was a trend toward higher prevalence of renal failure in the multivessel PCI group; however, it was nonsignificant (OR, 1.30; 95% CI, 0.98-1.72; *P* = .06).[15]

Non-ST-Elevation MI

As compared to STEMI patients with multivessel CAD, data are limited in patients with non-ST-elevation myocardial infarction (NSTEMI). There are trials that have evaluated multivessel PCI strategies in patients with NSTEMI. The SMILE (Impact of Difference Treatment in Multivessel Non-ST-Elevation Myocardial Infarction Patients: One Stage Vs Multistaged Percutaneous Coronary Intervention) trial addressed a one-stage versus a multistage PCI approach with respect to major adverse cardiovascular event (MACE) (cardiac death, reinfarction, rehospitalization for unstable angina, repeat coronary revascularization, and stroke at 1 year).[16] In the multistage PCI arm, the second-stage procedure was performed between 3 and 7 days after the index procedure. The occurrence of MACE was significantly lower in the one-stage group (13.63%) compared to the multistage PCI group (23.19%) (HR, 0.549; 95% CI,

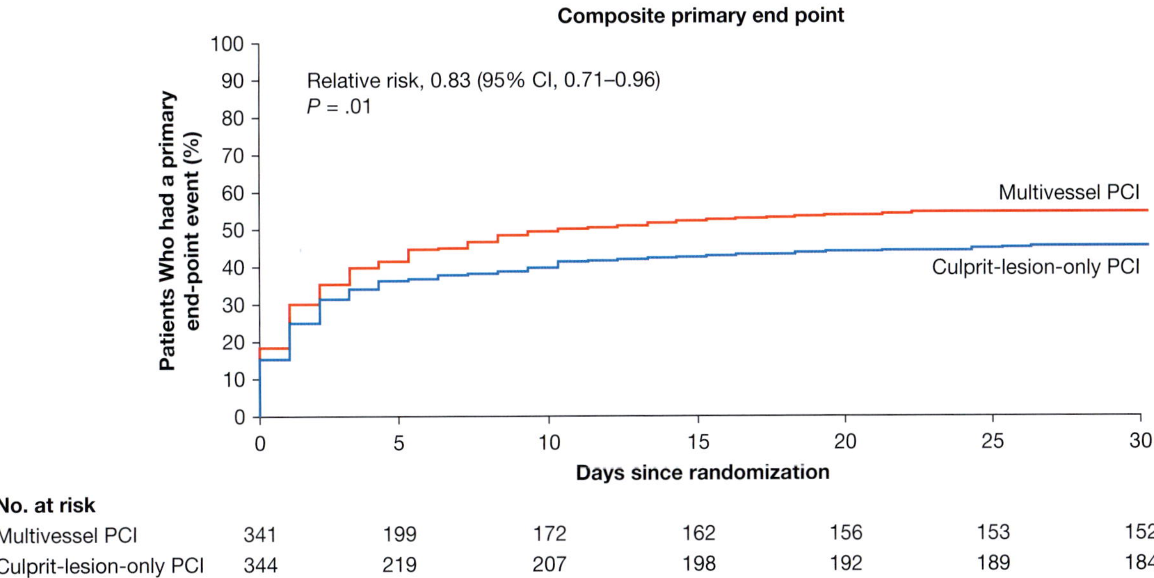

FIGURE 21.2 Event rates of the primary endpoint at 30 days in CULPRIT-SHOCK trial.[12] CI, confidence interval; PCI, percutaneous coronary intervention. (From Gershlick AH, Khan JN, Kelly DJ, et al. Randomized trial of complete versus lesion-only revascularization in patients undergoing primary percutaneous coronary intervention for STEMI and multivessel disease: the CvLPRIT trial. *J Am Coll Cardiol.* 2015;65(10):963-972.)

0.363-0.828, *P* = .004). These differences were driven in part by lower repeat revascularization in patients undergoing one-stage PCI, with no difference observed between groups with regard to cardiac death and MI.[16]

The BIOVASC trial was a prospective noninferiority RCT including both STEMI and NSTEMI patients that were randomized to immediate (*n* = 764) or staged (*n* = 761) complete revascularization with respect to the composite outcome of all-cause mortality, MI, any unplanned ischemia-driven revascularization, or cerebrovascular events.[17] At 1 year, the primary outcome occurred in 7.6% of patients in the immediate CR group versus 9.4% in the staged CR group. Notably, as compared to patients undergoing staged CR, immediate CR was associated with a reduction in MI (4.5% vs 1.9%; HR, 0.41; 95% CI, 0.22-0.76; *P* = .0045) and unplanned ischemia-driven revascularization (6.7% vs 4.2%; HR, 0.61; 95% CI, 0.39-0.95; *P* = .030).[17]

In case of cardiogenic shock, CULPRIT-SHOCK trial enrolled ~40% of patients with NSTEMI, and those randomized to culprit-only PCI had lower rates of meeting the primary endpoint (composite of death and renal-replacement therapy at 30 days).[13] The 2021 revascularization guidelines provide a class 3 (harm) recommendation against routine multivessel PCI of nonculprit lesions in patients with non-ST-elevation acute coronary syndromes (ACSs) who present in cardiogenic shock.[5]

Stable Ischemic Heart Disease

Clinical practice guideline recommendations addressing multivessel PCI in stable ischemic heart disease (SIHD) are summarized in **Table 21.1**. These guidelines provide class I recommendations for CABG in patients with multivessel CAD and LV dysfunction (left ventricular ejection fraction [LVEF] <35%) and those with LM CAD. In patients with SIHD and multivessel CAD appropriate for either CABG or PCI, clinical practice guidelines indicate that revascularization is reasonable to lower the risk of cardiovascular events, such as spontaneous MI, unplanned urgent revascularization, or cardiac death (class 2a, B-R). There are several SIHD scenarios in which multivessel PCI is considered, particularly in those who are poor candidates for surgery.

For patients with SIHD, data from trials such as ISCHEMIA (International Study of Comparative Health Effectiveness with Medical and Invasive Approaches)[18] and COURAGE (Clinical Outcomes Utilizing Revascularization and Aggressive Drug Evaluation)[19] do not support routine revascularization to improve clinical outcomes. In ISCHEMIA trial, which randomized 5179 patients with moderate or severe ischemia on stress testing to an initial invasive strategy (angiography and revascularization when feasible) and medical therapy or to an initial medical therapy alone and angiography if medical therapy failed, an initial invasive did not reduce the risk of ischemic cardiovascular events or death from any cause over a median of 3.2 years (invasive strategy: 318 primary outcome events vs conservative strategy: 352 events). In the invasive-strategy group, 145 deaths occurred versus 144 deaths in the conservative-strategy group (HR, 1.05; 95% CI, 0.83-1.32).[18] Similar results were observed in the COURAGE trial that randomized 2287 patients with ischemia to medical therapy or PCI. COURAGE trial showed no significant differences between the two groups in the composite of death, MI, and stroke (PCI group 20.0% vs medical-therapy group 19.5%; HR, 1.05; 95% CI, 0.87-1.27; *P* = .62), hospitalization for ACS (12.4% vs 11.8%; HR, 1.07; 95% CI, 0.84-1.37; *P* = .56); or MI (13.2% vs 12.3%; HR, 1.13; 95% CI, 0.89-1.43; *P* = .33).[19] An extended follow-up of up to 15 years did not find any difference in survival.[20] These trials, however, had multiple exclusion criteria. For example, in the COURAGE trial, patients with persistent class IV angina, markedly positive stress tests, refractory heart failure, LVEF <30%, and revascularization within the previous 6 months were excluded. Similarly, in the ISCHEMIA trial, patients with recent ACS, unprotected LM stenosis of at least 50%, an LVEF <35%, New York Heart Association class III or IV heart failure, and unacceptable angina despite medical therapy were excluded. In routine clinical practice, several of these scenarios may involve multivessel CAD and have a CABG indication; however, surgical ineligibility or patient preference when there is equipoise between PCI and CABG may lead to PCI as an alternative option.

In patients with multivessel CAD, a complete revascularization strategy is associated with improved outcomes irrespective of revascularization modality. In a meta-analysis of 89,883 patients

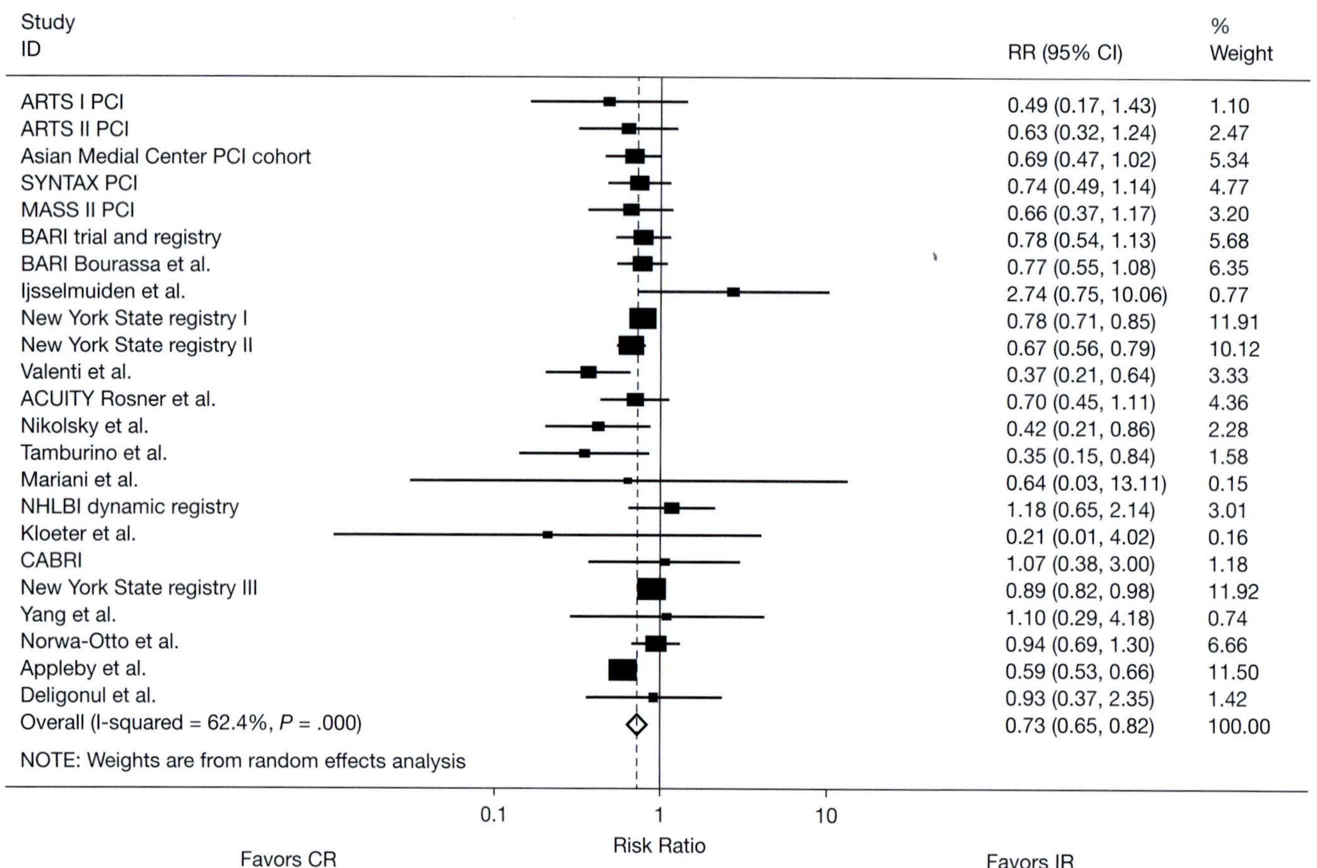

FIGURE 21.3 Pooled analyses with RR and 95% CI for the occurrence of total mortality in PCI studies. *Boxes* are the RR estimates from each study, the *horizontal bars* are 95% CI. The size of the box is proportional to the weight of the study in the pooled analysis.[21] ACUITY, Acute Catheterization and Urgent Intervention Triage Strategy; ARTS, Arterial Revascularization Therapies Study; BARI, Bypass Angioplasty Revascularization Investigation; CABG, coronary artery bypass graft; CABRI, Coronary Angioplasty Versus Bypass Revascularization Investigation; CI, confidence interval; NHLBI, National Heart, Lung, and Blood Institute; PCI, percutaneous coronary intervention; RR, risk ratio or relative risk; SYNTAX, Synergy Between PCI With Taxus and Cardiac Surgery. (From Garcia S, Sandoval Y, Roukoz H, et al. Outcomes after complete versus incomplete revascularization of patients with multivessel coronary artery disease: a meta-analysis of 89,883 patients enrolled in randomized clinical trials and observational studies. *J Am Coll Cardiol.* 2013;62(16):1421-1431. Figure 4.)

enrolled in randomized clinical trials and observational studies, relative to incomplete revascularization, complete revascularization (CABG or PCI) was associated with a lower long-term mortality (RR, 0.71; 95% CI, 0.65-0.77; $P < .001$), MI (RR, 0.78; 95% CI, 0.68-0.90; $P = .001$), and repeat coronary revascularization (RR, 0.74; 95% CI, 0.65-0.83; $P < .001$).[21] Similar findings were observed for PCI with respect to mortality (RR, 0.72; 95% CI, 0.64-0.81; $P < .001$) (**Fig. 21.3**), MI (RR, 0.80; 95% CI, 0.71-0.91; $P = .001$), and repeat revascularization (RR, 0.74; 95% CI, 0.65-0.83; $P < .001$).[21] Based on these findings, the likelihood of achieving complete revascularization should influence the decision to proceed with CABG or PCI. The most common reasons for not achieving complete revascularization with PCI are CTO, bifurcation disease, and diffuse disease or small vessels. While complete revascularization is a reasonable goal, reasonably acceptable incomplete revascularization is also an acceptable strategy in multiple scenarios.[22] For example in patients with frailty, advanced age, or those in which the procedural risks outweigh the benefits.

COMPLEXITY GRADING AND RISK STRATIFICATION

The SYNTAX Score

To quantify the complexity of multivessel CAD and inform decisions about revascularization, scores such as the SYNTAX score can be used. The SYNTAX score was developed for the SYNTAX trial[23] (**Fig. 21.4**) to grade the anatomical complexity of coronary lesions in patients with LM or three-vessel disease.[24] In the study population of the SYNTAX trial, and later in external validation cohorts, the SYNTAX score was demonstrated to be an independent predictor of long-term major adverse cardiac and cerebrovascular events and of death in patients treated with PCI but not CABG.[24-28] The SYNTAX score can be calculated with the following online calculator http://www.syntaxscore.com. It takes into account the dominance of the coronaries, the coronary segment of the lesions, diameter stenosis (extra points for CTOs and their characteristics), trifurcation lesions, bifurcation lesions, aorto-ostial lesions, severe tortuosity, lesion length, calcification, thrombus, and diffuse disease. Adequate training should decrease interobserver variability of the score. The SYNTAX II score was developed to provide a more individualized approach to guide decision making between CABG and PCI, including not only the anatomical SYNTAX score but also clinical variables. SYNTAX score II contains 8 variables: anatomical SYNTAX score, age, creatinine clearance, LVEF, the presence of unprotected LM CAD, peripheral vascular disease, female sex, and chronic obstructive pulmonary disease. In the original study, 4-year mortality in patients with CAD disease could be well predicted by the SYNTAX score II,[29] although the SYNTAX II score failed to predict the outcome of the EXCEL trial.[30]

The 2018 European Society of Cardiology and the European Association for Cardio-Thoracic Surgery (ESC/EACTS) Guidelines on myocardial revascularization provide a class I LOE A

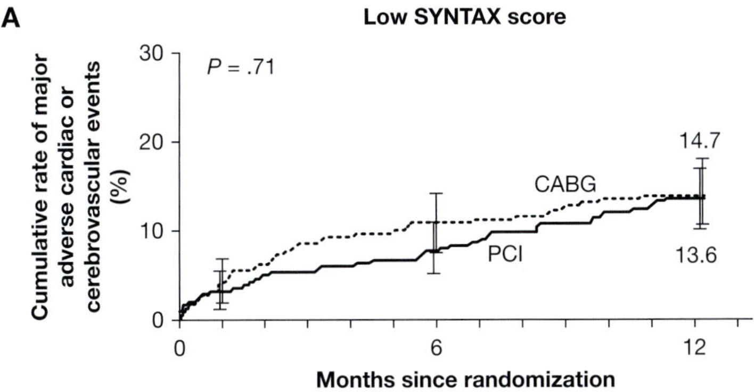

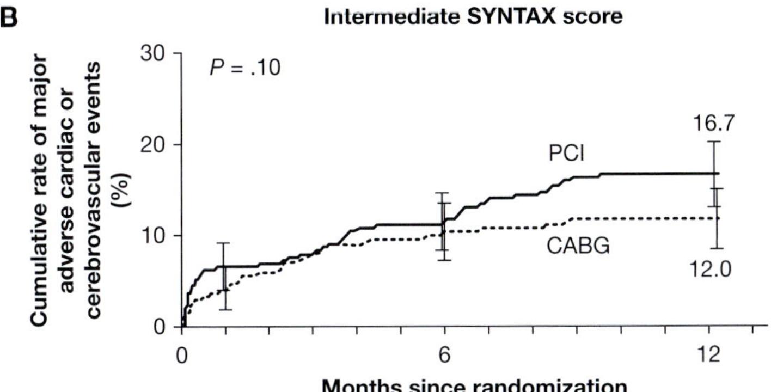

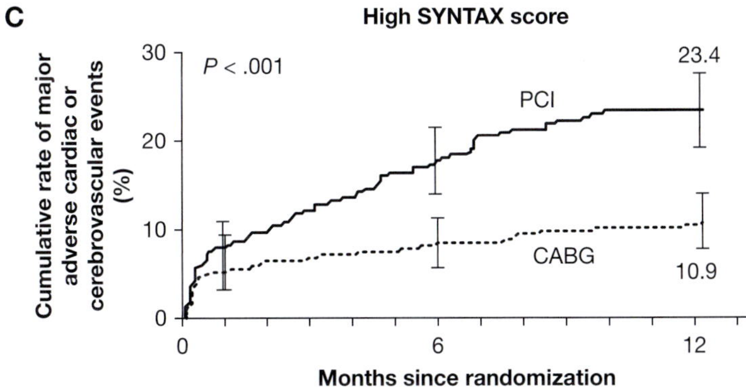

FIGURE 21.4 Rates of major adverse cardiac or cerebrovascular events among the study patients according to treatments group and SYNTAX score category.[23] CABG, coronary artery bypass graft; PCI, percutaneous coronary intervention; SYNTAX, Synergy Between PCI With TAXUS and Cardiac Surgery. (From Serruys PW, Morice MC, Kappetein AP, et al. Percutaneous coronary intervention versus coronary-artery bypass grafting for severe coronary artery disease. *N Engl J Med.* 2009;360(10):961-972. Copyright © 2009 Massachusetts Medical Society. Reprinted with permission from Massachusetts Medical Society.)

recommendation for PCI in patients with three-vessel CAD and low SYNTAX score (0-22) without diabetes mellitus (CABG gets the same recommendation in this group). In patients with three-vessel CAD and intermediate or high SYNTAX score (>22) without diabetes mellitus, CABG is recommended (class I, LOE A), while PCI is class III (harm) LOE A.[25] In patients with three-vessel CAD, low SYNTAX score (0-22) and diabetes mellitus CABG is recommended with class I, LOE A, while PCI has a class IIb LOE A recommendation. Similar patients (three-vessel CAD, diabetes mellitus) but intermediate or high SYNTAX score (>22) are recommended to receive CABG (class I, LOE A), meanwhile PCI is class III (harm) LOE A recommendation.[25]

Clinical characteristics that favor PCI are the presence of severe comorbidity (not adequately reflected by scores), advanced age, frailty, reduced life expectancy, restricted mobility, and conditions that affect rehabilitation. Anatomical characteristics that favor PCI include multivessel disease with SYNTAX score 0 to 22, anatomy likely resulting in incomplete revascularization with CABG (poor quality or missing conduits), severe chest deformation or scoliosis, sequelae of chest radiation, and porcelain aorta.[25] Conversely, the clinical characteristics of patients favoring CABG are diabetes, reduced LVEF (LVEF ≤ 35%), contraindication to dual antiplatelet therapy, and recurrent diffuse in-stent restenosis. The anatomical and technical characteristics that favor CABG are multivessel disease with SYNTAX score ≥23, LM CAD, anatomy likely resulting in incomplete revascularization with PCI, and severely calcified lesions limiting lesion expansion. In addition to these ascending aortic pathology with indication for surgery and concomitant cardiac surgery also favor revascularization with CABG.[25]

Predicted Surgical Mortality

There are two scores available to assist decision making and can be applied as a guide within the context of a multidisciplinary heart team to assess patients who are eligible for both CABG and PCI to predict surgical mortality. The European System for Cardiac Operative Risk Evaluation (EuroSCORE II: www.euroscore.org/calc.html)[31] as well as the Society of Thoracic Surgeons score (http://riskcalc.sts.org) were both created using clinical variables to estimate the operative in-hospital or 30-day mortality risk.[32,33]

European guidelines also emphasize that there is not a single risk model that provides perfect risk assessment because the scores are limited by the following factors: the specific definitions used or the methodology applied, the absence of important variables such as frailty, the practicability of calculation, a failure to reflect all relevant mortality and morbidity endpoints, and limited external validation.[25]

PATIENT COMORBIDITIES AND MULTIVESSEL PCI

LV Dysfunction, Viability, and Mechanical Circulatory Support

Reduced LV function is an independent predictor of worse outcomes in patients undergoing coronary revascularization.[34] Among patients with mild-to-moderate systolic dysfunction, CABG is associated with improved survival and LV function (meta-analysis including 7 randomized trials).[35] The STICH trial that enrolled patients with symptomatic ischemia from multivessel CAD and LVEF <35% did not show improved survival with CABG compared with medical therapy at 5 years. At 10 years, however, there was lower cardiovascular and all-cause mortality and composite outcome for CABG (58.9% vs 66.1%; HR, 0.84; 95% CI, 0.73-0.97; $P = .02$).[36]

In the Revascularization for Ischemic Ventricular Dysfunction (REVIVED) trial,[34] 700 patients with LVEF ≤35%, extensive CAD amenable to PCI, and demonstrable myocardial viability were randomized to either PCI plus optimal medical therapy or optimal medical therapy alone to evaluate the primary composite outcome of death for any cause or hospitalization for heart failure. Multivessel CAD was frequent in this trial, with 38% and 51% of those randomized to PCI having 2- and 3-vessel CAD. At a median of 41 months, the primary outcome occurred in 37.2% in the PCI group and 38.0% in the optimal medical therapy group and the LVEF was similar between groups at 6 and 12 months. In this trial, the median percentage of completeness of revascularization was 71% in the PCI group.[34]

With respect to complete revascularization, in the PROTECT II study, 452 symptomatic patients with complex three-vessel disease or unprotected LM CAD and severely depressed LV function (EF < 35%) were randomized to ventricular support using an intra-aortic balloon pump or Impella 2.5 device (Abiomed, Danvers, MA) during nonemergent high-risk PCI. The study showed no difference in 30-day incidence of MACE between the two groups; however, a trend for improved outcomes was observed in the Impella 2.5 group at 90 days.[37] In a substudy of PROTECT II trial, among 182 patients with quantitative echocardiography (LV volumes and biplane EF), Daubert et al assessed the extent and predictors of reverse LV remodeling, defined as improved systolic function with an absolute increase in EF >5%. Reverse LV remodeling occurred more frequently in patients with more extensive revascularization (OR, 7.52; 95% CI, [1.31-43.25]) and was associated with significantly fewer major adverse events (composite of death/MI stroke/transient ischemic attack): 9.7% versus 24.2% ($P < .01$). There was also a greater reduction in New York Heart Association class III/IV heart failure among reverse LV remodelers. These results suggest that selected patients may benefit from high-risk PCI with hemodynamic support who have multivessel CAD, reduced EF, and who are not candidates for CABG.[38] The PROTECT III study demonstrated improved completeness of revascularization and improved 90-day outcomes compared to PROTECT II study. In patients with severely depressed EF, Impella supported high-risk PCI.[39] The PROTECT IV trial will randomize patients undergoing high-risk PCI for complex CAD and reduced EF to Impella 2.5 or CP supported PCI versus IABP supported PCI (ClinicalTrials.gov Identifier: NCT04763200).

DIABETES

Diabetic patients represent 20% to 25% of patients undergoing revascularization, and they are more likely to have diffuse CAD, multivessel involvement, and LV dysfunction.[40] The mortality rate of diabetics following PCI is almost twice as high as that of nondiabetics.[41] The BARI trial (Bypass Angioplasty Revascularization Investigation) compared angioplasty with CABG in the management of patients with multivessel disease and found a survival advantage with surgical revascularization among diabetic patients (although the trial was conducted before the introduction of coronary stents).[42] Five-year survival for diabetics assigned to percutaneous transluminal coronary angioplasty was 65.5% compared with 80.6% for those assigned to CABG. The survival benefit was evident in patients who had at least one internal mammary artery used as a conduit. In contrast, ARTS,[43] MASS II,[44] ERACI/ERACI II,[45] and SOS[46] studies addressing PCI versus CABG showed statistically equivalent outcomes in their diabetic subsets. Among diabetics in the SYNTAX trial, the composite major adverse cardiac, cerebrovascular, and revascularization event rate was significantly higher for patients receiving PCI (46.5% in the PCI group vs 29.0% in the CABG group; $P < .01$).

The FREEDOM trial (Future Revascularization Evaluation in Patients with Diabetes Mellitus: Optimal Management of Multivessel Disease) was a multicenter prospective randomized trial comparing CABG with PCI stenting using sirolimus-eluting stents in diabetic patients with multivessel disease.[47] Patients in the CABG group had significantly lower rates of the composite endpoint of all-cause death, cerebrovascular accident, or MI compared with patients in the first-generation deug-eluting stent group (18.7% in the CABG group vs 26.6% in the PCI group; $P < .01$). Similar to the results from the SYNTAX study, among patients with SYNTAX scores <22, the FREEDOM trial reported no difference between treatment groups for the composite endpoint. There was a mortality benefit associated with CABG in patients with SYNTAX scores of 23 to 32, but not for patients with SYNTAX scores of 33 or higher, which may in part be related to statistical power given that fewer than 20% of patients in the FREEDOM trial had a SYNTAX score of 33 or higher.[47]

The 2021 ACCF/AHA guidelines recommend CABG with class I LOE A in patients with diabetes and multivessel CAD with involvement of the LAD, who are appropriate candidates for CABG. Prognostically, CABG with left internal mammary artery to LAD is superior to PCI to reduce mortality and repeat revascularizations. In patients who are poor candidates for CABG and amendable to PCI, revascularization with PCI is recommended with class 2a LOE B-NR to reduce long-term ischemic outcomes.

In patients with diabetes and LM stenosis and low- or intermediate complexity CAD in the rest of the coronaries, PCI may be considered as an alternative to CABG to reduce major adverse cardiovascular outcomes (class 2b, LOE B-R).[5]

The 2018 ESC/EACTS guidelines on myocardial revascularization recommend CABG in patients with three-vessel CAD, low SYNTAX score (0-22), and diabetes mellitus with class I, LOE A, while PCI has a class IIb LOE A recommendation. Patients with three-vessel CAD, diabetes mellitus, but intermediate or high SYNTAX score (>22) are recommended to receive CABG (class I, LOE A), meanwhile PCI is class III (harm) LOE A recommendation.[25]

ANATOMICAL FACTORS AND MULTIVESSEL PCI

There are multiple anatomical factors that can influence multivessel PCI. In elective cases, disease complexity and patient comorbidities such as LV dysfunction and heart failure are important considerations for vascular access. In patients with LV dysfunction and complex CAD undergoing high-risk interventions, there may be consideration for mechanical circulatory with devices such as Impella. In such cases, noninvasive imaging, for example with computed tomography, may be favored to inform vascular access site planning. The presence of bifurcation lesions, CTOs, and coronary calcification may favor the use of larger sheath sizes. Many of these interventions can be performed via the radial approach, but complex CAD requiring certain bifurcation techniques (eg, mini-crush) or atherectomy may be facilitated with the upfront use of larger sheaths, in which case, slender sheaths or sheathless guides may be used for transradial PCI.

PROCEDURAL FACTORS AND MULTIVESSEL PCI

There are multiple procedural factors and comorbidities that should also be considered when performing multivessel PCI. For nonemergent cases, elective and planned multivessel PCI should be performed following a heart team approach as appropriate and shared decision making as well as in the background of optimal guideline-directed medical therapy (including preloading).[5]

In patients with impaired renal function, low-dose contrast strategies can be planned upfront to minimize contrast. This include the use of a radial approach, biplane coronary angiography, liberal use of intracoronary physiology and imaging with intravascular ultrasound to guide PCI, and techniques to minimize contrast utilization. For patients with multivessel CAD, functional complete revascularization is a reasonable objective, for which reason noninvasive or invasive assessments of ischemia and functional significance can be used to improve the selection of lesions that warrant PCI over those in which PCI can be deferred and medical therapy favored. Likewise, coronary physiology and imaging can be used to guide decisions about stent size and length and facilitate PCI. Among patients with multivessel CAD, while same-sitting multivessel PCI aimed at complete revascularization is a reasonable objective, radiation and contrast dose are important metrics that should be assessed regularly during the case as they can inform decisions about when to pause and consider staged PCI.

SUMMARY

The decision to perform multivessel PCI requires careful consideration of complex clinical, anatomic, and technical variables. It is important to consider patient factors, such as age, frailty, diabetes, renal dysfunction, myocardial viability, extent of ischemia, and LV dysfunction that may influence decisions about revascularization as well as anatomical factors such as the presence of LM disease, bifurcation lesions, coronary calcification, and coronary CTOs, and the degree to which each revascularization modality can achieve complete revascularization. A heart team approach and shared decision making are important to guide decisions about revascularization.

References

1. Anderson HV, Shaw RE, Brindis RG, et al. A contemporary overview of percutaneous coronary interventions. The American College of Cardiology-National Cardiovascular Data Registry (ACC-NCDR). *J Am Coll Cardiol*. 2002;39(7):1096-1103.
2. Frutkin AD, Lindsey JB, Mehta SK, et al. Drug-eluting stents and the use of percutaneous coronary intervention among patients with class I indications for coronary artery bypass surgery undergoing index revascularization: analysis from the NCDR (National Cardiovascular Data Registry). *JACC Cardiovasc Interv* 2009;2(7):614-621.
3. Gogo PB Jr, Dauerman HL, Mulgund J, et al. Changes in patterns of coronary revascularization strategies for patients with acute coronary syndromes (from the CRUSADE Quality Improvement Initiative). *Am J Cardiol*. 2007;99(9):1222-1226.
4. Sandoval Y, Brilakis ES, Canoniero M, Yannopoulos D, Garcia S. Complete versus incomplete coronary revascularization of patients with multivessel coronary artery disease. *Curr Treat Options Cardiovasc Med*. 2015;17(3):366.
5. Lawton JS, Tamis-Holland JE, Bangalore S, et al. 2021 ACC/AHA/SCAI guideline for coronary artery revascularization: executive summary—a report of the American College of Cardiology/American Heart Association Joint Committee on Clinical Practice Guidelines. *Circulation*. 2022;145(3):e4-e17.
6. Patel MR, Calhoon JH, Dehmer GJ, et al. ACC/AATS/AHA/ASE/ASNC/SCAI/SCCT/STS 2017 appropriate use criteria for coronary revascularization in patients with stable ischemic heart disease: a report of the American College of Cardiology appropriate use criteria task force, American Association for Thoracic Surgery, American Heart Association, American Society of Echocardiography, American Society of Nuclear Cardiology, Society for Cardiovascular Angiography and Interventions, Society of Cardiovascular Computed Tomography, and Society of Thoracic Surgeons. *J Am Coll Cardiol*. 2017;69(17):2212-2241.
7. O'Gara PT, Kushner FG, Ascheim DD, et al. 2013 ACCF/AHA guideline for the management of ST-elevation myocardial infarction: a report of the American College of Cardiology Foundation/American Heart Association Task Force on Practice Guidelines. *Circulation*. 2013;127(4):e362-e425.
8. Wald DS, Morris JK, Wald NJ, et al. Randomized trial of preventive angioplasty in myocardial infarction. *N Engl J Med*. 2013;369(12):1115-1123.
9. Engstrøm T, Kelbaek H, Helqvist S, et al. Complete revascularisation versus treatment of the culprit lesion only in patients with ST-segment elevation myocardial infarction and multivessel disease (DANAMI-3-PRIMULTI): an open-label, randomised controlled trial. *Lancet*. 2015;386(9994):665-671.
10. Smits PC, Abdel-Wahab M, Neumann FJ, et al. Fractional flow reserve-guided multivessel angioplasty in myocardial infarction. *N Engl J Med*. 2017;376(13):1234-1244.
11. Mehta SR, Wood DA, Storey RF, et al. Complete revascularization with multivessel PCI for myocardial infarction. *N Engl J Med*. 2019;381(15):1411-1421.
12. Gershlick AH, Khan JN, Kelly DJ, et al. Randomized trial of complete versus lesion-only revascularization in patients undergoing primary percutaneous coronary intervention for STEMI and multivessel disease: the CvLPRIT trial. *J Am Coll Cardiol*. 2015;65(10):963-972.

13. Thiele H, Akin I, Sandri M, et al.. PCI strategies in patients with acute myocardial infarction and cardiogenic shock. *N Engl J Med.* 2017;377(25):2419-2432.
14. Thiele H, Akin I, Sandri M, et al. One-year outcomes after PCI strategies in cardiogenic shock. *N Engl J Med.* 2018;379(18):1699-1710.
15. Kolte D, Sardar P, Khera S, et al. Culprit vessel-only versus multivessel percutaneous coronary intervention in patients with cardiogenic shock complicating ST-segment-elevation myocardial infarction: a collaborative meta-analysis. *Circ Cardiovasc Interv.* 2017;10(11):e005582.
16. Sardella G, Lucisano L, Garbo R, et al. Single-staged compared with multi-staged PCI in multivessel NSTEMI patients: the SMILE trial. *J Am Coll Cardiol.* 2016;67(3):264-272.
17. Diletti R, den Dekker WK, Bennett J, et al. Immediate versus staged complete revascularisation in patients presenting with acute coronary syndrome and multivessel coronary disease (BIOVASC): a prospective, open-label, non-inferiority, randomised trial. *Lancet.* 2023;401(10383):1172-1182.
18. Maron DJ, Hochman JS, Reynolds HR, et al. Initial invasive or conservative strategy for stable coronary disease. *N Engl J Med.* 2020;382(15):1395-1407.
19. Boden WE, O'Rourke RA, Teo KK, et al. Optimal medical therapy with or without PCI for stable coronary disease. *N Engl J Med.* 2007;356(15):1503-1516.
20. Sedlis SP, Hartigan PM, Teo KK, et al. Effect of PCI on long-term survival in patients with stable ischemic heart disease. *N Engl J Med.* 2015;373(20):1937-1946.
21. Garcia S, Sandoval Y, Roukoz H, et al. Outcomes after complete versus incomplete revascularization of patients with multivessel coronary artery disease: a meta-analysis of 89,883 patients enrolled in randomized clinical trials and observational studies. *J Am Coll Cardiol.* 2013;62(16):1421-1431.
22. Dauerman HL. Reasonable incomplete revascularization. *Circulation.* 2011;123(21):2337-2340.
23. Serruys PW, Morice MC, Kappetein AP, et al. Percutaneous coronary intervention versus coronary-artery bypass grafting for severe coronary artery disease. *N Engl J Med.* 2009;360(10):961-972.
24. Sianos G, Morel MA, Kappetein AP, et al. The SYNTAX Score: an angiographic tool grading the complexity of coronary artery disease. *EuroIntervention.* 2005;1(2):219-227.
25. Neumann FJ, Sousa-Uva M, Ahlsson A, et al. 2018 ESC/EACTS Guidelines on myocardial revascularization. *EuroIntervention.* 2019;14(14):1435-1534.
26. Wykrzykowska JJ, Garg S, Girasis C, et al. Value of the SYNTAX score for risk assessment in the all-comers population of the randomized multicenter LEADERS (Limus Eluted from A Durable versus ERodable Stent coating) trial. *J Am Coll Cardiol.* 2010;56(4):272-277.
27. Garg S, Serruys PW, Silber S, et al. The prognostic utility of the SYNTAX score on 1-year outcomes after revascularization with zotarolimus- and everolimus-eluting stents: a substudy of the RESOLUTE All Comers Trial. *JACC Cardiovasc Interv.* 2011;4(4):432-441.
28. Cavalcante R, Sotomi Y, Mancone M, et al. Impact of the SYNTAX scores I and II in patients with diabetes and multivessel coronary disease: a pooled analysis of patient level data from the SYNTAX, PRECOMBAT, and BEST trials. *Eur Heart J* 2017;38(25):1969-1977.
29. Farooq V, van Klaveren D, Steyerberg EW, et al. Anatomical and clinical characteristics to guide decision making between coronary artery bypass surgery and percutaneous coronary intervention for individual patients: development and validation of SYNTAX score II. *Lancet.* 2013;381(9867):639-650.
30. Campos CM, van Klaveren D, Farooq V, et al. Long-term forecasting and comparison of mortality in the evaluation of the Xience everolimus eluting stent vs. coronary artery bypass surgery for effectiveness of left main revascularization (EXCEL) trial: prospective validation of the SYNTAX score II. *Eur Heart J.* 2015;36(20):1231-1241.
31. Nashef SA, Roques F, Sharples LD, et al. EuroSCORE II. *Eur J Cardio Thorac Surg.* 2012;41(4):734-745; discussion 44-45.
32. Shahian DM, O'Brien SM, Filardo G, et al.. The Society of Thoracic Surgeons 2008 cardiac surgery risk models: part 1—coronary artery bypass grafting surgery. *Ann Thorac Surg.* 2009;88(1 suppl):S2-S22.
33. Shahian DM, O'Brien SM, Filardo G, et al. The Society of Thoracic Surgeons 2008 cardiac surgery risk models: part 3—valve plus coronary artery bypass grafting surgery. *Ann Thorac Surg.* 2009;88(1 suppl):S43-S62.
34. Perera D, Clayton T, O'Kane PD, et al. Percutaneous revascularization for ischemic left ventricular dysfunction. *N Engl J Med.* 2022;387(15):1351-1360.
35. Yusuf S, Zucker D, Peduzzi P, et al. Effect of coronary artery bypass graft surgery on survival: overview of 10-year results from randomised trials by the Coronary Artery Bypass Graft Surgery Trialists Collaboration. *Lancet.* 1994;344(8922):563-570.
36. Velazquez EJ, Lee KL, Jones RH, et al. Coronary-artery bypass surgery in patients with ischemic cardiomyopathy. *N Engl J Med.* 2016;374(16):1511-1520.
37. O'Neill WW, Kleiman NS, Moses J, et al. A prospective, randomized clinical trial of hemodynamic support with Impella 2.5 versus intra-aortic balloon pump in patients undergoing high-risk percutaneous coronary intervention: the PROTECT II study. *Circulation.* 2012;126(14):1717-1727.
38. Daubert MA, Massaro J, Liao L, et al. High-risk percutaneous coronary intervention is associated with reverse left ventricular remodeling and improved outcomes in patients with coronary artery disease and reduced ejection fraction. *Am Heart J.* 2015;170(3):550-558.
39. O'Neill WW, Anderson M, Burkhoff D, et al. Improved outcomes in patients with severely depressed LVEF undergoing percutaneous coronary intervention with contemporary practices. *Am Heart J.* 2022;248:139-149.
40. Ammann P, Brunner-La Rocca H, Fehr T, et al. Coronary anatomy and left ventricular ejection fraction in patients with type 2 diabetes admitted for elective coronary angiography. *Catheter Cardiovasc Interv.* 2004;62(4):432-438.
41. Laskey WK, Selzer F, Vlachos HA, et al. Comparison of in-hospital and one-year outcomes in patients with and without diabetes mellitus undergoing percutaneous catheter intervention (from the National Heart, Lung, and Blood Institute Dynamic Registry). *Am J Cardiol.* 2002;90(10):1062-1067.
42. Bypass Angioplasty Revascularization Investigation (BARI) Investigators. Comparison of coronary bypass surgery with angioplasty in patients with multivessel disease. *N Engl J Med.* 1996;335(4):217-225.
43. Serruys PW, Ong AT, van Herwerden LA, et al. Five-year outcomes after coronary stenting versus bypass surgery for the treatment of multivessel disease: the final analysis of the Arterial Revascularization Therapies Study (ARTS) randomized trial. *J Am Coll Cardiol.* 2005;46(4):575-581.
44. Hueb W, Lopes NH, Gersh BJ, et al. Five-year follow-up of the Medicine, Angioplasty, or Surgery Study (MASS II): a randomized controlled clinical trial of 3 therapeutic strategies for multivessel coronary artery disease. *Circulation.* 2007;115(9):1082-1089.
45. Rodriguez AE, Baldi J, Fernández Pereira C, et al. Five-year follow-up of the Argentine randomized trial of coronary angioplasty with stenting versus coronary bypass surgery in patients with multiple vessel disease (ERACI II). *J Am Coll Cardiol.* 2005;46(4):582-588.
46. Booth J, Clayton T, Pepper J, et al. Randomized, controlled trial of coronary artery bypass surgery versus percutaneous coronary intervention in patients with multivessel coronary artery disease: six-year follow-up from the Stent or Surgery Trial (SoS). *Circulation.* 2008;118(4):381-388.
47. Farkouh ME, Domanski M, Sleeper LA, et al. Strategies for multivessel revascularization in patients with diabetes. *N Engl J Med.* 2012;367(25):2375-2384.

22 Bifurcation and Left Main Lesions

Max W. Maffey, Carlos E. Uribe, and Luiz F. Ybarra

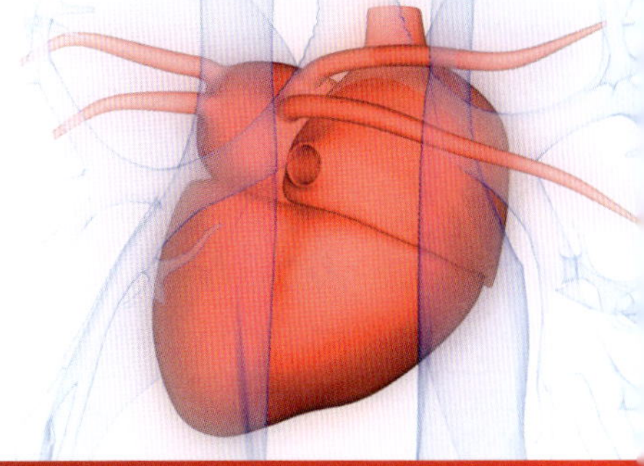

INTRODUCTION

Bifurcation percutaneous coronary intervention (PCI) is one of the most technically challenging, controversial, and interesting aspects of interventional cardiology. Arterial bifurcations produce areas of variable endothelial shear stress. Areas such as the lateral wall of the main vessel and side branch are exposed to low endothelial stress and, as a result, are particularly prone to atherosclerotic plaque formation. Conversely, areas of high endothelial shear stress, such as the carina, are relatively spared.[1] As a result, bifurcation lesions are common and comprise approximately 20% of all PCI procedures.[2] Prior to the stent era, there was general concern as there were no modalities to adequately deal with dissection or abrupt closure of the main vessel or side branch. With the advent and subsequent development of stent technology, tools were developed to help address these complex lesions. However, bifurcation PCI remains associated with a higher risk of procedural complications and short- and long-term clinical sequalae.[3]

Any discussion of bifurcation lesion PCI is incomplete without a thorough discussion of left main (LM) PCI and vice versa. The LM bifurcation is involved in 61% of all LM lesions.[4] For several decades, coronary artery bypass grafting (CABG) remained the mainstay of treatment for both simple and complex LM disease. With the progression of percutaneous techniques and devices and the advent of several landmark randomized clinical trials, PCI offers an excellent alternative for appropriately selected patients. However, given the large amount of myocardium at risk, LM lesions also comprise the highest risk lesion subset, and several unique considerations must be made when planning and performing PCI.

Despite marked advances, both bifurcation and LM PCI remain controversial topics. Several trials have been completed in recent years, providing further evidence to help inform clinical decision making. As new techniques are developed, classification schemes are made, and as technology progresses, it is clear that there is marked heterogeneity within both groups. Not all bifurcation and LM lesions are created equal, and because of this, it is important to review the literature on both topics, including classification schemes, seminal trials, advice from current guidelines, and some potential approaches for dealing with these patient populations in clinical practice.

BIFURCATION DEFINITION AND CLASSIFICATION

In general, a coronary bifurcation can be conceptualized as three different diameter vessels: the proximal main vessel (PMV), the distal main vessel (DMV), and the side branch. Murray's law defines the relationship of the diameters of the PMV, DMV, and side branch. This relationship is summarized by Finet's formula: PMV diameter = 0.678 (DMV diameter + side-branch diameter).[5]

Historically, defining what actually constitutes a bifurcation lesion has been controversial. Randomized trials and registries used variable definitions and classification schemes, which resulted in significant difficulties when applying this literature to clinical practice. In 2007, Louvard et al published a consensus group statement, which defined a bifurcation lesion as "a coronary artery narrowing occurring adjacent to, and/or involving, the origin of a significant side branch."[6] The same authors defined a significant side branch as one that "you do not want to lose in the global context of a particular patient (symptoms, location of ischemia, branch responsible for symptoms of ischemia, viability, collateralizing vessel, left ventricular function, and so forth)."[6]

What actually constitutes a "significant" side branch has been a focus of much debate and research. A clinically significant vessel has been defined as a vessel that subtends >10% of myocardial mass.[7] By this definition, only a minority (~20%) of non-LM side branches are considered clinically significant. Side branches >73 mm in length meet this definition.[7] Angiographic scoring systems such as the SNuH score, which takes into account the diameter of a side branch, the number of other side branches, and height of a side branch, can also help predict whether a side branch is significant.[8] Additional data from functional testing and cardiac computed tomography (CT) may also be of use.

Several systems exist for classifying bifurcation lesions. However, in large part due to its simplicity, the Medina classification has become the most prevalent in both the literature and clinical practice (see **Fig. 22.1**). In this classification system, a stenosis greater than 50% is considered significant. The number one (1) is used to denote the presence of a significant stenosis, whilst zero (0) is used to denote the absence of a significant stenosis. The classification uses this binary notation to record the presence or the absence of a significant stenosis within the three main segments of a bifurcation lesion in the following order: the PMV, the DMV, and the side branch.[9] As an example, a lesion that involves both the PMV and DMV but not the side branch would be recorded as 1,1,0. Angiographic examples of lesions with their associated Medina classifications can be seen in **Figs. 22.2** and **22.3**.

Though the Medina classification is straightforward and user friendly, it is by no means a comprehensive anatomical classification system. It does not provide information regarding several lesion characteristics that predict both short- and long-term complications, including the bifurcation angle, the size of the side branch, length of the side-branch lesion, and the presence or absence of calcification.[10–12] These characteristics also provide an operator with crucial information that may assist in procedural planning.

The concept of a "true bifurcation" is also used frequently in trials and clinical practice, although with variable definitions (such as Medina 1,1,1, 1,0,1, or 0,1,1). It should be noted, however, that not all trials were strict in the lesions included.

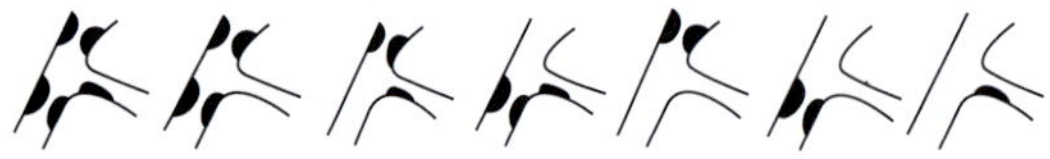

Medina	1,1,1	1,1,0	1,0,1	0,1,1	1,0,0	0,1,0	0,0,1
Duke (modified)	D	C	F	G	A	B	E
Sanborn	I	-	-	III	IV	II	IV
Lefevre	1	2	-	4	3	4a	4b
Safian	IA	IB	IIA	IIIA	IIB	IIIB	IV
Movahed	L	S	2	1m	1s	V	T
Staico-Feres	3	2A	2B	2C	1A	1B	1C

FIGURE 22.1 Bifurcation classifications. (Courtesy of Dr. Issam Moussa.)

PCI TECHNIQUES

When approaching bifurcation lesions, adequate planning and a thorough understanding of the available evidence are crucial for achieving procedural success and optimizing long-term outcomes. Current consensus documents promote an ethos that favors approaches, which are simple and safe, respect the original bifurcation anatomy, minimize the number of stents, and optimize the flow and function of the bifurcation after PCI.[13] In general, there are two major methods of bifurcation stenting: provisional and two-stent. Provisional stenting involves the intention of stenting the main vessel across the side-branch ostium. Further side-branch intervention would only occur if the side branch is significantly compromised. The two-stent strategy is an umbrella term that encompasses a varying range of techniques but, in essence, involves the intention of upfront stenting of both the main vessel and side branch. The following section will explore technical aspects of bifurcation PCI including access and equipment selection, lesion preparation, provisional and two-stent approaches, imaging, and physiology and will examine the current evidence available in the literature.

Equipment and Access

The radial approach has been shown to reduce bleeding complications and improve outcomes in both acute coronary syndrome (ACS) and stable coronary artery disease populations.[14] Radial access also carries a class I recommendation for both these patient groups.[15,16] Bifurcation or LM PCI is not an exception to this recommendation. The vast majority of bifurcation PCI (including two-stent techniques) can also be performed via a 6-French guiding catheter with some exceptions (see "*Planning and Lesion Preparation*" below). Therefore, larger access is infrequently required.

Planning and Lesion Preparation

Given the three-dimensional structure of bifurcations, multiple angiographic angulations are required to obtain a clear understanding of all three segments of the bifurcation. A clear view of the side-branch ostium is crucial, and multiple angiographic images may need to be explored to find a "working view." A recent paper based on coronary CT and fluoroscopy gantry angle extrapolation demonstrated the ideal coronary angiography projections for most coronary bifurcations (see **Fig. 22.4**).

If a decision has been made that a side branch is significant, wiring of both the main vessel *and* side branch is recommended.[13] As a general rule, the most difficult branch to wire should be wired first. The second wire should be minimally manipulated to avoid "wire wrap." The need for a side-branch wire is self-explanatory when a two-stent approach is adopted. However, wiring the side branch is also thought to have several benefits when adopting a provisional approach (see "*Provisional Stenting Technique*" below). One no exception to this rule is if rotational atherectomy is required to prepare either limb of the bifurcation. In this circumstance, a second wire is likely to be damaged by the rotational atherectomy burr if it is left in situ. This presents a challenge as rotational atherectomy may lead to dissection, which can result in significant challenges

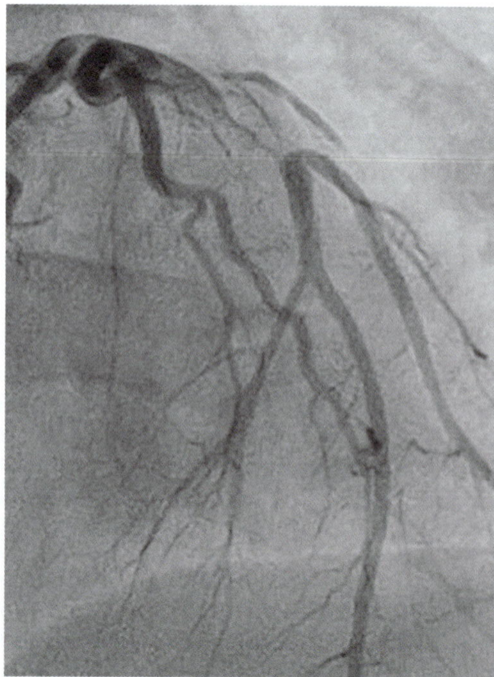

FIGURE 22.2 An example of a Medina 1,0,0 lesion involving the LAD and diagonal vessel. LAD, left anterior descending artery.

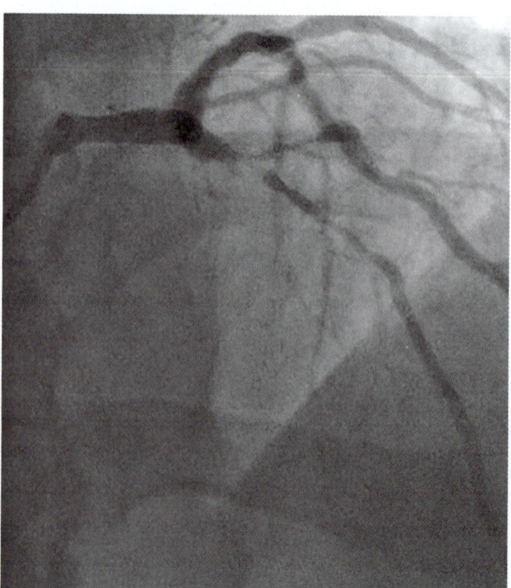

FIGURE 22.3 A Medina 1,1,1 bifurcation lesion involving the LAD and first diagonal. LAD, left anterior descending artery.

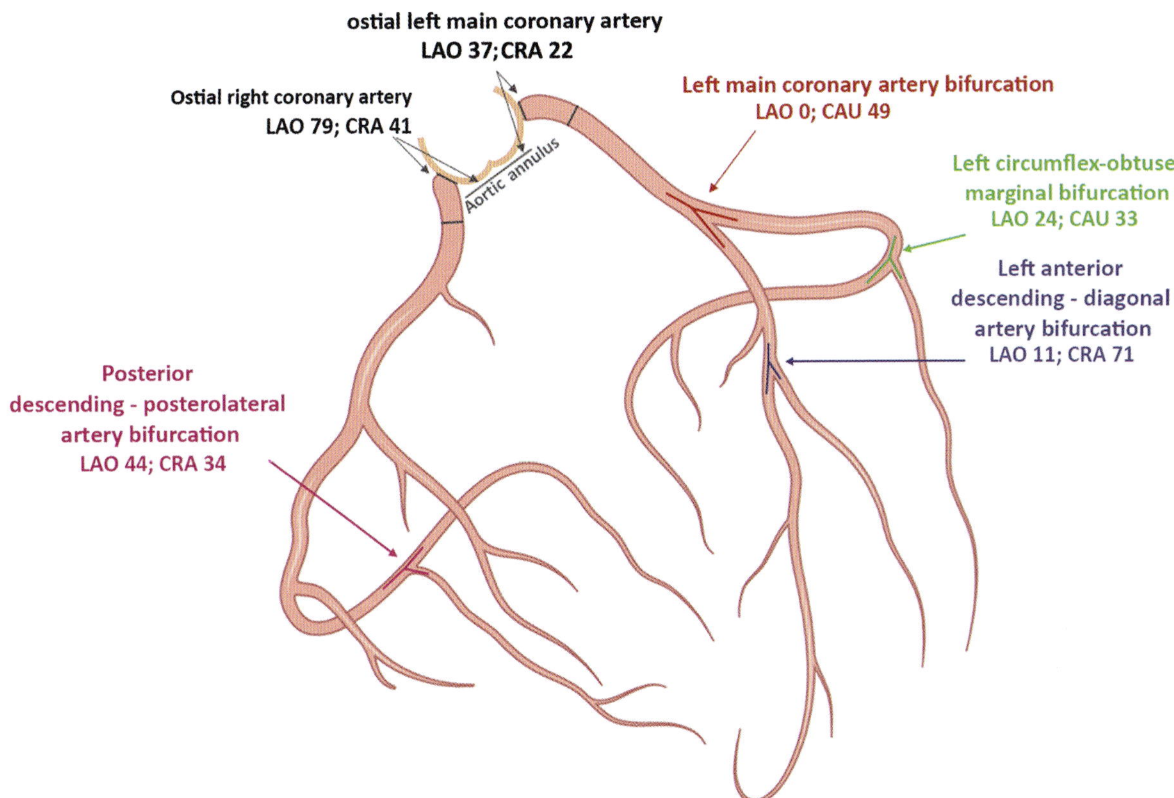

FIGURE 22.4 Optimal fluoroscopic viewing angles of coronary ostia and bifurcations. CAU, caudal; CRA, cranial; LAO, left anterior oblique. (Reproduced with permission from Kočka V, Thériault-Lauzier P, Xiong TY, et al. Optimal fluoroscopic projections of coronary ostia and bifurcations defined by computed tomographic coronary angiography. *JACC Cardiovasc Interv*. 2020;13(21):2560-2570.[68])

rewiring the side branch. In some circumstances, it may be highly desirable to leave a second wire in situ. This includes side branches that are very difficult to wire or very anatomically or clinically important side branches such as the left circumflex in LM PCI. In these circumstances, using a large French guide catheter (≥8 Fr), a microcatheter can be advanced over the second wire to protect it from the rotational atherectomy burr. If multiple rotational atherectomy runs are performed, the microcatheter should be advanced or retracted a small amount to reduce the risk of damaging the microcatheter.

Preparation of the main vessel with balloon angioplasty should be performed in most cases. However, if a provisional approach is adopted, preparation of the side branch should be avoided as this may lead to dissection and necessitate transition to a two-stent approach.[17] If a decision is made to adopt an up-front two-stent approach, both the main vessel and side branch should be prepared. Other methods of lesion preparation such as rotational atherectomy should be employed as required.

Provisional Versus Two-Stent Approach

When determining how best to treat a bifurcation lesion, one of the first decisions that must be made is between a provisional or two-stent strategy. Several studies have been performed to address this question (see **Table 22.1**). In short, current evidence suggests equal or better outcomes with provisional stenting in simple bifurcation lesions. Provisional stenting has also been demonstrated to have significantly shorter procedure times and fluoroscopy times and lower contrast volumes.[21,23,26] Complex lesions are defined by the DEFINITION criteria, which utilizes a set of angiographic characteristics that predict major adverse events post-PCI (see **Table 22.2**).[29] Importantly, the DEFINITION II study established that, in complex lesions that meet these criteria, upfront two-stent strategies have reduced rates of target lesion revascularization, target vessel myocardial infarction (MI), and target vessel failure.[19] Based on the available evidence, current consensus documents recommend provisional stenting as the standard approach with upfront two-stent strategies reserved for those lesions with complex anatomy.[13]

Provisional Stenting Technique

As previously noted, wires are usually placed in both the side branch and main vessel when performing provisional stenting. Keeping a wire in the side branch has several potential benefits including (1) to provide a marker for rewiring in the event of side-branch occlusion; (2) to assist in anchoring of the guiding catheter providing better support for equipment delivery; (3) to facilitate access to the side branch by altering the bifurcation angle; and (4) in extreme situations, to allow the passage of a small balloon behind the main vessel stent struts in order to restore side-branch flow.[17] In practice, the decision to wire a side branch is based on a number of factors, including the area of myocardium supplied by the side branch, lesion complexity, and the degree of disease in the ostial/proximal side branch.

After the lesion has been prepared (see "*Planning and Lesion Preparation*" above), a stent is then deployed in the main vessel. This stent should be sized to the distal vessel, and stent selection should take into account the need for postdilation of the stent proximal to the bifurcation – the so-called "Proximal Optimization Technique" or POT. Stent expansion diameters are fixed, and excessive dilatation may result in deformation of the stent architecture. Maximal

TABLE 22.1 Studies Comparing Provisional With Two-Stent Techniques in Bifurcation PCI

STUDY	STUDY TYPE	N	PATIENT COHORT	TWO-STENT TECHNIQUE	PRIMARY ENDPOINT	RESULTS
EBC Main (2021)[18]	Prospective, randomized, multicenter	467	LM; Medina 1,1,1 or 0,1,1	Culotte, DK-minicrush, T-stent, TAP	Composite of all-cause death, MI, and TLR at 12 mo.	Fewer events in the provisional group but did not reach statistical significance
DEFINITION II (2020)[19]	Prospective, randomized, multicenter	653	Non-LM or LM; complex Medina 1,1,1 or 0,1,1	DK crush (78%), culotte (17.9%), TAP (3.3%), other	Composite of TLR, TVMI, and TLF (including cardiac death) at 12 mo	Significantly lower rates of primary endpoint in 2-stent group
DK crush V (2017)[20]	Prospective, randomized, multicenter	482	Unprotected LM; Medina 1,1,1 or 0,1,1	DK crush	Composite rate of TLF: cardiac death, TVMI, or clinically driven TLR	Significantly lower rate of the primary endpoint in DK crush group
PERFECT (2015)[21]	Prospective, randomized, multicentre	419	Non-LM; Medina 1,0,1; 1,1,1; 0,1,1; or 0,0,1.	Crush	% Diameter stenosis and overall restenosis rate at 8-mo angiography. MACE (death, MI, and TVR) at 12 mo	No difference in angiographic or clinical endpoints
EBC TWO (2016)[22]	Prospective, randomized, multicenter	200	Non-LM; Medina 1,1,1; 1,0,1; 0,1,1	Culotte	Composite of all cause death, MI, TVR at 12 mo	No significant difference in the primary endpoint
BBC ONE/ NORDIC I 5-y follow-up (2016)[23]	Pooled data from two randomized studies	890	Bifurcation disease – all Medina classifications	Crush, T-stent, culotte	All-cause mortality at 5 y	Significantly lower mortality with provisional stenting vs two-stent techniques
DK crush II (2011)[24]	Prospective, randomized, multicenter	370	Non-LM; Medina 1,1,1 or 0,1,1	DK crush	MACE (cardiac death, MI, and TVR)	No difference in MACE. Higher rates of angiographic restenosis and TVR in provisional group
BBC ONE (2010)[25]	Prospective, randomized, multicentre	500	Non-LM bifurcation disease – all Medina classifications	Crush, culotte	Composite of all-cause death, MI, TVF by 9 mo	Significantly lower rate of the primary endpoint with provisional stenting
CACTUS (2009)[26]	Prospective, randomized, multicentre	350	Non-LM; Medina 1,1,1; 1,0,1; 0,1,1	Crush	Angiographic: In-segment restenosis rate at 6 mo Clinical: MACE (cardiac death, MI, and TVR) at 6 mo	No significant difference in the primary angiographic or clinical endpoints
BBK (2008)[27]	Prospective, randomized	202	Non-LM; all Medina classifications; >50% stenosis in main vessel OR side branch	T stent	Angiographic in-segment % stenosis of side-branch at 9 mo	No significant difference
NORDIC I (2006)[28]	Prospective, randomized, multicentre	413	All Medina classifications excluding left-dominant LM disease	Crush (50%), culotte (21%), other (29%)	MACE (cardiac death, MI, TVR, and stent thrombosis) at 6 mo	No significant difference in the primary endpoint

DK crush, double kissing crush; LM, left main; MACE, major adverse cardiovascular event; MI, myocardial infarction; PCI, percutaneous coronary intervention; TAP, T and Protrude; TLF, target lesion failure; TLR, target lesion revascularization; TVMI, target vessel myocardial infarction.

stent expansion diameters are available in the manufacturers' product information. Furthermore, the proximal edge of the stent should be placed so that enough stent length is present to allow for POT to be performed. The minimum length is determined by the shortest available balloon length (usually 6-8 mm). The proximal vessel size and, therefore, POT balloon size, can be determined by a number of means including quantitative coronary angiography, intravascular imaging when available, or Finet's formula (see "*Bifurcation Definition and Classification*" above). POT should be performed with a noncompliant balloon, and caution should be taken to ensure that the distal edge of the balloon is inflated just proximal to the carina.[17] A recent study has shown that POT may also reduce the need for additional side vessel intervention.[30]

Another consideration is whether the side-branch wire should be left in place whilst main vessel stenting and POT take place – a process known as "jailing." As previously mentioned, a wire left in situ behind stent struts may have significant benefits. However, concern exists regarding the possibility of wire damage and fracture when removing jailed wires. These concerns are supported by a study that performed microscopic evaluation of jailed wires.

TABLE 22.2 The DEFINTION Criteria for Complex Bifurcation Lesions[29]

One of the Following Major Criteria
Distal LM bifurcation: SB ≥ 70% and SB lesion length ≥10 mm
OR
Non-LM bifurcations: SB ≥ 90% and SB lesion length ≥10 mm
Plus Any Two of the Following Minor Criteria
Moderate-to-severe calcification
Multiple lesions
Bifurcation angle <45° or >70°
Main vessel reference vessel diameter <2.5 mm
MV lesion length ≥25 mm
Thrombus-containing lesions

LM, left main; MV, main vessel; SB, side branch.
From Chen SL, Sheiban I, Xu B, et al. Impact of the complexity of bifurcation lesions treated with drug-eluting stents: the DEFINITION study (Definitions and impact of complEx biFurcation lesIons on clinical outcomes after percutaNeous coronary IntervenTIOn using drug-eluting steNts). *JACC Cardiovasc Interv*. 2014;7:1266-1276.

This study also suggested that polymer-coated wires are more resistant to retrieval damage and are more efficient in crossing the side-branch ostium than nonpolymer-coated wires.[31] However, a study using data from the COBIS III registry suggested a possible benefit of wire jailing with significantly lower rates of side-branch occlusion in patients with a side branch or main vessel stenosis ≥60%.[32]

After POT, angiography is performed and the side branch is assessed. Side-branch compromise has been defined variably in the literature. In clinical practice, assessing side-branch compromise is complex and considers a variety of factors including the diameter and length of the side branch, the degree of angiographic stenosis, the presence or the absence of symptoms, electrocardiogram (ECG) changes, and thrombolysis in myocardial infarction (TIMI) flow. The decision on whether to "rescue" a compromised side branch by further intervention is equally complex. For example, a relatively short side branch of 2 mm in diameter with a 90% stenosis and TIMI 2 flow with no associated symptoms or ECG changes after main vessel stenting may not be intervened on any further. On the other hand, a long, 3.5-mm side branch with a 95% ostial stenosis and TIMI 3 flow with associated chest pain and ECG changes post-main vessel stenting is likely to be rescued. Functional assessment of the side branch using fractional flow reserve (FFR) may also be of use in situations where side-branch compromise is unclear and has been demonstrated to be a viable alternative to angiographic assessment with comparable clinical outcomes.[33]

If "rescuing" the side branch has been deemed necessary, the side branch is then rewired through a distal stent strut. This allows for better strut clearance from the side-branch ostium and allows stents scaffold to be positioned opposite to the carina.[17] The jailed side-branch wire is then removed. What should follow in the sequence of side-branch rescue is a current matter of debate. Regardless, the overall goal is to use a balloon to restore flow to the side branch whilst maintaining the architectural integrity of the main vessel stent. Some operators achieve this using a kissing balloon inflation (KBI). KBI is a process of inflating two balloons – one across the side-branch ostium and the other in the main vessel which "kiss" in the PMV. In provisional stenting, routine KBI, regardless of side-branch compromise, has not demonstrated clear clinical benefits and may cause greater harm.[34] Therefore, selective use of KBI when needed is recommended. If KBI is performed, noncompliant balloons should be used as they have been associated with a reduction in side-vessel stenting and periprocedural MI.[30] A process of sequential POT-side-branch-POT dilatations has also been proposed, which appears to offer a simpler alternative that may reduce strut malapposition and reduces elliptical deformation of the main vessel stent.[35] However, this approach has also been scrutinized due to reported main vessel stent distortion, reduced ostial side-branch area especially with narrow bifurcation angles, and a lack of complete correction of main vessel distortion with the final rePOT step.[36]

If an acceptable result is achieved with balloon dilatation, no further intervention may be required. If side-branch results are suboptimal after balloon dilatation, a decision may be made to insert a second stent. The exact technique used depends on the anatomy of the bifurcation. Bifurcation angles close to 90° may be suitable for a T-stent strategy, whereas more acute angles may be best suited to a reverse crush, culotte, or TAP (T and Protrusion) technique.

Two-Stent Techniques

If a decision is made to perform an upfront two-stent intervention, the choices of method are many and varied. Several studies have been published attempting to determine which strategy has superior clinical outcomes (see **Table 22.3**). However, as bifurcation

TABLE 22.3 Studies Comparing Two-Stent Techniques in Bifurcation PCI

STUDY	STUDY TYPE	N	PATIENT COHORT	DK CRUSH	CULOTTE	TAP	CRUSH
BBK II (2016)[37]	Prospective, randomized, single center	300	LM and non-LM; ~97% Medina 1,1,1 or 1,0,1 or 0,1,1		Angiographic restenosis ↓	Angiographic restenosis ↑	
DK crush III (2013)[38]	Prospective, randomized, multicenter	419	Unprotected LM; medina 1,1,1 or 0,1,1	MACE TLR ↓	MACE TLR ↑		
Nordic II (2009)[39]	Prospective, randomized, multicenter	424	~78% Medina 1,1,1 or 1,0,1 or 0,1,1 (significantly more in culotte group)		MACE ↔		MACE ↔
DK crush I (2008)[40,41]	Prospective, randomized, multicenter	311	"True bifurcation lesions"	MACE TLR-free survival ↓			MACE TLR-free survival ↑

LM, left main; MACE, major adverse cardiovascular event; TLR, target lesion revascularization.

lesions are as anatomically diverse as the clinical scenarios they are associated with, knowledge of a variety of techniques is required.

The European Bifurcation Club have proposed a classification to help describe and further define two-stent techniques: the MADS classification.[17] This classification groups the aforementioned two-stent strategies based on the position of the first stent – **M**ain proximal first (eg, Skirt stent); main **A**cross the side branch (eg, TAP, culotte); **D**ouble proximal lumen (eg, simultaneous kissing stents [SKSs]); and **S**ide-branch first (eg, DK crush). This classification was further amended in 2019 to include a coded description of subsequent balloon techniques – P for postdilation of the PMV; S for balloon dilatation of the side-branch ostium; and K for KBI.[17]

Crush

This technique involves stenting the side-branch first, with some degree of proximal stent hanging from the side branch into the main branch. The next step is deploying the main-branch stent, which "crushes" the proximal side-branch stent to the artery wall. The "mini" crush is the same procedure, but with less of the proximal side-branch stent hanging into the main branch. This technique is no longer recommended due to the greater risk of failed KBI, which may lead to worse clinical outcomes.[42]

Reverse Crush

This technique is often used as a part of an initial provisional technique. When it is realized that the side branch requires stenting, a stent is positioned in the side branch. A balloon is placed in the main branch, and the side-branch stent is then pulled back 2 to 3 mm across the ostium and deployed. The side-branch stent balloon is removed, and the main-branch balloon is deployed at high pressure.

Double Kissing Crush

In the double kissing (DK) crush technique, the side branch is stented, followed by a balloon inflation in the main branch (balloon crush). Kissing balloons in the side and main branch are then performed. Next, the main vessel is stented, and a POT is performed. A second KBI is then performed followed by a final POT.

Culotte

In this technique, two stents are used to create "pant legs." First, both branches are individually predilated. Next, a stent is deployed across the side branch with the proximal portion positioned into the main branch. A POT is then performed, and the main branch is rewired through the first stent and predilated. A stent is then positioned through the first stent into the main branch. A POT is then performed, and the jailed side-branch wire is removed. The side branch is rewired, and KBI is performed followed by a final POT (see **Fig. 22.5**). This technique is best utilized in bifurcations that meet in which the side branch and DMV have similar diameters (up to 0.5 mm difference) and those with narrow (<70°) bifurcation angles.[42]

T and Protrusion

This technique consists of several steps. The first step involves stenting the main branch while jailing the guide wire in the side branch. Next, the side branch is rewired, and then KBI is performed. Next, a stent is placed in the side branch and a balloon is kept in the main branch. The side-branch stent is pulled back just enough to cover the ostium. The stent is then deployed. Next, the stent balloon is pulled back slightly into the main branch. Finally, kissing balloon is performed with the side-branch and main-branch balloons.

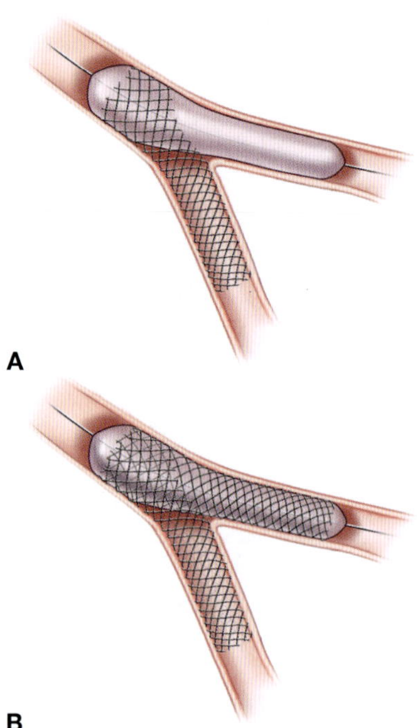

FIGURE 22.5 Culotte stenting. In this technique, the main-branch and side-branch vessels are wired. Diagram **A** shows the main-branch stent deployed and the side-branch stent rewired and ballooned. Diagram **B** shows the side-branch stent being deployed in a "pants leg" type fashion with proximal overlap. As a final step, the main branch would be rewired and the final "kissing balloon" would be performed followed by a POT.

T Stent

In this technique, a stent is placed in the side branch and positioned right at the ostium with no protrusion into the main branch. A balloon in the main branch is helpful in positioning the side-branch balloon. After side-branch deployment, a stent is placed in the main branch. The "modified" T stent involves positioning of the side-branch and main-branch stents simultaneously. The side-branch stent is then deployed first, and equipment is removed before deploying the main-branch stent (see **Fig. 22.6**).

V Stenting

A method where two stents are deployed simultaneously in both a main branch and a side branch such that the stents touch at their proximal portions forming a "carina." It should be noted that this requires a ≥7 Fr guiding catheter (see **Fig. 22.7**).

Simultaneous Kissing Stents

SKS is a process similar to V stenting, except that the proximal stents hang back into the main vessel >5 mm or more. Some operators also refer to this as the "double barrel" technique, especially when this is performed in left-main bifurcation stenting. The advantage of both the V and the SKS techniques is that neither branch access is lost nor "recrossing" is required. Like the V stenting technique, this requires a ≥7 Fr guiding catheter (see **Fig. 22.8**).

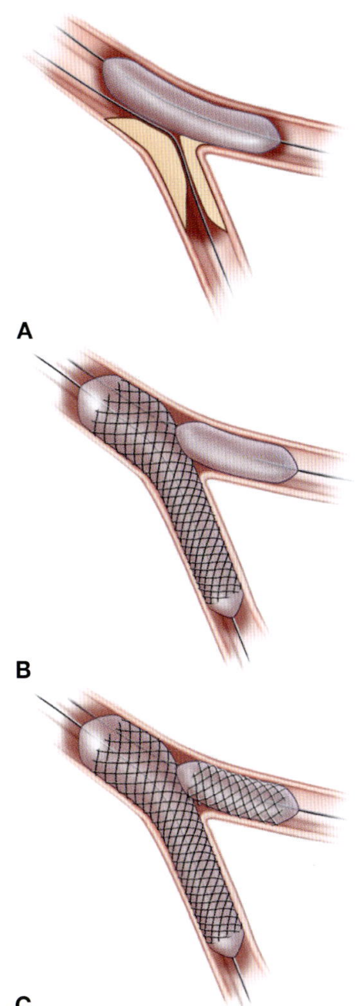

FIGURE 22.6 In this technique, the main branch and side branch are both wired. Diagram **A** shows the side branch being ballooned first. Diagram **B** shows a stent being deployed in the main branch. The side branch is rewired through the main-branch stent strut. Sometimes a balloon in the side branch can help estimate where the side branch stent will be placed. Diagram **C** shows a stent being deployed in the side branch. A final "kissing balloon" inflation (in which balloons are deployed simultaneously in both stents) is performed.

LEFT MAIN OSTIUM AND MIDSHAFT

As previously noted, the majority of LM disease involves the distal bifurcation (**Fig. 22.9**). However, disease can also involve the ostium (23%) and midshaft (15%).[4] It is important to note that patients who undergo PCI of the LM ostium and midshaft appear to have better clinical outcomes than those who undergo PCI to the LM bifurcation. In a subanalysis of the EXCEL trial, distal LM PCI was associated with higher rates of target-vessel revascularization at 3 years compared with CABG, whereas patients who underwent PCI with disease at the ostium of midshaft have similar outcomes to CABG.[43] Therefore, lesion location should be a decisive factor when selecting a revascularization strategy.

As a result of observations that patients with LM stenoses between 50% and 70% derive benefit from CABG, intervention is indicated for stenoses >50%.[15,16] A study utilizing intravascular ultrasound (IVUS) has demonstrated the average LM diameter to be 5 mm with ranges between 3.5 and 6.5 mm.[44] Larger-size guiding catheters (ie, ≥7 Fr) should be considered if rotational atherectomy is required as these are needed for the larger burr sizes that are often required to adequately prepare calcified LM lesions. A more passive guide (such as the Judkins left) may be of use for ostial LM lesions. This has the benefit of being easier to retract and advance and thus accurately position an ostial stent. The decision to wire one or both left anterior descending artery (LAD) and LCx is a matter of debate. Some operators argue that wiring of only one vessel (usually the LAD) is necessary as side-branch loss is unlikely, and removal of the trapped wire may lead to the guide being pulled into the LM with consequent deformation of the proximal stent architecture. Others argue that wiring of both vessels is important as this can facilitate prompt side-branch rescue in the event of LM

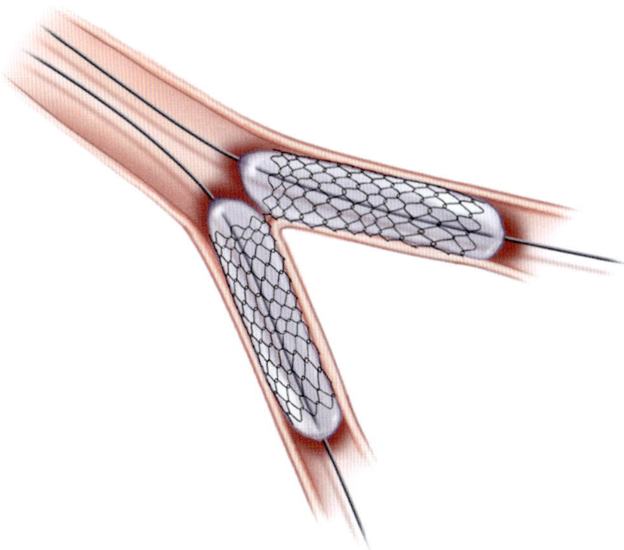

FIGURE 22.7 V stenting. In this technique, two stents are deployed simultaneously, creating a "carina" at the site of the bifurcation.

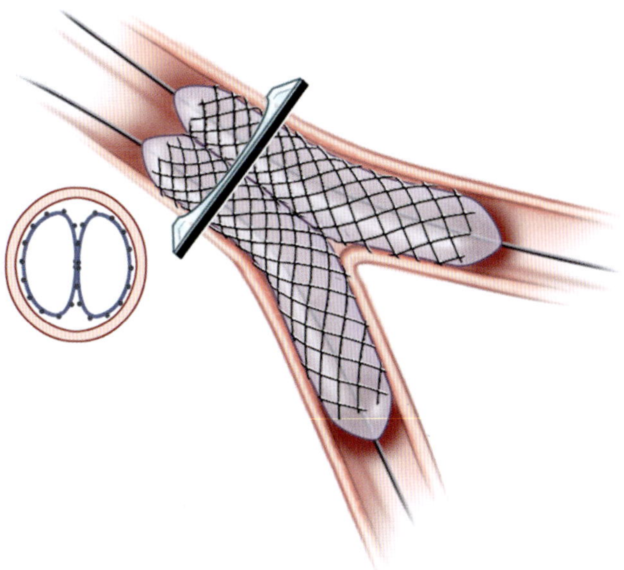

FIGURE 22.8 Simultaneous kissing stents (SKSs). In this technique, both stents are deployed simultaneously, but a portion of the stents overlap in the proximal main vessel.

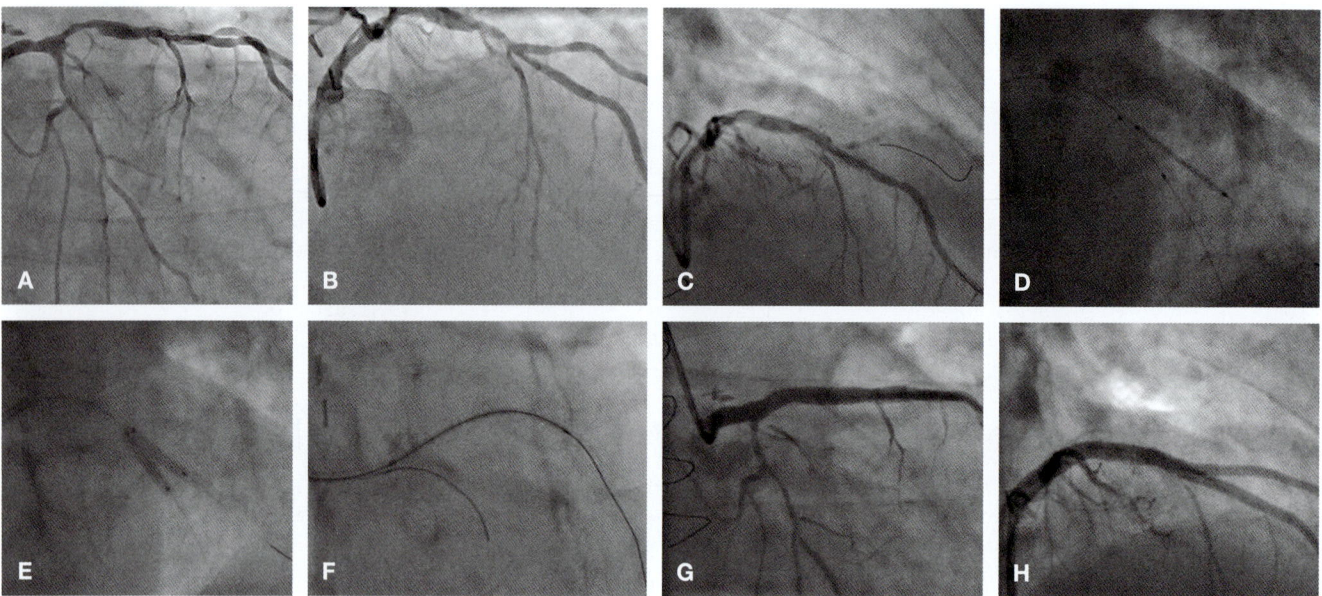

FIGURE 22.9 An example of bifurcation and left main PCI. Panel **A** shows RAO caudal projection of the left coronary system of a patient post-cardiac transplant. There is a severe stenosis of the ostial and proximal LAD. A chronic total occlusion of the ramus intermedius and moderate left main disease are also present. Panel **B** shows RAO cranial projection of the LAD. There is Medina 1,1,0 disease at the bifurcation with a large first diagonal. The primary strategy was provisional stenting to the LAD and left main bifurcations with IVUS guidance. Panel **C** demonstrates TIMI 1 flow in the diagonal after both vessels were wired and the LAD predilated. At this point, a decision was made to convert to a two-stent approach with a DK crush technique. Panel **D** shows positioning of the diagonal stent prior to deployment. A balloon is in place in the LAD to facilitate crush. Panel **E** demonstrates the first kissing balloon inflation. The remainder of the LAD/diagonal DK crush was completed. Panel **F** shows a stent being positioned at the ostium of the left main which overlap with the previously deployed LAD stent. A second wire has been placed in the aortic root to help guide stent placement at the ostium. Postdilatation of the left main and LAD stents was guided by IVUS. Panel **G** shows the final result in the RAO caudal projection. There was TIMI 3 flow in the left circumflex. Panel **H** shows the final results of the LAD/diagonal DK crush in the RAO cranial projection. DK, double kissing; IVUS, intravascular ultrasound; LAD, left anterior descending artery; PCI, percutaneous coronary intervention; RAO, right anterior oblique; TIMI, thrombolysis in myocardial infarction.

dissection. Intracoronary imaging is also an important adjunct to LM PCI providing useful information prestenting and poststenting (see "*Imaging and Physiology*" below).

IMAGING AND PHYSIOLOGY

The use of IVUS and optical coherence tomography (OCT) can provide import information prestenting and poststenting. IVUS can be particularly useful in determining the severity of LM stenosis. A minimum luminal area (MLA) of <6 mm^2 on IVUS strongly predicts the physiological significance of LM disease.[45] Deferring revascularization in patients with an MLA ≥6 mm^2 has also been demonstrated to result in similar rates of cardiac death-free survival and event-free survival compared with revascularized patients.[46] In Asian populations, an MLA of 4.5 mm^2 may be acceptable.[47] Plaque configuration, including side-branch involvement, can also be delineated, which may assist when deciding on the most appropriate stenting strategy. Intracoronary imaging can also be used to evaluate stent expansion, edge dissections, or malapposition. In addition, OCT can be utilized to confirm side-branch wire crossing location (proximal or distal struts) and to guide positioning of the side-branch stent.

Intracoronary imaging as an adjunct to PCI has also been demonstrated to have significant clinical benefits. The ULTIMATE trial, which included approximately 25% bifurcation lesions, demonstrated significantly lower rates of target vessel failure compared to angiography alone.[41] Furthermore, a prospective study of complex bifurcation lesions demonstrated reduced major adverse cardiovascular event (MACE) with IVUS guidance up to 7 years post-PCI.[48]

In LM PCI, the use of intracoronary imaging is of particular importance with the MAIN-COMPARE registry study demonstrating lower mortality in patients undergoing IVUS-guided LM PCI versus angiography alone.[49] Additionally, a substudy of the NOBLE trial demonstrated significantly less target lesion revascularization in patients who underwent IVUS post-PCI.[50]

Pressure wire-based functional assessment can also be of vital importance in bifurcation and LM PCI. As previously mentioned, FFR has been demonstrated to be a viable alternative to angiographic assessment of the side branch after main vessel stenting when performing provisional PCI.[33] As angiography tends to underestimate or overestimate the severity of LM disease, pressure wire-based assessments can be of use. In fact, up to 40% of patients with LM stenoses of <50% are found to have hemodynamically significant disease by pressure-wire assessment.[51] Deferring revascularization in patients with FFR-negative (<0.80) intermediate angiographic stenoses (30%-49%) has also been demonstrated to have favorable outcomes.[52]

ANTIPLATELETS

Currently, dual antiplatelet therapy (DAPT) is recommended for 6 months after PCI in stable coronary artery disease and for 12 months in ACSs with allowances to prolong or truncate this based on the relative risks of bleeding and ischemia.[15,53] The 2016 AHA/ACC focused update on DAPT duration does not provide specific recommendations for duration of therapy in patients undergoing LM or bifurcation PCI.[54] The 2017 European Society of Cardiology (ESC) focused update on DAPT grants a class IIb level or recommendation for prolonged DAPT in patients undergoing complex PCI including patients with bifurcation stenting with two stents implanted.[53]

The optimum duration of DAPT in patients after bifurcation PCI is a current topic of debate. What is clear is that all two-stent techniques carry an increased risk of stent thrombosis and ischemic events.[17] Therefore, meticulous attention to PCI techniques to optimize stent apposition and expansion is crucial. In addition, patient adherence to DAPT is vital. One pooled patient-level analysis of patients undergoing complex PCI (including bifurcation lesions treated with a two-stent technique) demonstrated that truncated DAPT of 3 or 6 months was associated with a higher incidence of 1-year major adverse cardiac events.[55] DAPT for ≥12 months is supported by a retrospective multicenter registry study of patients undergoing both provisional and two-stent bifurcation techniques, which demonstrated an increased risk of death or MI at 4 years post-PCI in patients receiving <12 months of DAPT.[56] Importantly, it should be noted that approximately 60% of this population were treated for an ACS. Conversely, a substudy of the GLOBAL LEADERS trial did not demonstrate any benefit of prolonged ticagrelor monotherapy in reducing all-cause death or new Q-wave MI in patients undergoing bifurcation PCI.[57]

The optimum duration of DAPT after LM PCI is also controversial. In general, the LM is a large-caliber short vessel and, therefore, rates of restenosis and thrombosis are relatively low, especially if the distal bifurcation is not involved.[58] However, this must be balanced against the potential consequences of these complications given the large amount of myocardium supplied by this vessel. Prolonged DAPT is supported by a retrospective analysis of the PRODIGY trial, which demonstrated a 50% reduction in definite, probable, or possible stent thrombosis with 24 months of DAPT compared with 6 months in patients with LM or proximal LAD disease regardless of whether PCI was performed to these vessels.[59] On the other hand, a recently published prospective randomized study comparing a novel biodegradable polymer stent followed by 4 months of DAPT to a standard durable polymer followed by 12 months of DAPT found that the biodegradable stent followed by truncated DAPT was noninferior at 2 years with respect to MACEs.[60]

PCI VERSUS CABG

Deciding on the most appropriate method of revascularization (PCI or CABG) in patients with LM disease is often complex and considers a number of anatomical and clinical characteristics. Several randomized trials have been published comparing the efficacy of CABG and PCI in LM disease, which have yielded conflicting results (see **Table 22.4**). What is clear is that the overall complexity of coronary artery disease, as measured by the SYNTAX score, is an important factor in guiding revascularization strategy. This score utilizes several anatomical variables and distributes patients

TABLE 22.4 Studies Comparing CABG and PCI in Left Main Disease

	SYNTAX SUBSTUDY (2010)[4]	PRECOMBAT (2011)[61]	EXCEL (2016)[62]	NOBLE (2016)[63]
Trial design	Subgroup analysis of multicenter RCT	Multicenter RCT, noninferiority	Multicenter RCT, noninferiority	Multicenter RCT, noninferiority
Follow-up	1 y	1 y	3 y	Median 3.1 y
n	705	600	1905	1201
Anatomical inclusion criteria	>50% stenosis	>50% stenosis	>70% or 50%-69% with demonstrable hemodynamic significance by invasive or noninvasive testing Low or intermediate anatomical complexity (SYNTAX score ≤32)	>50% or FFR ≤ 0.80
Primary endpoint	Composite: all-cause death, stroke, myocardial infarction, or repeat revascularization	Composite: all-cause death, stroke, MI, ischemia-driven TVR	Composite: all-cause death, stroke MI	Composite: all-cause death, stroke, MI, repeat revascularization
Result	No significant difference – 13.7% CABG vs 15.8% PCI (*P* = .44) Repeat revascularization significantly higher with PCI (11.8% vs 6.5%, *P* = .02) Stroke significantly higher with CABG (2.7% vs 0.3%, *P* = .03)	6.7% CABG vs 8.7% PCI (*P* = .01 for noninferiority)	14.7% CABG vs 15.4% PCI (*P* = .02 for noninferiority)	28% for PCI vs 18% for CABG (HR = 1.51 [95% CI 1.13-2.00]) – exceeded the limit for noninferiority
Conclusion	Substudy only – hypothesis – generating	Rates of primary endpoint similar but study underpowered due to low event rate – hypothesis-generating	PCI noninferior to CABG	PCI inferior to CABG
Additional note				Biolimus-eluting biodegradable stent used for majority of patients

CABG, coronary artery bypass grafting; MI, myocardial infarction; n, number of patients; PCI, percutaneous coronary intervention; RCT, randomized control trial; TVR, target-vessel revascularization.

into low- (≤22), intermediate- (23-32), and high-complexity (≥33) terciles. The SYNTAX trial demonstrated significantly higher cardiovascular events in patients with high syntax scores undergoing PCI whilst equipoise was demonstrated in those with scores <33.[64] Subsequent studies of PCI and CABG in LM disease subsequently excluded those with highly complex disease.[62,63] As a result of this evidence, both the current European and American revascularization guidelines recommend CABG over PCI in patients with significant LM and highly complex disease.[15,16]

Longer term follow-up of trials comparing CABG and PCI for LM disease have also been published. Ten-year mortality data from the SYNTAX trial demonstrated similar rates of all-cause death in those undergoing PCI or CABG for LM disease.[65] Five-year outcome data from the EXCEL trial also demonstrated no significant difference in the combined primary endpoint of death, stroke, or MI.[66] Updated 5-year follow-up data of the NOBLE trial demonstrated persistent superiority of CABG over PCI.[67]

CURRENT GUIDELINES

Both the 2018 ESC/European Association for cardiothoracic Surgery (EACTS) and the 2021 ACC/AHA/Society for Cardiovascular Angiography and Interventions (SCAI) revascularization guidelines do not provide explicit classes of recommendation regarding bifurcation PCI.[15,16] The 2018 ESC/EACTS guidelines do note that provisional stenting should be the preferred approach for most bifurcation lesions with up-front two-stent strategies reserved for more complex lesions and true distal LM bifurcations. The document also notes that there is no compelling evidence to favor one technique over another when a two-stent strategy is required in non-LM lesions. In true LM lesions, it is noted that DK crush has the most favorable outcome data.[16]

Current ESC/EACTS and ACC/AHA/SCAI revascularization guideline recommendations for LM disease are summarized in **Table 22.5**.

CONCLUSIONS

Bifurcation and LM lesions are some of the most heterogenous and challenging in PCI. As such, a thorough understanding of the techniques involved and the clinical literature are vital tools in an interventionalist's skillset. There continues to be much debate and conjecture within both fields, and this will only continue as new technologies are developed and further research is published.

TABLE 22.5 Guideline Recommendations for Left Main Disease

TOPIC	ACC/AHA/SCAI[15]	COR	LOE	ESC/EACTS[16]	COR	LOE
Assessment of left main disease	In patients with intermediate stenosis of the left main artery, IVUS is reasonable to help define lesion severity	2a	B-NR	IVUS should be considered to assess the severity of unprotected left main lesions	IIa	B
Revascularization to improve survival vs medical therapy	In patients with SIHD and significant left main stenosis, CABG is recommended to improve survival	1	B-R	In patients with stable angina or silent ischemia with left main disease with stenosis >50% with documented ischemia OR hemodynamically significant stenosis (FFR ≤ 0.80 OR iwFR ≤ 0.89 or > 90% stenosis), revascularization is recommended to improve prognosis	I	A
	In selected patients with SIHD, significant left main stenosis for whom PCI can provide equivalent revascularization to that possible with CABG, PCI is reasonable to improve survival	2a	B-NR			
CABG vs PCI	In patients who require revascularization for significant left main CAD with high-complexity CAD, it is recommended to choose CABG over PCI to improve survival	I	B-R	Left main disease with low SYNTAX score (0-22) – CABG and PCI equally recommended	I vs I	A vs A
				Left main disease with intermediate SYNTAX score (23-32) – CABG higher COR than PCI	I vs IIa	A vs A
				Left main disease with high SYNTAX (≥33) – CABG recommended; PCI not recommended	I vs III	A vs B
Use of IVUS to guide PCI	In patients undergoing coronary stent implantation, IVUS can be useful for procedural guidance, particularly in cases of left main or complex coronary artery stenting, to reduce ischemic events	2a	B-R	IVUS should be considered to optimize treatment of unprotected left main lesions	IIa	B

ACC, American College of Cardiology; AHA, American Heart Association; CABG, coronary artery bypass grafting; COR, Class of Recommendation; EACTS, European Association for Cardiothoracic Surgery; ESC, European Society of Cardiology; FFR, fractional flow reserve; IVUS, intravascular ultrasound; iwFR, instantaneous wave-free ratio; LOE, Level of Evidence; NR, nonrandomized; PCI, percutaneous coronary intervention; R, randomized; SCAI, Society for Cardiovascular Angiography and Interventions.

Acknowledgments

We acknowledge the contributions of the previous authors: Michael S. Lee, MD, MPH, SCAI, FACC, Gopi Manthripragada, MD, Alaa S. Ayoub, MD and Michael S. Levy, MD, MPH.

For further review and interactivities, please see the chapter-based multiple choice questions and videos accessible in the complimentary eBook bundled with this text. Access instructions are located in the inside front cover.

References

1. Chatzizisis YS, Jonas M, Coskun AU, et al. Prediction of the localization of high-risk coronary atherosclerotic plaques on the basis of low endothelial shear stress: an intravascular ultrasound and histopathology natural history study. *Circulation*. 2008;117(8):993-1002.
2. Tsuchida K, Colombo A, Lefevre T, et al. The clinical outcome of percutaneous treatment of bifurcation lesions in multivessel coronary artery disease with the sirolimus-eluting stent: insights from the Arterial Revascularization Therapies Study part II (ARTS II). *Eur Heart J*. 2007;28(4):433-442.
3. Redfors B, Genereux P, Witzenbichler B, et al. Percutaneous coronary intervention of bifurcation lesions and platelet reactivity. *Int J Cardiol*. 2018;250:92-97.
4. Morice MC, Serruys PW, Kappetein AP, et al. Outcomes in patients with de novo left main disease treated with either percutaneous coronary intervention using paclitaxel-eluting stents or coronary artery bypass graft treatment in the Synergy Between Percutaneous Coronary Intervention with TAXUS and Cardiac Surgery (SYNTAX) trial. *Circulation*. 2010;121(24):2645-2653.
5. Sawaya FJ, Lefevre T, Chevalier B, et al. Contemporary approach to coronary bifurcation lesion treatment. *JACC Cardiovasc Interv*. 2016;9(18):1861-1878.
6. Louvard Y, Thomas M, Dzavik V, et al. Classification of coronary artery bifurcation lesions and treatments: time for a consensus! *Catheter Cardiovasc Interv*. 2008;71(2):175-183.
7. Lunardi M, Louvard Y, Lefèvre T, et al. Definitions and standardized endpoints for treatment of coronary bifurcations. *J Am Coll Cardiol*. 2022;80(1):63-88.
8. Koo BK, Lee SP, Lee JH, et al. Assessment of clinical, electrocardiographic, and physiological relevance of diagonal branch in left anterior descending coronary artery bifurcation lesions. *JACC Cardiovasc Interv*. 2012;5(11):1126-1132.
9. Medina A, Suarez de Lezo J, Pan M. A new classification of coronary bifurcation lesions. *Rev Esp Cardiol*. 2006;59(2):183.
10. Seo JB, Shin DH, Park KW, et al. Predictors for side branch failure during provisional strategy of coronary intervention for bifurcation lesions (from the Korean bifurcation registry). *Am J Cardiol*. 2016;118(6):797-803.
11. Freixa X, Almasood AA, Asif N, et al. Long-term outcomes using a two-stent technique for the treatment of coronary bifurcations. *Int J Cardiol*. 2013;168(1):446-451.
12. Zimarino M, Barbato E, Nakamura S, et al. The impact of the extent of side branch disease on outcomes following bifurcation stenting. *Catheter Cardiovasc Interv*. 2020;96(1):E84-E92.
13. Albiero R, Burzotta F, Lassen JF, et al. Treatment of coronary bifurcation lesions, part I: implanting the first stent in the provisional pathway. The 16th expert consensus document of the European Bifurcation Club. *EuroIntervention*. 2022;18(5):e362-e376.
14. Ferrante G, Rao SV, Juni P, et al. Radial versus femoral access for coronary interventions across the entire spectrum of patients with coronary artery disease: a meta-analysis of randomized trials. *JACC Cardiovasc Interv*. 2016;9(14):1419-1434.
15. Lawton JS, Tamis-Holland JE, Bangalore S, et al. 2021 ACC/AHA/SCAI guideline for coronary artery revascularization: a report of the American College of Cardiology/American Heart Association Joint Committee on clinical practice guidelines. *Circulation*. 2022;145(3):e18-e114.
16. Neumann FJ, Sousa-Uva M, Ahlsson A, et al. 2018 ESC/EACTS Guidelines on myocardial revascularization. *Eur Heart J*. 2019;40(2):87-165.
17. Banning AP, Lassen JF, Burzotta F, et al. Percutaneous coronary intervention for obstructive bifurcation lesions: the 14th consensus document from the European Bifurcation Club. *EuroIntervention*. 2019;15(1):90-98.
18. Hildick-Smith D, Egred M, Banning A, et al. The European bifurcation club Left Main Coronary Stent study: a randomized comparison of stepwise provisional vs. systematic dual stenting strategies (EBC MAIN). *Eur Heart J*. 2021;42(37):3829-3839.
19. Zhang JJ, Ye F, Xu K, et al. Multicentre, randomized comparison of two-stent and provisional stenting techniques in patients with complex coronary bifurcation lesions: the DEFINITION II trial. *Eur Heart J*. 2020;41(27):2523-2536.
20. Chen SL, Zhang JJ, Han Y, et al. Double kissing crush versus provisional stenting for left main distal bifurcation lesions: DKCRUSH-V randomized trial. *J Am Coll Cardiol*. 2017;70(21):2605-2617.
21. Kim Y, Lee J, Roh J, et al. Randomized comparisons between different stenting approaches for bifurcation coronary lesions with or without side branch stenosis. *JACC Cardiovasc Interv*. 2015;8(4):550-560.
22. Hildick-Smith D, Behan MW, Lassen JF, et al. The EBC TWO study (European bifurcation coronary TWO): a randomized comparison of provisional T-stenting versus a systematic 2 stent culotte strategy in large caliber true bifurcations. *Circ Cardiovasc Interv*. 2016;9:e003643.
23. Behan MW, Holm NR, de Belder AJ, et al. Coronary bifurcation lesions treated with simple or complex stenting: 5-year survival from patient-level pooled analysis of the Nordic Bifurcation Study and the British Bifurcation Coronary Study. *Eur Heart J*. 2016;37(24):1923-1928.
24. Chen SL, Santoso T, Zhang JJ, et al. A randomized clinical study comparing double kissing crush with provisional stenting for treatment of coronary bifurcation lesions: results from the DKCRUSH-II (Double Kissing Crush versus Provisional Stenting Technique for Treatment of Coronary Bifurcation Lesions) trial. *J Am Coll Cardiol*. 2011;57(8):914-920.
25. Hildick-Smith D, de Belder AJ, Cooter N, et al. Randomized trial of simple versus complex drug-eluting stenting for bifurcation lesions: the British Bifurcation Coronary Study—old, new, and evolving strategies. *Circulation*. 2010;121(10):1235-1243.
26. Colombo A, Bramucci E, Sacca S, et al. Randomized study of the crush technique versus provisional side-branch stenting in true coronary bifurcations: the CACTUS (coronary bifurcations—application of the crushing technique using sirolimus-eluting stents) study. *Circulation*. 2009;119(1):71-78.
27. Ferenc M, Gick M, Kienzle RP, et al. Randomized trial on routine vs. provisional T-stenting in the treatment of de novo coronary bifurcation lesions. *Eur Heart J*. 2008;29(23):2859-2867.
28. Steigen TK, Maeng M, Wiseth R, et al. Randomized study on simple versus complex stenting of coronary artery bifurcation lesions: the Nordic bifurcation study. *Circulation*. 2006;114(18):1955-1961.
29. Chen SL, Sheiban I, Xu B, et al. Impact of the complexity of bifurcation lesions treated with drug-eluting stents: the DEFINITION study (Definitions and impact of complEx biFurcation lesIons on clinical outcomes after percutaNeous coronary IntervenTIOn using drug-eluting steNts). *JACC Cardiovasc Interv*. 2014;7(11):1266-1276.
30. Arunothayaraj S, Lassen JF, Clesham GJ, et al. Impact of technique on bifurcation stent outcomes in the European bifurcation club left main coronary trial. *Catheter Cardiovasc Interv*. 2023;101(3):553-562.
31. Pan M, Ojeda S, Villanueva E, et al. Structural damage of jailed guidewire during the treatment of coronary bifurcation lesions: a microscopic randomized trial. *JACC Cardiovasc Interv*. 2016;9(18):1917-1924.
32. Choi YJ, Lee SJ, Kim BK, et al. Effect of wire jailing at side branch in 1-stent strategy for coronary bifurcation lesions. *JACC Cardiovasc Interv*. 2022;15(4):443-455.
33. Chen SL, Ye F, Zhang JJ, et al. Randomized comparison of FFR-guided and angiography-guided provisional stenting of true coronary bifurcation lesions: the DKCRUSH-VI trial (double kissing crush versus provisional stenting technique for treatment of coronary bifurcation lesions VI). *JACC Cardiovasc Interv*. 2015;8(4):536-546.

34. Gwon HC, Hahn JY, Koo BK, et al. Final kissing ballooning and long-term clinical outcomes in coronary bifurcation lesions treated with 1-stent technique: results from the COBIS registry. *Heart*. 2012;98(3):225-231.
35. Foin N, Torii R, Mortier P, et al. Kissing balloon or sequential dilation of the side branch and main vessel for provisional stenting of bifurcations: lessons from micro-computed tomography and computational simulations. *JACC Cardiovasc Interv*. 2012;5(1):47-56.
36. Andreasen LN, Holm NR, Webber B, Ormiston JA. Critical aspects of balloon position during final proximal optimization technique (POT) in coronary bifurcation stenting. *Catheter Cardiovasc Interv*. 2020;96(1):31-39.
37. Ferenc M, Gick M, Comberg T, et al. Culotte stenting vs. TAP stenting for treatment of de-novo coronary bifurcation lesions with the need for side-branch stenting: the Bifurcations Bad Krozingen (BBK) II angiographic trial. *Eur Heart J*. 2016;37(45):3399-3405.
38. Chen SL, Xu B, Han YL, et al. Comparison of double kissing crush versus Culotte stenting for unprotected distal left main bifurcation lesions: results from a multicenter, randomized, prospective DKCRUSH-III study. *J Am Coll Cardiol*. 2013;61(14):1482-1488.
39. Erglis A, Kumsars I, Niemela M, et al. Randomized comparison of coronary bifurcation stenting with the crush versus the culotte technique using sirolimus eluting stents: the Nordic stent technique study. *Circ Cardiovasc Interv*. 2009;2(1):27-34.
40. Chen SL, Zhang JJ, Ye F, et al. Study comparing the double kissing (DK) crush with classical crush for the treatment of coronary bifurcation lesions: the DKCRUSH-1 Bifurcation Study with drug-eluting stents. *Eur J Clin Invest*. 2008;38(6):361-371.
41. Zhang J, Gao X, Kan J, et al. Intravascular ultrasound versus angiography-guided drug-eluting stent implantation: the ULTIMATE trial. *J Am Coll Cardiol*. 2018;72(24):3126-3137.
42. Burzotta F, Lassen JF, Louvard Y, et al. European Bifurcation Club white paper on stenting techniques for patients with bifurcated coronary artery lesions. *Catheter Cardiovasc Interv*. 2020;96(5):1067-1079.
43. Gershlick AH, Kandzari DE, Banning A, et al. Outcomes after left main percutaneous coronary intervention versus coronary artery bypass grafting according to lesion site: results from the EXCEL trial. *JACC Cardiovasc Interv*. 2018;11(13):1224-1233.
44. Oviedo C, Maehara A, Mintz GS, et al. Intravascular ultrasound classification of plaque distribution in left main coronary artery bifurcations: where is the plaque really located? *Circ Cardiovasc Interv*. 2010;3(2):105-112.
45. Jasti V, Ivan E, Yalamanchili V, Wongpraparut N, Leesar MA. Correlations between fractional flow reserve and intravascular ultrasound in patients with an ambiguous left main coronary artery stenosis. *Circulation*. 2004;110(18):2831-2836.
46. de la Torre Hernandez JM, Hernandez Hernandez F, Alfonso F, et al. Prospective application of pre-defined intravascular ultrasound criteria for assessment of intermediate left main coronary artery lesions results from the multicenter LITRO study. *J Am Coll Cardiol*. 2011;58(4):351-358.
47. Park SJ, Ahn JM, Kang SJ, et al. Intravascular ultrasound-derived minimal lumen area criteria for functionally significant left main coronary artery stenosis. *JACC Cardiovasc Interv*. 2014;7(8):868-874.
48. Chen L, Xu T, Xue XJ, et al. Intravascular ultrasound-guided drug-eluting stent implantation is associated with improved clinical outcomes in patients with unstable angina and complex coronary artery true bifurcation lesions. *Int J Cardiovasc Imaging*. 2018;34(11):1685-1696.
49. Park SJ, Kim YH, Park DW, et al. Impact of intravascular ultrasound guidance on long-term mortality in stenting for unprotected left main coronary artery stenosis. *Circ Cardiovasc Interv*. 2009;2(3):167-177.
50. Ladwiniec A, Walsh SJ, Holm NR, et al. Intravascular ultrasound to guide left main stem intervention: a NOBLE trial substudy. *EuroIntervention*. 2020;16(3):201-209.
51. Park SJ, Kang SJ, Ahn JM, et al. Visual-functional mismatch between coronary angiography and fractional flow reserve. *JACC Cardiovasc Interv*. 2012;5(10):1029-1036.
52. Hamilos M, Muller O, Cuisset T, et al. Long-term clinical outcome after fractional flow reserve–guided treatment in patients with angiographically equivocal left main coronary artery stenosis. *Circulation*. 2009;120(15):1505-1512.
53. Valgimigli M, Bueno H, Byrne RA, et al. 2017 ESC focused update on dual antiplatelet therapy in coronary artery disease developed in collaboration with EACTS: the Task Force for dual antiplatelet therapy in coronary artery disease of the European Society of Cardiology (ESC) and of the European Association for Cardio-Thoracic Surgery (EACTS). *Eur Heart J*. 2018;39(3):213-260.
54. Levine GN, Bates ER, Bittl JA, et al. 2016 ACC/AHA guideline focused update on duration of dual antiplatelet therapy in patients with coronary artery disease: a report of the American College of Cardiology/American Heart Association task force on clinical practice guidelines—an update of the 2011 ACCF/AHA/SCAI guideline for percutaneous coronary intervention, 2011 ACCF/AHA guideline for coronary artery bypass graft surgery, 2012 ACC/AHA/ACP/AATS/PCNA/SCAI/STS guideline for the diagnosis and management of patients with stable ischemic Heart disease, 2013 ACCF/AHA guideline for the management of ST-elevation myocardial infarction, 2014 AHA/ACC guideline for the management of patients with non–ST-elevation acute coronary syndromes, and 2014 ACC/AHA guideline on perioperative cardiovascular evaluation and management of patients undergoing noncardiac surgery. *Circulation*. 2016;134(10):e123-e155.
55. Giustino G, Chieffo A, Palmerini T, et al. Efficacy and safety of dual antiplatelet therapy after complex PCI. *J Am Coll Cardiol*. 2016;68(17):1851-1864.
56. Jang WJ, Ahn SG, Song YB, et al. Benefit of prolonged dual antiplatelet therapy after implantation of drug-eluting stent for coronary bifurcation lesions: results from the coronary bifurcation stenting registry II. *Circ Cardiovasc Interv*. 2018;11(7):e005849.
57. Kogame N, Chichareon P, De Wilder K, et al. Clinical relevance of ticagrelor monotherapy following 1-month dual antiplatelet therapy after bifurcation percutaneous coronary intervention: insight from GLOBAL LEADERS trial. *Catheter Cardiovasc Interv*. 2020;96(1):100-111.
58. Stone GW, Bohra C. In search of the "IDEAL" left main coronary stent and DAPT regimen. *EuroIntervention*. 2022;17(18):1457-1459.
59. Costa F, Adamo M, Ariotti S, et al. Left main or proximal left anterior descending coronary artery disease location identifies high-risk patients deriving potentially greater benefit from prolonged dual antiplatelet therapy duration. *EuroIntervention*. 2015;11:e1222-e1230.
60. van Geuns RJ, Chun-Chin C, McEntegart MB, et al. Bioabsorbable polymer drug-eluting stents with 4-month dual antiplatelet therapy versus durable polymer drug-eluting stents with 12-month dual antiplatelet therapy in patients with left main coronary artery disease: the IDEAL-LM randomised trial. *EuroIntervention*. 2022;17(18):1467-1476.
61. Park SJ, Kim YH, Park DW, et al. Randomized trial of stents versus bypass surgery for left main coronary artery disease. *N Engl J Med*. 2011;364(18):1718-1727.
62. Stone GW, Sabik JF, Serruys PW, et al. Everolimus-Eluting stents or bypass surgery for left main coronary artery disease. *N Engl J Med*. 2016;375(23):2223-2235.
63. Makikallio T, Holm NR, Lindsay M, et al. Percutaneous coronary angioplasty versus coronary artery bypass grafting in treatment of unprotected left main stenosis (NOBLE): a prospective, randomised, open-label, non-inferiority trial. *Lancet*. 2016;388(10061):2743-2752.
64. Serruys PW, Morice MC, Kappetein AP, et al. Percutaneous coronary intervention versus coronary-artery bypass grafting for severe coronary artery disease. *N Engl J Med*. 2009;360(10):961-972.
65. Thuijs D, Kappetein AP, Serruys PW, et al. Percutaneous coronary intervention versus coronary artery bypass grafting in patients with three-vessel or left main coronary artery disease: 10-year follow-up of the multicentre randomised controlled SYNTAX trial. *Lancet*. 2019;394(10206):1325-1334.
66. Stone GW, Kappetein AP, Sabik JF, et al. Five-year outcomes after PCI or CABG for left main coronary disease. *N Engl J Med*. 2019;381(19):1820-1830.
67. Holm NR, Makikallio T, Lindsay MM, et al. Percutaneous coronary angioplasty versus coronary artery bypass grafting in the treatment of unprotected left main stenosis: updated 5-year outcomes from the randomised, non-inferiority NOBLE trial. *Lancet*. 2020;395(10219):191-199.
68. Kočka V, Thériault-Lauzier P, Xiong TY, et al. Optimal fluoroscopic projections of coronary ostia and bifurcations defined by computed tomographic coronary angiography. *JACC Cardiovasc Interv*. 2020;13(21):2560-2570.

Small Vessel and Diffuse Disease

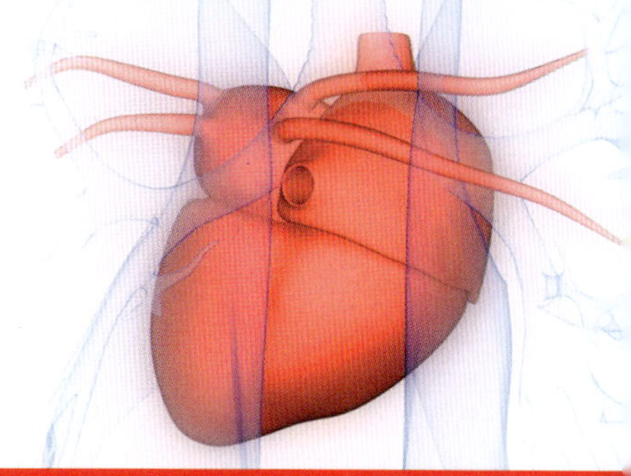

Owais S. Abdul-Kafi and Mladen I. Vidovich

Percutaneous coronary interventions (PCIs) in small vessels (SVs) remains one of the most challenging aspects of interventional cardiology practice. Along with diabetes mellitus and diffuse disease (DD) in coronary arteries, PCI for SVs has traditionally been associated with increased rates of in-stent restenosis (ISR), stent thrombosis (ST), reduced success rates, and overall increased complications including higher levels of target lesion revascularization (TLR) and higher rates of major adverse cardiac events (MACEs).[1-5] Similar to percutaneous revascularization, in-hospital mortality after coronary artery bypass grafting (CABG) is higher in patients with small coronary arteries.[6] The ISCHEMIA trial[7] suggests that conservative medical management could also be considered a viable therapeutic alternative to invasive management for patients with stable coronary artery disease (CAD).

The field of SV PCI has grown tremendously over the past 5 to 10 years as advances in angiographic techniques, intravascular imaging, functional testing, drug-eluting stents (DESs), drug-coated balloons (DCBs), cutting balloons, intravascular calcium modification, and operator familiarity with these techniques have led to lower ISR, ST, and target vessel revascularization (TVR) in these patients. This chapter will discuss these techniques and advances specifically as they apply to SV PCI, and because there is significant overlap of SV disease with DD, we will also discuss advances in these techniques for diffuse CAD.

DEFINITION

Similar to the last iteration of this chapter that was published in 2018, there is still no agreed-upon consensus for what defines SV CAD. Most interventional cardiologists would agree that vessel size <2.5 mm is an SV[8]; however, trials have had varying definitions of what constitutes an SV, from as small as 2.0 mm[9] to as large as 3.0 mm,[10,11] and some classified vessels <2.25 mm that are still amenable to intervention as "very small."[12] SV disease is classified in a different category from microvascular disease such as that found in patients who have myocardial infarction with nonobstructive coronary arteries (MINOCA)[13] or coronary microvascular dysfunction.[14] SV disease is obstructive disease (>70% stenosis visually or positive functional testing) amenable to PCI, but microvascular disease is too small for PCI.

Historically, SV PCI was performed in 30% to 50% of interventions,[3,15] especially in patients with older age,[16,17] chronic kidney disease,[18] diabetes mellitus,[17] poorly controlled hypertension, smokers, and those who have bifurcation lesions with a small side branch;[19] however, more recent trials enrolled substantially more patients with SV disease than previously as patients with these and other chronic diseases live longer. These trials included patients who had SV PCI performed for "off-label use" and may be more representative of lesions encountered in current clinical practice. Sixty-two percent of participants in the TWENTE trial,[20] which compared zotarolimus-eluting versus everolimus-eluting cobalt-chromium stents in patients with non-ST segment myocardial infarction or stable angina, had at least one SV (defined as ≤2.75 mm in diameter), and 47% of the patients in the RESOLUTE-US[5] trial had PCI for a vessel with diameter ≤2.5 mm. As stent technology and interventional cardiology techniques evolve, our definition for what constitutes an "SV" will continue to progress in an effort to provide the best care for this growing population.

Late Loss in SV PCI

After the initial success of percutaneous transluminal coronary angioplasty (PTCA) and PCI with bare-metal stent (BMS) in large vessels, it was quickly recognized that PTCA for SV disease is associated with technical challenges and more frequent restenosis and thrombosis requiring repeat interventions. SV size is a known independent risk factor contributing to vessel restenosis;[2] however, the degree of neointimal hyperplasia is independent of vessel size,[21] so late loss is similar in SVs and large vessels.[22] Conversely to late loss, which is the absolute amount of restenosis, the relative degree of restenosis is directly dependent on vessel size as the same amount of restenosis constitutes a higher percentage of lumen diameter in a SV as compared to a large vessel. As a result, the percent net lumen loss is higher in SVs, resulting in a higher rate of restenosis[23] (**Fig. 23.1**).

IMAGING & FUNCTIONAL TESTING OF SVS

Numerous trials have shown the benefits of intravascular imaging and functional testing to determine lesion characteristics and degree of calcification, lumen diameter, other lesion anatomical features to help guide PCI, as well as guide post-PCI evaluation and stent optimization in patients with CAD.[24-26] Because the acute gain in lumen diameter and area is smaller in patients with SV disease, intravascular imaging and functional testing is thought to be more important in patients undergoing PCI for SV disease as compared to large vessels to help provide the best short- and long-term outcomes.

Intravascular Ultrasound

Because the lumen diameter is smaller in SVs and relative loss of luminal area much higher with restenosis, the use of intravascular ultrasound (IVUS) and IVUS-guided stent postdilation is expected to provide better outcomes in patients undergoing SV PCI as opposed to normal vessel diameter. A retrospective study[27] of patients who underwent IVUS-guided SV PCI (diameter <2.75 mm) showed significantly lower rates of TLR (39% vs 26%, $P = .01$) in patients who had a luminal area by IVUS >6.0 mm^2 as opposed to those who had an area less than 6.0 mm^2. MACE was not significantly reduced (44% vs 34%, $P = .07$), and death and myocardial infarction similar. A more recent prospective randomized trial

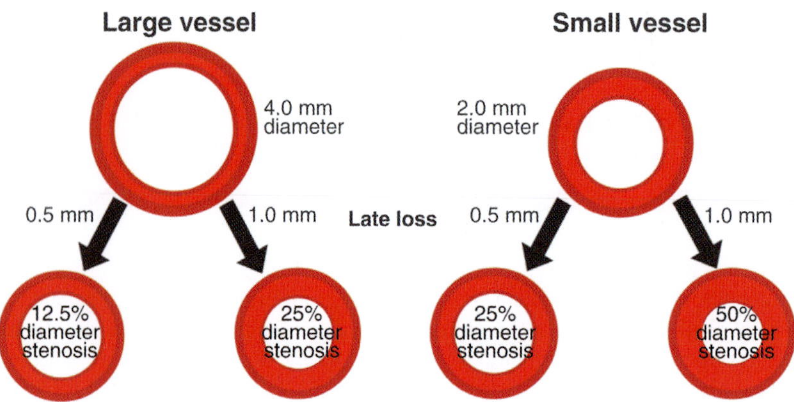

FIGURE 23.1 Impact of late loss on diameter stenosis in large and small vessels. Equivalent late loss in different sized vessels causes significantly different percent diameter stenosis.

to determine the clinical utility of IVUS in patients with diabetes undergoing SV PCI showed that the use of IVUS was associated with increased lesion length ($P \leq .001$) and decreased number of implanted stents ($P = .002$), diameter size ($P = .001$) and proportion of ISR ($P = .001$). The IVUS-guided SV PCI group had significantly lower incidence of MACE at 2 years (Kaplan-Meier curve log-rank $P = .029$) mostly due to decreased risk of TLR.

Optical Coherence Tomography and Optical Frequency Domain Imaging

Optical coherence tomography (OCT) and optical frequency domain imaging (OFDI) are light-based intravascular imaging technologies with higher axial resolution than IVUS (10-20 µm vs 60-150 µm), allowing for more detailed visualization of stent undersizing and complications, such as dissection, tissue protrusion, or stent malapposition.[28] A small study of 69 patients undergoing OCT-guided SV PCI with 2.5 mm DES showed that a minimal stent area of 3.5 mm^2 or higher as seen on OCT predicted ISR and TLR at 9 months (1.4% vs 7.2%).[29] Another study that was performed to assess vessel healing response and cross-sectional level by OCT after implantation of the ultrathin strut, everolimus-eluting stent (EES) with a biodegradable polymer showed no significant difference in the early (3 months) or long-term neointimal hyperplasia response between stents placed in small- and medium-vessel diameter (≤3.0 mm^2) as opposed to large vessels (≥3.0 mm^2).[30]

The MISTIC-1 (Multimodality Imaging Study in Cardiology cohort 1) trial[31] found that OFDI-guided PCI was noninferior to IVUS-guided PCI in patients with stable CAD in terms of in-stent minimal lumen area (MLA) at 8 months (primary endpoint) and device-related composite endpoints at 3 years. This trial, though not technically an SV CAD trial, included most patients with SV CAD as the mean reference vessel diameter was 2.69 mm (range 2.41-3.09 mm).

Near-Infrared Spectroscopy Imaging

Near-infrared diffuse reflectance spectroscopy (NIRS) is an imaging modality that uses the absorbance and reflective properties of substances when exposed to near-infrared light (wavelength 800-2500 nm).[32] In coronary atherosclerotic disease specifically, this imaging modality is combined with IVUS in a single catheter (NIRS-IVUS) and can be used to detect the presence of lipid-core plaque[25] (vulnerable plaque) that may not be causing flow-limiting stenosis but may be predictive of future coronary events. While there are no studies for NIRS imaging in patients specifically undergoing SV PCI, the PROSPECT-ABSORB[33] trial studied the effect of PCI on angiographically nonobstructive stenosis but with IVUS plaque burden >65% and included patients with reference vessel diameter 2.73 ± 0.51 mm and minimal luminal diameter 2.29 ± 0.46 mm. This trial found significantly higher MLA in patients who underwent PCI at 25 months (6.9 ± 2.6 mm^2 vs 3.0 ± 1.0 mm^2, $P < .0001$), lower rates of lesion-related MACE (4.3% vs 10.7%, $P = .12$), and significantly lower rates of maximal lipid content as detected by NIRS (6.2% vs 26.9%, $P < .0001$).

INTRACORONARY FUNCTIONAL TESTING OF SV DISEASE

Several trials have shown that fractional flow reserve (FFR)-guided PCI is superior to coronary angiography for intermediately stenotic (40%–70%) lesions[34,35] in stable ischemic heart disease, and the FLAVOR[36] trial showed that FFR-guided PCI was noninferior to IVUS-guided PCI with respect to the composite endpoint of death, myocardial infarction, or revascularization at 24 months. For intermediate left main disease, IVUS-measured MLA of 6.0 to 7.5 mm^2 (4.5-4.8 mm^2 for patients of Asian descent[37]) has been shown to be equivalent to FFR in determining significance of lesions;[38,39] however, IVUS is only moderately correlated with FFR in nonleft main disease, especially smaller-sized vessels less than 3 mm in diameter.[40]

FFR and Instantaneous Wave-Free Ratio in SV Disease

The previously mentioned FLAVOR trial excluded patients who had a lesion diameter of <2.5 mm by visual estimation on coronary angiogram. Another trial[41] that evaluated long-term (median follow-up of 3.3 years) outcomes in patients who underwent FFR-guided or coronary angiography-guided SV PCI (lesion diameter of ≤3 mm) found that patients in the FFR-guided group had significantly lower MACE (hazard ratio [HR], 0.458; 95% confidence interval [CI], 0.310-0.679; $P < .001$) and procedure costs (3253 ± 102 Euros vs 4714 ± 37 Euros; $P < .0001$) but not mortality (HR, 0.684; 95% CI, 0.355-1.316; $P = .255$).

The instantaneous wave-free ratio (iFR)-SWEDEHEART trial randomly assigned patients with stable angina or acute coronary syndrome (ACS) to undergo iFR-guided PCI or FFR-guided PCI and found iFR to be noninferior to FFR in 12-month MACE.[42]

Although this was not specifically a trial for patients with SV CAD, the mean stent diameter used was 2.97 ± 0.47 mm suggesting that about half the participants had SV CAD (using a cutoff of 3.0 mm). Some stratification was performed to assess for clinical differences among different clinical subgroups; however, vessel size was not one of the subgroups that was studied.

Quantitative Flow Ratio in SV Disease

Quantitative flow ratio (QFR) is a less-invasive method that uses 3-dimensional quantitative coronary angiography to measure flow through a coronary artery lesion without use of a pressure wire or need for hyperemia.[43] An observational single-center study of 436 consecutive patients with 516 different coronary lesions who had FFR and QFR performed were dichotomized based on reference vessel diameter (≤2.8 mm vs >2.8 mm).[44] Although the smaller-sized vessel group had a higher percent of functionally significant lesions, there was no significant difference between QFR measurement accuracy when compared to FFR in determining that a coronary lesion is significant, irrespective of lesion diameter.

Lesion Modification in SV Disease

Before the introduction of DES, research focused on alternative strategies such as atherectomy to reduce the high rates of ISR and ST in SV CAD. A 1993 landmark study[45] suggested that the late (>6 month) outcome after PTCA, BMS, and directional atherectomy depended mostly on the immediate result and not due to specific long-term (late loss) differences in these techniques, and this was confirmed in a large meta-analysis in 2004.[46] Smaller subsequent studies that were performed to assess the use of lesion modification in SV CAD will be described in this section.

Orbital Atherectomy

The ORBIT II study was a prospective single-arm multicenter trial that enrolled patients with severely calcified lesions (defined as angiographic radio-opacities lacking cardiac motion prior to contrast injection, total calcium length ≥15 mm that extends into the target lesion, or the presence of ≥270° of calcium on IVUS) to undergo orbital atherectomy prior to stent delivery and compared safety and efficacy at 30 days and 3 years. A subgroup analysis[47] was performed to assess the safety and efficacy of orbital atherectomy in patients with SVs, defined as ≤2.5 mm in diameter, accounting for 12.4% of the original trial. The subanalysis showed no significant difference in the primary outcome of severe angiographic complications defined as type C to F dissection, perforation, persistent slow flow or no-reflow, and acute vessel closure (30.6% vs 22.5%, P = .22), and no difference in the secondary outcomes of cardiac death (9.8% vs 6.3%, P = .33) and MI (12.8% vs 10.9%, P = .67). There was a nonsignificantly significant higher rate of TVR in the SV group (16.8% vs 9.3%, P = .13). Another retrospective study[48] of orbital atherectomy found no significant difference in the primary outcome of MACE (composite of death, MI, TVR, and stroke) at 30 days (0.0% vs 1.9%; P = 0.40) in patients who had SV PCI defined as stent diameter 2.5 mm (n = 38) compared to the control group with larger stent sizes (n = 382).

Rotational Atherectomy

The 2003 Dilation verses Ablation Revascularization Trial Targeting Restenosis (DART)[49] trial randomized 446 patients with myocardial ischemia associated with an angiographic stenosis of a vessel measuring 2.0 to 3.0 mm in diameter to either rotational atherectomy (RA) or PTCA. The mean reference diameter was 2.46 ± 0.40 mm, and the mean lesion length was 9.97 ± 5.59 mm. There was no significant difference in acute procedural success, target vessel failure, MLA, percent diameter stenosis, and non-Q-wave MI between the two groups. Acute gain and late loss were similar between both groups. Another 2003 study[50] randomized patients with symptomatic diffuse stenosis of the LAD with vessel diameter 2.0 to 2.9 mm to RA (n = 21) or balloon dilation (n = 20) before stenting. Acute lumen gain was greater in the RA group (P = .038), but net gain at follow-up was similar in both groups (P = .24). There was no significant difference in angiographic restenosis rate, TVR, and event-free survival at 1 year.

Since then, there were no subsequent trials or registries comparing RA specifically for SVs. The two largest registries of patients undergoing RA (J-PCI[51] and ROTATE[52]) stratify patients according to lesion length, but not lesion diameter, so the knowledge of safety and efficacy of RA in the DES era is limited.

Intravascular Lithotripsy

Since the Food and Drug Administration (FDA) approval of intravascular lithotripsy (IVL) for CAD in 2021 based on the Disrupt CAD III trial,[53] IVL has been used in an increasing number of patients with calcified CAD to modify vessel calcification, facilitate stent implantation, and reduce rates of underexpansion and malapposition. The currently approved IVL system (by Shockwave) is available in 2.5- to 4-mm diameter balloons. The reference vessel diameter in the Disrupt CAD III trial was 3.03 ± 0.47 mm, suggesting that about half of the participants had a diameter ≤3.0 mm; however, there was no subgroup analysis comparing outcomes for this group. The Disrupt CAD IV trial[54] performed in 2021 for Japanese regulatory approval of coronary IVL included patients with slightly smaller diameter vessels (mean diameter of 2.9 ± 0.4 mm) and demonstrated high freedom from 30-day MACE (93.8%) and high procedural success (93.8%). No subgroup analysis was published for smaller vessel diameter as compared to normal vessel diameter, although there was discussion that procedural success was similar in each IVL balloon size (2.5, 3, 3.5, and 4 mm).

Cutting Balloons

Cutting balloons are coronary balloons with three or four microsurgical blades along their surface and apply a focused force on these blades, effectively "cutting" calcified plaque and exposing more of the vessel's elastic intimal tissue in an attempt to increase stent expansion. Cutting balloon angioplasty (CBA) was compared to balloon angioplasty in patients with SV CAD defined as vessel diameter <3.0 mm.[55] Procedural success and the rate of coronary dissection was similar between the two groups, although rate of severe dissection (type E and F) occurred in 2.5% of patients in the balloon angioplasty group and none in the CBA group, and in-hospital complications were also higher in the balloon angioplasty group. The restenosis rate at 6 months was lower but not statistically significantly lower in the CBA compared to the balloon angioplasty group (37.5% vs 48.1%); however, in patients with very SVs (≤2.75 mm), the rate of restenosis was statistically significantly lower in the CBA group (36.9% vs 62.7%, P = .05). Another study that compared CBA, balloon angioplasty, or stenting (BMS) in SVs (≤2.5 mm) found significantly lower rates of MACE (death, MI, and TLR) in the CBA group as opposed to the two other groups.[56]

Historically, cutting balloons were more bulky and more difficult to deliver (Flextome, by Boston Scientific); however, the newer-generation Wolverine cutting balloon (also by Boston Scientific) released in 2016 has a lower profile and a more deliverable catheter with improved flexibility at the tip, allowing it to be used for smaller lesions.[57] No specific trials have been performed for the Wolverine cutting balloon in patients undergoing SV PCI; however, extrapolation from studies of the Wolverine cutting balloon in all-comers undergoing PCI suggests it is safe and effective for heavily calcified lesions.[58,59]

Scoring Balloons

Scoring balloons consist of three to four rectangular nitinol-based struts that wrap around a semicompliant balloon in a helical pattern.[60] They include the AngioSculpt (Phillips) and Lacrosse NSE (Asomedica) and were initially more deliverable than first-generation cutting balloons;[57] however, a recent trial comparing the Wolverine cutting balloon to the Lacrosse NSE showed significantly higher delivery success rate in the Wolverine group compared to the Lacrosse NSE group (90.8% vs 79.5%, P = .006).[58] Although this was not technically an SV PCI trial, the mean reference diameter of the arteries prior to either intervention was 2.56 ± 0.67 mm, and the mean diameter of the first predilation balloon used (prior to passage of the cutting or scoring balloon) was 1.99 ± 0.41 mm, suggesting that the majority of the vessels in this trial were small.

Super High-Pressure Balloons

Super high-pressure dual-layer balloons such as the OPN balloon (SIS Medical) are an additional tool that can be used to uniformly expand a lesion, with low rates of dissection, perforation, or balloon rupture.[57] These balloons are rated to 35 atm, and while most of the data are from small observational case series or retrospective analysis, their clinical utility is mostly limited to unexpanded stents, ISR, and severe plaque preparation before stent implantation. No specific data exist to compare the use of the OPN balloon specifically in SV CAD; however, the balloon is available in 1.5- to 4-mm diameter sizes and has been demonstrated to be safe and effective in a case series that evaluated 326 consecutive balloon-undilatable resistant lesions, achieving adequate expansion in >90% of these lesions with 0.9% 30-day MACE.[61]

Comparison of Lesion Modification Techniques in SV PCI

Direct comparison between RA, orbital atherectomy, IVL, and cutting balloons is difficult as the patients, operators, and lesions have varying characteristics that would warrant one lesion modification strategy over another. In addition, costs may favor one strategy over another. A meta-analysis of the PREPARE-CALC and ISAR-CALC randomized controlled trials was performed to assess the safety and efficacy of RA, modified balloon (cutting or scoring balloons), and super high-pressure balloons and found no significant difference in stent expansion or stent asymmetry.[62] Strategy success was higher in the RA group compared to the other two groups, but overall clinical events were low and similar between the groups. The mean vessel diameter was 3.0 ± 0.43 mm, suggesting that about half the participants underwent SV PCI in this meta-analysis.

Drug-Eluting Stents

The three key components of DESs are the metal struts (platform), polymer coating that acts as a reservoir for the drug, and the specific antiproliferative drug released into the vessel.[63] Each of these components has been improved upon over the past two decades, leading to thinner struts, polymers that hold onto the drugs for longer, and drugs that are less proliferative and maintain efficacy over time.

Multiple studies have demonstrated the safety, efficacy, and decreased risk of ISR, ST of all-comers who had DESs as compared to BMSs in the entire spectrum of CAD,[64-66] and is discussed in more detail in another chapter. Specifically for patients with SV disease, the NHLBI Dynamic Registry[67] evaluated real-world patients in the United States and found that those treated with DES had significantly lower rates of repeat revascularization and MACE (HR, 0.59; 95% CI, 0.42-0.83; P = .001) at 1 year compared to patients with BMS, with similar risks of death and MI. The DES group had longer lesions (16.7 vs 13.1 mm; P < .001) and slightly smaller vessel size (2.6 vs 2.7 mm; P < .001). In addition, the use of DES in SV lesions was associated with lower risk of 1-year CABG (HR, 0.40; 95% CI, 0.17-0.95; P = .04).

Strut Thickness and Metallurgy in DES

Stent technology has significantly improved since the development of the first-generation DESs. Strut thickness has significantly decreased, and the metals used for the platform have significantly improved over the past two decades, leading to an easier ability to perform PCI in SVs with less ISR and ST compared to previous generations of DES or BMS.

The TAXUS ATLAS SV[68] study was a nonrandomized trial that compared a thin-strut (97 μm) 2.25 mm paclitaxel-eluting stent (PES) with historical controls of the thick-strut (132 μm) first-generation PES. Unlike the RESOLUTE-US trial,[69] which compared the same stent and the same drug delivered on a different polymer, the TAXUS ATLAS SV trial compared identical polymer, drug dosage, and elution kinetics on different strut-thickness stent platforms. The thin-strut stainless-steel stent significantly reduced 9-month angiographic restenosis (18.5% vs 32.7%, P = .0219) and 12-month TLR (6.1% vs 16.9%, P = .0039). The importance of this trial is that these findings were concordant with previous data obtained with the thin-strut BMS, suggesting that thinner struts were associated with better outcomes. This confirms the concept that even with antiproliferative agents, strut thickness plays a central role in SV PCI outcomes.

This concept of even thinner struts being better was further tested in a randomized controlled trial that compared ultrathin (60 μm for stent diameter ≤3.0 mm and 80 μm for stent diameter ≥3.5 mm) bioresorbable polymer sirolimus-eluting stents (BP SESs) to thin-strut (81 μm) durable polymer EESs in patients in the BIOFLOW-V study.[70] This study followed patients for 5 years and found nonstatistically significantly reduced risk of target lesion failure (12.3% vs 15.3%, P = .108); however, statistically significantly reduced risk of target-vessel-related MI (6.6% vs 10.3%, P = .015), late, and very late ST (0.3% vs 1.6%, P = .021). There was no statistically significant difference between these two stents for patients with SV CAD (vessel diameter ≤2.75 mm) (HR, 0.80 favoring BP SES, 95% CI, 0.57-1.13).

BIO-RESORT[71] was a three-arm noninferiority trial of different strut thickness and metals that had a prespecified subgroup performed for patients with SV CAD (diameter ≤2.5 mm). This subgroup included 1452 patients who were randomly assigned to ultrathin strut (60 μm) cobalt-chromium BP SESs (Orsiro, Biotronik) or very thin-strut (74 μm) platinum-chromium biodegradable polymer EESs (Synergy, Boston Scientific) to the previous-generation thin-strut (91 μm) cobalt-chromium durable polymer zotarolimus-eluting stents (ZESs; Resolute Integrity, Medtronic). There was a lower but not statistically significantly lower rate of target lesion failure in the BP SES as compared to EES or ZES;

however, there was a difference between BP SES and ZES in TLR at 1 year (HR, 0.40, 95% CI, 0.20-0.81; *P* = .009) and 3 years (HR, 0.42, 95% CI, 0.20-0.85; *P* = .02). There was no significant between-stent difference in cardiac death, target vessel MI, or ST.

ST in DES After SV PCI

There are conflicting data in the literature regarding the impact of SV disease as an ***independent*** risk factor for ST.[72] The most important cause for this incongruence in the literature is that ST is a complex phenomenon and is associated with numerous covariates that include patient comorbidities (eg, diabetes, renal insufficiency), lesion characteristics (eg, SV, long lesions [LLs], bifurcation disease), device types (eg, polymer type, strut thickness, antiproliferative drug), dual antiplatelet therapy (DAPT) considerations (eg, various drugs, patient compliance, DAPT duration), and clinical syndrome (eg, stable coronary disease).[73,74] As a result, it is difficult to associate SV PCI with an increased risk of ST in the same way stent length diabetes have been clearly associated. Although many retrospective analyses have adjusted for multiple patient and lesion characteristics, it remains difficult to separate small-sized diameter vessel and long-vessel disease from comorbid diabetes because they frequently tend to occur simultaneously.[75]

An important study that deserves special mention is that at the beginning of the DES era, it was observed that ST was associated with small minimum stent size at the end of PCI.[76] Small minimum stent area, in turn, is most commonly associated with stent underexpansion and SV size. As such, this IVUS study elegantly summarizes the difficulty in separating the aforementioned factors coexisting with SV CAD that may contribute to ST.

As stent polymer, strut thickness, and drug characteristics continued to improve over the past two decades, the rates of ST have continued to decrease.[77-81] The most recent trials comparing contemporary polymers, strut thicknesses, and drugs in DES have shown very low rates of ST in all-comers,[63,65,70] including patients who underwent SV PCI.[17,44,47,71,82] The differences in ST nowadays likely have more to do with antiplatelet therapy and clinical syndrome (stable angina, ACS) rather than differences between stent characteristics or vessel size.[83,84]

DCBs for SV CAD

Although DCBs have been used for peripheral artery disease (PAD) in the United States and for CAD and PAD outside the United States for several years, their use for CAD in the United States is still undergoing clinical trials and yet to be approved. Outside the United States, DCBs[85-87] are well established for the treatment of coronary ISR as they allow delivery of an antiproliferative drug without the need for multiple layers of stents. Another advantage of DCB is the ability to significantly shorten the duration of DAPT to as little as 4 weeks,[88] which is especially useful for patients at high bleeding risk. One early trial[16] of DCB in SV CAD studied elderly patients who underwent SV PCI (vessel diameter <2.8 mm) and found no significant difference in clinical outcomes between older and younger patients despite the more complex coronary anatomy in older patients. Another trial of patients undergoing SV PCI with paclitaxel-coated balloons (vessel diameter of 2.0-2.75 mm)[89] and short DAPT duration found no significant difference in clinical outcomes between patients who had stable CAD and ACS.

Three contemporary trials compared DCB and DES for patients with de novo SV CAD. BASKET-SMALL 2 was an open-label noninferiority randomized controlled trial that compared a paclitaxel-eluting balloon to a second-generation paclitaxel or EES in patients undergoing SV PCI with vessel diameter 2.0 to 3.0 mm and found DCB to be noninferior to DES in MACE at 12 months.[11] The RESTORE CVD China[10] trial compared a paclitaxel-eluting balloon to an ZES for patients undergoing SV PCI with vessel diameter 2.25 to 2.75 mm and found the DCB to be noninferior to DES for in-segment restenosis at 9 months and noninferior rates of target lesion failure at 1 year. Finally, a second-generation DCB was compared to an EES in patients undergoing SV PCI (vessel diameter of 2.0-2.75 mm) in the PICCOLETO II trial[9] and found the DCB to be superior to the EES in terms of late-lumen loss with similar rates of MACE. Further studies are needed to determine long-term outcomes in patients undergoing SV PCI with DCB.

DIFFUSE DISEASE

Similarly to SV disease, DD, also frequently referred to as LLs, has been associated with worse outcomes when compared with shorter lesions and lesions in larger vessels. Both DD and SV disease are frequently seen in diabetic populations. DD frequently requires multiple overlapping stents, which may be associated with worse clinical outcomes.[90,91]

Definition

The traditional ACC/AHA definition from the PTCA era classified lesions >20 mm in length as type C lesions with an anticipated success rate of <60%.[92] With the advances in stenting technology and adjunctive pharmacology, the definition has undergone significant modification and a contemporary definition, developed for the SYNTAX trial, defines a "DD/SV" category when "75% length of the segment distal to the lesion has a vessel diameter of <2 mm irrespective of absence of disease at that distal segment."[93] Hence, from the standpoint of nomenclature, "DD" is different from "multivessel" disease as DD refers to LL in one specific vessel. As previously shown, the shift in overall perception regarding "SVs" has similarly changed for "DD," with current clinical PCI practice addressing ever-longer lesions than in the PTCA era. Many diffuse and LL also meet criteria for SV, especially in the distal vessel segments.

DES in DD

Second-generation DESs have provided a major advance in the treatment of DD. EES was compared with PES (first-generation stent) in a pooled analysis of the SPIRIT and COMPARE trials, and three groups were studied: short lesions in large vessels, LL or SVs, and finally LL in SVs. Two-year MACEs were similar in the lower risk group comprising short lesions in large vessels (4.8% vs 7.0%, *P* = .11). However, EES ***outperformed*** SES in the high-risk groups: lower MACE in the LL or SV group (6.6% vs 11.2%, *P* < .01) and in the LL in SV group (9.1% vs 12.7%). EES had lower MACE compared with PES regardless of lesion length or reference vessel diameter. ST was low and similar, 0.5%, 0.8%, and 0.9%, respectively.[94]

In a pooled analysis of 13,266 patients receiving Xience EES, two groups were compared—very LLs (35 mm) and control (>24 to <35 mm). The mean lesion length in the very LL group was 47.1 mm. There was no difference in target lesion failure, MACE nor ST at 1 year.[95] This trial is important as it shows that improvement in stent technology has resulted in better outcomes in LL.

The current improvement with the availability of 48 mm stents has provided further important advances in treatment of LLs. In several trials, the use of 48 mm EES was found to be safe and effective and with comparable clinical outcomes with multiple overlapping stents.[96-98]

Prior to the introduction of 48-mm DES, it was estimated that stent overlap occurred in approximately 10% of PCI. The reasons for this are multifold and are mainly due to LL, incomplete lesion coverage, or technical issues, such as edge dissections.[99] With the increasing complexity of PCI, aging population with more comorbidities, lesions longer than 40 mm are found in at least 25% of patients in current practice.[98]

Overlapping stents present several technical and clinical challenges—side-branch compromise due to multiple stent layers, altered stent healing due to different antiproliferative drug and polymer kinetics, and potential for geographic miss between stents due to technical considerations.[100]

Long stents eliminate the aforementioned downsides of overlapping stents but present other challenges. Due to the tapering nature of coronary arteries, the minimal lumen diameter of the vessel almost invariably decreases over the 48 mm stent length and may present sizing difficulties. While the proximal vessel segment may be undersized, there is a risk of distal edge dissection and oversizing of the distal segment. Meticulous postdilatation and imaging-guided PCI are nearly indispensable when placing 48-mm stents. IVUS-guided LL PCI is associated with reduced MACE[101] and improved long-term patient survival.[102]

There are few studies in the literature directly comparing overlapping stents with 48-mm stents, and all present comparable safety and efficacy.[97,103-105] As indicated previously, overlapping stents and 48-mm stents presents each its unique technical challenges. Continuous improvement in stent design (polymer, drug, and cell geometry) along with improved implantation techniques (image guidance with IVUS and OCT) have allowed for improved outcomes in these highly complicated lesions.

"Full-Metal Jacket"

With first-generation DES, long-term outcomes of "full metal jacket" stenting were investigated in a retrospective study with 357 patients. The follow-up was 8 years, and 90.5% were alive at the end of the observation period. ST occurred in 12 patients. Left ventricular dysfunction, stent length >80 mm were major predictors of MACE.[106]

Second-generation DES were compared to first-generation DES in a retrospective study. At the 2 years, MACE was lower in second-generation DES group (9.8% vs 20.4%, $P = .03$). Overall, "full metal jacket" outcomes with second-generation DES were improved compared to first-generation DES.[107]

These trials suggest that further improvements in stent technology and adjunctive pharmacology are needed to address very LL ("full metal jacket") that very frequently may involve chronic totally occlusions.

Hybrid revascularization with DCBs has been proposed as an alternative to very LLs stenting,[108] and the results appear promising while awaiting larger and long-term outcome trials.[109]

At the present time, DCBs are not approved for use by the FDA in the United States (March 2023). Multiple trials are ongoing or have been proposed to further elucidate the role of DCBs in LLs.[110]

SV CAD IN WOMEN AND DIFFERENT ETHNIC GROUPS

Despite the significant amount of research that has been performed to understand the pathophysiology and best treatment strategies for CAD and specifically SV CAD, there is still a lack of high-quality clinical trials that enrolled enough women and patients from under-represented ethnic groups in these trials to be able to make these same high-quality conclusions.[111] It has long been known that women have different disease mechanisms that lead to atherosclerosis,[112] and women have a higher burden of SV CAD as well as microvascular disease compared to men.[113] A study from as early as 1993[114] found that women who underwent CABG with at least two arterial grafts and had SV CAD faced higher early mortality within 30 days than those who did not have SV CAD (even higher than those who were undergoing repeat CABG), suggesting that the mechanism for CAD and mechanism for restenosis of grafts in women with SVD CAD is different. Despite these differences and knowledge that women have higher rates of SV CAD, the trials that have been performed for SV CAD have not enrolled a proportionally appropriate number of women. A 1998 study on PCI in SV CAD enrolled 14% women,[3] the TAXUS trials on SV and LLs had 35% women,[68] a meta-analysis on 12 RCTs for SV CAD by in 2012 had a mean female enrollment of 30%,[77] a 2016 study on very small CAD enrolled 22% women,[17] ORBIT II in 2018 had 35% women,[47] BIO-RESORT in 2019 enrolled 30% women,[71] COMBO in 2020 had 28% women,[115] PICOLETTO II in 2020 had 27% women,[9] BASKET-SMALL 2 in 2020 had 27% women,[116] a meta-analysis comparing DCB to DES in 2022 had 26% women.[117] Even studies that were performed to evaluate the correlation between diagnostic modalities to evaluate SV CAD had a significant male majority (the FFR study in SV CAD in 2012 had 37% women[41] and the FFR vs QFR SV CAD study in 2019 had 32% women[44]), and a study that was done to identify risk factors for early cardiac events after SV PCI had only 25% women among >3000 patients enrolled.[4] Needless to say, further studies are needed to determine the optimal diagnostic and treatment strategies for SV CAD in women.

In addition to the lack of enrollment of women in clinical trials for SV CAD (and CAD in general), most clinical trials reviewed in this chapter did not report specific ethnic groups for their patient populations. There is evidence that White and Non-Hispanic African American patients not only have different risk factors and rates of cardiovascular disease[118] but also have different results on cardiac imaging and diagnostic studies[119,120] and different responses to intervention such as PCI and CABG;[121] however, there is dearth of data for Hispanic patients and even less data for other ethnic minorities.[122-124] A systematic review[125] of PCI trials in North America, Europe, and Asia between 1990 and 2014 found major differences in risk factors among enrolled patients between the different continents, clearly suggesting that disease mechanisms that contributed to CAD in these patients was different. Because there is lack of data on specific ethnic groups in most of the clinical trials for CAD and SV CAD specifically, the best diagnostic modalities, measurement cutoffs, and interventional techniques in different ethnic groups are unknown and deserves further study.

Key Points

General

- No standardized definition of "SV" exists for coronary disease. Most trials use cutoffs between 2.5 and 3.0 mm to define an SV.
- Women are known to have different atherosclerotic disease mechanisms than men; however, there are not enough data in the literature regarding optimal diagnostic and imaging modalities, size cutoffs, intervention strategies in women with SV CAD as women only represented 14% to 37% of participants in the trials.

- Even less data exist on ethnic minorities with SV CAD as most trials did not report ethnicity and racial demographics.

Imaging and Functional Testing of SV CAD

- In nonleft main SV CAD, functional testing (FFR, iFR) is better than IVUS in determining lesion significance.

Lesion Modification in SV CAD

- Difficult to compare different lesion modification techniques and devices as the indications, contraindications, technical factors are different.
- All lesion modification techniques including orbital and RA, IVL, scoring and cutting balloons were shown in multiple trials to be safe and effective in heavily calcified SV CAD.

DESs in SV CAD

- Multiple large trials showed DES to be better than BMS and PTCA in SV CAD.
- As technology improved, DES struts became thinner over time and the polymer coating became better, leading to insignificant between-stent differences.
- Differences in ISR and ST nowadays likely have to do with clinical syndrome and antiplatelet strategy.

DCBs in SV CAD

- Novel drug-delivery system that can lead to significantly shorter DAPT duration (4 weeks).
- Recent trials show DCB are noninferior to DES in SV CAD.

DD and LLs

- Treated lesion length has been increasing over time due to increased patient age and comorbidities.
- DDs/LLs are estimated at least at 25% of all PCIs.
- Second-generation DESs lower restenosis, MACE and ST compared with first-generation DES.
- Overlapping DES may be associated with worse outcomes.
- 48-mm stents have demonstrated safety and efficacy in LLs compared with overlapping DES.
- "Full-metal jacket" PCI is associated with high MACE; second-generation DESs have improved overall outcomes in this high-risk subgroup.
- DCBs are currently being evaluated in LLs (not approved for use in the United States, March 2023).

References

1. Saucedo JF, Popma JJ, Kennard ED, et al. Relation of coronary artery size to one-year clinical events after new device angioplasty of native coronary arteries (a New Approach to Coronary Intervention [NACI] Registry Report). *Am J Cardiol*. 2000;85(2):166-171.
2. Schunkert H, Harrell L, Palacios IF. Implications of small reference vessel diameter in patients undergoing percutaneous coronary revascularization. *J Am Coll Cardiol*. 1999;34(1):40-48.
3. Akiyama T, Moussa I, Reimers B, et al. Angiographic and clinical outcome following coronary stenting of small vessels: a comparison with coronary stenting of large vessels. *J Am Coll Cardiol*. 1998;32(6):1610-1618.
4. Hausleiter J, Kastrati A, Mehilli J, et al. Predictive factors for early cardiac events and angiographic restenosis after coronary stent placement in small coronary arteries. *J Am Coll Cardiol*. 2002;40(5):882-889.
5. Kirtane AJ, Yeung AC, Ball M, et al. Long-term (5-year) clinical evaluation of the Resolute zotarolimus-eluting coronary stent: the RESOLUTE US clinical trial. *Catheter Cardiovasc Interv*. 2020;95(6):1067-1073.
6. O'Connor NJ, Morton JR, Birkmeyer JD, Olmstead EM, O'Connor GT. Effect of coronary artery diameter in patients undergoing coronary bypass surgery. Northern New England Cardiovascular Disease Study Group. *Circulation*. 1996;93(4):652-655.
7. Maron DJ, Hochman JS, Reynolds HR, et al. Initial invasive or conservative strategy for stable coronary disease. *N Engl J Med*. 2020;382(15):1395-1407.
8. Sanz-Sánchez J, Chiarito M, Gill GS, et al. Small vessel coronary artery disease: rationale for standardized definition and critical appraisal of the literature. *J Soc Cardiovasc Angiogr Interv*. 2022;1:100403.
9. Cortese B, Di Palma G, Guimaraes MG, et al. Drug-coated balloon versus drug-eluting stent for small coronary vessel disease: PICCOLETO II randomized clinical trial. *JACC Cardiovasc Interv*. 2020;13(24):2840-2849.
10. Tang Y, Qiao S, Su X, et al. Drug-coated balloon versus drug-eluting stent for small-vessel disease: the RESTORE SVD China randomized trial. *JACC Cardiovasc Interv*. 2018;11(23):2381-2392.
11. Jeger RV, Farah A, Ohlow MA, et al. Drug-coated balloons for small coronary artery disease (BASKET-SMALL 2): an open-label randomised non-inferiority trial. *Lancet*. 2018;392(10150):849-856.
12. Biondi-Zoccai G, Moretti C, Abbate A, Sheiban I. Percutaneous coronary intervention for small vessel coronary artery disease. *Cardiovasc Revasc Med*. 2010;11(3):189-198.
13. Abdu FA, Mohammed AQ, Liu L, Xu Y, Che W. Myocardial infarction with Nonobstructive Coronary Arteries (MINOCA): a review of the current position. *Cardiology*. 2020;145(9):543-552.
14. Del Buono MG, Montone RA, Camilli M, et al. Coronary microvascular dysfunction across the spectrum of cardiovascular diseases: JACC state-of-the-art review. *J Am Coll Cardiol*. 2021;78(13):1352-1371.
15. Biondi-Zoccai GG, Sangiorgi GM, Antoniucci D, et al. Testing prospectively the effectiveness and safety of paclitaxel-eluting stents in over 1000 very high-risk patients: design, baseline characteristics, procedural data and in-hospital outcomes of the multicenter Taxus in Real-life Usage Evaluation (TRUE) Study. *Int J Cardiol*. 2007;117(3):349-354.
16. Sinaga DA, Ho HH, Zeymer U, et al. Drug coated balloon angioplasty in elderly patients with small vessel coronary disease. *Ther Adv Cardiovasc Dis*. 2015;9(6):389-396.
17. Ismail MD, Ahmad WA, Leschke M, et al. The outcomes of patients with very small coronary artery disease treated with thin strut cobalt chromium bare metal stents: an observational study. *SpringerPlus*. 2016;5(1):1668.
18. Scholz SS, Lauder L, Ewen S, et al. One-year clinical outcomes in patients with renal insufficiency after contemporary PCI: data from a multicenter registry. *Clin Res Cardiol*. 2020;109(7):845-856.
19. Cassese S, Byrne RA, Tada T, et al. Incidence and predictors of restenosis after coronary stenting in 10 004 patients with surveillance angiography. *Heart*. 2014;100(2):153-159.
20. von Birgelen C, van der Heijden LC, Basalus MW, et al. Five-year outcome after implantation of zotarolimus- and everolimus-eluting stents in randomized trial participants and nonenrolled eligible patients: a secondary analysis of a randomized clinical trial. *JAMA Cardiol*. 2017;2(3):268-276.
21. Hoffmann R, Mintz GS, Pichard AD, Kent KM, Satler LF, Leon MB. Intimal hyperplasia thickness at follow-up is independent of stent size: a serial intravascular ultrasound study. *Am J Cardiol*. 1998;82(10):1168-1172.
22. Mauri L, Orav EJ, Kuntz RE. Late loss in lumen diameter and binary restenosis for drug-eluting stent comparison. *Circulation*. 2005;111(25):3435-3442.
23. Pocock SJ, Lansky AJ, Mehran R, et al. Angiographic surrogate end points in drug-eluting stent trials: a systematic evaluation based on individual patient data from 11 randomized, controlled trials. *J Am Coll Cardiol*. 2008;51(1):23-32.

24. Schuurman AS, Vroegindewey MM, Kardys I, et al. Prognostic value of intravascular ultrasound in patients with coronary artery disease. *J Am Coll Cardiol*. 2018;72(17):2003-2011.
25. Groves EM, Seto AH, Kern MJ. Invasive testing for coronary artery disease: FFR, IVUS, OCT, NIRS. *Cardiol Clin*. 2014;32(3):405-417.
26. Case BC, Yerasi C, Forrestal BJ, et al. Intravascular ultrasound guidance in the evaluation and treatment of left main coronary artery disease. *Int J Cardiol*. 2021;325:168-175.
27. Iakovou I, Mintz GS, Dangas G, et al. Optimal final lumen area and predictors of target lesion revascularization after stent implantation in small coronary arteries. *Am J Cardiol*. 2003;92(10):1171-1176.
28. Mintz GS, Guagliumi G. Intravascular imaging in coronary artery disease. *Lancet*. 2017;390(10096):793-809.
29. Matsuo Y, Kubo T, Aoki H, et al. Optimal threshold of postintervention minimum stent area to predict in-stent restenosis in small coronary arteries: an optical coherence tomography analysis. *Catheter Cardiovasc Interv*. 2016;87(1):E9-E14.
30. Kaul U, Abhyankar A, K Abhaichand R, et al. Serial evaluation of vascular responses after implantation of everolimus-eluting coronary stent by optical coherence tomography. *Catheter Cardiovasc Interv*. 2022;99(2):381-390.
31. Muramatsu T, Ozaki Y, Nanasato M, et al. Comparison between optical frequency domain imaging and intravascular ultrasound for percutaneous coronary intervention guidance in biolimus A9-eluting stent implantation: a randomized MISTIC-1 non-inferiority trial. *Circ Cardiovasc Interv*. 2020;13(11):e009314.
32. Kuku KO, Singh M, Ozaki Y, et al. Near-infrared spectroscopy intravascular ultrasound imaging: state of the art. *Front Cardiovasc Med*. 2020;7:107.
33. Stone GW, Maehara A, Ali ZA, et al. Percutaneous coronary intervention for vulnerable coronary atherosclerotic plaque. *J Am Coll Cardiol*. 2020;76(20):2289-2301.
34. Tonino PA, De Bruyne B, Pijls NH, et al. Fractional flow reserve versus angiography for guiding percutaneous coronary intervention. *N Engl J Med*. 2009;360(3):213-224.
35. De Bruyne B, Pijls NH, Kalesan B, et al. Fractional flow reserve-guided PCI versus medical therapy in stable coronary disease. *N Engl J Med*. 2012;367(11):991-1001.
36. Koo BK, Hu X, Kang J, et al. Fractional flow reserve or intravascular ultrasonography to guide PCI. *N Engl J Med*. 2022;387(9):779-789.
37. Park SJ, Ahn JM, Kang SJ, et al. Intravascular ultrasound-derived minimal lumen area criteria for functionally significant left main coronary artery stenosis. *JACC Cardiovasc Interv*. 2014;7(8):868-874.
38. de la Torre Hernandez JM, Hernández Hernandez F, Alfonso F, et al. Prospective application of pre-defined intravascular ultrasound criteria for assessment of intermediate left main coronary artery lesions results from the multicenter LITRO study. *J Am Coll Cardiol*. 2011;58(4):351-358.
39. Fassa AA, Wagatsuma K, Higano ST, et al. Intravascular ultrasound-guided treatment for angiographically indeterminate left main coronary artery disease: a long-term follow-up study. *J Am Coll Cardiol*. 2005;45(2):204-211.
40. Waksman R, Legutko J, Singh J, et al. FIRST: fractional flow reserve and intravascular ultrasound relationship study. *J Am Coll Cardiol*. 2013;61(9):917-923.
41. Puymirat E, Peace A, Mangiacapra F, et al. Long-term clinical outcome after fractional flow reserve-guided percutaneous coronary revascularization in patients with small-vessel disease. *Circ Cardiovasc Interv*. 2012;5(1):62-68.
42. Götberg M, Christiansen EH, Gudmundsdottir IJ, et al. Instantaneous wave-free ratio versus fractional flow reserve to guide PCI. *N Engl J Med*. 2017;376(19):1813-1823.
43. Ties D, van Dijk R, Pundziute G, et al. Computational quantitative flow ratio to assess functional severity of coronary artery stenosis. *Int J Cardiol*. 2018;271:36-41.
44. Erbay A, Steiner J, Lauten A, Landmesser U, Leistner DM, Stähli BE. Assessment of intermediate coronary lesions by fractional flow reserve and quantitative flow ratio in patients with small-vessel disease. *Catheter Cardiovasc Interv*. 2020;96(4):743-751.
45. Kuntz RE, Gibson CM, Nobuyoshi M, Baim DS. Generalized model of restenosis after conventional balloon angioplasty, stenting and directional atherectomy. *J Am Coll Cardiol*. 1993;21(1):15-25.
46. Bittl JA, Chew DP, Topol EJ, Kong DF, Califf RM. Meta-analysis of randomized trials of percutaneous transluminal coronary angioplasty versus atherectomy, cutting balloon atherotomy, or laser angioplasty. *J Am Coll Cardiol*. 2004;43(6):936-942.
47. Lee MS, Shlofmitz RA, Shlofmitz E, et al. Orbital atherectomy for the treatment of small (2.5mm) severely calcified coronary lesions: ORBIT II subanalysis. *Cardiovasc Revasc Med*. 2018;19(3 pt A):268-272.
48. Lee MS, Shlofmitz E, Shlofmitz R. Outcomes of orbital atherectomy in severely calcified small (2.5 mm) coronary artery vessels. *J Invasive Cardiol*. 2018;30(8):310-314.
49. Mauri L, Reisman M, Buchbinder M, et al. Comparison of rotational atherectomy with conventional balloon angioplasty in the prevention of restenosis of small coronary arteries: results of the Dilatation vs Ablation Revascularization Trial Targeting Restenosis (DART). *Am Heart J*. 2003;145(5):847-854.
50. Kwon K, Choi D, Choi SH, et al. Coronary stenting after rotational atherectomy in diffuse lesions of the small coronary artery: comparison with balloon angioplasty before stenting. *Angiology*. 2003;54(4):423-431.
51. Sakakura K, Inohara T, Kohsaka S, et al. Incidence and determinants of complications in rotational atherectomy: insights from the national clinical data (J-PCI registry). *Circ Cardiovasc Interv*. 2016;9(11):e004278.
52. Iannaccone M, Barbero U, D'ascenzo F, et al. Rotational atherectomy in very long lesions: results for the ROTATE registry. *Catheter Cardiovasc Interv*. 2016;88(6):E164-E172.
53. Hill JM, Kereiakes DJ, Shlofmitz RA, et al. Intravascular lithotripsy for treatment of severely calcified coronary artery disease. *J Am Coll Cardiol*. 2020;76(22):2635-2646.
54. Saito S, Yamazaki S, Takahashi A, et al. Intravascular lithotripsy for vessel preparation in severely calcified coronary arteries prior to stent placement - primary outcomes from the Japanese Disrupt CAD IV study. *Circ J*. 2021;85(6):826-833.
55. Muramatsu T, Tsukahara R, Ho M, et al. Effectiveness of cutting balloon angioplasty for small vessels less than 3.0 mm in diameter. *J Interv Cardiol*. 2002;15(4):281-286.
56. Iijima R, Ikari Y, Wada M, Shiba M, Nakamura M, Hara K. Cutting balloon angioplasty is superior to balloon angioplasty or stent implantation for small coronary artery disease. *Coron Artery Dis*. 2004;15(7):435-440.
57. Shah M, Najam O, Bhindi R, De Silva K. Calcium modification techniques in complex percutaneous coronary intervention. *Circ Cardiovasc Interv*. 2021;14(5):e009870.
58. Ishihara T, Iida O, Takahara M, et al. Improved crossability with novel cutting balloon versus scoring balloon in the treatment of calcified lesion. *Cardiovasc Interv Ther*. 2021;36(2):198-207.
59. Tsujimura T, Ishihara T, Takahashi K, et al. Cutting balloons versus conventional balloons for treating patients with coronary artery disease presenting with moderate-to-severely calcified lesions: impact on post-interventional minimum stent area. *Cardiovasc Interv Ther*. 2022;37(4):700-709.
60. Gershony G., Virmani R., Lotan C., Konstantino E., Leon M. A novel angioplasty catheter for the treatment of complex coronary artery disease: AngioSculpt. *Am J Cardiol*.2003;92:166L.
61. Secco GG, Buettner A, Parisi R, et al. Clinical experience with very high-pressure dilatation for resistant coronary lesions. *Cardiovasc Revasc Med*. 2019;20(12):1083-1087.
62. Rheude T, Fitzgerald S, Allali A, et al. Rotational atherectomy or balloon-based techniques to prepare severely calcified coronary lesions. *JACC Cardiovasc Interv*. 2022;15(18):1864-1874.
63. O'Brien B, Zafar H, Ibrahim A, Zafar J, Sharif F. Coronary stent materials and coatings: a technology and performance update. *Ann Biomed Eng*. 2016;44(2):523-535.
64. Zbinden R, von Felten S, Wein B, et al. Impact of stent diameter and length on in-stent restenosis after DES vs BMS implantation in patients needing large coronary stents-A clinical and health-economic evaluation. *Cardiovasc Ther*. 2017;35(1):19-25.
65. Volodarskiy A, Kumar S, Pracon R, et al. Drug-eluting vs bare-metal stents in patients with chronic kidney disease and coronary artery disease: insights from a systematic review and meta-analysis. *J Invasive Cardiol*. 2018;30(1):10-17.
66. Capodanno D, Di Salvo ME, Capranzano P, et al. Long term results of unprotected left main percutaneous coronary intervention with DES versus BMS. *Minerva Cardioangiol*. 2009;57:1-6.

67. Parikh SV, Luna M, Selzer F, et al. Outcomes of small coronary artery stenting with bare-metal stents versus drug-eluting stents: results from the NHLBI dynamic registry. *Catheter Cardiovasc Interv*. 2014;83(2):192-200.
68. Turco MA, Ormiston JA, Popma JJ, et al. Reduced risk of restenosis in small vessels and reduced risk of myocardial infarction in long lesions with the new thin-strut TAXUS Liberté stent: 1-year results from the TAXUS ATLAS program. *JACC Cardiovasc Interv*. 2008;1(6):699-709.
69. Yeung AC, Leon MB, Jain A, et al. Clinical evaluation of the Resolute zotarolimus-eluting coronary stent system in the treatment of de novo lesions in native coronary arteries: the RESOLUTE US clinical trial. *J Am Coll Cardiol*. 2011;57(17):1778-1783.
70. Kandzari DE, Koolen JJ, Doros G, et al. Ultrathin bioresorbable polymer sirolimus-eluting stents versus durable polymer everolimus-eluting stents: BIOFLOW V final 5-year outcomes. *JACC Cardiovasc Interv*. 2022;15(18):1852-1860.
71. Buiten RA, Ploumen EH, Zocca P, et al. Outcomes in patients treated with thin-strut, very thin-strut, or ultrathin-strut drug-eluting stents in small coronary vessels: a prespecified analysis of the randomized BIO RESORT trial. *JAMA Cardiol*. 2019;4(7):659-669.
72. Baran KW, Lasala JM, Cox DA, et al. A clinical risk score for prediction of stent thrombosis. *Am J Cardiol*. 2008;102:541-545.
73. Holmes DR, Kereiakes DJ, Laskey WK, et al. Thrombosis and drug-eluting stents: an objective appraisal. *J Am Coll Cardiol*. 2007;50(2):109-118.
74. Brodie B, Pokharel Y, Garg A, et al. Predictors of early, late, and very late stent thrombosis after primary percutaneous coronary intervention with bare-metal and drug-eluting stents for ST-segment elevation myocardial infarction. *JACC Cardiovasc Interv*. 2012;5(10):1043-1051.
75. Kuramitsu S, Sonoda S, Ando K, et al. Drug-eluting stent thrombosis: current and future perspectives. *Cardiovasc Interv Ther*. 2021;36(2):158-168.
76. Okabe T, Mintz GS, Buch AN, et al. Intravascular ultrasound parameters associated with stent thrombosis after drug-eluting stent deployment. *Am J Cardiol*. 2007;100(4):615-620.
77. Cortese B, Bertoletti A, De Matteis S, Danzi GB, Kastrati A. Drug-eluting stents perform better than bare metal stents in small coronary vessels: a meta-analysis of randomised and observational clinical studies with mid-term follow up. *Int J Cardiol*. 2012;161(2):73-82.
78. Biondi-Zoccai GG, Sangiorgi GM, Chieffo A, et al. Validation of predictors of intraprocedural stent thrombosis in the drug-eluting stent era. *Am J Cardiol*. 2005;95(12):1466-1468.
79. Daemen J, Wenaweser P, Tsuchida K, et al. Early and late coronary stent thrombosis of sirolimus-eluting and paclitaxel-eluting stents in routine clinical practice: data from a large two-institutional cohort study. *Lancet*. 2007;369(9562):667-678.
80. Naidu SS, Krucoff MW, Rutledge DR, et al. Contemporary incidence and predictors of stent thrombosis and other major adverse cardiac events in the year after XIENCE V implantation: results from the 8,061-patient XIENCE V United States study. *JACC Cardiovasc Interv*. 2012;5(6):626-635.
81. Ito H, Hermiller JB, Yaqub M, et al. Performance of everolimus-eluting versus paclitaxel-eluting coronary stents in small vessels: results from the SPIRIT III and SPIRIT IV clinical trials. *J Interv Cardiol*. 2011;24(6):505-513.
82. Murphy G, Naughton A, Durand R, et al. 50 Drug-eluting balloons and drug-eluting stents in the treatment of small coronary arteries: a systematic review and meta-analysis of long-term clinical outcomes. *Heart*. 2022;108:A43-A46.
83. Wiviott SD, Braunwald E, McCabe CH, et al. Intensive oral antiplatelet therapy for reduction of ischaemic events including stent thrombosis in patients with acute coronary syndromes treated with percutaneous coronary intervention and stenting in the TRITON-TIMI 38 trial: a subanalysis of a randomised trial. *Lancet*. 2008;371(9621):1353-1363.
84. Chen W, Zhang C, Zhao J, et al. Effects of clopidogrel, prasugrel and ticagrelor on prevention of stent thrombosis in patients underwent percutaneous coronary intervention: a network meta-analysis. *Clin Cardiol*. 2021;44(4):488-494.
85. Arslani K, Jeger R. Drug-coated balloons for small coronary disease-A literature review. *Curr Cardiol Rep*. 2021;23(11):173.
86. Byrne RA, Cassese S, Windisch T, et al. Differential relative efficacy between drug-eluting stents in patients with bare metal and drug-eluting stent restenosis; evidence in support of drug resistance: insights from the ISAR-DESIRE and ISAR-DESIRE 2 trials. *EuroIntervention*. 2013;9(7):797-802.
87. Mauler-Wittwer S, Garot P. The Biolimus A9-coated BioFreedom™ stent: from clinical efficacy to real-world evidence. *Future Cardiol*. 2021;17(2):239-255.
88. Bonaventura K, Sonntag S, Kleber FX. Antiplatelet therapy in the era of percutaneous coronary intervention with drug-eluting balloons. *EuroIntervention*. 2011;7:K106-K111.
89. Mahmood Zuhdi AS, Zeymer U, Waliszewski M, et al. The use of paclitaxel coated balloon (PCB) in acute coronary syndrome of small vessel de novo lesions: an analysis of a prospective 'real world' registry. *SpringerPlus*. 2016;5:373.
90. Hara H, Ono M, Kawashima H, et al. Impact of stent length and diameter on 10-year mortality in the SYNTAXES trial. *Catheter Cardiovasc Interv*. 2021;98(3):E379-E387.
91. Kong MG, Han J-K, Kang J-H, et al. Clinical outcomes of long stenting in the drug-eluting stent era: patient-level pooled analysis from the GRAND-DES registry. *EuroIntervention*. 2021;16:1318-1325.
92. Ryan TJ, Bauman WB, Kennedy JW, et al. Guidelines for percutaneous transluminal coronary angioplasty. A report of the American heart Association/American College of Cardiology task force on assessment of diagnostic and therapeutic cardiovascular procedures (Committee on percutaneous transluminal coronary angioplasty). *Circulation*. 1993;88(6):2987-3007.
93. Sianos G, Morel MA, Kappetein AP, et al. The SYNTAX Score: an angiographic tool grading the complexity of coronary artery disease. *EuroIntervention*. 2005;1(2):219-227.
94. Claessen BE, Smits PC, Kereiakes DJ, et al. Impact of lesion length and vessel size on clinical outcomes after percutaneous coronary intervention with everolimus-versus paclitaxel-eluting stents: pooled analysis from the SPIRIT (clinical evaluation of the XIENCE V everolimus eluting coronary stent system) and COMPARE (second-generation everolimus-eluting and paclitaxel-eluting stents in real-life practice) randomized trials. *JACC Cardiovasc Interv*. 2011;4(11):1209-1215.
95. Bouras G, Jhamnani S, Ng VG, et al. Clinical outcomes after PCI treatment of very long lesions with the XIENCE V everolimus eluting stent; Pooled analysis from the SPIRIT and XIENCE V USA prospective multicenter trials. *Catheter Cardiovasc Interv*. 2017;89(6):984-991.
96. Hsiao FC, Tsai CT, Hsu LA, et al. Procedural and one-year clinical outcomes of long 48 mm Xience Xpedition everolimus-eluting stent in complex long diffuse coronary artery lesions. *J Invasive Cardiol*. 2022;34(2):E80-E86.
97. Gautier A, Hovasse T, Arroyo D, et al. Safety and efficacy of 48 mm Xience Xpedition everolimus-eluting stent for the treatment of long coronary lesions. *Catheter Cardiovasc Interv*. 2022;100(2):179-187.
98. Youn YJ, Jeon HS, Kim YI, et al. Impact of the ultra-long 48 mm drug-eluting stent on procedural and clinical outcomes in patients with diffuse long coronary artery disease. *Clin Cardiol*. 2023;46(4):416-424.
99. Räber L, Jüni P, Löffel L, et al. Impact of stent overlap on angiographic and long-term clinical outcome in patients undergoing drug-eluting stent implantation. *J Am Coll Cardiol*. 2010;55(12):1178-1188.
100. Sakamoto A, Torii S, Jinnouchi H, Virmani R, Finn AV. Histopathologic and physiologic effect of overlapping vs single coronary stents: impact of stent evolution. *Expert Rev Med Devices*. 2018;15(9):665-682.
101. Hong SJ, Mintz GS, Ahn CM, et al. Effect of intravascular ultrasound–guided drug-eluting stent implantation: 5-year follow-up of the IVUS-XPL randomized trial. *JACC Cardiovasc Interv*. 2020;13(1):62-71.
102. Hong SJ, Zhang JJ, Mintz GS, et al. Improved 3-year cardiac survival after IVUS–guided long DES implantation: a patient-level analysis from 2 randomized trials. *JACC Cardiovasc Interv*. 2022;15:208-216.
103. Tan C, Tin Z, Arshad M, et al. Treatment with 48-mm everolimus-eluting stents: procedural safety and 12-month patient outcome. *Herz*. 2019;44(5):419-424.
104. El Amrawy AM, Loutfi MI, El Tahan SM, Ayad SW. Feasibility and clinical outcomes of 48 mm drug-eluting stents in the management of patients with coronary artery disease. *J Invasive Cardiol*. 2021;33(12):E960-E967.
105. Sim HW, Thong EH, Loh PH, et al. Treating very long coronary artery lesions in the contemporary drug-eluting-stent era: single long 48 mm stent versus two overlapping stents showed comparable clinical outcomes. *Cardiovasc Revasc Med*. 2020;21(9):1115-1118.

106. Lee CW, Ahn JM, Lee JY, et al. Long-term (8-year) outcomes and predictors of major adverse cardiac events after full metal jacket drug-eluting stent implantation. *Catheter Cardiovasc Interv*. 2014;84(3):361-365.
107. Yoshioka G, Kuriyama N, Watanabe N, Ashikaga K, Shibata Y, Node K. Full-metal jacket technique using second-generation drug-eluting stent: clinical and angiographic follow-up in 2 years. *Cardiovasc Interv Ther*. 2019;34(4):305-311.
108. Yang X, Lu W, Pan L, et al. Long-term outcomes of drug-coated balloons in patients with diffuse coronary lesions. *Front Cardiovasc Med*. 2022;9:935263.
109. Costopoulos C, Latib A, Naganuma T, et al. The role of drug-eluting balloons alone or in combination with drug-eluting stents in the treatment of de novo diffuse coronary disease. *JACC Cardiovasc Interv*. 2013;6(11):1153-1159.
110. Yerasi C, Case BC, Forrestal BJ, et al. Drug-coated balloon for De Novo Coronary artery disease: JACC state-of-the-art review. *J Am Coll Cardiol*. 2020;75(9):1061-1073.
111. Iribarren A, Diniz MA, Merz CNB, Shufelt C, Wei J. Are we any WISER yet? Progress and contemporary need for smart trials to include women in coronary artery disease trials. *Contemp Clin Trials*. 2022;117:106762.
112. Bairey Merz CN, Shaw LJ, Reis SE, et al. Insights from the NHLBI-Sponsored Women's Ischemia Syndrome Evaluation (WISE) Study: Part II—gender differences in presentation, diagnosis, and outcome with regard to gender-based pathophysiology of atherosclerosis and macrovascular and microvascular coronary disease. *J Am Coll Cardiol*. 2006;47 (3 suppl):S21-S29.
113. Patel H, Aggarwal NT, Rao A, et al. Microvascular disease and small-vessel disease: the nexus of multiple diseases of women. *J Womens Health (Larchmt)*. 2020;29(6):770-779.
114. Ramström J, Lund O, Cadavid E, Thuren J, Oxelbark S, Henze A. Multiarterial coronary artery bypass grafting with special reference to small vessel disease and results in women. *Eur Heart J*. 1993;14(5):634-639.
115. Chandrasekhar J, Zeebregts D, Kalkman DN, et al. 1-Year outcomes with COMBO stents in small-vessel coronary disease: subgroup analysis from the COMBO collaboration. *Cardiovasc Revasc Med*. 2020;21(12):1542-1547.
116. Jeger RV, Farah A, Ohlow MA, et al. Long-term efficacy and safety of drug-coated balloons versus drug-eluting stents for small coronary artery disease (BASKET-SMALL 2): 3-year follow-up of a randomised, non-inferiority trial. *Lancet*. 2020;396(10261):1504-1510.
117. Megaly M, Buda K, Saad M, et al. Outcomes with drug-coated balloons vs. Drug-eluting stents in small-vessel coronary artery disease. *Cardiovasc Revasc Med*. 2022;35:76-82.
118. Benjamin EJ, Muntner P, Alonso A, et al. Heart disease and stroke statistics-2019 update: a report from the American Heart Association. *Circulation*. 2019;139(10):e56-e528.
119. Zhang L, Olalere D, Mayrhofer T, et al. Differences in cardiovascular risk, coronary artery disease, and cardiac events between black and white individuals enrolled in the PROMISE trial. *JAMA Cardiol*. 2022;7(3):259-267.
120. Tang W, Detrano RC, Brezden OS, et al. Racial differences in coronary calcium prevalence among high-risk adults. *Am J Cardiol*. 1995;75(16):1088-1091.
121. Leigh JA, Alvarez M, Rodriguez CJ. Ethnic minorities and coronary heart disease: an update and future directions. *Curr Atheroscler Rep*. 2016;18(2):9.
122. Orimoloye OA, Budoff MJ, Dardari ZA, et al. Race/ethnicity and the prognostic implications of coronary artery calcium for all-cause and cardiovascular disease mortality: the coronary artery calcium consortium. *J Am Heart Assoc*. 2018;7(20):e010471.
123. Budoff MJ, Young R, Burke G, et al. Ten-year association of coronary artery calcium with atherosclerotic cardiovascular disease (ASCVD) events: the multi-ethnic study of atherosclerosis (MESA). *Eur Heart J*. 2018;39(25):2401-2408.
124. McClelland RL, Jorgensen NW, Budoff M, et al. 10-Year coronary heart disease risk prediction using coronary artery calcium and traditional risk factors: derivation in the MESA (Multi-Ethnic study of atherosclerosis) with validation in the HNR (Heinz Nixdorf Recall) study and the DHS (Dallas heart Study). *J Am Coll Cardiol*. 2015;66(15):1643-1653.
125. Liu E, Hsueh L, Kim H, Vidovich MI. Global geographical variation in patient characteristics in percutaneous coronary intervention clinical trials: a systematic review and meta-analysis. *Am Heart J*. 2018;195:39-49.

Bypass Graft Intervention and Embolic Protection

Salman S. Allana and Emmanouil S. Brilakis

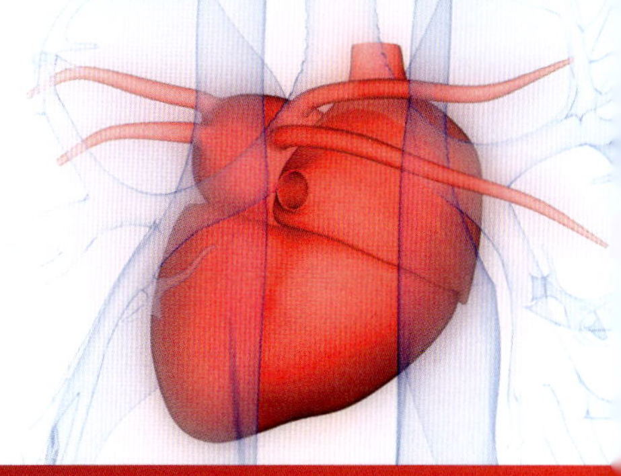

EPIDEMIOLOGY

In the National Cardiovascular Data Registry (NCDR) registry, between 2004 and 2009, 17.5% of all percutaneous coronary interventions (PCIs) were performed in patients with prior coronary artery bypass graft (CABG) surgery[1]: 11% were performed in native coronary arteries, 6.1% in saphenous vein grafts (SVGs), 0.4% in arterial grafts, and 0.04% in both arterial grafts and SVGs.[1] Bypass graft PCI constituted 6.0% of the total NCDR PCI volume from January 2010 through June 2011.

PATENCY OF BYPASS GRAFTS

There are two types of bypass grafts used for CABG: SVGs and arterial grafts that include internal mammary artery (IMA), radial artery, and gastroepiploic artery. Although only a minority of cases are clinically apparent, early graft failure after CABG is reported in up to 12% of grafts as evaluated by intraoperative angiography.[2] These likely result from technical surgical issues, poor quality of the bypass conduit, competitive flow in the native vessel, or poor native vessel runoff.

SVGs have high failure rates: approximately 40% to 50% are occluded 10 years post-CABG.[3] With a longer time from CABG, proportionately more interventions are required in SVGs, which is consistent with the accelerated atherosclerotic process of these grafts. In the PRAGUE-4 trial,[4] 1-year SVG patency rate was 59% in patients receiving on-pump CABG and 49% in patients receiving off-pump CABG; the arterial graft patency rate at 1 year was high at 91% in both groups. Left internal mammary graft (LIMA) to left anterior descending artery (LAD) grafts have high patency rates and have been associated with better survival.[5] Use of the radial artery as a bypass conduit has been associated with better mid- and long-term patency rates and improved cardiac outcomes when compared with SVGs.[6] The current 2021 American College of Cardiology/American Heart Association/Society for Cardiovascular Angiography and Interventions (ACC/AHA/SCAI) guidelines for coronary revascularization recommend the use of the IMA, preferably left to bypass the LAD and use of the radial artery in preference to SVG to the second most important, significantly stenosed non-LAD vessel for improvement in long-term cardiac outcomes as class 1 indications.[7] Use of bilateral mammary arteries and complete arterial revascularization instead of SVG use has also been associated with better long-term outcomes in observational studies.[8-10] Bilateral IMA grafting carries a class 2a recommendation in the 2021 ACC/AHA/SCAI guidelines for coronary artery revascularization to improve long-term cardiac outcomes if performed by experienced operators but has been associated with higher risk of sternal wound infections.[7,11]

INDICATIONS FOR BYPASS GRAFT INTERVENTIONS

In patients with prior CABG presenting with recurrent anginal symptoms, management options include medical therapy, redo CABG, and PCI (native vessel or bypass graft). LIMA grafts often have significant tortuosity that may hinder revascularization attempts. Moreover, proximal subclavian stenoses could affect flow through the LIMA. Intervention in SVG bypass grafts is challenging because of (1) difficulties in graft localization and engagement; (2) high rates of periprocedural myocardial infarction due to distal embolization in SVGs; and (3) high restenosis rates. Prior CABG patients undergoing PCI of a native coronary artery have better outcomes compared with those undergoing bypass graft PCI.[1,12] In a meta-analysis of 22 studies including 40,984 patients, compared with bypass graft PCI, native artery PCI was associated with lower major adverse cardiac events (MACEs) (odds ratio [OR], 0.51; 95% confidence interval [CI], 0.45-0.57; $P < .001$), lower all-cause death (OR, 0.65; 95% CI, 0.49-0.87; $P = .004$), lower myocardial infarction (OR, 0.56; 95% CI, 0.45-0.69; $P < .001$), and lower target vessel revascularization (TVR) (OR, 0.62; 95% CI, 0.51-0.76; $P < .001$) during a median follow-up of 2 years.[13] Hence, when feasible, it is reasonable to choose PCI of the native coronary artery over PCI of the severely diseased SVG (class 2a recommendation in the ACC/AHA/SCAI coronary revascularization guidelines).[7] In patients presenting with acute coronary syndrome secondary to an acute graft occlusion or stenosis with native vessel being chronically occluded, PCI of the culprit SVG is urgently performed to minimize myocardial injury, but the long-term graft patency is poor. Staged revascularization of the corresponding native coronary artery could provide superior long-term patency.

Percutaneous revascularization is generally preferred over surgical revascularization in patients with prior CABG, given the higher risk of repeat CABG compared with first CABG and comparable postprocedural outcomes.[14] Factors favoring repeat CABG include vessels unsuitable for PCI, multiple diseased bypass grafts, availability of the IMA for grafting chronically occluded coronary arteries, and good distal targets for bypass graft placement.[15] In contrast, factors favoring PCI over CABG include limited areas of ischemia-causing symptoms, suitable PCI targets, a patent graft to the LAD, poor CABG targets, and comorbid conditions.[15] Additional contraindications to redo CABG are porcelain aorta and IMA bypass conduit course under the sternum.

BYPASS GRAFT ANATOMY AND ENGAGEMENT

Knowledge of bypass graft anatomy is critical for optimizing cardiac catheterization and interventions among prior CABG patients. When the anatomy is not known, more contrast, fluoroscopy time, and catheters are needed to identify all patent grafts.[16] Graft markers are very helpful for engaging bypass grafts but are not used in most patients. Review of prior coronary and bypass graft angiograms is extremely helpful. In nonurgent cases, multidetector computed tomography (MDCT) can provide adequate visualization of SVGs given their reduced motion and large lumens. MDCT has 96% sensitivity and 95% specificity for evaluating graft patency.[17,18]

In the left anterior oblique view, SVGs to the left coronary artery usually arise from the left and to the right coronary artery from the right side of the aorta. The SVG to the obtuse marginal artery is likely to be the highest graft originating from the left side of the aorta, and SVG to the LAD is usually the lowest.

In patients with unknown CABG anatomy, performance of bilateral subclavian artery angiography can help assess whether one or both IMAs are utilized as grafts, and whether proximal subclavian artery stenosis is present, which could lead to subclavian steal.[19] Alternatively, the pressure gradient on pull back from the subclavian artery into the aorta can be used to evaluate for proximal subclavian artery stenosis supplying the IMA. In some patients when grafts arising in the aorta cannot be engaged, aortography is performed, usually in the left anterior oblique projection to evaluate for graft patency and assist with graft localization.

Engagement of SVGs for angiography and/or PCI can be performed using either a femoral or a radial approach; femoral access makes engagement easiest and was associated with lower utilization of contrast and radiation in one of the two randomized trials performed to date.[20] The RADIAL Versus Femoral Access for Coronary Artery Bypass Graft Angiography and Intervention (RADIAL CABG) trial reported that diagnostic coronary angiography via radial access was associated with a higher mean contrast volume (142 ± 39 mL vs 171 ± 72 mL, $P < .01$), longer procedure time (21.9 ± 6.8 minutes vs 34.2 ± 14.7 minutes, $P < .01$), greater patient air kerma radiation exposure (1.08 ± 0.54 Gy vs 1.29 ± 0.67 Gy, $P = .06$), and higher operator radiation doses (first operator: 1.3 ± 1.0 mrem vs 2.6 ± 1.7 mrem, $P < .01$), as compared with femoral access.[20] In contrast, the Left Radial comparEd to Femoral Approach for COronary Angiography in Patients With Previous CABG StuDy (L-RECORD) trial did not show significant differences in procedure time, radiation, and fluoroscopy dose for radial versus femoral access.[21] When radial access is utilized and graft engagement is challenging, early conversion to femoral access should be considered.[22]

If graft intervention is needed, obtaining adequate guide catheter support is critical. This can be accomplished by using larger-sized guide catheters (7 or 8 Fr), supportive guide catheter shapes (such as Amplatz), or by employing deep graft intubation – for example, using a guide catheter extension.[23] The multipurpose guide is most commonly used for SVGs to the right coronary/posterior descending artery and the Amplatz left for left-sided grafts.

ADJUNCTIVE PHARMACOTHERAPY

Anticoagulation can be achieved with either unfractionated heparin or bivalirudin. A significant difference between native vessel and SVG PCI is that glycoprotein (GP) IIb/IIIa inhibitors are not beneficial in SVG PCI[24] and may be harmful.[25] Hence, GP IIb/IIIa inhibitors should not be used in SVG interventions, with the possible exception of heavily thrombotic lesions. However, in the NCDR, GP IIb/IIIa inhibitors were used in 40% of SVG PCI in the United States between 2004 and 2009.[26] The 2011 ACC/AHA PCI guidelines state that "platelet GP IIb/IIIa inhibitors are not beneficial as adjunctive therapy during SVG PCI" (class III, level of evidence B).[15]

Prehospital administration of antiplatelet therapy (single or dual) has been associated with lower MACE after SVG intervention compared with placebo.[27] In one study, higher rates of death and myocardial infarction were observed after clopidogrel discontinuation at 12 months, suggesting that prolonged dual antiplatelet therapy may be beneficial in these patients.[28] DAPT has been associated with benefit in SVG lesions and is part of the DAPT score[29] that can help select patients likely to derive benefit from prolonged (30-month) versus standard (12-month) DAPT duration.

Intragraft vasodilators, such as adenosine,[30] nitroprusside,[31] nicardipine,[32] and verapamil,[33] might also be useful in preventing no-reflow and periprocedural myocardial infarction during SVG interventions and are often used due to low cost and risk, but they have not been proven to be effective in randomized controlled trials.

CHOICE OF STENTS IN SVGS

Several studies have compared various PCI techniques in SVGs (**Table 24.1**).

The Saphenous Vein De Novo (SAVED) trial compared bare-metal stent (BMS) implantation to balloon angioplasty. Although the study missed its primary angiographic endpoint (6-month binary angiographic restenosis), it demonstrated that compared with balloon angioplasty, BMS implantation was associated with improved procedural success and lower incidence of the composite endpoint of death, myocardial infarction, and TVR at 6 months.[34] Similar results were observed in the Venestent trial,[35] and stent implantation became the standard of care for the percutaneous treatment of SVG lesions. Stenting is overall recommended in SVG PCI, although in the cases of distal anastomotic lesions, balloon angioplasty may suffice, especially if the graft may be needed for retrograde option for recanalization of the chronically occluded native vessel in the future.

Covered stents were subsequently developed and tested in SVGs in an attempt to reduce the rates of distal embolization and periprocedural myocardial infarction. Nevertheless, none of four randomized trials showed a decrease in the incidence of periprocedural myocardial infarction,[36-39] and covered stents also had higher risk for subsequent myocardial infarction and thrombotic occlusion.[39] As a result, covered stents are currently used in SVGs only for the treatment of perforations.

The 2011 ACC/AHA guidelines state, "Drug eluting stents (DES) are generally preferred over bare metal stents (BMS)" for SVG lesions.[15] Whether drug-eluting stents (DESs) provide better outcomes in SVGs has been controversial for several years. Five randomized controlled trials have compared DES with BMS in SVG lesions (**Table 24.1**).

The Reduction of Restenosis in Saphenous Vein Grafts with Cypher (RRISC) sirolimus-eluting stent trial compared a sirolimus-eluting stent (SESCypher, Cordis, Warren, NJ) with a BMS of similar design in 75 patients[40,41] and reported lower rates of angiographic restenosis and lower incidence of target lesion revascularization at 6 months with the use of SES. Nevertheless, during long-term follow-up (median, 32 months), mortality was higher in the SES group (29% vs 0%, $P = .001$), and there was no reduction with DES in the incidence of TVR.[41] The RRISC study raised concerns about the long-term safety of DES in SVGs, but these results have not been replicated in subsequent studies, and it is highly

TABLE 24.1 Large Published Trials of Stenting for Saphenous Vein Graft Lesions

TRIAL	YEAR	N	PRIMARY ENDPOINT	BARE-METAL STENT EVENT RATE (%)	OTHER GROUP EVENT RATE (%)	P
BMSs vs Balloon Angioplasty						
SAVED[34]	1997	220	6-mo angiographic restenosis	37	46	.24
Venestent[35]	2003	150	6-mo angiographic restenosis	19.1	32.8	.069
BMSs vs Covered Stents						
RECOVERS[36]	2003	301	6-mo angiographic restenosis	24.8	24.2	.237
STING[37]	2003	211	6-mo angiographic restenosis	20	29	.15
SYMBIOT III[38]	2006	700	8-mo angiographic percent diameter stenosis	30.9	31.9	.80
BARRICADE[39]	2011	243	8-mo angiographic restenosis	28.4	31.8	.63
BMSs vs DESs						
RRISC	2006[40]	75	6-mo angiographic restenosis	32.6	13.6	.031
	2007[41]		MACE at 32 mo	41	58	.13
SOS	2009[42]	80	12-mo angiographic restenosis	51	9	<.001
	2010[43]	80	Target vessel failure at 35 mo	72	34	.001
ISAR-CABG	2011[44]	610	12-mo composite of death, MI and TLR	22	15	.02
	2018[45]	610	5 y composite of death, MI and TLR	53.6	55.5	.89
BASKET-SAVAGE[46]	2016	173	12-mo composite of cardiac death, MI, and TVR	17.9	2.3	<.001
	2020	173	5 y composite of cardiac death, MI, and TVR	56.1	35.5	<.001
DIVA[47]	2017	597	12-mo composite of cardiac death, target vessel MI, and TLR	19%	17%	.67

BARRICADE, Barrier Approach to Restenosis: Restrict Intima to Curtail Adverse Events Trial; BASKET-SAVAGE, Study to Test the Efficacy and Safety of Drug Eluting Versus Bare-Metal Stents for Saphenous Vein Graft Interventions; BMS, bare-metal stent; DES, drug-eluting stent; ISAR-CABG, Is Drug-Eluting-Stenting Associated with Improved Results in Coronary Artery Bypass Grafts? trial; MACE, major adverse cardiac event; MI, myocardial infarction; RECOVERS, European multicenter Randomized Evaluation of polytetrafluoroethylene COVERed stent in Saphenous vein grafts Trial; RRISC, Reduction of Restenosis In Saphenous vein grafts with Cypher sirolimus-eluting stent Trial; SAVED, Saphenous Vein De Novo trial; SOS, Stenting Of Saphenous vein grafts trial; STING, Stents IN Grafts trial; SYMBIOT III, A Prospective, Randomized Trial of a Self-Expanding PTFE Stent Graft During SVG Intervention; TLR, target lesion revascularization; TVR, target vessel revascularization.

unusual for patients undergoing SVG PCI with BMSs to have 0% mortality for nearly 3 years (mortality during the first-year post-SVG PCI is approximately 5% in most series). Also, most patients in the study died due to noncardiac causes or cardiac causes unrelated to the target SVG.

The Stenting of Saphenous Vein Grafts (SOS) trial compared a paclitaxel-eluting stent (Taxus, Boston Scientific, Natick, MA) with a similar BMS in 80 patients and reported reduced angiographic stenosis and lower incidence of repeat revascularization and myocardial infarction with DESs during early and long-term follow-up.[42,43]

Both the RRISC and SOS trials had a primary angiographic endpoint and were underpowered for clinical events. The "Is Drug-Eluting-Stenting Associated with Improved Results in Coronary Artery Bypass Grafts?" (ISAR-CABG) study was the largest randomized controlled trial performed to date in SVGs and demonstrated that implantation of first-generation DESs (sirolimus eluting and paclitaxel eluting) significantly reduced the incidence of target lesion revascularization (7% vs 13%, $P = .01$) compared with BMSs, without significant differences in the incidence of all-cause death (5% vs 5%, $P = .83$), myocardial infarction (5% vs 6%, $P = .27$), and definite or probable stent thrombosis (1% vs 1%, $P = .99$).[44] However, the advantage of DESs over BMSs demonstrated at 1 year was lost at 5 years due to higher attrition of efficacy in the DES group.[45] The Basel Kosten Effektivitäts Trial-SAphenous Venous Graft Angioplasty Using GP IIa/IIIb Receptor Inhibitors and Drug-Eluting Stents (BASKET-SAVAGE, $n = 173$) revealed a lower incidence of MACEs with the Taxus DES, compared with BMS at 12 months (2.3% vs 17.9%, $P < .001$) and 3 years (12.4% vs 29.8%, $P = .0012$), driven mainly by lower TVR in the DES group (19.1% vs 4.5% at 3 years).[46] Five-year MACE rates remained lower in the DES compared with the BMS arm (35.5% vs 56.1%, hazard ratio, 0.40; 95% CI, 0.23-0.68, $P < .001$); a landmark analysis from 1 to 5 years revealed a persistent benefit of DES over BMS (hazard ratio, 0.33; 95% CI, 0.13-0.74, $P = .007$) in terms of TVR.[46] The Drug-Eluting Stents versus Bare Metal Stents in Saphenous Vein Graft Angioplasty (DIVA) trial was a double-blind randomized controlled trial including 599 patients with significant SVG lesion requiring PCI with intent-to-use embolic protection. At 12 months and over a median follow-up of 2.7 years, the study showed similar incidence of target vessel failure with DES (88% second generation) and BMS (37% for DES and 34% for BMS over entire length of follow-up; adjusted hazard ratio of 1.10; $P = .44$).[47] In contrast to ISAR-CABG, DIVA used second-generation DESs in most patients, was a blinded study, and did not have routine angiographic follow-up.

In summary, based on the results of ISAR-CABG and DIVA, BMS and DES have similar outcomes in de novo SVG lesions.

EMBOLIC PROTECTION DEVICES

SVG lesions are complex. Morphologically, SVG atherosclerosis tends to be diffuse, concentric, and friable with a poorly developed or absent fibrous cap and little evidence of calcification. Intimal hyperplasia, defined as the accumulation of smooth muscle cells and extracellular matrix in the intima, is the major disease process in SVGs between 1 month and 1 year after implantation. This process, in itself, rarely produces significant stenosis but creates the foundation for later development of SVG atheroma. Histologically, SVG atheromas have more foam cells and inflammatory cells, including multinucleate giant cells, than native coronary atheromas with appearance similar to experimental models of immune-mediated atherosclerosis and are associated with severe angiographic degeneration and friable atheroma.[48] Thus, SVG interventions may be complicated by distal embolization causing periprocedural myocardial infarction and no reflow.

Potential interventions to reduce distal embolization and no reflow include the use of embolic protection devices (EPDs), intragraft vasodilator administration such as adenosine, nitroprusside, nicardipine, and verapamil, use of GP IIb/IIIa inhibitors, direct stenting without predilatation, use of excimer laser atherectomy, and implantation of undersized stents.[49] High-pressure balloon inflations should be avoided in SVGs due to the risk of distal embolization and perforation. The only strategy, however, that has been shown to reduce the risk of no reflow and improved outcomes in a randomized controlled trial is the use of EPD.[50] EPDs capture the debris from friable atheromas during PCI before it enters the microcirculation (**Fig. 24.1** and **Table 24.2**).

The Saphenous vein graft Angioplasty Free of Emboli Randomized (SAFER) trial[50] randomized 801 patients undergoing SVG PCI to stenting over a standard wire versus PCI with the use of a distal occlusion balloon EPD (GuardWire, Medtronic Vascular, Santa Rosa, CA; **Fig. 24.2**). In the SAFER trial, the primary endpoint (a composite of death, myocardial infarction, emergency bypass, or target lesion revascularization by 30 days) occurred in 65 patients (16.5%) assigned to control versus 39 patients (9.6%) assigned to the EPD (P = .004). This 42% relative reduction in

Embolic Protection Devices available in the US for SVG interventions in 2012

Device	Manufacturer	Approval date
Guardwire	Medtronic	6/2001
Filterwire	Boston Scientific	6/2003
Spider	ev3	6/2006

FIGURE 24.1 Embolic protection devices available in the United States for SVG interventions in 2023. SVG, saphenous vein graft.

MACEs was driven by a reduction in the incidence of myocardial infarction (8.6% vs 14.7%, P = .008) and the "no-reflow" phenomenon (3% vs 9%, P = .02).

Given the results of SAFER trial, subsequent EPD studies utilized a noninferiority design, because it was considered unethical denying patients the benefits associated with EPD use.[51-56] Several devices were shown to be noninferior to the GuardWire (**Table 24.2**), yet only two of those are currently available in the United States: the FilterWire (Boston Scientific, Natick, MA, **Fig. 24.3**), and the Spider (ev3, Plymouth, MN). A proximal occlusion device (Proxis, St Jude) was clinically available in the past, but production was discontinued in 2012.

Based on the results of these studies, the 2011 ACC/AHA PCI guidelines recommended routine use of EPD in SVG lesions as a class I indication, level of evidence B.[15] Despite these recommendations, EPDs are underutilized in SVG interventions. In the NCDR Cath PCI Registry and British Cardiovascular Intervention Society

TABLE 24.2 Major Published Trials of Embolic Protection in SVGs

TRIAL	YEAR	N	PRIMARY ENDPOINT			
EPD VS NO EPD				**EPD EVENT RATE (%)**	**CONTROL GROUP EVENT RATE (%)**	***P* SUPERIORITY**
SAFER[50]	2002	801	30-d composite of death, MI, emergency CABG, or TLR	(GuardWire) 9.6	16.5	0.004
EPD vs Another EPD				**Test EPD event rate (%)**	**Control EPD Event Rate (%)**	**p Noninferiority**
FIRE[51]	2003	651	30-d composite of death, MI, or TVR	(FilterWire) 9.9	(GuardWire) 11.6	0.0008
SPIDER[52]	2005	732	30-d composite of death, MI, urgent CABG, or TVR	(Spider) 9.1	(GuardWire 24% or FilterWire 76%) 8.4	0.012
PRIDE[53]	2005	631	30-d composite of cardiac death, MI, or TLR	(Triactiv) 11.2	(FilterWire) 10.1	0.02
CAPTIVE[54]	2006	652	30-d composite of death, MI, or TVR	(Cardioshield) 11.4	(GuardWire) 9.1	0.057
PROXIMAL[55]	2007	594	30-d composite of death, MI, or TVR	(Proxis) 9.2	(GuardWire 19% or FilterWire 81%) 10.0	0.006
AMETHYST[56]	2008	797	30-d composite of death, MI, or urgent repeat revascularization	(Interceptor Plus) 8.0	(GuardWire 72% or FilterWire 18%) 7.3	0.025

GuardWire, Medtronic Vascular, Santa Rosa, CA; FilterWire, Boston Scientific, Natick, MA; SPIDER, ev3, Plymouth, MN; Triactive, Kensey Nash Corp, Exton, PA; Cardioshield, MedNova, Galway; Proxis, St Jude Medical, Minneapolis, MN; Interceptor Plus, Medtronic Vascular.

AMETHYST, Assessment of the Medtronic AVE Interceptor Saphenous Vein Graft Filter System; CABG, coronary artery bypass graft surgery; CAPTIVE, CardioShield Application Protects during Transluminal Intervention of Vein grafts by reducing Emboli; EPD, embolic protection device; FIRE, FilterWire EX Randomized Evaluation; MI, myocardial infarction; PRIDE, Protection During Saphenous Vein Graft Intervention to Prevent Distal Embolization; PROXIMAL, Proximal Protection During Saphenous Vein Graft Intervention; SAFER, Saphenous vein graft Angioplasty Free of Emboli Randomized; SPIDER, Saphenous Vein Graft Protection in a Distal Embolic Protection Randomized Trial; TLR, target lesion revascularization; TVR, target vessel revascularization.

databases, in contemporary PCI, EPDs were being used in only 14% to 21% of patients.[57,58] In the ISAR CABG trial, an EPD was used in less than 1% of the study patients. Subsequent observational studies exploring the "real-world" benefits of EPDs provided conflicting findings.[59,60] A meta-analysis of 2 randomized studies and six observational reports showed no benefit with the use of EPDs in SVG PCI.[59] There was no significant difference in all-cause mortality, MACE, TVR, periprocedural MI, and late MI (OR, 0.80; CI, 0.52-1.23; $P = .30$) between the two groups. Based on these data, the recommendation for routine use of EPD in SVG PCI was downgraded to class 2a in the 2021 ACC/AHA/SCAI guideline for coronary artery revascularization.[7]

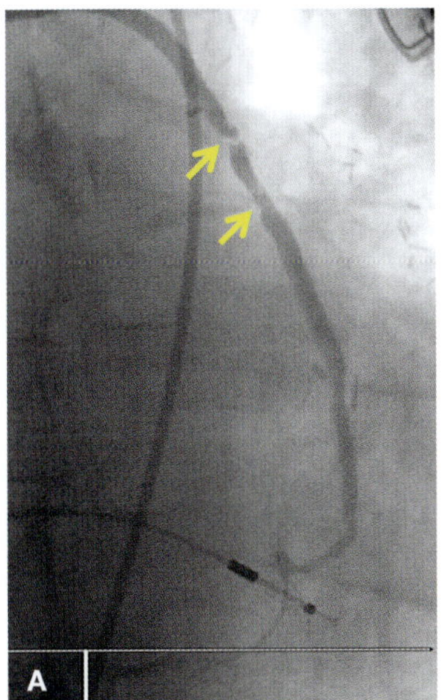

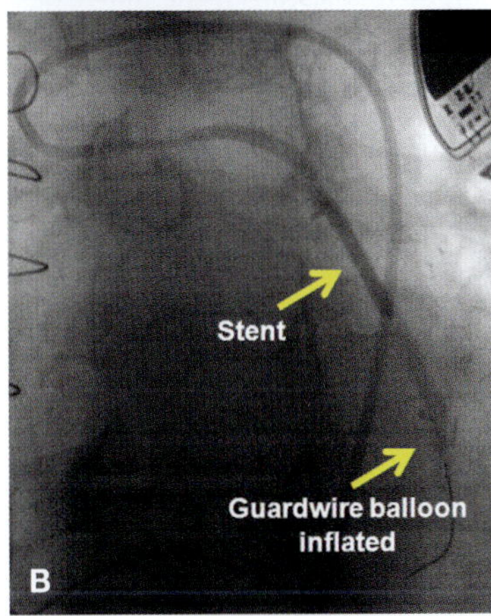

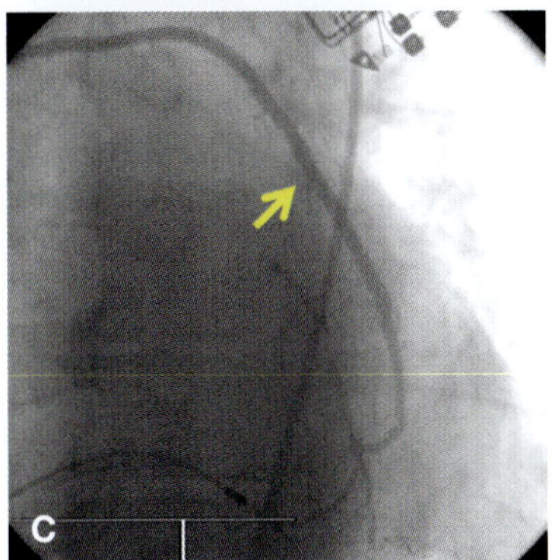

FIGURE 24.2 Saphenous vein graft intervention using the GuardWire (Medtronic Vascular, Santa Rosa, CA). Coronary angiography demonstrating a lesion in the body of the saphenous vein graft (*arrows*, **panel A**). A stent was implanted after inflation of the GuardWire balloon distally (**panel B**), with an excellent final angiographic result (**panel C**).

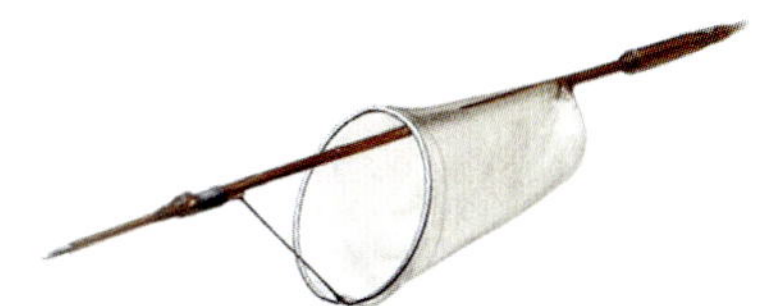

Filterwire	
Design	Polyurethane filter basket
Guide catheter	6 French
Pore size	110 µm
Diameters	2.25-3.5 and 3.5-5.5
Length	300 cm, 190 cm
Crossing profile	3.2 French
Landing zone	>25 mm (2.25) or >30 mm (3.5)

110-micron-pore polyurethane filter
Nosecone
Catheter stop
Spinner tube
Radiopaque spring coil tip
PTFE coated wire 0.014"
Suspension arm
Radiopaque NiTi Loop

FIGURE 24.3 Description of the FilterWire (Image provided courtesy of Boston Scientific. ©2024 Boston Scientific Corporation or its affiliates. All rights reserved.)

Ostial, proximal, and SVG body lesions can be protected with a filter, whereas distal anastomotic lesions cannot be protected with any of the currently available devices (**Fig. 24.4**). Use of a filter requires the presence of an adequately long landing zone. EPDs may not be necessary for the treatment of SVG in-stent restenotic lesions because these fibrotic lesions are less likely to cause distal embolization and myocardial infarction.[60] Use of a buddy wire should be avoided when using a filter due to risk of inadvertent stenting over the buddy wire leading to filter entrapment.[61]

SPECIAL LESION SUBSETS

SVG Acute Occlusions

Acute SVG thrombosis can be challenging to treat due to large thrombus burden, diffuse SVG degeneration, and high recurrent SVG failure rates.[62] Aggressive use of thrombectomy and EPDs is often required to restore luminal patency. Excimer laser can cause thrombus vaporization, with low risk of distal embolization.[63] If thrombectomy fails, one approach is to perform balloon angioplasty with an undersized balloon to restore TIMI 1-2 flow followed by anticoagulation for 1 to 2 weeks in addition to antiplatelet therapy before proceeding with stent implantation.[64] Even if acute recanalization is achieved, long-term SVG patency is low.[62] Alternative revascularization approaches, such as PCI of the bypassed native coronary artery,[65] may provide better outcomes,[1,12] but these can be challenging procedures, requiring dedicated equipment and expertise.[66]

SVG Chronic Total Occlusions

In chronic occlusion of an SVG, PCI of the SVG has been associated with low success rates and high likelihood of requiring repeat intervention

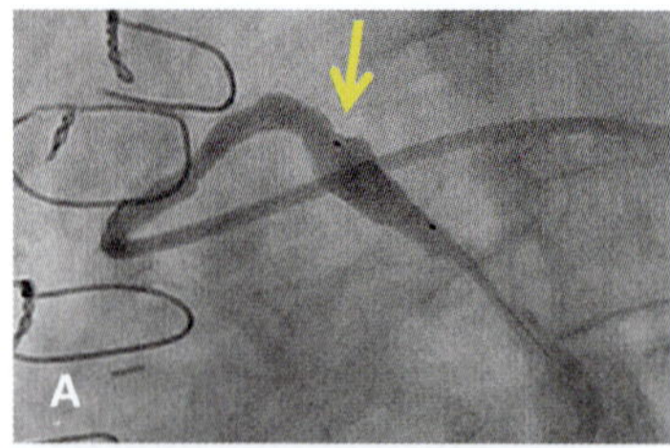

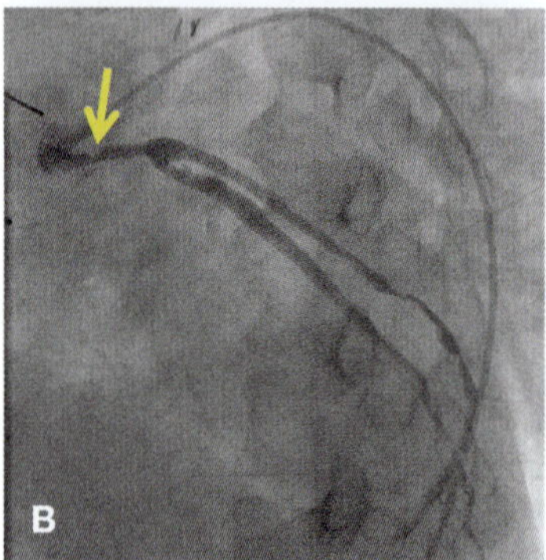

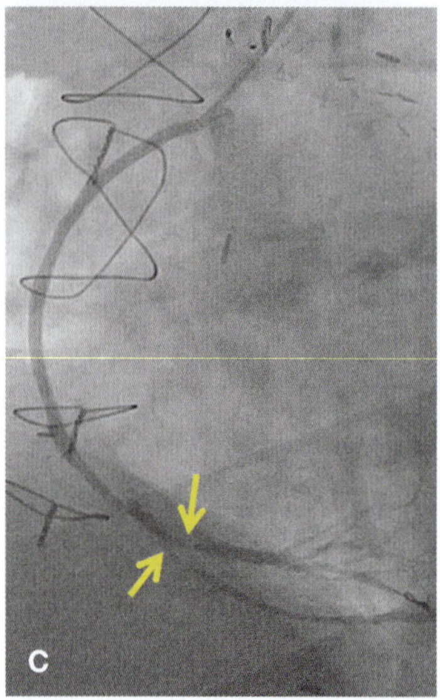

FIGURE 24.4 Saphenous vein graft lesions in which an embolic protection device could not be used because of the large caliber of the graft (**panel A**), lesion located proximal to a Y-graft bifurcation (**panel B**), or because of lesion location at the distal SVG anastomosis (**panel C**).

and is a class III recommendation in the 2021 ACC/AHA/SCAI coronary revascularization guidelines.[7] In a series of 34 patients undergoing SVG chronic total occlusion PCI, procedural success was achieved in 23 patients (68%); during a median follow-up of 18 months, 68% developed in-stent restenosis and 61% required TVR.[67]

Intermediate SVG Lesions

Unlike native coronary arteries, SVG intermediate lesions have high rates of progression.[68] Prophylactic stenting of such lesions with DES was associated with a lower rate of SVG disease progression and a trend toward a lower incidence of MACEs at 1-year follow-up compared with medical treatment alone in the Moderate *VE*in Graft *LE*sion Stenting With the *T*axus Stent and *I*ntravascular Ultrasound (VELETI) Pilot trial.[69] The VELETI trial was underpowered for clinical endpoints with a small sample size (*n* = 57). Nevertheless, the subsequent VELETI II study did not demonstrate benefit with prophylactic SVG stenting and was stopped prematurely for futility after randomizing 125 patients.[70] More studies are needed to justify routine stenting of intermediate SVG lesions.

Physiologic assessment using hyperemic or resting indices is used to determine the significance of native coronary vessel stenosis but has not been well studied in SVG lesions. Limited studies show that FFR has low sensitivity, but an acceptable specificity and negative predictive value compared with stress myocardial perfusion imaging in assessing the significance of SVG lesions[71]

ARTERIAL GRAFTS

PCI of arterial grafts is infrequent,[1] especially for IMA grafts that have high long-term patency rates.[3] PCI of IMA grafts is most commonly required at the distal anastomotic site and can be challenging due to (1) difficulty engaging the graft, especially in the presence of proximal subclavian artery tortuosity, (2) difficulty wiring and delivering equipment through the graft due to "pseudolesion" formation, and (3) difficulty reaching the target lesion, due to long graft length. Specialized catheters, such as the internal mammary VB (IM VB1) catheter, can facilitate IMA graft engagement, but occasionally using the ipsilateral radial access may be required. Using soft guide wires may decrease the risk for IMA kinking, and occasional use of shortened guide catheters may be required to allow balloon or stent delivery to a distal anastomotic lesion or to a lesion in the native vessel distal to the IMA anastomosis. Semicompliant balloons with a lower crossing profile are more likely to cross tortuous segments than noncompliant balloons.

INTRAVASCULAR ULTRASOUND

Use of intravascular ultrasound (IVUS) can assess thrombus burden and help with decision of performing thrombectomy or use of an EPD. Considering that SVGs have thin walls and are at higher risk of perforation with high-pressure predilatation or postdilatation, appropriate stent sizing is key and is facilitated by the use of IVUS. With coronary or graft perforation, patients with prior CABG do not normally develop circumferential effusions but are prone to developing localized effusions due to the presence of adhesions, which may not be amenable to percutaneous drainage. Saphenous vein or arterial graft perforation may occasionally cause hemoptysis, likely due to the proximity of the grafts with the lung parenchyma. Many operators prefer the use of an appropriately sized stent in the SVG based on IVUS and avoid or minimize stent postdilatation. On the contrary, stent undersizing in SVG PCI can hinder further equipment delivery and may result in stent deformation during attempts to pass equipment through it.

SVG ANEURYSMS

SVG aneurysm is defined as a focal dilatation of SVG greater than 1.5 times the proximal reference diameter (**Fig. 24.5**).[72] Although the mechanism of SVG aneurysm is poorly defined, it is postulated to result from wall stress in the setting of high pulsatile flow.[72-75] Risk of complications from SVG aneurysm range from 33.3% in

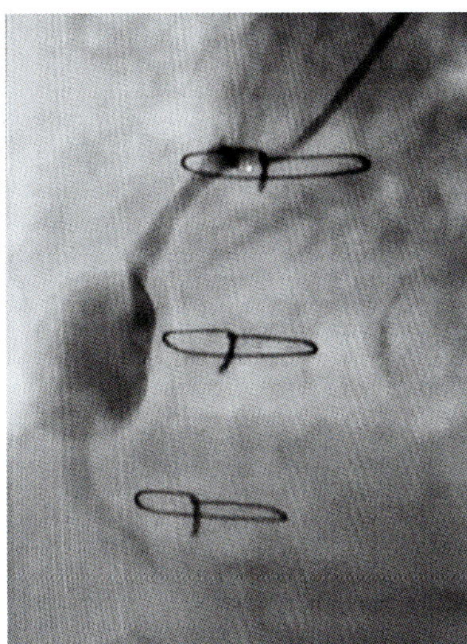

FIGURE 24.5 Aneurysm of the saphenous vein graft to the right coronary artery.

small aneurysms to 69.2% in large (>100 mm diameter) aneurysms and include angina, dyspnea, orthopnea, myocardial infarction from thrombus formation in the aneurysm with distal embolization, compression of surrounding structures, and sudden death from rupture.[76] SVG aneurysms can be treated surgically or percutaneously using covered stents. Alternatively, the corresponding native coronary artery can be recanalized followed by percutaneous closure of the aneurysm using vascular plugs or coils. Both the proximal and the distal segment of the aneurysmal SVG should be occluded to prevent continued blood flow and expansion of the SVG aneurysm.

Key Points

- SVG interventions currently account for approximately 6% of PCIs performed in the United States.
- GP IIb/IIIa inhibitors should not be used in SVG interventions.
- DESs are associated with similar clinical outcomes as BMSs in SVG lesions.
- In contrast to the SAFER trial that showed better outcomes with EPD use during SVG PCI, more recent observational studies did not show benefit (EPD use in SVG PCI carries a level IIa recommendation) during SVG PCI.
- Two EPDs are available for clinical use in SVGs in the United States in 2023: the FilterWire (Boston Scientific) and Spider (ev3).

For further review and interactivities, please see the chapter-based multiple choice questions and videos accessible in the complimentary eBook bundled with this text. Access instructions are located in the inside front cover.

References

1. Brilakis ES, Rao SV, Banerjee S, et al. Percutaneous coronary intervention in native arteries versus bypass grafts in prior coronary artery bypass grafting patients a report from the national cardiovascular data registry. *JACC Cardiovasc Interv*. 2011;4(8):844-850.
2. Zhao DX, Leacche M, Balaguer JM, et al. Routine intraoperative completion angiography after coronary artery bypass grafting and 1-stop hybrid revascularization results from a fully integrated hybrid catheterization laboratory/operating room. *J Am Coll Cardiol*. 2009;53(3):232-241.
3. Goldman S, Zadina K, Moritz T, et al. Long-term patency of saphenous vein and left internal mammary artery grafts after coronary artery bypass surgery results from a Department of Veterans Affairs Cooperative Study. *J Am Coll Cardiol*. 2004;44(11):2149-2156.
4. Widimsky P, Straka Z, Stros P, et al. One-year coronary bypass graft patency. A randomized comparison between off-pump and on-pump surgery angiographic results of the PRAGUE-4 trial. *Circulation*. 2004;110(22):3418-3423.
5. Cameron A, Davis KB, Green G, Schaff HV. Coronary bypass surgery with internal-thoracic-artery grafts — effects on survival over a 15-year period. *N Engl J Med*. 1996;334(4):216-219.
6. Guadino M, Benedetto U, Fremes S, et al. Radial-artery or saphenous-vein grafts in coronary-artery bypass surgery. *N Engl J Med*. 2018;378:2069-2077.
7. Writing Committee Members; Lawton JS, Tamis-Holland JE, Bangalore S, et al. 2021 ACC/AHA/SCAI guideline for coronary artery revascularization: a report of the American College of Cardiology/American Heart Association Joint Committee on clinical practice guidelines. *J Am Coll Cardiol*. 2022;79(2):e21-e129.
8. Gaudino M, Di Franco A, Rahouma M, et al. Un-measured confounders in observational studies comparing bilateral versus single internal thoracic artery for coronary artery bypass grafting: a meta-analysis. *J Am Heart Assoc*. 2018;7(1):e008010.
9. Gaudino M, Puskas JD, Di Franco A, et al. Three arterial grafts improve late survival: a meta-analysis of propensity-matched studies. *Circulation*. 2017;135(11):1036-1044.
10. Yanagawa B, Verma S, Mazine A, et al. Impact of total arterial revascularization on long term survival: asystematic review and meta-analysis of 130,305 patients. *Int J Cardiol*. 2017;233:29-36.
11. Schwann TA, Habib RH, Wallace A, et al. Operative outcomes of multiple-arterial versus single-arterialcoronary bypass grafting. *Ann Thorac Surg*. 2018;105(4):1109-1119.
12. Brilakis ES, O'Donnell CI, Penny W, et al. Percutaneous coronary intervention in native coronary arteries versus bypass grafts in patients with prior coronary artery bypass graft surgery: insights from the Veterans Affairs Clinical Assessment, Reporting, and Tracking Program. *JACC Cardiovasc Interv*. 2016;9:884-893.
13. Farag M, Gue YX, Brilakis ES, Egred M. Meta-analysis comparing outcomes of percutaneous coronary intervention of native artery versus bypass graft in patients with prior coronary artery bypass grafting. *Am J Cardiol*. 2021;140:47-54.
14. Morrison DA, Sethi G, Sacks J, et al. Percutaneous coronary intervention versus repeat bypass surgery for patients with medically refractory myocardial ischemia: AWESOME randomized trial and registry experience with post-CABG patients. *J Am Coll Cardiol*. 2002;40(11):1951-1954.
15. Levine GN, Bates ER, Blankenship JC, et al. 2011 ACCF/AHA/SCAI guideline for percutaneous coronary intervention. A report of the American College of Cardiology Foundation/American Heart Association task force on practice guidelines and the society for cardiovascular angiography and interventions. *J Am Coll Cardiol*. 2011;58(24):e44-e122.
16. Varghese I, Boatman DM, Peters CT, et al. Impact on contrast, fluoroscopy, and catheter utilization from knowing the coronary artery bypass graft anatomy before diagnostic coronary angiography. *Am J Cardiol*. 2008;101(12):1729-1732.
17. Kohsaka S, Makaryus AN. Coronary angiography using noninvasive imaging techniques of cardiac CT and MRI. *Curr Cardiol Rev*. 2008;4:323-330.
18. Schlosser T, Konorza T, Hunold P, Kühl H, Schmermund A, Barkhausen J. Noninvasive visualization of coronary artery bypass grafts using 16-detector row computed tomography. *J Am Coll Cardiol* 2004;44(6):1224-1229.

19. Dimas B, Lindsey JB, Banerjee S, Brilakis ES. ST-segment elevation acute myocardial infarction due to severe hypotension and proximal left subclavian artery stenosis in a prior coronary artery bypass graft patient. *Cardiovasc Revasc Med.* 2009;10(3):191-194.
20. Michael TT, Alomar M, Papayannis A, et al. A randomized comparison of the transradial and transfemoral approaches for coronary artery bypass graft angiography and intervention: the RADIAL-CABG trial (RADIAL versus Femoral Access for Coronary Artery Bypass Graft Angiography and Intervention). *JACC Cardiovasc Interv*. 2013;6(11):1138-1144.
21. Tsigkas G, Makris A, Tsiafoutis I, et al. The L-RECORD study. *JACC Cardiovasc Interv*. 2020;13(8):1014-1016.
22. Cooper L, Banerjee S, Brilakis ES. Crossover from radial to femoral access during a challenging percutaneous coronary intervention can make the difference between success and failure. *Cardiovasc Revasc Med.* 2010;11(4):266.e5-266.e8.
23. Farooq V, Mamas MA, Fath-Ordoubadi F, Fraser DG. The use of a guide catheter extension system as an aid during transradial percutaneous coronary intervention of coronary artery bypass grafts. *Catheter Cardiovasc Interv*. 2011;78(6):847-863.
24. Roffi M, Mukherjee D, Chew DP, et al. Lack of benefit from intravenous platelet glycoprotein IIb/IIIa receptor inhibition as adjunctive treatment for percutaneous interventions of aortocoronary bypass grafts: a pooled analysis of five randomized clinical trials. *Circulation*. 2002;106(24):3063-3067.
25. Coolong A, Baim DS, Kuntz RE, et al. Saphenous vein graft stenting and major adverse cardiac events: a predictive model derived from a pooled analysis of 3958 patients. *Circulation*. 2008;117(6):790-797.
26. Brilakis E, Wang TY, Rao SV, et al. Frequency and predictors of drug-eluting stent use in saphenous vein bypass graft percutaneous coronary interventions: a report from the American College of Cardiology National Cardiovascular Data CathPCI Registry. *JACC Cardiovasc Interv*. 2010;3(10):1068-1073.
27. Harskamp RE, Beijk MA, Damman P, Tijssen JG, Lopes RD, de Winter RJ. Prehospitalization antiplatelet therapy and outcomes after saphenous vein graft intervention. *Am J Cardiol*. 2013;111(2):153-158.
28. Sachdeva A, Bavisetty S, Beckham G, et al. Discontinuation of long term clopidogrel therapy is associated with death and myocardial infarction after saphenous vein graft percutaneous coronary intervention. *J Am Coll Cardiol*. 2012;60(23):2357-2363.
29. Yeh RW, Secemsky EA, Kereiakes DJ, et al. Development and validation of a prediction rule for benefit and harm of dual antiplatelet therapy beyond 1 year after percutaneous coronary intervention. *JAMA*. 2016;315(16):1735-1749.
30. Sdringola S, Assali A, Ghani M, et al. Adenosine use during aortocoronary vein graft interventions reverses but does not prevent the slow-no reflow phenomenon. *Catheter Cardiovasc Interv*. 2000;51(4):394-399.
31. Zoghbi GJ, Goyal M, Hage F, et al. Pretreatment with nitroprusside for microcirculatory protection in saphenous vein graft interventions. *J Invasive Cardiol*. 2009;21(2):34-39.
32. Fischell TA, Subraya RG, Ashraf K, Perry B, Haller S. "Pharmacologic" distal protection using prophylactic, intragraft nicardipine to prevent no-reflow and non-Q-wave myocardial infarction during elective saphenous vein graft intervention. *J Invasive Cardiol*. 2007;19(2):58-62.
33. Michaels AD, Appleby M, Otten MH, et al. Pretreatment with intragraft verapamil prior to percutaneous coronary intervention of saphenous vein graft lesions: results of the randomized, controlled vasodilator prevention on no-reflow (VAPOR) trial. *J Invasive Cardiol*. 2002;14(6):299-302.
34. Savage MP, Douglas JS Jr, Fischman DL, et al. Stent placement compared with balloon angioplasty for obstructed coronary bypass grafts. Saphenous Vein De Novo Trial Investigators. *N Engl J Med*. 1997;337(11):740-747.
35. Hanekamp CE, Koolen JJ, Den Heijer P, et al. Randomized study to compare balloon angioplasty and elective stent implantation in venous bypass grafts: the Venestent study. *Catheter Cardiovasc Interv*. 2003;60(4):452-457.
36. Stankovic G, Colombo A, Presbitero P, et al. Randomized evaluation of polytetrafluoroethylene-covered stent in saphenous vein grafts: the randomized evaluation of polytetrafluoroethylene COVERed stent in Saphenous vein grafts (RECOVERS) Trial. *Circulation*. 2003;108(1):37-42.
37. Schachinger V, Hamm CW, Münzel T, et al. A randomized trial of polytetrafluoroethylene-membrane-covered stents compared with conventional stents in aortocoronary saphenous vein grafts. *J Am Coll Cardiol*. 2003;42(8):1360-1369.
38. Turco MA, Buchbinder M, Popma JJ, et al. Pivotal, randomized U.S. study of the Symbiot™ covered stent system in patients with saphenous vein graft disease: eight-month angiographic and clinical results from the Symbiot III trial. *Catheter Cardiovasc Interv*. 2006;68(3):379-388.
39. Stone GW, Goldberg S, O'Shaughnessy C, et al. 5-year follow-up of polytetrafluoroethylene-covered stents compared with bare-metal stents in aortocoronary saphenous vein grafts the randomized BARRICADE (barrier approach to restenosis: restrict intima to curtail adverse events) trial. *JACC Cardiovasc Interv*. 2011;4(3):300-309.
40. Vermeersch P, Agostoni P, Verheye S, et al. Randomized double-blind comparison of sirolimus-eluting stent versus bare-metal stent implantation in diseased saphenous vein grafts: six-month angiographic, intravascular ultrasound, and clinical follow-up of the RRISC Trial. *J Am Coll Cardiol*. 2006;48(12):2423-2431.
41. Vermeersch P, Agostoni P, Verheye S, et al. Increased late mortality after sirolimus-eluting stents versus bare-metal stents in diseased saphenous vein grafts: results from the randomized DELAYED RRISC Trial. *J Am Coll Cardiol*. 2007;50(3):261-267.
42. Brilakis ES, Lichtenwalter C, de Lemos JA, et al. A randomized controlled trial of a paclitaxel-eluting stent versus a similar bare-metal stent in saphenous vein graft lesions the SOS (Stenting of Saphenous Vein Grafts) trial. *J Am Coll Cardiol*. 2009;53(11):919-928.
43. Brilakis ES, Lichtenwalter C, Abdel-karim AR, et al. Continued benefit from paclitaxel-eluting compared with bare-metal stent implantation in saphenous vein graft lesions during long-term follow-up of the SOS (Stenting of Saphenous Vein Grafts) trial. *JACC Cardiovasc Interv*. 2011;4(2):176-182.
44. Mehilli J, Pache J, Abdel-Wahab M, et al. Drug-eluting versus bare-metal stents in saphenous vein graft lesions (ISAR-CABG): a randomised controlled superiority trial. *Lancet*. 2011;378(9796):1071-1078.
45. Colleran R, Kufner S, Mehilli J, et al. Efficacy over time with drug-eluting stents in saphenous vein graft lesions. *J Am Coll Cardiol*. 2018;71(18):1973-1982.
46. Fahrni G, Farah A, Engstrøm T, et al. Long-term results after drug-eluting versus bare-metal stent implantation in saphenous vein grafts: randomized controlled trial. *J Am Heart Assoc*. 2020;9(20):e017434.
47. Brilakis ES, Edson R, Bhatt DL, et al. Drug-eluting stents versus bare-metal stents in saphenous vein grafts: a double-blind, randomised trial. *Lancet*. 2018;391(10134):1997-2007.
48. Motwani JG, Topol EJ. Aortocoronary saphenous vein graft disease. Pathogenesis, predisposition, and prevention. *Circulation*. 1998;97(9):916-931.
49. Bhatt DL. ***Cardiovascular Intervention: A Companion to Braunwalkd's Heart Disease***. 1st ed. Elsevier; 2015.
50. Baim DS, Wahr D, George B, et al. Randomized trial of a distal embolic protection device during percutaneous intervention of saphenous vein aorto-coronary bypass grafts. *Circulation*. 2002;105(11):1285-1290.
51. Stone GW, Rogers C, Hermiller J, et al. Randomized comparison of distal protection with a filter-based catheter and a balloon occlusion and aspiration system during percutaneous intervention of diseased saphenous vein aorto-coronary bypass grafts. *Circulation*. 2003;108(5):548-553.
52. Dixon SR. *Saphenous vein graft protection in a distal embolic protection randomized trial*. Paper presented at *Transcatheter Cardiovascular Therapeutics 2005*; October 18, 2005;Washington, DC.
53. Carrozza JP Jr, Mumma M, Breall JA, et al. Randomized evaluation of the TriActiv balloon-protection flush and extraction system for the treatment of saphenous vein graft disease. *J Am Coll Cardiol*. 2005;46(9):1677-1683.
54. Holmes DR, Coolong A, O'Shaughnessy C, et al. Comparison of the CardioShield filter with the guardwire balloon in the prevention of embolisation during vein graft intervention: results from the CAPTIVE randomised trial. *EuroIntervention*. 2006;2:161-168.
55. Mauri L, Cox D, Hermiller J, et al. The PROXIMAL trial: proximal protection during saphenous vein graft intervention using the Proxis embolic protection system—a randomized, prospective, multicenter clinical trial. *J Am Coll Cardiol*. 2007;50(15):1442-1449.
56. Kereiakes DJ, Turco MA, Breall J, et al. A novel filter-based distal embolic protection device for percutaneous intervention of saphenous vein

graft lesions: results of the AMEthyst randomized controlled trial. *JACC Cardiovasc Interv*. 2008;1(3):248-257.
57. Brennan JM, Al-Hejily W, Dai D, et al. Three-year outcomes associated with embolic protection in saphenous vein graft intervention: results in 49 325 senior patients in the medicare-linked national cardiovascular data registry cath PCI registry. *Circ Cardiovasc Interv*. 2015;8(3):e001403.
58. Shoaib A, Kinnaird T, Curzen N, et al. Outcomes following percutaneous coronary intervention in saphenous vein grafts with and without embolic protection devices. *JACC Cardiovasc Interv*. 2019;12(22):2286-2295.
59. Paul TK, Bhatheja S, Panchal HB, et al. Outcomes of saphenous vein graft intervention with and without embolic protection device: a comprehensive review and meta-analysis. *Circ Cardiovasc Interv*. 2017;10(12): e005538.
60. Ashby DT, Dangas G, Aymong EA, et al. Effect of percutaneous coronary interventions for in-stent restenosis in degenerated saphenous vein grafts without distal embolic protection. *J Am Coll Cardiol*. 2003;41(5):749-752.
61. Gutierrez A, Chugh Y, Kostantinis S, Brilakis ES. The perils of buddy wire use with a filterwire. *Cardiovasc Revasc Med*. 2022;40S:214-217.
62. Abdel Karim AR, Banerjee S, Brilakis ES. Percutaneous intervention of acutely occluded saphenous vein grafts: contemporary techniques and outcomes. *J Invasive Cardiol*. 2010;22(6):253-257.
63. Ebersole D, Dahm JB, Das T, et al. Excimer laser revascularization of saphenous vein grafts in acute myocardial infarction. *J Invasive Cardiol*. 2004;16(4):177-180.
64. Fiorina C, Meliga E, Chizzola G, et al. Early experience with a new approach for percutaneous of totally occluded saphenous vein graft: is the flow the best thrombolytic? *Eurointervention*. 2010;6(4):461-466.
65. Nguyen-Trong PK, Alaswad K, Karmpaliotis D, et al. Use of saphenous vein bypass grafts for retrograde recanalization of coronary chronic total occlusions: insights from a Multicenter Registry. *J Invasive Cardiol*. 2016;28(6):218-224.
66. Brilakis ES, Banerjee S, Lombardi WL. Retrograde recanalization of native coronary artery chronic occlusions via acutely occluded vein grafts. *Catheter Cardiovasc Interv*. 2010;75(1):109-113.
67. Al-Lamee R, Ielasi A, Latib A, et al. Clinical and angiographic outcomes after percutaneous recanalization of chronic total saphenous vein graft occlusion using modern techniques. *Am J Cardiol*. 2010;106(12):1721-1727.
68. Ellis SG, Brener SJ, DeLuca S, et al. Late myocardial ischemic events after saphenous vein graft intervention—importance of initially "nonsignificant" vein graft lesions. *Am J Cardiol*. 1997;79(11):1460-1464.
69. Rodes-Cabau J, Bertrand OF, Larose E, et al. Comparison of plaque sealing with paclitaxel-eluting stents versus medical therapy for the treatment of moderate nonsignificant saphenous vein graft lesions. The moderate VEin Graft LEsion stenting with the Taxus stent and Intravascular Ultrasound (VELETI) Pilot Trial. *Circulation*. 2009;120(20):1978-1986.
70. Rodes-Cabau J, Jolly SS, Cairns J, et al. Sealing intermediate nonobstructive coronary saphenous vein graft lesions with drug-eluting stents as a new approach to reducing cardiac events: a randomized controlled trial. *Circ Cardiovasc Interv*. 2016;9(11): e004336.
71. Aqel R, Zoghbi GJ, Hage F, Dell'Italia L, Iskandrian AE. Hemodynamic evaluation of coronary artery bypass graft lesions using fractional flow reserve. *Catheter Cardiovasc Interv*. 2008;72(4):479-485.
72. Memon AQ, Huang RI, Marcus F, Xavier L, Alpert J. Saphenous vein graft aneurysm: case report and review. *Cardiol Rev*. 2003;11(1):26-34.
73. Liang BT, Antman EM, Taus R, Collins JJ Jr, Schoen FJ. Atherosclerotic aneurysms of aortocoronary vein grafts. *Am J Cardiol*. 1988;61(1):185-188.
74. Teja K, Dillingham R, Mentzer RM. Saphenous vein aneurysms after aortocoronary bypass grafting: postoperative interval and hyperlipidemia as determining factors. *Am Heart J*. 1987;113(6):1527-1529.
75. McGeachie JK, Prendergast FJ, Morris PJ. Vein grafts for arterial repair: an experimental study of the histological development of the intima. *Ann R Coll Surg Engl*. 1983;65(2):85-89.
76. Ramirez FD, Hibbert B, Simard T, et al. Natural history and management of aortocoronary saphenous vein graft aneurysms: a systematic review of published cases. *Circulation*. 2012;126(18):2248-2256.

Complications of Coronary Intervention

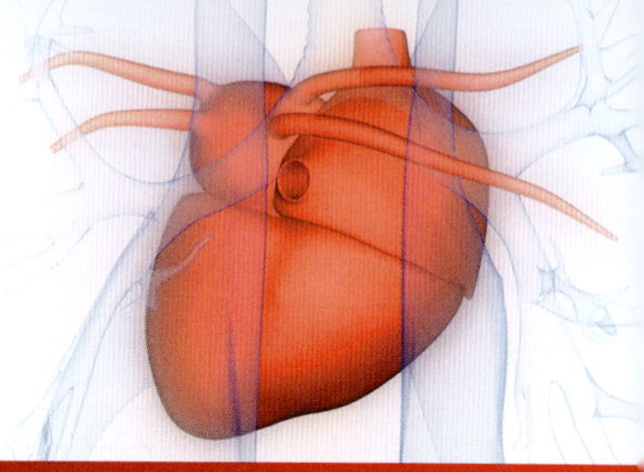

Perwaiz M. Meraj

Planning a percutaneous coronary intervention (PCI) requires an understanding of potential complications that may arise. Addressing these complications is critical to the practice of interventional cardiology. During the informed consent to patients, it is critical to appreciate and explain the possible complications of PCI. Recognition of potential complications at an early stage of the procedure and the techniques necessary to try to reverse an adverse outcome are of paramount importance. The most common cause of post-PCI deaths is from a procedural complication rather than from a preexisting cardiac condition.[1] Some of the complications are generic to all coronary angiography procedures, while others are specific to coronary intervention. Events such as death, myocardial infarction (MI), and bleeding occur at higher rates for interventional procedures because there is direct manipulation of the coronary arteries, often accompanied by prolonged procedural time, complexity, and the use of higher-intensity anticoagulation (**Tables 25.1** and **25.2**). Complications of PCI can occur at any step of the procedure, from the administration of sedation to transfer as the patient leaves the laboratory. The goal of this chapter is to incorporate the latest statistics and guidelines regarding the diagnosis and management of complications of PCI.

MORTALITY

Mortality is the most serious complication of PCI. The cause can be secondary to any of the other complications listed in this chapter. In-hospital mortality is very rare with diagnostic angiography (<0.1%), but the rate increases exponentially with the addition of coronary intervention. The mortality rate greatly varies, depending on the urgency of PCI, with a range of 0.2% in elective PCI to up to 66% in the highest-risk patients with ST-segment elevation myocardial infarction (STEMI) in myocardial shock.[2,3]

The most comprehensive risk prediction tool for in-hospital mortality is the CathPCI registry. Version 4 was updated in 2009 to include extreme-risk patients, such as those with cardiogenic shock and preoperative cardiac arrest. Data from 1.2 million procedures were used to develop both a full (precatheterization and postcatheterization data) and a precatheterization-only risk prediction model for PCI in-hospital mortality. These models show that increasing clinical acuity is the strongest predictor of mortality. In the absence of cardiogenic shock, the risk of in-hospital mortality for elective, urgent, and emergent cases was 0.2%, 0.6%, and 2.3%, respectively. In the presence of transient shock but not salvage status, the risk of in-hospital mortality was 15.1%; with sustained shock or salvage, the risk was 33.8%; and, with sustained shock and salvage, the risk was 65.9%.[3]

Besides clinical acuity, higher age (especially >70 years), history of renal disease, history of cerebrovascular disease, history of peripheral arterial disease, history of chronic obstructive pulmonary disease, history of diabetes, history of heart failure, lower ejection fraction, cardiac arrest within 24 hours, having a STEMI, or body mass index >30 kg were all independent predictors of mortality. After diagnostic catheterization, the full model also predicts higher mortality if there was recent (<30 days) in-stent thrombosis, proximal left anterior descending disease, left main disease, multivessel disease, or a chronic total occlusion. These anatomic

TABLE 25.1 Event Rates of Common Complications Diagnostic Versus PCI

COMPLICATION	EVENT RATE DIAGNOSTIC PROCEDURE	EVENT RATE INTERVENTIONAL PROCEDURE
Death	0.1%	1.27%
Significant bleed	0.5%	5%-12%
AV fistula	0.75%	1.1%
Pseudoaneurysm	0.2%	1%-2%
Periprocedural MI (>3 × ULN cardiac enzyme)	0.1%	16%-18%
Air embolism	0.1%-0.3%	0.1%-0.3%
Cerebrovascular accident	0.3%	0.3%
Ventricular fibrillation	0.4%	0.84%
Coronary dissection	0.06%	29%
Aortic dissection	<0.01%	0.02%
Infection/bacteremia	0.11%	0.64%
Anaphylactoid reaction to contrast	0.23%	0.23%
Cholesterol embolization	0.8%-1.4%	0.8%-1.4%

AV, arteriovenous; MI, myocardial infarction; PCI, percutaneous coronary intervention; ULN, upper limit of normal

risks correlate to increased SYNTAX scores, another anatomic risk prediction model that can assess preoperative major adverse cardiac events when treating complicated coronary anatomy.

COMPLICATIONS OF VASCULAR ACCESS/BLEEDING

A great cardiac catheterization procedure begins with perfect access. The major complications are femoral artery pseudoaneurysm, arteriovenous fistula, and bleeding (including retroperitoneal hemorrhage). As seen in **Table 25.1**, the incidence of these complications is increased in procedures in which PCI is performed compared with that in a strictly diagnostic procedure.[4] Specific discussion of each of these complications of vascular access is beyond the scope of this chapter.

While bleeding can be a complication of vascular access, it can be a general complication of PCI, and the current guidelines recommend as a class I indication that all patients should be evaluated for risk of bleeding for PCI given that periprocedural bleeding is a major risk factor for subsequent mortality.[5] Risk scores/calculators can be used to assess the risk of bleeding with independent predictors, including advanced age, smaller body mass index, chronic kidney disease, baseline anemia, vascular access site (femoral vs radial), sheath size, and the number and type of antiplatelet agents and anticoagulants used.

COMPLICATIONS OF ATHEROEMBOLISM (STROKE, PERIPROCEDURAL MI, CHOLESTEROL EMBOLIZATION)

Advancing large-bore guiding catheters or even 6-Fr catheters across a diseased aorta (either abdominal or thoracic) heavily burdened with atherosclerotic plaque may cause thromboembolic events, resulting in peripheral ischemia, renal failure, or stroke. Peripheral atheroembolism with obstruction of small arteries and arterioles by cholesterol crystals is known as cholesterol embolization syndrome (CES). This is relatively rare (incidence of 0.75%-1.4%). This is diagnosed by one of three typical cutaneous signs: livedo reticularis, blue toe syndrome/trash foot, or frank digital gangrene, in addition to laboratory evidence of an elevated eosinophil count. In-hospital mortality is as high as 16% in those patients with definite CES, because multiorgan embolization can often lead to multiorgan failure.[6]

Atheroemboli can also obstruct the arteries of the brain, causing a cerebral vascular accident (CVA) or transient ischemic attack (TIA). The overall incidence of TIA or CVA is quite low after PCI.[5] There are various multivariate predictors of in-hospital CVA (**Table 25.3**). The most common symptoms of a perioperative TIA or CVA are motor or speech deficits. In-hospital death can occur in up to 25% of those with a CVA, but increased mortality is not expected with a TIA.[7] Intravenous thrombolytic therapy is the treatment of choice if the stroke occurs within 4.5 hours of the procedure if there are no absolute contraindications to thrombolysis.[8] For patients ineligible for intravenous thrombolytic therapy, neurointervention with intra-arterial mechanical thrombectomy or intra-arterial thrombolytic therapy can be administered within 6 hours of onset or even as an adjunct in select patients with large vessel occlusions (especially in the proximal anterior circulation) that have already received intravenous thrombolytic therapy. Before intravenous thrombolytic therapy can be considered, typically a noncontrast computed tomography (CT) scan is first done to rule out hemorrhagic stroke or hemorrhagic conversion of an ischemic stroke. In rare cases, if the stroke occurs and is recognized during the procedure in a hybrid room with appropriate personnel capable of cerebral angiography, consideration should be given for emergent cerebral angiography and intervention if an ischemic stroke with large arterial occlusion is found.[9]

Intracoronary atheroembolism is one mechanism of periprocedural MI. Periprocedural MI is considered a major adverse cardiac event and a core measure in the recent society of cardiovascular angiography and interventions quality assessment and improvement position statement.[10] A meta-analysis of 15 observational studies found that periprocedural MIs were linked with worse in-hospital and long-term outcomes.[11] According to the new universal definitions of MI, a PCI-related MI is the increase of biomarkers greater than three times the 99th percentile of the upper reference limit.[12] While it is common (24%) to have some evidence of myonecrosis (any enzyme level above the upper limits of normal) after a percutaneous intervention, it is rarer (8%) to have a true periprocedural MI.[13] Besides intracoronary atheroembolism, other causes of periprocedural MI include occluded side branches, no-reflow, vessel perforation, vasospasm, acute stent thrombosis, and dissection. The management of the periprocedural MI depends on its underlying cause.

CONTRAST MEDIA REACTIONS

Angiography with radiocontrast media is the first step to every intervention. The most severe contrast media reactions include anaphylactoid reactions and acute renal failure from contrast-induced

TABLE 25.2 Complications Specific to PCI

COMPLICATION	EVENT RATE
No-reflow phenomenon	2%
Stent thrombosis	1%
Vessel perforation	0.4%
Stent embolization	0.4%-1.7%
Need for emergent bypass surgery	0.15%-0.3%
Wire fracture	<0.1% (case reports only)
Stent infection	<0.1% (case reports only)

PCI, percutaneous coronary intervention.

TABLE 25.3 Independent Predictors of In-Hospital CVA

PREDICTOR OF CVA	ODDS RATIO
Thrombolytics prior to PCI	4.7
Creatinine clearance <40 mL/min	3.1
Urgent or emergent PCI	2.7
Unplanned intra-aortic balloon pump	2.3
IV heparin prior to PCI	1.9
Hypertension	1.9
Diabetes	1.8

CVA, cerebral vascular accident; IV, intravenous; PCI, percutaneous coronary intervention.

Adapted from Dukkipati S, O'Neill WW, Harjai KJ, et al. Characteristics of cerebrovascular accidents after percutaneous coronary interventions. *J Am Coll Cardiol.* 2004;43(7):1161-1167, with permission.

nephropathy (CIN). Anaphylactoid reactions are rare, occurring in only 0.23% of procedures.[14] The 2011 PCI guidelines[5] list two recommendations regarding anaphylactoid reactions.

1. It is a class I recommendation with patients with prior evidence of an anaphylactoid reaction to contrast media to receive appropriate steroid (60 mg prednisone night before and morning of procedure) and antihistamine prophylaxis (50 mg 1 hour prior) before repeat contrast administration.
2. It is a class III recommendation (no benefit) in patients with a prior history of allergic reactions to shellfish or seafood to give prophylaxis for a contrast reaction as iodine does not mediate seafood, shellfish, or contrast media reactions.

To prevent acute renal failure from contrast-induced nephropathy, the 2011 guidelines state:

1. It is recommended that patients be assessed for CIN before PCI.
2. Patients undergoing cardiac catheterization with contrast should receive adequate preparatory hydration (normal saline has been shown to be more ideal than ½ normal saline).
3. In patients with creatinine clearance <60 mL/min, the volume of contrast media should be minimized.

AIR EMBOLISM

With contrast administration, another potential complication is air embolization, which can be a cause of periprocedural MI or stroke. This is always an iatrogenic complication caused by failure to clear the air from the manifold system. Automatic injection systems have a lower rate of air embolism because of their air sensors, which prevent injection of air if detected in the system. Nevertheless, their air detection systems do not fully eliminate the incidence of air embolisms and should be considered another safety mechanism, not a replacement, for good technique of aspiration and visual inspection (especially at the Y-connector). Treatment of coronary air embolism consists of immediate initiation of 100% oxygen by facemask. The oxygen helps to minimize ischemia and to produce a diffusion gradient, which helps with reabsorption. If large air bubbles persist, the air can then be aspirated by various aspiration catheters. Further general complications of PCI that might occur at any time during the procedure include arrhythmias and the "no-reflow" phenomenon.

ARTERIAL DISSECTION

The guide catheter itself can cause coronary dissection with or without extension to the aortic root. More commonly, coronary dissection is caused by advancement of the coronary guide wire or by balloon inflation. Large visible dissections have been described in up to 30% of all angioplasty procedures.[15] Previously, this was a significant risk factor for acute/abrupt vessel closure, which occurs rarely in the era of coronary stenting. The National Heart, Lung, and Blood Institute classifications of coronary dissections are seen in **Table 25.4**.[16] Types E and F may represent the additional complication of intracoronary thrombus.

Catheter-related dissection is a much rarer event, with a reported incidence of 0.06%.[17] The mechanism of the dissection is likely because of mechanical trauma to the intima of the vessel (either normal or with plaque) from a catheter that is wedged into the wall rather than lying coaxial. A jet of contrast from an abnormally seated catheter might also cause or worsen a coronary dissection. Risk factors for catheter-induced coronary artery dissection include left main disease, use of Amplatz-shaped catheters, acute MI, extensive catheter manipulation, vigorous contrast injection, deep intubation of the catheter within the coronary artery (sometimes caused by deep inspiration by the patient), and variant anatomy of the coronary ostia.[18] Careful monitoring of catheter pressure and avoidance of injection when pressure damping occurs is critical.

TABLE 25.4 Classification of Coronary Dissection

TYPE OF DISSECTION	DESCRIPTION
Type A	Luminal haziness
Type B	Linear dissection
Type C	Extraluminal contrast staining
Type D	Spiral dissection
Type E	Dissection with persistent filling defects
Type F	Dissection with total occlusion

Stenting the dissected area remains the standard of treatment. If a guide catheter–induced dissection is noticed, this should be fixed before the initial intended lesion that prompted the PCI. If the dissection is not fixed, it can propagate forward and cause abrupt vessel closure or propagate backward and cause aortic dissection. Caution must be taken as contrast injections alone can extend the dissection and should be avoided.

The incidence of aortic dissection caused by catheter trauma is very rare, 0.02%. **Table 25.5** shows a classification scheme for extension of an aortic dissection.[19] Almost all cases of retrograde extension of dissection are from the right coronary artery (RCA). Class I and II lesions have a good prognosis and just require stenting of the coronary dissection with close clinical follow-up.

It is reasonable to follow the evolution of the dissection with imaging modalities (CT or transesophageal echocardiography). If the patient remains stable over the next 24 to 48 hours of hospitalization, then they can be safely discharged without the expectation for further complication.[19] To reduce the chance of extension, the systolic blood pressure must be optimally controlled. Nevertheless, antiplatelet therapy should not be suspended with a freshly placed coronary stent. Class III aortic dissections generally should be treated surgically and are associated with a much higher mortality rate. If surgery is not a possibility, then the entrance of the dissection in the coronary should be stented to avoid further propagation of the aortic dissection.

TABLE 25.5 Classification of Coronary Dissection With Retrograde Extension Into the Aortic Root

CLASSIFICATION	EXTENT OF AORTIC INVOLVEMENT IN THE DISSECTION
Class I	Involving the ipsilateral cusp
Class II	Involving cusp and extending up the aorta <40 mm
Class III	Involving cusp and extending up the aorta >40 mm

ARRHYTHMIA

Arrhythmias can consist of tachycardia or bradycardia. Typically, the unstable tachycardias such as ventricular tachycardia or ventricular fibrillation are more commonly seen in the setting of an acute MI (up to 4%) compared with elective PCI (0.8%).[20,21] Bradycardia can be seen in the case of RCA occlusion, use of rotational atherectomy in the RCA, or use of rheolytic thrombectomy catheters. For treatment, adherence to standard Adult Cardiovascular Life Support (ACLS) protocols is recommended. In general, for unstable patients, it is always good practice to electrically cardiovert tachycardic arrhythmias. For unstable bradycardia, atropine can be given and transcutaneous pacing can be initiated. These measures can buy some time to set up for temporary transvenous balloon flotation pacemaker placement. Transvenous pacemakers should be placed prophylactically for cases of rotational atherectomy in the RCA and in all cases of rheolytic thrombectomy. If transvenous pacing is not readily available, then guide wire pacing (hooking a negative lead to the guide wire and a positive lead to the patient) has been shown to be a viable alternative.

NO-REFLOW PHENOMENON

An acute onset of TIMI 0 flow in a coronary vessel during PCI is known as abrupt vessel closure. It may be because of dissection, thrombus, spasm, or the no-reflow phenomenon. There can be some confusion in nomenclature because some authors only use the term no-reflow in conjunction with microembolization during primary PCI leading to microvascular obstruction or vasospasm, whereas others use the term loosely to describe the sudden absence of flow during any PCI procedure. Intravascular ultrasonography is the gold standard to help discern the cause of no-reflow if not already obvious by clinical suspicion or angiographic appearance. If closure is caused by thrombus or new plaque rupture, then manual aspiration with an aspiration catheter is appropriate. Additional anticoagulation with glycoprotein IIb/IIIa inhibitors by either the intravenous or the intracoronary route should be started if there is no contraindication. Rechecking activated clotting time levels is prudent. Additional angioplasty and stenting might be necessary. If closure is because of dissection, then additional stenting is necessary. If closure is caused by severe spasm, then intracoronary nitroglycerin doses at a concentration of 100 µg/mL are given until the vasospasm is relieved.

Although intracoronary nitroglycerin can help relieve vasospasm, it has not been shown to be effective in relief of the no-reflow phenomenon from distal microembolization.[22] The 2011 ACC PCI guidelines give a class IIa recommendation for administration of an intracoronary vasodilator (specifically, adenosine, calcium channel blocker, or nitroprusside) to treat PCI-related no-reflow that occurs during primary or elective PCI.[5] Often, several grams of these agents, ideally delivered distally in the vessel, in small 100-µg intracoronary boluses will be necessary. No-reflow from embolization to the microvasculature is most commonly seen in interventions on saphenous vein grafts and in primary PCI for acute MIs. Prophylactic distal filters can help reduce the microembolic burden in saphenous vein graft interventions. In fact, embolic protection devices are considered a class I indication in PCI of saphenous vein grafts when technically feasible. On the other hand, recent guidelines list glycoprotein IIb/IIIa inhibitors as a class III recommendation in saphenous vein graft interventions because they have shown no benefit.[5] Initially, based on earlier studies, aspiration thrombectomy prior to primary PCI was initially a class IIa recommendation in the 2011 PCI guidelines.[5] Nevertheless, with additional evidence from larger trials, the 2015 focused update moved routine aspiration thrombectomy to a class III (no benefit) recommendation, with limited use in bailout scenarios as a class IIb recommendation.[23]

CORONARY PERFORATION

Finally, as seen in **Table 25.2**, there are more technically specific complications that can occur with the intracoronary use of wires and stents. These complications include coronary perforation, wire fracture, stent dislodgement with or without embolization, stent infection, and stent thrombosis. Nearly all of these complications are rare and may not be seen during a training fellowship. Coronary perforation happens in 0.4% of PCI cases.[24] Coronary perforation can be caused by a wire "exiting" the vessel or by a tear in the vessel from angioplasty or stenting or rotational atherectomy. **Table 25.6** shows the Ellis classification of coronary perforations.[25]

Class I and II perforations are usually just managed conservatively without any specific treatment. They have a low incidence of tamponade (0.4% and 3.3%, respectively). Class III perforations, however, have a much higher rate of tamponade (45.7%) and a high mortality rate (21.2%).[24] As little as 100 mL of an acute pericardial effusion can cause chamber compression and hemodynamic collapse. To minimize the chance of wire exit, hydrophilic-tipped or stiff wires that are used to get through difficult lesions should be exchanged for typical workhorse wires with softer hydrophobic tips. Also, it is good practice to always have the tip of the wire in the radiographic plane of view at all times. If a distal perforation from a wire tip occurs, the initial step should be balloon tamponade of the vessel at the perforation site. Prolonged (several minutes) inflations with test deflations can be tried over an hour. If balloon tamponade is not successful, then consideration must be given for distal coil placement.[26] Anticoagulation should *not* be immediately reversed with the wire and balloon in the vessel during the attempted perforation occlusion. Immediate reversal could lead to thrombosis throughout the whole vessel along the length of the wire or in recently stented segments, which could lead to a higher degree of mortality than the perforation itself.[27,28] Reversal of anticoagulation should be reserved until the PCI equipment is removed from the coronary vessel. If a GP IIb–IIIa inhibitor is in use, it should be turned off during the case. Platelet transfusions may only be beneficial in patients receiving large molecule, noncompetitive inhibitors of the IIb/IIIa receptor. Covered stents are not helpful at the site of distal wire perforations because of the tapered vessel size at its end. Nevertheless, if a branch of a main

TABLE 25.6 Ellis Classification of Coronary Perforations

CLASS	DESCRIPTION
I	Extraluminal crater without extravasation
II	Pericardial or myocardial blush/staining without contrast jet extravasation
III	Perforation >1 mm in diameter with contrast streaming or cavity spilling

From Ellis SG, Ajluni S, Arnold AZ, et al. Increased coronary perforation in the new device era: incidence, classification, management, and outcome. *Circulation*. 1994;90:2725-2730, with permission.

vessel is the one that is leaking, the whole branch can be excluded with a covered stent.

For larger perforations, placement of a polytetrafluoroethylene-covered stent is often the best choice of treatment. After every balloon inflation or atherectomy run, a puff of contrast should be given to assess the vessel for perforation. This will allow for immediate recognition of perforation, because delay in recognition could lead to cardiovascular collapse. If the perforation occurred after a balloon inflation or stent placement, the balloon should be immediately reintroduced and reinflated to stop further extravasation of blood into the pericardial space. At this point, if tamponade has occurred, a pericardial drain should be placed to relieve any tamponade, while more definitive measures to control the perforation are instituted. Again, if heparin is used, immediate reversal with heparin should not be done as long as equipment remains in the artery.[27,28] Bivalirudin should be discontinued immediately as it will take up to 2 hours to decrease the anticoagulation status to a normal level. GP IIb–IIIa inhibitors should also be discontinued.

RETAINED PCI EQUIPMENT COMPONENTS

Rarely, fragments of interventional equipment may be broken and remain in a coronary artery. This may occur with guide-wire tips, fragments of various other catheters, or stents. These retained intravascular fragments carry the risk of coronary artery occlusion because of thrombus formation, distal embolization of clot, and vessel perforation.

Guide-wire fracture has an incidence of less than 0.1% according to very rare case reports in the literature compared with the number of interventions done worldwide. More cases of guide-wire fracture have been reported with the rotational atherectomy wires. There are multiple options to deal with a retained wire fragment. If the retained fragment is very small, it can be left in place and allowed to endothelialize, as a stent would. Nevertheless, a balloon should be used to position the fragment against the wall rather than intraluminally, which would be a risk for thrombosis. Dual antiplatelet therapy should be initiated for 1 month in this circumstance.

Alternatively, a stent can be deployed to trap the wire in place and avoid any possibility of further migration.[29] If the wire fragment is very long and extends into the guiding catheter, then a balloon can be advanced to the end of the guide catheter and inflated, thereby trapping the wire against the side of the guide.[30] At this point, the guide, balloon, and retained wire can be removed all at once. If a longer wire is retained but does not extend into the guide, then removal with a microsnare is the best choice.[31] If a microsnare is not readily available, then using two new guide wires through one torquing device can create an effective helical snare to entrap the retained wire.[32]

Stent dislodgement and embolization is much rarer with contemporary premounted balloons. Nevertheless, the incidence remains at ~0.36%, typically because of dislodgement in tortuous, calcified vessels.[33] Management includes retrieval, deployment in place, or crushing against the wall of the vessel with a balloon or new stent. Ideally, retrieval should be tried first so you can avoid placing a stent in an unintended position. Mortality rates have been reported as high as 17% for stent embolizations that are unsuccessfully managed (usually requiring emergent surgery), but they are as low as 0.9% in patients who have successful retrieval of a stent.[34] Retrieval methods are similar to those discussed with fractured wire retrieval. Microsnares or dual wires can be used to ensnare and remove the loose stent. Additional methods include advancing a small balloon over the same wire upon which the undeployed stent is sitting, inflating the balloon past the stent, and then pulling back the balloon, which should shift the free stent into the guide. If the stent is dislodged in a large proximal vessel, then retrieval with myocardial biopsy forceps can be considered as well. If retrieval is not possible, then "playing the stent where it lies" (ie, deploying or crushing the stent at that site) is the best option. First, place a small balloon (similar to the stent length) over the wire and through the uninflated stent. Initially, this can be attempted with a small 1.5-mm balloon blown up to 1 to 2 atm; this might be enough to capture the stent and move the system as a whole to a more desirable spot (to the initial lesion or at least out of the left main). If it cannot be moved, then deploy the balloon at full atmospheres to dilate the stent as much as possible. A second deflated balloon equal to the vessel diameter can then be placed to assure adequate stent apposition. Rarely, a small-diameter balloon will not recross the stent. In this case, another stent is placed adjacent to the embolized stent and is used to crush the loose stent against the wall of the artery. In up to 50% of embolization cases, the stent might be embolized outside the coronary artery. In these situations, snares or forceps can be used to retrieve the stent if it can be visualized in the periphery.[34] If it cannot be retrieved or even visualized, this is usually not a concern regarding adverse events, as reported by a large case series.[33]

STENT THROMBOSIS

Stent thrombosis is a rare but devastating complication of PCI. Mortality rates are reported from 25% to 40%.[35-37] Stent thrombosis is defined as acute (<24 hours), subacute (within 30 days), late (between 1 month and 1 year), or very late (>1 year). In an attempt to standardize the definition of stent thrombosis, the academic research consortium divided the criteria for stent thrombosis into definite, probable, or possible (**Table 25.7**).[38]

Both bare-metal stent and drug-eluting stent thromboses occur most commonly in the acute or subacute time frame. First-generation drug-eluting stents also carried a higher risk of thrombosis in the late and very late period because of incomplete

TABLE 25.7 Academic Research Consortium Criteria for Stent Thrombosis

DEFINITION	CRITERIA
Definite stent thrombosis	Angiographic confirmation of thrombus that originates inside or within 5 mm of the stent, which is associated with symptoms, ECG changes, or biomarker elevation, or pathologic confirmation of stent thrombosis determined at autopsy or from tissue obtained following thrombectomy
Probable stent thrombosis	Unexplained death occurring within 30 d after the index procedure, or a myocardial infarction occurring at any time after the index procedure that was documented by ECG or imaging to occur in an area supplied by the stented vessel in the absence of angiographic confirmation of stent thrombosis or other culprit lesion
Possible stent thrombosis	Unexplained death occurring more than 30 d after the index procedure

ECG, electrocardiogram.

TABLE 25.8 Risk Factors for Stent Thrombosis

Premature discontinuation of antiplatelet therapy
Renal failure
Bifurcation lesion
Left ventricular ejection fraction
Stent length

Adapted from Lakovou I, Schmidt T, Bonizzoni E, et al. Incidence, predictors and outcome of thrombosis after successful implantation of drug-eluting stents. *JAMA*. 2005;293(17):2126-2130, with permission.

endothelialization of the target vessel, but current third-generation stents with biocompatible polymers are considered to have a lower risk of stent thrombosis than bare-metal stents, thus obviating the use of bare metal stents in the vast majority of cases. Premature discontinuation of dual antiplatelet therapy is the greatest risk factor for stent thrombosis (with up to a 29% incidence of stent thrombosis), although the safety of shortened dual antiplatelet durations has become recently more established. Other risk factors are listed in **Table 25.8**.[39]

Stent Infection

The rarest complication of PCI is stent infection. Less than 15 case reports of intracoronary stent infection are presented in the literature.[40] Both drug-eluting stents and bare-metal stents have been associated with stent infection. In some cases, mycotic aneurysms are formed at the site of stenting, but other cases just present with persistent bacteremia. *Staphylococcus aureus* is the most common microorganism implicated. Stent infection presents within 4 weeks after stent implantation with fever and bacteremia. Chest pain, ECG changes, and troponin elevation might be absent, so a high degree of suspicion must be raised for any fever occurring within 1 month of PCI. Diagnosis can be confirmed by angiography, CT, or magnetic resonance imaging. Besides antibiotic therapy, most cases (>60%) will require surgery. In general, there is up to a 40% mortality rate with stent infection.[41] Strict infection control measures must be adhered to in the catheterization laboratory to avoid bacteremia. Risk factors for bacteremia associated with cardiac catheterization are shown in **Table 25.9**.

TABLE 25.9 Risk Factors for Bacteremia After Cardiac Catheterization

Avoidable Risk Factors
Difficult vascular access
Multiple skin punctures
Repeated catheterization at the same vascular access site
Extended duration of the procedure
Use of multiple PTCA balloons
Deferred removal of the arterial sheath
Unavoidable Risk Factors
Presence of congestive heart failure
Patient's age >60 y

PTCA, percutaneous transluminal coronary angioplasty.
Derived from Kaufman BA, Kaiser C, Pfisterer ME, Bonetti PO. Coronary stent infection: a rare but severe complication of percutaneous coronary intervention. *Swiss Med Weekly*. 2005;135:483-487.

Key Points

- CES is rare, but if extensive, it can be associated with high mortality because of multiorgan showering/failure. Livedo reticularis is a common physical finding in this syndrome.
- Periprocedural MI is currently defined as a biomarker increased greater than three times the 99th percentile of the upper reference limit.
- Periprocedural MI has been associated with worse short-term and long-term prognosis.
- Periprocedural CVA must be identified quickly. Acute thrombolysis or neurointervention must be considered depending on the timing of recognition of the stroke and/or exclusion criteria for thrombolytics.
- Coronary dissection is extremely common with angioplasty but usually easily fixed with stenting.
- Limited aortic dissection from catheter trauma is usually well tolerated and does not require surgery.
- Extensive iatrogenic aortic dissections >40 mm in length generally require cardiothoracic surgery and are associated with a high mortality rate.
- Reduce CIN with adequate hydration and decreased contrast use.
- Intravenous normal saline is the hydration fluid of choice. It has proven benefits compared with 1/2 normal saline.
- Follow current ACLS protocols for arrhythmia.
- Prophylactic transvenous pacing should be done in rotational atherectomy cases of the RCA.
- Adenosine, nitroprusside, and calcium channel blockers (verapamil was studied the most) are effective for the no-reflow phenomenon because of microembolization.
- Nitroglycerin is *not* useful for the no-reflow phenomenon because of microembolization.
- Intracoronary thrombectomy with thrombus aspiration devices (not rheolytic thrombectomy) has shown improved outcomes in primary PCI.
- The initial treatment of any perforation is immediate balloon inflation.
- Immediate pericardiocentesis should follow balloon inflation.
- Covered stents are necessary for those perforations that are not resolved by balloon inflation.
- Immediate reversal of anticoagulation with PCI equipment in the artery can lead to acute thrombosis—wait until all equipment is out before reversal, if necessary.
- Retained PCI equipment is a rare phenomenon.
- Stent embolization can usually be resolved percutaneously.
- The mortality rate is 25% to 40% with stent thrombosis.
- Stent infection is very rare (only case reports).

References

1. Malenka DJ, O'Rourke D, Miller MA, et al. Cause of in-hospital death in 12,232 consecutive patients undergoing percutaneous transluminal coronary angioplasty. The Northern New England Cardiovascular Disease Study Group. *Am Heart J*. 1999;137(4 pt 1):632-638.
2. Peterson ED, Dai D, DeLong ER, et al. Contemporary mortality risk prediction for percutaneous coronary intervention: results from 588,398 procedures in the National Cardiovascular Data Registry. *J Am Coll Cardiol*. 2010;55(18):1923-1932.
3. Brennan JM, Curtis JP, Dai D, et al. Enhanced mortality risk prediction with a focus on high-risk percutaneous coronary intervention: results from 1,208,137 procedures in the NCDR (National Cardiovascular Data Registry). *JACC Cardiovasc Interv*. 2013;6(8):790-799.
4. Messina LM, Brothers TE, Wakefield TW, et al. Clinical characteristics and surgical management of vascular complications in patients undergoing cardiac catheterization: interventional versus diagnostic procedures. *J Vasc Surg*. 1991;13(5):593-600.
5. Levine G, Bates ER, Blankenship JC, et al. ACCF/AHA/SCAI guideline for percutaneous coronary intervention: a report of the American College of Cardiology Foundation/American Heart Association Task Force on Practice Guidelines and the Society for Cardiovascular Angiography and Interventions. *J Am Coll Cardiol*. 2011;58(24):e44-e122.
6. Fukumoto Y, Tsutsui H, Tsuchihashi M, Masumoto A, Takeshita A, Cholesterol Embolism StudyCHEST Investigators. The incidence and risk factors of cholesterol embolization syndrome, a complication of cardiac catheterization: a prospective study. *J Am Coll Cardiol*. 2003;42(2):211-216.
7. Dukkipati S, O'Neill WW, Harjai KJ, et al. Characteristics of cerebrovascular accidents after percutaneous coronary interventions. *J Am Coll Cardiol*. 2004;43(7):1161-1167.
8. Khatri P, Taylor RA, Palumbo V, et al. The safety and efficacy of thrombolysis for strokes after cardiac catheterization. *J Am Coll Cardiol*. 2008;51(9):906-911.
9. Hamon M, Baron JC, Viader F, Hamon M. Periprocedural stroke and cardiac catheterization. *Circulation*. 2008;118(6):678-683.
10. Bashore TM, Balter S, Barac A, et al. 2012 American College of Cardiology Foundation/Society for Cardiovascular Angiography and Interventions expert consensus document on cardiac catheterization laboratory standards update: a report of the American College of Cardiology Foundation Task Force on Expert Consensus documents developed in collaboration with the Society of Thoracic Surgeons and Society for Vascular Medicine. *J Am Coll Cardiol*. 2012;59(24):2221-2305.
11. Testa L, Van Gaal WJ, Biondi Zoccai GGL, et al. Myocardial infarction after percutaneous coronary intervention: a meta analysis of troponin elevation applying the new universal definition. *QJM*. 2009;102(6):369-378.
12. Thygesen K, Alpert JS, White HD, Joint ESC/ACCF/AHA/WHF Task Force for the Redefinition of Myocardial Infarction. Universal definition of myocardial infarction. *Eur Heart J*. 2007;28(20):2525-2538.
13. Wang T, Peterson ED, Dai D, et al. Patterns of cardiac marker surveillance after elective percutaneous coronary intervention and implications for the use of periprocedural myocardial infarction as a quality metric: a report from the National Cardiovascular Data Registry (NCDR). *J Am Coll Cardiol*. 2008;51(21):2068-2074.
14. Goss JE, Chambers CE, Heupler FA. Systemic anaphylactoid reactions to iodinated contrast media during cardiac catheterization procedures: guidelines for prevention, diagnosis, and treatment. *Cathet Cardiovasc Diagn*. 1995;34(2):99-104.
15. Bredlau CE, Roubin GS, Leimgruber PP, Douglas JS Jr, King SB III, Gruentzig AR. In-hospital morbidity and mortality in patients undergoing elective coronary angioplasty. *Circulation*. 1985;72(5):1044-1052.
16. Huber M, Mooney JF, Madison J, Mooney MR. Use of a morphologic classification to predict clinical outcome after dissection from coronary angioplasty. *Am J Cardiol*. 1991;68(5):467-471.
17. Knight C, Stables R, Sigwart U. Emergency coronary artery stenting for coronary dissection complicating diagnostic cardiac catheterisation. *Br Heart J*. 1995;74(2):199-201.
18. Boyle A, Chan M, Dib J, Resar J. Catheter-induced coronary artery dissection: risk factors, prevention, and management. *J Invasive Cardiol*. 2006;18(10):500-503.
19. Dunning DW, Kahn JK, Hawkins ET, O'Neill WW. Iatrogenic coronary artery dissections extending into and involving the aortic root. *Catheter Cardiovasc Interv*. 2000;51(4):387-393.
20. Addala S, Kahn JK, Moccia TF, et al. Outcome of ventricular fibrillation developing during percutaneous coronary interventions in 19,497 patients without cardiogenic shock. *Am J Cardiol*. 2005;96(6):764-765.
21. Mehta R, Harjai KJ, Grines L, et al. Sustained ventricular tachycardia or fibrillation in the cardiac catheterization laboratory among patients receiving primary percutaneous coronary intervention: incidence, predictors, and outcomes. *J Am Coll Cardiol*. 2004;43(10):1765-1772.
22. Werner GS, Lang K, Kuehnert H, Figulla HR. Intracoronary Verapamil for reversal of no-reflow during coronary angioplasty for acute myocardial infarction. *Catheter Cardiovasc Interv*. 2002;57(4):444-451.
23. Levine GN, Bates ER, Blankenship JC, et al. 2015 ACC/AHA/SCAI focused update on primary percutaneous coronary intervention for patients with ST-elevation myocardial infarction: an update of the 2011 ACCF/AHA/SCAI guideline for percutaneous coronary intervention and the 2013 ACCF/AHA guideline for the management of ST-elevation myocardial infarction. *J Am Coll Cardiol*. 2016;67(10):1235-1250.
24. Shimony A, Joseph L, Mottillo S, Eisenberg MJ. Coronary artery perforation during percutaneous coronary intervention: a systematic review and meta-analysis. *Can J Cardiol*. 2011;27(6):843-850.
25. Ellis SG, Ajluni S, Arnold AZ, et al. Increased coronary perforation in the new device era: incidence, classification, management, and outcome. *Circulation*. 1994;90(6):2725-2730.
26. Pershad A, Yarkoni A, Biglari D. Management of distal coronary perforations. *J Invasive Cardiol*. 2008;20(6):E187-E191.
27. Cosgrave J, Qasim A, Latib A, Aranzulla TC, Colombo A. Protamine usage following implantation of drug-eluting stents: a word of caution. *Catheter Cardiovasc Interv*. 2008;71(7):913-914.
28. Wilsmore B, Gunalingam B. Iatrogenic coronary arteriovenous fistula during percutaneous coronary intervention: unique insight into intra-procedural management. *J Interv Cardiol*. 2009;22(5):460-465.
29. Kilic H, Akdemir R, Bicer A. Rupture of guide wire during percutaneous transluminal coronary angioplasty, a case report. *Int J Cardiol*. 2008;128(3):e113-e114.
30. Patel T, Shah S, Pandya R, Sanghvi K, Fonseca K. Broken guidewire fragment: a simplified retrieval technique. *Catheter Cardiovasc Interv*. 2000;51(4):483-486.
31. Gavlick K, Blankenship JC. Snare retrieval of the distal tip of a fractured rotational atherectomy guidewire: roping the steer by its horns. *J Invasive Cardiol*. 2005;17(12):E55-E58.
32. Gurley J, Booth DC, Hixson C, Smith MD. Removal of retained intracoronary percutaneous transluminal coronary angioplasty equipment by a percutaneous twin guidewire method. *Cathet Cardiovasc Diagn*. 1990;19(4):251-256.
33. Dunning DW, Kahn JK, O'Neill WW. The long-term consequences of lost intracoronary stents. *J Interv Cardiol*. 2002;15(5):345-348.
34. Bolte J, Neumann U, Pfafferott C, et al. Incidence, management, and outcome of stent loss during intracoronary stenting. *Am J Cardiol*. 2001;88(5):565-567.
35. Spertus JA, Kettelkamp R, Vance C, et al. Prevalence, predictors, and outcomes of premature discontinuation of thienopyridine therapy after drug-eluting stent placement: results from the PREMIER registry. *Circulation*. 2006;113(24):2803-2809.
36. Pfisterer M, Brunner-La Rocca HP, Buser PT, et al. Late clinical events after clopidogrel discontinuation may limit the benefit of drug-eluting stents: an observational study of drug-eluting versus bare-metal stents. *J Am Coll Cardiol*. 2006;48(12):2584-2591.
37. Eisenstein EL, Anstrom KJ, Kong DF, et al. Clopidogrel use and long-term clinical outcomes after drug-eluting stent implantation. *JAMA*. 2007;297(2):159-168.
38. Cutlip DE, Windecker S, Mehran R, et al. Clinical end points in coronary stent trials: a case for standardized definitions. *Circulation*. 2007;115(17):2344-2351.
39. Iakovou I, Schmidt T, Bonizzoni E, et al. Incidence, predictors and outcome of thrombosis after successful implantation of drug-eluting stents. *JAMA*. 2005;293(17):2126-2130.
40. Viola GM, Darouiche RO. Cardiovascular implantable device infections. *Curr Infect Dis Rep*. 2011;13(4):333-342.
41. Kaufmann BA, Kaiser C, Pfisterer ME, Bonetti PO. Coronary stent infection: a rare but severe complication of percutaneous coronary intervention. *Swiss Med Wkly*. 2005;135(33-34):483-487.

Chronic Total Occlusion Percutaneous Coronary Intervention (CTO PCI)

Megha Prasad, Katherine J. Kunkel, and Mir Basir

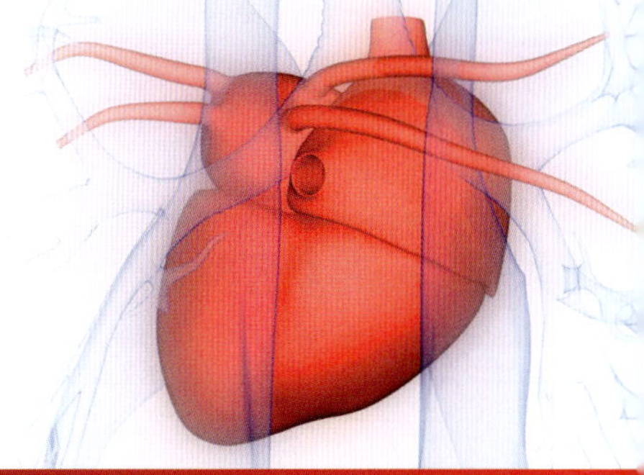

DEFINITION & INCIDENCE

A chronic total occlusion (CTO) is defined as a complete (100% occlusion) in a coronary artery with a thrombolysis in myocardial infarction (TIMI) flow of 0, present for at least 3 months duration.[1] While the true timing of occlusion is often difficult to determine in the absence of prior angiograms, it can often be deduced angiographically or in combination with clinical symptoms and presentation. It has been estimated that coronary CTOs are present in 5% to 30% of patients who undergo diagnostic coronary angiography.[1]

INDICATIONS FOR REVASCULARIZATION

The decision to revascularize a CTO is often based on several factors. It is important to begin by assessing the risks and benefits of revascularization, as should be done with any invasive procedure. Clinicians should attempt to apply what is known from existing data within the field and provide patients an assessment of their individual and the institution's success and complication rates.[2] Emphasis should be placed on efforts to engage patients in shared decision making, based on the individual needs of the patient.[3]

Management of CTOs is similar to the management of coronary artery disease (CAD) without a CTO and includes optimal medical therapy (OMT), percutaneous coronary intervention (PCI), or coronary artery bypass grafting (CABG).[3,4] Once an indication for revascularization is established, the decision as to whether to pursue CTO PCI or CABG is based on the complexity of disease, the perceived risk and benefits, and shared decision making namely patient preference. In those with multivessel disease, CABG is often considered, but in patients with single-vessel disease, PCI is often the preferred strategy.[5-11]

The indications for revascularization of a CTO are also similar to the indications for revascularization in patients with CAD without a CTO. The primary indication for revascularization is to provide symptom relief in patients experiencing ischemic symptoms such as angina or dyspnea despite OMT. Other indications include inducible ischemia on noninvasive testing, left ventricular dysfunction, and arrhythmias, which are attributed to the CTO. Since the main goal of CTO PCI is to provide symptom relief in an effort to improve a patient's quality of life and reduce their ischemic symptoms, when possible, it is important to obtain objective assessment of a patient's degree of symptoms. Objective testing can include exercise testing as well as angina, symptom, or quality-of-life questionnaires. These tests can be quite helpful in understanding the impact of ischemic symptoms on a patient's quality of life.[5-9]

Once symptoms are identified, the benefits of revascularization must be weighed against acute and long-term risks associated with CTO PCI. In patients in whom the likelihood of procedural success is high and the risk/benefit profile is favorable, CTO-PCI may be considered (see **Table 26.1**).

EVIDENCE DEFINING THE ROLE OF CTO PCI

Randomized Clinical Trials

To define the role of CTO PCI in clinical practice, several randomized trials have evaluated the effect of CTO PCI on mortality, morbidity, and quality of life. However, differences in inclusion criteria, study protocols (namely the timing of PCI of non-CTO lesions), and endpoints make comparison between trials challenging.

The EXPLORE trial was the first randomized control trial to evaluate the impact of CTO PCI on left ventricular function and clinical outcomes in ST elevation myocardial infarction (STEMI) patients.[12] Investigators hypothesized that early revascularization of coronary CTO would improve myocardial perfusion in overlapping territories with the infarct-related vessel and protect against negative remodeling. To evaluate this, 304 patients with STEMI treated with primary PCI who were found to have a non-infarction-related CTO were randomized to CTO PCI or no CTO PCI within 7 days of STEMI. The technical success rate of CTO PCI was 72%. Periprocedural complications were more common among patients who underwent CTO PCI. Overall, the study found no difference in left ventricle ejection fraction (LVEF) or left ventricle end-diastolic volume at 4 months in the patients who underwent CTO PCI compared to those who received OMT alone. There was no significant difference in major adverse cardiac event (MACE) between the two groups. While subgroup analysis showed a significant interaction between left anterior descending CTO revascularization and improvement in LVEF, this should be interpreted with caution given then overall negative trial findings. When interpreting EXPLORE, it is important to consider that the trial was not powered to detect differences in clinical endpoints.

The DECISION CTO trial was a prospective open-label randomized trial designed to compare the outcomes of OMT versus PCI and OMT in patients with coronary CTOs.[13] Patients with silent ischemia, stable angina, or ACS were eligible for inclusion. Patients assigned to CTO PCI underwent revascularization within 30 days of randomization. Revascularization of all significant non-CTO lesions was recommended. Investigators found that there was no difference in the primary endpoint of death, TIMI, stroke, or any repeat revascularization at 3 years. No differences were seen in symptoms or quality of life between the two groups. The trial had several important limitations; the study was stopped prematurely and underpowered for the primary outcome, with most patients coming from a single center. Non-CTO PCI was included after randomization, limiting the interpretation of baseline characteristics. Additionally, there was a high crossover rate, with 18% of patients in the OMT arm undergoing CTO PCI and 15% of patients in the CTO PCI arm undergoing OMT (half due to a failed PCI).

To further examine the role of CTO PCI on the quality of life, the EuroCTO trial compared the effects of PCI versus OMT on the health status of patients with CTO at 1 year.[14] Symptomatic patients with at least one CTO found on routine angiography judged to be appropriate for PCI by the operator were eligible

TABLE 26.1 Approach to Percutaneous Revascularization of CTO

APPROACH TO PERCUTANEOUS REVASCULARIZATION OF CTO
1. Patient identified as having a CTO
1. If not already known, assess the patient's symptoms and prior testing. Common symptoms that may warrant revascularization include: • Angina • Shortness of breath • Identification of large ischemic burden • Left ventricular failure • Arrhythmias When possible, symptoms should be assessed objectively using objectives methods such as exercise capacity or scientifically validated questionnaires

1. Assess the risks and benefits of CTO PCI based on the patient's anatomy and comorbidities.
• Outline the benefits of CTO PCI
  • Predominantly symptom relief
  • Explicitly define the lack of mortality benefit or myocardial infarction reduction, in an effort to reassure patients wishing for a conservative approach
• Provide both contemporary as well as personal and institutional experience and risk of CTO PCI
  • Contemporary MACCE rate of ~3%-7%
  • Contemporary success rate >85%

1. Patient-centric discussion on the role of CTO PCI, individualized to the patient's risk and symptoms • Start by optimize medical therapy, if not already done so • Reassure patients on their diagnosis and explicitly discuss the frequency of CTO • Provide patients and families time to research and educate themselves on the topic • Reassure families that revascularization can be provided in the future if symptoms are not yet significant or refractory to medical therapy • For patient wishing to pursue revascularization, provide an outline of events and typical experiences.

CTO, chronic total occlusion; MACCE, major adverse cardiac and cerebrovascular event; PCI, percutaneous coronary intervention.

for randomization. All patients with multivessel coronary disease had their non-CTO lesions treated before randomization at least 4 weeks prior to baseline assessment. The trial included 396 patients randomized in a 2:1 fashion to PCI versus OMT. PCI success rate was 86%, and 7% of patients in the OMT arm crossed over to CTO PCI due to severe symptoms. At 12 months, Seattle Angina Questionnaire in the intention-to-treat populations demonstrated that patients who underwent CTO PCI had statistically less frequent angina, less physical limitations, and improved quality of life compared to those randomized to OMT. More patients in the PCI group had complete freedom from angina. The EQ-5D index showed significantly improved mobility and activity as well as less pain/discomfort in the PCI group. Canadian Cardiovascular Society (CCS) classification improved considerably in the PCI group. The overall 1-year MACE rate was comparable (6.7% in the OMT group and 5.2% in the PCI group), with a PCI complication rate of 2.9%. The major limitation of EuroCTO is that the trial did not reach the prespecified target of patients enrolled. Additionally, blinding was not possible as there was no sham procedure.

The IMPACTOR-CTO trial was a single-center randomized trial designed to evaluate the impact of inducible ischemia with PCI versus OMT on functional status and quality of life in patients with right coronary artery CTO.[15] About 94 patients were randomized to PCI versus OMT. The overall success rate of CTO PCI was 83%. Following PCI, patients had a significant decrease in myocardial-inducible ischemia compared to those randomized to OMT. Patients who underwent CTO PCI had improved 6-minute walk test and quality of life compared to those who received OMT. The procedural complication rate was 8.5%. The generalizability of this study is limited as it was performed at a single center, and the primary analysis was performed using a per protocol (not an intention-to-treat) analysis.

The REVASC trial examined the effect of CTO PCI on left ventricular function.[16] About 205 patients with CTO were randomized to PCI or OMT. All coexisting non-CTO lesions were treated. Patients underwent cardiac magnetic resonance imaging at baseline and 6 months. No difference was seen in the CTO PCI arm versus the OMT arm at 6 months with respect to change in segmental wall thickening or LV function in the CTO territory. In patients with the highest burden of coronary disease (obstructive lesions in non-CTO territory), CTO PCI was associated with greater improvement in segmental wall thickening than no CTO PCI. MACE rates were lower in the CTO PCI arm, primarily driven by a lower rate of repeat intervention in the PCI arm.

Overall, randomized clinical trials of CTO PCI have been limited due to poor enrollment, lack of standardized outcome measures, and variations in investigator expertise. Going forward, the CTO-ARC consortium has worked to standardize procedural definitions, endpoints, and clinical trial design.[17] Implementation of a more uniform approach to trials of CTO PCI will allow more meaningful comparisons between trials and aggregation of data.

Observational Studies

The largest contemporary databases examining real-world CTO PCI experience are the OPEN-CTO and PROGRESS-CTO registries. The OPEN-CTO was an investigator-initiated, multicenter, prospective observational registry of patients undergoing CTO PCI at 12 high-volume US centers.[18] CTO PCI was performed using the hybrid algorithm. In OPEN-CTO, the most common indication for CTO PCI was symptom relief (72% of patients had CCS class III or IV angina). Among those with stress tests, 41% had high-risk findings. Half of the lesions in OPEN-CTO had a J-CTO score of 2 or higher. The core laboratory adjudicated technical success rate was 86%. The most common complication was perforations, which occurred in 8.8% of patients, 48% of which were clinically significant. The overall major adverse cardiac and cerebrovascular event rate was 7.0%, with an in-hospital death rate of 0.9% and a 2.6% rate of periprocedural TIMI. When compared to the National Cardiovascular Data Registry risk prediction tool, the observed to expected ratio for mortality was 2.3. The Society of Thoracic Surgeons predicted mortality with CABG of the entire cohort was 1.7%. At 1 month, Seattle angina questionnaire, Rose dyspnea score, and PHQ-8 scores had improved significantly after CTO PCI. Changes in scores for angina frequency, physical limitation, and quality of life were all statistically significant. Improvements in symptoms were significantly greater following successful CTO PCI than unsuccessful procedures. Overall, the high technical success rate in OPEN-CTO was counterbalanced by a higher than expected complication rate. Patients with successful CTO PCI demonstrated significant health benefits at 1 month.

The PROGRESS-CTO registry is an ongoing multicenter, prospective, international investigator-initiated study. As of the end of 2022, there are over 7000 patients enrolled in PROGRESS-CTO registry. Data from this registry have led to the development of the PROGRESS-CTO score, which estimates the likelihood of technical success based on lesion characteristics, the PROGRESS-CTO complication score, and the PROGRESS-perforation score.[5,19] It has also led to numerous insights on procedural techniques and factors influencing procedural success rates in CTO PCI, such as proximal cap ambiguity, lesion length, number of operators, access site, and patient factors including gender and body mass index.

Guidelines

CTO PCI has a IIA recommendation from the European Society of Cardiology for patients with expected ischemia reduction in a corresponding myocardial territory and/or angina relief.[20] The use of retrograde techniques in the event of failed antegrade techniques has a class IIB recommendation. While the US guidelines had a class IIA recommendation for CTO PCI in the 2011 guideline document, this recommendation was downgraded to a IIB recommendation in the latest guidelines.[21] This change in the guidelines was primarily due to lack of mortality benefit to CTO PCI in randomized trials as well as conflicting data on the effect of CTO PCI on angina and quality of life. Additionally, the consistently higher rate of complications in CTO compared to standard PCI was cited as a reason for the downgrade in recommendation from IIA to IIB with the 2022 US guidelines.

PLANNING & TECHNIQUE

CTO-PCI planning includes assessing indications, patient-specific risk factors, and the overall health status of the patient, as well as careful examination of the CTO anatomy. Ideally, this should result in a clear and distinct plan to achieve a successful and safe outcome. In general, CTO-PCI should not be performed ad hoc, to allow for preprocedural planning, and preparation of the operator and catheterization laboratory staff. This can also help to minimize patient and operator fatigue, contrast use, and allow time to obtain all appropriate noninvasive testing including viability testing or computed tomography (CT). Most importantly, this also allows a robust discussion with patients and their families to ensure understanding of risks, alternatives, and shared decision making.

Intraprocedurally operation should begin with dual injection angiography to better understand coronary anatomy. Dual angiography should be performed by taking a lone cine acquisition on low magnification where the donor vessel is injected first followed by injection of the occluded vessel. The dual injection provides improved visualization of the CTO segment and allows the operator to assess the proximal and distal cap, collateral circulation, and occlusion length. This allows for a crossing strategy to be chosen according to patient-specific anatomy. In select cases, the use of CT angiography may be useful to provide an assessment of the proximal cap location, degree of tortuosity, vessel course, the presence of calcification, and the length of the occluded segment.

Intraprocedural planning should also include an understanding of the patient's hemodynamic status and the potential risk inducing ischemia, particularly if a retrograde approach is needed. For example, patients with elevated filling pressures, a reduced ejection fraction, who require a last remaining conduit to be used as a donor vessel may require medical optimization or consideration of mechanical circulatory support.

EQUIPMENT

While there is some overlap between equipment used in standard PCI and CTO PCI, a variety of specialty equipment is required to successfully complete CTO PCI (**Table 26.2**). Coronary guide catheters used in CTO PCI are often 7 and 8 Fr to provide adequate support while advancing equipment into the CTO body, through significant calcification, and across collaterals. Additionally, side hole guide catheters may be preferred with ostial occlusions to reduce the risk of hydraulic dissection. About 90 cm guides are often used in place of standard guides so as to reduce the risk of being limited by microcatheter crossing length. Due to the frequent use of microcatheters with multiple exchanges during CTO PCI, a "trapper" balloon is often used to maintain wire position while exchanging microcatheters and balloons. This facilitates rapid and reliable equipment exchange while using short coronary wires. Guide catheter extensions are also frequently used in CTO PCI to provide additional support, a target for wiring in reverse-controlled antegrade and retrograde subintimal tracking (R-CART), and selective injections. In the event that trapping is also needed, a TrapLiner can also be used.

Coronary microcatheters are a critical piece of equipment in CTO PCI. They provide support for wires, allow for rapid wire exchange and reshaping, perform selective contrast injections, and protect the proximal vessel from wire-related injuries. Compared to over the wire balloons, microcatheters are preferred as they allow for better distal tip visualization, are more flexible and trackable, and are less likely to kink. Microcatheters are typically made in 135 and 150 cm lengths. About 150 cm microcatheters are generally reserved for retrograde conduits and collateral crossing. The most utilized microcatheters are low profile-braided microcatheters, which are lubricious and can be rapidly spun to facilitate forward movement and lesion crossing (Corsair, Turnpike, etc). There are also low profile hydrophilic-coated microcatheters, which are typically used for retrograde collateral crossing as they are not able to be spun (Caravel, Finecross, etc). Lastly there are stiffer more aggressive microcatheters, which are designed to be spun through calcified and balloon uncrossable lesions (Turnpike Spiral/Gold, etc). Additional specialized microcatheters include angled and steerable microcatheters as well as dual lumen microcatheters, which can be used to facilitate wiring branching vessels, provide additional support when wiring through the over the wire port, and administer intracoronary medications (Twinpass, Sasuke, etc).

TABLE 26.2 Equipment Needed for CTO PCI

CATEGORY NO.	EQUIPMENT	MUST HAVE	GOOD TO HAVE
1.	Sheaths		45-cm long sheaths
2.	Guides	• XB/EBU 3.0, 3.5, 3.75, 4.0 • AL1, AL0.75 • JR4 • Y-connector with hemostatic valve (such as Co-pilot or Guardian) • Guide catheter extensions (Guideliner and Guidezilla)	• 90-cm long • Side hole guides, especially AL1
3.	Microcatheters	• Finecross (150 cm for retrograde—135 cm for antegrade) • Corsair or TurnPike (150 cm for retrograde—135 cm for antegrade) • Small (1.20, 1.25, or 1.5 mm diameter), 20-mm long, over-the-wire balloons of 145 cm or longer total length	• Venture • TwinPass • SuperCross • MultiCross and CenterCross (increase support)
4.	Guidewires[a]	Fielder XT, Fighter Confianza Pro 12 Pilot 200 Gaia 1, 2, and 3 Sion Fielder FC RG3 (for externalization)	Miracle 3 or 12
5.	Dissection/e-entry equipment	CrossBoss catheter Stingray balloon and wire	
6.	Snares	Ensnare or Atrieve 18-30 mm or 27-45 mm	Amplatz Gooseneck snares
7.	Balloon "uncross-able-undilatable" lesion equipment	Small, 20-mm long, over-the-wire and rapid-exchange balloons Threader Turnpike Spiral or Gold Laser	Rotablator AngioSculpt Tornus
8.	Intravascular imaging	IVUS (any)	IVUS (solid state)
9.	Complication management	Covered stents Coils + delivery microcatheters (such as Renegade or Progreat) Pericardiocentesis tray	Pericardiocentesis tray
10.	Radiation protection		Radiation scatter shields X-ray machine with radiation-reduction protocols

CTO, chronic total occlusion; IVUS, intravascular ultrasound; PCI, percutaneous coronary intervention.
[a]For radial operators, 300-cm wires are required because the trapping technique cannot be used through a 6-French guide catheter for trapping over-the-wire balloons, the CrossBoss catheter, and the Stingray balloon.

Specialized coronary guidewires distinguish CTO PCI from traditional PCI. When performing CTO PCI, the specific properties of a guidewire are selected to perform a specific portion of the CTO PCI procedure. Coronary wires are engineered with individual characteristics determined by the wire's tip taper, core material, lubricious coating, polymer jacket, and tip load. After performing a specific task, the guidewire is rapidly exchanged for the next wire to perform the next task. In general, there are four major categories of wires (wires for crossing microchannels, wires for penetration and knuckling, wires for crossing collateral channels, and wires for externalization). There are many wires commercially available in each category. Operators are encouraged to limit their use of wires to one to two wires per category, avoiding multiple wires with similar properties in their early experience.

Microchannel tracking is best performed with a tapered polymer jacketed wire (Fielder XT, Fighter, etc). These wires can also be knuckled and given their low tip load, preferentially form small knuckles. Wires for penetration include medium tip load polymer jacketed wires (Mongo, Pilot 200, etc) as well as stiff tapered-tip wires (Gaia Next, Confiaza Pro 12, Hornet 14, etc). There are also specialized wires for collateral crossing, which have been engineered to have extremely low tip loads (Sion, Sion Black, Suoh 03, etc). Finally, wires for externalization (RG3, R350, etc) are needed for selected cases of retrograde CTO PCI.

Specialized equipment for dissection/re-entry technique includes the CrossBoss and Stingray balloon. Endovascular snares are often needed in retrograde CTO PCI to facilitate guidewire externalization. Ensnares are preferred over goose neck snares as the multiple loops on the snare make wire capture easier.

Advanced atherectomy tools including balloons, specialty balloons, laser atherectomy, rotational/orbital atherectomy, and Shockwave lithotripsy are frequently used in CTO PCI.

Intravascular imaging is also critical to the long-term patency of CTO PCI. Intravascular ultrasound is preferred as OCT requires contrast injection for visualization, which is discouraged during CTO PCI given the presence of coronary dissections. Hemodynamic support equipment may also be used in CTO PCI to support the procedure or in the event of hemodynamic collapse due to procedural complications.

Complications are more common in CTO PCI than standard PCI. To be prepared for possible complications, a cart with emergency supplies should be kept in the room where CTO PCI is being performed. This should include equipment, such as covered stents, coils, and pericardiocentesis trays.

Antegrade Wire Escalation

Perhaps the most widely used crossing strategy is antegrade wire escalation due to its simplicity and relative safety profile.[22] This strategy has thought to be one on which the foundation of CTO-PCI is based. While widely used, it is important to recognize that antegrade wire escalation is most useful in short occlusions less than 20 mm of length, longer occlusions of straight segments of a vessel, in select cases of in-stent restenosis, and in those occlusions where a microchannel is suspected (**Fig. 26.1**). Antegrade wire escalation can be approached via a stepwise algorithmic approach:[23,24]

1. *Choose a microcatheter*
2. First, a microcatheter is selected to support the guidewire and allow for changing of the tip without needing to recross vessel that has already been traversed. The main goals of a microcatheter are to enhance the penetrating capacity of the wire, allow wire tip reshaping without needing to recross the vessel due to loss of wire position, and allow for ease of wire exchanges.
3. *Access proximal cap*
4. The next step is to use a workhouse guide wire to the proximal cap of the CTO. A soft-tipped workhorse wire should be chosen and advanced through the microcatheter. The operator should then advance the microcatheter as needed for support. Once the microcatheter is positioned just proximal to the proximal cap, the workhorse guidewire can be removed.

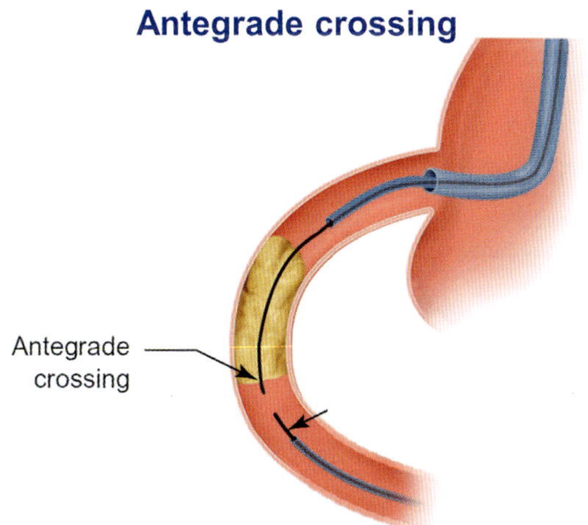

FIGURE 26.1 Illustration of antegrade wire escalation. (Reproduced with permission from Brilakis ES, (ed). *Manual of Coronary Chronic Total Occlusion Interventions. A Step-By-Step Approach.* Waltham, MA: Elsevier; 2013.)

5. *Select and shape Guidewire*
6. After the microcatheter is appropriately positioned, the next step is to select and shape an appropriate guidewire for initial antegrade CTO guidewire crossing. This decision is guided by a risk-benefit analysis, and with each wire escalation, the operator must weigh the risks of potential harm from a more penetrating wire compared with the chance of crossing the total occlusion.
7. The first wire to be chosen is generally a tapered polymer-jacketed wire to track a microchannel. If this fails, then the operator should assess if the course of the occluded vessel is known and proceed with a stiff-tapered wire if the course is known or a stiff-polymer jacketed wire if the course is not known.
8. Shaping of the guidewire is important to maximize the likelihood of successful CTO crossing. The wire should be shaped with a small 1 mm long, 30° to 45° distal bend to enhance penetrating capacity and sheering of the wire allowing it to enter microchannels while reducing the likelihood of deflection outside of the vessel architecture.
9. *Advancing Guidewire*
10. The wire can then be advanced by either sliding, drilling, or penetration. Sliding should be implemented first with the aim of tracking the microchannels within the CTO with gentle tip rotation and probing. Drilling is controlled rotation of the guidewire in each direction, generally used with moderate tip polymer jackets wire. Lastly, penetration involves forward guide advancement directing the wire and pushing using a stiff guidewire.
11. *CTO crossing*
12. Once the proximal cap is penetrated, the occlusion can be navigated with a softer guidewire. This is referred to as escalation followed by de-escalation. The Gaia series wires or a FielderXT or Pilot 200 may be used for traversing the occlusion. As the distal cap is penetrated, a retrograde injection should be used to ensure positioning of the wire.
13. *Confirm distal wire position*
14. Retrograde injection and distal wiring with a workhorse guidewire may be useful to ensure that the distal wire is intraplaque.
15. *Advance microcatheter and complete case*
16. If the wire is true lumen distally, the microcatheter can be advanced and the case can be completed with balloon dilatation and PCI. If the wire is not intraplaque, various techniques can be used to secure intraplaque wire position including parallel wiring and redirecting.
17. Thus, antegrade wire escalation is a commonly used technique in CTO-PCI. The operator should be comfortable with both wire escalation as well as de-escalation to safely cross and traverse a total occlusion. Additionally, use of a contralateral injection to help with visualization of the distal wire is important to ensure appropriate wire positioning and to avoid complications. While antegrade wire escalation is generally successful in shorter occlusions, and straighter segment longer lesions or those with in-stent restenosis, it is the most widely used crossing strategy.

Antegrade Dissection/Re-entry

Antegrade dissection re-entry (ADR) is an important strategy, especially useful for crossing long, calcified, or tortuous CTOs (**Fig. 26.2**). ADR involves working in the extraplaque space, which takes advantage of the distensibility of the vessel architecture allowing for safe crossing.

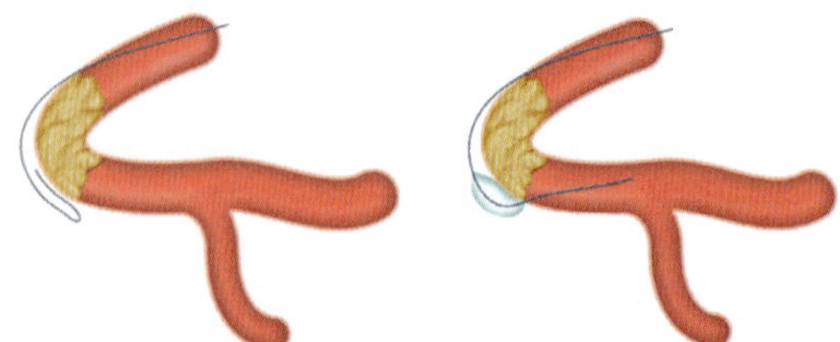

FIGURE 26.2 Illustration of antegrade dissection and re-entry. (Reproduced with permission from Brilakis ES, (ed). *Manual of Coronary Chronic Total Occlusion Interventions. A Step-By-Step Approach.* Waltham, MA: Elsevier; 2013.)

While ADR is generally safe and not associated with significant complications, it is important to recognize that it does often result in loss of branches and a potential increase in rates of in-stent restenosis. Thus, the goal is to minimize size of dissection plane allowing re-entry.

Dissection

While often an ADR approach may be chosen when a wire becomes subintimal, there are situations especially with a calcified tortuous vessel or a proximal ambiguous cap for example where one way may want to intentionally dissect the vessel.

Generally, a polymer jacketed wire such as a Pilot 200 or Mongo wire may be used to initiate a dissection plane. The wire is shaped like a knuckle and then advanced through a microcatheter and pushed to initiate a dissection plane. Several additional steps are often taken if this is not successful including using an appropriately sized balloon to cause injury to the vessel wall also known as balloon assisted subintimal entry. A power knuckle may be used that involves using the balloon as an anchor and pushing a knuckle into the subintimal space. Lastly, contrast modulation with a Carlino maneuver may be used with a forceful small <3 mL injection through a microcatheter into the proximal cap. This can help resolve proximal cab ambiguity and may help disrupt the proximal cap. When intentionally dissecting the coronary, it is important that the operator has a plan for re-entry or a plan for plaque modification and staged PCI.

Re-entry

There are several techniques that can be used for re-entry, and these can largely be divided into wire-based strategies and catheter-based strategies.[25]

Wire-based strategies involve advancing the knuckled guidewire until spontaneous re-entry occurs. This technique has been called the STAR technique. The STAR technique has several limitations including loss-of-side branches and higher rates of reocclusion. For these reasons, it is often considered a bail-out strategy when there are limited other options.

Mini-STAR or limited antegrade subintimal tracking may be used to attempt re-entry into the true lumen earlier after the occlusion. These techniques may be challenging largely because of extensive uncontrolled dissection and compression of the true lumen and thus may have lower success rates. Because of the limitations of wire-based approaches to re-entry, there is a need for dedicated re-entry devices. The Stingray balloon is a widely used approach that is reproducible and reliable and the current standard mode of re-entry.

Successful use of the Stingray device involves appropriately preparing the balloon, delivering the balloon to the re-entry zone, and then inflating the balloon assessing the orientation of the balloon relative to the true lumen by viewing the balloon in different angiographic projections. At that point, re-entry may be achieved using a stick and drive technique using a stiff guide wire or may be performed using a stiff guidewire for puncture followed by exchange to polymer-jacketed guidewire, referred to as a stick and swap technique. Alternatively, this may be done without angiographic guidance in an effort to minimize use of contrast and radiation. As the wire exits the correct port, it is advanced without rotation to puncture back into the true lumen, often creating a popping sensation followed by a contralateral injection to determine whether the distal wire is intraplaque.

Retrograde

Retrograde coronary techniques were first described in 1990 by Kahn and Hartzler.[26] This technique involves accessing the distal cap of a CTO via a collateral channel or bypass graft and crossing the body of the CTO in a distal to proximal fashion. Retrograde crossing can be done in a true lumen to true lumen fashion or using dissection re-entry techniques (**Fig. 26.3**).

Collateral Crossing

The first step in retrograde CTO PCI is identifying and crossing a retrograde conduit. The most commonly used collaterals are septal collaterals followed by epicardial collaterals and bypass grafts. The technical difficulty of collateral crossing can be estimated with the J-channel score.[27] In general, collaterals that are larger and have less tortuosity are more favorable for crossing.

Collateral crossing is performed with specialized microcatheters and wires. In general, low-profile flexible microcatheters are preferred for collateral crossing. Specialized wires with high lubricity, flexibility, and low tip load facilitate collateral channel tracking. Technique to cross collaterals involves rapid wire advancement and withdrawal, guided by wire movement commonly referred to as the "surfing" technique. Contrast-guided "surfing" involved selectively injecting contrast into a collateral using a microcatheter to help guide collateral wiring.

Retrograde True Lumen Crossing

After reaching the distal cap with a wire and microcatheter, the CTO is accessed using a medium tip load polymer jacketed wire or a higher tip load torqueable wire. In retrograde CTO crossing, the

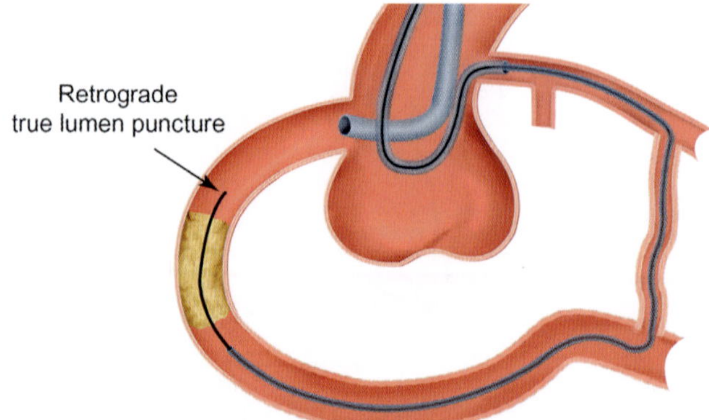

FIGURE 26.3 Illustration of the retrograde approach. (Reproduced from Brilakis ES (ed). *Manual of Coronary Chronic Total Occlusion Interventions. A Step-By-Step Approach.* Waltham, MA: Elsevier; 2013.)

retrograde wire is advanced across the CTO and crosses into the true lumen. After advancing the retrograde wire and microcatheter across the CTO, the retrograde wire is exchanged for a specialized externalization wire. Wire externalization can be performed in several ways, including advancing the retrograde microcatheter into the antegrade guide or guide extension, snaring the externalization wire in the aorta, or using a "tip in" technique with a microcatheter. Once externalized, the wire provides a rail for plaque modification and stenting of the lesion.

Retrograde Dissection/Re-entry

The most common method of retrograde CTO crossing is with a retrograde dissection/re-entry technique, commonly referred to as R-CART. To perform R-CART, the CTO body must be accessed from both the proximal and distal caps. Wires and microcatheters are then advanced into the CTO until the antegrade and retrograde gear is overlapping. This is commonly achieved using a knuckled polymer jacketed wire. As the antegrade and retrograde gear could be in the intraplaque or subintimal space, the goal of R-CART is to create fenestrations in the intima, allowing a connection to be formed between the subintimal and intraplaque spaces. This is achieved by performing balloon angioplasty within the CTO over the antegrade wire in the location of the overlapped antegrade and retrograde gear. Ultimately, the retrograde wire is advanced through the fenestration into the proximal true lumen. The retrograde microcatheter is then advanced across the CTO and the wire exchanged for a specialized externalization wire.

There are multiple variations of R-CART. In conventional R-CART, a 1:1 sized balloon is used in the CTO to make the antegrade/retrograde connection. Directed R-CART uses a smaller balloon in the CTO segment to minimize the size of subintimal hematoma formation. Guide extension-assisted R-CART uses an antegrade guide extension to minimize the distance traversed by the retrograde equipment to the guide. Extended R-CART involves making the connection between the intraplaque and subintimal space outside the CTO body, typically proximal to the proximal cap. Finally, cutting balloon-assisted R-CART uses a cutting balloon to perform angioplasty, maximizing the fenestrations between the subintimal and intraplaque spaces. A variation of R-CART is the CART technique in which the angioplasty balloon is delivered to the CTO segment over the retrograde wire. Use of CART is limited by technical challenges associated with delivering a bulky balloon through small tortuous collateral channels.

CTO PCI Algorithms

Multiple algorithms have been developed to aid in the planning and execution of CTO PCI. Different algorithms highlight historical differences in the approach to CTO PCI in different regions of the world. These include the hybrid algorithm, Asia Pacific CTO Algorithm, Euro CTO Club algorithm, CTO Club China algorithm, and Japan CTO Club.[24,28-31] While these algorithms have many similarities, there are subtle but important differences among the algorithms including the use of preprocedural CTA, the role of IVUS in CTO PCI, and when to transition between antegrade and retrograde strategies.

In an effort to facilitate CTO PCI decision making and teaching across geographies, the global algorithm was developed.[32] In the global algorithm, dual injection angiography is performed with careful analysis of the angiogram. The first major decision point is the presence or the absence of proximal cap ambiguity. In the presence of proximal cap ambiguity, the operator has the option to move the cap, use IVUS for an IVUS-guided puncture if a side branch is present, or transition to a retrograde approach. If there is no proximal cap ambiguity, the next decision point is an assessment of the distal vessel quality. In the event of poor distal vessel quality, a retrograde approach is preferred if feasible. If there is good distal vessel quality, the preferred strategy is antegrade wiring. In the event that antegrade wiring fails, the operator can choose to attempt parallel wiring or antegrade dissection/re-entry techniques. When one strategy fails, the operator is encouraged to quickly change techniques to maximize procedural efficiency. In the event of multiple failed strategies, the global algorithm provides direction on investment procedures as well as when to stop an unsuccessful procedure based on time, radiation, and contrast use.

There are several important differences when comparing the global algorithm to the hybrid algorithm. Antegrade wiring is favored as the initial strategy more strongly in the global algorithm than the hybrid algorithm. The global algorithm gives the operator more options for dealing with proximal cap ambiguity, whereas the hybrid algorithm will move more quickly to a retrograde strategy in the face of proximal cap ambiguity. The global algorithm also introduces investment procedures and provides specific guidance regarding stopping a procedure, namely procedure duration more than 3 hours, three times the glomerular filtration rate in contrast, or Air Kerma greater than 5 Gy unless the procedure is well advanced.

Lesion Preparation

Lesion preparation is similar to standard PCI with a few important exceptions. Orbital atherectomy should be avoided in the presence of significant coronary dissections with preference for intravascular lithotripsy or rotational atherectomy, which have been shown to be safe in the subintimal space.[33,34] Adequate balloon expansion and image-guided lesion preparation is critical to insure a high-quality and durable CTO PCI result.

Image Guidance

Intravascular imaging is critical to both success of CTO-PCI and also durability. Intravascular imaging has several important uses in CTO-PCI. First, it can be useful for CTO crossing by resolving proximal cap ambiguity and facilitating proximal cap puncture as well as true lumen wire re-entry especially if the wire is initially extraplaque. A short tipped IVUS catheter may be useful to place in a side branch and use to visualize a proximal cap. Severe calcification may obscure the proximal cap and CTO entry, and by increasing the field of view in large vessels, a CTO may be punctured using direct visualization of the cap. When there is difficulty with antegrade wire escalation, visualization of the ambiguous cap and assessment of the morphology may be useful in choosing and shaping the guidewire.

If a wire is advanced extraplaque during crossing of the CTO, re-entry may be facilitated by not only various wire and device-based strategies discussed earlier but also can be attempted with direct penetration into the true lumen under visualization by IVUS. It may also be useful in appropriate balloon sizing when performing antegrade and retrograde tracking (reverse CART). It is important to recognize potential pitfalls of this technique, however. At times, advancing the IVUS catheter may be difficult and may require dilation of the extraplaque space. Retrograde crossing may also be facilitated by antegrade visualization of the cap during crossing. Additionally, it is important to recognize that the IVUS catheter itself may extend the dissection and increase the size of the extraplaque space. As such, IVUS-guided re-entry is often considered a last resort after difficulty crossing.

Additionally, intravascular imaging is critical to optimize the results of CTO-PCI by ensuring adequate stent expansion, especially in calcified vessels, to help minimize rates of in-stent restenosis and stent thrombosis. Lastly, this may help evaluate and treat complications. For example, identification of distal or proximal edge dissections after stent placement can be critical to ensuring vessel patency and long-term durability.

COMPLICATIONS AND MANAGEMENT

As with all PCIs, there is a risk of complications that must be weighed against potential benefits of revascularization. There are several potential complications that may result from CTO-PCI (see **Fig. 26.4**).[35,36]

Donor Vessel Injury

During retrograde CTO-PCI, the donor vessel may become injured or may thrombose leading to extensive ischemia and hemodynamic collapse. This may occur due to catheter-induced injury or donor vessel thrombosis. Prevention involves ensuring adequate anticoagulation and careful attention to guide and wire position in not only the occluded artery but also the donor vessel. High activated clotting time of at least >350 during retrograde CTO-PCI may help prevent donor vessel thrombosis.

In patients who are high risk for donor vessel injury or ischemia such as patients where the retrograde donor vessel is the last remaining conduit, there should be strong consideration for use of mechanical circulatory support devices.

Treatment of donor vessel thrombosis or injury largely involves hemodynamic stabilization of the patient, treatment of the abrupt occlusion with ballooning or PCI as indicated, aspiration of thrombus, and consideration of intravenous antiplatelet therapies in the setting of donor vessel thrombosis.

Aortocoronary Dissection

While aortocoronary dissection can occur with all PCI, it is more common in patients undergoing CTO PCI, especially when using a retrograde approach. Guide catheters with side holes may decrease the risk of trauma, but this must be weighed against the false sense of security provided by the wave form in patients being treated with a guide catheter with side holes. This generally occurs secondary to deep coronary engagement and aggressive guide catheters, which are often used for CTO-PCI. Additionally, contrast injections through a dampened pressure wave form may result in a dissection. During retrograde crossing, when attempting externalization of the wire, the retrograde wire may be advanced into the subintimal and subaortic space.

Management involves stopping injection into the coronary artery, use of IVUS to place a stent and ensure ostial coverage, followed by serial noninvasive imaging test to ensure stabilization or resolution of aortic dissection. Early involvement of cardiac surgery is advised although rarely necessary.

Side Branch Occlusion

Side branch occlusion is another complication during CTO-PCI and is especially common when antegrade dissection re-entry strategies are used. This may result in an increased risk of periprocedural TIMI. To avoid this, antegrade dissection/re-entry strategies should be used strategically and involve re-entry prior to the bifurcation with side-branch protection with a second guidewire.

Perforation

Perforation is another common complication in CTO-PCI, and there are various strategies described to help reduce risk of perforation including use of intravascular imaging to size balloons, rapid

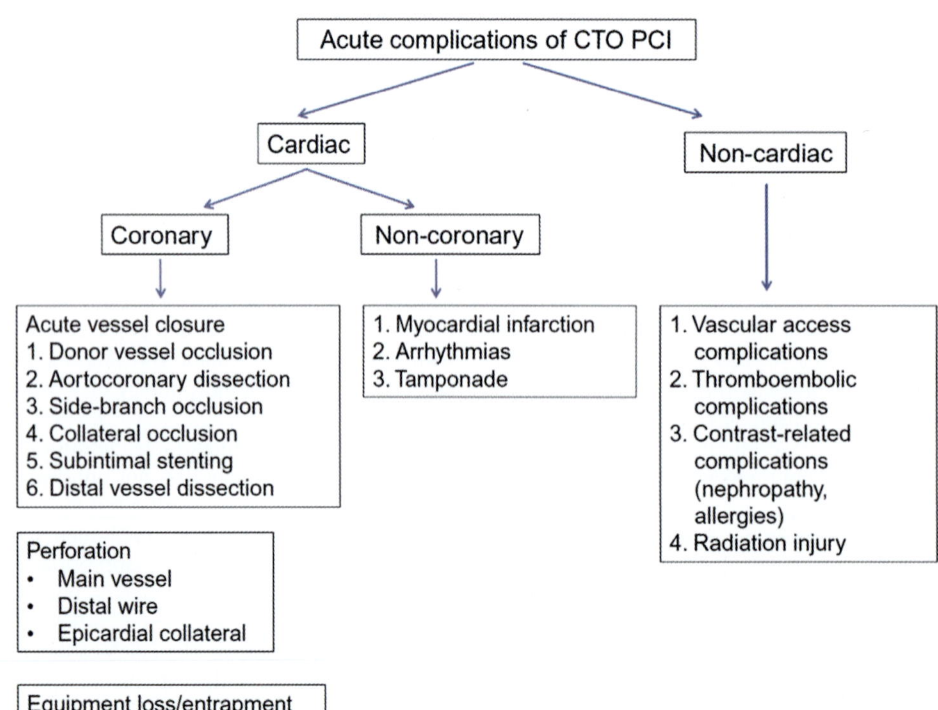

FIGURE 26.4 Classification of acute complications of CTO PCI. CTO PCI, chronic total occlusion percutaneous coronary intervention.

wire de-escalation to avoid excessive use of stiff wires that may cause injury, and visualization of distal wire position with contralateral injection in multiple views prior to microcatheter advancement to ensure adequate distal wire position.[37]

Perforation can lead to pericardial effusion and tamponade and may necessitate surgery, and thus, rapid management via an algorithmic structured approach is necessary. Perforations may be graded according to Ellis classification describing the extent of the perforation with one extending just outside the lumen with no staining to class 3 involving perforation into an anatomic cavity chamber. Perforations may occur of the main vessel, the distal vessel, or the collateral and each involve varying methods to treat.

Generally, perforations are treated with balloon inflammation immediately to avoid accelerated accumulation of blood in the pericardial space and tamponade. Hemodynamic stabilization is achieved with intravenous fluids, pressors, and support as needed with pericardiocentesis being performed immediately in the setting of hemodynamic compromise. Various tools are available to help with management of a perforation including covered stents, which can be used in a large main vessel and coils and or fat for distal vessel perforations. Collateral vessel perforation is a serious complication that may result when performing retrograde CTO-PCI and can lead to rapid hemodynamic compromise and is generally managed with prolonged inflation of a small balloon with consideration of embolization/coiling from both directions as blood flow can continue retrogradely despite antegrade occlusion of a collateral. Early involvement of cardiac surgery is advisable to help with the acute and long-term management of the patients. Anticoagulation should not be reversed until all equipment has been removed.

Equipment Loss or Entrapment

Equipment delivery is often challenging especially in calcified and tortuous occlusions, and stent loss or wire entrapment may be a complication of complex anatomy especially in a total occlusion. Prevention includes limiting overtorquing of equipment, especially wires and microcatheters, avoiding microcatheter tips of antegrade and retrograde gear from meeting, minimizing decelerations when performing rotational atherectomy, and appropriate preparation of the vessel and delivery via a guide extension catheter as needed especially in tortuous and calcified vessels to avoid stent loss. There are a variety of described ways to manage lost equipment. The operator must first decide if the equipment should be retrieved or crushed, and this can be determined by weighing risks and benefits. If the device is to be retrieved, the use of balloons, snares, guide extension, and/or turning multiple wires to entrap the equipment and pull back may help in retrieval.

Radiation Injury

As CTO-PCI may involve extended length of time and amount of radiation, it is important for operators to keep in mind the amount of radiation administered during a procedure and monitor for long-term complications of radiation injury with skin checks. Minimizing radiation injury through radiation safety techniques as well as minimizing duration of procedure are important to minimize radiation to the patient.

Complication Management

Thus, management of complications is a critical skill for CTO-PCI operators. Prevention through careful techniques, constant attention to guide catheter position and distal wire position, liberal use of contralateral injection to ensure appropriate distal guide wire positioning during crossing as well as use of intravascular imaging to appropriately size balloon inflations may be helpful in minimizing risk of perforations. Lastly, use of guide extension catheters and adequate preparation of the vessel may help reduce risk of loss of equipment especially in tortuous/calcified vessels. With the occurrence of complications, however, the operator must be facile in managing patients who may decompensate quickly, ensuring rapid hemodynamic stabilization while addressing the underlying etiology with a systematic algorithmic approach.

CONCLUSIONS

Coronary CTOs are frequently identified on coronary angiography and are often the source of ischemic symptoms for patients. As with any invasive procedures, shared decision making with a careful analysis of the risks and benefits of revascularization is necessary. Clinical trials have not demonstrated reductions in death or TIMI with CTO-PCI, and refractory ischemic symptoms are the main reason to consider CTO-PCI. Operators must be facile in multiple crossing strategies to facilitate successful and safe CTO-PCI.

Disclosures

KK reports receiving funds from Abiomed, Bristol Myers Squibb, CSI, Janssen, Medtronic, and Shockwave. MB reports receiving funds from Abiomed, Boston Scientific, Chiesi, Saranas, and Zoll.

Acknowledgments

The authors thank Drs Brilakis, Burke, and Banerjee for allowing to use figures from their previous work.

References

1. Azzalini L, Vo M, Dens J, Agostoni P. Myths to debunk to improve management, referral, and outcomes in patients with chronic total occlusion of an epicardial coronary artery. *Am J Cardiol*. 2015;116(11):1774-1780. doi:10.1016/j.amjcard.2015.08.050
2. Basir MB, Karatasakis A, Alqarqaz M, et al. Further validation of the hybrid algorithm for CTO PCI; difficult lesions, same success. *Cardiovasc Revasc Med*. 2017;18(5):328-331.
3. Hamzaraj K, Kammerlander A, Gyongyosi M, Frey B, Distelmaier K, Graf S. Patient selection and clinical indication for chronic total occlusion revascularization—a workflow focusing on non-invasive cardiac imaging. *Life*. 2022;13(1):4.
4. Barbarawi M, Kheiri B, Zayed Y, et al. Meta-analysis of percutaneous coronary intervention versus medical therapy in the treatment of coronary chronic total occlusion. *Am J Cardiol*. 2019;123(12):2060-2062.
5. Christopoulos G, Kandzari DE, Yeh RW, et al. Development and validation of a novel scoring system for predicting technical success of chronic total occlusion percutaneous coronary interventions: the PROGRESS CTO (prospective global registry for the study of chronic total occlusion intervention) score. *JACC Cardiovasc Interv*. 2016;9(1):1-9.
6. Choi SY, Choi BG, Rha SW, et al. Percutaneous coronary intervention versus optimal medical therapy for chronic total coronary occlusion with well-developed collaterals. *J Am Heart Assoc*. 2017;6(9):e006357.
7. Choo EH, Koh YS, Seo SM, et al. Comparison of successful percutaneous coronary intervention versus optimal medical therapy in patients with coronary chronic total occlusion. *J Cardiol*. 2019;73(2):156-162.
8. Flores-Umanzor EJ, Cepas-Guillen PL, Vazquez S, et al. Survival benefit of revascularization versus optimal medical therapy alone for chronic total occlusion management in patients with diabetes. *Catheter Cardiovasc Interv*. 2021;97(3):376-383.

9. Flores-Umanzor EJ, Vazquez S, Cepas-Guillen P, et al. Impact of revascularization versus medical therapy alone for chronic total occlusion management in older patients. *Catheter Cardiovasc Interv*. 2019;94(4):527-535.
10. Galassi AR, Sucato V, Diana D, Novo G. Medical therapy or revascularization for patients with chronic total occlusion? A dilemma almost solved. *Hellenic J Cardiol*. 2020;61(4):272-273.
11. Mohr FW, Morice MC, Kappetein AP, et al. Coronary artery bypass graft surgery versus percutaneous coronary intervention in patients with three-vessel disease and left main coronary disease: 5-year follow-up of the randomised, clinical SYNTAX trial. *Lancet*. 2013;381(9867):629-638.
12. Henriques JP, Hoebers LP, Råmunddal T, et al; EXPLORE Trial Investigators. Percutaneous intervention for concurrent chronic total occlusions in patients with STEMI: the EXPLORE trial. *J Am Coll Cardiol*. 2016;68(15):1622-1632.
13. Lee SW, Lee PH, Ahn JM, et al. Randomized trial evaluating percutaneous coronary intervention for the treatment of chronic total occlusion. *Circulation*. 2019;139(14):1674-1683.
14. Werner GS, Martin-Yuste V, Hildick-Smith D, et al; EUROCTO trial investigators. A randomized multicentre trial to compare revascularization with optimal medical therapy for the treatment of chronic total coronary occlusions. *Eur Heart J*. 2018;39(26):2484-2493.
15. Obedinskiy AA, Kretov EI, Boukhris M, et al. The IMPACTOR-CTO trial. *JACC Cardiovasc Interv*. 2018;11(13):1309-1311.
16. Mashayekhi K, Nührenberg TG, Toma A, et al. A randomized trial to assess regional left ventricular function after stent implantation in chronic total occlusion: the REVASC trial. *JACC Cardiovasc Interv*. 2018;11(19):1982-1991.
17. Ybarra LF, Rinfret S, Brilakis ES, et al; Chronic Total Occlusion Academic Research Consortium. Definitions and clinical trial design principles for coronary artery chronic total occlusion therapies: CTO-ARC consensus recommendations. *Circulation*. 2021;143(5):479-500.
18. Sapontis J, Salisbury AC, Yeh RW, et al. Early procedural and health status outcomes after chronic total occlusion angioplasty: a report from the OPEN-CTO registry (outcomes, patient health status, and efficiency in chronic total occlusion hybrid procedures). *JACC Cardiovasc Interv*. 2017;10(15):1523-1534.
19. Simsek B, Kostantinis S, Karacsonyi J, et al. Predicting periprocedural complications in chronic total occlusion percutaneous coronary intervention: the PROGRESS-CTO complication scores. *JACC Cardiovasc Interv*. 2022;15(14):1413-1422.
20. Authors/Task Force members; Windecker S, Kolh P, Alfonso F, et al. 2014 ESC/EACTS guidelines on myocardial revascularization: the task force on myocardial revascularization of the European Society of Cardiology (ESC) and the European Association for Cardio-Thoracic Surgery (EACTS) developed with the special contribution of the European Association of Percutaneous Cardiovascular Interventions (EAPCI). *Eur Heart J*. 2014;35(37):2541-2619.
21. Lawton JS, Tamis-Holland JE, Bangalore S, et al. 2021 ACC/AHA/SCAI guideline for coronary artery revascularization: a report of the American College of Cardiology/American Heart Association Joint Committee on clinical practice guidelines. *Circulation*. 2022;145(3):e18-e114.
22. Maeremans J, Knaapen P, Stuijfzand WJ, et al. Antegrade wire escalation for chronic total occlusions in coronary arteries: simple algorithms as a key to success. *J Cardiovasc Med*. 2016;17(9):680-686.
23. Wu EB, Tsuchikane E, Ge L, et al. Retrograde versus antegrade approach for coronary chronic total occlusion in an algorithm-driven contemporary Asia-Pacific multicentre registry: comparison of outcomes. *Heart Lung Circ*. 2020;29(6):894-903.
24. Harding SA, Wu EB, Lo S, et al. A new algorithm for crossing chronic total occlusions from the Asia Pacific chronic total occlusion club. *JACC Cardiovasc Interv*. 2017;10(21):2135-2143.
25. Wu EB, Brilakis ES, Lo S, et al. Advances in CrossBoss/stingray use in antegrade dissection reentry from the Asia Pacific chronic total occlusion club. *Catheter Cardiovasc Interv*. 2020;96(7):1423-1433.
26. Kahn JK, Hartzler GO. Retrograde coronary angioplasty of isolated arterial segments through saphenous vein bypass grafts. *Cathet Cardiovasc Diagn*. 1990;20(2):88-93.
27. Nagamatsu W, Tsuchikane E, Oikawa Y, et al. Successful guidewire crossing via collateral channel at retrograde percutaneous coronary intervention for chronic total occlusion: the J-Channel score. *EuroIntervention*. 2020;15(18):e1624-e1632.
28. Brilakis ES, Grantham JA, Rinfret S, et al. A percutaneous treatment algorithm for crossing coronary chronic total occlusions. *JACC Cardiovasc Interv*. 2012;5(4):367-379.
29. Galassi AR, Werner GS, Boukhris M, et al. Percutaneous recanalisation of chronic total occlusions: 2019 consensus document from the EuroCTO Club. *EuroIntervention*. 2019;15(2):198-208. doi:doi: 10.4244/EIJ-D-18-00826
30. Ge JB, Ge L, Huo Y, et al. Updated algorithm of chronic total occlusion percutaneous coronary intervention from chronic total occlusion club China. *Cardiology*. 2021;6(2):81.
31. Tanaka H, Tsuchikane E, Muramatsu T, et al. A novel algorithm for treating chronic total coronary artery occlusion. *J Am Coll Cardiol*. 2019;74(19):2392-2404. doi:10.1016/j.jacc.2019.08.1049
32. Wu EB, Brilakis ES, Mashayekhi K, et al. Global chronic total occlusion crossing algorithm: JACC state-of-the-art review. *J Am Coll Cardiol*. 2021;78(8):840-853. doi:10.1016/j.jacc.2021.05.055
33. Yeoh J, Hill J, Spratt JC. Intravascular lithotripsy assisted chronic total occlusion revascularization with reverse controlled antegrade retrograde tracking. *Catheter Cardiovasc Interv*. 2019;93(7):1295-1297. doi: 10.1002/ccd.28165
34. Cosgrove C, Mahadevan K, Spratt JC, McEntegart M. The impact of calcium on chronic total occlusion management. *Interv Cardiol*. 2021;16:e30. doi:10.15420/icr.2021.01
35. Riley RF, Sapontis J, Kirtane AJ, et al. Prevalence, predictors, and health status implications of periprocedural complications during coronary chronic total occlusion angioplasty. *EuroIntervention*. 2018;14(11):e1199-e1206.
36. Riley RF, Walsh SJ, Kirtane AJ, et al. Algorithmic solutions to common problems encountered during chronic total occlusion angioplasty: the algorithms within the algorithm. *Catheter Cardiovasc Interv*. 2019;93(2):286-297.
37. Azzalini L, Poletti E, Ayoub M, et al. Coronary artery perforation during chronic total occlusion percutaneous coronary intervention: epidemiology, mechanisms, management, and outcomes. *EuroIntervention*. 2019;15(9):e804-e811.

Contemporary Techniques for Forearm Arterial Access: Radial, Distal Radial, and Ulnar Approach

Marco Shaker, Anshul Pranva, Olivia Zurawska, and Adhir Shroff

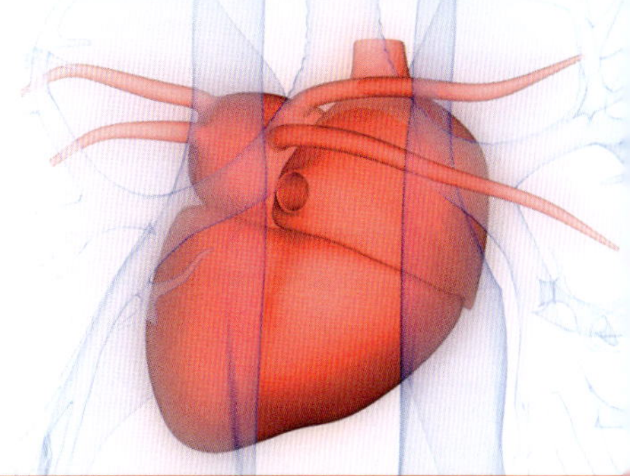

Arterial vascular access for percutaneous coronary intervention (PCI) can be obtained through various sites. The femoral artery had been the predominant access site for many years, but there has been a significant increase in the use of the radial artery given lower rates of access-site complications, less bleeding, and improved patient comfort. Alternatives to the traditional radial artery access have also been developed including the distal-radial artery approach[1] and ulnar artery access.[2]

In this chapter, we put forward the clinical data, anatomy, contemporary access, and closure techniques that incorporate best practices for each of these access sites. We will touch on common complications of each of these access sites as well.

RADIAL ARTERY ACCESS

Clinical Trial Data

Radial artery access has become a common approach for intervention in acute coronary syndrome (ACS) and stable ischemic heart disease. The past decade has seen several clinical trials that have helped to shape this transformation in access site for PCI. While the details of each trial are beyond the scope of this review, **Table 27.1** includes an overview of some of the largest, pivotal, randomized trials of radial access for PCI.

The European Society of Cardiology has recommended transradial access (TRA) as the preferred approach in ST-segment elevation myocardial infarction (STEMI)/non-ST-segment elevation ACS (NSTE-ACS), and the Society for Cardiovascular Angiography and Intervention has suggested that operators with appropriate expertise may choose a default TRA approach to reduce vascular complications and bleeding.[8,9] A recent expert consensus document from the American Heart Association has advocated for a "radial first" strategy for ACS patients.[10] This recommendation has been incorporated into most recent US coronary revascularization guidelines for patients presenting with STEMI or NSTE-ACS.[11]

Anatomy

The radial artery originates from the division of the brachial artery in front of the head of the radius. It runs along the lateral aspect of the forearm and splits into its superficial and palmar branches just distal to the wrist. When it reaches the wrist, the radial artery is easily palpated above the trapezium and scaphoid bones and the external lateral ligament. The radial artery is conventionally punctured 1 to 2 cm proximal to the wrist joint, and the distal-radial artery is approached in the proximal part of the anatomical snuff box. Common anatomical variants include (a) radial artery with a high takeoff, (b) the presence of radial and/or brachial loops, and (c) excessive tortuosity (**Fig. 27.1**).

The ulnar artery is the larger of the two branches of the brachial artery; typically originating 5 to 7 cm distal to the elbow, and it progresses along the medial portion of the forearm and runs distally adjacent to the ulnar nerve. At the level of the wrist, it divides into two branches that join the radial artery and its superficial branch to form the deep and superficial palmar arches (**Fig. 27.2**). The ulnar artery is best palpated on the anteromedial aspect of the proximal wrist fold when the wrist is hyperextended. Puncture of the ulnar artery most often occurs in the proximal wrist fold. Anatomical variations are relatively rare and when seen, are similar to the ones seen with the radial artery such as a superficial ulnar artery, ulnar loops, and high take-off origin.[12]

Use of Ultrasound

Ultrasound guidance in aiding vascular access has helped with regard to increasing the first attempt success rate and decreases the number of attempts required to successfully place a sheath.[13] It can guide the selection of an appropriately sized sheath so as to prevent placing an oversized sheath into an artery. Ultrasound may also delineate anatomical variants.

The mean internal diameter of the radial artery is usually greater than the ulnar artery (3.0 ± 0.6 vs 2.7 mm ± 0.6) and greater in men as compared to women.[14,15] Diameters of the radial artery of people of South Asian descent are smaller as compared to their Caucasian counterparts.[16] There is no direct correlation between vessel diameters and body mass index (BMI).[17]

Radial Artery Puncture Technique

1. The hand is supinated so both the radial and ulnar artery are exposed at the level of the wrist joint. Gentle hyperextension can be helpful. Use of a towel or a gauze is usually sufficient. In our practice, connecting the pulse oximeter to the same hand is standard practice so we can observe the plethysmographic tracing during and after the case. The hand and fingers are usually taped to the arm board so the supination position is maintained during access but can be released once the access sheath is in place for patient comfort.
2. Use of a dedicated sterile radial drape or a multiaccess drape is preferred to maintain an uninterrupted sterile field for the procedure.
3. The radial artery is then palpated. Ultrasound can be utilized as per above.
4. The entry site is typically 1 to 1.5 cm proximal to the wrist crease. The artery is straight at this location while remaining over the radial bone.
5. There are two common access techniques for radial artery puncture:
   a. The front-wall or "bare needle" approach involves using 20 or 21G needle with a 0.021- or 0.025-in wire. The needle is advanced until it punctures the front wall of the artery. Once pulsatile blood flow is observed, the wire is advanced into the artery. The needle is removed, and the access sheath is placed into the vessel. This method is similar to the traditional femoral artery approach.

TABLE 27.1 Overview of the Landmark Clinical Trials of Radial Access for PCI

	RIVAL[3]	RIFLE-STEACS[4]	STEMI-RADIAL[5]	MATRIX[6]	SAFARI-STEMI[7]
Author	Jolly et al	Romagnoli et al	Bernat et al	Valgimigli et al	Le May et al
Indication	ACS	STEMI	STEMI	ACS	STEMI
Population	7021	1001 STEMI	707	8404	2292
Enrollment period	2006-2010	2009-2011	2009-2012	2011-2014	2011-2018
Trial design	Multicenter 158 international sites 1:1 randomization open label	Multicenter 4 European sites 1:1 randomization open label	Multicenter 4 international sites 1:1 randomization open label	Multicenter 78 European sites 1:1 randomization open label	Multicenter 5 Canadian sites 1:1 randomization open label
Primary outcome	NACE Composite of death, MI, stroke, or non-CABG major bleeding at 30 d	NACE Composite of cardiac death, MI, stroke, TLR, or non-CABG major bleeding at 30 d	Composite of major bleeding and vascular complications	MACE + NACE coprimary Composite of (1) death, MI, stroke, or (2) death, MI, stroke, or BARC non-CABG major bleeding at 30 d	Death at 30 d
Bleeding definition	ACUITY major and access site bleeding	Hemorrhage with unplanned diagnostics, prolonged hospitalization, or life-saving drug discontinuation	HORIZONS-AMI trial, major bleeding	BARC 3 or 5 bleeding	TIMI major or minor bleeding
Main findings	Radial and femoral approaches are safe for PCI, but the lower incidence of local vascular complications may be a reason to use the radial approach	Radial access has lower cardiac mortality and morbidity in STEMI-ACS patients	In STEMI-ACS, radial access is associated with significant lower major bleeding or access site complications and superior net clinical benefits	Radial access was associated with lower NACEs compared with femoral access. Radial access should become the default approach in ACS patients undergoing invasive management	There are no significant differences in survival or other clinical end points at 30 d between the radial access vs femoral access in patients with STEMI referred for primary PCI. However, small absolute differences in end points cannot be definitively refuted given the premature termination of the trial

ACS, acute coronary syndrome; AMI, acute myocardial infarction; BARC, Bleeding Academic Research Consortium; CABG, coronary artery bypass graft; MACE, major adverse clinical event; MI, myocardial infarction; NACE, net adverse clinical event; PCI, percutaneous coronary intervention; STEMI, ST-segment elevation myocardial infarction; TIMI, thrombolysis in myocardial infarction; TLR, target vessel revascularization.

b. The back-wall or "cannula over needle" or "through and through" technique involved using a 20 or 22G needle with a plastic cannula. In this approach, the needle/cannula system is advanced until blood is seen entering the cannula chamber. At this point, in contrast to the bare needle approach, the needle and cannula are advanced further into the patient until blood is no longer flowing (through the back wall of the radial artery). At this point, the needle is removed, leaving the plastic cannula through both walls of the artery. A 0.021 or 0.025 wire is then kept near the mouth of the cannula as it is withdrawn slowly. When the tip of the cannula is pulled back into the lumen of the vessel, there will be brisk flow noted and the wire can be advanced into the vessel. The cannula is then removed, and the access sheath is placed into the vessel (**Fig. 27.3**).

3. The access sheath is secured with a clear adhesive dressing and flushed with sterile saline.
4. It is reasonable to administer a vasodilator cocktail at this point.
5. Administration of systemic anticoagulation is considered a best practice for radial artery procedures. Dosing, timing, and route of administration have been studied, and the current recommendations are listed (**Table 27.2**).

Radial Artery Hemostasis Technique

At the end of the procedure, the catheters should be removed and the sheath should be flushed with saline. While manual compression is an effective method to achieve hemostasis, use of a compression device or system is commonly employed. There are multiple devices in the US market approved for this indication, ie, TR band, VasoStat, PreludeSync, Zephyr, etc.[24] Use of the patent hemostasis method is the

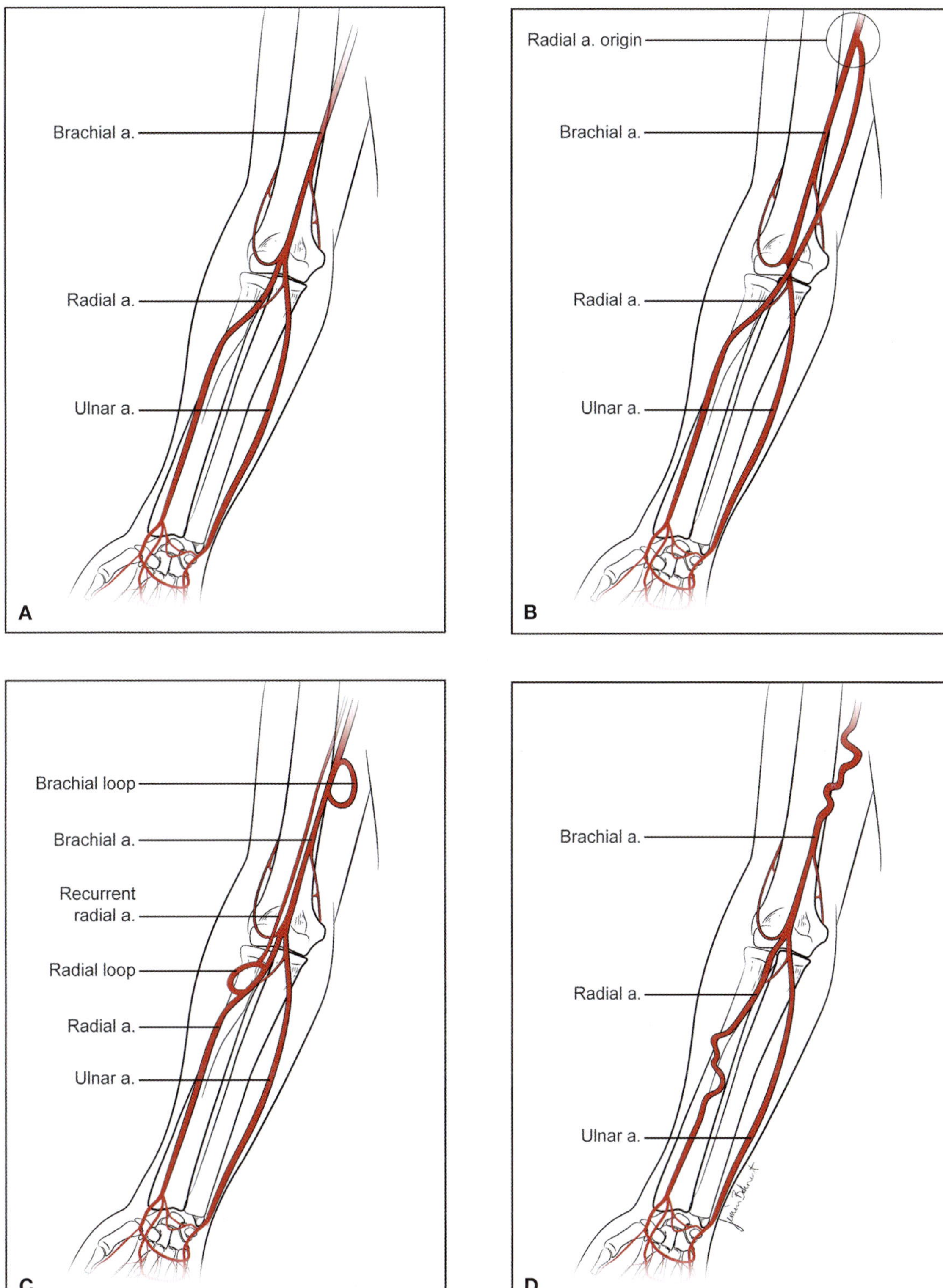

FIGURE 27.1 Variations of radial artery anatomy. **A,** Normal or most common anatomy. **B,** High (proximal) origin of the radial artery. **C,** Radial and brachial artery loops. **D,** Tortuosity of the radial and brachial arteries.

best way to minimize radial artery occlusion (RAO).[25] Use of prophylactic ulnar artery compression can further lower the rate of RAO.[26] Use of hemostatic pads has been recently shown to decrease compression time without an increase in bleeding complications.[27] The optimal duration of compression appears to be approximately 2 hours,[28] and prolonged compression only serves to increase the rate of RAO.

Complications

Although forearm arterial access has decreased complications, operators must be aware of some adverse events that can occur with this access approach (**Table 27.3**). In this brief chapter, we will cover a few of the most common complications, including radial artery spasm, RAO, and entrapped catheters.

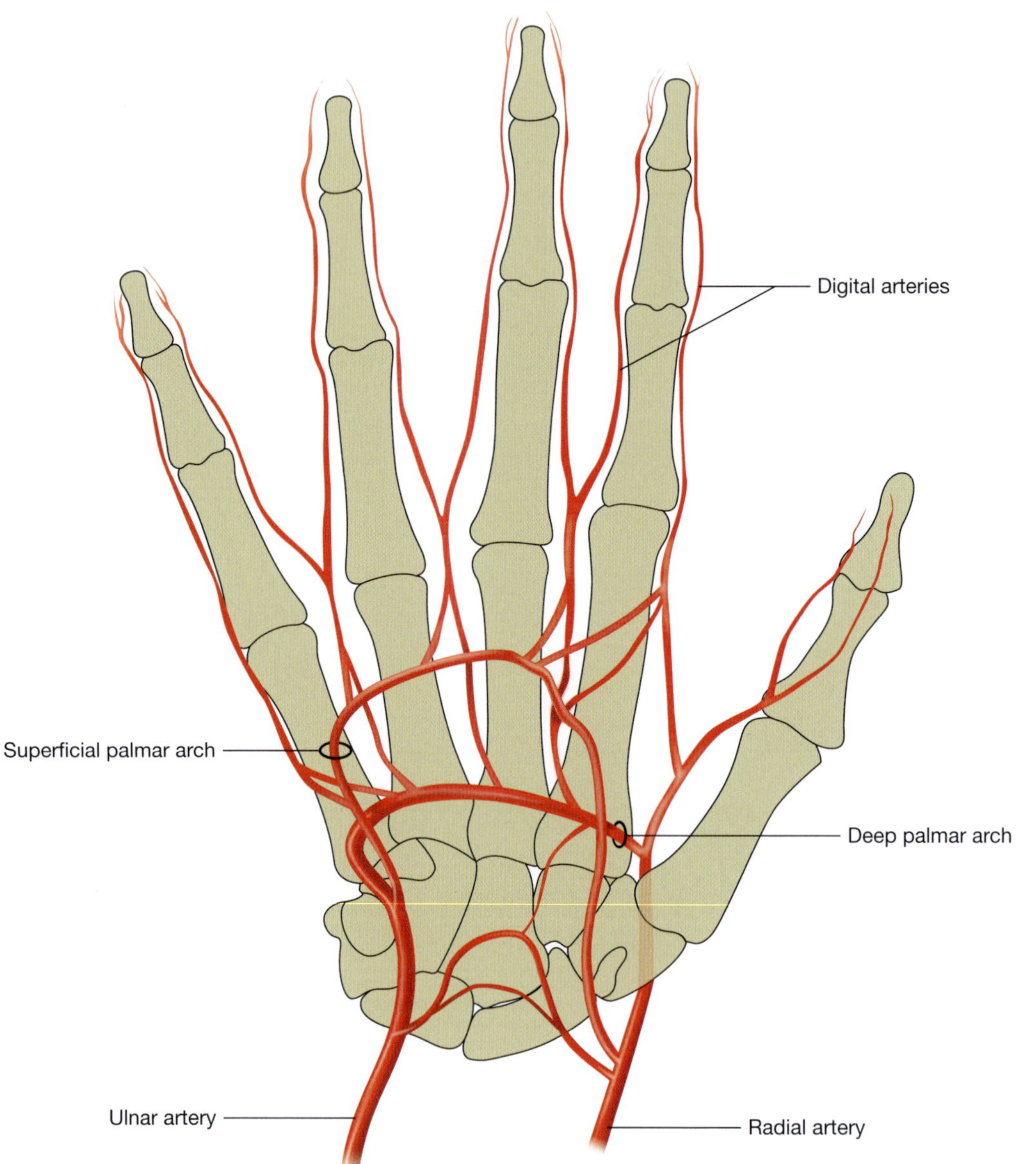

FIGURE 27.2 Arterial blood supply to the hand.

Radial Artery Spasm

The reported incidence of radial artery spasm ranges from 4% to 20%, partly due to lack of a uniform definition of this complication.[29] The pathophysiology of the radial artery spasm is that the manipulation of the catheter and stretching of the arterial wall stimulates the adrenoreceptors in the radial artery wall, which will cause the vasoconstriction.[29]

Operators should take into consideration some factors such as history of coronary artery bypass graft, female sex, low body mass, small radial artery diameter, and large caliber of catheters used, all of which will increase the risk of spasm. The use of smaller caliber catheters, ultrasound, sedatives, local analgesics, and spasmolytics decreases the risk of radial artery spasm.[30]

Symptoms: Arm pain is the most common symptom of radial artery spasm. Rarely does the pain become significant enough that it requires pausing or abandoning the procedure from this access site. Anatomical variants including branching of the radial artery from a more proximal location of the brachial or axillary artery are more prone to spasm as are accessory radial branches commonly seen with radial-ulnar loops.

Treatment: Pausing the procedure for a few minutes, pressure-mediated vasodilation or administration of vasodilators such as nitroglycerin or verapamil will help relieve the spasm.[29,31] If the radial artery spasm is severe enough to cause catheter or sheath entrapment, local ultrasound-guided radial nerve block, deep sedation with propofol, or general anesthesia have been reported but are rarely needed. Vascular surgery consultation is needed only in the most exceptional circumstances. The most frequent consequence of severe nonresolving spasm is the need to crossover to an alternate vascular access site.

Radial Artery Occlusion

In a systematic review of 66 studies, the incidence of RAO was 4.4% when defined by the absence of radial pulse and 10.5% when

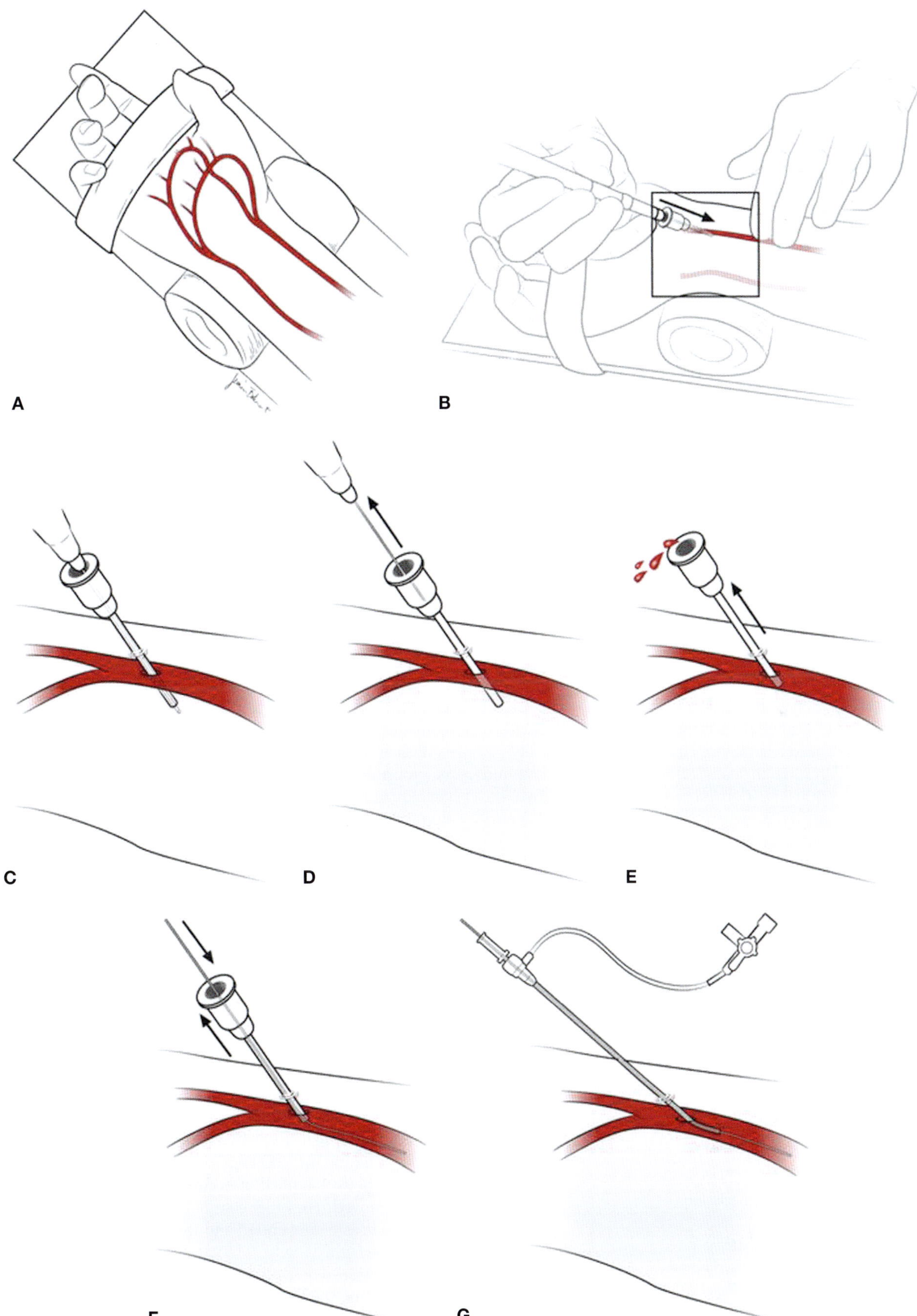

FIGURE 27.3 Back-wall puncture technique. **A,** Wrist in extension position. **B,** Insert needle with cannula. **C,** Advance needle and cannula through the front and back wall of the vessel. **D,** Remove the needle. **E,** Withdraw the cannula until pulsatile blood blood flow is seen. **F,** Advance the guidewire into the radial artery. **G,** Place radial sheath over wire into the vessel.

TABLE 27.2 Dosing, Timing, and Route of Anticoagulant Administration

ANTICOAGULANT DOSE AND CHOICE			
Heparin	SPIRIT OF ARTEMIS Trial (RCT; 3102 patients)	100 U/kg UFH had lower rate of RAO than 50 U/kg (3.0% vs 8.1%, $P < .001$) Similar rate of complications	*JACC Cardiovasc Interv.* 2018;11(22):2241-2250[18]
	Aykan et al (RCT; 459 patients)	5000 U UFH had a lower rate of RAO than 2500 U (1.2% vs 5.5%, $P = .01$)	*Int J Cardiol.* 2015;187:389-392[19]
LMWH (enoxaparin)	Feray et al. (case series, 50 cases)	Postprocedural RAO noted in two cases (4%)	*J Thromb Thrombolysis.* 2010;29(3):322-325[20]
Bivalirudin	Plante et al (case series, 400 consecutive cases)	Bivalirudin given prior to PCI provided similar rate of RAO as UFH (3.5% vs 7.0%, $P = .18$)	*Catheter Cardiovasc Interv.* 2010;76(5):654-658[21]
Timing of anticoagulation administration	PHARAOH (RCT; 400 patients)	As compared to patients getting UFH upon sheath insertion, administration of UFH at the time of sheath removal showed similar rate of RAO (early 7.5% vs 7.0% or late 4.5% vs 5.0%)	*Am J Cardiol.* 2012;110(2):173-176[22]
Route of anticoagulation administration	Pancholy (RCT; 500 patients)	There was no difference in RAO among patients receiving UFH via the intra-arterial vs intravenous routes (6.0% vs 5.6%, p = ns)	*Am J Cardiol.* 2009;104(8):1083-1085[23]

defined by the absence of radial flow assessed by ultrasound. Thus, the presence of a radial pulse does not preclude a diagnosis of RAO, and ultrasound examination is the preferred diagnostic test, although reverse Barbeau test may be equivalent diagnostically.[32]

RAO appears to resolve in many instances over the days and weeks following a catheterization procedure. In a meta-analysis, the rate of RAO was 7.7% when measured within 24 hours and it decreased to 5.5% at 1 month likely due to spontaneous recanalization.[32] Owing to the rich collateral circulation in the hand, RAO in clinical practice is nearly universally asymptomatic. Acute hand ischemia has certainly been reported, however.

TABLE 27.3 Radial Artery Access—Intra- and Postprocedural Complications

Intraprocedural Complications
Radial artery spasm
Catheter entrapment
Arterial dissection
Arterial perforation
Postprocedural Complications:
Radial artery occlusion
Bleeding
Forearm hematoma
Compartment syndrome
Arteriovenous fistula
Nerve injury
Hand dysfunction
Complex regional pain syndrome
Pseudoaneurysm

Pathophysiology: Sheath insertion leads to endothelial damage and stasis of the blood flow, which can promote thrombus formation.

Risk factors for RAO: Female sex, old age, low BMI, as well as procedure-related factors such as low artery-to-sheath ratio, inadequate anticoagulation, and duration of radial artery compression following the procedure. Some of the factors that have shown to improve or reduce the rate of RAO include use of hydrophilic sheaths, administration of full-dose systemic anticoagulation, patent hemostasis, ulnar artery compression, and shorter compression times.[32]

Treatment: In the setting of a recent RAO, ulnar artery compression for 1 hour may help the recanalization as it will facilitate the flow in the radial artery.[5] Use of ulnar compression has also been studied as a prophylactic measure to prevent RAO.[26] Low molecular weight heparin for up to 90 days and direct oral anticoagulants may be used to treat the RAO. Angioplasty is rarely necessary to treat hand ischemia.[33]

Catheter Entrapment

How does it happen? Excessive manipulation of the catheter might lead to kinking the catheter especially with tortuous anatomy. Once a catheter is kinked, it becomes difficult to remove until the kink is removed. The other common cause of entrapment is related to arterial spasm. Prevention and treatment of spasm is covered in an earlier section.

How to resolve it?Untwisting the catheter in the opposite direction should be the first strategy to resolve the kink. If that is not successful, then passing a stiffer wire or microcatheter to strengthen the catheter can be attempted. Blood pressure cuff inflation to attempt clamping of the distal portion of the catheter could allow untwisting of the proximal portion of the catheter and resolve the kink. In refractory cases, contralateral TRA or transfemoral access can be obtained, and a snare is advanced in order to capture the distal end of the catheter. Then, by applying tension to the snare and the proximal end of the catheter, the catheter can be unwound. The need for surgical intervention is extremely rare.

Alternative Approaches to Forearm Radial Access

Distal Radial Approach

The distal radial artery (DRA) access approach offers some potential advantages compared to traditional radial access. Proponents of this approach via the anatomic "snuffbox" suggest that it is a more ergonomic position for the patient and operator especially for left arm cases.[34] It also avoids repeated puncture in the traditional location, which may preserve this access site. In a recently completed, large, randomized trial, investigators demonstrated that DRA did not differ in RAO, bleeding, or vascular complications as compared to forearm radial access. The DRA group did have a higher crossover rate and more spasm, but hemostasis time was shorter.[35] In a meta-analysis, there was evidence for lower rates of proximal RAO in the DRA group as compared to traditional radial access without any increase in hematoma or radial artery spasm.[36]

Anatomy

The anatomical snuffbox (radial fossa) is a triangular-shaped space on the dorsum of the hand. Its medial border is formed by the tendon of extensor pollicis longus, and its lateral border is formed by the tendons of extensor pollicis brevis and the abductor pollicis longus. The floor of the anatomical snuffbox is formed by the scaphoid and the trapezium bones. The radial artery, reaching the wrist level, twists posterolaterally, crossing the anatomical snuffbox (**Fig. 27.4**).

Access Technique

1. The forearm is placed in a midway position between prone and supine over the left groin in case of left radial access or by the side of the right hip in case of right radial access (**Fig. 27.5**).
2. It has been suggested that the patient could grasp his/her thumb under the other 4 fingers or grasp a roll of gauge in order to bring the artery to the surface of the radial fossa.
3. Using ultrasound and the front-wall approach, puncture the artery and advance the access sheath wire. Deliver your access sheath over the wire.
4. Administer vasodilator cocktails and anticoagulation as per standard forearm access cases.

Closure Technique

- Given the geometry of the snuffbox, some changes to the traditional hemostasis band positioning are necessary, or dedicated bands for this access site are also available (**Fig. 27.6**).
- Patent hemostasis continues to be the best practice.

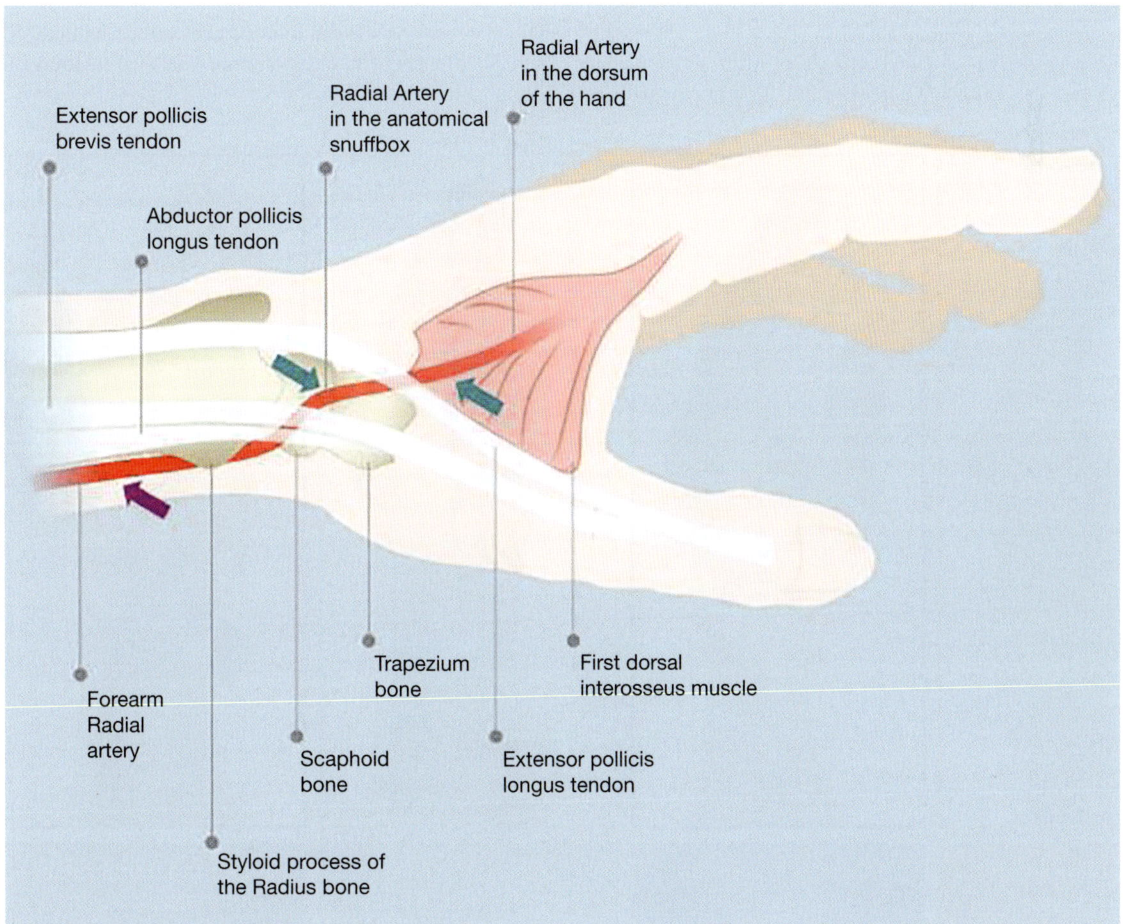

FIGURE 27.4 Anatomical illustration of the anatomical snuffbox and the relations to the hand bones. (From Aminian A, Sgueglia GA, Wiemer M, et al. Distal versus conventional radial access for coronary angiography and intervention: the DISCO RADIAL trial. *JACC Cardiovasc Interv.* 2022;15:1191-1201.)[35]

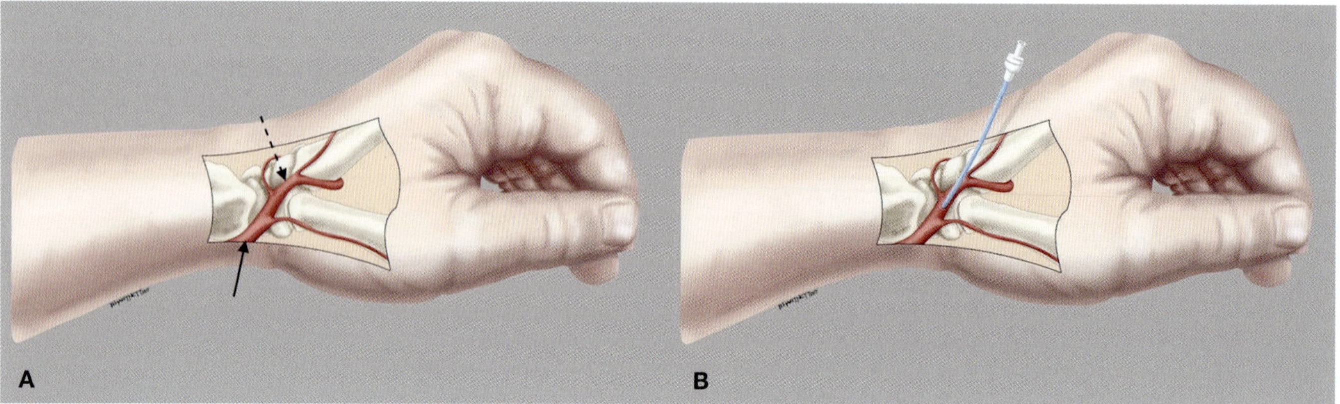

FIGURE 27.5 **A,** Arterial anatomy demonstrating the puncture site in the distal radial artery at the anatomical snuffbox (*dotted arrow*) versus the conventional radial artery at the wrist (*solid arrow*). **B,** Position of vascular sheath inserted in the distal radial artery. (Reprinted by permission from Hadjivassiliou A, Cardarelli-Leite L, Jalal S, et al. Left distal transradial access (ldTRA): a comparative assessment of conventional and distal radial artery size. *Cardiovasc Intervent Radiol.* 2020;43:850-857.)[37]

Ulnar Artery Approach

The ulnar artery can also be used as an arterial access site for coronary procedures. In some individuals, the ulnar artery is larger than the radial artery. In contrast to the radial artery, the ulnar artery at the level of the wrist does not pass over a bone. The ulnar nerve also runs very close to the artery. Despite these differences, there is good clinical evidence to support its use.

In a meta-analysis, the transulnar approach (TUA) was compared with transradial approach and showed similar risks of major adverse cardiovascular event and access-related complications. TUA resulted in higher rates of access crossover (risk ratio: 2.31 [1.07-4.98]; $P = .003$) and more number of punctures (1.57 vs 1.4; $P = .0002$). There was no difference in arterial access time (12.8 vs 10.9 min), fluoroscopy time (7.6 vs 7.2 min), and contrast volume (151 vs 153.7 mL). The authors concluded that TUA compared with TRA has similar efficacy and safety except for higher puncture attempts and access site crossover.[39]

At the current time, use of the ulnar artery is considered a secondary access choice if the radial artery is not available or diminutive.

Technique for Ulnar Artery Access

The approach is similar to the front wall or bare needle approach described earlier for radial access. Use of ultrasound may help to avoid injuring the ulnar nerve.

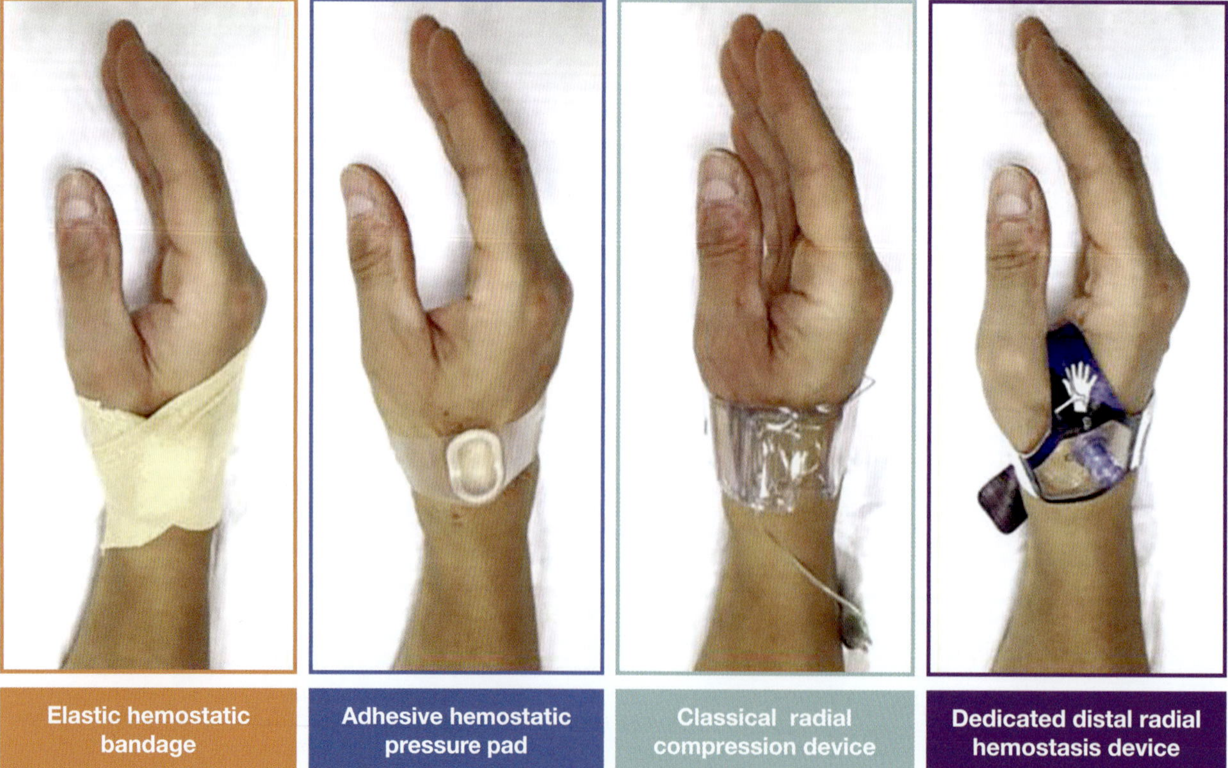

FIGURE 27.6 Distal radial artery closure devices. (From Sgueglia GA, Lee BK, Cho BR, et al. Distal radial access: consensus report of the first Korea-Europe transradial intervention meeting. *JACC Cardiovasc Interv.* 2021;14:892-906. Copyright 2021, with permission from Elsevier.)[38]

Ulnar Artery Hemostasis Techniques

The approach to ulnar artery hemostasis is similar to radial artery closure. For some bands, the application will have to be altered to allow the compressive surface to be centered over the ulnar puncture site. Beware of access site bleeding as the ulnar artery does not course over a bony surface. In clinical trials, hemostasis and vascular complications appear to occur at a similar rate as with radial access.

CONCLUSIONS

Forearm arterial access is gradually becoming the predominant vascular access site for coronary diagnostic and interventional procedures. Patients experience lower vascular complications, less bleeding, and improved comfort with radial access as compared to femoral access, particularly when performing PCI in the setting of ACS.[9] Alternatives to radial access including distal radial and ulnar artery access are emerging as other suitable options for certain clinical scenarios. Each of these access approaches has unique challenges and complications that must be recognized. An evidence-based approach to one's technique will result in the best patient outcomes.

Key Points

- PCI using radial artery access as compared to femoral artery access is associated with lower rates of access site complications, less bleeding, and improved patient comfort.
- Radial artery access is the preferred access approach for patients suffering from ACSs.
- Distal radial access and ulnar artery access are alternatives to the radial artery access.
- Best practices to reduce RAO include systemic anticoagulation, maintaining a low sheath:artery diameter ratio, patent hemostasis, and avoiding prolonged compression times.

Disclosures

Shaker, Doctor, Zurawska: None to disclose. Shroff: Medtronic, CSI, and Terumo—consultant.

For further review and interactivities, please see the chapter-based multiple choice questions and videos accessible in the complimentary eBook bundled with this text. Access instructions are located in the inside front cover.

References

1. Nairoukh Z, Jahangir S, Adjepong D, Malik BH. Distal radial artery access: the future of cardiovascular intervention. *Cureus*. 2020;12(3):e7201.
2. Fernandez R, Zaky F, Ekmejian A, Curtis E, Lee A. Safety and efficacy of ulnar artery approach for percutaneous cardiac catheterization: systematic review and meta-analysis. *Catheter Cardiovasc Interv*. 2018;91(7):1273-1280.
3. Jolly SS, Yusuf S, Cairns J, et al; RIVAL trial group. Radial versus femoral access for coronary angiography and intervention in patients with acute coronary syndromes (RIVAL): a randomised, parallel group, multicentre trial. *Lancet*. 2011;377(9775):1409-1420.
4. Romagnoli E, Biondi-Zoccai G, Sciahbasi A, et al. Radial versus femoral randomized investigation in ST-segment elevation acute coronary syndrome: the RIFLE-STEACS (radial versus femoral randomized investigation in ST-elevation acute coronary syndrome) study. *J Am Coll Cardiol*. 2012;60(24):2481-2489.
5. Bernat I, Bertrand OF, Rokyta R, et al. Efficacy and safety of transient ulnar artery compression to recanalize acute radial artery occlusion after transradial catheterization. *Am J Cardiol*. 2011;107(11):1698-1701.
6. Valgimigli M, Frigoli E, Leonardi S, et al. Radial versus femoral access and bivalirudin versus unfractionated heparin in invasively managed patients with acute coronary syndrome (MATRIX): final 1-year results of a multicentre, randomised controlled trial. *Lancet*. 2018;392(10150):835-848.
7. Le May M, Wells G, So D, et al. Safety and efficacy of femoral access vs radial access in ST-segment elevation myocardial infarction: the SAFARI-STEMI randomized clinical trial. *JAMA Cardiol*. 2020;5(2):126-134.
8. Ibanez B, James S, Agewall S, et al. 2017 ESC Guidelines for the management of acute myocardial infarction in patients presenting with ST-segment elevation: the Task Force for the management of acute myocardial infarction in patients presenting with ST-segment elevation of the European Society of Cardiology (ESC). *Eur Heart J*. 2018;39(2):119-177.
9. Shroff AR, Gulati R, Drachman DE, et al. SCAI expert consensus statement update on best practices for transradial angiography and intervention. *Catheter Cardiovasc Interv*. 2020;95(2):245-252.
10. Mason PJ, Shah B, Tamis-Holland JE, et al. An update on radial artery access and best practices for transradial coronary angiography and intervention in acute coronary syndrome: a scientific statement from the American Heart Association. *Circ Cardiovasc Interv*. 2018;11(9):e000035.
11. Lawton JS, Tamis-Holland JE, Bangalore S, et al. 2021 ACC/AHA/SCAI guideline for coronary artery revascularization: executive summary—a Report of the American College of Cardiology/American Heart Association Joint Committee on clinical practice guidelines. *Circulation*. 2022;145(3):e4-e17.
12. Sattur S, Singh M, Kaluski E. Transulnar access for coronary angiography and percutaneous coronary intervention. *J Invasive Cardiol*. 2014;26:404-408.
13. Seto AH, Roberts JS, Abu-Fadel MS, et al. Real-time ultrasound guidance facilitates transradial access: RAUST (Radial Artery access with Ultrasound Trial). *JACC Cardiovasc Interv*. 2015;8(2):283-291.
14. Roberts JS, Niu J. An ultrasound survey of the radial and ulnar arteries in an American population: implications for transradial access. *J Invasive Cardiol*. 2023;35(3):E143-E150.
15. Meo D, Falsaperla D, Modica A, et al. Proximal and distal radial artery approaches for endovascular percutaneous procedures: anatomical suitability by ultrasound evaluation. *Radiol Med*. 2021;126(4):630-635.
16. Kotowycz MA, Johnston KW, Ivanov J, et al. Predictors of radial artery size in patients undergoing cardiac catheterization: insights from the Good Radial Artery Size Prediction (GRASP) study. *Can J Cardiol*. 2014;30(2):211-216.
17. Dharma S, Kedev S, Patel T, Rao SV, Bertrand OF, Gilchrist IC. Radial artery diameter does not correlate with body mass index: a duplex ultrasound analysis of 1706 patients undergoing trans-radial catheterization at three experienced radial centers. *Int J Cardiol*. 2017;228:169-172.
18. Hahalis GN, Leopoulou M, Tsigkas G, et al. Multicenter randomized evaluation of high versus standard heparin dose on incident radial arterial occlusion after transradial coronary angiography: the SPIRIT OF ARTEMIS study. *JACC Cardiovasc Interv*. 2018;11(22):2241-2250.
19. Aykan AC, Gokdeniz T, Gul I, et al. Comparison of low dose versus standard dose heparin for radial approach in elective coronary angiography? *Int J Cardiol*. 2015;187:389-392.
20. Feray H, Izgi C, Cetiner D, et al. Effectiveness of enoxaparin for prevention of radial artery occlusion after transradial cardiac catheterization. *J Thromb Thrombolysis*. 2010;29(3):322-325.
21. Plante S, Cantor WJ, Goldman L, et al. Comparison of bivalirudin versus heparin on radial artery occlusion after transradial catheterization. *Catheter Cardiovasc Interv*. 2010;76(5):654-658.
22. Pancholy SB, Bertrand OF, Patel T. Comparison of a priori versus provisional heparin therapy on radial artery occlusion after transradial coronary angiography and patent hemostasis (from the PHARAOH Study). *Am J Cardiol*. 2012;110(2):173-176.

23. Pancholy SB. Comparison of the effect of intra-arterial versus intravenous heparin on radial artery occlusion after transradial catheterization. *Am J Cardiol*. 2009;104(8):1083-1085.
24. Device Guide. *US Edition. Bryn Mawr Communications II*. LLC; 2023. https://citoday.com/device-guide/us
25. Pancholy S, Coppola J, Patel T, Roke-Thomas M. Prevention of radial artery occlusion-Patent hemostasis evaluation trial (PROPHET study): a randomized comparison of traditional versus patency documented hemostasis after transradial catheterization. *Catheter Cardiovasc Interv*. 2008;72(3):335-340.
26. Pancholy SB, Bernat I, Bertrand OF, Patel TM. Prevention of radial artery occlusion after transradial catheterization: the PROPHET-II randomized trial. *JACC Cardiovasc Interv*. 2016;9(19):1992-1999.
27. Safirstein JG, Tehrani DM, Schussler JM, et al. Radial hemostasis is facilitated with a potassium ferrate hemostatic patch: the STAT2 trial. *JACC Cardiovasc Interv*. 2022;15(8):810-819.
28. Maqsood MH, Pancholy S, Tuozzo KA, Moskowitz N, Rao SV, Bangalore S. Optimal hemostatic band duration after transradial angiography or intervention: insights from a mixed treatment comparison meta-analysis of randomized trials. *Circ Cardiovasc Interv*. 2023;16(2):e012781.
29. Roy S, Kabach M, Patel DB, Guzman LA, Jovin IS. Radial artery access complications: prevention, diagnosis and management. *Cardiovasc Revasc Med*. 2022;40:163-171.
30. Ho HH, Jafary FH, Ong PJ. Radial artery spasm during transradial cardiac catheterization and percutaneous coronary intervention: incidence, predisposing factors, prevention, and management. *Cardiovasc Revasc Med*. 2012;13(3):193-195.
31. Collet C, Corral JM, Cavalcante R, et al. Pressure-mediated versus pharmacologic treatment of radial artery spasm during cardiac catheterisation: a randomised pilot study. *EuroIntervention*. 2017;12(18):e2212-e2218.
32. Rashid M, Kwok CS, Pancholy S, et al. Radial artery occlusion after transradial interventions: a systematic review and meta-analysis. *J Am Heart Assoc*. 2016;5(1):e002686.
33. Zankl AR, Andrassy M, Volz C, et al. Radial artery thrombosis following transradial coronary angiography: incidence and rationale for treatment of symptomatic patients with low-molecular-weight heparins. *Clin Res Cardiol*. 2010;99(12):841-847.
34. Kiemeneij F. Left distal transradial access in the anatomical snuffbox for coronary angiography (ldTRA) and interventions (ldTRI). *EuroIntervention*. 2017;13:851-857.
35. Aminian A, Sgueglia GA, Wiemer M, et al. Distal versus conventional radial access for coronary angiography and intervention: the DISCO RADIAL trial. *JACC Cardiovasc Interv*. 2022;15(12):1191-1201.
36. Rigatelli G, Zuin M, Daggubati R, et al. Distal snuffbox versus conventional radial artery access: an updated systematic review and meta-analysis. *J Vasc Access*. 2022;23(4):653-659.
37. Hadjivassiliou A, Cardarelli-Leite L, Jalal S, et al. Left distal transradial access (ldTRA): a comparative assessment of conventional and distal radial artery size. *Cardiovasc Intervent Radiol*. 2020;43(6):850-857.
38. Sgueglia GA, Lee BK, Cho BR, et al. Distal radial access: consensus Report of the first Korea-Europe transradial intervention meeting. *JACC Cardiovasc Interv*. 2021;14(8):892-906.
39. Dahal K, Rijal J, Lee J, Korr KS, Azrin M. Transulnar versus transradial access for coronary angiography or percutaneous coronary intervention: a meta-analysis of randomized controlled trials. *Catheter Cardiovasc Interv*. 2016;87(5):857-865.

28 Femoral Approaches

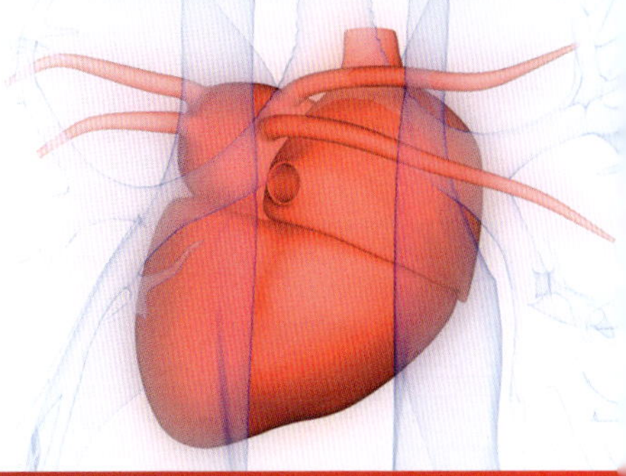

Mazen Abu-Fadel

Invasive cardiac and endovascular procedures are increasing in number and complexity in cardiac catheterization laboratories and endovascular suites across the world. The initial approach to all these procedures requires vascular access into the arterial or venous circulation. While access is just a means to an end, it remains one of the most challenging and life-threatening steps we perform. Newer procedures and techniques require larger sheaths and equipment; thus, optimal access and closure techniques are crucial not only for the success of any of these procedures but also to decrease patients' mortality and morbidity. Accordingly, it is crucial that optimal technique and best practices be employed when gaining vascular access, and when obtaining hemostasis of the access site. The majority of such procedures are performed from the radial and femoral arteries. Each access site has its own advantages and disadvantages. The "radial-first" strategy in cardiac and peripheral catheterization procedures has caused an increase in transradial access as the primary approach in most cardiac catheterization laboratories. However, mastery of femoral access is critical for any interventionalist since it remains necessary for procedures with radial access failure and for procedures requiring larger sheaths. In addition, transradial approaches are not feasible for many peripheral and structural interventions. This chapter will review femoral artery anatomy, access techniques, and best practices to obtain safe femoral access and regress.

ANATOMY OF THE COMMON FEMORAL ARTERY

The common femoral artery (CFA) is the continuation of the external iliac artery after it traverses the inguinal ligament. From there, the artery follows the medial side of the head and neck of the femur inferiorly and laterally before splitting into the superficial and deep femoral artery. The CFA artery traverses medial to the anterior crural nerve and lateral to the femoral vein in the femoral or Scarpa triangle comprising what is commonly referred to as the "groin" area. The artery is covered anteriorly with the inferior extension of the fascia of the transverse abdominal and iliac muscle. The most superficial part of the CFA is the section of the artery that traverses over the head of the femur.[1] The diameter of the CFA varies according to age, body size, and sex. The most recent studies in subjects coming to the cath lab for various procedures showed the mean diameter of the CFA to be 6.9 ± 1.4 mm in both males and females.[2]

CFA bifurcation may occur at any level along the course of the vessel. In a study that analyzed 972 femoral angiograms for the level of the CFA bifurcation, it was observed that in 64.8% of patients the bifurcation occurred below the inferior border of the head of the femur. In addition, the bifurcation was at or below the middle of the head of the femur in 98.5% of the study population.[3] This information is important to know when accessing the CFA without any previous imaging to define the location of the bifurcation or without ultrasound guidance for direct visualization. Another important anatomic landmark is the takeoff and course of the inferior epigastric artery (IEA) and its relation to the arteriotomy site. The IEA originates from the external iliac, immediately above the inguinal ligament. It curves forward in the subperitoneal tissue and then ascends obliquely along the medial margin of the abdominal inguinal ring and continues its course cranially. Multiple variations exist, and the origin may take place from any part of the external iliac between the inguinal ligament and a point 6 cm above it; or less frequently it may arise below this ligament, from the CFA. Patients' demographics are of limited utility for predicting anatomic variants of the CFA bifurcation and the course of the IEA. The IEA origin has a more variable anatomic pattern, with high body surface area, male gender, and white race associated with a low IEA origin.[4]

The ideal access site into the CFA should be below the most inferior point of the IEA and above the CFA bifurcation anterior to the femoral head (**Fig. 28.1**). As such, in the majority of patients, the ideal access site falls midway between the superior and the inferior borders of the head of the femur.[5,6] Access sites below the CFA bifurcation or below the inferior border of the femoral head (whichever is higher) are associated with increased rates of pseudoaneurysms and hematomas and limit the ultimate size of a sheath that can be used. Access sites above the most inferior deflection of the IEA are problematic in that the EIA is in a retroperitoneal

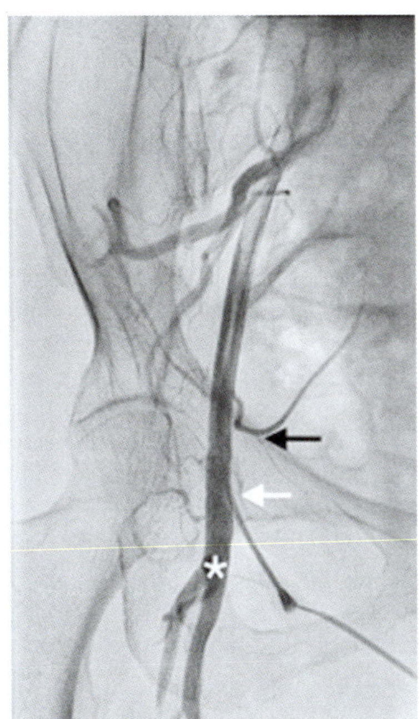

FIGURE 28.1 Ideal access site. Site of arteriotomy (*white arrow*) at the level of the mid femoral head, above the CFA bifurcation (*asterisk*) and below the most inferior border of the inferior epigastric artery (*black arrow*). CFA, common femoral artery.

TABLE 28.1 Considerations Prior to CFA Access

- Patient preference
- Body habitus, especially severe obesity
- Inability to lie flat during or after the procedure
- Prior femoral access site complications
- Presence of a femoral bruit on examination
- Peripheral arterial disease of the lower extremities
- Prior bypass surgery, especially fem-fem bypass
- Prior radiation or surgery to the groin area
- Anticoagulation, bleeding, and transfusion considerations
- Severe vessel tortuosity or aneurysmal dilatation
- Active infection in the groin area or skin breakdown
- Nonpalpable femoral pulse
- Recent use of some vascular closure devices such as a collagen plug

CFA, common femoral artery.

location and can be associated with increased rates of bleeding especially retroperitoneal hemorrhage.[7,8] In addition to minimizing access site complications, CFA access through the anterior wall in an ideal location is necessary for optimal utilization of vascular closure devices.

Considerations Prior to CFA Access

Prior to attaining CFA access, it is prudent to obtain a thorough history and physical as well as review previous femoral angiograms and imaging available. Even though CFA access can be achieved on almost all patients, it should be reconsidered in patients who may have features that predispose them to an increased risk of CFA access complications. These considerations are presented in **Table 28.1**.

Techniques for CFA Access

The original percutaneous method of obtaining vascular access was pioneered by Seldinger in the 1950s. The original method involved performing a posterior wall stick with a needle and stylet, removal of the stylet, and withdrawal of the needle until blood exited the hub of the needle, followed by introduction of a wire into the vascular space. Over time, the technique for femoral artery access has been modified with emphasis on obtaining an anterior wall stick (modified Seldinger technique) to help minimize potential complications arising from posterior wall access and/or injury. Traditionally, after local anesthesia with 1% lidocaine, an 18-gauge needle has been used to gain access, which can accommodate a 0.038″ guidewire. More recently, micropuncture techniques have been popularized, which involve the use of small initial access needles and wires, <21 gauge, with upsizing catheters that ultimately allow placement of a standard guidewire and sheath.

Sedation and Local Anesthesia

The first step in obtaining access at any site is appropriate sedation and local anesthesia. Vascular access, especially in the CFA area, is usually uncomfortable for the patient, who may remember and fixate on the discomfort they experienced during the first couple minutes of the procedure. Thus, sedation should be given 3 to 5 minutes prior to starting the procedure and attempting vascular access. Once well sedated, and after identifying the point of needle entry by one of the methods described later, local anesthetic is given. Many ways have been described, but in general, while the pulse is located between your index and middle finger, local anesthesia is given below the skin to form a wheel or bleb followed by advancing the needle deeper into the tissue toward the CFA. It is important to draw back on the plunger before injecting in the subcutaneous space to avoid injecting into a vascular structure. This is followed by injecting lidocaine at a constant rate while drawing the needle backward toward the skin thus anesthetizing the track that the access needle is going to take into the CFA.

If using ultrasound-guided access, first start by locating the ideal access and skin entry site with the ultrasound probe then use the local anesthesia needle to deliver the medication as described previously. With ultrasound imaging, the operator can actually observe in real time the lidocaine being injected and will be able to give it just on top of the CFA without entering the artery and then all the way back to the skin.

Ideal Puncture Site of the CFA

Ideally, the anterior wall of the CFA should be punctured 1 to 2 cm below the inguinal ligament but proximal to its bifurcation into the superficial femoral and deep femoral arteries. At this site, the CFA can be easily compressed against the femoral head to achieve manual hemostasis. Access below the CFA bifurcation, even if the bifurcation is anterior to the femoral head, will increase the risk of vascular complications such as hematomas and pseudoaneurysms and may prevent the use of larger sheaths if needed. In addition, the ideal access site should be below the level of the most inferior horizontal reflection of the IEA. Entry above the most inferior point of the course of the IEA can be used to define an unmistakably high puncture. Thus, access should be below that point but above the CFA bifurcation (**Fig. 28.1**). A puncture above the level of the most inferior horizontal reflection of the IEA will predispose patient to an increased risk of potentially life-threatening retroperitoneal hemorrhage due to the lack of an underlying bony structure to help with hemostasis during compression.[9] In a review of 989 femoral angiograms from the Femoral Arterial Access with Ultrasound Trial (FAUST), the CFA bifurcation occurs consistently (95%) below the middle third of the femoral head and no patient factors were predictive of a high bifurcation. The IEA origin had a more variable anatomic pattern (11% in the middle third of the femoral head), with high body surface area, male gender, and white race associated with a low IEA origin. The most inferior reflection of the IEA occurred 92.2% of the time below the superior border of the head of the femur.[4,10] In addition, in almost 65% of patients the CFA bifurcated was below the most inferior border of the head of the femur.[3] In this case, the length of the CFA that extends from the inferior border of the femoral head to its bifurcation is considered a suboptimal access site since there is no bony structure to help compress the CFA after the sheath is pulled, increasing the risk of hematomas and pseudoaneurysms (**Fig. 28.1**).

Accessing the CFA in an ideal location may be accomplished more easily in patients with previous femoral angiography where the relationship between the head of the femur, the CFA bifurcation, and the most inferior border of the IEA can be seen. In patients with no previous invasive or noninvasive femoral angiography, multiple methods have been described to assist the operator achieve an ideal access site. Some of the techniques employed to guide femoral artery access include the use of anatomic landmarks, palpation of the strongest femoral pulse, fluoroscopy, and ultrasound imaging. While all of the other techniques rely on extrapolating the relationship between the CFA and the femoral head, only ultrasound imaging allows visualization of the CFA and its bifurcation.

Traditional Anatomic Landmarks to Access the CFA

Anatomic landmarks that have been utilized to identify the CFA include the inguinal skin crease, maximal femoral pulse, and bony landmarks. Many operators use the inguinal skin crease as a starting point for CFA access and are under the impression that the skin crease overlies the inguinal ligament. In fact, the inguinal skin crease is the least reliable among the anatomic landmarks. In patients with lean body habitus, the skin crease may be on top of the inguinal ligament; however, in the majority of patients, especially the obese, it may be as low as 11 cm (mean 6.5 cm) from the ligament and below the CFA bifurcation in as many as 75.6% of patients.[11] Using the point of maximal femoral pulsation to access the CFA is more reliable. The site of maximal pulsation is over the CFA in 92.7% of patients.[12] It is important to keep in mind that in obese patients the point of maximal pulse may be below the CFA since this is the only area that a pulse can be palpated due to the thickness of the subcutaneous tissues more cranially. In addition, up to 20% of patients who require femoral access do not have a strong or even palpable pulse to start with making the point of maximal impulse useless. The third commonly used anatomic landmark is the imaginary line connecting the anterior superior iliac spine and the pubic tubercle. This line represents the outline of the inguinal ligament. Accessing the CFA 2 to 3 cm below the midpoint of this landmark has been used by many as a guide for arterial sheath insertion. This, however, is still a problem in obese patients, where the bony landmarks are not as prominent or palpable. In the Fluoro Access study, it was shown that using the bony landmarks to obtain access into the CFA led to the arteriotomy site to be at the mid-level of the head of the femur in 20.4% of patients only. In addition, the access site was below the middle of the femoral head in 36.8% of patients. Among these low arteriotomies, 17.4% were below the inferior border of the femoral head thus making the bony landmark technique a suboptimal one as well. Arteriotomies below the femoral head were seen more frequently in obese patients with body mass indexes over 32 kg/m^2.[3]

Fluoroscopy Use to Access the CFA

When originally described, fluoroscopy-guided access (indirect fluoroscopy technique) involved placing a straight tip hemostat or radiopaque marker on the skin to mark the lower edge of the femoral head under fluoroscopy in the posterior-anterior projection. This was considered the skin entry level for retrograde femoral access. From that level, the needle would then be advanced at 45° angle into the subcutaneous tissue toward the pulse until the needle crosses the anterior wall of the CFA. This technique was tested in a prospective randomized study against the use of bony anatomic landmarks. In this study, fluoroscopy-guided access decreased arterial punctures below the femoral head especially in obese patients (3.3% vs 6.4% in the traditional arm P = .03); however, fluoroscopy did not increase the percentage of patients with an ideal access site in the CFA.[3] It is now obvious that the skin entry site should vary depending on the amount of subcutaneous tissue between the skin and the CFA (**Fig. 28.2**).

Some operators use the direct fluoroscopy technique that goes multiple steps beyond the indirect technique that just locates the bottom of the femoral head. After fluoroscopically locating the inferior border of the femoral head, repeat fluoroscopy is performed after the needle (usually a micropuncture needle) has been advanced into the subcutaneous tissue but has not entered the CFA. This will help the operator guide the tip of the needle toward the middle of the femoral head to achieve an ideal puncture site.[5,6] Under fluoroscopy, the transition between the micropuncture needle and its wire (needle-wire interface) will represent the site of entry into the CFA (**Fig. 28.3**).

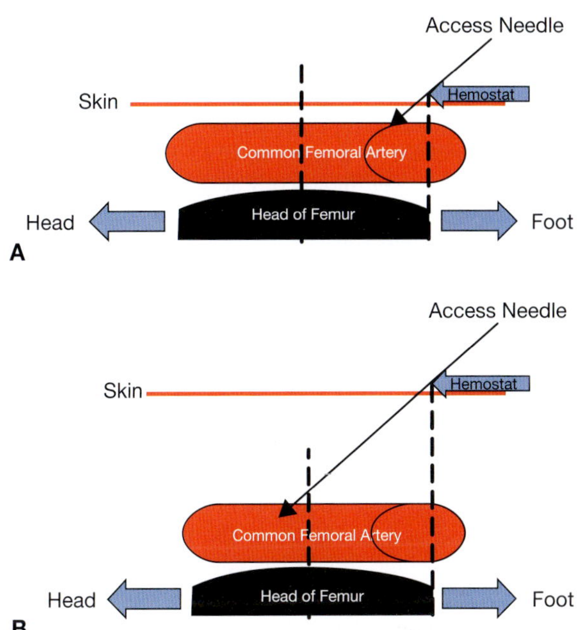

FIGURE 28.2 Illustration showing how the distance between the skin and the common femoral artery can affect the location of the arteriotomy even when the access needle is advanced at the same angle. In both illustrations A and B, the skin entry site is at the level of the inferior border of the femoral head. (From Abu-Fadel MS, ed. Common femoral artery access. In: *Arterial and Venous Access in the Cardiac Catheterization Lab.* 1st ed. New Brunswick, NJ: Rutgers University Press; 2016:1-20.)

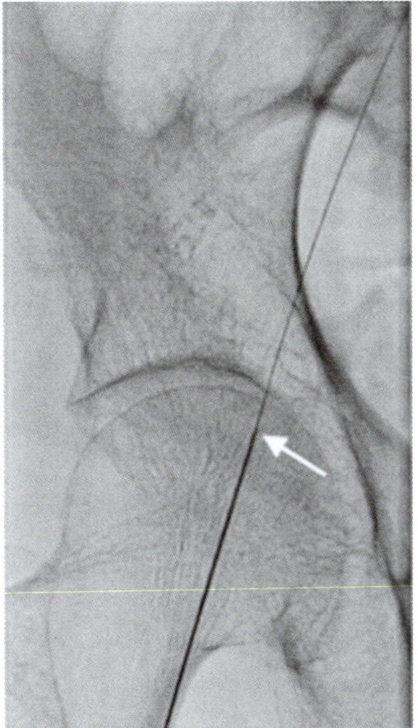

FIGURE 28.3 Fluoroscopy showing the interface or transition between the micropuncture needle and its 0.018-in wire (*arrow*). This interface represents the site at which the needle entered the artery. In this case, the access was above the ideal position, so the needle/wire were removed and manual pressure was applied for 3 minutes to obtain hemostasis before reattempting access.

Ultrasound-Guided CFA Access

Fluoroscopy has multiple limitations when obtaining femoral artery access mainly due to the anatomic variation in the CFA and its bifurcation. Ultrasound-guided access has emerged as an efficient and safe method to access the CFA. This technique offers multiple advantages over fluoroscopy alone including direct visualization of the CFA, needle advancement into a healthy part of the CFA through the anterior wall, prevention of accidental venous puncture, and a decrease in the radiation dose to both the patient and the operator. See **Table 28.2** for advantages and limitations to using ultrasound imaging for vascular access.

There are multiple options of portable ultrasound machines that can be used in the catheterization laboratory to assist in vascular access. In choosing an ultrasound machine for vascular access procedures it is critical that (1) the image is of high quality, (2) the depth of the display can be reduced to show shallow vessels easily, and (3) the display is large enough to be viewed from a distance. Cost, startup time, and durability are also important to consider. The ultrasound machine should have the ability to record, save, and export images and clips to external drives or databases, which is required for reimbursement of ultrasound guidance. Other materials include disposable sterile ultrasound probe cover kits containing ultrasound transmission gel. Needle guides are optional and tend to be most useful for deep and critical areas.[13]

The basic anatomic views of a tubular vascular structure that can be obtained with ultrasound imaging are transverse/cross-sectional (axial), longitudinal (sagittal), and oblique (a mix between axial and sagittal).

The axial view is the basic and most frequently used ultrasound view for vascular access. This view is easily obtained by orienting the long axis of the probe perpendicular to the axis of the vessel. This generates a circular, cross-sectional image of the vessel and provides information about the diameter of the vessel and relationship with other structures especially adjacent vessels (artery or vein). Its advantages include the ease of maintaining the image position and a wide field of view of adjacent structures. Its main disadvantage is difficulty in visualizing the needle or track, which appears as a small echogenic dot, with the risk that the puncture will be more superior or out of plane than expected. With practice in jabbing of the needle and adjustment of probe angles, the needle tip can be imaged effectively. As a result, the axial view is the standard view for ultrasound guidance.[13]

TABLE 28.2 Advantages and Limitations to Using Ultrasound for Vascular Access

Advantages of Ultrasound-Guided Access
Real-time visualization of vessel
Improved success rate
Decrease complications
Decrease accidental venous punctures
Decrease time to sheath insertion
Identifies adjacent structures
Identifies calcifications and plaque in vessel
Accurately determine vessel size and depth
Observe real-time anterior wall vessel puncture
Limitations of Ultrasound Usage
Small learning curve
Equipment availability
Equipment expense
Limited reimbursement

The longitudinal view is obtained by orienting the long axis of the probe in line with the vessel (90° from the axial view). This generates a linear (sagittal) image of length of the vessel but provides no imaging of the surrounding medial or lateral structures. When used for vascular access, the longitudinal view has the advantage of continuous visualization of the needle as it is advanced toward the vessel. This view and the oblique view have multiple challenges that make their use infrequent for vascular access.[13]

Ultrasound guidance can provide clear evidence of the location of veins relative to arteries using gentle compression of the transducer against the skin. This collapses the vein and reveals the pulsations of the artery, thereby distinguishing the two vascular structures. With the axial approach, the center of the image matches the center of the probe. Moving the transducer until the vessel is in the center of the image ensures that the vessel lies beneath the center of the transducer. Insertion of the needle just below the center of the transducer should thus ensure that the needle is directly above the anterior wall of the CFA. Although the needle is echogenic, it is not visible until it crosses the plane of the ultrasound. Short back-and-forth movements of the needle (jabbing) can help visualize and identify the needle tip compared with other echogenic structures. This enables the operator to make small adjustments in either the insertion location or angulation of the needle to successfully cannulate the CFA. The needle should be inserted into the skin underneath the center marking of the probe at about a 45° to 60° angle. If the vessel is not superficial, the needle can be inserted some distance from the probe to match the depth of the vessel, so that a 45° angled needle intersects the ultrasound plane at the depth of the vessel.[13] One important risk in using ultrasound is that the operator may go too cranial with the probe or angulate the probe to look more cranial than needed and thus access the artery above the middle of the femoral head or even access the external iliac artery. In order to avoid this mistake, the operator can use anatomic and fluoroscopic guidance to help. As the probe is moved cranially, the CFA starts to dive into the pelvic rim as it transitions into the external iliac artery. The CFA should be accessed above the femoral head at its shallowest point and before it starts to dive into the pelvis (**Fig. 28.4**). In addition, by increasing ultrasound depth, the femoral head can also be observed and be used to guide needle access over the middle of the bony structure. The most contemporary way to access the CFA is to use a combination of fluoroscopy and ultrasound guidance as described later in this chapter.

In the 1004-patient FAUST study,[10] we demonstrated that ultrasound guidance reduced the number of attempts required to successfully cannulate the femoral artery (1.3 vs 3; $P < .001$), increased the first-pass success rate (82.7% vs 46.4%; $P < .001$), and reduced the risk of accidental venipuncture (2.4% vs 15.8%; $P < .001$). As a result, the incidence of any vascular complications was reduced with ultrasound guidance (1.4% vs 3.4%; $P = .041$). In addition, the average time to access was reduced with ultrasound guidance from 213 to 185 seconds ($P = .016$), excluding time to set up the device. In the FAUST trial, the overall rate of CFA cannulation was not significantly different with ultrasound guidance compared with fluoroscopy (86.4% vs 83.3%; $P = .17$) but was higher in the 31% of patients with high CFA bifurcations (82.6% vs 69.8%; $P < .01$).

These findings were more recently redemonstrated in the UNIVERSAL trial.[14] The results of this trial show that, among patients undergoing coronary angiography or intervention, routine ultrasonography with fluoroscopy-guided femoral artery access did not reduce a composite of major bleeding and major vascular complications versus fluoroscopic guidance alone. The trial did

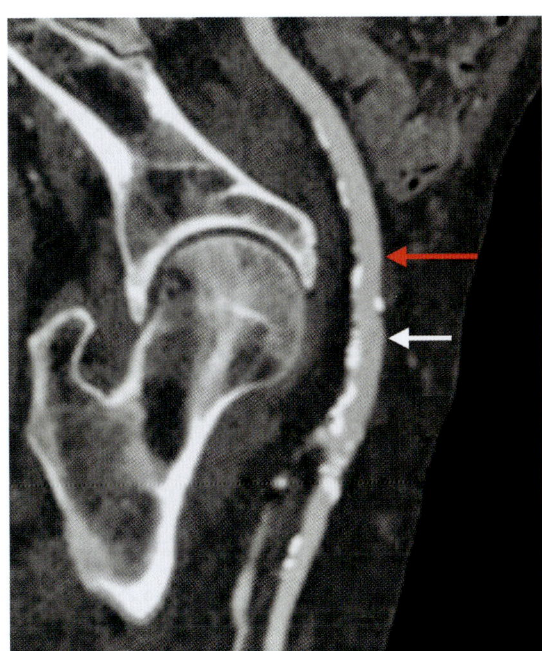

FIGURE 28.4 Sagittal CT angiography images of the external iliac and common femoral arteries showing the relationship of the CFA with the femoral head. The CFA is shallowest over the middle aspect of the femoral head and as we go cranially and transition into the external iliac artery, the artery dives into the pelvic rim and the distance from the skin is increased (red vs white arrows).

show that the ultrasonography group had less accidental venipuncture and greater first-pass success without a significant difference in time to obtain femoral artery access.

A meta-analysis of seven randomized control trials (prior to the publication of the UNIVERSAL trial) comparing transfemoral ultrasound-guided cannulation versus standard approach in patients undergoing percutaneous cardiovascular interventions showed that the use of ultrasound-guided cannulation is associated with a higher rate of cannulation at the first attempt, a lower total number of attempts, as well as shorter time to access compared with the standard approach to accessing the CFA. In addition, patients undergoing transfemoral ultrasound-guided cannulation of the CFA experienced a lower rate of vascular complications, including hematomas and venipunctures.[15]

Ultrasound guidance for femoral arterial access thus reduces vascular complications, number of attempts, accidental venipunctures, and time to access. It is a straightforward technique that is relatively easy to learn and utilizes equipment that is readily available in most hospitals. With some experience (ie, after 10 procedures), it facilitates precise CFA cannulation regardless of anatomic variation, which may decrease access site complications and increase the success of closure device placement. Ultrasound guidance has particular utility in patients with challenging femoral access, feeble femoral pulses, or high bleeding risk.

Use of a Micropuncture Needle for CFA Access

The micropuncture needle has been widely used to obtain access into the CFA with or without ultrasound guidance. It is especially helpful for smaller calcified arteries or in coagulopathic patients in an attempt to decrease access site complications. As compared with the regular 18-gauge needle, the micropuncture needle is a 21-gauge access needle that decreases the size of the CFA arteriotomy by 56%. It also decreases the blood flow through the hole in the CFA by six-fold resulting in decreased bleeding in cases of a failed attempt or posterior wall puncture.[16] More recently, the micropuncture system has been more widely used despite having no strong data to show that it decreases vascular access site complications. In the FEMORIS single-center trial with 402 patients randomized to 18-gauge versus 21-gauge micropuncture access needle, there was no difference in the primary endpoint of composite bleeding, but the study was underpowered and terminated prematurely. However, lower bleeding rates were seen in the prespecified subgroups such as women (17.4% vs 5.8%; P = .05) and those with final sheath size ≤6 Fr (15.1% vs 6.4%; P = .02).[17] Nevertheless, the micropuncture system makes it easier to obtain hemostasis and reattempt access on the same site if the original arteriotomy in the CFA is not at the ideal level or if it is in one of the CFA branches.

The micropuncture kit comes with a 21-gauge needle, 0.018″ guidewire, and 4 or 5F micropuncture sheath with a respective dilator for initial access and exchange to 0.035″ system. Some micropuncture kits come with a hydrophilic-coated guidewire, but these are better used in non-CFA access such as radial and tibial vessels. The guidewire used for CFA is usually the stainless-steel soft-tip tapered wire. If using micropuncture with ultrasound, a micropuncture needle with an echogenic tip can be used, which is more visible, especially the tip of the needle to visualize access through the anterior wall of the CFA. After locating the skin entry site and injecting local anesthetic, the micropuncture needle is advanced into the CFA. When a flash of bright red blood comes out of the back end of the needle, the 0.018″ guidewire is advanced into the CFA/iliac arteries. It is very important to visualize the wire advancing into the iliac arteries under live fluoroscopy since this wire tends to enter small branches without much resistance and may lead to wire perforation and potentially retroperitoneal bleeds. As a matter of fact, a single-center study that evaluated complication rates between the micropuncture system and usual 18-gauge needle access into the CFA showed no difference in the overall complication rates but the risk of retroperitoneal bleed, even though small, was significantly higher in the micropuncture group due to wire migration (and perforation) into smaller pelvic arteries if not visualized while being advanced under fluoroscopy (**Fig. 28.5**).[18]

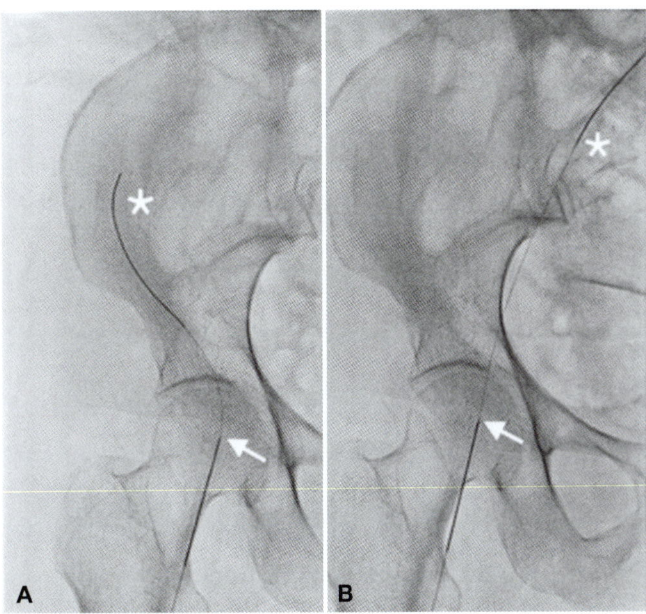

FIGURE 28.5 **A:** Fluoroscopy showing appropriate access using a micropuncture needle/wire at the level of the middle of the femoral head (*arrow*); however, the micropuncture wire traversed small pelvic arteries (*asterisk*), which may increase the risk of perforation and retroperitoneal bleeding. **B:** Redirecting the wire into the external iliac artery (*asterisk*) prior to dilating the access site and inserting the sheath into the common femoral artery.

Confirming Access Site

After the needle enters the artery, multiple techniques have been used to confirm the arteriotomy site in the CFA. The first technique involves advancing the wire through the micropuncture needle into the iliac vessels and then examining the needle-wire interface under fluoroscopy. This locates precisely the relationship of the puncture site to the femoral head (**Fig. 28.3**).[16] The second technique involves injecting contrast through the micropuncture needle and recording an angiogram of the entry site. We do not recommend this technique since there are multiple risks involved with it, including a risk of losing access to the vessel lumen, dissecting the

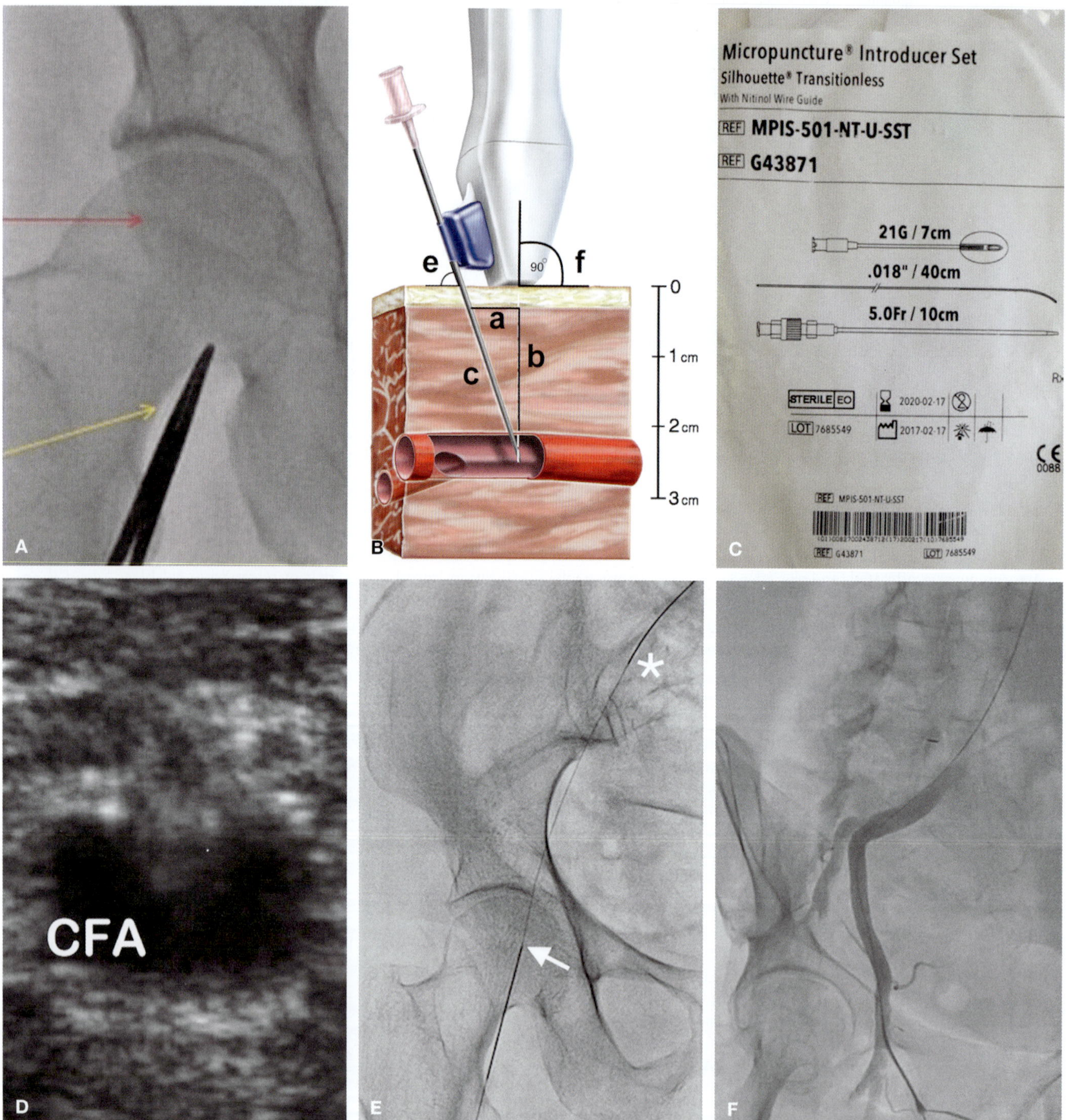

FIGURE 28.6 Contemporary femoral arterial access utilizes fluoroscopy, micropuncture, and ultrasonography as well as visualization of the needle and sheath entry site into the CFA. **A:** Locating the inferior border of the femoral head (Red arrow) with a hemostat (Yellow arrow) and fluoroscopy in the AP projection. **B:** Real-time ultrasonography is used with or without a needle guide to access the CFA above the bifurcation at its shallowest point above the femoral head. **C:** Micropuncture needle with or without echogenic tip should be used with real-time ultrasound guidance for access. Image shows an echogenic tip package of a micropuncture needle. **D:** Real-time visualization of the needle tip accessing the anterior wall of the CFA. **E:** Fluoroscopy showing the needle-wire interface and confirming access into the CFA over the middle third of the femoral head (arrow) as well as the micropuncture wire course in the iliac artery and not in pelvic branches (star). **F:** Femoral angiogram done in the ipsilateral oblique projection with a J-wire through the sheath to prevent iliac artery dissection.

CFA, and direct radiation to the operator hands. The third method involves advancing the 0.018″ wire through the micropuncture needle, removing the needle, and then advancing the inner dilator of the micropuncture sheath over the 0.018″ wire and using this small dilator for femoral angiography rather than injecting directly through the micropuncture needle.[5] While this is a safer way to perform the femoral angiogram, there is still a possibility to dissect the iliac artery with the tip of the inner dilator of the micropuncture sheath especially if the iliac artery is tortuous. On the other hand, transducing a pressure with an extension tubing to ensure an appropriate waveform may reduce the risk of inadvertently injecting contrast into the suboptimal plane. The most commonly used technique and likely the safest is to perform femoral angiography through the access sheath with the J-wire in place to deflect the sheath from the vessel wall and maintain vessel control should complications occur. CFA access is not complete without angiography of the access site preferably before anticoagulation is given to the patient.

Contemporary CFA Access

Contemporary femoral access[19] involves the utilization of all the steps discussed previously including reviewing previously available imaging, palpation of anatomic landmarks, fluoroscopic localization of the femoral head by placing a radiopaque marker such as a hemostat at the lower edge of the femoral head, and marking that location. Ultrasonography is then used to locate the most superficial part of the CFA above the bifurcation. Ultrasonography will also help identify and avoid access into any calcification or diseased segments of the CFA. Lidocaine is then injected at this site while holding the vascular probe steady in place. Depending on the depth of the CFA from the surface of the skin, the access needle, preferably a micropuncture needle with an echogenic tip, should be advanced starting caudal to the ultrasound probe toward the CFA at approximately a 45° angle in a jabbing fashion to visualize the needle tip above the CFA in the ultrasound plane. When blood flashes out of the needle, the micropuncture wire is advanced into the CFA ideally under fluoroscopic guidance to prevent it from going into the small pelvic arteries and cause microperforations. While the wire is through the needle, fluoroscopic assessment of the needle entry site should be performed. If the wire-needle interface is not at the ideal access location in the middle third of the femoral head then the needle and wire may be removed and manual pressure applied for few minutes to achieve hemostasis and then reattempt access. When the ideal arteriotomy location is achieved, the micropuncture sheath and then eventually the desired sheath can be advanced into the CFA and an angiogram in 30° ipsilateral view should be performed with the 0.035-in wire through the sheath (**Fig. 28.6**).

CONCLUSION

The most common vascular access sites for angiography and interventions include the femoral and radial arteries. Best practice techniques differ for each vascular access site and must be utilized to minimize difficulties and complications. The femoral artery remains an important access site, especially for peripheral and structural interventions. Knowledge of the anatomy and the course of the CFA, as well as the use of ultrasound guidance, may facilitate better and safer femoral access and decrease complication rates.

Key Points

- Femoral access remains necessary for procedures requiring larger sheaths and because transradial approaches are not feasible for many peripheral and structural interventions.
- The ideal access site into the CFA should be below the most inferior point of the IEA and above the CFA bifurcation anterior to the femoral head.
- Even though femoral access can be achieved on almost all patients, it should be reconsidered in patients who may have features that predispose them to an increased risk of femoral artery access complications.
- Anatomic landmarks and fluoroscopy have multiple limitations when obtaining femoral artery access, mainly due to the patient's body habitus as well as anatomic variation in the CFA and its bifurcation.
- Ultrasound-guided access has emerged as an efficient and safe method to access the CFA and should be considered for all patients.
- The use of micropuncture may facilitate safer access into the CFA.
- Contemporary CFA access can decrease patients' access site complications and improve arteriotomy location by utilizing anatomy, fluoroscopy, ultrasonography, as well as micropuncture and access site angiography.

For further review and interactivities, please see the chapter-based multiple choice questions and videos accessible in the complimentary eBook bundled with this text. Access instructions are located in the inside front cover.

References

1. Spijkerboer AM, Scholten FG, Mali WP, van Schaik JP. Antegrade puncture of the femoral artery: morphologic study. *Radiology*. 1990;176(1):57-60.
2. Schnyder G, Sawhney N, Whisenant B, Tsimikas S, Turi ZG. Common femoral artery anatomy is influenced by demographics and comorbidity: implications for cardiac and peripheral invasive studies. *Catheter Cardiovasc Interv*. 2001;53(3):289-295.
3. Abu-Fadel MS, Sparling JM, Zacharias SJ, et al. Fluoroscopy vs. traditional guided femoral arterial access and the use of closure devices: a randomized controlled trial. *Catheter Cardiovasc Interv*. 2009;74(4):533-539.
4. Seto AH, Tyler J, Suh WM, et al. Defining the common femoral artery: Insights from the femoral arterial access with ultrasound trial. *Catheter Cardiovasc Interv*. 2017;89(7):1185-1192.
5. Cilingiroglu M, Feldman T, Salinger MH, Levisay J, Turi ZG. Fluoroscopically-guided micropuncture femoral artery access for large-caliber sheath insertion. *J Invasive Cardiol*. 2011;23(4):157-161.
6. Abu-Fadel MS, ed. Common femoral artery access. *Arterial and Venous Access in the Cardiac Catheterization Lab*. 1st ed. Rutgers University Press; 2016:1-20.
7. Sherev DA, Shaw RE, Brent BN. Angiographic predictors of femoral access site complications: implication for planned percutaneous coronary intervention. *Catheter Cardiovasc Interv*. 2005;65(2):196-202.

8. Tiroch KA, Matheny ME, Resnic FS. Quantitative impact of cardiovascular risk factors and vascular closure devices on the femoral artery after repeat cardiac catheterization. *Am Heart J*. 2010;159(1):125-130.
9. Ellis SG, Bhatt D, Kapadia S, Lee D, Yen M, Whitlow PL. Correlates and outcomes of retroperitoneal hemorrhage complicating percutaneous coronary intervention. *Catheter Cardiovasc Interv*. 2006;67(4):541-545.
10. Seto AH, Abu-Fadel MS, Sparling JM, et al. Real-time ultrasound guidance facilitates femoral arterial access and reduces vascular complications: FAUST (Femoral Arterial Access with Ultrasound Trial). *JACC Cardiovasc Interv*. 2010;3(7):751-758.
11. Lechner G, Jantsch H, Waneck R, Kretschmer G. The relationship between the common femoral artery, the inguinal crease, and the inguinal ligament: a guide to accurate angiographic puncture. *Cardiovasc Intervent Radiol*. 1988;11(3):165-169.
12. Grier D, Hartnell G. Percutaneous femoral artery puncture: practice and anatomy. *Br J Radiol*. 1990;63(752):602-604.
13. Abu-Fadel MS, ed. Ultrasound guided arterial and venous access. *Arterial and Venous Access in the Cardiac Catheterization Lab*. 1st ed. Rutgers University Press; 2016:117-151.
14. Jolly SS, AlRashidi S, d'Entremont M, et al. Routine ultrasonography guidance for femoral vascular access for cardiac procedures: the UNIVERSAL randomized clinical trial. *JAMA Cardiol*. 2022;7(11):1110-1118.
15. Sorrentino S, Nguyen P, Salerno N, et al. Standard versus ultrasound-guided cannulation of the femoral artery in patients undergoing invasive procedures: a meta-analysis of randomized controlled trials. *J Clin Med*. 2020;9(3):677.
16. Turi ZG. Overview of vascular closure. *Endovasc Today*. 2009;8:24-32.
17. Ambrose JA, Lardizabal J, Mouanoutoua M, et al. Femoral micropuncture or routine Introducer Study (FEMORIS). *Cardiology*. 2014;129(1):39-43.
18. Ben-Dor I, Maluenda G, Mahmoudi M, et al. A novel, minimally invasive access technique versus standard 18-gauge needle set for femoral access. *Catheter Cardiovasc Interv*. 2012;79(7):1180-1185.
19. Sandoval Y, Burke MN, Lobo AS, et al. Contemporary arterial access in the cardiac catheterization laboratory. *JACC Cardiovasc Interv*. 2017;10(22):2233-2241.

Alternative Large Bore Access: Axillary, Transcaval

Hussein Rahim, Sumit Sohal, and Raj Tayal

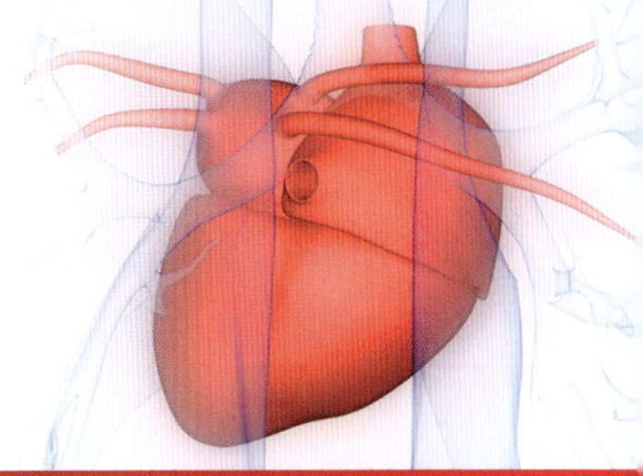

The need for large bore percutaneous access continues to increase as procedures such as transcatheter aortic valve replacement (TAVR), endovascular aortic aneurysm repair (EVAR), and the insertion of temporary mechanical circulatory support (MCS) for shock or complex coronary intervention continue to become more readily adopted throughout the world. Recent data suggest over a 1500% increase in the use of MCS over the last two decades alone.[1] In parallel with this, the expansion of TAVR into low-risk cohorts is projected to increase the procedural volumes exponentially.[2] While transfemoral access remains the preferred approach for most procedures requiring large bore access, its availability may be compromised by the presence of prohibitive iliofemoral disease in 13% to 20% of the population.[3,4] Owing to technological advancements that have led to a reduction in the profile of many of these devices, and the availability of tools such as intravascular lithotripsy to facilitate large bore access in the setting of calcific peripheral arterial disease,[5] the rate of transfemoral access continues to increase. In fact, the STS-ACC TVT Registry of Transcatheter Aortic Valve Replacement reported 95.3% of all TAVR cases performed were done via a transfemoral approach in 2021.[6]

Despite this, several scenarios remain where alternative access either is necessary due to anatomical limitations, such as severe obstructive peripheral arterial disease and the presence of aortic dissection, or may be preferred such as in the setting of prolonged MCS. The use of transapical access has largely been abandoned due to data suggesting poorer outcomes compared with transfemoral access.[7] Similarly, although transcarotid access was initially presented as an attractive alternative access in TAVR due to lower stroke rates, it requires the use of general anesthesia and surgical instrumentation, and more recent data including a meta-analysis show no difference in overall stroke rates between a transaxillary and transcarotid approach.[8]

In this chapter, we describe the indications, techniques, and common complications associated with two of the most commonly utilized methods of alternative access: transaxillary and transcaval access.

TRANSAXILLARY ACCESS

Percutaneous axillary access is an attractive alternative access option for both TAVR and percutaneous MCS such as Impella (Abiomed, MA, USA) and intra-aortic balloon pumps as it utilizes the same technical skills used during transfemoral access; therefore, it is easy to learn for most interventional cardiologists.[9,10] However, there are specific anatomic and technical aspects that are critical for success. In the following discussion we describe a step-by-step approach to successful transaxillary access. The Society for Cardiovascular Angiography and Interventions recently published a position statement on best practices for percutaneous axillary arterial access and training, which can be referenced for further details.[3]

Step-by-Step Transaxillary Access

Step 1: Selecting the Patient

In patients who are deemed to require alternative access, the axillary artery is typically a suitable site because even in patients with severe peripheral arterial disease it is relatively free of calcification and atherosclerosis. This was illustrated in an analysis of 208 patients undergoing routine computed tomographic angiography (CTA) prior to TAVR, which demonstrated that less than 2% of patients had significant stenosis and less than 9% had significant calcification. The average minimal lumen diameter was 6.0 mm ± 1.1 mm, which is large enough to accommodate up to an 18 French sheath. The axillary artery therefore provides a suitable conduit for most percutaneous procedures such as TAVR or Impella CP insertion without the need for surgical graft placement.[11] While having advanced imaging such as CTA can be advantageous for preprocedural planning, as most patients have a suitable axillary artery it is possible to use this site on an emergent basis for MCS, with some experienced operators reporting insertion times as short as 7 to 10 minutes.[12,13] In this emergent setting, ultrasound evaluation or angiography of the axillary artery can be performed at the time of the procedure to confirm its suitability for access. If preprocedural imaging is available, inadequate vessel size, severe calcification, steep subclavian angulation, extreme aortic root angulation, prior dissection, presence of an ipsilateral internal mammary graft, or arteriovenous fistula can be considered relative contraindications.[14]

Step 2: Understanding the Anatomy of Axillary Artery

The axillary and subclavian arteries have different histopathological characteristics compared with the femoral artery (**Fig. 29.1**).[10] The axillary artery has multiple layers of elastic fibers while the femoral artery has a thicker media consisting of mostly smooth muscle cells. The adventitia of the femoral artery is also more fibrous, providing more support for the use of closure devices. In early experience, there were multiple failures with the ProStar (Abbott, IL, USA) closure device in the axillary site due to its stiffer body and likely greater distortion of the elastic vessel.[10] Therefore, most operators today typically use the Proglide Perclose (Abbott) device for closure.

Anatomically, the axillary artery has three segments (**Fig. 29.2**).[15] The first segment is medial to pectoralis minor, the second segment is posterior to pectoralis minor, and the third segment is lateral to the pectoralis minor. The phrenic nerve, brachial plexus, and long thoracic nerve are in close proximity to the axillary artery. The median and ulnar nerves are at high risk for injury if the third segment is chosen for puncture as they pass anterior to the third segment and are encompassed within the brachial fascial sheath, making the risk of creating a compression syndrome or plexopathy higher with any extravasation from the access site during catheter exchanges or after closure. The anterior circumflex and humeral arteries also arise from the third segment of the vessel, disruption of which either by dissection or occlusion by placement of a covered

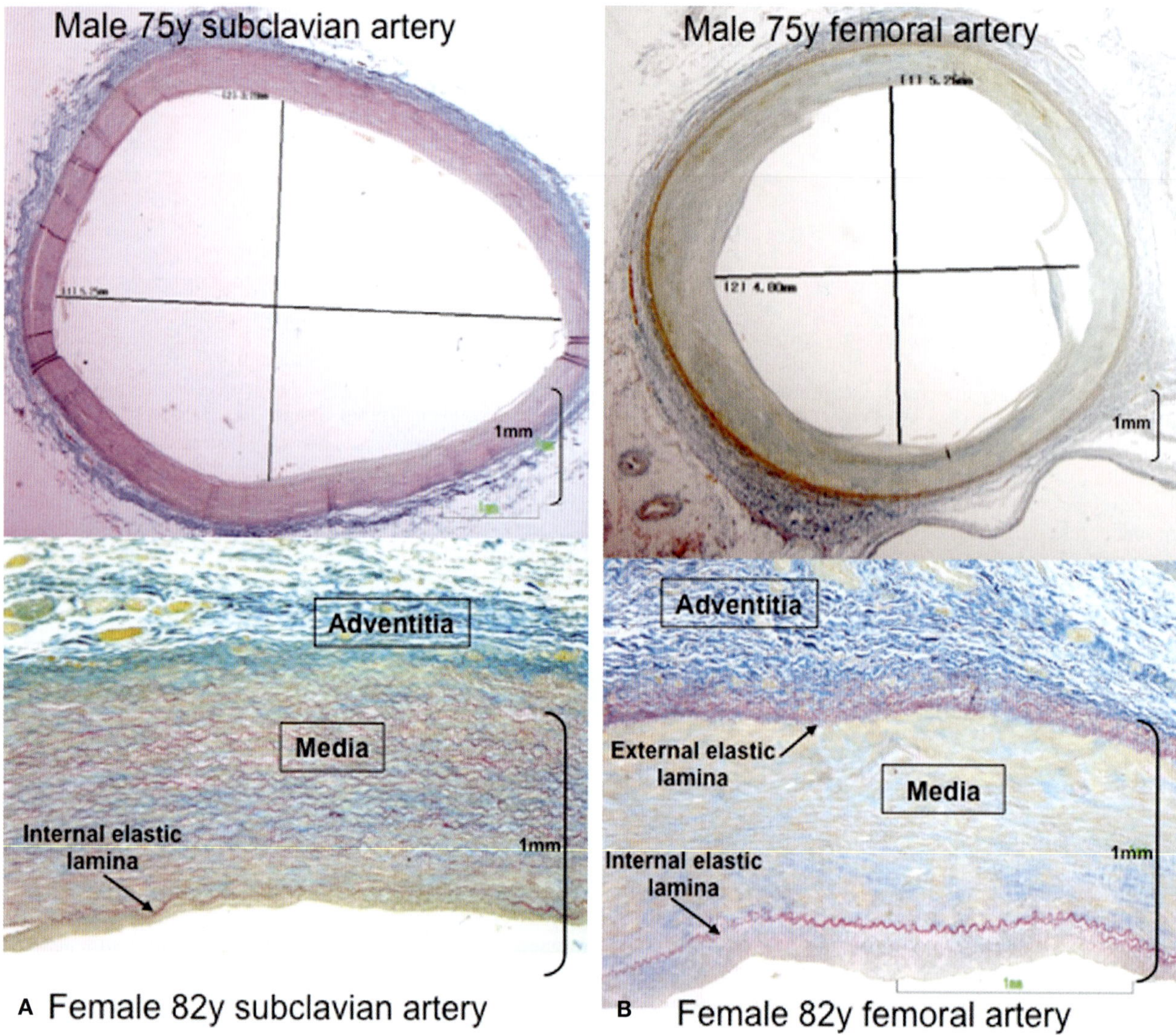

FIGURE 29.1 Histological sections of the subclavian and femoral arteries. **A:** Subclavian artery. **B:** Femoral artery. These histological sections demonstrate significantly more elastic fibers in the subclavian artery compared with the femoral artery. (Reprinted from Schafer U, Ho Y, Frerker C, et al. Direct percutaneous access technique for transaxillary transcatheter aortic valve implantation: "the Hamburg Sankt Georg approach". *JACC Cardiovasc Interv*. 2012;5(5):477-486, Copyright (2012), with permission from Elsevier.)

stent if needed as a bail out strategy to obtain hemostasis increases the risk for the development of avascular necrosis of the humeral head. Use of the first segment of the axillary artery has been well described in the literature; however, due to its proximity to the intrathoracic space, access in this region increases the risk for the development of a pneumothorax or hemothorax and leaves almost no options for surgical bailout. Therefore, the multidisciplinary SCAI consensus document recommends the second segment of the axillary artery as the safest target for puncture. The second segment is devoid of any brachial plexus elements on its anterior surface, is easily compressed against the chest wall using manual pressure to obtain hemostasis, and is free of meaningful vascular branches making placement of covered stents safe if necessary.[3]

Step 3: Preparation and Room Setup

Typically, transaxillary procedures can be done with conscious sedation. The patient is placed in a supine position and prepped in the usual manner. The arm may be kept at the patient's side or abducted at 90°. An additional access site, whether that be femoral or ipsilateral radial, is typically obtained to be used for baseline angiography and for placement of a 0.18′ wire as a target for vascular access, which may be identified fluoroscopically as well as under ultrasound evaluation. This wire further serves as a mechanism to maintain bidirectional control of the vessel, for advancement of a peripheral balloon to perform dry closure, and for placement of a covered stent if needed as a bailout strategy. An additional sterile table is placed adjacent to the site of axillary access as well as another table parallel to the patient on the patient's right side as is standard (**Fig. 29.3**). If possible, the monitors can be placed at the foot of the bed to allow for visualization from both sides.

Step 4: Access

While both axillary arteries can be used, the left axillary artery carries a lower theoretical risk of stroke as direct crossing of the right common carotid can be avoided. In addition, left-sided access is also favored in elderly patients due to predilection for the development of type II and III aortic arches with time, as well as for TAVR given coplanar alignment. Valve deployment is often easier from

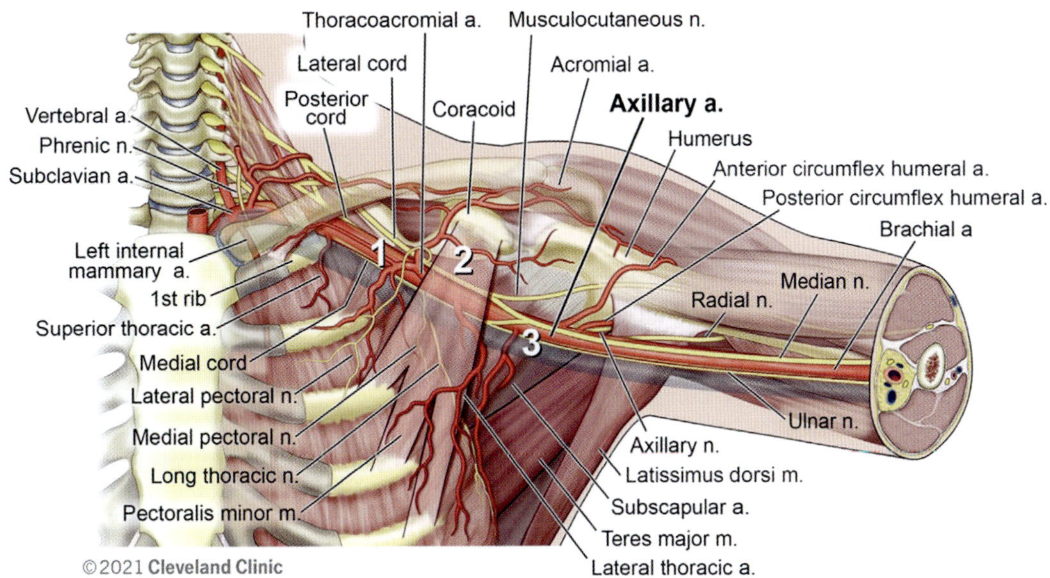

FIGURE 29.2 Anatomy of the axillary artery. Axillary artery and surrounding structures including vessels, bones, nerves, and muscles. The three segments of the axillary artery are marked relative to the pectoralis minor muscle. (Reprinted from Seto AH, Estep JD, Tayal R, et al. SCAI position statement on best practices for percutaneous axillary arterial access and training. *JSCAI*. 2022;1(3):100041, Copyright (2022), with permission from Elsevier.)

the left versus the right axillary, although the right may be preferred in the setting of shock as it requires less time and almost no reorientation of the room or equipment. Handedness and vertebral dominance should also be considered in this decision given the risk of median nerve palsy with prolonged device implantation.[16] After obtaining either femoral access or ipsilateral radial access, selective angiography of the axillary artery is performed (**Fig. 29.4**). The angiogram allows one to assess vessel caliber, tortuosity, and degrees of stenosis just prior to access. Most importantly, this allows one to identify the borders of the second segment of the

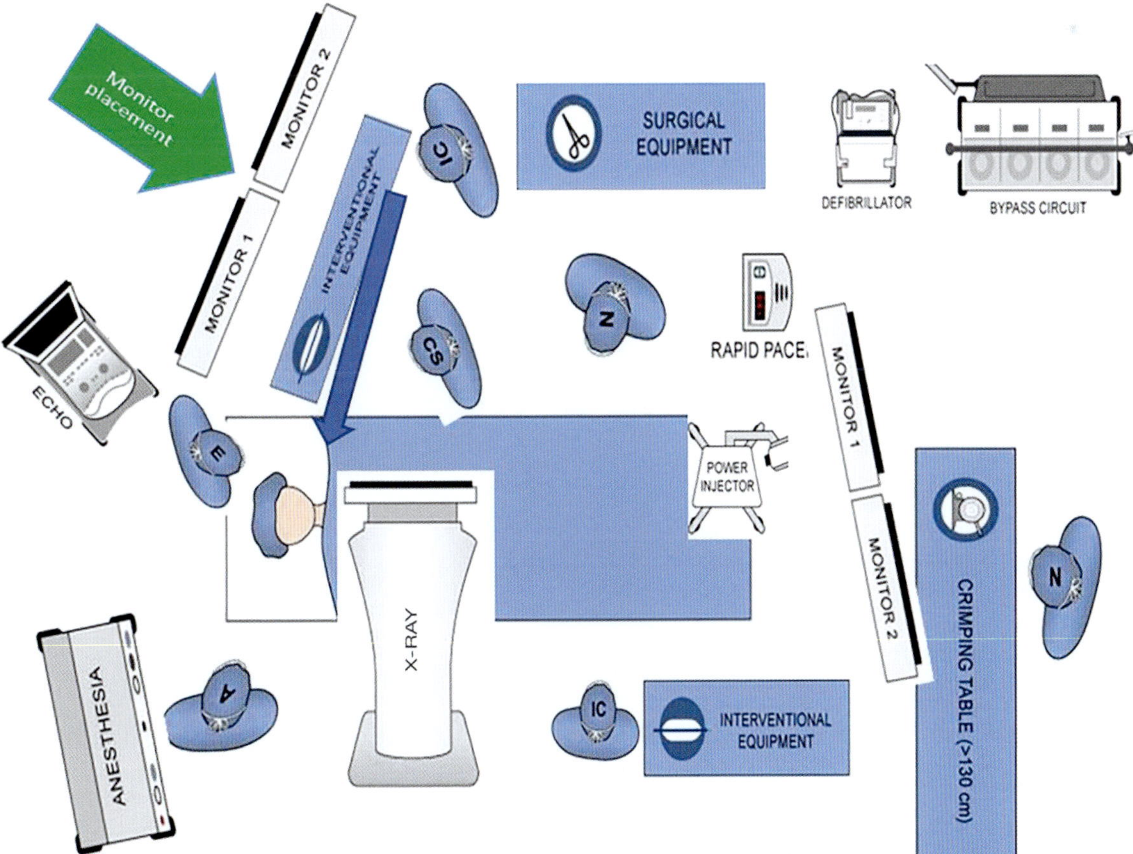

FIGURE 29.3 Hypothetical room set up. While some operators report obtaining access with the arm at the side, abduction of the arm 90° is most common. Tables and monitors need to be positioned carefully to facilitate the procedure.

axillary artery. The medial border will be identified by the ribcage, as anything medial to this will be within the thorax. Bleeding complications within the thorax are difficult to both identify and treat. The lateral border will be the subscapular artery and the anterior circumflex humeral artery. Any puncture distal to this will be in the third segment of the axillary artery. Operators should aim to identify a segment free of disease between these two borders for puncture.

After a site for puncture is identified a supportive 0.18″ wire is placed for protection and bailout across the axillary artery into the brachial artery or descending aorta if ipsilateral radial access is used. The wire can also be used as a marker for fluoroscopic puncture in conjunction with ultrasound. Of utmost importance is the angle of needle entry for axillary access. Compared with femoral access, axillary access requires a much shallower angle of entry ~25° to 30°. This decreases the risk of kinking during sheath insertion. Typically, access is obtained through the pectoralis minor. The use of a micropuncture technique is strongly recommended.[3]

Step 5: "Preclose"

Once access is obtained a 5-French sheath can be inserted. An angiogram through the sheath can be performed to confirm location. Once location of the puncture is confirmed, most operators utilize suture-mediated closure devices such as the Perclose Proglide. The access site is preclosed with two Perclose devices at the 10- and 2-o'clock positions. The sutures are deployed but not cinched down onto the vessel. In contradistinction to femoral access, axillary access is typically obtained by puncture directly through the pectoralis minor muscle rather than through only subcutaneous tissue and fascia. Accordingly, care must be taken to ensure an adequate tract is made using blunt dissection or serial dilation in order to ensure the Percloses are deployed into the arterial wall and not in the muscle itself. This is the primary cause of Perclose failure and persistent postprocedural extravasation. Similarly, due to the more elastic nature of the axillary artery due to the presence of a larger proportion of elastic lamina and less muscular lamina relative to the femoral artery, care must be taken during deployment to not overtighten the sutures as this may cause an iatrogenic stenosis or closure of the vessel. In patients who are receiving 9Fr or smaller sheaths for devices such as an intra-aortic balloon pump a preclose may not be necessary as manual hemostasis may suffice.[17]

After preclosure is performed, a 6- to 8-French sheath is inserted and a standard 0.35″ wire advanced into the ascending aorta via a JR4 diagnostic catheter or similar. The wire is then exchanged out for a stiff 0.35″ wire. Over the stiff wire, serial dilations can be performed followed by insertion of a large-bore sheath. If a large bore sheath is to be left in place for a long period, a repeat angiogram to ensure flow to the distal extremity is imperative; however, if access is obtained in the second portion of the vessel, the need for distal perfusion of the upper extremity is extremely rare even if the sheath is occlusive due to the robust nature of subscapular collateral vessels. Serial assessment of the distal extremity is recommended. Flow may not be pulsatile; however, it is typically sufficient. If ischemia is noted, assessment of collateral vessel flow or the creation of external or internal bypass circuit may be necessary.[18]

Step 6: Closure

After the procedure is completed, closure should be performed under fluoroscopic guidance. Use of a "dry closure" technique is imperative. The dry closure technique involves utilizing the previously placed 0.18″ wire from the secondary access (typically femoral) across the axillary artery into the brachial artery (**Fig. 29.5**). An appropriately sized (1:1) 7-10 × 40 mm, 0.35′ compatible balloon is placed proximal to the arteriotomy, most commonly in the subclavian artery. The balloon is inflated to low pressure, typically no greater than four to six atmospheres, once the sheath has been withdrawn distal to it and prior to its removal from the arteriotomy. The previously deployed Perclose sutures are cinched into place. After the sutures are deployed the balloon can be gently deflated and bleeding can be assessed. If there is obvious bleeding from the site, the balloon can be advanced to the arteriotomy site and reinflated to maintain hemostasis. Concomitant application of external manual hemostasis is recommended for 5 minutes after which the balloon may be moved proximal to the site, a Touhy-Borst attached to the balloon, and a

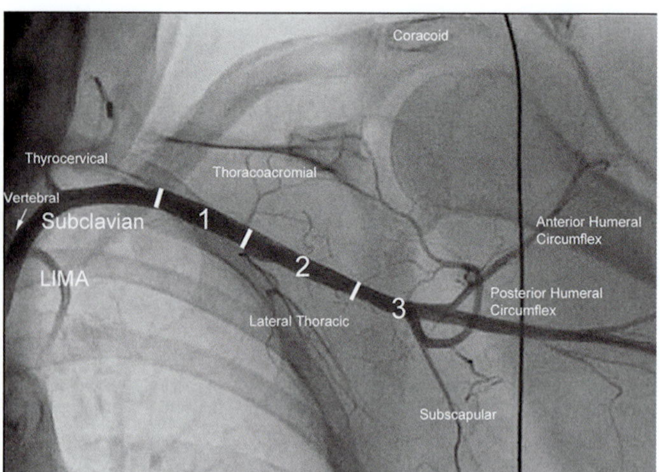

FIGURE 29.4 Angiography of the axillary artery and clinically relevant branches. LIMA, left internal mammary artery. (Reprinted from Seto AH, Estep JD, Tayal R, et al. SCAI position statement on best practices for percutaneous axillary arterial access and training. *JSCAI*. 2022;1(3):100041, Copyright (2022), with permission from Elsevier.)

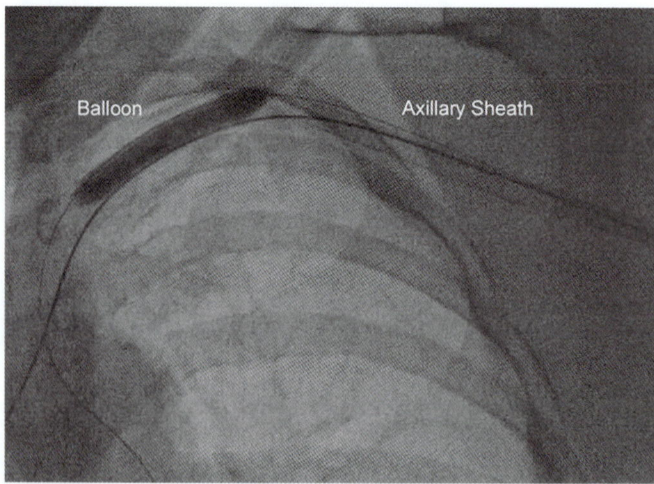

FIGURE 29.5 Dry closure. Dry closure of the axillary artery, utilizing a balloon advanced from the femoral artery. The balloon is positioned proximal to the arteriotomy and inflated to facilitate a bloodless field for closure. (Reprinted from Seto AH, Estep JD, Tayal R, et al. SCAI position statement on best practices for percutaneous axillary arterial access and training. *JSCAI*. 2022;1(3):100041, Copyright (2022), with permission from Elsevier.)

repeat angiogram performed with the wire still in place. If bleeding persists, it is recommended the balloon be readvanced and the internal balloon tamponade with external manual compression be repeated for an additional 5 minutes. If bleeding persists, protamine and continued manual pressure or use of a covered stent may be considered. Once the operators are satisfied with the closure, a final digital subtraction angiogram should be taken with a slight caudal or cranial angulation to demonstrate adequate closure has been achieved without compromise of the distal limb.[3]

Safety and Management of Complications

While the safety profile of transaxillary access is excellent, vascular issues are the most common complication. The Axillary Access Registry to Monitor Safety (ARMS) was a prospective, observational multicenter registry to evaluate the safety of axillary access for mechanical support.[19] A total of 102 patients were enrolled with 10 minor bleeding events noted, only 4 of which required transfusion. In a recent report from the TVT registry the rate of vascular complications from axillary access during TAVR was reported to be 2.5%.[20]

Bleeding is another common complication from transaxillary access. Most episodes of bleeding are minor and if proper technique is followed can be avoided. However, major bleeding can carry the consequences of compression of the adjacent brachial plexus, nerve injury, or compartment syndrome. Therefore, a final angiogram after closure is imperative. If there is residual bleeding, manual hemostasis coupled with balloon tamponade is usually sufficient to control the bleeding. If there is continued bleeding despite these efforts, the implantation of a covered stent is recommended. We recommend the deployment of self-expanding Viabahn stents (Gore, DE, USA) over balloon expandable stents as the axillary artery is a flexion point and self-expanding stents are less likely to get kinked.[3] Prior to deployment care must be taken to ensure no major branches are covered. If access was obtained appropriately in the second segment of the artery this should not be a problem. In rare instances surgical cutdown may be necessary to control the bleeding if the above method fails. Bleeding may not be immediately apparent especially if access was obtained close to the first segment, as it may be intrathoracic in this segment. Similarly, bleeding can frequently track along the flanks causing significant bruising (**Fig. 29.6**) and can be missed if only the access site is assessed for hematoma. Other vascular complications noted in the ARMS registry included pseudoaneurysm, dissection, and upper extremity ischemia but were all rare.[19]

Neurological complications are probably the most feared complications of transaxillary access. Owing to its proximity to the internal carotid arteries and plausible relationship of catheter course to differential plaque distribution in the aortic arch, there is an increased risk of stroke compared with transfemoral access, although the exact risk is unclear.[21] In the ARMS registry there was only one stroke in the 102 patients enrolled.[19] In a recent report from the TVT registry the stroke rate for axillary access was reported to be 6.3%.[20] No differences were noted in stroke rates associated with percutaneous versus surgical cutdown.[22] The other neurological complication unique to transaxillary access is brachial plexus injury. In the ARMS registry there were three patients with brachial plexus–related symptoms all consisting of paresthesias in the distribution of the median nerve after multiple days of support, most likely due to inflammation or mild extravasation at the arteriotomy.[19]

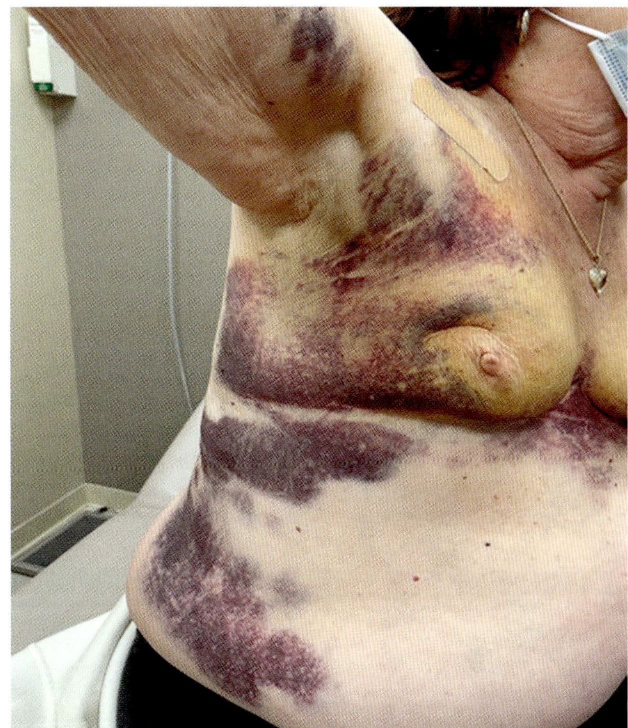

FIGURE 29.6 Large bruise after axillary access. Major bleeding complications after axillary access typically do not always present as large hematomas at the site of access, as blood may track into the intrathoracic cavity or along the ipsilateral flank of the patient.

TRANSCAVAL ACCESS

When transfemoral access is not feasible due to small or diseased peripheral arteries, transcaval access is another alternative access technique. Transcaval access may be performed under moderate sedation and utilizes an electrified wire to access the infrarenal aorta from an initial percutaneous transfemoral venous access. Transcaval access was first performed in 2013 as part of an alternative access strategy for TAVR.[23] Since then, it has grown in popularity and has been performed in thousands of patients at multiple institutions in a variety of scenarios for multiple indications. Some of the benefits of transcaval access include reduced radiation exposure to the operator as compared with transaxillary, transcarotid, or transapical approaches and the ability to deliver up to a 26-French device into the aorta without risk of distal limb ischemia or disruption of the iliofemoral arteries. That said, widespread adoption of transcaval remains somewhat limited and it remains among the less common alternative access strategies[24,25] utilized globally due to procedural costs, limited bailout options, lack of familiarity with components of electrosurgery, and relatively steep learning curve.

Technique

A preprocedural CT is imperative to successful transcaval access, although its feasibility using simultaneous angiography and venography has been demonstrated by operators well versed with the technique.[26] Objectives of the preprocedural CT include finding a calcium-free crossing target of 10 mm in at least one dimension, evaluating the distance from the groin to determine the length of the introducer sheath, avoiding interposed bowel between the inferior vena cava (IVC) and aorta, identifying and avoiding vascular branches, and planning a bailout strategy including the use of covered stents if necessary.[27] The CT is also used to "coregister" the crossing site. Utilizing anatomic landmarks such as the superior margin of the iliac crests and nearest lumbar vertebrae the site of crossing identified in the CT can be identified under fluoroscopy intraprocedure. Targeting an appropriate, calcium-free site in the aorta is important as well because unsuccessful punctures dramatically increase the risk of complications.[28,29] Once the procedure is adequately planned, percutaneous femoral venous and arterial access are obtained.

From the venous access site, a JR4 guide catheter is advanced to the identified crossing site in the IVC. A gooseneck snare (Medtronic, MN, USA) is positioned in the abdominal aorta across from the JR4 guide. A stiff 0.14″ wire such as an Astato XS20 (Asahi-Intecc, Tokyo, Japan) is loaded onto a Piggyback microcatheter (Teleflex, PA, USA) and Navicross microcatheter (Terumo, Tokyo, Japan). A brief electric current at 30-50W is applied to the 0.14″ wire, and it is advanced through the IVC and aortic walls into the snare (**Fig. 29.7**). Once the wire is snared, the microcatheters are advanced from the IVC to the aorta. The 0.14″ wire is exchanged for a stiff 0.35″ wire such as a Lunderquist guidewire (Cook Medical, IN, USA). A large-bore sheath is then advanced over this wire. Once the procedure is completed, heparin is reversed and the site of arterial access is typically closed with a cardiac occluder such as an Amplatzer Duct Occluder (Abbott). After deployment an aortogram is necessary to ensure no further extravasation or residual aortocaval fistula. If there is residual bleeding balloon tamponade or a covered stent may be required.[26,27,30]

Clinical Experience

The first prospective trial for transcaval access enrolled 100 patients undergoing evaluation for TAVR who were found to have anatomy unsuitable for traditional transfemoral access.[31] Technical success was defined as access and closure without intraprocedural mortality or emergent surgery and was achieved in 98% of patients. Major vascular complications occurred in 13% of patients with a median length of stay of 4 days. All aortic access points were closed with Amplatzer nitinol cardiac occluders (Abbott). At 1-year follow-up there were no new vascular complications related to the transcaval access. Only one patient had a patent aortocaval fistula, and no patients were found to have evidence of occluder fracture, dislocation, or migration.[31] Since this initial description there have been multiple studies from centers describing their own experiences that mirror the safety and efficacy described earlier.[32-34] However,

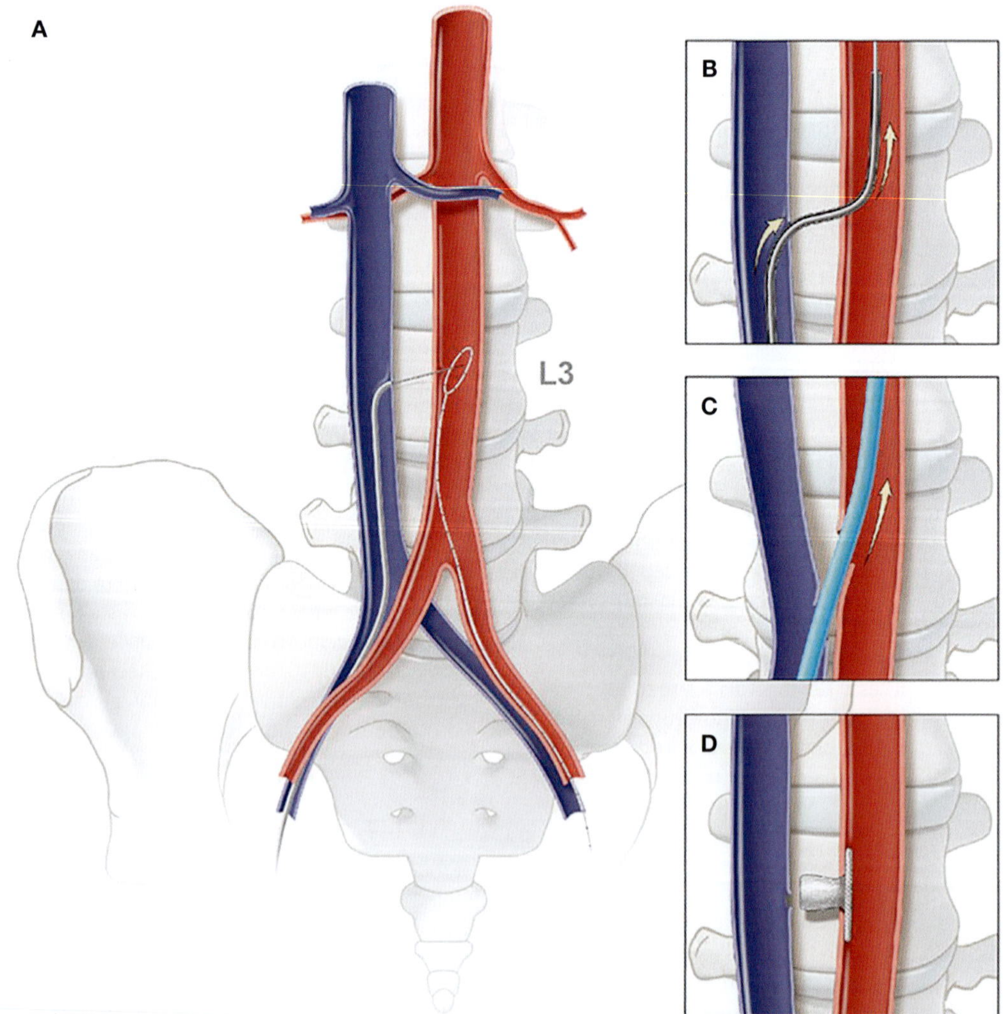

FIGURE 29.7 Transcaval access. **A:** An electrified guidewire is directed from the IVC to a snare in the aorta. **B:** Microcatheters are advanced into the aorta. **C:** A large sheath is introduced. **D:** The aortotomy is closed with a nitinol device. (Reprinted from Khan JM, Rogers T, Greenbaum AB, et al. Use of electrosurgery in interventional cardiology. *Interv Cardiol Clin.* 11(3):257-266, Copyright (2022), with permission from Elsevier.)

caution must be noted that these studies were conducted at centers with highly experienced operators familiar with the technique.

The indications and anatomies for which transcaval access have been performed continue to expand beyond TAVR. Transcaval access for the placement of hemodynamic support in the setting of cardiogenic shock has been described in several case reports.[35-38] In one report, 10 patients underwent placement of an Impella 5.0 device via transcaval access without prior CT guidance. Seven patients survived to device explant. Other authors have described use of the technique for embolization of type 2 endoleaks.[39] Another case report describes the successful use of transcaval access for TEVAR.[40] Although initially thought to be prohibitive, there have also been reports of transcaval access being performed successfully in hostile anatomies such as calcified aortas, existing abdominal aortic aneurysms, or even in patients with prior abdominal aortic aneurysm repair.[41,42]

There have been no randomized trials comparing transcaval access and transaxillary access; however, each technique has its own risks and benefits (**Table 29.1**). Both procedures require technical skill and a fundamental understanding of anatomy, risks and benefits, and bailout strategies. Outcomes associated with either procedure have been shown to improve linearly with increased operator experience. While the skill set required for traditional transfemoral approach may be translatable to transaxillary access, the technique remains limited by the increased risk of stroke rate in patients undergoing TAVR at 6.3% versus 3.1% for femoral access.[24] Transaxillary access has been shown to have shorter insertion times, is able to readily be performed in emergent settings without advanced imaging, allows for early patient ambulation, and has been shown to have lower major bleeding risks but typically remains limited to devices 18 French or less. Transcaval access allows for insertion of larger-caliber devices and reduced radiation exposure to the operator and may be associated with a lower stroke risk; however, it remains limited by the cost of the occluder devices required for the procedure and complexity of bailout strategies, if needed.[43]

In closing, while the use of alternative access for TAVR remains an attractive option, more head-to-head studies are needed to compare the outcomes among these strategies. Operator experience plays a great role in optimizing these procedures, and the use of a new alternative access site should be undertaken with caution and in the presence of an experienced proctor.

TABLE 29.1 Comparison of Advantages and Disadvantages of Transcaval Versus Transaxillary Access

	AXILLARY ACCESS	TRANSCAVAL ACCESS
Easier to learn	X	
Faster insertion time	X	
Lower stroke risk		X
Lower bleeding risk	X	
Shorter time to ambulation	X	
Percutaneous solutions to complications	X	X
Lower cost	X	
Percutaneous insertion of Impella 5.0		X

For further review and interactivities, please see the chapter-based multiple choice questions and videos accessible in the complimentary eBook bundled with this text. Access instructions are located in the inside front cover.

References

1. Stretch R, Sauer CM, Yuh DD, Bonde P. National trends in the utilization of short-term mechanical circulatory support: incidence, outcomes, and cost analysis. *J Am Coll Cardiol*. 2014;64(14):1407-1415. doi:10.1016/j.jacc.2014.07.958
2. Durko AP, Osnabrugge RL, Van Mieghem NM, et al. Annual number of candidates for transcatheter aortic valve implantation per country: current estimates and future projections. *Eur Heart J*. 2018;39(28):2635-2642. doi:10.1093/eurheartj/ehy107
3. Seto AH, Estep JD, Tayal R, et al. SCAI position statement on best practices for percutaneous axillary arterial access and training. *J Soc Cardiovasc Angiogr Interv*. 2022;1(3):100041. doi:10.1016/j.jscai.2022.100041
4. Beurtheret S, Karam N, Resseguier N, et al. Femoral versus nonfemoral peripheral access for transcatheter aortic valve replacement. *J Am Coll Cardiol*. 2019;74(22):2728-2739. doi:10.1016/j.jacc.2019.09.054
5. Tayal R, Sohal S, Okoh A, Wasty N, Waxman S, Salemi A. Intravascular lithotripsy enabled transfemoral transcatheter aortic valve implantation via percutaneous axillary access approach. *Cardiovasc Revasc Med*. 2021;28S:89-93. doi:10.1016/j.carrev.2020.12.018
6. Carroll JD, Mack MJ, Vemulapalli S, et al. STS-ACC TVT registry of transcatheter aortic valve replacement. *Ann Thorac Surg*. 2021;111(2):701-722. doi:10.1016/j.athoracsur.2020.09.002
7. Sohal S, Mehta H, Kurpad K, et al. Declining trend of transapical access for transcatheter aortic valve replacement in patients with aortic stenosis. *J Interv Cardiol*. 2022;2022:5688026. doi:10.1155/2022/5688026
8. Amer MR, Mosleh W, Megaly M, Shah T, Ooi YS, McKay RG. Outcomes of transcarotid versus trans-subclavian transcatheter aortic valve replacement: a systematic review and meta-analysis. *Cardiovasc Revasc Med*. 2021;33:20-25. doi:10.1016/j.carrev.2021.01.001
9. Tayal R, Hirst CS, Garg A, Kapur NK. Deployment of acute mechanical circulatory support devices via the axillary artery. *Expert Rev Cardiovasc Ther*. 2019;17(5):353-360. doi:10.1080/14779072.2019.1606712
10. Schäfer U, Ho Y, Frerker C, et al. Direct percutaneous access technique for transaxillary transcatheter aortic valve implantation: "the Hamburg Sankt Georg approach." *JACC Cardiovasc Interv*. 2012;5(5):477-486. doi:10.1016/j.jcin.2011.11.014
11. Arnett DM, Lee JC, Harms MA, et al. Caliber and fitness of the axillary artery as a conduit for large-bore cardiovascular procedures. *Catheter Cardiovasc Interv*. 2018;91(1):150-156. doi:10.1002/ccd.27416
12. Tayal R, Barvalia M, Rana Z, et al. Totally percutaneous insertion and removal of Impella device using axillary artery in the setting of advanced peripheral artery disease. *J Invasive Cardiol*. 2016;28(9):374-380.
13. Mathur M, Hira RS, Smith BM, Lombardi WL, McCabe JM. Fully percutaneous technique for transaxillary implantation of the Impella CP. *JACC Cardiovasc Interv*. 2016;9(11):1196-1198. doi:10.1016/j.jcin.2016.03.028
14. Harloff MT, Percy ED, Hirji SA, et al. A step-by-step guide to transaxillary transcatheter aortic valve replacement. *Ann Cardiothorac Surg*. 2020;9(6):510-521. doi:10.21037/acs-2020-av-79
15. Thawabi M, Tayal R, Khakwani Z, Sinclair M, Cohen M, Wasty N. Suggested bony landmarks for safe axillary artery access. *J Invasive Cardiol*. 2018;30(3):115-118.
16. Cheney AE, McCabe JM. Alternative percutaneous access for large bore devices. *Circ Cardiovasc Interv*. 2019;12(6):e007707. doi:10.1161/CIRCINTERVENTIONS.118.007707
17. Tayal R, DiVita M, Sossou CW, et al. Efficacy of manual hemostasis for percutaneous axillary artery intra-aortic balloon pump removal. *J Interv Cardiol*. 2020;2020:8375878. doi:10.1155/2020/8375878
18. Kaki A, Alraies MC, Kajy M, et al. Large bore occlusive sheath management. *Catheter Cardiovasc Interv*. 2019;93(4):678-684. doi:10.1002/ccd.28101

19. McCabe JM, Kaki AA, Pinto DS, et al. Percutaneous axillary access for placement of microaxial ventricular support devices: the axillary Access Registry to Monitor Safety (ARMS). *Circ Cardiovasc Interv*. 2021;14(1):e009657. doi:10.1161/CIRCINTERVENTIONS.120.009657
20. Dahle TG, Kaneko T, McCabe JM. Outcomes following subclavian and axillary artery access for transcatheter aortic valve replacement: society of the thoracic Surgeons/American College of Cardiology TVT registry report. *JACC Cardiovasc Interv*. 2019;12(7):662-669. doi:10.1016/j.jcin.2019.01.219
21. Sohal S, Khakwani MZ, Sandhu Z, et al. Coronary catheter course via the left radial approach is diametrically opposed to the course via the femoral approach: a stroke paradox. *CJC Open*. 2023;5(2):164-166. doi:10.1016/j.cjco.2022.11.017
22. Christine CJ, Tsuyoshi K, Rajiv T, Thom DG, James MM. Percutaneous versus surgical transaxillary access for transcatheter aortic valve replacement: a propensity-matched analysis of the US experience. *EuroIntervention*. 22AD;17(18):1514-1522. https://eurointervention.pcronline.com/article/percutaneous-versus-surgical-transaxillary-access-for-transcatheter-aortic-valve-replacement-a-propensity-matched-analysis-of-the-us-experience
23. Greenbaum AB, O'Neill WW, Paone G, et al. Caval-aortic access to allow transcatheter aortic valve replacement in otherwise ineligible patients: initial human experience. *J Am Coll Cardiol*. 2014;63(25 pt A):2795-2804. doi:10.1016/j.jacc.2014.04.015
24. Dahle TG, Kaneko T, McCabe JM. Outcomes following subclavian and axillary artery access for transcatheter aortic valve replacement: Society of the Thoracic Surgeons/American College of Cardiology TVT registry report. *JACC Cardiovasc Interv*. 2019;12(7):662-669. doi:10.1016/j.jcin.2019.01.219
25. Van Mieghem NM, Tijssen J. Alternative access for TAVR: see the forest for the trees. *JACC Cardiovasc Interv*. 2022;15(9):976-978. doi:10.1016/j.jcin.2022.04.001
26. Lederman RJ, Greenbaum AB, Rogers T, Khan JM, Fusari M, Chen MY. Anatomic suitability for transcaval access based on computed tomography. *JACC Cardiovasc Interv*. 2017;10(1):1-10. doi:10.1016/j.jcin.2016.09.002
27. Lederman RJ, Greenbaum AB, Khan JM, Bruce CG, Babaliaros VC, Rogers T. Transcaval access and closure best practices. *JACC Cardiovasc Interv*. 2023;16(4):371-395. doi:10.1016/j.jcin.2022.12.005
28. Bruce CG, Khan JM, Rogers T, et al. Transcatheter electrosurgery: a narrative review. *Circ Cardiovasc Interv*. 2023;16(3):e012019. doi:10.1161/CIRCINTERVENTIONS.122.012019
29. Khan JM, Rogers T, Greenbaum AB, Babaliaros VC, Bruce CG, Lederman RJ. Use of electrosurgery in interventional cardiology. *Interv Cardiol Clin*. 2022;11(3):257-266. doi:10.1016/j.iccl.2022.01.004
30. Lederman RJ, Babaliaros VC, Greenbaum AB. How to perform transcaval access and closure for transcatheter aortic valve implantation. *Catheter Cardiovasc Interv*. 2015;86(7):1242-1254. doi:10.1002/ccd.26141
31. Greenbaum AB, Babaliaros VC, Chen MY, et al. Transcaval access and closure for transcatheter aortic valve replacement: a prospective investigation. *J Am Coll Cardiol*. 2017;69(5):511-521. doi:10.1016/j.jacc.2016.10.024
32. Michail M, Cockburn J, Tanseco KVP, et al. Feasibility of transcaval access TAVI in morbidly obese patients: a single-center experience. *Catheter Cardiovasc Interv*. 2022;100(7):1302-1306. doi:10.1002/ccd.30465
33. Giulia C, Ole de B, Thomas P, et al. Feasibility and safety of transcaval transcatheter aortic valve implantation: a multicentre European registry. *EuroIntervention*. 7AD;15(15):e1319-e1324. https://eurointervention.pcronline.com/article/initial-european-experience-with-transcaval-transcatheter-aortic-valve-implantation
34. Barbash IM, Segev A, Berkovitch A, et al. Clinical outcome and safety of transcaval access for transcatheter aortic valve replacement as compared to other alternative approaches. *Front Cardiovasc Med*. 2021;8:731639. doi:10.3389/fcvm.2021.731639
35. Cui CQ, Cook BS, Cauchi MP, Foerst JR. A case series: alternative access for refractory shock during cardiac arrest. *Eur Heart J Case Rep*. 2019;3(3):ytz101. doi:10.1093/ehjcr/ytz101
36. Cheney AE, McCabe JM. Alternative access for mechanical circulatory support. *Interv Cardiol Clin*. 2021;10(2):257-268. doi:10.1016/j.iccl.2020.12.001
37. Chiang M, Gonzalez PE, Basir MB, et al. Modified transcaval left atrial venoarterial extracorporeal membrane oxygenation without preplanning contrast CT: step-by-step guide. *JACC Cardiovasc Interv*. 2022;15(16):e181-e185. doi:10.1016/j.jcin.2022.05.033
38. Afana M, Altawil M, Basir M, et al. Transcaval access for the emergency delivery of 5.0 liters per minute mechanical circulatory support in cardiogenic shock. *Catheter Cardiovasc Interv*. 2021;97(3):555-564. doi:10.1002/ccd.29235
39. Van Sickler AP, Smith AH, Ellis RC, et al. A novel technique and outcomes for transcaval endoleak embolization. *Ann Vasc Surg*. 2023;93:300-307. doi:10.1016/j.avsg.2023.01.013
40. Fanari Z, Hammami S, Goswami NJ, Goldstein JA. Percutaneous thoracic aortic aneurysm repair through transcaval aortic access. *Catheter Cardiovasc Interv*. 2017;90(5):806-808. doi:10.1002/ccd.27130
41. Baz Alonso JA, Jiménez-Díaz VA, Dominguez-Erquicia P, Puga L, Barreiro-Perez M, Íñiguez-Romo A. Facilitated transcaval access by shockwave lithoplasty and conscious sedation for transcatheter aortic valve replacement. *JACC Cardiovasc Interv*. 2022;15(23):e241-e244. doi:10.1016/j.jcin.2022.09.012
42. Vuruşkan E, Kaplan M, Altunbaş G, Düzen İV, Yılmaz Coşkun F, Sucu MM. Transcaval transcatheter aortic valve replacement through abdominal aortic aneurysm in a patient with no option for other vascular access. *Anatol J Cardiol*. 2021;25(6):456-457. doi:10.5152/AnatolJCardiol.2021.91
43. Lederman RJ, Babaliaros VC, Lisko JC, et al. Transcaval versus transaxillary TAVR in contemporary practice: a propensity-weighted analysis. *JACC Cardiovasc Interv*. 2022;15(9):965-975. doi:10.1016/j.jcin.2022.03.014

Vascular Access Site Management (Closure Devices and Complications)

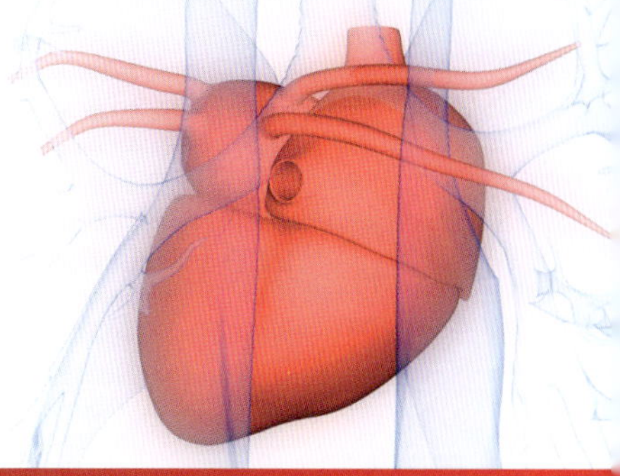

Sridevi R. Pitta and Jun Li

Transfemoral vascular access is still the most commonly used access site and remains necessary for numerous procedures, requiring large-bore access, including complex high-risk coronary interventions, structural procedures, and procedures involving mechanical circulatory support. Although access itself is simply a means to an end, unfortunately potentially life-threatening complications can arrive at the access site independent of the outcomes of the actual endovascular procedure.[1] Utilizing safe femoral access techniques, particularly ultrasound (US) guidance, reduces the potential for multiple punctures and allows the operator to identify a puncture site free of calcium and disease, making closure devices safer.[2,3] Traditionally, femoral artery access hemostasis has been achieved by manual compression (MC); however, vascular closure devices (VCDs) have been shown to increase efficacy with earlier ambulation, reduce time to hemostasis, aid in patient comfort, and in safety with reduced vascular and bleeding complications at the access site.[4,5] These have led to a gradual shift from MC to using VCDs. Insights from the Veterans Affairs Healthcare System demonstrate that VCD utilization has increased from 60.4% in fiscal year 2006 to 75.3% in fiscal year 2018, consistent with an average increase of 1.2% each year.[6] Globally, the VCD market has reached $1.3 billion in 2021 and is expected to continue expanding due to an increasing prevalence of cardiovascular disease, advances in innovative medical technologies, and preference for minimally invasive procedures. This chapter will review the indications, contraindications, types of closure devices, and techniques and complications associated with femoral vascular access closure devices.

RECOMMENDATIONS FOR VCD USE

VCDs have been Food and Drug Administration (FDA)-approved since 1993 for use in closure of femoral artery access sites following diagnostic or interventional endovascular procedures. In 2011, the American college of cardiology/American heart association/Society of coronary angiography and intervention (ACCF/AHA/SCAI)/percutaneous coronary intervention (PCI) guideline update outlined several indications for VCD use.[7,8]

1. Performing femoral angiography prior to the use of a VCD was given a Class I indication (Level of evidence C). The safety and efficacy of these devices are optimized when the common femoral artery (CFA) access site has a landing zone of adequate diameter (from 4 to 6 mm) without atherosclerotic disease or calcification (**Fig. 30.1** and **Table 30.1**).
2. The use of VCDs for the purposes of achieving faster hemostasis and earlier ambulation compared with the use of MC was given Class IIa recommendation (Level of evidence B). Recommendations were based on existing clinical trial data comparing the safety and efficacy of VCDs to MC, showing that VCDs consistently reduced time to hemostasis and ambulation compared to MC[4,9] (**Table 30.2**).
3. Routine use of VCDs for the purpose of decreasing vascular complications, including bleeding, received a Class III indication (Level of evidence B), since VCDs have not been shown to reduce the incidence of vascular complications.[10]

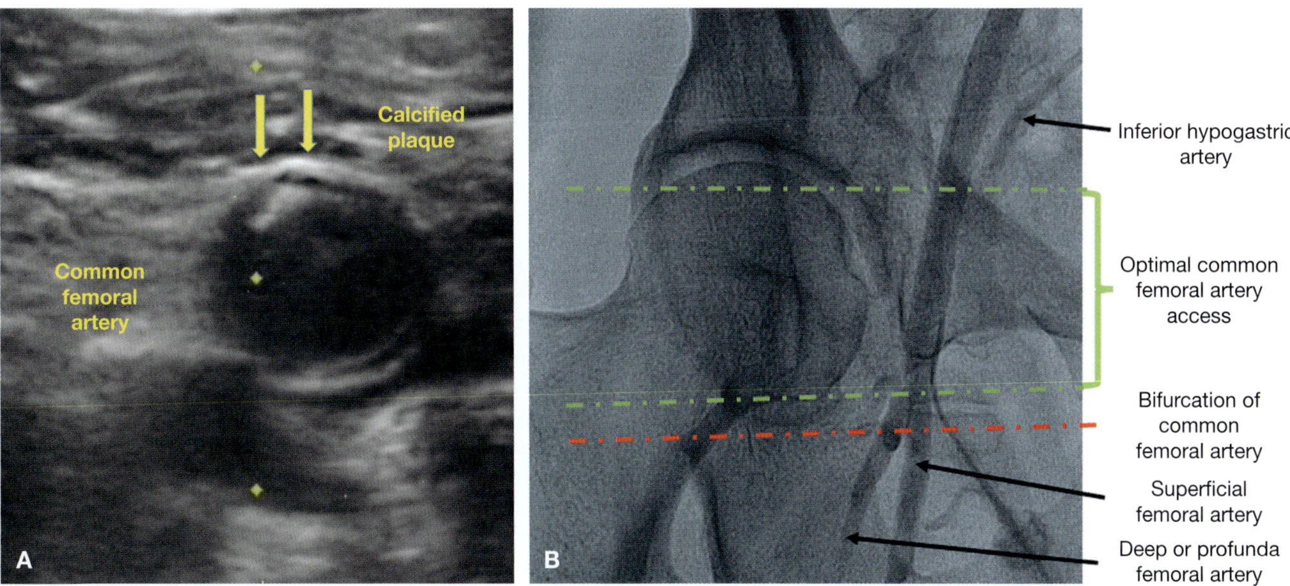

FIGURE 30.1 **A,** Ultrasound-guided common femoral artery (CFA) access identifies landing zone (from 4 to 6 mm), bifurcation, and atherosclerotic disease or calcification. **B,** Performing femoral angiography prior to the use of a vascular closure device using micropuncture technique to assess optimal anatomic suitability for deployment and hemostasis.

TABLE 30.1 VCD Instructions for Use

Indications
• For use in closing and reducing time to hemostasis at the femoral artery puncture site for cardiac catheterization or interventional procedures. • For use to allow ambulation as soon as possible after sheath removal.
Contraindications
• None
Warnings
• Do not use if the puncture site is at or distal to the common femoral artery bifurcation or is proximal to the inguinal ligament. • Do not use if there is posterior wall or multiple punctures.
Precautions
• Maintain sterility at all times during the use of the devices. • See specific device instructions.

VCD, vascular closure device.

LIMITATIONS TO VCD USE

- High stick: Expert consensus suggests that VCDs should not be routinely used in high sticks into the external iliac artery (above the CFA angiographically demarcated by the inferior most border of the inferior epigastric artery), or in low sticks (ie, below the bifurcation of the CFA into the profunda and superficial femoral arteries). In three independent registries, the use of a VCD was associated with a 1.4- to 2.3-fold higher odds ratio of a vascular complication in patients when it was used in the presence of a high stick, although in two of these studies, the confidence intervals crossed 0 and were not statistically significant.
- Alternate access: Small registries have evaluated the use of VCDs for brachial, axillary, antegrade femoral, and popliteal artery access.[11] Nevertheless, the data are limited, and firm understanding of their safety and effectiveness in these alternative arterial access sites is lacking.
- Venous access: VCDs have been used to close large venous access sites, but the data are extremely limited concerning the safety and efficacy of this procedure.

TABLE 30.2 2011 ACCF/AHA/SCAI PCI Guidelines

VASCULAR CLOSURE DEVICES: RECOMMENDATIONS

• Class I
  • Patients considered for vascular closure devices should undergo a femoral angiogram to ensure their anatomic suitability for deployment (level of evidence: C).
• Class IIa
  • The use of vascular closure devices is reasonable for the purposes of achieving faster hemostasis and earlier ambulation than the use of manual compression (level of evidence: B).
• Class III: No benefit
  • The routine use of vascular closure devices is not recommended for the purpose of decreasing vascular complications, including bleeding (level of evidence: B).

PCI, percutaneous coronary interventions.

- Re-access after use of VCD: Limited observational data suggest re-access is safe and effective. Applegate et al evaluated the safety of re-access in 181 patients following placement of an Angio-Seal device 1 day to 180 days after the initial VCD was placed and observed three hematomas >5 cm as the only adverse outcome of this practice.[12] Although other clinical data are lacking, re-access using other VCDs is commonly performed in routine practice.
- Infection control and antibiotic use: Several early-generation suture-based devices were associated with access-site infections.[13] These most likely arose from the considerable tissue tract manipulation required for placement of these devices, as well as the "foreign body" left in the vessel itself. Nevertheless, because of these reports, VCDs are discouraged in the presence of active local groin infections. In addition, all the device manufacturers strongly recommend complete re-prepping of the access site, as well as re-gloving of the operators, prior to the deployment of a VCD. The use of prophylactic antibiotics has been advocated by some in analogy to the recommendations for other minor surgical procedures, but there are no clinical data to guide practice.

LEARNING CURVE FOR VCDS

From the outset of clinical introduction of VCDs, it was recognized that there was a learning curve associated with achieving optimal outcomes with these devices.[14] Proficiency was dependent on both operator and institutional VCD and femoral artery experience and also varied by device. Each currently available device has its own unique delivery system and requires specific training to achieve proficiency. Resnic et al quantified the learning curve associated with the use of the StarClose closure device from the National Cardiovascular Data Registry (NCDR) Cath/PCI registry.[15] In 107,710 procedures with at least one VCD deployment, they found device success of 93% increasing to 97% at the end of the 2-year study period (2006-2007). They identified a triphasic learning curve: initial rapid learning from 0 to 22 cases followed by declining success rate in the next 23 to 50 cases with a final recovery to improved device success, requiring more than 50 cases[15] (**Fig. 30.2**). A similar learning curve for Angio-Seal device deployment was observed in the first 50 cases (14% nondeployment vs 3.5% for the subsequent 202 procedures, $P = .009$); failure to deploy was independent of sheath size used.[14] Balzer et al also noted suture-based closure devices have steeper and longer learning curve for technical success.[16]

CLASSIFICATION OF VCDS

Currently, several types of VCDs are FDA-approved for use in the United States (**Table 30.3**).[14] A variety of methods are used for vascular closure, from collagen plugs to suture to nitinol clip application. VCDs are categorized as either active or passive approximators, or/and external hemostatic devices by their mechanism of hemostasis, as well as whether or not there is any permanent intravascular element. The term "active approximation" is used to indicate that a mechanical seal of the opening of the arterial wall is achieved with the closure device. Active approximation devices include Angio-Seal, FISH, Perclose, and StarClose (**Fig. 30.3A**). The term "passive approximation" is used to indicate that hemostasis is achieved by tamponading the arterial access site just above the

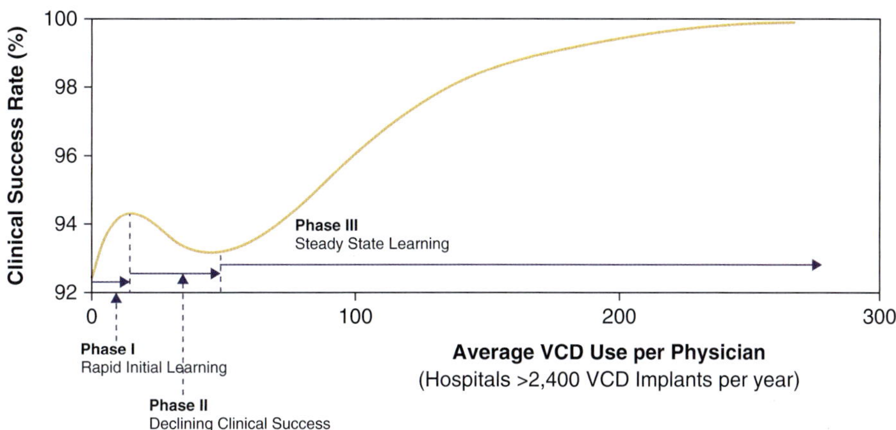

FIGURE 30.2 Graph of clinical success rate of use of the StarClose device as a function of average vascular closure device (VCD) use per physician. (Adapted from Resnic FS, Wang TY, Arora N, et al. Quantifying the learning curve in the use of a novel vascular closure device: an analysis of the NCDR (National Cardiovascular Data Registry) CathPCI registry. *JACC Cardiovasc Interv.* 2012;5(1):82-89.)

artery. Passive approximation devices include the Exoseal, Mynx, and Vascade VCD (**Fig. 30.3B**). Passive approximation devices are also known as extravascular sealants because there is no intravascular element present at the completion of the closure. Each of the passive approximation devices utilize a vessel locator system using an intravascular identification system that is subsequently removed at completion of the closure. The Angio-Seal, FISH, and Perclose devices all have an intravascular component (with Angio-Seal and FISH bioresorbable), and at times, the StarClose device may have a tine that is intravascular as well. These intravascular components theoretically constitute a risk of infection but also provide for a more secure closure. Each manufacturer has guidelines for the puncture site size range of use for their device, although in clinical practice, any of these devices can be used for sheath sizes up to 8 Fr. Prostar XL (Abbott Vascular, Redwood City, CA) and two ProGlides, MANTA VCD (Essential Medical),[17] are currently

TABLE 30.3 Vascular Closure Devices FDA Approved 2023

CLOSURE DEVICE	TYPE	PRODUCTS	COMMENTS
Active Approximation Devices			
Angio-Seal	Bioresorbable intraluminal, anchor, suture, and collagen form arteriotomy sandwich	Evolution	Automated compaction
		STS Plus	Self-tightening suture
		VIP	V twist collagen
FISH	Small intestinal mucosa (SIS) plug pulled against vessel wall creates mechanical seal	CombiClose	Combined working sheath and closure device
		ControlClose	
Perclose	Suture-based "surgical" arterial wall closure	Perclose A-T	Braided suture with preformed knot
		ProGlide	Monofilament suture with preformed knot
		ProStar XL	Two braided and untied sutures
		Prostyle	Monofilament polypropylene suture
StarClose	Nitinol clip delivered onto vessel creates "purse string" closure	StarClose SE	Two major and four minor tissue tines
Manta	Bio-resorbable hemostatic plug (collagen) outside of the artery, held by suture linked to a small molded polymer toggle positioned inside the artery.	MANTA	Resorbable collagen with anchor sandwich access site
Passive Approximation Devices (Extravascular)			
EXOSEAL	Extravascular polyglycolic acid plug	EXOSEAL	Accurate extravascular placement
MYNX	Extravascular sealant	MYNX ACE	Seals arteriotomy and expands to fill tissue track
		MYNXGRIP	Active tissue adherence of sealant
		MYNX CONTROL	Active extravascular sealant
Cardiva Catalyst	Collapsible disc with collagen patch (Vascade)	Cardiva Catalyst II	Collapsible disc with procoagulant material
		Cardiva Catalyst III	Additional thrombogenic material for anticoagulated patients
		Vascade	Collapsible disc with extravascular patch

available devices for closure of large-bore arterial sheaths and ranges from 10 to 25 Fr. The lower limit of a suitable vessel size for closure has not been rigorously studied, although it is generally accepted that vessels smaller than 4 to 5 mm are not optimal for VCD use and do not typically require closure.

SPECIFIC VCDS—ACTIVE APPROXIMATION

Angio-Seal

The Angio-Seal device (St. Jude Medical, St. Paul, MN) consists of an intraluminal polylactic-polyglycolic acid polymer anchor (2 × 11 mm) attached to a bioresorbable suture over which a collagen plug is compressed against the external wall of the artery and is ultimately secured by a knot, forming an "arteriotomy sandwich" at the access site (**Fig. 30.3A**). The anchor is non-thrombogenic, and all the components are bioresorbable, with chemically complete bioresorption occurring by 3 months. The device is introduced with its own delivery sheath and is available in 6 and 8 Fr sizes. The most recent iteration of the device, "Evolution," uses an automated tamping mechanism designed to optimize site closure.

Fish

The FISH device (Morris Innovative, Bloomington, IN) incorporates a sleeve of small intestinal mucosa (SIS) within the closure sheath (**Fig. 30.3A**). Hemostasis is attained immediately after sheath removal when the SIS is pulled up against the inner surface of the arterial wall at the access site and embedded into the arterial wall at the access site, secured by a bioresorbable extravascular plug. It is fully bioresorbable. The device can be either a standalone closure device (ControlClose) or a combination of working sheath and closure device (CombiClose).

Perclose

The Perclose devices (Abbott Vascular, Redwood City, CA) ProGlide and ProStar and newer Prostyle achieve percutaneous suture-mediated closure in a fashion analogous to that obtained by direct surgical closure of a vessel. The ProGlide device deploys two sutures through the anterior wall of the artery, which is received by the footplate within the artery and then exteriorized (**Fig. 30.3A**). The device is then removed from the artery, leaving a pretied suture knot, with hemostasis achieved by tightening

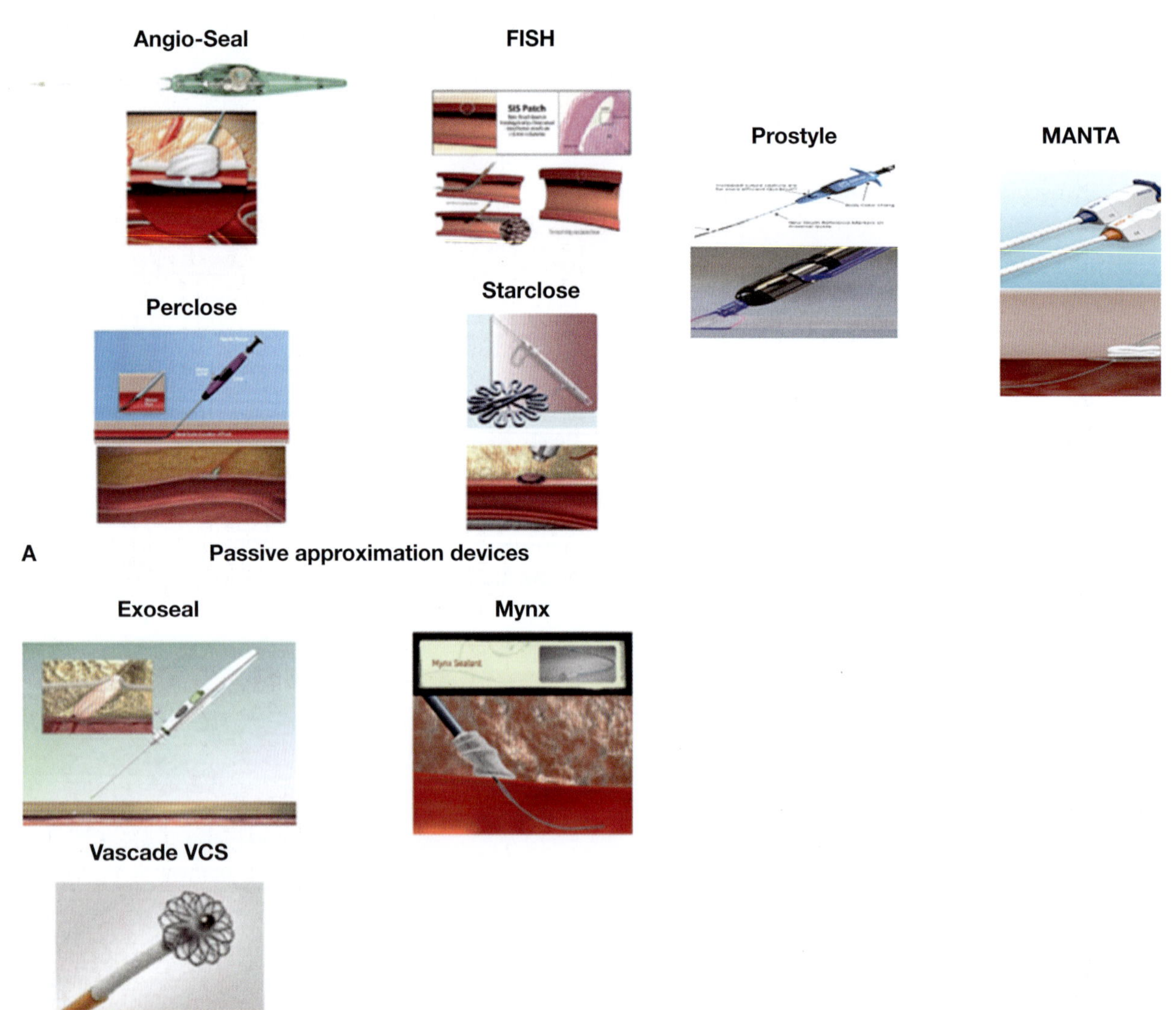

FIGURE 30.3 **A,** Active approximation devices. **B,** Passive approximation devices.

of the knot onto the surface of the artery. ProStyle is the next-generation design evolution of the Proglide and features higher-tensile-strength needles for more reliability in challenging anatomy. The 10-Fr ProStar device requires tissue track manipulation to position the barrel of the receiving portion of the device with needles from inside the vessel wall into the receiving barrels, followed by exteriorization of the sutures. The sutures then are used to tie knots that are pushed down onto the artery's surface, achieving hemostasis. It is generally accepted that these devices can be used for closures of sheath size <10 Fr or smaller. These devices can additionally be used for preclosure of large-bore arteriotomies with more than one device.

StarClose

The StarClose device (Abbott Vascular. Redwood City, CA) delivers a nitinol clip to close the arteriotomy from the extravascular side to achieve hemostasis (**Fig. 30.3A**). The nitinol clip has two major and four minor tines that create a "purse string" type of closure at the surface of the arterial wall, with the tines secured within the arterial wall itself. The StarClose device is inserted over a wire through a sheath that comes with the device, which is specifically designed and required for this use. A retractable anchor is used to ensure satisfactory positioning at the arteriotomy site, and then the clip is deployed on the exterior surface of the vessel.

Manta

The Manta system is a collagen-based VCD similar to the Angio Seal but is much larger and designed specifically for large-bore femoral arterial access-site closure following the use of 10 to 20 Fr devices or sheaths (12-25 Fr outer diameter).[18,19] The SAFE MANTA IDE clinical trial, the largest US prospective multicenter, single-arm trial, demonstrated that the Manta device successfully achieves fast reliable biomechanical closure with rapid hemostasis (**Fig. 30.3A**).

PASSIVE APPROXIMATION DEVICES

EXOSEAL

The EXOSEAL device (Cordis, Miami, FL) delivers an extravascular plug to the arteriotomy site. The plug consists of completely bioresorbable polyglycolic acid and achieves hemostasis by MC of the arteriotomy site under the femoral sheath (**Fig. 30.3B**). A vessel locator system prevents intravascular insertion of the plug and allows very accurate placement of the plug.

MYNX

The MYNX VCD (Cordis, Miami, FL) utilizes an extravascular polyethylene glycol (PEG) sealant, which is completely bioresorbable, to achieve hemostasis. An intravascular balloon is pulled up against the inner surface of the artery through a delivery sheath, anchoring the device while the PEG plug is positioned on the exterior surface of the vessel (**Fig. 30.3B**). Within minutes, the plug hydrates and expands to form an extravascular seal above the vessel and within the tissue tract.

Vascade Vascular Closure System

The Vascade vascular closure system (Cardiva Medical Inc., Santa Clara, CA) incorporates an extravascular collagen plug to the traditional Vascade footplate-facilitated MC system (**Fig. 30.3B**). After being put in place, the collagen plug is positioned in the track above the access site; the footplate is then removed, creating an external seal.

External Hemostatic Devices

Compression devices: Passive closure devices also include assisted compression devices that provide hands-free mechanical compression. FDA-approved devices include FemoStop (Abbott Vascular), QuicKlamp (TZ Medical), CompressAR (Advanced vascular) have been evaluated in small randomized or observational studies in limited risk population.

Hemostasis patches: Assisted coagulant patches and sealants such as the D-stat patch (Vascular Solutions), Syvek Patch (Marine Polymer Technologies), and StatSeal (Biolife LLC) hasten initial hemostasis when used as an adjunct to MC.

CLINICAL EVALUATION OF SAFETY AND EFFICACY OF VCDS

The first-generation VCDs, Angio-Seal and Perclose, as well as the VCDs most recently introduced into the market, have undergone a series of modifications designed to enhance their effectiveness and ease of use. Some of these modifications include downsizing of devices, streamlining of transitioning points into and out of the artery, simplifying and ensuring suture capture for the Perclose device, and standardized device-deployment techniques. As a reflection of these changes, the VCD deployment success rate increased from approximately 88% seen in the original randomized clinical trials to over 95% in the two most recent randomized trials.

Randomized Clinical Trials

ISAR CLOSURE compared the safety and efficacy of two closure devices, FemoSeal (St. Jude Medical, St Paul, MN) and EXOSEAL (Cordis, Miami, FL), used for MC in patients undergoing transfemoral angiography[20] A total of 1509 patients received the FemoSeal device, 1506 the EXOSEAL device, and 1509 patients underwent MC. The primary endpoint of the study was access-site complications at 30 days (**Table 30.4**). The overall rate of access-site complications for VCDs was 6.9% compared to 7.9% for MC, with P for non-inferiority <0.01. However, rates of hematoma >5 cm were higher in the MC group (6.8%) than in VCD (4.8%), $P = .06$. The authors concluded that, in patients undergoing transfemoral angiography, the use of VCDs was non-inferior but not superior to MC for overall vascular closure rates, although there were lower rates of hematoma >5 cm with VCD use.

The CLOSE UP Study compared the FemoSeal VCD to MC in 1001 patients undergoing diagnostic angiography.[21] The primary endpoint was groin hematoma >5 cm, which occurred in 2.2% of the FemoSeal group compared to 6.7% of the MC group, $P = .002$ (**Table 30.5**). All major adverse vascular events at 14 days occurred in 0.6% of the FemoSeal group, and 1.0% of the manual group, P = NS (**Table 30.6**). Similar to the ISAR CLOSURE Study, the authors concluded that, in patients undergoing diagnostic angiography via the femoral artery, the use of a VCD resulted in similar overall rates of vascular complication but reduced the incidence of hematoma >5 cm.

A network meta-analysis of the safety of VCDs obtained from randomized clinical trials conducted from 1992 to 2014 has been

TABLE 30.4 Outcomes at 30 days

	NO. (%) OF PATIENTS			
	VASCULAR CLOSURE DEVICE (*N* = 3015)	MANUAL COMPRESSION (*N* = 1509)	DIFFERENCE IN PROPORTIONS, % (95% CI)	*P* VALUE
Vascular access site complications (primary endpoint)[a]	208 (6.9)	119 (7.9)	−1 (−2.7-0.7)	<.001[b]
Hematoma >5 cm	145 (4.8)	102 (6.8)	−2 (−3.4 to −0.4)	.006
Pseudoaneurysm	53 (1.8)	23 (1.5)	0.3 (−0.5-1.1)	.56
Arteriovenous fistula	12 (0.4)	2 (0.1)	0.3 (−0.1-0.6)	.13
Access site–related major bleeding[c]	3 (0.1)	3 (0.2)	−0.1 (−0.4-0.2)	.39
Acute ipsilateral leg ischemia	0	0		
Need for vascular surgical or interventional treatment	0	0		
Local infection	1	0		.48
Secondary Endpoints				
Time to hemostasis, median (IQR), min	1 (0.5-2.0)	10 (10-15)		<.001
Repeat manual compression	53 (1.8)	10 (0.7)		.003

[a]Primary endpoint defined as the composite of hematoma at least 5 cm in size, pseudoaneurysm, arteriovenous fistula, access site–related major bleeding, acute ipsilateral leg ischemia, need for vascular surgical or interventional treatment, or local infection.
[b]*P* value from the noninferiority analysis.
[c]Based on criteria form REPLACE-2 (Randomized Evaluation in PCI Linking Angiomax to Reduced Clinical Events).
IQR, interquartile range; PCI, percutaneous coronary interventions.

TABLE 30.5 The Individual Components of Major Adverse Vascular Events (MAVE)

	MANUAL COMPRESSION (*N* = 500)	FEMOSEAL (*N* = 501)	*P* VALUE
Pseudoaneurysm	1 (0.2)	2 (0.4)	1.00
Infection	2 (0.4)	1 (0.2)	1.00
Need for vascular surgery	0 (0)	0 (0)	1.00
Major bleeding	2 (0.4)	0 (0)	.50
Retroperitoneal bleeding	0 (0)	0 (0)	1.00

Values are *n* (%). Fisher's exact test was used.
Adapted from Holm NR, Sindberg B, Schou M, et al. Randomised comparison of manual compression and FemoSeal vascular closure device for closure after femoral artery access coronary angiography: the CLOSure dEvices Used in everyday Practice (CLOSE-UP) study. *EuroIntervention*. 2014;9:183-190.

TABLE 30.6 Individual Rates of Hematoma >5 cm

	MANUAL COMPRESSION (*N* = 500)	FEMOSEAL (*N* = 501)	*P* VALUE
In-hospital (primary endpoint)	31 (6.2)	11 (2.2)	.002
At 14 d (self-reporting)	38 (8.7)	29 (6.4)	.20
14-d total (self-reporting)	38 (8.7)	29 (6.4)	.20

Values are *n* (%). Fisher's exact test or chi-square test was used.
Used with permission of Europa Group, from Holm NR, Sindberg B, Schou M, et al. Randomised comparison of manual compression and FemoSeal™ vascular closure device for closure after femoral artery access coronary angiography: the CLOSure dEvices Used in everyday Practice (CLOSE-UP) study. *EuroIntervention*. 2014;9:183-190; permission conveyed through Copyright Clearance Center, Inc.

published.[22] They identified 40 randomized trials comprising 16,868 patients undergoing either diagnostic angiography or PCI from a transfemoral approach. Twenty-eight of the trials were performed before 2005, while 12 of the trials were performed after 2005. The risk ratio for vascular complications of VCD compared to MC was 1.05 (95% CI, 0.83-1.32) for those studies before 2005, while the risk ratio was 0.64 (95% CI, 0.46-0.89) after 2005 (**Fig. 30.4**). The authors concluded that there was substantial heterogeneity in study design and outcomes among the studies. Despite this, there appeared to be a temporal trend toward lower rates of vascular complication with VCD use compared to MC after 2005, as opposed to those before 2005. Whether these results will change the guidelines outlining the indications for VCD use for improving safety remains to be determined.

Registries

Three very large contemporary registries merit mention. An instrumental variable analysis from the American college of cardiology (ACC) NCDR Cath/PCI registry of cases performed between 2009 and 2013 identified 1,053,155 VCDs used during 2,056,585 PCIs.[23] The overall absolute rate of vascular complication was 1.5%, with

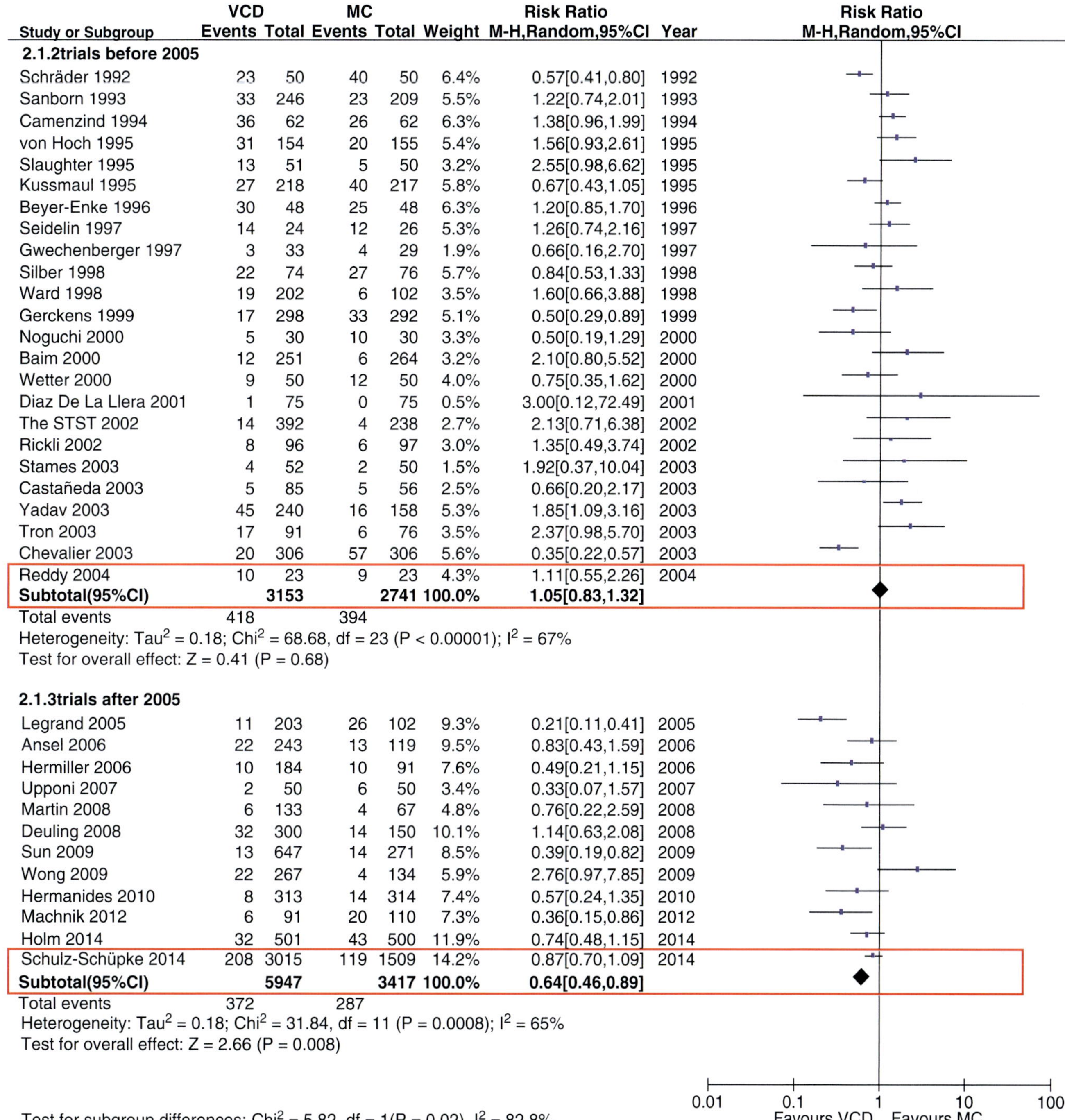

FIGURE 30.4 Forest plot of rates of vascular complications with vascular closure device (VCD) use or manual compression (MC) in studies before 2005 (*upper panel*) and after 2005 (*lower panel*). (Adapted from Jiang J, Zou J, Ma H, et al. Network meta-analysis of randomized trials on the safety of vascular closure devices for femoral arterial puncture site haemostasis. *Sci Rep*. 2015;5:13761.)

VCD use associated with a 0.4% absolute reduction in vascular complications (95% CI, 0.31-0.42); the number needed to treat to prevent one vascular complication: 250. The authors concluded that VCD use after PCI is associated with a significant but very small reduction in overall major bleeding compared to MC. The British Cardiovascular Intervention Society identified 271,845 patients undergoing PCI between 2006 and 2011.[24] They evaluated 30-day mortality stratified by VCD use or MC. VCD use was associated with 1.8% mortality at 30 days compared to 2.0% for MC, with a hazard ratio of 0.91 (95% CI, 0.86-0.97, $P < .01$); after propensity score–matching adjustment. The authors concluded that the use of a VCD was associated with a significant but small reduction in 30-day all-cause mortality. Finally, the Blue Cross Blue Shield Cardiovascular Consortium of Michigan identified 85,048 PCIs occurring between 2007 and 2009 with VCD use in 28,528.[20] A vascular complication occurred in 1.9% of the overall study. After propensity score–matching adjustment, the odds ratio of a vascular complication was 0.78 for VCD use compared to MC (95% CI, 0.67-0.90), $P = .01$. The odds ratio of transfusions for VCD use compared to MC was 0.85 (95% CI, 0.74-0.96), $P = .011$. The authors concluded that the use of a VCD was associated with a modest relative decrease in overall vascular complications and transfusions compared to MC, which was attenuated if glycoprotein IIb/IIIa inhibitors were used. They also noted that VCD use was associated with a small but significant relative increase in retroperitoneal bleeding compared to MC.

Head-To-Head Comparisons of VCD Types

There have been multiple small registries, and more than 10 randomized clinical trials, that have compared the safety and efficacy of one closure device to another.[22] These studies have been limited by small study size and heterogeneity in study design and outcomes, weakening the strength of conclusions that can be reached from the comparisons. The current expert consensus opinion suggests that currently there are no definitive data showing that one device is superior to others with regard to safety and efficacy.

CLINICAL UTILITY OF VCDS

With a growing emphasis on outpatient management of PCI patients, the use of VCDs to facilitate same-day PCI discharge has been evaluated in several small studies and found to be both safe and efficacious. Rao et al. evaluated clinical outcomes of 107,018 patients aged 65 years or older undergoing PCI from the ACC NCDR Cath/PCI registry.[25] They identified 1339 patients who underwent same-day PCI discharge, with femoral access used in 96% and VCD used in 65% of those patients. The authors found no difference in the rates of death or re-hospitalization in the same-day discharge group (0.37%; 95% CI, 0.16-0.87) versus overnight stay (0.5%; 95% CI, 0.46-0.54, $P = .51$). Although the use of transradial interventions has grown, principally because of the appeal of this access site for same-day PCI discharge, there are currently no conclusive data comparing outcomes of the radial artery to femoral artery access with VCD use on the safety and efficacy of these different access approaches.

The recent tremendous growth in the use of large-bore (ie, >10 Fr) sheaths for both structural heart and endovascular procedures has spurred interest in the percutaneous management of access sites. Currently, only the Perclose suture-based device allows preclosure of large-bore access sites. Preclosure is achieved by the use of either one ProStar or two ProGlides through smaller procedural sheaths (typically, 6 Fr), with the sutures exteriorized but without tying the knots down to the surface of the artery. In the case of the use of two ProGlides, they are typically oriented 30° to 60° apart (on a clock face). At the end of the case, a number of strategies have been used to minimize bleeding while the preclosed sutures are tightened, allowing hemostasis. The preclosure technique, eliminating the need for surgical cut down, has allowed transition from general anesthesia to deep sedation and earlier ambulation of patients. The PEVAR trial (Percutaneous Access vs Open Femoral Exposure for Endovascular Aortic Aneurysm Repair) compared clinical outcomes of 30 days using preclosure with ProGlide ($n = 50$), preclosure with ProStar ($n = 51$), or open femoral exposure ($n = 101$).[26] The primary endpoint of treatment success (composite of procedural technical success and absence of vascular complications) occurred in 88% of ProGlide patients, 78% of ProStar patients, and 78% of femoral exposure patients. ProGlide treatment success was non-inferior to femoral exposure, but ProStar was not non-inferior to femoral exposure.

COMPLICATIONS OF FEMORAL ACCESS AND VCDS

Regardless of the mechanism utilized to achieve hemostasis (eg, variety of VCD or MC), complications can occur. The first step for prevention is meticulous, US-guided access to target entry point, as discussed in Chapters 27 and 28. Potential femoral artery access related complications includes[27] hematoma, pseudoaneurysm (PSA), arteriovenous fistula (AVF), dissection, thrombosis and occlusion, nerve injury, and infection.

The rates of vascular complications vary widely based on reporting methodology, time of assessment, and definitions used (**Table 30.7**)[28]; rates of complication are increased in large-bore access.[27] Regardless of type of procedure or VCD chosen, hematoma formation remains the most common access site complication.[29,30] Fortunately, major vascular complications requiring surgical or endovascular intervention occur in less than 1% of patients overall.[27,29,30] Although many coronary interventionists have adopted a radial-first approach, femoral access remains mainstay of therapy for large-bore access and many endovascular procedures. Thus, the ability to provide rescue therapy remains a critical skillset to maintain in the interventional cardiologist's armamentarium (**Fig. 30.5**).

Bleeding

The most frequent complication, hematoma formation, can typically be managed conservatively. Frequent and fastidious monitoring of the femoral access point is key in early identification of hematoma formation in the periprocedural phase. In circumstances where a hematoma is too large for effective MC or in the presence of rapidly

TABLE 30.7 Vascular Closure Device Complications[a]

- Deployment failure with immediate bleeding (3.9%-6.7%)
- Leg ischemia and/or occlusion requiring surgery (0%-0.1%)
- Vessel dissection (not reported in studies)
- Bleeding including retroperitoneal hemorrhage (0.7%)
- Pseudoaneurysm (0.7%-1.6%)
- Arterio-venous fistulae (0.2%-0.3%)
- Hematoma (5.4%)
- Infection (0.2%-0.3%)
- Nerve injury (<0.1%)

[a]Abstracted from Robertson L, Andras A, Colgan F, Jackson R. Vascular closure devices for femoral arterial puncture site hemostasis. *Cochrane Database Syst Rev.* 2016;3:CD009541. doi:10.1002/14,651,858.CD009541.pub2, for collagen-based, and suture-based device studies.

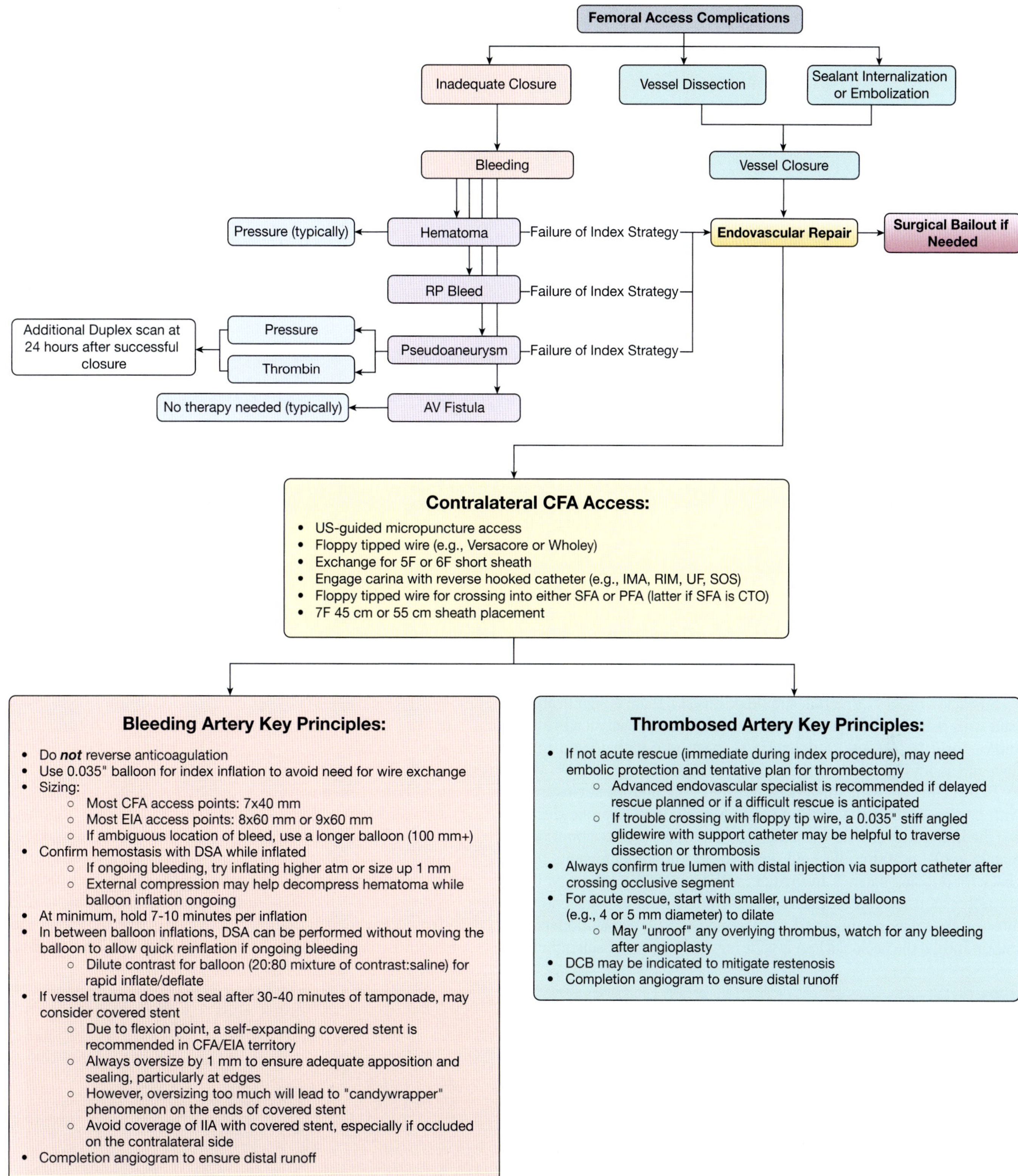

FIGURE 30.5 A proposed algorithm for femoral access complications. If common femoral contralateral access is not possible, brachial arterial access may be appropriate to reach the treatment zone and to deliver appropriate therapies. AV, arteriovenous; CFA, common femoral artery; CTO, chronic total occlusion; DCB, drug coated balloon; DSA, digital subtraction angiography; EIA, external iliac artery; IIA, internal iliac artery; PFA, profunda femoris artery; RP, retroperitoneal; SFA, superficial femoral artery.

expanding hematoma despite MC, an emergent return to the angiography suite is indicated to ensure adequate hemostasis.

Retroperitoneal (RP) bleeding is typically the result of a high access point into the external iliac artery with inadequate vessel closure by VCD or MC, or may be due to vessel trauma during the procedure. Most RP-associated bleeding will tamponade on their own with appropriate volume and/or blood resuscitation, assuming a lack of active antithrombotic agents. In the event of ongoing deterioration despite resuscitation, an emergent return to the angiography suite is also indicated (**Fig. 30.6**). In the rare patient with

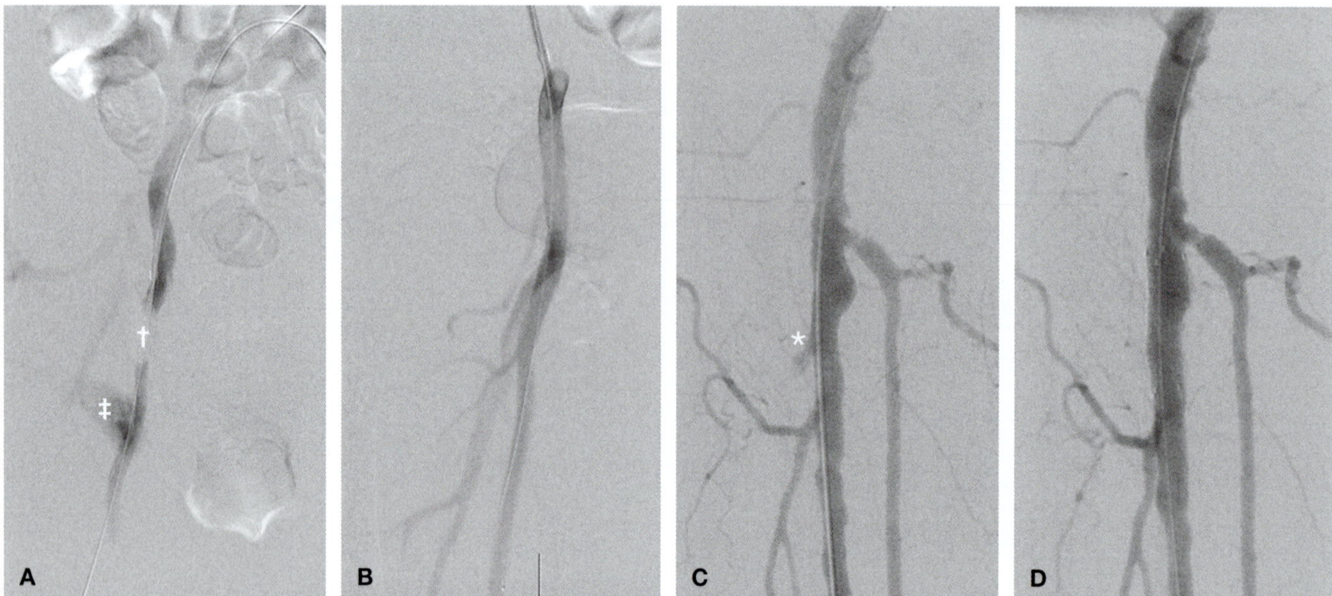

FIGURE 30.6 Angiographic examples of endovascular rescues for femoral access complications. **A,** A patient with post-TAVR deployment with nose-cone-associated damage at the site of arteriotomy. †Site of balloon tamponade, which is well sized and apposed to the wall but is inappropriately positioned. ‡Site of ongoing extravasation. A longer balloon with appropriate positioning resulted in complete hemostasis **(B)**. **C,** An obese patient with postendovascular procedure underwent manual compression of access site. Developed difficult-to-control bleeding (marked by *) with very large hematoma, unable to compress for hemostasis reliably. **D,** A self-expanding covered stent was deployed, with care taken not to occlude any of the branches.

inferior epigastric artery perforation, coil or thrombin embolization is indicated of the vessel. While surgical repair is feasible in patients with bleeding complications, it is often impractical because of the time required to mobilize a surgical team; thus, an endovascular-first approach is oftentimes a more favorable option (**Fig. 30.6A-D**).

Suspicion of PSA formation should be raised if there is significant pain with palpation of a patient with hematoma, especially if a bruit and/or thrill is present. Doppler US is diagnostic with to-and-fro flow and should be performed in a timely fashion. For small PSA (1- to 2-cm diameter) with small neck (≤2 mm), an attempt at closure with compression at the neck of the PSA using the US probe during the index scan should be made. Typically, this requires approximately a 20- to 30-minute hold, in 5- to 10-minute increments to check for ongoing patency. In a patient with larger PSA, or those who are nonresponsive to compression, US-guided thrombin injection into the PSA may be indicated with trained vascular practitioners. Importantly, if the neck of a PSA is wide (eg, ≥5-8 mm), consideration for open vs. endovascular repair may be needed to prevent thrombin embolization and distal extremity occlusion. A technique of balloon-assisted occlusion at the level of PSA during thrombin injection has been described to help prevent thrombin embolization, which can be utilized in a patient with a wide PSA neck.[31] Approximately 24 hours after PSA closure via either compression or thrombin injection, a repeat Duplex is indicated to ensure sustained closure and to ensure a lack of inadvertent deep venous thrombosis formation from compression. If systemic antithrombotic agents can be avoided for approximately 1 week, it will allow for better sealing.

AVF typically do not result in symptoms, but a thrill or bruit may be appreciated on examination. Doppler typically shows continuous flow across AVF and into the venous outflow. In the absence of antithrombotic agents, many AVF will close on their own and pose no clinical consequence. If there is significant pain associated with an AVF, or persistent AVF with high-outflow heart failure suspected, either surgical or endovascular repair may be indicated (**Fig. 30.7A and B**).

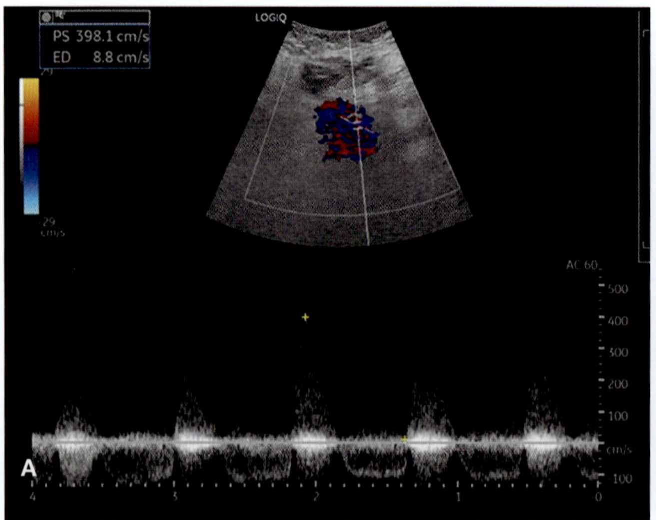

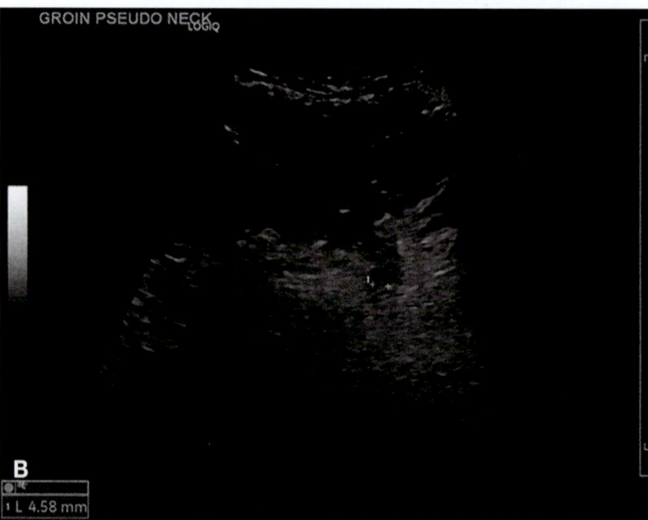

FIGURE 30.7 Duplex **(A)** and Doppler **(B)** examples of a femoral artery pseudoaneurysm.

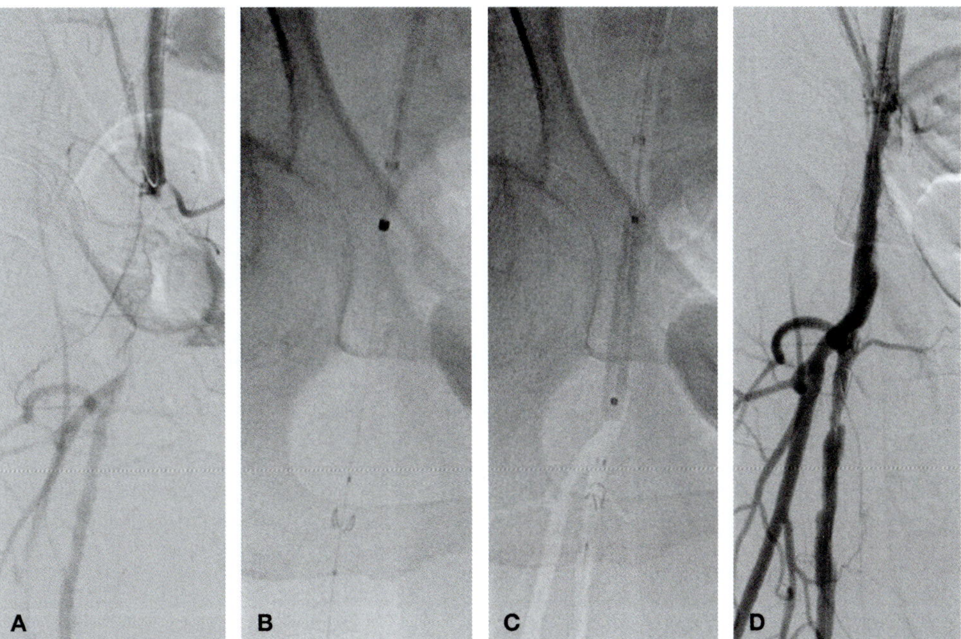

FIGURE 30.8 A patient who underwent endovascular procedure of the left lower extremity with deployment of a collagen plug for hemostasis **(A)**. Developed symptomatic rest pain on the right lower extremity at 1 week postoperatively. Radial access was obtained, with angiogram showing complete occlusion of the common femoral artery. **B,** Laser atherectomy and **(C)** drug-coated balloon yielded improved flow through the access point **(D)**. A small amount of residual thrombus abutting the medial wall, treated medically.

Vessel Closure

Dissection of the vessel can occur during the initial access or from multiple failed suture-mediated VCD. As a result of dissection, vessel closure and thrombosis may ensue, resulting in acute limb ischemia. Vessel closure may also occur from inadvertent intra-arterial shifting of an extravascular plug or sealant. Recognition of vessel closure is important, as emergent rescue is indicated to minimize significant tissue loss. Majority of these rescues can be accomplished endovascularly (**Fig. 30.8E-H**)

Allergic Reactions and Infection Risk

Local allergic reactions have also been reported after VCD use. The Angio-Seal device has a bovine collagen component that may elicit a localized inflammatory reaction manifesting as a small red bump at the access site. No specific management is usually necessary. Infections may also arise following VCD use. Fortunately, the overall incidence appears to be less than 0.1%. The organism responsible is generally *Staphylococcus aureus*, as would be expected from a skin source. There have been case fatalities associated with abscess formation in the subcutaneous base overlying the femoral artery associated with infectious arteritis itself.

CONCLUSIONS

MC has been the gold standard for achieving hemostasis over 50 years. Nevertheless, limitations of MC including delayed time to hemostasis and ambulation, as well as patient discomfort, led to the development of VCDs. VCDs achieve hemostasis by both active and passive approximation at the access site and require training and education to achieve competency in their use. First-generation VCDs carried complication rates similar to those of MC, leading to a Class III 2011 PCI guideline for use of VCDs to reduce complications. Nonetheless, more recent randomized clinical trials and large registries suggest a decrease in the rate of vascular complications with VCDs, which may lead to a modification of these recommendations. VCDs have been used clinically to achieve same-day discharge and allow percutaneous management of large-bore access sheaths using a preclosure technique. Access-site complications, although infrequent, can be potentially life-threatening, and meticulous attention to detail is warranted to optimize the safe use of these devices.

Key Points

- Hemostasis of femoral artery access can be achieved with either MC or VCDs.
- VCDs reduce time to hemostasis and ambulation but have not been shown to definitively reduce overall rates of vascular complications compared with MC, although two recent randomized trials (ISAR-CLOSURE and CLOSE UP) showed reduced rates of hematoma >5 cm with VCDs compared to MC.
- VCDs are classified as either active approximation (mechanical seal of the arterial wall) or passive approximation (external tamponade of the arterial access site).
- No VCD has been shown to be definitively more efficacious than another in reducing rates of vascular complications.
- Substantial improvements in the design of VCDs have improved deployment success and reduced failures.
- There is a significant learning curve associated with the use of VCDs, with a recent NCDR registry indicating "competence" after deployment of >50 VCDs.

- VCD use is optimal when used to close CFA access sites, avoiding both "high" (EIA access) and "low" (superficial) femoral or profunda femoral artery access.
- Specific VCD complications—including embolization of the device, device-mediated leg ischemia, and access-site infection—are uncommon but potentially life-threatening.

For further review and interactivities, please see the chapter-based multiple choice questions and videos accessible in the complimentary eBook bundled with this text. Access instructions are located in the inside front cover.

References

1. Lee MS, Applegate B, Rao SV, Kirtane AJ, Seto A, Stone GW. Minimizing femoral artery access complications during percutaneous coronary intervention: a comprehensive review. *Catheter Cardiovasc Interv*. 2014;84(1):62-69.
2. Sandoval Y, Burke MN, Lobo AS, et al. Contemporary arterial access in the cardiac catheterization laboratory. *JACC Cardiovasc Interv*. 2017;10(22):2233-2241.
3. Pitta SR, Bagai J. *Safe Femoral Access: Using All the Tools in the Toolbox*; 2020. https://scai.org/safe-femoral-access-using-all-tools-toolbox
4. Gewalt SM, Helde SM, Ibrahim T, et al. Comparison of vascular closure devices versus manual compression after femoral artery puncture in women. *Circ Cardiovasc Interv*. 2018;11(8):e006074.
5. Schroff A, Pinto D, *Vascular Access, Management, and Closure: Best Practices*. Accessed August 12, 2020. https://scai.org/publications/vascular-access-management-andclosure-best-practices
6. Prouse A, Gunzburger E, Yang F, et al. Contemporary use and outcomes of arterial closure devices after percutaneous coronary intervention: insights from the veterans affairs clinical assessment, reporting, and tracking program. *J Am Heart Assoc*. 2020;9(4):e015223.
7. Levine GN, Bates ER, Blankenship JC, et al. 2011 ACCF/AHA/SCAI guideline for percutaneous coronary intervention. A report of the American College of Cardiology Foundation/American Heart Association Task Force on practice guidelines and the Society for Cardiovascular Angiography and Interventions. *J Am Coll Cardiol*. 2011;58(24):e44-e122.
8. Patel MR, Jneid H, Derdeyn CP, et al. Arteriotomy closure devices for cardiovascular procedures: a scientific statement from the American Heart Association. *Circulation*. 2010;122(18):1882-1893.
9. Koreny M, Riedmüller E, Nikfardjam M, Siostrzonek P, Müllner M. Arterial puncture closing devices compared with standard manual compression after cardiac catheterization: systematic review and meta-analysis. *JAMA*. 2004;291(3):350-357.
10. Biancari F, D'Andrea V, Di Marco C, Savino G, Tiozzo V, Catania A. Meta-analysis of randomized trials on the efficacy of vascular closure devices after diagnostic angiography and angioplasty. *Am Heart J*. 2010;159(4):518-531.
11. Sheth RA, Ganguli S. Closure of alternative vascular sites, including axillary, brachial, popliteal, and surgical grafts. *Tech Vasc Interv Radiol*. 2015;18(2):113-121.
12. Applegate RJ, Rankin KM, Little WC, Kahl FR, Kutcher MA. Restick following initial angioseal use. *Catheter Cardiovasc Interv*. 2003;58(2):181-184.
13. Sohail MR, Khan AH, Holmes DR Jr, Wilson WR, Steckelberg JM, Baddour LM. Infectious complications of percutaneous vascular closure devices. *Mayo Clin Proc*. 2005;80(8):1011-1015.
14. Warren BS, Warren SG, Miller SD. Predictors of complications and learning curve using the Angio-Seal closure device following interventional and diagnostic catheterization. *Catheter Cardiovasc Interv*. 1999;48(2):162-166.
15. Resnic FS, Wang TY, Arora N, et al. Quantifying the learning curve in the use of a novel vascular closure device: an analysis of the NCDR (National Cardiovascular Data Registry) CathPCI registry. *JACC Cardiovasc Interv*. 2012;5(1):82-89.
16. Balzer JO, Scheinert D, Diebold T, Haufe M, Vogl TJ, Biamino G. Postinterventional transcutaneous suture of femoral artery access sites in patients with peripheral arterial occlusive disease: a study of 930 patients. *Catheter Cardiovasc Interv*. 2001;53(2):174-181.
17. van Wiechen MP, Ligthart JM, Van Mieghem NM. Large-bore vascular closure: new devices and techniques. *Interv Cardiol*. 2019;14(1):17-21.
18. Abdel-Wahab M, Hartung P, Dumpies O, et al. Comparison of a pure plug-based versus a primary suture-based vascular closure device strategy for transfemoral transcatheter aortic valve replacement: the CHOICE-CLOSURE randomized clinical trial. *Circulation*. 2022;145(3):170-183.
19. Wood DA, Krajcer Z, Sathananthan J, et al. Pivotal clinical study to evaluate the safety and effectiveness of the MANTA percutaneous vascular closure device. *Circ Cardiovasc Interv*. 2019;12(7):e007258.
20. Schulz-Schüpke S, Helde S, Gewalt S, et al. Comparison of vascular closure devices vs manual compression after femoral artery puncture: the ISAR-CLOSURE randomized clinical trial. *JAMA*. 2014;312(19):1981-1987.
21. Holm NR, Sindberg B, Schou M, et al. Randomised comparison of manual compression and FemoSeal™ vascular closure device for closure after femoral artery access coronary angiography: the CLOSure dEvices Used in everyday Practice (CLOSE-UP) study. *EuroIntervention*. 2014;10(2):183-190.
22. Jiang J, Zou J, Ma H, et al. Network meta-analysis of randomized trials on the safety of vascular closure devices for femoral arterial puncture site haemostasis. *Sci Rep*. 2015;5:13761.
23. Wimmer NJ, Secemsky EA, Mauri L, et al. Effectiveness of arterial closure devices for preventing complications with percutaneous coronary intervention: an instrumental variable analysis. *Circ Cardiovasc Interv*. 2016;9(4):e003464.
24. Farooq V, Goedhart D, Ludman P, de Belder MA, Harcombe A, El-Omar M. Response by Farooq et al to Letter Regarding Article, "Relationship Between Femoral Vascular Closure Devices and Short-Term Mortality From 271 845 Percutaneous Coronary Intervention Procedures Performed in the United Kingdom Between 2006 and 2011: A Propensity Score-Corrected Analysis From the British Cardiovascular Intervention Society". *Circ Cardiovasc Interv*. 2016;9(9):e004321.
25. Rao SV, Kaltenbach LA, Weintraub WS, et al. Prevalence and outcomes of same-day discharge after elective percutaneous coronary intervention among older patients. *JAMA*. 2011;306(13):1461-1467.
26. Nelson PR, Kracjer Z, Kansal N, et al. A multicenter, randomized, controlled trial of totally percutaneous access versus open femoral exposure for endovascular aortic aneurysm repair (the PEVAR trial). *J Vasc Surg*. 2014;59(5):1181-1193.
27. Mach M, Okutucu S, Kerbel T, et al. Vascular complications in TAVR: incidence, clinical impact, and management. *J Clin Med*. 2021;10(21):5046. doi:10.3390/jcm10215046.
28. Robertson L, Andras A, Colgan F, Jackson R. Vascular closure devices for femoral arterial puncture site haemostasis. *Cochrane Database Syst Rev*. 2016;3:Cd009541.
29. Pok J, Lavingia KS, Amendola MF. Close versus seal? MAUDE database analysis of the angio-seal and Perclose ProGlide system. *J Vasc Surg/Society for Vascular Surgery (SVS)*. 2020;72(1):E118-E119. doi:10.1016/j.jvs.2020.04.210
30. Alhusain R, Awadelkarim A, Bishop P, Sattar Y, Lakkis NM, Alraies MC. D-51 Complications and failure methods of the MYNX vascular closure devices: insights from MAUDE database. *Journal of the Society for Cardiovascular Angiography & Interventions (JSCAI)*. 2022;1(3):100256.
31. Al-Thani H, Hussein A, Sadek A, Barah A, El-Menyar A. Balloon-assisted percutaneous thrombin injection for treatment of Iatrogenic left subclavian artery pseudoaneurysm in a critically ill COVID-19 patient. *Case Rep Vasc Med*. 2021;2021:4245484.

Women and Percutaneous Coronary Intervention

Alexandra J. Lansky, Suzanne J. Baron, and J. Dawn Abbott

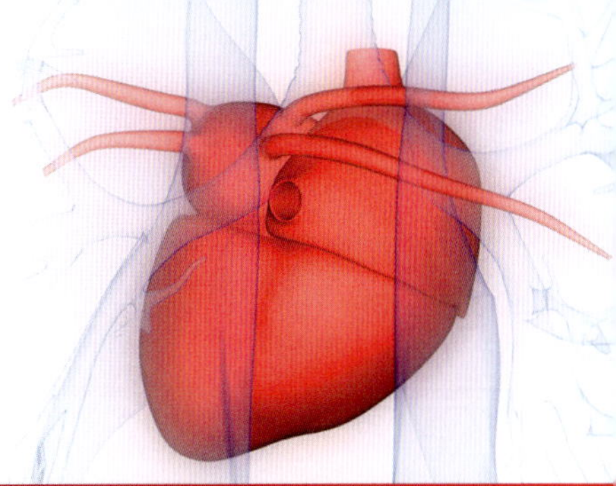

Cardiovascular disease (CVD) is the leading cause of death for women worldwide, with an estimated 8.5 million deaths worldwide[1,2] and 400,000 in the United States annually.[1-3] While mortality rates have declined in the past two decades, delays in the diagnosis and delivery of optimal treatment for women persist, resulting in worse outcomes.[4] Cardiovascular procedures, including cardiac catheterization, percutaneous coronary intervention (PCI), coronary artery bypass grafting (CABG), mechanical circulatory support (MCS), and implantable defibrillators, continue to be underutilized in women compared with men, independent of clinical indication. Underuse of these procedures predicts a higher morality in women.[5,6] This chapter will summarize the available literature on myocardial revascularization in women.

EPIDEMIOLOGY OF ISCHEMIC HEART DISEASE

CVD affects an estimated 422.7 million worldwide and is the cause of death of 17.9 million (47.5% women), with marked regional variation.[2] In the United States, the overall prevalence of CVD is estimated to be 37.4% for men and 35.9% for women older than 20 years of age, and the prevalence increases with age in both sexes.[3] Women older than 60 years have a lower prevalence of coronary artery disease (CAD) and myocardial infarction (MI) compared with age-matched men. In patients younger than 60 years, however, there is a similar and lower prevalence of CAD 6% and 2.5% MI in women and men, contributing to the underdiagnosis and delayed diagnosis in this age group. Women presenting with obstructive CAD are typically older than men, with the most common underlying mechanism of MI caused by atherosclerotic plaque rupture or erosion.[7] While traditional atherosclerotic CVD risk factors, such as diabetes mellitus, hypertension, dyslipidemia, smoking, and obesity, remain critical targets for primary and secondary prevention for both women and men, nontraditional risk factors specific to women also contribute to their risk of CVD. These include preterm delivery,[8] gestational diabetes, breast cancer therapy, autoimmune diseases,[9] hypertensive pregnancy disorders,[10,11] and anxiety and depression.[12,13]

Nonobstructive and/or nonatherosclerotic CAD is increasingly recognized as an underlying etiology of ischemia or MI, particularly younger women (<55 years) as summarized in two recent consensus statements.[14,15] MI with nonobstructive coronary arteries (MINOCA) is up to 5-fold more common in women compared with men.[16] Underlying causes of MINOCA include nonocclusive plaque rupture/erosion, embolism/thrombosis, vasospasm, coronary microvascular dysfunction, spontaneous coronary artery dissection (SCAD), and takotsubo cardiomyopathy and should be suspected when caring for women presenting with MI.[17,18]

Anatomic and Diagnostic Considerations

Women have a smaller heart size and coronary arteries than men. Based on coronary angiography, the average coronary diameter in women is about 0.5 mm smaller.[19] Intravascular ultrasound (IVUS) measures of cross-sectional vessel wall, mean vessel area, and mean lumen area are also smaller in women than in men and translate into comparable plaque burden (plaque area normalized to vessel area) despite lower absolute plaque volume.[20] Despite these anatomical differences, there are no sex-specific recommendations for invasive optical coherence tomography or IVUS guidance of PCI, although some evidence suggest greater utility of intravascular imaging for women in detecting and managing stent edge dissections, which tend to be more common and complex in women.[21]

Invasive Physiology for Ischemia Testing

Fractional flow reserve (FFR) and nonhyperemic pressure ratios, such as instantaneous wave-free ratio (iFR) and resting full-cycle ratio, are commonly used invasive diagnostic tools for the functional assessment of angiographically intermediate coronary lesions and post-PCI outcomes. There are currently no data to support sex-specific cutoffs for invasive functional assessments; however, lesions of similar angiographic severity are less likely to be ischemia producing in women.[22,23] In a subanalysis of the Fractional Flow Reserve Versus Angiography for Multivessel Evaluation (FAME) trial, the proportion of functionally significant lesions (FFR ≤ 0.80) was lower in women than in men for lesions with a 50% to 70% stenosis (21.1% vs 39.5%, $P < .001$) and for lesions with a 70% to 90% stenosis (71.9% vs 82.0%, $P = .019$). Possible explanations include higher rates of microvascular dysfunction in women, smaller areas of compromised myocardial territory, or less accurate stenosis severity estimation in women due to smaller vessels.[24] Another plausible explanation is that the higher resting coronary blood flow observed in women could affect any index that is dependent on resting flow or a net change in flow.[25] This hypothesis is supported by the finding that an FFR-guided strategy based on the clinically validated threshold (≤0.80) is associated with a higher rate of revascularization than an iFR-guided strategy (≤0.89) in men but not in women.[26] Importantly, the clinical benefit of an FFR-versus iFR-guided strategy is similar for both women and men, supporting the use of both FFR and iFR in guiding revascularization, regardless of sex. Studies on diastolic pressure ratio during the diastolic wave-free period (dPR_{WFP}) are discordant between the sexes when compared with FFR, suggesting that optimal thresholds for some physiologic indices may need to be sex based.[27]

Revascularization Versus Optimal Medical Therapy in Chronic Coronary Syndromes

The updated revascularization guidelines emphasize angina relief (class 1) and improved morality and prognosis (recommendation based on anatomic subset) as primary goals of revascularization in chronic coronary syndromes (CCSs).[28] Therefore, when considering medical or PCI treatment options, consideration should be given to women's higher burden and frequency of angina (**Table 31.1**). The Clinical Outcomes Utilizing Revascularization

TABLE 31.1 Sex-Based Substudies of Randomized Clinical Trials in Chronic Coronary Syndromes

TRIAL	FOLLOW-UP	POPULATION	STUDY INTERVENTION	MAIN STUDY FINDINGS	SUMMARY
FAME[23]	2-y	744 men and 261 women with multivessel CAD	Intervention: FFR-guided PCI (384 vs 125) Comparator: Angiography-guided PCI (360 vs 136)	The proportion of functionally significant lesions (FFR ≤ 0.80) was lower in women than in men for lesions with 50% to 70% stenosis (21.1% vs 39.5%, $P < .001$) and for lesions with 70% to 90% stenosis (71.9% vs 82.0%, $P = .019$). Although women were older and had significantly higher rates of hypertension than men, there were no differences in the rates of MACE (20.3% vs 20.2%, $P = .923$) or the individual components of MACE at 2 y, irrespective of treatment strategy	In women, angiographic lesions of similar severity were less likely to be ischemia producing than in men. FFR-guided PCI is equally beneficial in women and men
COURAGE[29]	Median 4.6-y	1949 men and 338 women with single, double, or triple vessel, stable CAD	Intervention: PCI and OMT (979 vs 169) Comparator: OMT (968 vs 169)	There was no difference in treatment effect by sex for the primary endpoint (death or MI; HR 0.89, 95% CI 0.77-1.03 for women and HR 1.02, 95% CI 0.96-1.10 for men; $p_{interaction} = 0.07$). Compared with men, women assigned to PCI had fewer hospitalizations for heart failure compared with OMT alone (HR 0.59; 95% CI 0.40-0.84, $P < .001$ for women and HR 0.86, 95% CI 0.74-1.01, $P = .47$ for men, $p_{interaction} = 0.02$). There was a sex-based differential treatment effect for randomization to PCI despite both sexes experiencing significantly reduced need for subsequent revascularization (HR 0.72; 95% CI 0.62-0.83, $P < .001$ for women; HR 0.84; 95% CI 0.79-0.89, $P < .001$ for men; $p_{interaction} = 0.02$).	There were no significant differences in treatment effect on major outcomes between men and women. Women assigned to PCI demonstrated a greater benefit compared with men, with a reduction in heart failure hospitalization and need for future revascularization
ISCHEMIA[30]	Enrollment data of participants	6256 men and 2262 women with CAD and moderate or severe ischemia	Intervention: Revascularization Comparator: OMT Analysis of combined treatment groups	Women were more likely to have no obstructive CAD (<50% stenosis in all vessels on CCTA; 353 of 1022 [34.4%] vs 378 of 3353 [11.3%]). Women had more angina at baseline than men (median [interquartile range] Seattle Angina Questionnaire Angina Frequency score: 80 [70-100] vs 90 [70-100]). Women had less severe ischemia on stress imaging (383 of 919 [41.7%] vs 1361 of 2972 [45.9%] with severe ischemia; 386 of 919 [42.0%] vs 1215 of 2972 [40.9%] with moderate ischemia; and 150 of 919 [16.4%] vs 394 of 2972 [13.3%] with mild or no ischemia). Female sex was independently associated with greater angina frequency (OR 1.41, 95% CI 1.13-1.76)	Women in the ISCHEMIA trial had more frequent angina, independent of having less extensive CAD, and less severe ischemia than men
EXCEL[31]	3-y	1464 men and 441 women with unprotected left main disease	Intervention: PCI (722 vs 226) Comparator: CABG (742 vs 215)	In multivariable analysis, sex was not independently associated with either the primary endpoint (HR 1.10; 95% CI 0.82-1.48, $P = .53$) or all-cause death (HR 1.39, 95% CI 0.92-2.10, $P = .12$) at 3 y. Women had a lower SYNTAX score at baseline vs men. (mean SYNTAX score 24.2 vs 27.2, $P < .001$). The 3-y rate of the composite primary endpoint in women was 19.7% with PCI vs 14.6% with CABG, and in men 13.8% with PCI vs 14.7% with CABG ($p_{interaction} = 0.06$).	In patients with unprotected left main disease in the EXCEL trial, sex was not an independent predictor of adverse outcome after revascularization. Women undergoing PCI had a trend for worse outcomes, related to associated comorbidities and increased periprocedural complications

TABLE 31.1 Sex-Based Substudies of Randomized Clinical Trials in Chronic Coronary Syndromes (*Continued*)

TRIAL	FOLLOW-UP	POPULATION	STUDY INTERVENTION	MAIN STUDY FINDINGS	SUMMARY
SYNTAX, PRECOMBAT, and BEST patient-level analysis[32]	Median 1806 d	2486 men and 794 women with MVD and unprotected LMD	Intervention: PCI (1222 vs 419) Comparator: CABG (1264 vs 375)	In SYNTAX, female sex favored CABG compared with PCI (HR for PCI: 2.213; 95% CI 1.242-3.943, *P* = .007). In trials performed in Asia (PRECOMBAT and BEST), the treatment effect was neutral between both strategies. Sex interaction with treatment strategy was evident in the SYNTAX (Western) trial ($p_{interaction}$ = 0.019) but not in the Asian trials (PRECOMBAT, $p_{interaction}$ = 0.469; BEST, $p_{interaction}$ = 0.472; I^2 = 58%)	This meta-analysis suggests the presence of heterogeneous sex–treatment interaction across Asian and Western trials
CARDia[33]	1-y	378 men and 132 women with diabetes and MVD or complex single-vessel disease	Intervention: CABG (197 M vs 57 F) Comparator: PCI (181 M vs 75 F)	There was no interaction between sex and combined outcome of death, MI, or stroke at 1 y (HR 2.13, 95% CI 0.68-6.68 for women; HR 1.07, 95% CI 0.59-1.93 for men, $p_{interaction}$ = 0.289). There was no interaction between sex and combined outcome of death, MI, stroke, or repeat revascularization (HR 2.4, 95% CI 0.87-6.61 for women; HR 1.62, 95% CI 0.95-2.74 for men, $p_{interaction}$ = 0.489)	There was no sex-based benefit for PCI or CABG on 1-y outcomes studied
BARI-2D[34]	5-y	759 men and 318 women with type 2 diabetes mellitus and stable coronary artery disease	PCI and CABG stratum with each stratum randomized to revascularization vs medical therapy and then insulin provision vs insulin sensitization	Women were more likely than men to have angina (67% vs 58%, *P* < .01) despite less disease on angiography (Myocardial Jeopardy Index 41 ± 24 vs 46 ± 24, *P* < .01; number of significant lesions 2.3 ± 1.7 vs 2.8 ± 1.8, *P* < .01). Over 5 y, no sex differences were observed in death/MI/cerebrovascular accident: HR 1.11, 99% CI 0.85-1.44) after adjustment for baseline variables. Women reported more angina than men (adjusted OR 1.51, 99% CI 1.21-1.89, *P* < .0001) and had lower scores for the Duke Activity Status Index (adjusted beta coefficient: −1.58, 99% CI: −2.84 to −0.32, *P* < .01)	There were no sex differences in outcomes in the BARI-2D trial. After 5 y of medical therapy with or without prompt revascularization, women had persistently higher angina rates and lower Duke Activity Status Index scores despite less anatomic disease at baseline
FREEDOM[35]	5-y	1356 men and 544 women with diabetes and multivessel CAD	Intervention: PCI (698 vs 255) Comparator: CABG (658 vs 289)	There was no interaction between sex and 5-y composite event rates for death, MI, or stroke (PCI vs CABG, 27% vs 18% for men and 26% vs 21% for women, $p_{interaction}$ = 0.46)	There was no sex-based benefit for PCI or CABG on 5-y outcomes studied

CABG, coronary artery bypass grafting; CAD, coronary artery disease; CCTA, coronary computed tomographic angiography; CI, confidence interval; FFR, fractional flow reserve; HR, hazard ratio; LMD, left main disease; MACE, major adverse cardiac event; MI, myocardial infarction; MVD, multivessel disease; OMT, optimal medical therapy; OR, odds ratio; PCI, percutaneous coronary intervention.

and Aggressive druG Evaluation (COURAGE) trial showed that PCI was more likely to result in lower rates of hospitalization for heart failure and repeat revascularization in women compared with men.[29] Recent meta-analyses of randomized trials evaluating routine revascularization with medical therapy compared with medical therapy alone in CCS have demonstrated that randomization to elective revascularization led to reduced cardiac mortality compared with medical therapy alone and lower rates of spontaneous MI.[36,37] The ISCHEMIA trial demonstrated that an invasive strategy reduced spontaneous MI, an independent predictor of mortality in the trial.[38] Whether sex-specific treatment differences will emerge from the recent ISCHEMIA trial is unknown, but results may provide needed insight into sex-specific options for treatment and diagnosis.[30]

PCI Versus CABG in Stable Chronic Multivessel CAD and Left Main Disease

CABG to improve survival is the guideline-recommended standard of care for patients with left main disease (LMD) (class I) and multivessel disease (MVD) with reduced left ventricular ejection fraction (LVEF < 35%) (class I).[28] PCI to improve survival carries a lower recommendation and has a class 2a for LMD and 2b for MVD and preserved LVEF. Women with MVD or LMD may benefit more from CABG than PCI compared with men (**Table 31.1**). Despite a lower anatomic burden of MVD, women in the SYNTAX trial had higher mortality rates with PCI compared with CABG at 5 years,[32] and similar trends were seen in women with LMD in the Evaluation of XIENCE Versus Coronary Artery Bypass Surgery for Effectiveness of Left Main Revascularization (EXCEL) trial.[31] These results are consistent with a recently published meta-analysis of 1909 women from six randomized trials, demonstrating that women with MVD and/or LMD had a 30% reduction in the composite of death, MI, or stroke 1 to 5 years after treatment with CABG compared with PCI.[39] This difference in outcomes for women is reflected in the SYNTAX II score, which adjusts female sex by a factor of 1.6 for PCI such that for any given set of criteria the SYNTAX II score will predict a higher 4-year mortality in women for PCI compared with CABG.[40] With significant underrepresentation of women, these trials and significant limitations of the original SYNTAX trial (<12% women and first-generation DES), contemporary studies are needed to evaluate the effects of sex on outcomes after CABG versus PCI for MVD or LMD and to determine whether sex-specific thresholds for judging anatomic complexity are needed.

REVASCULARIZATION FOR NON-ST-ELEVATION MI

An early invasive approach in patients with non-ST-elevation myocardial infarction (NSTEMI) improves outcomes and reduces mortality, particularly in high-risk patients.[41-44] Nevertheless, PCI is performed less often in younger (<55 years) women compared with men, contributing to a 50% higher risk of in-hospital and long-term mortality in women after an NSTEMI.[45-47] The introduction of high-sensitivity troponin assays with sex-specific thresholds has improved the diagnosis of NSTEMI (increase in acute MI detection by 11.5% in women and 9.8% in men compared with standard troponin assays) and the identification of high-risk patients in both sexes[48] and may improve some of the sex disparities observed in NSTEMI outcomes.

REVASCULARIZATION FOR ST-ELEVATION MI

Approximately 23% to 40% of patients presenting with ST-elevation myocardial infarction (STEMI) are women.[49-56] Female sex has been associated with delays in symptom onset to hospital presentation[49-52] and delays to intervention for STEMI,[50,51,53,54] which have been attributed, in part, to atypical symptoms in women.[57] Furthermore, women are significantly less likely to receive invasive therapies in STEMI, due in part to more comorbidities and frailty on admission and less obstructive CAD on angiography.[58,59] Together, these delays and disparities in care have contributed to worse in-hospital mortality in women presenting with STEMI, particularly in younger women although the gap in risk-adjusted mortality rates has narrowed over time especially with the adoption of primary angioplasty.[50,52,53,55,60-70] Once treatment has been initiated, rates of procedural success, postprocedural epicardial flow, myocardial perfusion, and ST-segment resolution are similar in both sexes after primary PCI.[54,71]

Revascularization for Women With STEMI

Primary PCI is the standard of care for all STEMI patients, and thrombolytic therapy should only be considered when primary PCI is not available. Women with STEMI are less likely to receive pharmacologic reperfusion therapy compared with men,[6,53,55,72,73] mainly due to delayed hospital presentation, older age, and the risk of bleeding.[72] While the treatment effect for thrombolysis is similar between women and men, women have a worse mortality and morbidity after thrombolytic therapy, due to advanced age, more comorbidities, and a higher risk of intracranial bleeding.[50,52,54,71,74-83]

The Complete versus Culprit-Only Revascularization Strategies to Treat Multivessel Disease after Early PCI for STEMI (COMPLETE) trial supports a strategy of complete revascularization and treatment of the nonculprit lesions at the time of primary PCI for STEMI or as a staged procedure[84]; however, subgroup analyses suggest less benefit of complete revascularization for women a trend (*P*-value for interaction = 0.08). Furthermore, sex-specific data are lacking regarding the differential effects of FFR guidance in nonculprit lesions in the setting of STEMI from the DANish Study of Optimal Acute Treatment of Patients With STEMI-3 (DANAMI-3) and COMPARE-ACUTE trials.[85,86]

Revascularization in Women With STEMI and Cardiogenic Shock

Cardiogenic shock and right ventricular infarction are more common in women with STEMI than in men (**Table 31.2**). Women also have lower blood pressures and lower cardiac outputs[87,92] compared with men in the setting of cardiogenic shock, although no clear sex-specific pattern in change in LV dysfunction has been identified.[79,81,95] Subanalyses of several trials, including the SHOCK trial and the CULPRIT-SHOCK trials, have failed to show a sex-specific benefit for intra-aortic balloon pump use or early multivessel revascularization in this setting.[87,92,96] Although randomized data on the use of MCS are lacking, one registry (*N* = 180) reported that women with cardiogenic shock (*n* = 49) had similar improvement in hemodynamics and derived greater clinical benefit than men with early initiation of MCS.[97] Nevertheless, studies continue to show that women presenting with acute MI and shock are less likely to receive MCS devices.[98-102]

Revascularization for Nonatherosclerotic Causes of STEMI

SCAD is a nonatherosclerotic and nontraumatic etiology of MI resulting from coronary obstruction by luminal compression caused by either a dissection flap or an extension of an intramural hematoma.[103] Although comprising less than 1% of all acute MIs, approximately 90% of patients with SCAD are women between 47 and 53 years of age[104] and accounts for 25% to 33% of MIs in women younger than 50 years and is the most common cause of pregnancy-associated MI (43%).[104] Approximately 15% of SCAD cases are pregnancy related, typically occurring in the postpartum period, suggesting hormonal shifts is a possible underlying mechanism with other possible triggers such as emotional and physical stress.[103] Fibromuscular dysplasia is commonly associated with SCAD, suggesting some aspect of vascular pathology or dysfunction in the etiology of SCAD.

Revascularization in the setting of SCAD is associated with increased complications, including a higher risk of dissection, abrupt vessel closure, and hematoma propagation. As a result, revascularization should be deferred when possible in patients with preserved coronary flow, minimal ischemia, and distal coronary

TABLE 31.2 Sex-Based Substudies of Randomized Clinical Trials and Registries in AMI Complicated by Cardiogenic Shock

STUDY	STUDY PERIOD	STUDY TYPE	STUDY POPULATION	N	% WOMEN	% PCI (WOMEN VS MEN)	% OTHER REVASCULARIZATION/ REPERFUSION (WOMEN VS MEN)	% MORTALITY (UNADJUSTED) (WOMEN VS MEN)
SHOCK[87]	1993-1997	Registry	Hospitalized with AMI with CS and LV failure	884	36%	Coronary angiogram: 62% both PCI: 35% vs 31%, p = NS	Lytics: 32% vs 36%, p = NS CABG:12% vs 17%, $P = .04$	Revascularized: 44% vs 38%, p = NS Not revascularized: 79% vs 78%, p = NS
Antoniucci et al[88]	1995-2001	Retrospective observational	Hospitalized with AMI with CS undergoing pPCI	208	31%	100%		6 mo: 42% vs 31%, p = NS
MITRA PLUS (2009)[89]	1992-2002	Registry	STEMI <24 h with CS	3857	41%		Early reperfusion: 50% vs 63%, $P < .0001$	68% vs 57%, $P < .0001$
Ontario MI Database (2013)[90]	1992-2008	Retrospective observational	Hospitalized with AMI with CS	9750	45%	11% vs 14%, $P < .001$	CABG: 2% vs 4%, $P < .001$	1 y: 80% vs 75%, $P < .001$
Kunadian et al (2013)[91]	2008-2011	Retrospective observational	Hospitalized with AMI with CS undergoing pPCI	141	43%	100%		35% vs 36%, p = NS
IABP-SHOCK II (2015)[92]	2009-2012	RCT	Hospitalized with AMI with CS undergoing early revascularization; randomized to IABP vs no IABP	600	31%	94% vs 97%, p = NS	CABG: 1.6% vs 0.7%, p = NS	Postprocedure: 18% vs 9%, $P = .004$ 30 d: 44% vs 39%, p = NS 6 mo: 54% vs 47%, p = NS 1 y: 57% vs 50%, p = NS
Nationwide Readmission Database (2018)[93]	2013-2014	Retrospective observational	Discharged posthospital-ization for AMI with CS	39,807	33%	57% vs 61%, $P < .01$	CABG: 31% vs 36%, $P < .01$	Sex-specific mortality not reported
FAST-MI (2018)[94]	1995, 2000, 2005, 2010	4 Registries	Hospitalized with AMI with CS	614	41%	PCI 1995: 15% vs 24% 2000: 28% vs 47% 2005: 36% vs 57% 2010: 69% vs 77% $P < .001$ for trend for both sexes	Lytics 1995: 19% vs 34% 2000: 20% vs 18% 2005: 18% vs 34% 2010: 2% vs10% P = NS for women $P = .02$ for men	30 d (1995): 77% vs 64% 30d (2010): 43% vs 35% 1y (1995): 81% vs 70% 1y (2010): 54% vs 48%

AMI, acute myocardial infarction; CABG, coronary artery bypass grafting; CS, cardiogenic shock; IABP, intra-aortic balloon pump; LV, left ventricular; NS, nonsignificant; PCI, percutaneous coronary intervention; pPCI, primary percutaneous coronary intervention; RCT, randomized controlled trial.

involvement,[103] particularly since spontaneous healing of the vessel has been shown to occur in 95% of patients after 30 days.[105] In the absence of high-risk clinical features (eg, left main and/or proximal LAD involvement, progression to occlusion after initial conservative therapy, unstable cardiac rhythm and/or hemodynamics), most patients can be managed with conservative therapy. While LV systolic dysfunction with SCAD should be treated with guideline-based heart failure medications, including beta-blockers, angiotensin receptor/neprilysin inhibitors, mineralocorticoid receptor antagonists, and sodium-glucose co-transporter 2 inhibitors,[106,107] the benefit of these agents in the setting of preserved LV function remains unclear, with the exception of beta-blockers, which may reduce recurrence of SCAD.[108] Scarce data exist regarding the benefit (or harm) of anticoagulants, antiplatelets, and statins in the setting of SCAD. Expert consensus recommends limiting anticoagulation to only those undergoing PCI.[106] Dual antiplatelet therapy (DAPT) is recommended during the acute phase of SCAD; however, the optimal duration of and aspirin monotherapy remains unclear.[106] Current consensus recommend that SCAD patients remain in hospital for 3 to 5 days due to a 5% to 10% in-hospital recurrence of MI or unplanned revascularization due to propagation of the dissection.[104]

Revascularization for Ischemic Cardiomyopathy

CABG improved survival in ischemic cardiomyopathy patients with LV dysfunction in trials conducted predominantly in men (>80%).[109,110] With advanced age and comorbidities, women undergoing cardiac surgery have a higher long-term mortality compared with men,[111] and the risk-benefit ratio of CABG is not well defined for women with ischemic cardiomyopathy. Less invasive revascularization strategies in this patient population have not been evaluated but may offer an advantage for women.

Revascularization in the Patient With Diabetes

Diabetes is more prevalent and a stronger risk factor for CAD in women than in men and is associated with worse outcomes after revascularization.[112] Randomized trials have demonstrated a benefit of CABG over PCI in diabetic patients with obstructive MVD.[35,113,114] While subgroup analyses have shown no treatment interaction by sex, women (25%) are under-represented in these studies.

Revascularization in the Setting of Chronic Kidney Disease

Chronic kidney disease (CKD) is more common in women than in men.[115] In the ISCHEMIA-CKD trial in patients with CCS, moderate-to-severe ischemia, and advanced CKD, an initial invasive strategy was not associated with a reduction in death or nonfatal MI compared with an initial conservative approach; however, no subgroup analysis reported based on sex.[116] Further studies are needed to identify the optimal revascularization strategy in women with CKD.

DEVICE CONSIDERATIONS DURING PERCUTANEOUS REVASCULARIZATION IN WOMEN

Drug-Eluting Stents

Drug-eluting stents (DESs) are well studied in women demonstrating similar outcomes between women and men. A patient-level pooled analysis of 26 randomized DES trials that included 43,904 patients and 11,557 women (26.3%) clearly demonstrated that DES, both first and newer generation, are associated with approximately 60% lower rates of target lesion revascularization compared with BMS in women and that the outcomes of death, MI, and stent thrombosis in women have improved with newer generation DES.[117]

Atherectomy Devices

There are three Food and Drug Administration-approved atherectomy devices: orbital atherectomy, rotational atherectomy (RA), and laser atherectomy. Retrospective analyses of trial data evaluating RA have demonstrated that women are at increased risk of procedural complications and major adverse cardiac events (MACEs) compared with men.[118] In a propensity matched series of 765 consecutive patients (37% women) undergoing RA followed for a median of 4.7 years, the primary endpoint of net adverse cardiac events (net adverse clinical events: all-cause death, MI, stroke, and target vessel revascularization plus any procedural complication) occurred more often in women (15.1 vs 9.0%; adjusted odds ratio [OR] 1.81, 95% confidence interval [CI] 1.04-3.13, $P = .037$). Women were at increased risk of procedural complications and were more likely to experience coronary dissection (4.6 vs 1.3%; $P = .008$), cardiac tamponade (2.1 vs 0.4%; $P = .046$), and significant bleeding (Bleeding Academic Research Consortium ≥2: 5.3 vs 2.3%; $P = .028$). Procedural complications during RA were associated with almost double the incidence of MACE at long-term follow-up (hazard ratio 1.92; 95% CI 1.34-2.77, $P < .001$). When RA was compared with modified balloon angioplasty for the treatment of severely calcified lesions, there was a significant interaction by sex, suggesting that RA may be beneficial in men but not women, although it is important to note that only 23 women were included in this study.[119] With insufficient data available to reliably determine the safety of atherectomy devices in women, and no data available on laser atherectomy in women, current limited evidence suggests that caution is needed when using atheroablative therapies in women.

Intravascular Lithotripsy

Intravascular lithotripsy (IVL) emits sonic pressure waves from an angioplasty balloon to fracture circumferential coronary calcium. The safety and effectiveness of IVL was evaluated in three single-arm studies, DISRUPT CAD I, II, and III, which enrolled a total of 631 patients.[120-122] In a patient-level pooled analysis of 628 patients (23% women), women had similar extent and severity of calcium compared with men. Despite women having more comorbidities and smaller vessel size (2.7 ± 0.4 mm vs 3.0 ± 0.5 mm, $P < .001$), there were no differences in the primary safety endpoint of 30-day MACE (8.3% vs 7.1%, $P = .61$) or the primary effectiveness endpoint defined as stent delivery with a residual in-stent stenosis ≤30% without in-hospital MACE (91.7% vs 92.6%, $P = .72$) between women and men. Importantly, IVL-related serious angiographic complications (flow-limiting dissection, perforation, abrupt closure, slow flow, and no reflow) were uncommon and similar for women and men (1.6% vs 2.3%, $P = .75$). The ongoing EMPOWER CAD trial will enroll 500 women with severely calcified lesions and will evaluate the acute and 3-year outcomes of an IVL first approach (ClinicalTrials.gov Identifier: NCT05755711).

LESION CONSIDERATIONS DURING PERCUTANEOUS REVASCULARIZATION IN WOMEN

Chronic Total Occlusions

Percutaneous revascularization of chronic total occlusions (CTOs) is complex and while women comprise less than 20% of trial participants, complications after CTO intervention, including coronary perforation, bleeding, and contrast-induced nephropathy, are observed more commonly in women.[123] A registry of 2002 patients (17% women) suggested that CTO procedural success and mortality reduction was similar in women and men.[124] A meta-analysis of 9 studies including 30,830 CTO patients treated with PCI found that female sex was not an independent risk factor for MACE or PCI success rate.[125] Overall, these nonrandomized studies suggest that female sex should not be a factor in withholding CTO PCI.

VASCULAR ACCESS IN WOMEN

Radial access is recommended in women to reduce bleeding and vascular complications including retroperitoneal hemorrhage (**Table 31.3**).[126-130] The MATRIX Access trial randomized 8404 patients (26.6% women) to femoral versus radial access for PCI.[126] Women had higher bleeding risk compared with men in this trial; however, the benefit of radial access was relatively greater in women for the primary endpoint of MACCE (composite of death, MI, or stroke; relative risk [RR] 0.73; *P* = .019) and net adverse events (composite of MACCE or major bleeding; RR 0.73, *P* = .012).[126] In contrast, the Safety and Efficacy of Femoral Access versus Radial Access in ST-Segment Elevation Myocardial Infarction (SAFARI) trial (*N* = 2292), which evaluated radial versus femoral access in the setting of STEMI, did not demonstrate a significant difference in the primary endpoint of all-cause mortality in either women or men.[131] Nevertheless, a meta-analysis of randomized controlled trials (RCTs) including the STEMI-RADIAL trial demonstrated that a radial approach was associated with decreased non-CABG-related bleeding (OR 0.56, 95% CI 0.44-0.72), vascular complications (OR 0.49, 95% CI 0.32-0.75), and MACCE (OR 0.73, 95% CI 0.58-0.93) in women,[129,132] suggesting that the radial artery should be the preferred access site for women to reduce procedural-related complications. Since women may be more prone to radial artery tortuosity or spasm (which could lead to unsuccessful radial access), administration of vasodilators and anxiolytics as well as procedural techniques to navigate the forearm vascular anatomy should be employed liberally.

Vascular complications with femoral vascular closure devices (VCDs) in women are inconsistent across studies.[133,134] The Instrumental Sealing of Arterial Puncture Site-CLOSURE Device versus Manual Compression (ISAR-CLOSURE) trial reported similar rates of vascular access-site complications in women receiving a VCD compared with those receiving manual compression (8.6% vs 9.8%; *P* = .451),[133] whereas other studies have reported reduced or even higher vascular complications with VCD in women.[135-137] As such, the optimal manner of achieving hemostasis at the access site in women undergoing transfemoral cardiac catheterization is not defined.

Antithrombotic Agents for the Treatment of Acute Coronary Syndromes

Antithrombotic therapy is the cornerstone of treatment in patients undergoing coronary revascularization, and women are undertreated with guideline-recommended therapies.[138,139] Although sex-specific differences in the pharmacokinetic (PK) profiles of antithrombotic drugs may cause variability in pharmacodynamic responses between women and men and may have a role in modulating bleeding risk, RCTs evaluating antithrombotic medications indicate that both women and men have similar therapeutic benefits.[140-142]

DAPT with aspirin and a P2Y12 inhibitor (clopidogrel, prasugrel, and ticagrelor) is the standard of care for preventing thrombotic events after PCI (**Table 31.4**). Although reduction in ischemic events has been shown to be greater in men with all oral $P2Y_{12}$ inhibitors, most studies have shown no significant interactions between specific P2Y12 inhibitor treatment and sex,[143] and sex has not been shown to be an independent predictor of bleeding complications with the use of specific agents.[144]

The minimum required duration of use for an oral $P2Y_{12}$ receptor inhibitor varies according to the clinical setting.[138] Prolongation of DAPT beyond this time frame reduces ischemic events and increases bleeding, and hence, this strategy is reserved for patients who remain at increased risk for ischemic recurrences but who are at low risk for bleeding.[138,145] Real-world registries have consistently shown increased bleeding among women with all $P2Y_{12}$ inhibitors[146,147] and may be attributed to factors modulating the

TABLE 31.3 Randomized Controlled Trials Comparing Sex-Specific Outcomes of Radial Versus Femoral Access

STUDY	POPULATION	N	% WOMEN	CLINICAL OUTCOMES: WOMEN: RADIAL VS FEMORAL AND MEN: RADIAL VS FEMORAL
MATRIX[126]	Patients with ACS undergoing cardiac catheterization	8402	27%	Mortality: Women: 2.4% vs 3.5%; Men: 1.3% vs 1.7%, p = NS all Any bleeding: Women: 10.7% vs 16.5%; Men: 7.6% vs 13.9%, *P* < .0001 all TIMI major bleed: Women: 0.7% vs 1.6%, *P* = .043; Men 0.6% vs 0.6%, p = NS
RIVAL[127]	Substudy of ACS patients undergoing cardiac catheterization	7021	27%	Primary outcome (death/MI/stroke/non-CABG bleeding): Women: 3.9% vs 5.0%, p = NS; Men: 3.5% vs 3.5%, p = NS ACUITY non-CABG bleed: Women: 3.7% vs 7.0%, *P* = .001; Men: 1.2% vs 3.3%, *P* < .0001 Major vascular complications: Women 3.1% vs 6.1%, *P* = .002; Men: 0.7% vs 2.8%, *P* < .0001
SAFE-PCI[128]	Women undergoing cardiac catheterization or elective PCI	1787	100%	BARC type 2,3, or 5 bleeding or vascular complications: 0.6% vs 1.7%, *P* = .03

ACS, acute coronary syndrome; BARC, Bleeding Academic Research Consortium; CABG, coronary artery bypass grafting; MI, myocardial infarction; NS, nonsignificant; PCI, percutaneous coronary intervention; TIMI, thrombolysis in myocardial infarction.

TABLE 31.4 Sex Differences in Clinical Trials of Adenosine Diphosphate $P2Y_{12}$ Inhibitors

DRUG	STUDY NAME, YEAR	POPULATION STUDIED	N	FEMALE (%)	OUTCOME	RESULTS				
						WOMEN		MEN		INTERACTION
						STUDY (%)	CONTROL (%)	STUDY (%)	CONTROL (%)	P VALUE
Clopidogrel	CURE, 2001	ACS	12,562	39	Efficacy	9.5	10.7	9.1	11.9	-
					Safety	4.0	2.4	3.5	2.9	-
	CREDO, 2003	PCI	2116	29	Efficacy	7.8	11.1	7.8	10.6	-
					Safety	9.1	6.1	8.7	6.9	-
	CLARITY, 2005	STEMI	3491	20	Efficacy	12.5	14.8	8.3	9.9	-
					Safety	3.1	3.3	1.6	1.4	-
	COMMIT, 2005	STEMI	45,852	28	Efficacy	13.3	14.0	7.7	8.6	-
					Safety	0.4	0.3	0.3	0.3	-
	CHARISMA, 2006	Secondary prevention	15,603	30	Efficacy	6.5	6.4	7.0	7.7	-
					Safety	1.5	1.3	1.7	1.4	-
	CURRENT, 2010	ACS	27,087	27	Efficacy	4.5	5.4	4.1	4.1	0.17
					Safety	-	-	-	-	-
	DAPT, 2014	PCI	9961	25	Efficacy	4.6	5.2	4.2	5.9	0.26
					Safety	2.6	1.8	2.3	1.3	0.50
Prasugrel	TRITON, 2007	ACS	13,608	26	Efficacy	11	12.6	9.5	11.9	>0.05
					Safety	-	-	-	-	-
	TRILOGY-ACS, 2012	ACS	9326	39	Efficacy	HR 1.00 [0.84-1.15]		HR 0.94 [0.81-1.08]		0.56
					Safety	HR 1.34 [0.77-2.33]		HR 1.26 [0.89-1.8]		0.51
	ACCOAST, 2013	ACS	4033	28	Efficacy	9.24	8.24	10.24	10.36	0.54
					Safety	3.8	1.08	2.09	1.46	0.09
	ISAR REACT 5, 2019	ACS	4018	24	Efficacy	8.3	8.9	6.5	9.4	-
					Safety	-	-	-	-	-
Ticagrelor	PLATO, 2009	ACS	18,624	28	Efficacy	11.2	13.2	9.4	11.1	0.78
					Safety	6.1	5.2	3.8	3.3	0.42
	ATLANTIC, 2014	STEMI	1862	20	Efficacy	7.5	6.1	3.8	4.0	0.87
					Safety	1.7	3.6	1.2	0.7	0.28

	PEGASUS, 2015	Secondary prevention	21,162	24	Efficacy	7.2	8.3	6.9	8.1	-
					Safety	1.5	0.7	1.8	0.8	-
	TREAT 2018	STEMI	3779	46	Efficacy	10.6	9.8	5.6	6.5	0.38
					Safety	-	-	-	-	-
	GLOBAL LEADERS, 2018	PCI	15,968	23	Efficacy	-	-	-	-	-
					Safety	-	-	-	-	-
	TWILIGHT, 2019	High-risk PCI	7119	24	Efficacy	3.5	3.5	4.0	4.1	0.97
					Safety	5.0	8.6	3.7	6,7	0.89
	THEMIS, 2019	Stable CAD/ diabetes	19,220	31	Efficacy	7.6	8.0	7.7	8.8	0.43
					Safety	1.7	0.4	2.3	1.3	**0.01**
Cangrelor	CHAMPION PHEONIX, 2013	PCI	11,145	28	Efficacy	4.75	6.9	4.68	5.51	0.23
					Safety	0.3	0.2	0.1	0.1	0.88

ACS, acute coronary syndrome; CAD, coronary artery disease; DAPT, dual antiplatelet therapy; HR, hazard ratio; PCI, percutaneous coronary intervention; STEMI, ST-elevation myocardial infarction.

PK effects of a drug such as a smaller volume of distribution, a lower glomerular filtration rate (by 10%-25%), and differential activity of hepatic enzymes.[140-142] Strategies to reduce bleeding complications include shortening DAPT duration, discontinuation of aspirin therapy and maintaining $P2Y_{12}$ inhibitor monotherapy after a brief period of DAPT, and de-escalation of $P2Y_{12}$ inhibiting therapy (ie, from prasugrel or ticagrelor to clopidogrel).[138,148-150] Discontinuation of aspirin therapy after the peri-PCI period (eg, time of discharge up to 1 week) has also emerged as a strategy to reduce the risk of bleeding among patients with atrial fibrillation requiring oral anticoagulation undergoing PCI.[151] Sex-based analyses of ongoing studies adopting such bleeding reduction strategies will provide important insights toward optimizing the choice and duration of antiplatelet therapy in women.

CONCLUSIONS

In many clinical situations, the level of evidence supporting clinical decisions in women is poor due to insufficient data. Continued efforts to evaluate sex-specific outcomes will continue to guide practice and additional investigations in women.

References

1. Sharma S, Wood MJ. The global burden of cardiovascular disease in women. *Curr Treat Options Cardiovasc Med*. 2018;20(10):81.
2. Roth GA, Johnson C, Abajobir A, et al. Global, regional, and national burden of cardiovascular diseases for 10 causes, 1990 to 2015. *J Am Coll Cardiol*. 2017;70:1-25.
3. Benjamin EJ, Virani SS, Callaway CW, et al. Heart disease and stroke statistics-2018 update: a report from the American Heart Association. *Circulation*. 2018;137(12):e67-e492.
4. Shiels MS, Chernyavskiy P, Anderson WF, et al. Trends in premature mortality in the USA by sex, race, and ethnicity from 1999 to 2014: an analysis of death certificate data. *Lancet*. 2017;389(10073):1043-1054.
5. Anand SS, Xie CC, Mehta S, et al. Differences in the management and prognosis of women and men who suffer from acute coronary syndromes. *J Am Coll Cardiol*. 2005;46(10):1845-1851.
6. Khera S, Kolte D, Gupta T, et al. Temporal trends and sex differences in revascularization and outcomes of ST-segment elevation myocardial infarction in younger adults in the United States. *J Am Coll Cardiol*. 2015;66(18):1961-1972.
7. Falk E, Nakano M, Bentzon JF, Finn AV, Virmani R. Update on acute coronary syndromes: the pathologists' view. *Eur Heart J*. 2013;34(10):719-728.
8. Kessous R, Shoham-Vardi I, Pariente G, Holcberg G, Sheiner E. An association between preterm delivery and long-term maternal cardiovascular morbidity. *Am J Obstet Gynecol*. 2013;209(4):368.e1-368.e3688.
9. Gianturco L, Bodini BD, Atzeni F, et al. Cardiovascular and autoimmune diseases in females: the role of microvasculature and dysfunctional endothelium. *Atherosclerosis*. 2015;241(1):259-263.
10. Bellamy L, Casas JP, Hingorani AD, Williams DJ. Pre-eclampsia and risk of cardiovascular disease and cancer in later life: systematic review and meta-analysis. *BMJ*. 2007;335(7627):974.
11. Bellamy L, Casas JP, Hingorani AD, Williams D. Type 2 diabetes mellitus after gestational diabetes: a systematic review and meta-analysis. *Lancet*. 2009;373(9677):1773-1779.
12. Elamragy AA, Abdelhalim AA, Arafa ME, Baghdady YM. Anxiety and depression relationship with coronary slow flow. *PLoS One*. 2019;14(9):e0221918.
13. Song X, Song J, Shao M, et al. Depression predicts the risk of adverse events after percutaneous coronary intervention: a meta-analysis. *J Affect Disord*. 2020;266:158-164.
14. Tamis-Holland JE, Jneid H, Reynolds HR, et al. Contemporary diagnosis and management of patients with myocardial infarction in the absence of obstructive coronary artery disease: a scientific statement from the American Heart Association. *Circulation*. 2019;139(18):e891-e908.
15. Kunadian V, Chieffo A, Camici PG, et al. An EAPCI expert consensus document on ischaemia with non-obstructive coronary arteries in collaboration with European Society of Cardiology Working group on coronary pathophysiology & microcirculation endorsed by coronary vasomotor disorders International study Group. *Eur Heart J*. 2020;41(37):3504-3520.
16. Safdar B, Spatz ES, Dreyer RP, et al. Presentation, clinical profile, and prognosis of young patients with Myocardial Infarction with Nonobstructive Coronary Arteries (MINOCA): results from the VIRGO study. *J Am Heart Assoc*. 2018;7(13):e009174.
17. Saw J, Aymong E, Mancini GB, Sedlak T, Starovoytov A, Ricci D. Nonatherosclerotic coronary artery disease in young women. *Can J Cardiol*. 2014;30(7):814-819.
18. Saw J, Aymong E, Starovoytov A, et al. Prospective Registry of Young women with MI: evaluating the prevalence and long-term impact of non-atherosclerotic CAD (PRYME). *J Am Coll Cardiol*. 2019;73:1033.
19. Yang F, Minutello RM, Bhagan S, Sharma A, Wong SC. The impact of gender on vessel size in patients with angiographically normal coronary arteries. *J Interv Cardiol*. 2006;19(4):340-344.
20. Lansky AJ, Ng VG, Maehara A, et al. Gender and the extent of coronary atherosclerosis, plaque composition, and clinical outcomes in acute coronary syndromes. *JACC Cardiovasc Imaging*. 2012;5(3 suppl):S62-S72.
21. Zeglin-Sawczuk M, Jang IK, Kato K, et al. Lipid rich plaque, female gender and proximal coronary stent edge dissections. *J Thromb Thrombolysis*. 2013;36(4):507-513.
22. Kim CH, Koo BK, Lee JM, et al. Influence of sex on relationship between total anatomical and physiologic disease burdens and their prognostic implications in patients with coronary artery disease. *J Am Heart Assoc*. 2019;8(5):e011002.
23. Kim HS, Tonino PA, De Bruyne B, et al. The impact of sex differences on fractional flow reserve-guided percutaneous coronary intervention: a FAME (Fractional Flow Reserve versus Angiography for Multivessel Evaluation) substudy. *JACC Cardiovasc Interv*. 2012;5(10):1037-1042.
24. Kang SJ, Ahn JM, Han S, et al. Sex differences in the visual-functional mismatch between coronary angiography or intravascular ultrasound versus fractional flow reserve. *JACC Cardiovasc Interv*. 2013;6:562-568.
25. Kobayashi Y, Fearon WF, Honda Y, et al. Effect of sex differences on invasive measures of coronary microvascular dysfunction in patients with angina in the absence of obstructive coronary artery disease. *JACC Cardiovasc Interv*. 2015;8(11):1433-1441.
26. Kim CH, Koo BK, Dehbi HM, et al. Sex differences in instantaneous wave-free ratio or fractional flow reserve-guided revascularization strategy. *JACC Cardiovasc Interv*. 2019;12(20):2035-2046.
27. Yonetsu T, Hoshino M, Lee T, et al. Impact of sex difference on the discordance of revascularization decision making between fractional flow reserve and diastolic pressure ratio during the wave-free period. *J Am Heart Assoc*. 2020;9(5):e014790.
28. Lawton JS, Tamis-Holland JE, Bangalore S, et al. 2021 ACC/AHA/SCAI guideline for coronary artery revascularization: a report of the American College of Cardiology/American Heart Association Joint Committee on clinical practice guidelines. *Circulation*. 2022;145(3):e18-e114.
29. Acharjee S, Teo KK, Jacobs AK, et al. Optimal medical therapy with or without percutaneous coronary intervention in women with stable coronary disease: a pre-specified subset analysis of the Clinical Outcomes Utilizing Revascularization and Aggressive druG Evaluation (COURAGE) trial. *Am Heart J*. 2016;173:108-117.
30. Reynolds HR, Shaw LJ, Min JK, et al. Association of sex with severity of coronary artery disease, ischemia, and symptom burden in patients with moderate or severe ischemia: secondary analysis of the ISCHEMIA randomized clinical trial. *JAMA Cardiol*. 2020;5(7):773-786.
31. Serruys PW, Cavalcante R, Collet C, et al. Outcomes after coronary stenting or bypass surgery for men and women with unprotected left main disease: the EXCEL trial. *JACC Cardiovasc Interv*. 2018;11(13):1234-1243.
32. Sotomi Y, Onuma Y, Cavalcante R, et al. Geographical difference of the interaction of sex with treatment strategy in patients with multivessel disease and left main disease: a meta-analysis from SYNTAX (synergy between PCI with Taxus and cardiac surgery), PRECOMBAT (bypass

surgery versus angioplasty using sirolimus-eluting stent in patients with left main coronary artery disease), and BEST (bypass surgery and everolimus-eluting stent implantation in the treatment of patients with multivessel coronary artery disease) randomized controlled trials. *Circ Cardiovasc Interv*. 2017;10(5):e005027.

33. Kapur A, Hall RJ, Malik IS, et al. Randomized comparison of percutaneous coronary intervention with coronary artery bypass grafting in diabetic patients. 1-year results of the CARDia (Coronary Artery Revascularization in Diabetes) trial. *J Am Coll Cardiol*. 2010;55(5):432-440.
34. Tamis-Holland JE, Lu J, Korytkowski M, et al. Sex differences in presentation and outcome among patients with type 2 diabetes and coronary artery disease treated with contemporary medical therapy with or without prompt revascularization: a report from the BARI 2D Trial (Bypass Angioplasty Revascularization Investigation 2 Diabetes). *J Am Coll Cardiol*. 2013;61(17):1767-1776.
35. Farkouh ME, Domanski M, Sleeper LA, et al. Strategies for multivessel revascularization in patients with diabetes. *N Engl J Med*. 2012;367(25):2375-2384.
36. Navarese EP, Lansky AJ, Kereiakes DJ, et al. Cardiac mortality in patients randomised to elective coronary revascularisation plus medical therapy or medical therapy alone: a systematic review and meta-analysis. *Eur Heart J*. 2021;42(45):4638-4651.
37. Bangalore S, Maron DJ, Stone GW, Hochman JS. Routine revascularization versus initial medical therapy for stable ischemic heart disease: a systematic review and meta-analysis of randomized trials. *Circulation*. 2020;142(9):841-857.
38. Chaitman BR, Alexander KP, Cyr DD, et al. Myocardial infarction in the ISCHEMIA trial: impact of different definitions on incidence, prognosis, and treatment comparisons. *Circulation*. 2021;143(8):790-804.
39. Gul B, Shah T, Head SJ, et al. Revascularization options for females with multivessel coronary artery disease: a meta-analysis of randomized controlled trials. *JACC Cardiovasc Interv*. 2020;13(8):1009-1010.
40. Farooq V, van Klaveren D, Steyerberg EW, et al. Anatomical and clinical characteristics to guide decision making between coronary artery bypass surgery and percutaneous coronary intervention for individual patients: development and validation of SYNTAX score II. *Lancet*. 2013;381(9867):639-650.
41. Navarese EP, Gurbel PA, Andreotti F, et al. Optimal timing of coronary invasive strategy in non-ST-segment elevation acute coronary syndromes: a systematic review and meta-analysis. *Ann Intern Med*. 2013;158(4):261-270.
42. Jobs A, Mehta SR, Montalescot G, et al. Optimal timing of an invasive strategy in patients with non-ST-elevation acute coronary syndrome: a meta-analysis of randomised trials. *Lancet*. 2017;390(10096):737-746.
43. Mehta SR, Granger CB, Boden WE, et al. Early versus delayed invasive intervention in acute coronary syndromes. *N Engl J Med*. 2009;360(21):2165-2175.
44. Milosevic A, Vasiljevic-Pokrajcic Z, Milasinovic D, et al. Immediate versus delayed invasive intervention for non-STEMI patients: the RIDDLE-NSTEMI study. *JACC Cardiovasc Interv*. 2016;9(6):541-549.
45. Mehilli J, Presbitero P. Coronary artery disease and acute coronary syndrome in women. *Heart*. 2020;106(7):487-492.
46. Udell JA, Fonarow GC, Maddox TM, et al. Sustained sex-based treatment differences in acute coronary syndrome care: insights from the American heart Association get with the guidelines coronary artery disease registry. *Clin Cardiol*. 2018;41(6):758-768.
47. Sabbag A, Matetzky S, Porter A, et al. Sex differences in the management and 5-year outcome of young patients (<55 years) with acute coronary syndromes. *Am J Med*. 2017;130(11):1324.e15-1324.e22.
48. Kimenai DM, Lindahl B, Jernberg T, Bekers O, Meex SJR, Eggers KM. Sex-specific effects of implementing a high-sensitivity troponin I assay in patients with suspected acute coronary syndrome: results from SWEDEHEART registry. *Sci Rep*. 2020;10(1):15227.
49. Yu J, Mehran R, Grinfeld L, et al. Sex-based differences in bleeding and long term adverse events after percutaneous coronary intervention for acute myocardial infarction: three year results from the HORIZONS-AMI trial. *Catheter Cardiovasc Interv*. 2015;85(3):359-368.
50. Lansky AJ, Pietras C, Costa RA, et al. Gender differences in outcomes after primary angioplasty versus primary stenting with and without abciximab for acute myocardial infarction: results of the Controlled Abciximab and Device Investigation to Lower Late Angioplasty Complications (CADILLAC) trial. *Circulation*. 2005;111(13):1611-1618.
51. Kaul P, Armstrong PW, Sookram S, Leung BK, Brass N, Welsh RC. Temporal trends in patient and treatment delay among men and women presenting with ST-elevation myocardial infarction. *Am Heart J*. 2011;161(1):91-97.
52. Kang SH, Suh JW, Yoon CH, et al. Sex differences in management and mortality of patients with ST-elevation myocardial infarction (from the Korean Acute Myocardial Infarction National Registry). *Am J Cardiol*. 2012;109(6):787-793.
53. Jneid H, Fonarow GC, Cannon CP, et al. Sex differences in medical care and early death after acute myocardial infarction. *Circulation*. 2008;118(25):2803-2810.
54. Tomey MI, Mehran R, Brener SJ, et al. Sex, adverse cardiac events, and infarct size in anterior myocardial infarction: an analysis of intracoronary abciximab and aspiration thrombectomy in patients with large anterior myocardial infarction (INFUSE-AMI). *Am Heart J*. 2015;169(1):86-93.
55. Heer T, Schiele R, Schneider S, et al. Gender differences in acute myocardial infarction in the era of reperfusion (the MITRA registry). *Am J Cardiol*. 2002;89(5):511-517.
56. Mega JL, Morrow DA, Ostor E, et al. Outcomes and optimal antithrombotic therapy in women undergoing fibrinolysis for ST-elevation myocardial infarction. *Circulation*. 2007;115(22):2822-2828.
57. Canto JG, Rogers WJ, Goldberg RJ, et al. Association of age and sex with myocardial infarction symptom presentation and in-hospital mortality. *JAMA*. 2012;307(8):813-822.
58. Shah P, Patel K, Vasudev R, et al. Gender differences in the revascularization rates and in-hospital outcomes in hospitalizations with ST segment elevation myocardial infarction. *Ir J Med Sci*. 2020;189(3):873-884.
59. Nanna MG, Hajduk AM, Krumholz HM, et al. Sex-based differences in presentation, treatment, and complications among older adults hospitalized for acute myocardial infarction: the SILVER-AMI study. *Circ Cardiovasc Qual Outcomes*. 2019;12(10):e005691.
60. Kyto V, Sipila J, Rautava P. Gender and in-hospital mortality of ST-segment elevation myocardial infarction (from a multihospital nationwide registry study of 31,689 patients). *Am J Cardiol*. 2015;115(3):303-306.
61. Wijnbergen I, Tijssen J, van't Veer M, Michels R, Pijls NH. Gender differences in long-term outcome after primary percutaneous intervention for ST-segment elevation myocardial infarction. *Catheter Cardiovasc Interv*. 2013;82(3):379-384.
62. Eitel I, Desch S, de Waha S, et al. Sex differences in myocardial salvage and clinical outcome in patients with acute reperfused ST-elevation myocardial infarction: advances in cardiovascular imaging. *Circ Cardiovasc Imaging*. 2012;5(1):119-126.
63. Jakobsen L, Niemann T, Thorsgaard N, et al. Sex- and age-related differences in clinical outcome after primary percutaneous coronary intervention. *EuroIntervention*. 2012;8:904-911.
64. Pancholy SB, Shantha GP, Patel T, Cheskin LJ. Sex differences in short-term and long-term all-cause mortality among patients with ST-segment elevation myocardial infarction treated by primary percutaneous intervention: a meta-analysis. *JAMA Intern Med*. 2014;174(11):1822-1830.
65. Suessenbacher A, Doerler J, Alber H, et al. Gender-related outcome following percutaneous coronary intervention for ST-elevation myocardial infarction: data from the Austrian acute PCI registry. *EuroIntervention*. 2008;4(2):271-276.
66. Berger JS, Elliott L, Gallup D, et al. Sex differences in mortality following acute coronary syndromes. *JAMA*. 2009;302(8):874-882.
67. Sjauw KD, Stegenga NK, Engstrom AE, et al. The influence of gender on short- and long-term outcome after primary PCI and delivered medical care for ST-segment elevation myocardial infarction. *EuroIntervention*. 2010;5(7):780-787.
68. Sadowski M, Gasior M, Gierlotka M, Janion M, Polonski L. Gender-related differences in mortality after ST-segment elevation myocardial infarction: a large multicentre national registry. *EuroIntervention*. 2011;6(9):1068-1072.
69. Corrada E, Ferrante G, Mazzali C, et al. Eleven-year trends in gender differences of treatments and mortality in ST-elevation acute myocardial infarction in northern Italy, 2000 to 2010. *Am J Cardiol*. 2014;114(3):336-341.
70. Murphy AC, Yudi MB, Farouque O, et al. Impact of gender and door-to-balloon times on long-term mortality in patients presenting with ST-elevation myocardial infarction. *Am J Cardiol*. 2019;124(6):833-841.

71. De Luca G, Suryapranata H, Dambrink JH, et al. Sex-related differences in outcome after ST-segment elevation myocardial infarction treated by primary angioplasty: data from the Zwolle Myocardial Infarction study. *Am Heart J*. 2004;148(5):852-856.
72. Cohen M, Gensini GF, Maritz F, et al. The role of gender and other factors as predictors of not receiving reperfusion therapy and of outcome in ST-segment elevation myocardial infarction. *J Thromb Thrombolysis*. 2005;19(3):155-161.
73. Liu J, Elbadawi A, Elgendy IY, et al. Age-stratified sex disparities in care and outcomes in patients with ST-elevation myocardial infarction. *Am J Med*. 2020;133(11):1293-1301.e1.
74. Bhan V, Cantor WJ, Yan RT, et al. Efficacy of early invasive management post-fibrinolysis in men versus women with ST-elevation myocardial infarction: a subgroup analysis from trial of routine angioplasty and stenting after fibrinolysis to enhance reperfusion in acute myocardial Infarction (TRANSFER-AMI). *Am Heart J*. 2012;164(3):343-350.
75. Jackson EA, Moscucci M, Smith DE, et al. The association of sex with outcomes among patients undergoing primary percutaneous coronary intervention for ST elevation myocardial infarction in the contemporary era: insights from the Blue Cross Blue Shield of Michigan Cardiovascular Consortium (BMC2). *Am Heart J*. 2011;161(1):106-112.e1.
76. De Luca G, Parodi G, Sciagra R, et al. Relation of gender to infarct size in patients with ST-segment elevation myocardial infarction undergoing primary angioplasty. *Am J Cardiol*. 2013;111(7):936-940.
77. El-Menyar A, Zubaid M, Rashed W, et al. Comparison of men and women with acute coronary syndrome in six Middle Eastern countries. *Am J Cardiol*. 2009;104(8):1018-1022.
78. Kaul P, Fu Y, Westerhout CM, Granger CB, Armstrong PW. Relative prognostic value of baseline Q wave and time from symptom onset among men and women with ST-elevation myocardial infarction undergoing percutaneous coronary intervention. *Am J Cardiol*. 2012;110(11):1555-1560.
79. Shacham Y, Topilsky Y, Leshem-Rubinow E, et al. Comparison of left ventricular function following first ST-segment elevation myocardial infarction treated with primary percutaneous coronary intervention in men versus women. *Am J Cardiol*. 2014;113(12):1941-1946.
80. Velders MA, Boden H, van Boven AJ, et al. Influence of gender on ischemic times and outcomes after ST-elevation myocardial infarction. *Am J Cardiol*. 2013;111(3):312-318.
81. Weissler-Snir A, Kornowski R, Sagie A, et al. Gender differences in left ventricular function following percutaneous coronary intervention for first anterior wall ST-segment elevation myocardial infarction. *Am J Cardiol*. 2014;114(10):1473-1478.
82. Tizon-Marcos H, Bertrand OF, Rodes-Cabau J, et al. Impact of female gender and transradial coronary stenting with maximal antiplatelet therapy on bleeding and ischemic outcomes. *Am Heart J*. 2009;157(4):740-745.
83. Diercks DB, Owen KP, Kontos MC, et al. Gender differences in time to presentation for myocardial infarction before and after a national women's cardiovascular awareness campaign: a temporal analysis from the can rapid risk stratification of unstable angina patients suppress ADverse Outcomes with Early Implementation (CRUSADE) and the National Cardiovascular Data Registry Acute Coronary Treatment and Intervention Outcomes Network-Get with the Guidelines (NCDR ACTION Registry-GWTG). *Am Heart J*. 2010;160(1):80-87.e3.
84. Mehta SR, Wood DA, Storey RF, et al. Complete revascularization with multivessel PCI for myocardial infarction. *N Engl J Med*. 2019;381(15):1411-1421.
85. Engstrøm T, Kelbaek H, Helqvist S, et al. Complete revascularisation versus treatment of the culprit lesion only in patients with ST-segment elevation myocardial infarction and multivessel disease (DANAMI-3-PRIMULTI): an open-label, randomised controlled trial. *Lancet*. 2015;386(9994):665-671.
86. Smits PC, Abdel-Wahab M, Neumann FJ, et al. Fractional flow reserve-guided multivessel angioplasty in myocardial infarction. *N Engl J Med*. 2017;376(13):1234-1244.
87. Wong SC, Sleeper LA, Monrad ES, et al. Absence of gender differences in clinical outcomes in patients with cardiogenic shock complicating acute myocardial infarction. A report from the SHOCK Trial Registry. *J Am Coll Cardiol*. 2001;38(5):1395-1401.
88. Antoniucci D, Migliorini A, Moschi G, et al. Does gender affect the clinical outcome of patients with acute myocardial infarction complicated by cardiogenic shock who undergo percutaneous coronary intervention?. *Catheter Cardiovasc Interv*. 2003;59(4):423-428.
89. Koeth O, Zahn R, Heer T, et al. Gender differences in patients with acute ST-elevation myocardial infarction complicated by cardiogenic shock. *Clin Res Cardiol*. 2009;98(12):781-786.
90. Abdel-Qadir HM, Ivanov J, Austin PC, Tu JV, Dzavik V. Sex differences in the management and outcomes of Ontario patients with cardiogenic shock complicating acute myocardial infarction. *Can J Cardiol*. 2013;29(6):691-696.
91. Kunadian V, Qiu W, Bawamia B, Veerasamy M, Jamieson S, Zaman A. Gender comparisons in cardiogenic shock during ST elevation myocardial infarction treated by primary percutaneous coronary intervention. *Am J Cardiol*. 2013;112(5):636-641.
92. Fengler K, Fuernau G, Desch S, et al. Gender differences in patients with cardiogenic shock complicating myocardial infarction: a substudy of the IABP-SHOCK II-trial. *Clin Res Cardiol*. 2015;104(1):71-78.
93. Mahmoud AN, Elgendy IY. Gender impact on 30-day readmissions after hospitalization with acute myocardial infarction complicated by cardiogenic shock (from the 2013 to 2014 national Readmissions Database). *Am J Cardiol*. 2018;121(5):523-528.
94. Isorni MA, Aissaoui N, Angoulvant D, et al. Temporal trends in clinical characteristics and management according to sex in patients with cardiogenic shock after acute myocardial infarction: the FAST-MI programme. *Arch Cardiovasc Dis*. 2018;111(10):555-563.
95. Guo RW, Yang LX, Liu B, et al. Effect of sex on recovery of ejection fraction in patients with anterior ST-segment elevation myocardial infarction undergoing primary percutaneous coronary intervention. *Coron Artery Dis*. 2014;25(2):133-137.
96. Rubini Gimenez M, Zeymer U, Desch S, et al. Sex-specific management in patients with acute myocardial infarction and cardiogenic shock: a substudy of the CULPRIT-SHOCK trial. *Circ Cardiovasc Interv*. 2020;13(3):e008537.
97. Joseph SM, Brisco MA, Colvin M, et al. Women with cardiogenic shock derive greater benefit from early mechanical circulatory support: an update from the cVAD registry. *J Interv Cardiol*. 2016;29(3):248-256.
98. Vallabhajosyula S, Dunlay SM, Barsness GW, et al. Sex disparities in the use and outcomes of temporary mechanical circulatory support for acute myocardial infarction-cardiogenic shock. *CJC Open*. 2020;2(6):462-472.
99. Yan I, Schrage B, Weimann J, et al. Sex differences in patients with cardiogenic shock. *ESC Heart Fail*. 2021;8(3):1775-1783.
100. Vallabhajosyula S, Vallabhajosyula S, Dunlay SM, et al. Sex and gender disparities in the management and outcomes of acute myocardial infarction-cardiogenic shock in older adults. *Mayo Clin Proc*. 2020;95(9):1916-1927.
101. Vallabhajosyula S, Ya'Qoub L, Singh M, et al. Sex disparities in the management and outcomes of cardiogenic shock complicating acute myocardial infarction in the young. *Circ Heart Fail*. 2020;13(10):e007154.
102. Ya'qoub L, Lemor A, Dabbagh M, et al. Racial, ethnic, and sex disparities in patients with STEMI and cardiogenic shock. *JACC Cardiovasc Interv*. 2021;14(6):653-660.
103. Hayes SN, Tweet MS, Adlam D, et al. Spontaneous coronary artery dissection: JACC state-of-the-art review. *J Am Coll Cardiol*. 2020;76(8):961-984.
104. Kim ESH. Spontaneous coronary-artery dissection. *N Engl J Med*. 2020;383(24):2358-2370.
105. Hassan S, Prakash R, Starovoytov A, Saw J. Natural history of spontaneous coronary artery dissection with spontaneous angiographic healing. *JACC Cardiovasc Interv*. 2019;12(6):518-527.
106. Adlam D, Alfonso F, Maas A, Vrints C, Writing Committee. European Society of Cardiology, acute cardiovascular care association, SCAD study group: a position paper on spontaneous coronary artery dissection. *Eur Heart J*. 2018;39(36):3353-3368.
107. Bauersachs J. Heart failure drug treatment: the fantastic four. *Eur Heart J*. 2021;42(6):681-683.
108. Saw J, Humphries K, Aymong E, et al. Spontaneous coronary artery dissection: clinical outcomes and risk of recurrence. *J Am Coll Cardiol*. 2017;70(9):1148-1158.
109. Velazquez EJ, Lee KL, Deja MA, et al. Coronary-artery bypass surgery in patients with left ventricular dysfunction. *N Engl J Med*. 2011;364(17):1607-1616.
110. Velazquez EJ, Lee KL, Jones RH, et al. Coronary-artery bypass surgery in patients with ischemic cardiomyopathy. *N Engl J Med*. 2016;374(16):1511-1520.

111. Johnston A, Mesana TG, Lee DS, Eddeen AB, Sun LY. Sex differences in long-term survival after major cardiac surgery: a population-based Cohort study. *J Am Heart Assoc*. 2019;8(17):e013260.
112. Kerkmeijer LS, Claessen BE, Baber U, et al. Incidence, determinants and clinical impact of definite stent thrombosis on mortality in women: from the WIN-DES collaborative patient-level pooled analysis. *Int J Cardiol*. 2018;263:24-28.
113. Detre KM, Rosen AD, Bost JE, et al. Contemporary practice of coronary revascularization in U.S. hospitals and hospitals participating in the bypass angioplasty revascularization investigation (BARI). *J Am Coll Cardiol*. 1996;28(3):609-615.
114. Dangas GD, Farkouh ME, Sleeper LA, et al. Long-term outcome of PCI versus CABG in insulin and non-insulin-treated diabetic patients: results from the FREEDOM trial. *J Am Coll Cardiol*. 2014;64(12):1189-1197.
115. Carrero JJ, Hecking M, Chesnaye NC, Jager KJ. Sex and gender disparities in the epidemiology and outcomes of chronic kidney disease. *Nat Rev Nephrol*. 2018;14(3):151-164.
116. Bangalore S, Maron DJ, O'Brien SM, et al. Management of coronary disease in patients with advanced kidney disease. *N Engl J Med*. 2020;382(17):1608-1618.
117. Stefanini GG, Baber U, Windecker S, et al. Safety and efficacy of drug-eluting stents in women: a patient-level pooled analysis of randomised trials. *Lancet*. 2013;382(9908):1879-1888.
118. Ford TJ, Khan A, Docherty KF, et al. Sex differences in procedural and clinical outcomes following rotational atherectomy. *Catheter Cardiovasc Interv*. 2020;95(2):232-241.
119. Abdel-Wahab M, Toelg R, Byrne RA, et al. High-speed rotational atherectomy versus modified balloons prior to drug-eluting stent implantation in severely calcified coronary lesions. *Circ Cardiovasc Interv*. 2018;11(10):e007415.
120. Brinton TJ, Ali ZA, Hill JM, et al. Feasibility of shockwave coronary intravascular lithotripsy for the treatment of calcified coronary stenoses. *Circulation*. 2019;139(6):834-836.
121. Ali ZA, Nef H, Escaned J, et al. Safety and effectiveness of coronary intravascular lithotripsy for treatment of severely calcified coronary stenoses: the disrupt CAD II study. *Circ Cardiovasc Interv*. 2019;12(10):e008434.
122. Hill JM, Kereiakes DJ, Shlofmitz RA, et al. Intravascular lithotripsy for treatment of severely calcified coronary artery disease. *J Am Coll Cardiol*. 2020;76(22):2635-2646.
123. Cheney A, Kearney KE, Lombardi W. Sex-based differences in chronic total occlusion management. *Curr Atheroscler Rep*. 2018;20(12):60.
124. Stahli BE, Gebhard C, Gick M, et al. Comparison of outcomes in men versus women after percutaneous coronary intervention for chronic total occlusion. *Am J Cardiol*. 2017;119(12):1931-1936.
125. Mannem S, Rattanawong P, Riangwiwat T, et al. Sex difference and outcome after percutaneous intervention in patients with chronic total occlusion: a systematic review and meta-analysis. *Cardiovasc Revasc Med*. 2020;21(1):25-31.
126. Gargiulo G, Ariotti S, Vranckx P, et al. Impact of sex on comparative outcomes of radial versus femoral access in patients with acute coronary syndromes undergoing invasive management: data from the randomized MATRIX-access trial. *JACC Cardiovasc Interv*. 2018;11(1):36-50.
127. Pandie S, Mehta SR, Cantor WJ, et al. Radial versus femoral access for coronary angiography/intervention in women with acute coronary syndromes: insights from the RIVAL trial (radial vs femorAL access for coronary intervention). *JACC Cardiovasc Interv*. 2015;8(4):505-512.
128. Rao SV, Hess CN, Barham B, et al. A registry-based randomized trial comparing radial and femoral approaches in women undergoing percutaneous coronary intervention: the SAFE-PCI for Women (Study of Access Site for Enhancement of PCI for Women) trial. *JACC Cardiovasc Interv*. 2014;7(8):857-867.
129. Al Halabi S, Burke L, Hussain F, et al. Radial versus femoral approach in women undergoing coronary angiography: a meta-analysis of randomized controlled trials. *J Invasive Cardiol*. 2019;31(11):335-340.
130. Tiroch KA, Arora N, Matheny ME, Liu C, Lee TC, Resnic FS. Risk predictors of retroperitoneal hemorrhage following percutaneous coronary intervention. *Am J Cardiol*. 2008;102(11):1473-1476.
131. Le May M, Wells G, So D, et al. Safety and efficacy of femoral access vs radial access in ST-segment elevation myocardial infarction: the SAFARI-STEMI randomized clinical trial. *JAMA Cardiol*. 2020;5(2):126-134.
132. Bernat I, Horak D, Stasek J, et al. ST-segment elevation myocardial infarction treated by radial or femoral approach in a multicenter randomized clinical trial: the STEMI-RADIAL trial. *J Am Coll Cardiol*. 2014;63(10):964-972.
133. Gewalt SM, Helde SM, Ibrahim T, et al. Comparison of vascular closure devices versus manual compression after femoral artery puncture in women. *Circ Cardiovasc Interv*. 2018;11(8):e006074.
134. Bogabathina H, Shi R, Singireddy S, et al. Reduction of vascular complication rates from femoral artery access in contemporary women undergoing cardiac catheterization. *Cardiovasc Revasc Med*. 2018;19(6S):27-30.
135. Daugherty SL, Thompson LE, Kim S, et al. Patterns of use and comparative effectiveness of bleeding avoidance strategies in men and women following percutaneous coronary interventions: an observational study from the National Cardiovascular Data Registry. *J Am Coll Cardiol*. 2013;61(20):2070-2078.
136. Chaudry HI, Lee J, Li SX, et al. Sex differences in acute bleeding and vascular complications following percutaneous coronary intervention between 2003 and 2016: trends from the dartmouth dynamic registry. *Cardiovasc Revasc Med*. 2021;28:32-38.
137. Eggebrecht H, von Birgelen C, Naber C, et al. Impact of gender on femoral access complications secondary to application of a collagen-based vascular closure device. *J Invasive Cardiol*. 2004;16(5):247-250.
138. Capodanno D, Alfonso F, Levine GN, Valgimigli M, Angiolillo DJ. ACC/AHA versus ESC guidelines on dual antiplatelet therapy: JACC guideline comparison. *J Am Coll Cardiol*. 2018;72(23 pt A):2915-2931.
139. Aggarwal NR, Patel HN, Mehta LS, et al. Sex differences in ischemic Heart Disease: advances, obstacles, and next steps. *Circ Cardiovasc Qual Outcomes*. 2018;11(2):e004437.
140. Capodanno D, Angiolillo DJ. Impact of race and gender on antithrombotic therapy. *Thromb Haemost*. 2010;104(3):471-484.
141. Romano S, Buccheri S, Mehran R, Angiolillo DJ, Capodanno D. Gender differences on benefits and risks associated with oral antithrombotic medications for coronary artery disease. *Expert Opin Drug Saf*. 2018;17(10):1041-1052.
142. Wang TY, Angiolillo DJ, Cushman M, et al. Platelet biology and response to antiplatelet therapy in women: implications for the development and use of antiplatelet pharmacotherapies for cardiovascular disease. *J Am Coll Cardiol*. 2012;59(10):891-900.
143. Berger JS, Bhatt DL, Cannon CP, et al. The relative efficacy and safety of clopidogrel in women and men a sex-specific collaborative meta-analysis. *J Am Coll Cardiol*. 2009;54(21):1935-1945.
144. Husted S, James SK, Bach RG, et al. The efficacy of ticagrelor is maintained in women with acute coronary syndromes participating in the prospective, randomized, PLATelet inhibition and patient Outcomes (PLATO) trial. *Eur Heart J*. 2014;35(23):1541-1550.
145. Berry NC, Kereiakes DJ, Yeh RW, et al. Benefit and risk of prolonged DAPT after coronary stenting in women. *Circ Cardiovasc Interv*. 2018;11(8):e005308.
146. Yu J, Baber U, Mastoris I, et al. Sex-based differences in cessation of dual-antiplatelet therapy following percutaneous coronary intervention with stents. *JACC Cardiovasc Interv*. 2016;9(14):1461-1469.
147. Grodecki K, Huczek Z, Scislo P, et al. Gender-related differences in post-discharge bleeding among patients with acute coronary syndrome on dual antiplatelet therapy: a BleeMACS sub-study. *Thromb Res*. 2018;168:156-163.
148. Capodanno D, Mehran R, Valgimigli M, et al. Aspirin-free strategies in cardiovascular disease and cardioembolic stroke prevention. *Nat Rev Cardiol*. 2018;15(8):480-496.
149. Angiolillo DJ, Rollini F, Storey RF, et al. International expert consensus on switching platelet P2Y(12) receptor-inhibiting therapies. *Circulation*. 2017;136(20):1955-1975.
150. Sibbing D, Aradi D, Alexopoulos D, et al. Updated expert consensus statement on platelet function and genetic testing for guiding P2Y(12) receptor inhibitor treatment in percutaneous coronary intervention. *JACC Cardiovasc Interv*. 2019;12(16):1521-1537.
151. Capodanno D, Huber K, Mehran R, et al. Management of antithrombotic therapy in atrial fibrillation patients undergoing PCI: JACC state-of-the-art review. *J Am Coll Cardiol*. 2019;74(1):83-99.

Primary and Secondary Coronary Prevention Guidelines

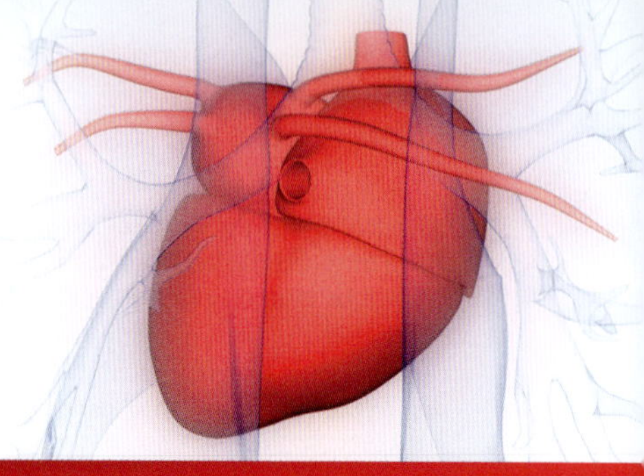

Faisal Latif

Emphasis on primary and secondary preventive cardiology is as important for the interventional community as it is for the general cardiovascular (CV) community, as majority of patients are followed by one or the other and not both. This chapter discusses many aspects of primary and secondary preventive cardiology, including some of the guidelines from the American Heart Association (AHA)/American College of Cardiology (ACC), as well as from other major organizations.[1]

ESTIMATION OF CV RISK

Ten-year and long-term estimation of atherosclerotic cardiovascular disease (ASCVD) risk forms the basis of primary prevention starting at age 20 years. Major risk factors include tobacco use, family history of premature ASCVD, dyslipidemia, type 2 diabetes mellitus (T2DM), elevated lipoprotein [a], and hypertension (HTN). For those aged 40 to 59 years, who are at elevated 10-year risk (>7.5%), aggressive risk factor modification with goal-directed treatment of aforementioned risk factors, optimizing lifestyle, is critical to mitigating the risk.[2]

No single risk estimation calculator is perfect. Therefore, additional tools such as coronary artery calcium (CAC) score can be used in selected patients at lower risk (<5% 10-year risk) or those with family history of premature ASCVD. The Multi-Ethnic Study of Atherosclerosis (MESA) and Astronaut Cardiovascular Health and Risk Modification (Astro-CHARM) risk scores incorporate both risk factors and CAC score to enhance patient-provider discussion and decision making.[3,4]

AHA/ACC GUIDELINES

During the past decade, major guidelines have emphasized several different classes of medications in addition to therapeutic lifestyle changes (TLCs). In interventional cardiology antiplatelet therapy has been emphasized for secondary prevention.

GENERAL CV RISK FACTOR INFORMATION

Dyslipidemia (DLP) and HTN produce a substantial burden in the United States and in most of Western civilization.[5,6] A substantial number of deaths each year are estimated to be caused by systolic blood pressure (SBP) that is higher than optimal (>115 mm Hg in epidemiologic studies) and by total cholesterol (TC) higher than optimal (estimated to be >150 mg/dL). In fact, almost 60% of the CV disease burden is caused by blood pressure (BP) and/or TC higher than optimal. In the United States, the combination of HTN and DLP was highly prevalent, with HTN affecting nearly one-quarter of the population, DLP impacting a third of the population, and both HTN and DLP impacting nearly 15%. Almost two-thirds of the patients with HTN also have DLP, and nearly half of those with DLP have HTN. Many studies suggest that most patients with HTN and DLP are not at both goals.

The risk of CHD events and strokes markedly rises with increasing age and increasing SBP. Likewise, there is a strong direct relationship between TC and low-density lipoprotein cholesterol (LDL-C) and major CV and CHD events. Although both SBP and TC markedly increase overall risk, as seen with other risk factors, often the individual risk factors are more than additive and actually potentiate each other in increasing overall risk, emphasizing the importance of multifactorial risk factor intervention.

Aspirin

Aspirin's role in secondary prevention of ASCVD is well established.[1] In the absence of contraindications, most patients should receive low doses of aspirin (81-325 mg) for life, and dual antiplatelet therapy (clopidogrel, prasugrel, ticagrelor) for at least 3 months, and probably for 12 months, in most patients following acute coronary syndrome (ACS) and percutaneous coronary intervention. This is discussed in detail elsewhere in this book.

One the other hand, while aspirin has been widely used for primary prevention of ASCVD,[7] its role in primary prevention of nonfatal myocardial infarction (MI) and stroke has been challenged due to lack of net benefit in more recent studies.[8-10] Particularly, it should be avoided in patients with history of gastrointestinal bleeding or significant bleeding from other source, age >70 years, thrombocytopenia, coagulopathy, chronic kidney disease (CKD), and concurrent use of anticoagulants, steroids, and nonsteroidal anti-inflammatory drugs.

HYPERTENSION

The lifetime incidence of HTN has been increasing during recent decades and has now reached nearly 90% in the United States.[1] Approximately 70% of individuals with HTN are aware of their condition, and nearly 60% are receiving treatment. Nevertheless, HTN is controlled in only 30% of patients. Large meta-analyses show nearly 50% increases in the long-term CV mortality for every 20 mm Hg increase in SBP above 115 mm Hg. Lowering elevated BP will decrease the risk of CV events regardless of age, race, gender, or other risk factors.

The recent HTN guidelines are based on the Joint National Commission (JNC) eight major recommendations,[5] as summarized in **Table 32.1**. In general, HTN therapy is recommended for BPs >140/90 mm Hg, but the current guidelines indicate that treatment in those 60 years and older is only definitively needed when BP is >150/90 mm Hg, although this has been questioned.[6] Based on the 2019 AHA/ACC guidelines, in adults with stage 1 HTN (BP 130-139/80-89 mm Hg) who have an estimated 10-year ASCVD risk of ≥10%, CKD, or diabetes mellitus (DM), an

TABLE 32.1 JNC 8's New HTN Guidelines

- 60 y and older, cut-point 150/90 mm Hg
- Under 60 y, cut-point 140/90 mm Hg
- 18 y and older with DM, cut-point 140/90
- 18 y and older with CKD, cut-point 140/90; use ACEI/ARB as first med
- Non-blacks, use thiazides, CCB, ACEI/ARB; in blacks, do not use ACEI/ARB (unless CKD)
- Increase dose or add med after 1 mo to reach goal
- No ACEI/ARB combination

ACEI, angiotensin-converting enzyme inhibitor; ARB, angiotensin receptor blocker; CCB, calcium channel blocker; CKD, chronic kidney disease; DM, diabetes mellitus; HTN, hypertension; JNC, Joint National Commission.
Adapted from: James PA, Oparil S, Carter BL, et al. 2014 evidence-based guideline for the management of high blood pressure in adults: report from the panel members appointed to the Eighth Joint National Committee (JNC 8). *JAMA*. 2014;311:507-520.

antihypertensive medication should be initiated with a target BP of <130/80 mm Hg.[11,12] Additionally, patients should be counseled to incorporate lifestyle changes that help lower BP (**Table 32.2**). Per JNC 8, beta-blockers (BBs) should be considered in patients with heart failure (HF), post-MI, and also certain tachyarrhythmias. Otherwise, BBs are not considered first-line therapy for routine HTN in JNC 8. In African American patients, angiotensin-converting enzyme inhibitors (ACEIs)/angiotensin receptor blockers (ARBs) are not considered first-line therapy unless there is CKD. In DM, ACEIs/ARBs are given equal status with diuretics and calcium channel blockers (CCBs). Also, ACEIs and ARBs should not generally be combined.

LIPID INTERVENTION

Substantial evidence from epidemiologic and lipid intervention trials demonstrate the importance of TC, LDL-C, high-density lipoprotein cholesterol (HDL-C), and triglycerides (TGs) in the development and progression of atherosclerosis, and especially in the risk of major CV and CHD events. Although levels of HDL-C and non-HDL-C actually correlate better with CHD than does LDL-C, the vast majority of the intervention data during the last two decades have focused on the role of LDL-C, especially with statins, which are emphasized in the guidelines.[13]

TABLE 32.2 Lifestyle Changes to Improve BP Control

	LIFESTYLE CHANGES
Weight loss	Generally, ~1 mm Hg BP reduction expected for 1-kg weight loss
Healthy diet	DASH (rich in fruits, vegetables, low-fat dairy)
Reduced salt intake	<1500 mg/d
Enhanced dietary potassium intake	3500-5000 mg/d
Physical activity	90-150 min/wk (aerobic)
	90-150 min/wk (dynamic resistance)
	4 × 2 min (hand grip); 3 sessions/wk (isometric)

The National Cholesterol Education Program (NCEP)-ATP III treatment algorithm was based on LDL-C and assessing for CHD, CHD risk equivalents, and common CHD risk factors (by assessing Framingham Risk Score [FRS] in patients with >2 risk factors).[14] According to these guidelines, CHD risk equivalents were considered to be DM, as well as other forms of atherothrombotic disease, such as peripheral arterial disease (PAD), abdominal aortic aneurysm, significant carotid disease, or having an FRS that suggests greater than 20% 10-year risk of CAD. Importantly, based on ACC/AHA guidelines, risk assessment has now changed from FRS to the Pooled Cohort Equation.[2] Also, DM is no longer considered a risk equivalent; risk is now calculated in patients with DM using the Pooled Cohort Equation.

Additional risk factors in diabetic patients include ≥10 years of T2DM, microalbuminuria, stage 3 CKD (glomerular filtration rate <60 mL/min/1.73 m^2), ankle brachial index <0.9, retinopathy, or neuropathy. In patients with multiple risk factors for ASCVD, aim should be to reduce LDL-C by ≥50%.

As discussed with MetS and HTN, TLCs are always recommended for treatment guidelines for lipids. Most of the prior emphasis was placed on the treatment of LDL-C and non-HDL-C (**Table 32.3**). The new ACC/AHA/NCEP IV guidelines[15] now focus on statins, especially in those with ASCVD or who are high risk.

For patients at 7.5% to 20% 10-year risk without DM, the CAC score can be used for decision making regarding use of statins: CAC score 0, statin can be avoided; CAC score 1 to 100, initiate moderate-intensity statin if age ≥55 years; CAC score >100 or ≥75th percentile, use statin regardless of age.

The current AHA/ACC guidelines focus on ASCVD (**Table 32.4**) and four major groups that benefit from statins (**Table 32.5**).[15] For many groups, intense statin therapy, especially those with ASCVD and LDL-C > 190 mg/dL, is defined as 40- and 80-mg doses of atorvastatin or 20 to 40 mg of rosuvastatin. For the elderly (>75 years), moderate doses of statins are generally recommended, despite data showing the efficacy and safety of higher doses in older patients. Nevertheless, the guidelines do state that clinicians should review and discuss the pros and cons of more aggressive treatments with their elderly patients. The AHA/ACC guidelines do not have definitive recommendations for DM < 40 years or >75 years, unless LDL-C is >190 mg/dL or there is an ASCVD. ACC has provided further guidance on use of non-statin therapies to lower LDL < 55 mg/dL or non-HDL-C < 85 mg/dL.[16] Non-statin options include ezetimibe, PCSK9 monoclonal antibodies (alirocumab, evolocumab), PCSK9 production inhibitor (inclisiran), bempedoic acid, and bile acid sequestrants (colesevelam). It is important to note that while other non-statin medications are

TABLE 32.3 ATP III LDL-C and Non-HDL-C Goals

RISK CATEGORY	LDL-C (MG/DL)	NON-HDL-C (MG/DL)
CHD or equivalent (10-y risk >20%)	<100	<130
>2 Risk factors (10-y risk <20%)	<130	<160
0-1 Risk factors	<160	<190

CHD, coronary heart disease; HDL-C, high-density lipoprotein cholesterol; LDL-C, low-density lipoprotein cholesterol.
Adapted from Expert Panel on Detection, Evaluation, and Treatment of High Blood Cholesterol in Adults. Executive summary of the third report of the National Cholesterol Education Program (NCEP) expert panel on detection, evaluation, and treatment of high blood cholesterol in adults (adult treatment panel III). *JAMA*. 2001;285:2486-2497.

TABLE 32.4 New ACC/AHA 2013 Cholesterol Guidelines. Emphasis on Clinical ASCVD

- ACS/MI
- Angina, stable or unstable
- Arterial revascularization, coronary and other
- Stroke/TIA
- PAD, presumably atherosclerotic

ACC/AHA, American College of Cardiology/American Heart Association; ACS, acute coronary syndrome; ASCVD, atherosclerotic cardiovascular disease; MI, myocardial infarction; PAD, peripheral arterial disease; TIA, transient ischemic attack.

Adapted from Stone NJ, Robinson JG, Lichtenstein AH, et al. 2013 ACC/AHA guideline on the treatment of blood cholesterol to reduce atherosclerotic cardiovascular risk in adults: a report of the American College of Cardiology/ American Heart Association Task Force on Practice Guidelines. *J Am Coll Cardiol.* 2014;63:2889-2934.

indicated for use along with maximally tolerated statin therapy, PCSK9 monoclonal antibodies (alirocumab, evolocumab) can be used either alone or in combination with other lipid-lowering therapies including statins.

METABOLIC SYNDROME

During the last decade, the NCEP–ATP III has emphasized the importance of MetS (previously referred to as insulin resistance syndrome or MetS X) in contributing to the overall risk of CHD.[14] As demonstrated in **Table 32.6**, the diagnosis depends on the parameters of obesity, TGs, HDL-C, BP, and fasting glucose. The prevalence of MetS markedly increases with age, and current statistics have determined the prevalence of MetS to be nearly one-quarter of the adult population and between 40% and 50% of older patients. Although in the general population the prevalence of MetS markedly increases with age, in patients with established CHD, the prevalence of MetS is actually inversely related to age.[17] The prevalence of MetS in older patients with CHD is similar to the prevalence in the general elderly population. Nevertheless, in younger patients with CHD (eg, those <60 years of age), the prevalence of MetS is nearly 75%, suggesting that three of every four younger patients with CHD meet the criteria for MetS.

Although many consider obesity, especially abdominal obesity, to be the major pathologic aspect of MetS, it should be emphasized that 5% of women and nearly 20% of men with MetS do not have a weight circumference that meets the current MetS criteria for abdominal obesity.

TABLE 32.5 New ACC/AHA 2013 Cholesterol Guidelines—Four Major Statin Benefit Groups

- ASCVD
- LDL-C 190 mg/dL and higher
- Diabetes, age 40-75 years
- 10-y risk of major ASCVD of 7.5% and higher, age 40-75 years

ACC/AHA, American College of Cardiology/American Heart Association; ASCVD, atherosclerotic cardiovascular disease; LDL-C, low-density lipoprotein cholesterol.

Adapted from Stone NJ, Robinson JG, Lichtenstein AH, et al. 2013 ACC/AHA guideline on the treatment of blood cholesterol to reduce atherosclerotic cardiovascular risk in adults: a report of the American College of Cardiology/ American Heart Association Task Force on Practice Guidelines. *J Am Coll Cardiol.* 2014;63:2889-2934.

Patients with MetS are at markedly increased risk of developing T2DM, so a major goal in the management of MetS is to prevent predictable complications, including T2DM, and, more importantly, major CV disease events. Therefore, many patients with MetS will require TLCs and pharmacotherapy. The major TLCs in MetS involve dietary restriction of calories, easily digestible and refined carbohydrates, saturated fats, and trans fatty acids. Increases in levels of soluble fiber and "good fats" (omega-9 and omega-3 fatty acids) in a diet are also beneficial. Additionally, achieving and maintaining ideal weight and waist circumference are also very important. Increasing aerobic exercise, which helps with weight reduction and maintenance of weight loss, as well as increasing cardiorespiratory fitness (CRF), which is a major predictor of long-term prognosis and survival, is a mainstay of therapy in patients with MetS. Several studies have demonstrated that TLCs consisting of dietary intervention, a small amount of weight loss, and moderate exercise training produced nearly 60% reductions in the subsequent development of T2DM. On the other hand, pharmacologic therapy, such as metformin or acarbose, reduces the prevalence in developing T2DM by only approximately 30%. Other pharmacologic agents that reduce development of T2DM are ACEIs and ARBs, which were shown to reduce T2DM by nearly 25%.[18,19] It should be emphasized that, even when pharmacologic therapy is needed in patients with MetS, concomitant TLCs are still important in long-term therapy.

NUTRITION

Healthy plant-based or Mediterranean-like diet high in fruits, vegetables, whole grains, nuts, lean vegetable, or animal protein (poultry or fish) has been shown to reduce CV mortality compared with standard diet. Long-term low-carbohydrate diet and high intake of animal fat and protein has been associated with increased CV and non-CV mortality, as is high-carbohydrate diet.[1]

OBESITY

Overweight conditions and obesity are strongly correlated with CV disease, because they adversely affect almost all of the major CHD risk factors, including (a) lipids (reducing HDL-C,

TABLE 32.6 Diagnosis of Metabolic Syndrome (MS)

RISK FACTOR	MEN	WOMEN
Waist circumference (inches)[a]	>40	>35
Triglycerides (mg/dL)	>150	>150
HDL-C (mg/dL)	<40	<50
BP (mm/Hg)	>130/85	>130/85
FBG (mg/dL)	>100	>100

Diagnosis of MS is made when >3 risk factors are present.

BP, blood pressure; FBG, fasting blood glucose; HDL-C, high-density lipoprotein cholesterol.

[a]Current level has been changed and is population/ethnicity specific (37 in or 94 cm men, and 31.5 in or 80 cm women in Middle East/Mediterranean).

Adapted from: Expert Panel on Detection, Evaluation, and Treatment of High Blood Cholesterol in Adults. Executive summary of the third report of the National Cholesterol Education Program (NCEP) expert panel on detection, evaluation, and treatment of high blood cholesterol in adults (adult treatment panel III). *JAMA.* 2001;285:2486-2497.

increasing TGs, slightly increasing LDL-C but changing LDL to a predominance of small dense particles that are more atherogenic); (b) HTN, by raising BP and promoting left ventricular hypertrophy, which is a potent independent risk factor for adverse CV events; (c) glucose, thus raising fasting and postprandial glucose levels, which are fundamentally pathophysiologic aspects of MetS and T2DM; (d) fitness, which reduces exercise capacity and CRF (also strongly related to increased CV disease); and (e) systolic and diastolic left ventricular function (obesity worsens both of these parameters).[20] Considering these myriad adverse effects on proven CV risk factors, it is not surprising that obesity is associated with almost all CV diseases, including HTN, CHD, and HF. TLCs for obese and overweight adults (body mass index >25 kg/m^2) include adherence to a low-calorie diet (decrease by 500 kcal or 800-1500 kcal/d) and high levels of physical activity (200-300 min/week). Weight loss of >5% of initial weight has been associated with improved BP and lipid and glycemic control and delays development of T2DM.

Nevertheless, despite a strong association with obesity, and with CV risk factors and the development of CV diseases, now numerous studies of cohorts with established CV diseases, including HTN, CHD, HF, atrial fibrillation (AF), and PAD, have demonstrated that overweight and obese persons have a better prognosis than do their leaner counterparts, which has been termed the "obesity paradox."[20,21] Although a detailed discussion of the obesity paradox and potential limitations for weight reduction and CV diseases is beyond the scope of this chapter, clearly the overall information available strongly supports efforts to prevent patients from becoming overweight or obese in the first place, something that should go a long way in the prevention of CV disease risk factors and many CV diseases. Additionally, despite the obesity paradox, the "weight" of information still strongly supports efforts at weight loss for most patients with advanced CV diseases, including HTN, CHD, and HF, although clearly better larger-scale outcome studies of significant weight loss is needed for all of these CV diseases.

DIABETES MELLITUS

Patients with DM are at a markedly increased risk of CHD, cerebrovascular disease, and PAD. CV disease continues to be the leading cause of morbidity and mortality among the population with DM, accounting for almost 70% of deaths among patients with T2DM.[1] Optimization of the dismal CV prognosis associated with DM requires aggressive, longitudinal, multifactorial CV risk factor treatment, including vigorous efforts at treating and/or preventing HTN, DLP, and obese and overweight conditions.

Dietary pattern, body weight, and less physical activity play an important role in development as well as progression of T2DM. Mediterranean, dietary approaches to stop hypertension (DASH), and vegetarian diets and at least 150 minutes of moderate to vigorous physical activity help improve glycemic control.

First-line medical therapy is metformin, found to be associated with a 39% reduction in risk of myocardial infraction. Sulfonylureas do not impact CV outcomes. Sodium-glucose cotransporter 2 (SGLT-2) inhibitors have been demonstrated to reduce ASCVD and HF, in patients with or without DM. Glucagon-like peptide-1 receptor (GLP-1R) agonists have been found to significantly reduce ASCVD events in patients with DM. Hence, consideration should be given to SGLT-2 inhibitors and GLP-1R agonists for primary prevention of CV events.

INFLAMMATION AND C-REACTIVE PROTEIN

Substantial evidence documents the central role of inflammation in the pathogenesis and progression of atherosclerosis and major CV events.[22] C-reactive protein (CRP) is a marker of systemic inflammation and has been implicated in the pathogenesis of many chronic diseases, including CV disease and CHD. While a value of CRP > 3 mg/L carries the highest relative risk for recurrent CV events, values >1 mg/L have been associated with increased risk compared with <1 mg/L. The JUPITER trial demonstrated benefit of statin therapy among individuals with LDL < 130 mg/dL and CRP > 2 mg/L.[23] Consideration should be made to retest CRP levels in 2 weeks and values averaged.[24] Even following CHD events, high CRP predicts further events. As observed in major statin trials following ACS, those patients with both low levels of LDL-C and low CRP have the lowest risk of recurrent CV events. Statins reduce CRP levels, and studies have shown this effect to be independent of reduction in LDL.[25] Recently, low-dose colchicine (a direct anti-inflammatory agent) has been approved for CV risk reduction.

Although the most recognized CV treatment for lowering levels of CRP is with the statin medications, particularly at higher doses, there is also substantial evidence that cardiac rehabilitation (CR) and exercise training, as well as increased levels of CRF, are associated with marked reductions in the levels of CRP, especially when exercise training is accompanied by significant weight loss.[26]

SMOKING

The toxic effects of long-term tobacco smoking on CV, CHD, and general health are well recognized and accounts for almost one-third of CHD deaths. A graded relationship exists between the number of cigarettes smoked and the risk of MI and ACS. Nevertheless, unlike the impact of smoking to increase the risk of lung cancer, which takes nearly 20 years of smoking cessation to reverse, adverse CV risk of past smoking is eliminated within 3 to 5 years after tobacco cessation.

Besides cigarettes, smokeless tobacco as well as secondhand smoking has been associated with increased risk of CHD. E-cigarettes and vaping are also highly likely to increase CV and pulmonary risk.[1]

Recommendations for smoking cessation are considered a quality measure following ACS and should be assessed and discussed at every clinical encounter. Several medications (nicotine, bupropion, and varenicline) are effective in improving the odds of smoking cessation.[1]

CR PROGRAMS, EXERCISE, AND FITNESS

CR programs have been neglected in preventive cardiology, with studies of Medicare beneficiaries showing that only 10% to 15% of covered participants actually attend these programs.[27] Considerable recent emphasis has been placed in making both the referral and participation in formal CR a performance measure. Clearly, CR programs have been proven to increase exercise capacity and CRF (a potent predictor of prognosis for almost all CV diseases and total mortality), improve CHD risk factors, reduce psychosocial stress (which also predicts recovery and prognosis), and, most importantly, reduce major morbidity and mortality.[27-29] Considering the importance of physical activity, exercise, and CRF in general health, the national guidelines for physical activity and exercise are approximately 150 min/wk of moderate exercise (eg, walking) or 75 min/wk of moderate- to high-intensity exercise (eg, running), and these recommendations are typically for both primary and secondary prevention. Many patients are unable to exercise longer duration in one instance; therefore, it should be emphasized that shorter duration of exercise seems to be as beneficial as longer ones (≥10 minute bouts).[30] Hence, focus should be on cumulative duration of weekly exercise rather than on individual bouts.

OTHER PREVENTIVE STRATEGIES

Long-term prevention also involves antiplatelet therapy in patients with established ASCVD or high risk. Although omega-3 fatty acids and prevention of vitamin D deficiency have potential medical benefits, there are no definitive cardiac guidelines regarding these agents. Small amounts of alcohol protect against most CVD, although any alcohol increases the risk of AF. Nevertheless, high alcohol use above two to three drinks per day increases the risk of HTN and hemorrhagic stroke. As mentioned previously, CR is indicated in patients after major CHD events and is now indicated in HF and PAD, although the AHA has recommended 1 gram of omega-3 after MI and for systolic HF.[31]

Key Points

- Estimation of CV risk using ACC/AHA or other risk calculators and use of CAC score when appropriate is the foundation of primary prevention of CHD.
- Role of aspirin in primary prevention is very limited.
- Current guidelines from JNC-8 recommend pharmacologic BP treatment when BP is >150/90 mm Hg in those 60 years and older. AHA/ACC guidelines recommend a target BP of <130/85 mm Hg in patients at elevated risk of CHD.
- ACEI/ARB, thiazide diuretics, or CCBs are all acceptable first-line antihypertensive therapy, even in diabetes.
- LDL < 55 mg/dL is the latest updated target based on ACC Expert Consensus in patients who are very high risk.
- Metabolic syndrome is the major component of diabetes associated with increased CHD risk.
- Healthy plant-based or Mediterranean-like diet has been shown to reduce CV mortality.
- In treating DM, strong consideration should be given to SGLT-2 inhibitors and GLP-1R agonists for primary prevention of CV events.
- All forms of tobacco products including e-cigarettes and vaping are associated with adverse CV events.

References

1. Arnett DK, Blumenthal RS, Albert MA, et al. 2019 ACC/AHA guideline on the primary prevention of cardiovascular disease: a report of the American College of cardiology/American Heart Association Task Force on clinical practice guidelines. *Circulation*. 2019;140(11):e596-e646. doi:10.1161/CIR.0000000000000678
2. American College of Cardiology, American Heart Association. ASCVD risk estimator. https://tools.acc.org/ldl/ascvd_risk_estimator/index.html#!/calulate/estimator.
3. Multi-Ethnic Study of Atherosclerosis. MESA 10-Year CHD risk with coronary artery calcification. https://www.mesa-nhlbi.org/MESACHDRisk/MesaRiskScore/RiskScore.aspx.
4. Astronaut Cardiovascular Health and Risk Modification (Astro-CHARM). 10-Year ASCVD Risk Calculator with Coronary Artery Calcium. http://astrocharm.org/calculator-working
5. James PA, Oparil S, Carter BL, et al. 2014 evidence-based guideline for the management of high blood pressure in adults: report from the panel members appointed to the Eighth Joint National Committee (JNC 8). *JAMA*. 2014;311(5):507-520.
6. Bangalore S, Gong Y, Cooper-DeHoff RM, Pepine CJ, Messerli FH. 2014 Eighth Joint National Committee panel recommendation for blood pressure targets revisited: results from the INVEST study. *J Am Coll Cardiol*. 2014;64(8):784-793.
7. U.S. Preventive Services Task Force. Aspirin for the prevention of cardiovascular disease: U.S. Preventive Services Task Force recommendation statement. *Ann Intern Med*. 150(6):396-404. doi:10.7326/0003-4819-150-6-200903170-00008
8. ASCEND Study Collaborative Group; Bowman L, Mafham M, Wallendszus K, et al. Effects of aspirin for primary prevention in persons with diabetes mellitus. *N Engl J Med*. 2018;379(16):1529-1539.
9. Gaziano JM, Brotons C, Coppolecchia R, et al. Use of aspirin to reduce risk of initial vascular events in patients at moderate risk of cardiovascular disease (ARRIVE): a randomised, double-blind, placebo-controlled trial. *Lancet*. 2018;392(10152):1036-1046.
10. McNeil JJ, Wolfe R, Woods RL, et al. Effect of aspirin on cardiovascular events and bleeding in the healthy elderly. *N Engl J Med*. 2018;379:1509.
11. Whelton PK, Carey RM, Aronow WS, et al. 2017 ACC/AHA/AAPA/ABC/ACPM/AGS/APhA/ASH/ASPC/NMA/PCNA guideline for the prevention, detection, evaluation, and management of high blood pressure in adults: a report of the American College of Cardiology/American Heart Association Task Force on Clinical Practice Guidelines. *J Am Coll Cardiol*. 2018;71(19):e127-e248.
12. Bundy JD, Li C, Stuchlik P, et al. Systolic blood pressure reduction and risk of cardiovascular disease and mortality: a systematic review and network meta-analysis. *JAMA Cardiol*. 2017;2(7):775-781.
13. Grundy SM, Stone NJ, Bailey AL, et al. 2018 AHA/ACC/AACVPR/AAPA/ABC/ACPM/ADA/AGS/APhA/ASPC/NLA/PCNA guideline on the management of blood cholesterol: a report of the American College of Cardiology/American Heart Association Task Force on clinical practice guidelines. *J Am Coll Cardiol*. 2019;73(24):e285-e350. [E-pub ahead of print].
14. Expert Panel on Detection, Evaluation, and Treatment of High Blood Cholesterol in Adults. Executive summary of the third report of the National Cholesterol Education Program (NCEP) expert panel on detection, evaluation, and treatment of high blood cholesterol in adults (adult treatment panel III). *JAMA*. 2001;285:2486-2497.
15. Stone NJ, Robinson JG, Lichtenstein AH, et al. 2013 ACC/AHA guideline on the treatment of blood cholesterol to reduce atherosclerotic cardiovascular risk in adults: a report of the American College of Cardiology/American Heart Association Task Force on Practice Guidelines. *J Am Coll Cardiol*. 2014;63(25 pt B):2889-2934.
16. Writing Committee; Lloyd-Jones DM, Morris PB, Ballantyne CM, et al. 2022 ACC expert consensus decision pathway on the role of nonstatin therapies for LDL-cholesterol lowering in the management of atherosclerotic cardiovascular disease risk: a report of the American College of Cardiology Solution Set Oversight Committee. *J Am Coll Cardiol*. 2022;80(14):1366-1418.
17. Milani RV, Lavie CJ. Prevalence and profile of metabolic syndrome in patients following acute coronary events and effects of therapeutic lifestyle change with cardiac rehabilitation. *Am J Cardiol*. 2003;92(1):50-54.
18. O'Keefe JH, Wetzel M, Moe RR, Bronsnahan K, Lavie CJ. Should an angiotensin-converting enzyme inhibitor be standard therapy for patients with atherosclerotic disease? *J Am Coll Cardiol*. 2001;37:1-8.
19. Abuissa H, Jones PG, Marso SP, O'Keefe JH Jr. Angiotensin-converting enzyme inhibitors or angiotensin receptor blockers for prevention of type

2 diabetes: a meta-analysis of randomized clinical trials. *J Am Coll Cardiol*. 2005;46(5):821-826.

20. Lavie CJ, De Schutter A, Parto P, et al. Obesity and prevalence of cardiovascular diseases and prognosis: the obesity paradox updated. *Prog Cardiovasc Dis*. 2016;58(5):537-547.
21. Lavie CJ, Sharma A, Alpert MA, et al. Update on obesity and obesity paradox in heart failure. *Prog Cardiovasc Dis*. 2016;58(4):393-400.
22. Lavie CJ, Milani RV, Verma A, O'Keefe JH. C-reactive protein and cardiovascular diseases: is it ready for primetime? *Am J Med Sci*. 2009;338(6):486-492.
23. Ridker PM, Danielson E, Fonseca FAH, et al. Rosuvastatin to prevent vascular events in men and women with elevated C-reactive protein. *N Engl J Med*. 2008;359(21):2195-2207.
24. Pearson TA, Mensah GA, Alexander RW, et al. Markers of inflammation and cardiovascular disease: application to clinical and public health practice—a statement for healthcare professionals from the Centers for Disease Control and Prevention and the American Heart Association. *Circulation*. 2003;107(3):499-511.
25. Plenge JK, Hernandez TL, Weil KM, et al. Simvastatin lowers C-reactive protein within 14 days: an effect independent of low-density lipoprotein cholesterol reduction. *Circulation*. 2002;106(12):1447-1452.
26. Lavie CJ, Church TS, Milani RV, Earnest CP. Impact of physical activity, cardiorespiratory fitness, and exercise training on markers of inflammation. *J Cardiopulm Rehabil Prev*. 2011;31(3):137-145.
27. Arena R, Williams M, Forman DE, et al. Increasing referral and participation rates to outpatient cardiac rehabilitation: the valuable role of healthcare professionals in the inpatient and home health settings—a science advisory from the American Heart Association. *Circulation*. 2012;125(10):1321-1329.
28. Menezes AR, Lavie CJ, Milani RV, Forman DE, King M, Williams MA. Cardiac rehabilitation in the United States. *Prog Cardiovasc Dis*. 2014;56(5):522-529.
29. Lavie CJ, Arena R, Franklin BA. Cardiac rehabilitation and healthy life-style interventions: rectifying program deficiencies to improve patient outcomes. *J Am Coll Cardiol*. 2016;67(1):13-15.
30. Vasankari V, Husu P, Vähä-Ypyä H, et al. Association of objectively measured sedentary behaviour and physical activity with cardiovascular disease risk. *Eur J Prev Cardiol*. 2017;24(12):1311-1318.
31. Siscovick DS, Barringer TA, Fretts AM, et al. Omega-3 polyunsaturated fatty acid (fish oil) supplementation and the prevention of clinical cardiovascular disease: a science advisory from the American Heart Association. *Circulation*. 2017;135(15):e867-e884.

PCI Guidelines for the Interventional Cardiology Boards

Jacqueline Tamis-Holland, MD, FSCAI, FACC, FAHA

In December 2021, the American College of Cardiology (ACC)/American Heart Association (AHA)/Society for Cardiovascular Angiography and Interventions (SCAI) published new guidelines for coronary revascularization.[1] These guidelines provide care recommendations for treating patients with acute coronary syndromes (ACSs) and chronic coronary syndromes. The focus of these guidelines have shifted from a "procedural-based" document to a "patient-centered" document. As such, the revascularization guidelines combined the recommendations for percutaneous coronary intervention (PCI) and coronary artery bypass graft (CABG) into one document. These guidelines replace the 2011 PCI Guidelines, the 2011 CABG Guidelines, and the 2015 PCI in ST elevation myocardial infarction (STEMI) update as well as the sections related to revascularization in the 2013 STEMI Guidelines, the 2014 Non ST Elevation Acute Coronary Syndrome (NSTE-ACS) Guidelines, and the 2014 Stable Ischemic Heart Disease Guidelines. These guidelines are intended to provide recommendations regarding the indications for revascularization in certain subgroups of patients, including patients with STEMI, NSTE-ACS, and chronic coronary artery disease (CCD). The guidelines also highlight clinical or anatomic situations in which one revascularization strategy is preferred (ie, CABG vs PCI).

Practice guidelines are the result of a thorough review of evidence with an aim to provide assistance to physicians to select the best management strategy for an individual patient undergoing revascularization. The guidelines are meant to improve quality of care and align with patients' interest. Despite the wide scope of these guidelines, in clinical practice, there can be great variability in patients' circumstances. As such, the guidelines are not intended to replace appropriate clinical judgment. In addition to clinical care, the guidelines can be quite useful for the clinician preparing for the interventional cardiology or general cardiology boards, as many questions on the board exams are derived from material contained in the guidelines.

Data on efficacy and outcomes represent the primary basis for the recommendations contained in the guidelines.[2] The Class of Recommendation (COR) is an estimate of the size of the treatment benefit, considering risks versus benefits. In general, class I recommendations are for the procedure/treatment that should be performed because the treatment is associated with a great benefit, which more than offsets the risk. Class IIa reflects a recommendation where there is likely benefit from the treatments/procedures to be performed and generally the procedure or treatment should be considered. Class IIb recommendations are made when the benefit-to-risk ratio is less certain. Class III denotes those treatments/procedures where the risks outweigh the benefits, and these therapies should not be provided. A class III recommendation can be one with "no benefit" or "harm." The latter of which represents great concern.

The Level of Evidence (LOE) provides information regarding the available data that was used to support a recommendation, with the weight of evidence, ranked as LOE A, B, or C. A recommendation with an LOE A is generally supported by the results of multiple randomized trials or a single "megatrial." An LOE B can be from one or more smaller randomized trials or a moderate sized randomized trial (B-R), or an LOE can be from nonrandomized studies (B-NR). An LOE C is either based on limited clinical data (case reports or case series or smaller studies) (C-LD) or expert opinion (C-EO), the latter of which is usually reserved for COR IIa or COR IIb recommendations. Board questions usually depict a clinical scenario looking for the correct answer based on the recommendations from the guidelines. When preparing for the interventional cardiology boards, one should primarily focus on class I (treatment/procedure that should be performed) and class III (treatment/procedure that should not be performed) recommendations, regardless of the LOE. For this reason, most of the discussion included in this chapter will be related to management options that are supported by class I or III recommendations in the guidelines. The chapter will also discuss the recommendations for medical therapies or procedural preferences for patients being considered or undergoing PCI. Since much of the rationale for specific recommendations are covered in other chapters of this text book, they will not always be included here.

IMPROVING EQUITY IN CARE AND EMPHASIZING SHARED DECISION MAKING

The first recommendation in the 2021 Revascularization Guidelines focuses on reducing disparities in care. The recommendation emphasizes the importance of deciding the optimal revascularization strategy based on a patient's clinical features and coronary anatomy, regardless of sex, race, or ethnicity (class I, LOE B-NR). This stems from data showing ongoing disparities in care for women and certain racial and ethnic groups[3,4] and little evidence to suggest differences in the relative benefit of revascularization for such groups. The subsequent recommendations provide guidance on the importance of shared decision making and informed consent. Physicians should thoughtfully explain the indications for a procedure and the pros and cons of each treatment option with the patient (class I, LOE C-LD). After a careful discussion, treatment decisions should be based on the best available option while incorporating the patient's beliefs, expectations, and priorities for defining a successful outcome (class I, LOE C-LD).

HEART TEAM APPROACH TO REVASCULARIZATION DECISIONS

The core composition for any heart team includes an interventional cardiologist, cardiac surgeon, and the patient's general cardiologist. Additional members of the heart team will depend on the clinical circumstances but may include other medical specialists (nephrology, endocrinology, oncology, or pulmonology), vascular

TABLE 33.1 Clinical Features and Lesion Characteristics Warranting a Heart Team Discussion

CLINICAL CHARACTERISTICS	ANATOMIC CHARACTERISTICS
Diabetes	Left main coronary artery disease
Frailty	Triple-vessel disease involving the left anterior descending artery
Severe lung disease	Multiple chronic total occlusions
Severe liver disease	Other complex coronary artery disease
Chronic kidney disease	Porcelain aorta
Other challenging issues	Severe left ventricular dysfunction

surgery, or social support staff. The foundation for a multidisciplinary approach to consideration for revascularization originates from earlier trials comparing PCI with CABG,[5] which required discussion among the interventional cardiologists and the cardiac surgeons to achieve consensus regarding appropriateness for inclusion within the trials. In patients with unprotected left main and/or complex coronary artery disease (CAD) or for patients with other clinical conditions for whom the optimal approach to revascularization is not clear (**Table 33.1**), the heart team should convene. In many cases, this may require terminating the procedure after diagnostic coronary angiography is performed. This "pause" allows a thorough review of the anatomy and clinical circumstances, and thoughtful input from team members affords both the interventional cardiologist and cardiac surgeon the opportunity to discuss revascularization options with the patient. Calculation of the Society of Thoracic Surgeons score and the SYNTAX score is often useful in making revascularization decisions because they have been shown to predict adverse outcomes in patients undergoing CABG and PCI.[6,7]

ASSESSING LESION SIGNIFICANCE

Despite its inherent limitations, coronary angiography is the default method for assessing the presence and extent of CAD. For lesions not involving the left main coronary artery, an angiographic stenosis of greater than or equal to 70% is considered severe. Lesions involving the left main artery with a 50% or greater diameter narrowing are also considered severe. Due to the eccentric nature of some lesions, these cutoffs become more meaningful when noted in multiple angiographic views. Over the past 10 years, intracoronary physiologic testing with fractional flow reserve (FFR) or instantaneous wave-free ratio (iFR) has emerged as an important tool for assessing lesion significance and to guide PCI. This is based on several studies demonstrating a reduction in clinical events when physiologic testing is used to guide PCI, with iFR showing similar benefits as FFR.[8,9] A large proportion of patients enrolled in the clinical trials to support FFR or iFR had angiographically intermediate lesions, and few patients had prior documented ischemia. For this reason, the assessment of physiologic significance in a patient with stable symptoms and CCD is often focused on the patients with intermediate disease or in patients without a prior stress test. In such cases, physiologic testing should be performed to guide PCI (class I, LOE A). When the results of physiologic testing is normal (ie, FFR > 0.80 or iFR > 0.89), PCI is not recommended (class III—no benefit, LOE-B-R) as prior studies have shown acceptable clinical outcomes with deferral of PCI.[10] Of note, the role of physiologic studies to guide CABG is less well understood.

REVASCULARIZATION IN STEMI

Reperfusion strategies in STEMI include primary PCI or fibrinolytic therapy. Of critical importance is that revascularization, via either modality, be undertaken in a timely fashion. The major challenges in primary PCI, which is the preferred modality, remains the achievement of rapid time to treatment and increased patient access to hospitals that provide primary PCI services. All communities should create and maintain a regional system of STEMI care that includes assessment and continuous quality improvement of emergency medical services (EMSs) and hospital-based activities.[11] Performance can be facilitated by participating in programs such as Mission: Lifeline.[12]

Primary PCI

Numerous trials have demonstrated an advantage of primary PCI to fibrinolytic therapy and a lower short- and long-term mortality with primary PCI even when patients are transferred from other institutions.[13] For this reason, primary PCI should be performed for patients with STEMI and symptom onset <12 hours (**Fig. 33.1**). The goal for treatment for patients presenting directly to a PCI center (either via EMS or walk-in) is <90 minutes from the first medical contact. This means that the time to device goal is 90 minutes beginning at the time that EMS first met the patient for those arriving via EMS and 90 minutes from hospital arrival for "walk-ins." For those patients undergoing interhospital transfer, the first door-to-device time goal is 120 minutes or less. It is important to note that the relative benefit of PCI to fibrinolytic therapy will decrease with increasing PCI-related time delay, but this benefit will also vary based on patient risk.[14] While there may be some benefit to proceeding with PCI in patients with symptom onset >12 hours with unstable features, or in stable patients who present between 12 and 24 hours after symptom onset, PCI of an occluded infarct artery 1 to 28 days after infarction in asymptomatic patients without evidence of severe myocardial ischemia has no incremental benefit beyond optimal medical therapy.[15] **Table 33.2** provides recommendations for primary PCI in patients with STEMI.

PCI After Fibrinolysis

A prolonged delay from hospital presentation to device (ie, >120 minutes for transfer patients) suggests that lytic therapy is preferred to primary PCI. Hospitals without immediate PCI capability should be equipped to provide fibrinolytic therapy (with or without a mechanism for early transfer after routine fibrinolytic therapy and with plans for immediate transfer in cases of failed fibrinolysis) if they anticipate that the average time to transfer their patients to a PCI-capable hospital will generally exceed 120 minutes. With fibrinolytic therapy, the key decision is for whom and when to perform coronary angiography. In cases of suspected fibrinolytic failure, a strategy of immediate coronary angiography followed by PCI improves outcomes.[16] The diagnosis of failed fibrinolysis is best made when there is ongoing chest pain and <50% ST-segment resolution 90 minutes after initiation of therapy in the lead showing the greatest degree of ST-segment elevation at presentation. In otherwise stable patients, studies have shown a lower rate of death or recurrent infarction when patients are routinely transferred to a PCI center for early angiography after fibrinolytic therapy.[17] Given

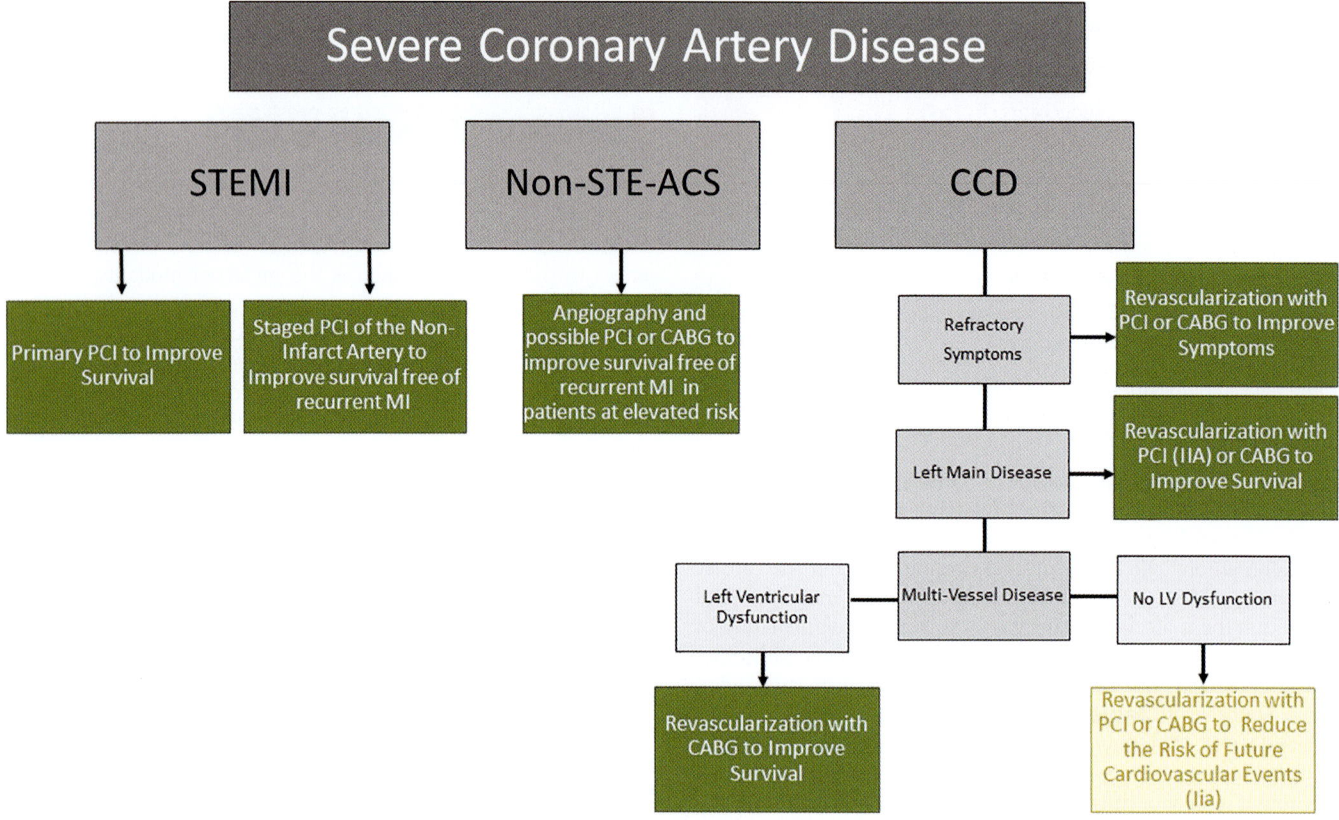

FIGURE 33.1 Indications for revascularization. The figure depicts the indications for revascularization in various clinical settings.

the higher risk of bleeding associated with invasive therapies after fibrinolysis, the greatest benefit from immediate transfer for early angiography and PCI is seen in patients who are at moderate and to high risk for adverse outcomes, such as those with anterior wall myocardial infarction (MI) or inferior wall MI with right ventricular involvement or precordial ST-segment depression as well as patients with ongoing pain. A leading cause of in-hospital mortality in STEMI is cardiogenic shock, and the only treatment proven to decrease mortality is revascularization, predominately through PCI. For this reason, patients who present to hospitals without primary PCI capabilities should be transferred to a PCI center for immediate PCI to improve their chances for survival.[18] **Table 33.2** highlights the recommendations for PCI after fibrinolytic therapy.

PCI of the Noninfarct Artery in STEMI

Over the past 10 years, there has been a greater focus on the utility and timing of PCI of the noninfarct artery in STEMI. Studies have shown safety and feasibility of proceeding with noninfarct artery PCI in STEMI, either at the time of primary PCI[19] or as a staged procedure[20] with a reduction in cardiovascular events when proceeding with complete revascularization. The most robust data supporting complete revascularization in STEMI comes from the Complete versus Culprit-Only Revascularization Strategies to Treat Multivessel Disease after Early PCI for STEMI (COMPLETE) trial, which reported a 24% reduction in the rate of death or recurrent MI at 3 years of follow-up with staged PCI of the noninfarct artery in patients with STEMI.[20] For this reason, in select patients with anatomy suitable for PCI, staged PCI of the noninfarct artery is recommended (**Fig. 33.1**). Contrary to expectations, multivessel PCI at the time of primary PCI in cases of acute MI complicated by cardiogenic shock is associated with a worse outcome.[21] **Table 33.2** provides key recommendations for managing the noninfarct artery in STEMI.

Early Angiography With Intent for Revascularization in NSTE-ACS

In patients with NSTE-ACS, early risk stratification is essential to help determine the best strategy (invasive or ischemia guided) and to determine the timing of coronary angiography. Various risk scores have been developed, but the TIMI risk score and GRACE score are most commonly used in clinical trials. Studies have shown a lower risk of cardiovascular events including lower rates of recurrent MI and the combined endpoint of death or recurrent MI and fewer symptoms in longer-term follow-up with a routine invasive strategy.[22] However, the benefits of an invasive strategy have not been reported in low-risk patients (ie, troponin-negative ACS). **Table 33.2** provides the key recommendations for invasive angiography with the intent to proceed with revascularization in NSTE-ACS. Unstable patients with NSTE-ACS who have cardiogenic shock, hemodynamic compromise, electrical instability, or refractory symptoms should be referred for immediate angiography with the intention of proceeding with early revascularization. In the absence of these features, an invasive strategy, with early angiography (within 12-24 hours) with the intention of proceeding with revascularization is indicated in patients who are at high risk for ischemic events (**Fig. 33.1**). For the remaining patients, angiography before discharge is a reasonable option. Unlike STEMI in which PCI is generally preferred, the choice of revascularization technique for patients with NSTE-ACS should be based on the anatomical considerations used for patients with CCD, with the caveat that PCI (particularly in the unstable patient) may be initially preferred regardless of anatomical characteristics to stabilize

TABLE 33.2 Key Guideline Recommendations for Angiography and/or PCI in Acute Coronary Syndromes

PCI of the infarct artery in STEMI	
Class I LOE A	In patients with STEMI and ischemic symptoms for <12 h, PCI should be performed to improve survival
Class I LOE B-R	In patients with STEMI and cardiogenic shock or hemodynamic instability, PCI or CABG (when PCI is not feasible) is indicated to improve survival, irrespective of the time delay from MI onset
Class I LOE C-LD	In patients with STEMI and evidence of failed reperfusion after fibrinolytic therapy, rescue PCI of the infarct artery should be performed to improve clinical outcomes
Class III—no benefit LOE B-R	In asymptomatic stable patients with STEMI who have a totally occluded infarct artery >24 h after symptom onset and are without evidence of severe ischemia, PCI should not be performed
PCI of the noninfarct artery in STEMI	
Class I LOE A	In selected hemodynamically stable patients with STEMI and multivessel disease, after successful primary PCI, staged PCI of a significant noninfarct artery stenosis is recommended to reduce the risk of death or MI
Class III—harm LOE B-R	In patients with STEMI complicated by cardiogenic shock, routine PCI of a noninfarct artery at the time of primary PCI should not be performed because of the higher risk of death or renal failure
Invasive angiography with intent for revascularization in NSTE-ACS	
Class I LOE A	In patients with NSTE-ACS who are at elevated risk of recurrent ischemic events and are appropriate candidates for revascularization, an invasive strategy with the intent to proceed with revascularization is indicated to reduce cardiovascular events
Class I LOE B-R	In patients with NSTE-ACS and cardiogenic shock who are appropriate candidates for revascularization, emergency revascularization is recommended to reduce the risk of death
Class I LOE C-LD	In appropriate patients with NSTE-ACS who have refractory angina or hemodynamic or electrical instability, an immediate invasive strategy with intent to perform revascularization is indicated to improve outcomes
Class IIa LOE B-R	In patients with NSTE-ACS who are initially stabilized and are at high risk of clinical events, it is reasonable to choose an early invasive strategy (within 24 h) over a delayed invasive strategy to improve outcomes
Class III—harm LOE B-R	In patients with NSTE-ACS who present in cardiogenic shock, routine multivessel PCI of nonculprit lesions in the same setting should not be performed

CABG, coronary artery bypass graft; LOE, Level of Evidence; MI, myocardial infarction; NSTE-ACS, non-ST elevation acute coronary syndrome; PCI, primary percutaneous intervention; STEMI, ST elevation myocardial infarction.

the patient. As was reported in patients with STEMI, single-setting multivessel PCI for patients with non-ST elevation infarction complicated by cardiogenic shock is associated with a worse outcome.[21]

REVASCULARIZATION IN CCD

The goals of revascularization for patients with CCD are to improve survival, reduce the risk of future cardiovascular events (such as but not limited to recurrent infarction, repeat revascularization, or hospitalization for unstable symptoms), and/or to relieve symptoms (**Table 33.3**; **Fig. 33.1**). When discussing options for revascularization with the patient, they should understand when the procedure is being performed in an attempt to improve overall outcomes, improve symptoms, or both.

Revascularization to Improve Survival in CCD

With a goal toward improving survival, there are a few important situations when revascularization has been associated with a reduction in all-cause mortality. These include patients with left ventricular (LV) dysfunction and patients with significant left main CAD.

Left Ventricular Dysfunction

Patients with multivessel CAD and LV dysfunction represent a high-risk subset with mortality rates of 33% in long-term follow-up.[23] An earlier report evaluating this subgroup of patients enrolled in the Coronary Artery Surgery Study demonstrated a survival advantage with CABG compared to conservative care in patients with triple-vessel disease and a left ventricular ejection fraction (LVEF) of 35% to 50%.[24] In the Surgical Treatment for Ischemic Heart Failure (STITCH) trial,[25] enrolling 1212 patients with multivessel CAD and an ischemic cardiomyopathy (LVEF ≤ 35%), the primary endpoint, all-cause survival at 5 years was not significantly different for the group of patients randomized to CABG versus medical therapy. However, at 10 years of follow-up, CABG was associated with a significant reduction in all-cause mortality.[26] For this reason, in appropriate candidates with a presumed ischemic cardiomyopathy and anatomy suitable for CABG, surgery is indicted to improve survival.

There are no recommendations in the 2021 Revascularization Guidelines regarding the role of PCI for patients with CAD and an ischemic cardiomyopathy. Since the publication of these guidelines, the Revascularization for Ischemic Ventricular Dysfunction (REVIVED-BCIS2) trial,[23] reported on 700 patients with an ischemic cardiomyopathy (LVEF ≤ 35%) and extensive CAD amenable to PCI, who were randomized to revascularization with PCI plus optimal medical therapy or optimal medical therapy alone. Over a mean follow-up of 41 months, the primary endpoint, all-cause mortality, or hospitalization for heart failure was not significantly different between the two groups. Additionally, there was no significant difference in the extent of improvement in LVEF in between the groups, although Kansas City Cardiomyopathy Questionnaire scores were slightly improved with PCI. This study is the only randomized trial evaluating the benefits of PCI on outcomes in patients with an ischemic cardiomyopathy. Given the absence of a clear benefit from revascularization with PCI, caution is warranted

TABLE 33.3 Key Guideline Recommendations for Revascularization in Chronic Coronary Syndromes

Revascularization to improve survival	
Class I LOE B-R	In patients with SIHD and multivessel CAD appropriate for CABG with severe left ventricular systolic dysfunction (left ventricular ejection fraction <35%), CABG is recommended to improve survival
Class I LOE B-R	In patients with SIHD and significant left main stenosis, CABG is recommended to improve survival
Class IIa LOE B-NR	In selected patients with SIHD and multivessel CAD appropriate for CABG and mild-to-moderate left ventricular systolic dysfunction (ejection fraction 35%–50%), CABG (to include a left internal mammary artery [LIMA] graft to the LAD) is reasonable to improve survival
Class IIa LOE B-NR	In selected patients with SIHD and significant left main stenosis for whom PCI can provide equivalent revascularization to that possible with CABG, PCI is reasonable to improve survival
Class III—no benefit LOE B-R	In patients with SIHD, normal left ventricular ejection fraction, and 1- or 2-vessel CAD not involving the proximal LAD, coronary revascularization is not recommended to improve survival
Class III—harm LOE B-NR	In patients with SIHD who have ≥1 coronary arteries that are not anatomically or functionally significant (<70% diameter stenosis of non-left main coronary artery or FFR >0.80), coronary revascularization should not be performed with the primary or sole intent to improve survival
Revascularization to reduce the risk of future cardiovascular events	
Class IIa LOE B-R	In patients with SIHD and multivessel CAD appropriate for either CABG or PCI, revascularization is reasonable to lower the risk of cardiovascular events, such as spontaneous MI, unplanned urgent revascularizations, or cardiac death
Revascularization to relieve symptoms	
Class I LOE A	In patients with refractory angina despite medical therapy and with significant coronary artery stenoses amenable to revascularization, revascularization is recommended to improve symptoms
Class III—harm LOE C-LD	In patients with angina but no anatomic or physiological criteria for revascularization, neither CABG nor PCI should be performed

CABG, coronary artery bypass graft; CAD, coronary artery disease; FFR, fractional flow reserve; LAD, left anterior descending artery; LOE, Level of Evidence; PCI, primary percutaneous intervention; SIHD, stable ischemic heart disease.

when proceeding with PCI in this subset of patients if the sole intent is to improve survival.

Left Main CAD

The prognosis for patients with untreated left main disease is poor with earlier registry data reporting 15-year mortality rates approaching 75%. The evidence to inform the recommendations for revascularization with CABG in patients with left main disease are derived from studies performed over 40 years ago but have reported a survival advantage with CABG.[27] Given the lack of clinical equipoise in this subset of patients, there are no contemporary randomized trials comparing revascularization with medical therapy for patients with left main CAD. However, in patients with low to intermediate left main disease, the studies comparing PCI to CABG demonstrated similar survival with PCI compared to CABG.[28] Therefore, PCI is also a reasonable option. It is important to recognize that when deciding between PCI and CABG, anatomic and clinical features remain an important determinant of strategy and the heart team should play a critical role in this decision making.[29]

Revascularization to Reduce the Risk of Future Cardiovascular Events

Traditionally, the guidelines have focused on the benefit of revascularization to improve mortality or improve symptoms. However, there are other clinical events that are important to patients that might warrant consideration for revascularization including a reduction in the risk of spontaneous MI, urgent revascularization, or the combined endpoint of death (or cardiac death) and spontaneous MI. No study has demonstrated a benefit in reducing the risk of these endpoints with revascularization for patients with single- or double-vessel disease.[30,31] And for this reason, there is no role for revascularization to improve cardiovascular outcomes in patients with single- or double-vessel disease not involving the left main and with normal LV function. However, in patients with extensive CAD, subgroup analyses of clinical studies have demonstrated a reduction in cardiovascular death, spontaneous infarction, or the combined endpoint of cardiovascular death or MI with revascularization.[32,33] For this reason, revascularization is reasonable in this subset of patients.

Revascularization to Improve Symptoms

Revascularization techniques and medical therapy have improved substantially during the last 40 years. The effectiveness in controlling symptoms has improved with both modalities. Despite the improvement in medical therapies, numerous studies have demonstrated superiority of revascularization over medical therapies.[34] While the gap between revascularization techniques and guideline-directed medical therapy (GDMT) is narrower, the failure of GDMT to provide symptomatic relief justifies the need for elective revascularization, and in these circumstances, revascularization is recommended.

CONSIDERATIONS ON THE CHOICE OF REVASCULARIZATION

While there are clear benefits to revascularization in patients with acute and chronic CAD, the decision to choose one strategy over another will often depend on the clinical presentation and

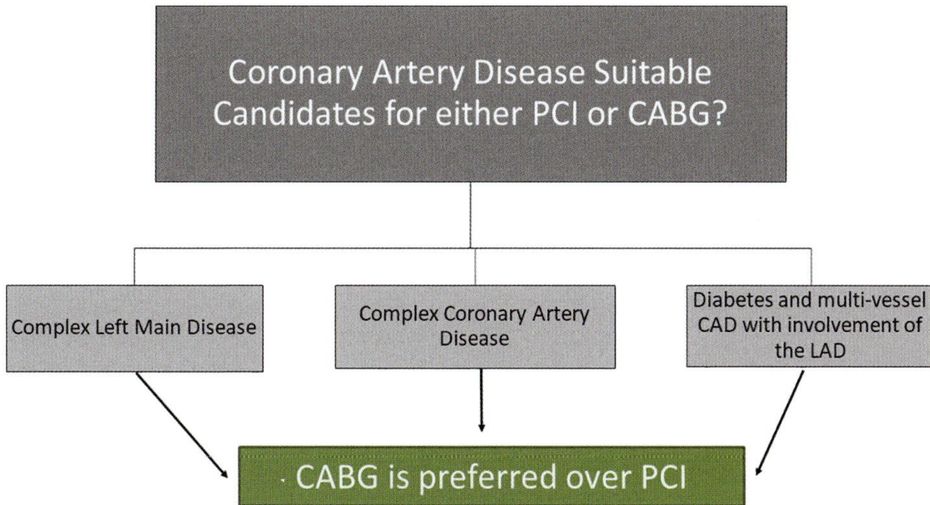

FIGURE 33.2 Choice of revascularization. The figure depicts the clinical and anatomic situations when CABG is preferred over PCI. For complex left main and for patients with diabetes, CABG is recommended over PCI to improve survival. For complex CAD, it is reasonable to choose CABG over PCI. CABG, coronary artery bypass graft; CAD, coronary artery disease; PCI, percutaneous coronary intervention.

the extent of disease (**Fig. 33.2**). **Table 33.4** provides the key guideline recommendations for choice of revascularization. PCI is typically reserved for those patients with single- or double-vessel disease, especially when there is no significant disease in the left anterior descending artery (LAD), while CABG is preferred for more complex disease, including complex left main disease, or complex triple-vessel disease. Additionally, studies have shown a benefit of revascularization with CABG (with an internal thoracic artery [IMA] to the LAD) over PCI for those patients with diabetes and multivessel disease involving the LAD.[35] In the Future Revascularization Evaluation in Patients with Diabetes Mellitus: Optimal Management of Multivessel Disease (FREEDOM) trial, which randomized 1900 patients with diabetes and multivessel disease to a strategy of CABG or PCI, CABG was associated with a significantly lower rate of the primary outcome of death, nonfatal infarction, and nonfatal stroke, as well as a lower all-cause mortality.[36] On the other hand, patients with diabetes and multivessel disease who are at high risk of CABG may be best treated with PCI providing the anatomy is suitable for PCI. In patients with prior CABG, if the IMA to the LAD is patent, then it is logical to attempt revascularization with PCI. However, if there is diffuse or complex disease without a patent IMA graft to the LAD, then revascularization with a reop CABG may be a more appropriate approach to care. Finally, in patients with multivessel disease suitable for either PCI or CABG, who cannot tolerate or will not be compliant with antiplatelet therapies, then it is logical to choose CABG over PCI.

TABLE 33.4 Key Guideline Recommendations for Choice of Revascularization

Class I LOE A	In patients with diabetes and multivessel CAD with the involvement of the LAD, who are appropriate candidates for CABG, CABG (with a LIMA to the LAD) is recommended in preference to PCI to reduce mortality and repeat revascularizations
Class I LOE B-R	In patients who require revascularization for significant left main CAD with high-complexity CAD, it is recommended to choose CABG over PCI to improve survival
Class IIa LOE B-R	In patients who require revascularization for multivessel CAD with complex or diffuse CAD (eg, SYNTAX score >33), it is reasonable to choose CABG over PCI to confer a survival advantage
Class IIa LOE B-NR	In patients with diabetes who have multivessel CAD amenable to PCI and an indication for revascularization and are poor candidates for surgery, PCI can be useful to reduce long-term ischemic outcomes
Class IIa LOE B-NR	In patients with previous CABG with a patent LIMA to the LAD who need repeat revascularization, if PCI is feasible, it is reasonable to choose PCI over CABG
Class IIa LOE C-LD	In patients with previous CABG and refractory angina on GDMT that is attributable to LAD disease, it is reasonable to choose CABG over PCI when an internal mammary artery (IMA) can be used as a conduit to the LAD
Class IIa LOE B-NR	In patients with multivessel CAD amenable to treatment with either PCI or CABG who are unable to access, tolerate, or adhere to DAPT for the appropriate duration of treatment, CABG is reasonable in preference to PCI

CABG, coronary artery bypass graft; CAD, coronary artery disease; GDMT, guideline-directed medical therapy; IMA, internal mammary artery; LAD, left anterior descending artery; LIMA, left internal mammary artery; LOE, Level of Evidence; PCI, primary percutaneous intervention.

SPECIAL POPULATIONS

There are various situations in which a patient's clinical circumstances may alter the way we manage a patient with CAD. For example, coronary angiography and revascularization has not been shown to be beneficial in patients with chronic kidney disease (CKD) and stable symptoms, and therefore, in patients with CKD, if there is no compelling reason to proceed with angiography and revascularization, a conservative approach is recommended. This is based on data from the International Study of Comparative Health Effectiveness with Medical and Invasive Approaches-CKD (ISCHEMIA-CKD) trial, which failed to demonstrate any benefit to angiography with the intent to proceed with revascularization in patients with CKD and intermediate- to high-risk findings on noninvasive stress testing.[37] Similarly while PCI is recommended in patients with ACSs, it is not recommended for patients who have ACSs due to spontaneous coronary artery dissection, if they are stable and do not have ongoing symptoms or evidence of hemodynamic compromise. There are a wide array of various patient subgroups that derive specific benefit or lack of benefit with revascularization that are discussed in this section. **Table 33.5** highlights the key guideline recommendations for revascularization in special populations. For a more detailed review, please refer to the Revascularization Guideline document.

PROCEDURAL CONSIDERATIONS FOR PCI

Radial Access

Radial artery access has become increasingly more popular due to the ease in access and avoidance of major vascular complications that can be encountered with femoral artery access. Over the past 10 years, numerous studies have explored the benefits of radial artery access and have demonstrated lower rates of bleeding and access site complications[38] with radial artery access. Additionally, in patients with ACS undergoing coronary angiography, pooled data have shown that radial artery access is associated with reduced mortality.[38] For this reason, when performing coronary angiography, radial artery access is recommended (**Table 33.6**). While there was a concern regarding the use of radial artery access and longer door to balloon times for patients with STEMI, studies have shown that it would require a very long delay in access site times to offset the benefits of radial artery access.[39] Despite the clear patient benefits, some studies have reported greater radiation dose for the operator with radial access even among experienced operators.[40] For this reason, the operator must pay particular attention to radiation safety in this setting.

TABLE 33.5 Key Guideline Recommendations for Revascularization in Special Populations

Older patients	
Class I LOE B-NR	In older adults, as in all patients, the treatment strategy for CAD should be based on an individual patient's preferences, cognitive function, and life expectancy
Patients with ventricular arrhythmias	
Class I LOE B-NR	In patients with ventricular fibrillation, polymorphic ventricular tachycardia, or cardiac arrest, revascularization of significant CAD is recommended to improve survival
Class III LOE C-LD	In patients with CAD and suspected scar-mediated sustained monomorphic VT, revascularization is not recommended for the sole purpose of preventing recurrent VT
Patients with chronic kidney disease	
Class I LOE C-LD	In patients with CKD undergoing contrast media injection for coronary angiography, measures should be taken to minimize the risk of contrast-induced AKI
Class I LOE C-EO	In patients with STEMI and CKD, coronary angiography and revascularization are recommended, with adequate measures to reduce the risk of AKI
Class III LOE B-R	In asymptomatic patients with stable CAD and CKD, routine angiography and revascularization are not recommended if there is no compelling indication
Patients with SCAD	
Class III—harm LOE C-LD	Routine revascularization for SCAD should not be performed
Patients undergoing noncardiac surgery	
Class III LOE B-R	In patients with non-left main or noncomplex CAD who are undergoing noncardiac surgery, routine coronary revascularization is not recommended solely to reduce perioperative cardiovascular events

AKI, acute kidney injury; CAD, coronary artery disease; CKD, chronic kidney disease; LOE, Level of Evidence; SCAD, spontaneous coronary artery dissection; STEMI, ST elevation myocardial infarction; VT, ventricular tachycardia.

Choice of Stents

Prior guidelines advised bare metal stents or balloon angioplasty over drug-eluting stents for those patients unable to tolerate longer dual antiplatelet therapy (DAPT) or if there was an anticipated future surgical procedure.[41] With the evolution of drug-eluting stent designs incorporating thinner stent struts, and various drug-delivery systems, the newer generation drug-eluting stents have been shown to have excellent safety and efficacy profiles and lower rates of stent thrombosis when compared to bare metal stents.[42] Drug-eluting stents have also been shown to be superior to other methods of treating restenosis.[43] For this reason, drug-eluting stents are recommended for treatment of de novo lesions and restenotic lesions (**Table 33.6**).

Use of Aspiration Thrombectomy in STEMI

Aspiration thrombectomy is a useful procedure when treating patients with refractory thrombus or no reflow. However, "routine" aspiration thrombectomy as a first-line agent in patients with STEMI has not been proven beneficial and is associated with a numerically increased risk of stroke.[44] For this reason, routine aspiration thrombectomy before primary PCI is not recommended (**Table 33.6**). It is important to recognize that this recommendation does not apply to selective or bailout aspiration thrombectomy, defined as thrombectomy that was initially unplanned but was later used during the procedure because of an unsatisfactory initial result or a procedural complication.

INTRAVASCULAR IMAGING

Intravascular imaging can be useful to allow a better understanding of lesion significance and lesion composition, including the presence and extent of coronary calcium, or to determine the mechanisms for stent failure.[45] For procedural planning, intravascular imaging allows for a more accurate measurement of reference vessel diameter and lesion length and provides information to optimally identify the "stent landing zones." Intravascular imaging also provides a more detailed assessment of the extent of stent expansion and apposition. Additionally, proximal and distal edge dissections are better identified with intravascular imaging.[45,46] Intravascular ultrasound (IVUS) can also be useful for assessing lesion significance in patients with intermediate left main disease in which there can be great variability in angiographic results. IVUS uses minimal luminal diameter to

TABLE 33.6 Key Guideline Recommendations Regarding Best Practices for PCI

Radial artery access	
Class I LOE A	In patients with ACS undergoing PCI, a radial approach is indicated in preference to a femoral approach to reduce the risk of death, vascular complications, or bleeding
Class I LOE A	In patients with SIHD undergoing PCI, the radial approach is recommended to reduce access site bleeding and vascular complications
Choice of stents	
Class I LOE A	In patients undergoing PCI, DES should be used in preference to BMS to prevent restenosis, MI, or acute stent thrombosis
Class I LOE A	In patients who develop clinical in-stent restenosis (ISR) for whom repeat PCI is planned, a DES should be used to improve outcomes if anatomic factors are appropriate and the patient is able to comply with DAPT
Thrombus aspiration	
Class III—no benefit LOE A	In patients with STEMI, routine aspiration thrombectomy before primary PCI is not useful
Class III—harm LOE B-R	In patients with STEMI complicated by cardiogenic shock, routine PCI of a noninfarct artery at the time of primary PCI should not be performed because of the higher risk of death or renal failure
Intravascular imaging	
Class IIa LOE B-R	In patients with intermediate stenosis of the left main artery, intravascular ultrasound (IVUS) is reasonable to help define lesion severity
Class IIa LOE B-R	In patients undergoing coronary stent implantation, IVUS can be useful for procedural guidance, particularly in cases of left main or complex coronary artery stenting, to reduce ischemic events
Class IIa LOE B-R	In patients undergoing coronary stent implantation, OCT is a reasonable alternative to IVUS for procedural guidance, except in ostial left main disease
Class IIa LOE C-LD	In patients with stent failure, IVUS or OCT is reasonable to determine the mechanism of stent failure
SVG PCI	
Class IIa LOE C-LD	In select patients with previous CABG undergoing PCI of a SVG, the use of an embolic protection device, when technically feasible, is reasonable to decrease the risk of distal embolization
Class IIa LOE B-NR	In patients with previous CABG, if PCI of a diseased native coronary artery is feasible, then it is reasonable to choose PCI of the native coronary artery over PCI of the severely diseased SVG
Class III—no benefit LOE C-LD	In patients with a chronic occlusion of a SVG, percutaneous revascularization of the SVG should not be performed

ACS, acute coronary syndromes; BMS, bare metal stent; CABG, coronary artery bypass graft; DES, drug-eluting stent; LOE, Level of Evidence; OCT, optimal coherence tomography; PCI, percutaneous coronary intervention; SVG, saphenous vein graft.

assess lesion severity, and in left main coronary artery, a variety of cutoffs have been advised including a minimum luminal area (MLA) of 6.0 mm^2 and an MLA of 7.5 mm^2. For these reasons, intravascular imaging is recommended as a reasonable option for lesion assessment (in cases of intermediate left main stenosis) or to guide PCI (**Table 33.6**).

It is important to note that since the publication of these guidelines various observational studies and meta-analyses have demonstrated a reduction in cardiovascular death and all-cause mortality with intravascular imaging to guide PCI, especially when used in complex lesions.[47,48] The Randomized Controlled Trial of Intravascular Imaging Guidance Versus Angiography-Guidance on Clinical Outcomes After Complex Percutaneous Coronary Intervention (RENOVATE-COMPLEX-PCI) trial[49] randomized 1639 patients undergoing complex PCI to a strategy of intravascular imaging-guided PCI or angiography-guided PCI. Imaging-guided PCI was associated with a 36% reduction in the primary composite endpoint of cardiovascular death, target vessel-related MI or clinically driven target vessel revascularization, and a lower rate of cardiovascular death.

TREATMENT OF SAPHENOUS VEIN GRAFTS

PCIs of saphenous vein grafts (SVGs) are associated with higher rates of ischemic events. Observational studies have reported an increased risk of no reflow and in-hospital mortality after SVG PCI as compared to PCI of the native vessel.[50] Embolic protection devices (EPDs) in SVG intervention had previously been recommended for SVG PCI[41]; however, more recent data have reported conflicting results with the use of EPDs,[51] and for this reason, the use of EPD in SVG PCI was downgraded to a IIA in the current guidelines (**Table 33.6**).[1] In cases where there is a chronic total occlusion of the SVG, PCI is not indicated because it is associated with low success rates and poor long-term patency rates.

MEDICAL THERAPIES

Anticoagulant Therapy

Anticoagulants have been used to support PCI since the introduction of PCI over 30 years ago. Unfractionated heparin remains the most commonly used anticoagulant for PCI. Other agents that can be used to support PCI include bivalirudin or enoxaparin. **Table 33.7** provides the key guideline recommendations for anticoagulant use in PCI. Enoxaparin is generally only used to support PCI in patients who are already on a therapeutic dose prior to PCI. For this reason, heparin should not be administered for PCI in patients who are already on a therapeutic dose of enoxaparin at the time of PCI. Bivalirudin and argatroban are also used to support PCI in patients with a history of heparin-induced thrombocytopenia.

Antiplatelet Therapy

Antiplatelet therapy remains a pivotal part of the treatment of patients with CAD undergoing PCI. Aspirin (325 mg) should be given before or at the time of PCI. The optimal chronic aspirin dose in patients treated with DAPT that provides protection from ischemic events while minimizing bleeding risk is 81 mg (range 75-100 mg).[52] Following PCI, aspirin (81 mg daily) should be continued indefinitely (**Table 33.7**).

P2Y12 receptor inhibitors should be given to all patients undergoing PCI. For those patients not already treated with a P2Y12 receptor inhibitor, a loading dose is recommended at the time of PCI followed by chronic therapies for 3 to 12 months (see section on *Duration of DAPTs* for details regarding DAPT duration). In patients undergoing elective PCI, clopidogrel is recommended. A loading dose of 600 mg allows for more rapid platelet inhibition compared to a 300-mg loading dose and has similar benefits to a 900-mg loading dose.[53] In patients with ACSs, prasugrel and ticagrelor are preferred over clopidogrel as they are associated with a lower rate of major cardiovascular events. In the TRial to Assess Improvement in Therapeutic Outcomes by Optimizing Platelet InhibitioN with Prasugrel-Thrombolysis In Myocardial Infarction (TRITON-TIMI 38),[54] prasugrel as

TABLE 33.7 Key Guideline Recommendations Regarding Anticoagulant and Antiplatelet Therapies for PCI

Anticoagulants	
Class I LOE C-EO	In patients undergoing PCI, administration of intravenous unfractionated heparin (UFH) is useful to reduce ischemic events
Class I LOE C-EO	In patients with heparin-induced thrombocytopenia undergoing PCI, bivalirudin or argatroban should be used to replace UFH to avoid thrombotic complications
Class III—harm LOE B-R	In patients on therapeutic subcutaneous enoxaparin, in whom the last dose was administered within 12 h of PCI, UFH should not be used for PCI and may increase bleeding
Antiplatelets	
Class I LOE B-R	In patients undergoing PCI, a loading dose of aspirin, followed by daily dosing, is recommended to reduce ischemic events
Class I LOE B-R	In patients with ACS undergoing PCI, a loading dose of P2Y12 inhibitor, followed by daily dosing, is recommended to reduce ischemic events
Class I LOE C-LD	In patients with SIHD undergoing PCI, a loading dose of clopidogrel, followed by daily dosing, is recommended to reduce ischemic events
Class I LOE C-LD	In patients undergoing PCI within 24 h after fibrinolytic therapy, a loading dose of 300 mg of clopidogrel, followed by daily dosing, is recommended to reduce ischemic events
Class IIa LOE B-R	In patients with ACS undergoing PCI, it is reasonable to use ticagrelor or prasugrel in preference to clopidogrel to reduce ischemic events, including stent thrombosis
Class III—harm LOE B-R	In patients undergoing PCI who have a history of stroke or transient ischemic attack, prasugrel should not be administered
Class III—no benefit LOE B-R	In patients with SIHD undergoing PCI, the routine use of an intravenous glycoprotein IIb/IIIA inhibitor agent is not recommended
Duration of DAPT	
Class I LOE B-R	In patients with SIHD treated with DAPT after DES implantation, P2Y12 inhibitor therapy (clopidogrel) should be given for at least 6 mo
Class I LOE B-R	In patients with ACS (NSTE-ACS or STEMI) treated with DAPT after BMS or DES implantation, P2Y12 inhibitor therapy (clopidogrel, prasugrel, or ticagrelor) should be given for at least 12 mo
Class IIa LOE B-A	In selected patients undergoing PCI, shorter-duration DAPT (1-3 mo) is reasonable, with subsequent transition to P2Y12 inhibitor monotherapy to reduce the risk of bleeding events
DAPT for patients with AF on anticoagulants	
Class I LOE B-R	In patients with atrial fibrillation who are undergoing PCI and are taking oral anticoagulant therapy, it is recommended to discontinue aspirin treatment after 1 to 4 wk while maintaining P2Y12 inhibitors in addition to a non-vitamin K oral anticoagulant (rivaroxaban, dabigatran, apixaban, or edoxaban) or warfarin to reduce the risk of bleeding

ACS, acute coronary syndrome; BMS, bare metal stent; DAPT, dual antiplatelet therapy; DES, drug-eluting stent; LOE, Level of Evidence; NSTE-ACS, non-ST elevation ACS; PCI, percutaneous coronary intervention; SIHD, stable ischemic heart disease; UFH, unfractionated heparin.

compared with clopidogrel was associated with a significant 19% reduction in relative risk of the composite endpoint of cardiovascular death, nonfatal MI, or nonfatal stroke. Somewhat offsetting this was a significant increase in the rate of TIMI major bleeding. Prasugrel is contraindicated in patients with a history of transient ischemic attack or stroke and should be used with caution in patients older than 75 years and in patients weighing less than 60 kg because of an increased risk of bleeding. Ticagrelor, unlike clopidogrel or prasugrel, is not a thienopyridine, and it also does not require metabolic conversion to an active metabolite. In ACS patients enrolled in the Platelet Inhibition and Patient Outcomes (PLATO) trial,[55] ticagrelor was associated with a significant 16% reduction in relative risk in the primary composite endpoint of vascular death, nonfatal MI, or nonfatal stroke compared to clopidogrel. Importantly, a significant reduction in vascular mortality and all-cause mortality was observed. In the PLATO trial, the key safety endpoint of major bleeding was not different between the two groups; however, the secondary safety endpoint of non-CABG major bleeding was significantly higher with ticagrelor as compared with clopidogrel. Ticagrelor and prasugrel have not been studied in elective PCI, thus no recommendation can be made regarding its use in this clinical setting. **Table 33.7** highlights the key recommendations for P2Y12 inhibitor use in patients undergoing PCI.

For patients not pretreated with oral P2Y12 inhibitors, in particular those at higher risk for ischemic events, intravenous antiplatelet agents targeting the glycoprotein IIB/IIIA receptor or the ADP receptor can be considered. However, with the institution of more potent oral agents with more rapid onset of platelet inhibition, there is no longer a role for intravenous glycoprotein IIB/IIIA receptor inhibitors in elective PCI (**Table 33.7**).

Duration of DAPTs

Over the years, the options for DAPTs and duration of use have greatly evolved. These regimens require a careful balance of the risks of thrombotic events and the potential for bleeding complications and should be individualized. A shorter duration of DAPT followed by aspirin monotherapy is associated with less bleeding when compared with DAPTs >12 months, while longer durations of DAPT are associated with a lower ischemic risk including the risk of MI or stent thrombosis but at the expense of more major bleeding.[56] The 2016 Guidelines for Duration of DAPT recommend 12 months of DAPT for patients undergoing PCI for ACS and 6 months of DAPT followed by aspirin monotherapy after elective PCI.[57] Since the publication of the 2016 DAPT guidelines, newer RCT and meta-analysis have demonstrated lower bleeding risk with shorter duration of DAPT (for 1-3 months) followed by P2Y12 monotherapy.[58-60] It is important to recognize that the trials exploring the benefits of P2Y12 monotherapy after a brief treatment with DAPT were not powered for ischemic endpoints including stent thrombosis. However pooled data of these trials have shown similar rates of stent thrombosis and major cardiovascular events with a shorter duration of DAPT followed by P2Y12 monotherapy when compared with standard DAPT.[61] The key guideline recommendations from the 2016 DAPT guidelines and the 2021 Revascularization guidelines related to the duration of DAPT after PCI are highlighted in **Table 33.7**.

The concomitant use of anticoagulant therapies with DAPT increases bleeding risk.[62] Over the past 5 years, several studies have explored a strategy of dual antithrombotic agents after a brief period of triple therapy following PCI.[63-66] Collectively, these studies have shown a reduction in bleeding events with dual therapies.[62] Importantly, these studies were not powered for ischemic events. A numerically higher rate of stent thrombosis in the first 30 days after cessation of aspirin has been reported,[67] and for this reason, concomitant aspirin therapy is generally advised for 1 to 4 weeks post PCI in patients treated with oral anticoagulants (**Table 33.7**).

POSTPROCEDURAL MANAGEMENT

Preventive therapies and lifestyle changes are a pivotal part of the management of patients with acute and chronic CAD undergoing PCI. This includes optimization of cholesterol, blood pressure, and blood glucose levels, smoking cessation, weight reduction for those who are overweight or obese, and the implementation of a regular exercise routine. To ensure patient compliance and participation in these lifestyle recommendations, it is important to understand the psychosocial factors that might impact patient participation and compliance with postprocedure care. Patient education (class I, LOE C-LD), smoking cessation counseling and treatment (class I, LOE A), management of depression (class I, LOE B-R), and participation in outpatient cardiac rehabilitation (class I, LOE A) will improve success in achieving these goals and are recommended.

ASSESSMENT OF OUTCOMES AFTER PCI

PCI quality and performance considerations are defined by attributes related to structure, processes, and risk-adjusted outcomes. They could be used for internal quality-improvement efforts and public reporting. Reporting of institutional risk-adjusted outcomes to allow the hospital system to benchmark their results with nationwide outcomes is becoming more common and is more reliable than operator-level outcomes due to lack of statistical power resulting from lower volumes. The 2021 Revascularization guidelines recommend PCI programs participate in state, regional, or national clinical data registries so that they may receive feedback regarding their risk-adjusted outcomes (class I, LOE B-NR).

SUMMARY

This chapter represents a summary of the ACC-AHA-SCAI Coronary Revascularization Guidelines published in 2021 along with a summary of the 2016 ACC-AHA Guidelines on the duration of DAPT after PCI. These recommendations should be used by the interventional and clinical cardiologist to guide management decisions for patients with CAD. The material covered here and in other chapters will be the foundation for a majority of interventional cardiology board questions, usually in the form of case scenarios. While this chapter highlighted some situations for which there are class IIa recommendations ("is reasonable"), when preparing for the boards, and in clinical practice, special attention should be placed on the class I and III recommendation for a particular topic because most of the questions will test a candidates' ability to identify "the most appropriate treatment" (class I) or one that is harmful or not useful (class III).

Key Points

- For the interventional cardiology boards (and in clinical practice), focus on class I and III recommendations.
- PCI is the preferred reperfusion strategy in STEMI, with the goal of first medical contact to balloon time <90 minutes for direct presenters and first door to device of <120 minutes for patients transferred from an outside institution.
- In select patients with STEMI, staged PCI of the noninfarct artery after successful primary PCI is recommended.
- An early invasive strategy is recommended in high-risk patients with non-STE ACS.
- The goals of PCI in patients with CCD are to improve MACE-free survival and/or symptoms.
- CABG is preferred over PCI in patients with complex disease, including complex left main disease and/or multivessel disease and in patients with diabetes and multivessel disease involving the LAD.
- Radial artery access is recommended.
- DAPT should be continued for at least 6 months after elective PCI and for 12 months following PCI for ACS.
- As an alternative, a shorter duration of DAPT followed by P2Y12 monotherapy is reasonable to reduce bleeding.
- In patients with atrial fibrillation undergoing PCI, dual antithrombotic therapy (after a brief period of triple therapy) is recommended over triple therapy.

References

1. Lawton JS, Tamis-Holland JE, Bangalore S, et al. 2021 ACC/AHA/SCAI guideline for coronary artery revascularization: a report of the American College of Cardiology/American Heart Association Joint Committee on Clinical Practice Guidelines. *Circulation*. 2022;145(3):e18-e114.
2. Halperin JL, Levine GN, Al-Khatib SM, et al. Further evolution of the ACC/AHA clinical practice guideline recommendation classification system: a report of the American College of Cardiology/American Heart Association Task Force on Clinical Practice Guidelines. *J Am Coll Cardiol*. 2016;67(13):1572-1574.
3. Arora S, Stouffer GA, Kucharska-Newton A, et al. Fifteen-year trends in management and outcomes of non-ST-segment-elevation myocardial infarction among black and white patients: the ARIC community surveillance study, 2000-2014. *J Am Heart Assoc*. 2018;7(19):e010203.
4. Gudnadottir GS, Andersen K, Thrainsdottir IS, James SK, Lagerqvist B, Gudnason T. Gender differences in coronary angiography, subsequent interventions, and outcomes among patients with acute coronary syndromes. *Am Heart J*. 2017;191:65-74.
5. Serruys PW, Morice MC, Kappetein AP, et al. Percutaneous coronary intervention versus coronary-artery bypass grafting for severe coronary artery disease. *N Engl J Med*. 2009;360(10):961-972.
6. Ad N, Holmes SD, Patel J, Pritchard G, Shuman DJ, Halpin L. Comparison of EuroSCORE II, original EuroSCORE, and the Society of Thoracic Surgeons risk score in cardiac surgery patients. *Ann Thorac Surg*. 2016;102(2):573-579.
7. Takahashi K, Serruys PW, Fuster V, et al. Redevelopment and validation of the SYNTAX score II to individualise decision making between percutaneous and surgical revascularisation in patients with complex coronary artery disease: secondary analysis of the multicentre randomised controlled SYNTAXES trial with external cohort validation. *Lancet*. 2020;396(10260):1399-1412.
8. Tonino PAL, De Bruyne B, Pijls NHJ, et al. Fractional flow reserve versus angiography for guiding percutaneous coronary intervention. *N Engl J Med*. 2009;360(3):213-224.
9. Davies JE, Sen S, Dehbi HM, et al. Use of the instantaneous wave-free ratio or fractional flow reserve in PCI. *N Engl J Med*. 2017;376(19):1824-1834.
10. Escaned J, Ryan N, Mejía-Rentería H, et al. Safety of the deferral of coronary revascularization on the basis of instantaneous wave-free ratio and fractional flow reserve measurements in stable coronary artery disease and acute coronary syndromes. *JACC Cardiovasc Interv*. 2018;11(15):1437-1449.
11. Jacobs AK, Antman EM, Ellrodt G, et al. Recommendation to develop strategies to increase the number of ST-segment-elevation myocardial infarction patients with timely access to primary percutaneous coronary intervention. *Circulation*. 2006;113(17):2152-2163.
12. Jollis JG, Al-Khalidi HR, Roettig ML, et al. Impact of regionalization of ST-segment-elevation myocardial infarction care on treatment times and outcomes for emergency medical services-transported patients presenting to hospitals with percutaneous coronary intervention: mission—lifeline accelerator-2. *Circulation*. 2018;137(4):376-387.
13. Keeley EC, Boura JA, Grines CL. Primary angioplasty versus intravenous thrombolytic therapy for acute myocardial infarction: a quantitative review of 23 randomised trials. *Lancet*. 2003;361(9351):13-20.
14. Pinto DS, Kirtane AJ, Nallamothu BK, et al. Hospital delays in reperfusion for ST-elevation myocardial infarction: implications when selecting a reperfusion strategy. *Circulation*. 2006;114(19):2019-2025.
15. Hochman JS, Lamas GA, Buller CE, et al. Coronary intervention for persistent occlusion after myocardial infarction. *N Engl J Med*. 2006;355(23):2395-2407.
16. Gershlick AH, Stephens-Lloyd A, Hughes S, et al. Rescue angioplasty after failed thrombolytic therapy for acute myocardial infarction. *N Engl J Med*. 2005;353(26):2758-2768.
17. Borgia F, Goodman SG, Halvorsen S, et al. Early routine percutaneous coronary intervention after fibrinolysis vs. standard therapy in ST-segment elevation myocardial infarction: a meta-analysis. *Eur Heart J*. 2010;31(17):2156-2169.
18. Babaev A, Frederick PD, Pasta DJ, et al. Trends in management and outcomes of patients with acute myocardial infarction complicated by cardiogenic shock. *JAMA*. 2005;294(4):448-454.
19. Wald DS, Morris JK, Wald NJ, et al. Randomized trial of preventive angioplasty in myocardial infarction. *N Engl J Med*. 2013;369(12):1115-1123.
20. Mehta SR, Wood DA, Storey RF, et al. Complete revascularization with multivessel PCI for myocardial infarction. *N Engl J Med*. 2019;381(15):1411-1421.
21. Thiele H, Akin I, Sandri M, et al. PCI strategies in patients with acute myocardial infarction and cardiogenic shock. *N Engl J Med*. 2017;377(25):2419-2432.
22. Mehta SR, Cannon CP, Fox KAA, et al. Routine vs selective invasive strategies in patients with acute coronary syndromes: a collaborative meta-analysis of randomized trials. *JAMA*. 2005;293(23):2908-2917.
23. Perera D, Clayton T, O'Kane PD, et al. Percutaneous revascularization for ischemic left ventricular dysfunction. *N Engl J Med*. 2022;387(15):1351-1360.
24. Passamani E, Davis KB, Gillespie MJ, Killip T. A randomized trial of coronary artery bypass surgery. Survival of patients with a low ejection fraction. *N Engl J Med*. 1985;312(26):1665-1671.
25. Velazquez EJ, Lee KL, Deja MA, et al. Coronary-artery bypass surgery in patients with left ventricular dysfunction. *N Engl J Med*. 2011;364(17):1607-1616.
26. Velazquez EJ, Lee KL, Jones RH, et al. Coronary-artery bypass surgery in patients with ischemic cardiomyopathy. *N Engl J Med*. 2016;374(16):1511-1520.
27. Yusuf S, Zucker D, Peduzzi P, et al. Effect of coronary artery bypass graft surgery on survival: overview of 10-year results from randomised trials by the Coronary Artery Bypass Graft Surgery Trialists Collaboration. *Lancet*. 1994;344(8922):563-570.
28. Sabatine MS, Bergmark BA, Murphy SA, et al. Percutaneous coronary intervention with drug-eluting stents versus coronary artery bypass grafting in left main coronary artery disease: an individual patient data meta-analysis. *Lancet*. 2021;398(10318):2247-2257.

29. Davidson LJ, Cleveland JC, Welt FG, et al. A practical approach to left main coronary artery disease: JACC state-of-the-art review. *J Am Coll Cardiol*. 2022;80(22):2119-2134.
30. Boden WE, O'Rourke RA, Teo KK, et al. Optimal medical therapy with or without PCI for stable coronary disease. *N Engl J Med*. 2007;356(15):1503-1516.
31. BARI 2D Study Group. A randomized trial of therapies for type 2 diabetes and coronary artery disease. *N Engl J Med*. 2009;360(24):2503-2515.
32. Chaitman BR, Hardison RM, Adler D, et al. The Bypass Angioplasty Revascularization Investigation 2 Diabetes randomized trial of different treatment strategies in type 2 diabetes mellitus with stable ischemic heart disease: impact of treatment strategy on cardiac mortality and myocardial infarction. *Circulation*. 2009;120(25):2529-2540.
33. Reynolds HR, Shaw LJ, Min JK, et al. Outcomes in the ISCHEMIA trial based on coronary artery disease and ischemia severity. *Circulation*. 2021;144(13):1024-1038.
34. Wijeysundera HC, Nallamothu BK, Krumholz HM, Tu JV, Ko DT. Meta-analysis: effects of percutaneous coronary intervention versus medical therapy on angina relief. *Ann Intern Med*. 2010;152(6):370-379.
35. Head SJ, Milojevic M, Daemen J, et al. Mortality after coronary artery bypass grafting versus percutaneous coronary intervention with stenting for coronary artery disease: a pooled analysis of individual patient data. *Lancet*. 2018;391(10124):939-948.
36. Farkouh ME, Domanski M, Sleeper LA, et al. Strategies for multivessel revascularization in patients with diabetes. *N Engl J Med*. 2012;367(25):2375-2384.
37. Bangalore S, Maron DJ, O'Brien SM, et al. Management of coronary disease in patients with advanced kidney disease. *N Engl J Med*. 2020;382(17):1608-1618.
38. Mason PJ, Shah B, Tamis-Holland JE, et al. An update on radial artery access and best practices for transradial coronary angiography and intervention in acute coronary syndrome: a scientific statement from the American Heart Association. *Circ Cardiovasc Interv*. 2018;11(9):e000035.
39. Wimmer NJ, Cohen DJ, Wasfy JH, Rathore SS, Mauri L, Yeh RW. Delay in reperfusion with transradial percutaneous coronary intervention for ST-elevation myocardial infarction: might some delays be acceptable? *Am Heart J*. 2014;168(1):103-109.
40. Sciahbasi A, Calabrò P, Sarandrea A, et al. Randomized comparison of operator radiation exposure comparing transradial and transfemoral approach for percutaneous coronary procedures: rationale and design of the minimizing adverse haemorrhagic events by TRansradial access site and systemic implementation of angioX—RAdiation Dose study (RAD-MATRIX). *Cardiovasc Revasc Med*. 2014;15(4):209-213.
41. Levine GN, Bates ER, Blankenship JC, et al. 2011 ACCF/AHA/SCAI guideline for percutaneous coronary intervention: a report of the American College of Cardiology Foundation/American Heart Association Task Force on Practice Guidelines and the Society for Cardiovascular Angiography and Interventions. *Circulation*. 2011;124(23):e574-e651.
42. Bangalore S, Kumar S, Fusaro M, et al. Short- and long-term outcomes with drug-eluting and bare-metal coronary stents: a mixed-treatment comparison analysis of 117 762 patient-years of follow-up from randomized trials. *Circulation*. 2012;125(23):2873-2891.
43. Siontis GC, Stefanini GG, Mavridis D, et al. Percutaneous coronary interventional strategies for treatment of in-stent restenosis: a network meta-analysis. *Lancet*. 2015;386(9994):655-664.
44. Jolly SS, James S, Džavík V, et al. Thrombus aspiration in ST-segment-elevation myocardial infarction: an individual patient meta-analysis—Thrombectomy Trialists Collaboration. *Circulation*. 2017;135(2):143-152.
45. Truesdell AG, Alasnag MA, Kaul P, et al. Intravascular imaging during percutaneous coronary intervention: JACC state-of-the-art review. *J Am Coll Cardiol*. 2023;81(6):590-605.
46. Räber L, Mintz GS, Koskinas KC, et al. Clinical use of intracoronary imaging. Part 1: guidance and optimization of coronary interventions. An expert consensus document of the European Association of Percutaneous Cardiovascular Interventions. *EuroIntervention*. 2018;14(6):656-677.
47. Darmoch F, Alraies MC, Al-Khadra Y, Moussa Pacha H, Pinto DS, Osborn EA. Intravascular ultrasound imaging–guided versus coronary angiography–guided percutaneous coronary intervention: a systematic review and meta-analysis. *J Am Heart Assoc*. 2020;9(5):e013678.
48. Hannan EL, Zhong Y, Reddy P, et al. Percutaneous coronary intervention with and without intravascular ultrasound for patients with complex lesions: utilization, mortality, and target vessel revascularization. *Circ Cardiovasc Interv*. 2022;15(6):e011687.
49. Lee JM, Choi KH, Song YB, et al. Intravascular imaging–guided or angiography-guided complex PCI. *N Engl J Med*. 2023;388(18):1668-1679.
50. Brilakis ES, Rao SV, Banerjee S, et al. Percutaneous coronary intervention in native arteries versus bypass grafts in prior coronary artery bypass grafting patients: a report from the National Cardiovascular Data Registry. *JACC Cardiovasc Interv*. 2011;4(8):844-850.
51. Shoaib A, Kinnaird T, Curzen N, et al. Outcomes following percutaneous coronary intervention in saphenous vein grafts with and without embolic protection devices. *JACC Cardiovasc Interv*. 2019;12(22):2286-2295.
52. Jolly SS, Pogue J, Haladyn K, et al. Effects of aspirin dose on ischaemic events and bleeding after percutaneous coronary intervention: insights from the PCI-CURE study. *Eur Heart J*. 2009;30(8):900-907.
53. von Beckerath N, Taubert D, Pogatsa-Murray G, Schömig E, Kastrati A, Schömig A. Absorption, metabolization, and antiplatelet effects of 300-600- and 900-mg loading doses of clopidogrel: results of the ISAR-CHOICE (intracoronary stenting and antithrombotic regimen—choose between 3 high oral doses for immediate clopidogrel effect) trial. *Circulation*. 2005;112(19):2946-2950.
54. Wiviott SD, Braunwald E, McCabe CH, et al. Prasugrel versus clopidogrel in patients with acute coronary syndromes. *N Engl J Med*. 2007;357(20):2001-2015.
55. Wallentin L, Becker RC, Budaj A, et al. Ticagrelor versus clopidogrel in patients with acute coronary syndromes. *N Engl J Med*. 2009;361(11):1045-1057.
56. Evidence Review Committee Members; Bittl JA, Baber U, Bradley SM, Wijeysundera DN. Duration of dual antiplatelet therapy: a systematic review for the 2016 ACC/AHA guideline focused update on duration of dual antiplatelet therapy in patients with coronary artery disease—a report of the American College of Cardiology/American Heart Association Task Force on Clinical Practice Guidelines. *Circulation*. 2016;134(10):e156-e178.
57. Levine GN, Bates ER, Bittl JA, et al. 2016 ACC/AHA guideline focused update on duration of dual antiplatelet therapy in patients with coronary artery disease: a report of the American College of Cardiology/American Heart Association Task Force on Clinical Practice Guidelines. An update of the 2011 ACCF/AHA/SCAI guideline for percutaneous coronary intervention, 2011 ACCF/AHA guideline for coronary artery bypass graft surgery, 2012 ACC/AHA/ACP/AATS/PCNA/SCAI/STS guideline for the diagnosis and management of patients with stable ischemic heart disease, 2013 ACCF/AHA guideline for the management of ST-elevation myocardial infarction, 2014 AHA/ACC guideline for the management of patients with non–ST-elevation acute coronary syndromes, and 2014 ACC/AHA guideline on perioperative cardiovascular evaluation and management of patients undergoing noncardiac surgery. *Circulation*. 2016;134(10):e123-e155.
58. Mehran R, Baber U, Sharma SK, et al. Ticagrelor with or without aspirin in high-risk patients after PCI. *N Engl J Med*. 2019;381(21):2032-2042.
59. Watanabe H, Domei T, Morimoto T, et al. Effect of 1-month dual antiplatelet therapy followed by clopidogrel vs 12-month dual antiplatelet therapy on cardiovascular and bleeding events in patients receiving PCI: the STOPDAPT-2 randomized clinical trial. *JAMA*. 2019;321(24):2414-2427.
60. Kim BK, Hong SJ, Cho YH, et al. Effect of ticagrelor monotherapy vs ticagrelor with aspirin on major bleeding and cardiovascular events in patients with acute coronary syndrome: the TICO randomized clinical trial. *JAMA*. 2020;323(23):2407-2416.
61. Giacoppo D, Matsuda Y, Fovino LN, et al. Short dual antiplatelet therapy followed by P2Y12 inhibitor monotherapy vs. prolonged dual antiplatelet therapy after percutaneous coronary intervention with second-generation drug-eluting stents: a systematic review and meta-analysis of randomized clinical trials. *Eur Heart J*. 2021;42(4):308-319.
62. Khan SU, Osman M, Khan MU, et al. Dual versus triple therapy for atrial fibrillation after percutaneous coronary intervention: a systematic review and meta-analysis. *Ann Intern Med*. 2020;172(7):474-483.

63. Lopes RD, Heizer G, Aronson R, et al. Antithrombotic therapy after acute coronary syndrome or PCI in atrial fibrillation. *N Engl J Med.* 2019;380(16):1509-1524.
64. Vranckx P, Valgimigli M, Eckardt L, et al. Edoxaban-based versus vitamin K antagonist-based antithrombotic regimen after successful coronary stenting in patients with atrial fibrillation (ENTRUST-AF PCI): a randomised, open-label, phase 3b trial. *Lancet.* 2019;394(10206):1335-1343.
65. Gibson CM, Mehran R, Bode C, et al. Prevention of bleeding in patients with atrial fibrillation undergoing PCI. *N Engl J Med.* 2016;375(25):2423-2434.
66. Cannon CP, Bhatt DL, Oldgren J, et al. Dual antithrombotic therapy with dabigatran after PCI in atrial fibrillation. *N Engl J Med.* 2017;377(16):1513-1524.
67. Lopes RD, Leonardi S, Wojdyla DM, et al. Stent thrombosis in patients with atrial fibrillation undergoing coronary stenting in the AUGUSTUS trial. *Circulation.* 2020;141(9):781-783.

Thoracic Aortic, Abdominal Aortic, and Lower Extremity Interventions

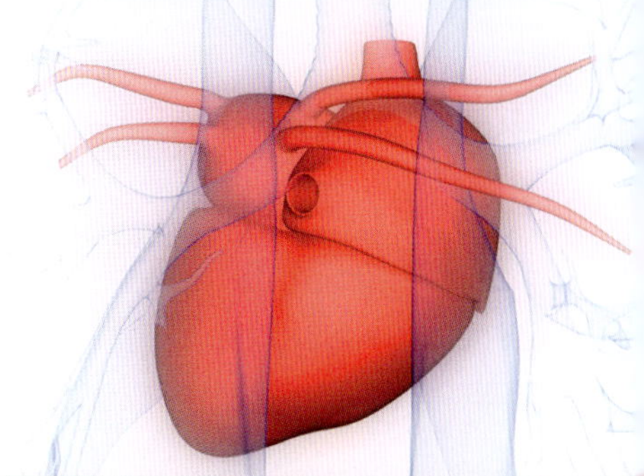

Sonal Pruthi, Sareena George, Daniel Snyder, Robert S. Zilinyi, Ari J. Mintz, Sanjum S. Sethi, and Sahil A. Parikh

Interventional cardiovascular specialists encounter peripheral artery disease (PAD) in all aspects of routine clinical practice. Even the most skilled operators will occasionally cause peripheral vascular complications that require interventional therapy. As such, an understanding of the basic principles and indications for peripheral revascularization is critical for all interventionalists, including those who do not routinely perform noncoronary interventions. Interventionalists are also increasingly involved in the treatment of all manifestations of PAD. This chapter succinctly summarizes thoracic, aortic, and lower extremity interventions, with an emphasis on what should be anticipated on the interventional cardiology board examination.

THORACIC AORTA

Subclavian and Brachiocephalic Intervention

Obstructive disease of the major aortic arch vessels supplying the upper extremities is a common condition affecting up to 7% of individuals in select populations.[1] When atherosclerotic in nature, subclavian and brachiocephalic disease is predominantly ostial or proximal in location, but other conditions—such as fibromuscular dysplasia, medium- and large-vessel vasculitides (eg, Takayasu arteritis, giant cell arteritis), thoracic outlet syndrome, or radiation-induced disease—may cause lesions in more distal locations.[2]

Symptoms of subclavian obstruction include arm claudication that manifests as fatigue, paresthesia, or pain during exertion. Proximal left subclavian artery stenosis may also impede antegrade flow through the left vertebral or internal mammary (LIMA) arteries, resulting in symptoms of vertebrobasilar insufficiency or angina when the LIMA has been used for coronary artery bypass grafting (CABG).

Revascularization of the brachiocephalic or subclavian arteries is indicated in the presence of significant symptoms, such as arm claudication, vertebrobasilar insufficiency, or angina. Additionally, when the LIMA is required as a conduit for CABG surgery, empiric revascularization of left subclavian artery stenosis is appropriate, even in the absence of symptoms. Importantly, isolated identification of flow reversal in the vertebral artery—a common finding on Doppler ultrasound examinations—should not prompt revascularization in asymptomatic patients unless the internal mammary is needed for arterial bypass.

Technically, percutaneous revascularization of the subclavian and brachiocephalic arteries is successful in >95% of cases and mostly used for atherosclerotic lesions.[3] In the presence of vasculitis, the most recent guidelines from the American College of Rheumatology guidelines recommend against invasive therapy and favor medical management and escalation of immunosuppression unless there is risk to life or organ function, refractory hypertension, or when a patient's activities are significantly affected, given elevated surgical risk given the nature of the disease.[4] Single-center data of endovascular treatment of Takayasu arteritis reported that subclavian lesions had lower late success rate and required more interventions when compared to other lesions (aortic, axillary, mesenteric, iliac, and renal), likely due to long and diffuse nature of disease in this segment. Thus, even when endovascular treatment of vasculitis is technically feasible, caution should be exercised in decision making.[4]

No randomized data exist comparing open surgical revascularization with stenting. The femoral approach is most often utilized, although brachial or radial access may facilitate treatment of chronic total occlusions (CTOs), where it may be difficult to localize the vessel's origin from the aortic arch or to maintain adequate catheter support to cross the occlusion.[5] Ostial and proximal lesions are generally treated with balloon-expandable stents (BESs) because radial force is desirable and this region is not exposed to extrinsic compression. For lesions located in the more distal portions of these vessels, self-expanding stents (SESs) may be preferred to accommodate for the increased mobility of the vessels in these regions. If, however, the lesion is just distal to the origin of the mammary or vertebral arteries, brachial or radial access should be considered to ensure that SES deployment does not inadvertently cover the origins of these vessels. Atheroembolization, while uncommon, represents a devastating potential complication and can occur due to the direct route to the cerebral circulation through the vertebral artery. Some operators advocate the use of cerebral embolic protection at the time of treatment of bulky or angiographically "worrisome" subclavian or brachiocephalic lesions,[6] but no convincing data are available to validate this strategy. **Fig. 34.1** shows stenting of a symptomatic right subclavian artery stenosis.

Coarctation

Aortic coarctation is a discrete narrowing of the thoracic aorta that preferentially occurs in proximity to the ligamentum arteriosum. It is the sixth most common form of congenital heart disease and commonly occurs with other congenital lesions, classically in association with bicuspid aortic valves. Coarctation in children and adults is most commonly manifested as hypertension and should be suspected in the presence of a brachial-femoral artery pulse delay. Individuals with unrepaired coarctation are at an increased risk of cardiovascular events, including stroke, heart failure, and death.

Endovascular or surgical repair is recommended in individuals with a gradient of >20 mm Hg across the segment of coarctation. Because collateralization may reduce the detectable gradient across the coarcted segment, intervention should also be considered in lower gradient states if diagnostic imaging demonstrates significant collateral flow. Surgical repair and endovascular angioplasty are both acceptable modes of therapy. In general, surgical repair is reserved for those with compelling anatomical indications such as branch artery involvement or associated large aneurysmal dilatation. Angioplasty is associated with significant recurrence rates; primary stenting is therefore generally preferred. The risk of aneurysm formation following surgical or endovascular treatment of

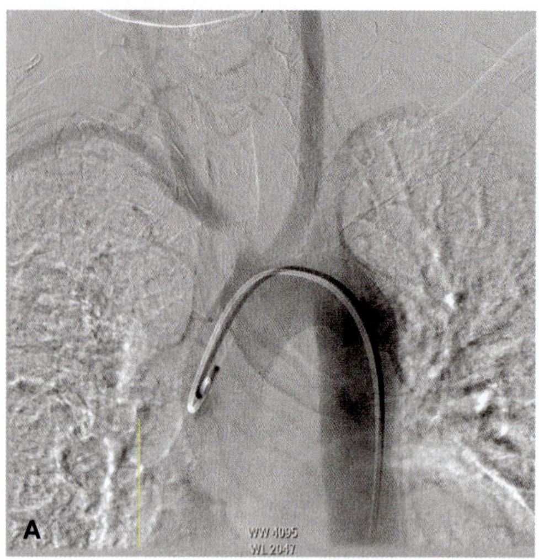

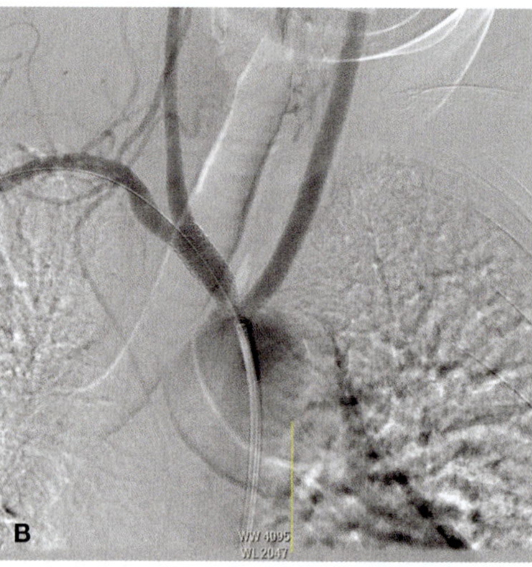

FIGURE 34.1 Subclavian intervention in a 46-year-old male with symptomatic subclavian artery stenosis. **A:** Severe stenosis is demonstrated in the proximal right subclavian artery. A 70 mm Hg gradient was present across this lesion. **B:** Following predilation, a 10.0 × 20 mm balloon-expandable stent was deployed with excellent angiographic results with no gradient postprocedure.

coarctation is significant, and patients with a history of coarctation repair should receive annual follow-up with thoracic aortic imaging at regular intervals.[7]

ACUTE AORTIC SYNDROMES

Acute aortic syndromes include aortic dissection, intramural hematoma, aortic pseudoaneurysm, and penetrating aortic ulcer.[8] Aortic dissections are classified as type A (occurring with the proximal tear in the ascending aorta or arch) or type B (occurring distal to the left subclavian artery). Intramural hematoma represents the presence of an aortic wall hematoma in the absence of an intimal tear. Aortic pseudoaneurysms and penetrating aortic ulcers represent an important subset of acute aortic pathologies. Most pseudoaneurysms occur as a result of blunt trauma (eg, following motor vehicle accident), whereas penetrating aortic ulcers tend to occur among patients with advanced atherosclerotic disease. The presence of a type A aortic dissection represents a surgical emergency; in contrast, the management of a type B dissection depends on the presence of distal organ malperfusion, such as renal dysfunction, mesenteric ischemia, or limb ischemia. In the absence of end-organ malperfusion, most cases of descending thoracic acute aortic syndromes are managed medically, with a focus on meticulous control of blood pressure to minimize subsequent extension of the dissection flap.[9] In the case of type B aortic dissection with malperfusion, thoracic endovascular aortic repair (TEVAR) with a covered stent graft may be considered to cover the site of the tear. Among patients with type B aortic dissection who are initially managed conservatively, approximately 25% to 30% develop aneurysmal degeneration of the aorta or extension of the dissection during the ensuing 5 years and consequently require endovascular repair.

THORACIC AORTIC ANEURYSM

Thoracic aortic aneurysms (TAAs) comprise approximately one-third of all aortic aneurysms. There are multiple etiologies of TAA, including atherosclerotic disease, aneurysmal progression at a site of prior dissection, and predisposing genetic disease states, such as Marfan syndrome. The majority of TAAs are asymptomatic and are detected on ultrasound or by computed tomography (CT) scan. The indications for repair include a symptomatic TAA, an asymptomatic ascending TAA of 5 to 6 cm, or an asymptomatic descending TAA of 6 to 7 cm diameter.[10] These thresholds for repair are a general guide for therapy because patients with genetic etiologies may benefit from earlier repair, due to the natural history of continued progression, while patients with significant comorbidities may be more favorably managed with continued monitoring until a higher threshold for repair is reached. The majority of ascending TAA are repaired surgically, although branched and fenestrated stent graft devices are being developed to promote future endovascular approaches. The majority of descending TAA may be repaired with TEVAR stent grafts.

ABDOMINAL AORTA

Abdominal aortic aneurysm (AAA) remains a prevalent condition that poses a significant risk of death from rupture. Tobacco use, Caucasian race, and male gender are the classic associated risk factors, while, interestingly, diabetes is associated with a reduced rate of AAA.[11] Current recommendations support a one-time ultrasound screening for AAA in males aged 65 to 74 with a history of smoking.[12] Other societal guidelines also suggest screening among patients with a family history of AAA, regardless of gender or smoking history. The most recent guidelines from the Society of Vascular Medicine suggested screening for AAA in first-degree relatives of patients who present with an AAA. Screening should be performed in first-degree relatives who are between 65 and 75 years of age or if older than 75 years and in good health.[13]

Open surgical repair was historically considered the standard of care, but more recently, endovascular aneurysm repair (EVAR) has been utilized in the majority of cases owing to its lower periprocedural risk.[14,15] Repair should be considered for the treatment of AAA larger than 5.5 cm, AAA that are expanding rapidly (>0.5 cm over 6 months), or for those of any size that are symptomatic. According to guidelines, ultrasound when feasible was recommended as preferred imaging modality for aneurysm screening and surveillance.

The most recent guidelines from the Society of Vascular surgery suggested the use of Vascular Quality Initiative (VQI) mortality risk score (class IIC) to be used as a basis of decision making in conjunction with mutual decision making with patients considering aneurysm repair.

In addition, they also specified that elective EVAR be limited to hospitals with a documented mortality and conversion rate to open surgical repair of <2% and perform at least 10 EVAR cases

TABLE 34.1 Randomized Trials of EVAR Versus Open Surgical Repair

TRIAL	PATIENTS	COMPARISON	FOLLOW-UP DURATION	PRIMARY ENDPOINT	SECONDARY ENDPOINTS
DREAM	351	EVAR vs open repair in surgically eligible patients	6 y	Cumulative survival, 69.9% vs 68.9%, *P* = NS	Freedom from reintervention, 81.9% vs 70.4% favoring open repair, *P* = .03
EVAR-1	1252	EVAR vs open repair in surgically eligible patients	6 y	Death, 7.5 vs 7.7 deaths per 100 patient-years, *P* = NS	Reintervention 5.1 vs 1.7 per 100 patient-years favoring open repair, *P* < .001
EVAR-2	404	EVAR vs no repair in surgically ineligible patients	6.1 y	Death, 21.0 vs 22.1 deaths per 100 patient-years, *P* = NS	Aneurysm-related mortality 3.6 vs 7.3 deaths per 1000 patient-years, *P* = .02

EVAR, endovascular aneurysm repair; NS, not significant.

each year. Similarly, open elective aneurysm repair be limited to hospitals with a mortality of <5% and perform at least 10 open aortic operations every year.[13]

EVAR is a reasonable option for those at high risk for open repair with suitable anatomy, and for other patients, the guidelines recommend decisions based on the VQI score. This is based on data from three major randomized trials summarized in **Table 34.1**. Overall, these trials indicate that EVAR is associated with lower short-term mortality than surgical revascularization, but long-term mortality is similar between treatment groups.[16-18] EVAR is associated with a higher rate of reintervention, approaching 25% at 5-year follow-up. These trials utilized older stent graft devices; newer-generation devices may improve technical success and are likely associated with lower rates of long-term reintervention.

Currently, the majority (approximately 80%) of patients with AAA in the United States are treated with EVAR. Factors that may favor open surgery include complex anatomy not amenable to endovascular repair, young age, and patients less willing to maintain close follow-up for surveillance and possible reintervention. There is a growing range of commercially available devices designed for the endovascular treatment of AAA. In general, these devices are comprised of SESs with interwoven fabric to exclude the aneurysmal segment and suprarenal fixation to prevent device migration. The sheath sizes of these devices have also decreased over time, and the majority of patients may now be treated using a fully percutaneous approach, including "preclosure" with a large suture-mediated closure device technique for management of the arteriotomy.

Importantly, patients who undergo EVAR require long-term surveillance in order to monitor for device failure, while such surveillance is generally not necessary for patients who undergo surgical repair. The major long-term complications associated with EVAR include the following: lack of an effective seal between the endograft and the aorta with consequent "type 1" endoleak and aneurysm expansion; or the persistent communication of collateral arteries and the aneurysm sac, resulting in "type II" endoleak and aneurysm expansion.

Endovascular repair is the preferred mechanism of repair in rupture aneurysms according to the current guidelines, and door to intervention time of <90 minutes is recommended.

LOWER EXTREMITY

General Overview

Lower extremity PAD is a highly prevalent condition and is estimated to affect ≈236 million adults (5.6%) worldwide. The prevalence of PAD has increased from 2000 to 2015 by ≈45% globally.[19] The majority of patients with PAD are asymptomatic, and most will not develop limb-threatening ischemia over time. Additionally, in symptomatic individuals, natural history studies suggest that most (70%-80%) will have stable claudication symptoms and that, fortunately, <4% will require amputation during long-term follow-up.[20] In patients who develop chronic limb-threatening ischemia (CLTI), 1-year cumulative incidence for mortality and amputation is ~20% with and ~50% at 5 years.[21] Occasionally, iliac revascularization is indicated to facilitate passage/placement of large bore devices (percutaneous left ventricular assist device, transcatheter aortic valve replacement, and endovascular aortic repair).

The mainstay of therapy for PAD includes risk factor modification to reduce the profound associated cardiovascular morbidity: smoking cessation, cholesterol reduction, treatment of diabetes, antihypertensive therapy, and antiplatelet therapy.[22]

Conservative management includes hygienic and supportive measures to prevent skin breakdown and infection, exercise conditioning, and pharmacotherapy for claudication.

Endovascular therapy is not indicated in patients with asymptomatic PAD. There is no evidence that symptomatic clinical outcome can be improved or averted by prophylactic revascularization (endovascular or surgical) and is not recommended in asymptomatic patients.[23]

Percutaneous revascularization of the lower extremities is commonly reserved for treatment of lifestyle-limiting symptoms that have persisted despite conservative measures, or for limb-threatening ischemia, namely rest pain or tissue loss.[23] As a general principle, inflow disease (ie, the more proximal segments) should be treated first for patients with claudication. In cases of critical limb ischemia (CLI), multilevel intervention is often necessary to establish straight-line flow to the affected limb.

Iliac Interventions

The TransAtlantic Inter-Society Consensus (TASC) document classification was developed to categorize aortoiliac lesions and guide therapy (**Table 34.2**).[24] In the TASC document, endovascular therapy was recommended for TASC A and B lesions, surgery was recommended for TASC D lesions, and individually tailored decisions were considered for TASC C lesions. While the TASC classification system provided a useful schema to categorize lesion complexity, the evolution of endovascular technology and techniques have permitted access to increasingly complex patients and lesions and have rendered the guidelines expressed in this landmark document less relevant to contemporary clinical practice. In

TABLE 34.2 TASC Lesion Classification

TASC CATEGORY	LESION CHARACTERISTICS
Aortoiliac	
A	Unilateral or bilateral stenosis of CIA, unilateral or bilateral stenoses of EIA (<3 cm)
B	Stenosis of infrarenal aorta (<3 cm), unilateral CIA occlusion, stenoses of EIA 3-10 cm in length not involving CFA, unilateral EIA occlusion not involving IIA or CFA
C	Bilateral CIA occlusions, bilateral EIA stenoses 3-10 cm in length, unilateral EIA stenosis extending into CFA, unilateral EIA occlusion involving IIA or CFA, heavily calcified unilateral EIA occlusion
D	Infrarenal aortoiliac occlusion, diffuse aortic and bilateral CIA disease requiring treatment, multiple stenoses involving CIA, EIA, and CFA, unilateral occlusion of CIA and EIA, bilateral EIA occlusions, iliac stenoses with AAA that are not amenable to endograft placement
Femoropopliteal	
A	Single stenosis <10 cm, occlusion <5 cm
B	Multiple stenoses each <5 cm, stenosis or occlusion <15 cm not involving infrageniculate popliteal artery, single or multiple lesions in the absence of continuous tibial vessel to improve distal bypass inflow, heavily calcified occlusion <5 cm, single popliteal stenosis
C	Multiple stenoses or occlusions >15 cm, recurrent disease needing treatment
D	Occlusions >20 cm of CFA or SFA involving popliteal artery, occlusion of popliteal and proximal trifurcation vessels
Infrapopliteal	
A	Single stenosis <5 cm in the target tibial artery
B	Multiple stenoses, each <5 cm in length, or total length <10 cm or single occlusion <3 cm in length in the target tibial artery
C	Multiple stenoses in the target tibial artery and/or single occlusion with total lesion length >10 cm
D	Multiple occlusions involving the target tibial artery with total lesion length >10 cm or dense lesion calcification or nonvisualization of collaterals. The other tibial arteries are occluded or have dense calcification

AAA, abdominal aortic aneurysm; CFA, common femoral artery; CIA, common iliac artery; EIA, external iliac artery; IIA, internal iliac artery; SFA, superficial femoral artery; TASC, TransAtlantic Inter-Society Consensus Document.

Adapted from: Jaff M, et al. An update on methods for revascularization and expansion of the TASC lesion classification to include below-the-knee arteries. *J Endovasc Ther.* 2015;22:663–677, with permission.

the current era, endovascular approaches are considered for most lesion subsets in most patients, because iliac artery stenting is associated with patency rates similar to that of surgery; however, it should be used in conjunction with exercise therapy.

In the CLEVER trial, 111 patients with symptomatic aortoiliac stenosis were randomized to treatment with a supervised exercise program, stenting, or optimal medical therapy. The primary endpoint, improvement in peak walking time at 6 months, was highest in those who underwent a supervised exercise program (5.8 ± 4.6 minutes greater than baseline), slightly lower for those treated with stenting (3.7 ± 4.9), and lowest for those randomized to treatment with optimal medical care (1.2 ± 2.6). Of interest, a secondary endpoint, including improvement in quality of life, was achieved in a greater number of patients treated with stenting than with those who underwent an exercise program, calling into question the generalizability and application to clinical practice of the study's primary finding.[25] In comparison, the recently published ERASE trial randomized 212 patients with aortoiliac or femoropopliteal (FP) disease and symptomatic claudication to exercise therapy alone or exercise therapy plus endovascular revascularization.[26] Patients randomized to combination therapy had a significantly improved maximum walking distance compared to supervised exercise therapy alone (264-1501 m vs 285-1240 m) and in pain-free walking distance. These results suggest that revascularization and supervised exercise therapy are complementary among patients with lifestyle-limiting claudication.

The optimal strategy for arterial access in patients undergoing intervention for aortoiliac disease depends on the characteristics and location of the lesion to be addressed. If entire reconstruction of the aortoiliac bifurcation is required, bilateral femoral access is employed to permit simultaneous bilateral iliac stent placement and "kissing" balloon postdilation. When treating unilateral disease within the proximal iliac system (eg, common iliac), ipsilateral access is desired to permit retrograde delivery of balloons and stents. In such cases, the contralateral approach may be more difficult because of the acute bend of the aortoiliac bifurcation and the associated challenges in establishing adequate coaxial support to deliver a balloon and stent to a lesion that is proximal in the common iliac artery. In contrast, if the target lesion is in the distal common or external iliac artery, contralateral access may be preferred, particularly in situations where the external iliac disease extends distally to the common femoral region, compromising ipsilateral sheath placement. With the advent of radial and pedal devices, in select cases, radial access can be sufficient for management of these lesions; however, one should be mindful of the limited bail out and covered stent options with adequate length to reach radial to peripheral.

The majority of iliac lesions are treated with stent placement; shorter and anatomically simple lesions may be treated with balloon angioplasty alone.[27] In simple TASC A and B lesion, percutaneous transluminal angioplasty (PTA) with provisional stenting versus primary stenting has similar technical success, symptomatic improvement, quality of life, and long-term patency.[28] A meta-analysis involving over 2000 patients revealed that stenting resulted in a 43% decrease in failure rates over a period of 4 years, in comparison to using PTA alone, and hence, primary stenting strategy is preferred.[29]

In the treatment of common iliac and proximal external iliac lesions, BESs are preferred, owing to their superior radial strength and more predictable delivery.[30] In vascular segments near the femoral region, which are inherently prone to flexion and extrinsic compression, the superior flexibility of SESs may outweigh the slightly inferior radial strength compared with BESs. ICE trial (iliac artery stents for common or external iliac artery occlusive disease) compared BES to SES and reported that SES had lower restenosis (6.1% vs 14.9%, P = .006) and target lesion revascularization (6.9% vs 3%, P = .041) at 12 months when compared to BES except in patients with heavy calcification.[31]

Available stents can also be classified as covered versus uncovered stents with covered stents comprising a metallic scaffold lined with polytetrafluoroethylene or Dacron material. Covered stents are preferred in calcific disease as they offer an added safety measure given the increased risk of arterial rupture from expansion of calcified segments. Covered stents have a decreased potential for restenosis by preventing intrusion of underlying plaque in the lumen.[32-34] On the contrary, they do carry higher risk of thrombosis, edge restenosis, and obliterating side branches.

Though drug-coated balloons (DCBs) and drug-eluting stents (DESs) could theoretically be beneficial in iliac lesions, they have not yet been evaluated systematically for the same. Moreover, we are currently limited by the size of DCB and DES with the largest available DCB being 7.0 mm and DES being 8.0 mm in diameter (**Fig. 34.2**).

FP Interventions

The FP arterial segment is long and relatively straight but is subjected to extrinsic compression from the thigh musculature and to flexion and torsion because of movement at the hip and knee joints. Disease within this segment is often calcific, diffuse, and frequently occlusive; endovascular interventions must be designed to confront these unique and formidable technical challenges. Similar to the schema developed to categorize iliac arterial disease, the TASC classification system describes FP lesions as type A, B, C, or D, corresponding to increasing anatomic complexity on the basis of length, the presence of occlusion, and territory involved (**Table 34.2**).[24] Virtually, all categories may be considered for an endovascular approach, although TASC C and D lesions have historically been regarded as "surgical disease" because the technical approach to complex stenoses and occlusions may be demanding.

Atherosclerotic disease in the common femoral artery represents a unique situation where endovascular therapy is most commonly avoided. Because the common femoral artery represents a valuable target for future peripheral bypass surgery, placing a stent in the vessel could potentially "burn a bridge" to important subsequent revascularization efforts. Moreover, the proximity of the hip joint and constant exposure to flexion increase the risk of stent fracture, and there is a paucity of data supporting balloon angioplasty for the treatment of common femoral disease. Open surgical interventions, including endarterectomy and bypass grafting, have been traditionally used for this segment.

In contrast, endovascular therapy of the FP segment is generally the first-line approach. Though endovascular intervention of stenotic lesions in FP lesions is relatively straight forward, restenosis remains the major limitation. With balloon angioplasty alone, restenosis rates as high as 63% at 1 year have been reported.[35] Similarly, poor outcomes were noted with the use of BESs in this territory, likely due to extrinsic compressive forces that characterize this arterial distribution.[36]

Newer devices have recently been developed to improve the long-term patency of endovascular interventions including DCBs and DES. Currently available DCBs deliver paclitaxel to the vessel

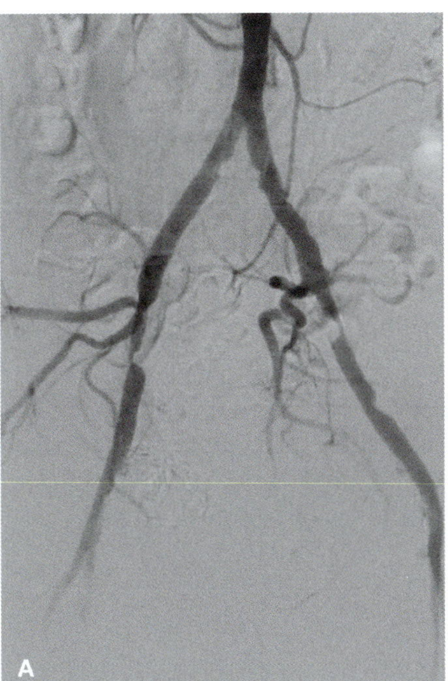

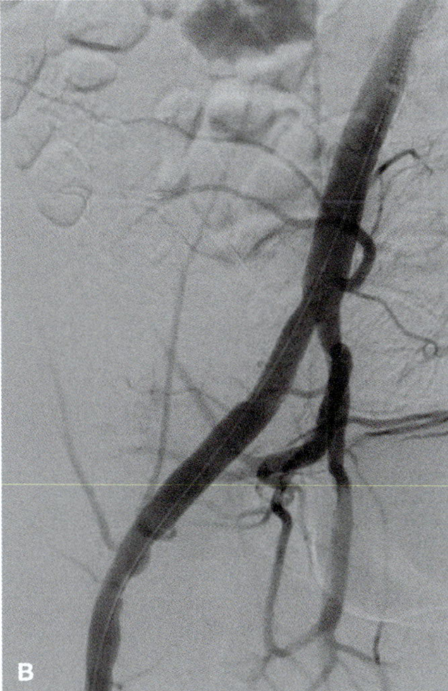

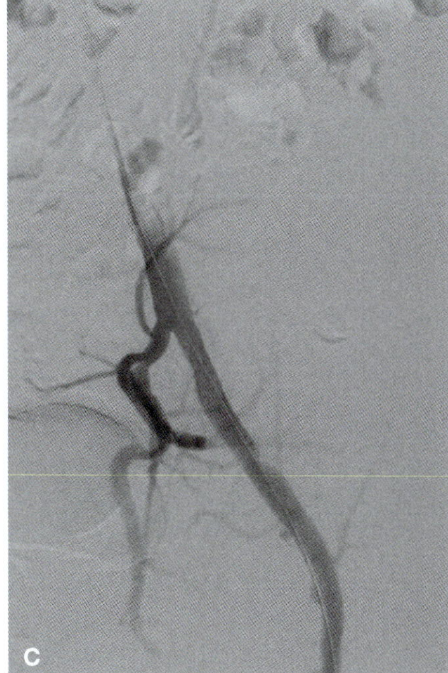

FIGURE 34.2 **A:** A 55-year-old male presenting with bilateral leg claudication (Rutherford class 3) refractory to medical therapy and exercise. Angiography demonstrated a severe stenosis in bilateral external iliac artery. After postdilation, he underwent placement of an SES stent (8.0 × 40 mm) on the right (**B**) and left (**C**) with excellent angiographic result. The procedure was performed with a left radial approach.

TABLE 34.3 Drug-Coated Balloon in FP Lesions

1. IN.PACT SFA trial:
   - Randomized controlled trial compared the IN.PACT Admiral DCB (Medtronic) with standard PTA in patients with FP lesions
   - Superior outcomes for DCB, with a significantly higher primary patency rate (82.2% vs 52.4% at 12 mo) and lower clinically driven target lesion revascularization (11.5% vs 20.6% at 12 mo) compared to PTA[39]
2. Lutonix Global SFA Registry:
   - Prospective multicenter registry evaluated the Lutonix DCB (Bard) in a real-world population with FP disease
   - Primary patency rate of 74.6% at 12 mo, with a low CD-TLR rate of 6.4%[38]
3. Levant 2 trial:
   - This randomized trial compared the Lutonix DCB with PTA in patients with FP disease
   - Higher primary patency rates for DCB at 12 mo (65.2% vs 52.6%) and lower rates of CD-TLR (12.7% vs 20.1%) compared to PTA[37]
4. Biolux P-I Trial:
   - This study evaluated the Passeo-18 Lux DCB (Biotronik) in patients with FP lesions
   - Primary patency rate of 91.3% at 12 mo, along with a low CD-TLR rate of 7.5%
5. Illumenate trial:
   - This trial evaluated the Stellarex DCB compared to balloon angioplasty for the treatment of SFA and popliteal artery
   - Superior primary patency rates for the Stellarex DCB group at 12 mo with primary patency: 82.2% vs 52.4% and lower rates of TLR (2.4% vs 20.6%)

CD-TLR, clinically driven target lesion revascularization; DCB, drug-coated balloon; FP, femoropopliteal; PTA, percutaneous transluminal angioplasty.

wall during balloon inflation, where the lipophilic nature of paclitaxel enables it to partition into the vessel wall, upon which it exerts its antirestenotic effect. DCBs have demonstrated patency rates similar to those historically garnered by nitinol SESs and superior primary patency, lower target lesion revascularization and need for repeat interventions as compared to primary angioplasty alone. Major trials in this segment are summarized in the table (**Table 34.3**).[4,37-40] After DCB angioplasty, focal stent placement may be necessary in cases of significant flow-limiting dissection or recoil; real-world studies suggest that the rates of bailout stenting are 10% to 20% and depend on the length of the lesion being treated.[41]

Paclitaxel-eluting nitinol stents have demonstrated superior patency to balloon angioplasty or older-generation bare nitinol stents, with a long-term reduction in the need for reintervention.[42] Advances in stent technology have led to the development of nitinol-based SESs that better resist the external forces generated by limb movement and muscle compression. For nonfocal disease (ie, longer than 40 mm), multiple randomized trials have now demonstrated the superiority of nitinol-based SESs compared with balloon angioplasty with provisional stenting and superiority to BMS in propensity matched analysis.[43] However, head-to-head comparisons of DESs and DCBs are still lacking.

Apart from restenosis, a major reason for failure and complications of endovascular therapy is failure to cross CTOs (~30%). Effective planning of CTO interventions in the FP and below the knee (BTK) arteries relies heavily on preintervention imaging and a comprehensive evaluation of the morphology. It is crucial to accurately determine the characteristics of the occlusion, including the location, lesion morphology, inflow and outflow vessels, and the arterial supply to the ischemic tissue. This meticulous assessment enables interventionalists to strategize and approach the procedure with precision, maximizing the chances of success and optimizing patient outcomes.

The CTOP classification system categorizes proximal CTO cap morphology into four types: type I with concave proximal and distal caps, type II with concave proximal and convex distal caps, type III with convex proximal and concave distal caps, and type IV with convex proximal and distal caps. In addition to cap morphology, factors such as occluded segment length, proximal cap ambiguity, vessel course, and target vessel quality impact the selection of the initial crossing strategy. Short or intermediate PCTOs with type I caps are typically crossed antegrade, while long PCTOs with type IV caps are often approached in a retrograde fashion. An initial antegrade approach is preferred for tapered PCTO caps, while retrograde crossing can be considered if antegrade dissection re-entry is unsuccessful, provided adequate distal access vessels or interventional collaterals are present.

Advanced methods such as re-entry devices, controlled dissection re-entry, and rendezvous techniques may be required in challenging cases. These techniques allow for accessing the true lumen and can be facilitated by re-entry devices or knuckle-wire manipulation. Atherectomy using intravascular lithotripsy, laser, orbital, rotational, or excisional means may be useful for debulking plaque in regions where stent placement is undesirable or in lesions with high calcific burden.

In contrast, surgical bypass in this segment is associated with marginally better durability but poses a much higher risk of global cardiovascular and local (wound-associated) adverse events (**Fig. 34.3**).[24,44]

Infrapopliteal Interventions and CLTI

The popliteal artery bifurcates BTK into the anterior tibial (AT) and tibioperoneal trunk; the tibioperoneal trunk gives rise to the posterior tibial (PT) and peroneal arteries. The AT, PT, and peroneal arteries form the major blood supply to the foot and, when diseased, may require endovascular therapy.

In contrast to iliac and FP disease, where the majority of interventions are performed for claudication, infrapopliteal revascularization is typically reserved for cases of CLTI. CLTI, defined as ischemic rest pain, tissue loss, or gangrene in the presence of PAD and hypoperfusion of the lower extremity >2 weeks duration. This is an important distinction because perfusion

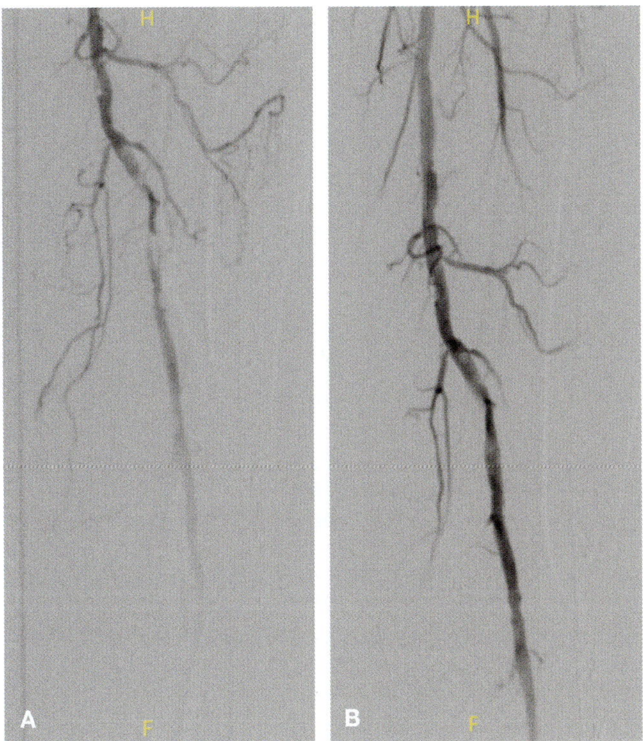

FIGURE 34.3 A 70-year-old male with Rutherford class 4 (rest pain). **A:** Angiogram demonstrated severe calcified distal SFA stenosis. **B:** Treated with intravascular lithotripsy and DCB, with subsequent angiogram with excellent result. DCB, drug-coated balloon; SFA, superficial femoral artery.

requirements for wound healing are much greater than those necessary to maintain tissue integrity. As a result, long-term tibial vessel patency following intervention is less important so long as patency has been durable enough to allow for ischemic ulcerations to heal. For a patient presenting with CLTI, it is imperative to consider a consultation with multidisciplinary care team and comprehensive imaging prior to the amputation and is recommended in the CLI Global Society guidelines to optimize limb salvage.[45] Endovascular therapy for CLI results in limb salvage for the majority of patients. In a study of 235 sequential patients undergoing angioplasty treatment for tibioperoneal stenosis in the context of CLI, 95% of patients were treated successfully, with a limb salvage rate of 91% among survivors at a mean follow-up of 34 months.[46]

A central principle in the treatment of CLTI is to re-establish a patent, straight line of blood flow from the heart to the foot, including at least one of the infrapopliteal vessels. A more contemporary concept correlates the area of tissue loss with the infrapopliteal artery that subtends the territory or "angiosome." An angiosome is a 3-dimensional anatomic block of tissue (including skin, subcutaneous tissue, fascia, muscle, and bone) fed by a source artery. A revascularization strategy that favors the infrapopliteal artery correlated with the angiosome of tissue loss may enhance wound healing.[47] When it is not possible to provide direct flow to the angiosome of interest, the goal should be to provide indirect flow via collaterals and optimize strategy to achieve maximum pedal reconstruction. It is unclear if the two strategies lead to change in limb salvage rate.

Given the comparable size of the infrapopliteal arteries to the coronaries, the majority of these interventions are performed utilizing equivalent narrow-caliber equipment compared to those used in coronary interventions, including 0.014-in wires, angioplasty balloons, and stent systems.

For infrapopliteal intervention, ipsilateral antegrade common femoral arterial access is often preferred. The relatively short distance and the straight access from groin to knee (and below) offer significant technical advantages for wire and catheter manipulation. The other preferred approach that has been increasingly used is "pedal" access (dorsalis pedis or PT) and has now become an important skill to master for treatment of FP or proximal infrapopliteal total occlusions. Such "ipsilateral retrograde" access may offer an advantage to cross recalcitrant occlusions where it is difficult to penetrate the proximal segments of occlusion using antegrade technique. Pedal access is often obtained using a narrow-caliber needle and wire systems (eg, micropuncture) and may be used in conjunction with an antegrade femoral sheath to permit wire snaring and exteriorization, followed by an antegrade approach to the lesion without the use of a large-caliber sheath in the pedal vessel. Pedal access carries a risk of compromising flow in the accessed vessel, which may represent the only outflow to the foot, although recent multicenter data have supported the overall safety of this approach.[48]

Similar to FP lesions, in infrapopliteal intervention, DCBs are superior to PTA alone in terms of angiographic results and wound healing.[49] Use of stents is generally reserved for rare cases of severely suboptimal angioplasty results or flow-limiting dissections, and when implanted, DESs are preferred (**Fig. 34.4**).[50]

SURGICAL BYPASS VERSUS ENDOVASCULAR THERAPY IN CLTI

Patients with CLTI may be treated with surgical bypass or endovascular techniques. The individual patient approach is based on several factors, including anatomic feasibility of revascularization, the presence of adequate vein for bypass, and patient comorbidities.

The BASIL trial was a randomized study of surgical bypass versus balloon angioplasty for patients with CLI and FP disease; with overall no significant difference in amputation-free survival or overall survival between the two strategies for the first 2 years. In fact, the curves started to separate in favor of bypass after 2 years. These results are however not generalizable to current endovascular techniques.[51]

The BEST CLI trial reported that in patients with CLTI, in which there was equipoise between surgical and endovascular intervention, surgical revascularization with a great saphenous venous conduit was superior to endovascular intervention in reducing major adverse limb events; however, this was mainly driven by need for repeat procedures in endovascular group. In patients without a suitable vein for bypass, endovascular revascularization is similar if not better.[51,52]

The BASIL-2 trial evaluated vein bypass compared with endovascular treatment among patients with CLTI due to infrapopliteal disease and reported superiority of endovascular treatment.[53]

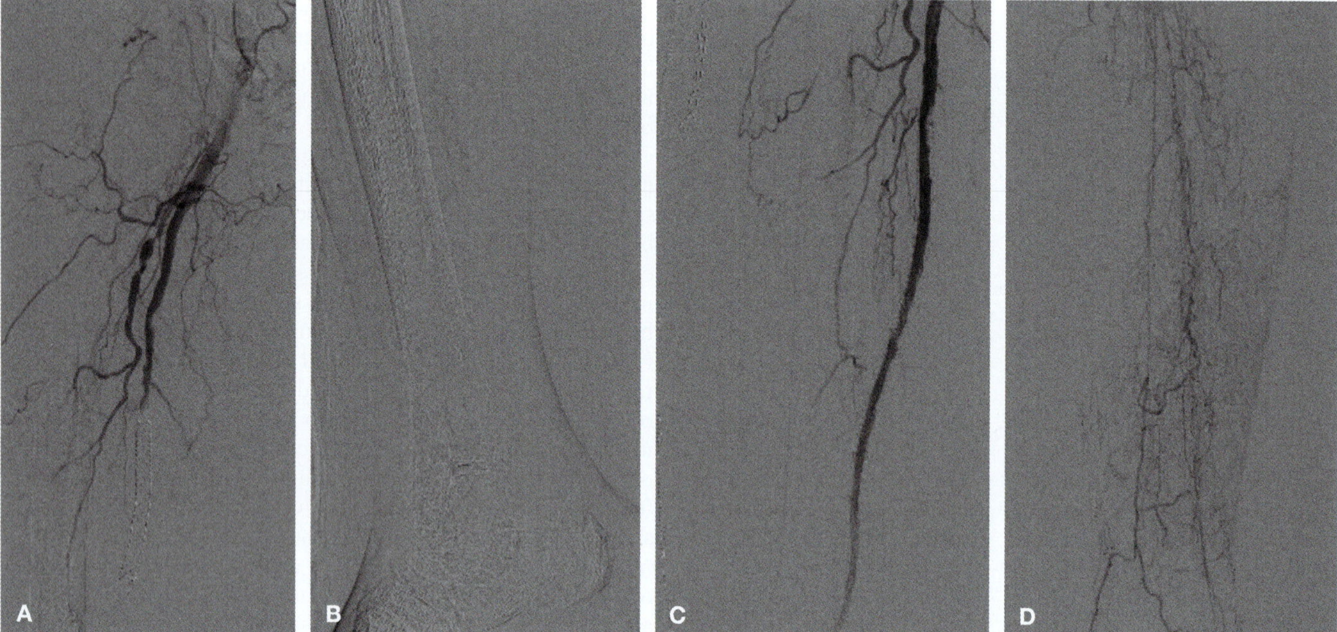

FIGURE 34.4 85F with prior right SFA, popliteal, TP trunk, and PT stents presenting with nonhealing ulcer in the PT angiosome (lateral heel). **A and B:** Runoff showed severe stenosis in the proximal SFA at the proximal edge of the previously placed SFA stent and occluded SFA, popliteal, TP trunk, and PT stents with reconstitution distally in the PT. The ATA and peroneal were occluded. **C and D:** Both up and over antegrade and retrograde pedal access via PT used. Occlusion crossed using a V18 wire and stents dilated with serial balloon dilation and treating resist areas with cutting balloons and subsequently DCB performed from SFATP trunk, with excellent angiographic result with patent PT stents and reconstitution of the peroneal and ATA via collaterals.ATA, anterior tibial artery; DCB, drug-coated balloon; PT, posterior tibial; SFA, superficial femoral artery; TP, tibioperoneal.

CONCLUSION

Endovascular therapy has emerged as a safe and less invasive alternative to surgery in most major peripheral vascular beds. Appropriate patient selection coupled with sound procedural technique offers many patients with PAD substantial benefit. With future research, we may refine our clinical insights, applying new technology to deliver optimal patient-centered lesion-specific care.

Key Points

Thoracic Aorta

- Arm claudication and symptomatic steal syndromes are indications for subclavian revascularization.
- Subclavian revascularization is indicated even in asymptomatic individuals if the disease subtends the internal mammary artery takeoff and the vessel is a required conduit for bypass surgery.
- In patients with disease secondary to vasculitis, escalation of immunosuppression is preferred over endovascular and surgical approach.
- Steal physiology detected on noninvasive testing should not be treated in asymptomatic patients.
- Patients with type A aortic dissection are usually treated with emergency surgery. Patients with uncomplicated type B aortic dissections may often be managed medically, although an increasing percentage are treated with TEVAR.

Abdominal Aorta

- Multiple trials have demonstrated similar long-term mortality with EVAR relative to open surgical repair.
- Reintervention rates are higher with EVAR, which also makes this a more expensive therapy that requires long-term surveillance.
- In patients with prohibitive surgical risk, EVAR does not appear to reduce all-cause mortality compared with no repair.

Lower Extremity

- Endovascular interventions for claudication should be performed only in individuals with lifestyle-limiting symptoms who have failed conservative measures, including risk-factor modification and exercise.
- All patients with CLTI require multidisciplinary care and evaluation of anatomy and attempt at revascularization (if feasible) to maximize limb salvage.
- Avoid angioplasty of the common femoral artery; disease in this segment should in most cases be reserved for surgery.
- Newer-generation nitinol stents and DCBs are each associated with improved patency in the superficial femoral artery.
- Infrapopliteal interventions are primarily reserved for patients with CLTI (eg, rest pain, tissue loss) with the therapeutic goal of restoring straight-line blood flow from the heart to the foot.

For further review and interactivities, please see the chapter-based multiple choice questions and videos accessible in the complimentary eBook bundled with this text. Access instructions are located in the inside front cover.

References

1. Shadman R, Criqui MH, Bundens WP, et al. Subclavian artery stenosis: prevalence, risk factors, and association with cardiovascular diseases. *J Am Coll Cardiol*. 2004;44(3):618-623. doi:10.1016/j.jacc.2004.04.044
2. Brott TG, Halperin JL, Abbara S, et al. 2011 ASA/ACCF/AHA/AANN/AANS/ACR/ASNR/CNS/SAIP/SCAI/SIR/SNIS/SVM/SVS guideline on the management of patients with extracranial carotid and vertebral artery disease: executive summary. A report of the American College of Cardiology Foundation/American Heart Association Task Force on Practice Guidelines, and the American Stroke Association, American Association of Neuroscience Nurses, American Association of Neurological Surgeons, American College of Radiology, American Society of Neuroradiology, Congress of Neurological Surgeons, Society of Atherosclerosis Imaging and Prevention, Society for Cardiovascular Angiography and Interventions, Society of Interventional Radiology, Society of NeuroInterventional Surgery, Society for Vascular Medicine, and Society for Vascular Surgery. *Circulation*. 2011;124(4):489-532. doi:10.1161/CIR.0b013e31820d8d78
3. Patel SN, White CJ, Collins TJ, et al. Catheter-based treatment of the subclavian and innominate arteries. *Catheter Cardiovasc Interv*. 2008;71(7):963-968. doi:10.1002/ccd.21549
4. Scheinert D, Schulte KL, Zeller T, Lammer J, Tepe G. Paclitaxel-releasing balloon in femoropopliteal lesions using a BTHC excipient: twelve-month results from the BIOLUX P-I randomized trial. *J Endovasc Ther*. 2015;22(1):14-21. doi:10.1177/1526602814564383
5. Yu J, Korabathina R, Coppola J, Staniloae C. Transradial approach to subclavian artery stenting. *J Invasive Cardiol*. 2010;22(5):204-206.
6. Michael TT, Banerjee S, Brilakis E. Subclavian artery intervention with vertebral embolic protection. *Catheter Cardiovasc Interv*. 2009;74(1):22-25. doi:10.1002/ccd.21959
7. Warnes CA, Williams RG, Bashore TM, et al. ACC/AHA 2008 guidelines for the management of adults with congenital heart disease: a report of the American College of Cardiology/American Heart Association Task Force on Practice Guidelines (Writing Committee to develop guidelines on the management of adults with congenital heart disease). Developed in collaboration with the American Society of Echocardiography, Heart Rhythm Society, International Society for Adult Congenital Heart Disease, Society for Cardiovascular Angiography and Interventions, and Society of Thoracic Surgeons. *J Am Coll Cardiol*. 2008;52(23):e143-e263. doi:10.1016/j.jacc.2008.10.001
8. Mussa FF, Horton JD, Moridzadeh R, Nicholson J, Trimarchi S, Eagle KA. Acute aortic dissection and intramural hematoma: a systematic review. *JAMA*. 2016;316(7):754-763. doi:10.1001/jama.2016.10026
9. Cooper M, Hicks C, Ratchford EV, Salameh MJ, Malas M. Diagnosis and treatment of uncomplicated type B aortic dissection. *Vasc Med*. 2016;21(6):547-552. doi:10.1177/1358863X16643601
10. Hiratzka LF, Bakris GL, Beckman JA, et al. 2010 ACCF/AHA/AATS/ACR/ASA/SCA/SCAI/SIR/STS/SVM guidelines for the diagnosis and management of patients with thoracic aortic disease: a report of the American College of Cardiology Foundation/American Heart Association Task Force on Practice Guidelines, American Association for Thoracic Surgery, American College of Radiology, American Stroke Association, Society of Cardiovascular Anesthesiologists, Society for Cardiovascular Angiography and Interventions, Society of Interventional Radiology, Society of Thoracic Surgeons, and Society for Vascular Medicine. *Circulation*. 2010;121(13):e266-e369. doi:10.1161/CIR.0b013e3181d4739e
11. Lederle FA, Johnson GR, Wilson SE, et al. The aneurysm detection and management study screening program: validation cohort and final results. Aneurysm Detection and Management Veterans Affairs Cooperative Study Investigators. *Arch Intern Med*. 2000;160(10):1425-1430. doi:10.1001/archinte.160.10.1425
12. Fleming C, Whitlock EP, Beil TL, Lederle FA. Screening for abdominal aortic aneurysm: a best-evidence systematic review for the U.S. Preventive Services Task Force. *Ann Intern Med*. 2005;142(3):203-211. doi:10.7326/0003-4819-142-3-200502010-00012
13. Chaikof EL, Dalman RL, Eskandari MK, et al. The Society for Vascular Surgery practice guidelines on the care of patients with an abdominal aortic aneurysm. *J Vasc Surg*. 2018;67(1):2-77.e2. doi:10.1016/j.jvs.2017.10.044
14. Ng TT, Mirocha J, Magner D, Gewertz BL. Variations in the utilization of endovascular aneurysm repair reflect population risk factors and disease prevalence. *J Vasc Surg*. 2010;51(4):801-809.e1. 801-809, 809 e801. doi:10.1016/j.jvs.2009.10.115
15. Kent KC. Clinical practice. Abdominal aortic aneurysms. *N Engl J Med*. 2014;371(22):2101-2108. doi:10.1056/NEJMcp1401430
16. De Bruin JL, Baas AF, Buth J, et al. Long-term outcome of open or endovascular repair of abdominal aortic aneurysm. *N Engl J Med*. 2010;362(20):1881-1889. doi:10.1056/NEJMoa0909499
17. United Kingdom EVAR Trial Investigators; Greenhalgh RM, Brown LC, et al. Endovascular versus open repair of abdominal aortic aneurysm. *N Engl J Med*. 2010;362(20):1863-1871. doi:10.1056/NEJMoa0909305
18. United Kingdom EVAR Trial Investigators; Greenhalgh RM, Brown LC, Powell JT, Thompson SG, Epstein D. Endovascular repair of aortic aneurysm in patients physically ineligible for open repair. *N Engl J Med*. 2010;362(20):1872-1880. doi:10.1056/NEJMoa0911056
19. Aday AW, Matsushita K. Epidemiology of peripheral artery disease and polyvascular disease. *Circ Res*. 2021;128(12):1818-1832. doi:10.1161/CIRCRESAHA.121.318535
20. Weitz JI, Byrne J, Clagett GP, et al. Diagnosis and treatment of chronic arterial insufficiency of the lower extremities: a critical review. *Circulation*. 1996;94(11):3026-3049. doi:10.1161/01.cir.94.11.3026
21. Abu Dabrh AM, Steffen MW, Undavalli C, et al. The natural history of untreated severe or critical limb ischemia. *J Vasc Surg*. 2015;62(6):1642-1651.e3. doi:10.1016/j.jvs.2015.07.065
22. Armstrong EJ, Chen DC, Westin GG, et al. Adherence to guideline-recommended therapy is associated with decreased major adverse cardiovascular events and major adverse limb events among patients with peripheral arterial disease. *J Am Heart Assoc*. 2014;3(2):e000697. doi:10.1161/JAHA.113.000697
23. Gerhard-Herman MD, Gornik HL, Barrett C, et al. 2016 AHA/ACC guideline on the management of patients with lower extremity peripheral artery disease: executive summary—a report of the American College of Cardiology/American Heart Association Task Force on Clinical Practice Guidelines. *Circulation*. 2017;135(12):e686-e725. doi:10.1161/CIR.0000000000000470
24. Norgren L, Hiatt WR, Dormandy JA, et al. Inter-Society Consensus for the Management of Peripheral Arterial Disease (TASC II). *J Vasc Surg*. 2007;45:S5-S67. doi:10.1016/j.jvs.2006.12.037
25. Murphy TP, Cutlip DE, Regensteiner JG, et al. Supervised exercise versus primary stenting for claudication resulting from aortoiliac peripheral artery disease: six-month outcomes from the claudication—exercise versus endoluminal revascularization (CLEVER) study. *Circulation*. 2012;125(1):130-139. doi:10.1161/CIRCULATIONAHA.111.075770
26. Fakhry F, Spronk S, van der Laan L, et al. Endovascular revascularization and supervised exercise for peripheral artery disease and intermittent claudication: a randomized clinical trial. *JAMA*. 2015;314(18):1936-1944. doi:10.1001/jama.2015.14851
27. Feldman DN, Armstrong EJ, Aronow HD, et al. SCAI guidelines on device selection in aorto-iliac arterial interventions. *Catheter Cardiovasc Interv*. 2020;96(4):915-929. doi:10.1002/ccd.28947
28. Bekken J, Jongsma H, Ayez N, Hoogewerf CJ, Van Weel V, Fioole B. Angioplasty versus stenting for iliac artery lesions. *Cochrane Database Syst Rev*. 2015;2015(5):CD007561. doi:10.1002/14651858.CD007561.pub2
29. Bosch JL, Hunink MG. Meta-analysis of the results of percutaneous transluminal angioplasty and stent placement for aortoiliac occlusive disease. *Radiology*. 1997;204(1):87-96. doi:10.1148/radiology.204.1.9205227
30. Aggarwal V, Waldo SW, Armstrong EJ. Endovascular revascularization for aortoiliac atherosclerotic disease. *Vasc Health Risk Manag*. 2016;12:117-127. doi:10.2147/VHRM.S98721

31. Krankenberg H, Zeller T, Ingwersen M, et al. Self-expanding versus balloon-expandable stents for iliac artery occlusive disease: the randomized ICE trial. *JACC Cardiovasc Interv*. 2017;10(16):1694-1704. doi:10.1016/j.jcin.2017.05.015
32. Mwipatayi BP, Sharma S, Daneshmand A, et al. Durability of the balloon-expandable covered versus bare-metal stents in the Covered versus Balloon Expandable Stent Trial (COBEST) for the treatment of aortoiliac occlusive disease. *J Vasc Surg*. 2016;64(1):83-94.e1. doi:10.1016/j.jvs.2016.02.064
33. Holden A, Merrilees S, Buckley B, Connor B, Colgan F, Hill A. First-in-human experience with the gore balloon-expandable covered endoprosthesis in iliac artery occlusive disease. *J Endovasc Ther*. 2017;24(1):11-18. doi:10.1177/1526602816680570
34. Piazza M, Squizzato F, Dall'Antonia A, et al. Editor's choice – outcomes of self expanding PTFE covered stent versus bare metal stent for chronic iliac artery occlusion in matched cohorts using propensity score modelling. *Eur J Vasc Endovasc Surg*. 2017;54(2):177-185. doi:10.1016/j.ejvs.2017.03.019
35. Ihnat DM, Duong ST, Taylor ZC, et al. Contemporary outcomes after superficial femoral artery angioplasty and stenting: the influence of TASC classification and runoff score. *J Vasc Surg*. 2008;47(5):967-974. doi:10.1016/j.jvs.2007.12.050
36. Surowiec SM, Davies MG, Eberly SW, et al. Percutaneous angioplasty and stenting of the superficial femoral artery. *J Vasc Surg*. 2005;41(2):269-278. doi:10.1016/j.jvs.2004.11.031
37. Rosenfield K, Jaff MR, White CJ, et al. Trial of a paclitaxel-coated balloon for femoropopliteal artery disease. *N Engl J Med*. 2015;373(2):145-153. doi:10.1056/NEJMoa1406235
38. Thieme M, Von Bilderling P, Paetzel C, et al. The 24-month results of the Lutonix Global SFA Registry: worldwide experience with Lutonix drug-coated balloon. *JACC Cardiovasc Interv*. 2017;10(16):1682-1690. doi:10.1016/j.jcin.2017.04.041
39. Tepe G, Laird J, Schneider P, et al. Drug-coated balloon versus standard percutaneous transluminal angioplasty for the treatment of superficial femoral and popliteal peripheral artery disease: 12-month results from the IN.PACT SFA randomized trial. *Circulation*. 2015;131(5):495-502. doi:10.1161/CIRCULATIONAHA.114.011004
40. Krishnan P, Faries P, Niazi K, et al. Stellarex drug-coated balloon for treatment of femoropopliteal disease: twelve-month outcomes from the randomized ILLUMENATE pivotal and pharmacokinetic studies. *Circulation*. 2017;136(12):1102-1113. doi:10.1161/CIRCULATIONAHA.117.028893
41. Micari A, Nerla R, Vadala G, et al. 2-Year results of paclitaxel-coated balloons for long femoropopliteal artery disease: evidence from the SFA-long study. *JACC Cardiovasc Interv*. 2017;10(7):728-734. doi:10.1016/j.jcin.2017.01.028
42. Dake MD, Ansel GM, Jaff MR, et al. Durable clinical effectiveness with paclitaxel-eluting stents in the femoropopliteal artery: 5-year results of the Zilver PTX randomized trial. *Circulation*. 2016;133(15):1472-1483. discussion 1483. doi:10.1161/CIRCULATIONAHA.115.016900
43. Armstrong EJ, Jeon-Slaughter H, Kahlon RS, Niazi KA, Shammas NW, Banerjee S. Comparative outcomes of supera interwoven nitinol vs bare nitinol stents for the treatment of femoropopliteal disease: insights from the XLPAD Registry. *J Endovasc Ther*. 2020;27(1):60-65. doi:10.1177/1526602819885652
44. Zlatanovic P, Mahmoud AA, Cinara I, Cvetic V, Lukic B, Davidovic L. Comparison of long term outcomes after endovascular treatment versus bypass surgery in chronic limb threatening ischaemia patients with long femoropopliteal lesions. *Eur J Vasc Endovasc Surg*. 2021;61(2):258-269. doi:10.1016/j.ejvs.2020.11.009
45. Mustapha JA, Saab FA, Martinsen BJ, et al. Digital subtraction angiography prior to an amputation for critical limb ischemia (CLI): an expert recommendation statement from the CLI global society to optimize limb salvage. *J Endovasc Ther*. 2020;27(4):540-546. doi:10.1177/1526602820928590
46. Dorros G, Jaff MR, Dorros AM, Mathiak LM, He T. Tibioperoneal (outflow lesion) angioplasty can be used as primary treatment in 235 patients with critical limb ischemia: five-year follow-up. *Circulation*. 2001;104(17):2057-2062. doi:10.1161/hc4201.097943
47. Spillerova K, Settembre N, Biancari F, Alback A, Venermo M. Angiosome targeted PTA is more important in endovascular revascularisation than in surgical revascularisation: analysis of 545 patients with ischaemic tissue lesions. *Eur J Vasc Endovasc Surg*. 2017;53(4):567-575. doi:10.1016/j.ejvs.2017.01.008
48. Stern JR, Cafasso DE, Connolly PH, Ellozy SH, Schneider DB, Meltzer AJ. Safety and effectiveness of retrograde arterial access for endovascular treatment of critical limb ischemia. *Ann Vasc Surg*. 2019;55:131-137. doi:10.1016/j.avsg.2018.08.072
49. Barbarawi M, Qazi AH, Lee J, et al. Meta-analysis comparing drug-coated balloons and percutaneous transluminal angioplasty for infrapopliteal artery disease. *Am J Cardiol*. 2022;183:115-121. doi:10.1016/j.amjcard.2022.08.007
50. Khalid CMP, Devarasetty PP, Royfman R, et al. Drug-eluting stents versus conventional endovascular therapies in symptomatic infrapopliteal peripheral artery disease: a meta-analysis. *J Soc Cardiovasc Angiogr Interv*. 2022;1:100024.
51. Bradbury AW, Adam DJ, Bell J, et al. Bypass versus Angioplasty in Severe Ischaemia of the Leg (BASIL) trial: an intention-to-treat analysis of amputation-free and overall survival in patients randomized to a bypass surgery-first or a balloon angioplasty-first revascularization strategy. *J Vasc Surg*. 2010;51(5 suppl):5S-17S. doi:10.1016/j.jvs.2010.01.073
52. Farber A, Menard MT, Conte MS, et al. Surgery or endovascular therapy for chronic limb-threatening ischemia. *N Engl J Med*. 2022;387(25):2305-2316. doi:10.1056/NEJMoa2207899
53. Bradbury AW, Moakes CA, Popplewell M, et al. A vein bypass first versus a best endovascular treatment first revascularisation strategy for patients with chronic limb threatening ischaemia who required an infra-popliteal, with or without an additional more proximal infra-inguinal revascularisation procedure to restore limb perfusion (BASIL-2): an open-label, randomised, multicentre, phase 3 trial. *Lancet*. 2023;401(10390):1798-1809. doi:10.1016/S0140-6736(23)00462-2

Carotid, Cerebrovascular, & Acute Stroke Intervention

Prateek Sharma, Jefferson T. Miley, and Peter P. Monteleone

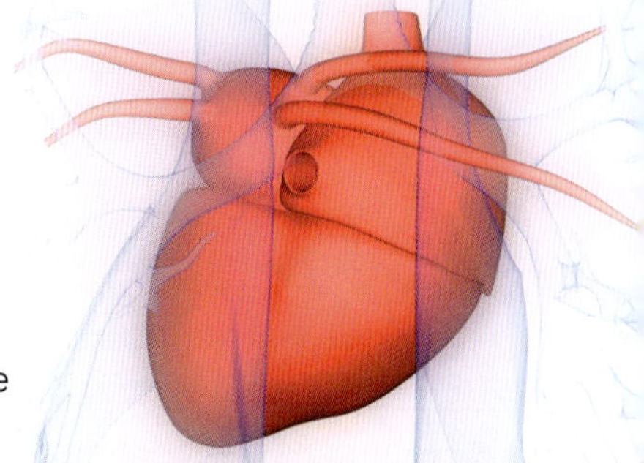

EXTRACRANIAL CAROTID INTERVENTIONS

Epidemiology and Natural History of Carotid Stenosis

Nearly 800,000 strokes occur each year in the United States, and over 160,000 Americans die annually from stroke. The estimated direct and indirect cost of stroke for 2019 was $56.5 billion, and it is expected that, between 2015 and 2035, total direct medical stroke-related costs will double, from $36.7 billion to $94.3 billion.[1] Stroke is the fifth-leading cause of mortality in the United States, and among survivors, 30% are permanently disabled (mean Rankin score >4).[1,2] Atherosclerotic carotid artery disease is the leading cause of noncardioembolic ischemic strokes.[3] Carotid plaque most often causes cerebrovascular events due to plaque rupture with atheroembolization, rather than carotid artery occlusion (<20% of ischemic strokes) with thrombosis.[4]

The natural history of carotid artery stenosis depends on the presence of symptoms (transient ischemic attack [TIA], stroke, and amaurosis fugax). Symptomatic patients have a 5- to 10-fold risk of stroke compared to asymptomatic patients. In a Medicare registry of patients who underwent carotid revascularization, asymptomatic patients with carotid artery stenosis outnumbered symptomatic patients 2.5:1.[5] Approximately 5% to 10% of patients over age 65 have a carotid stenosis >50%, with 1% having a stenosis >75%. Because the majority (>80%) of ischemic strokes have no warning symptoms, the management of asymptomatic carotid atherosclerosis with either revascularization and/or medical therapy is important.[6]

Transient focal neurologic symptoms are associated with a 30% risk of stroke within 6 months. TIA is currently defined as a transient episode of neurologic dysfunction caused by focal brain, spinal cord, or retinal ischemia, without acute infarction, based on pathologic, imaging, other objective evidence, and/or clinical evidence.[7] Stroke, central nervous system infarction, is defined by neuropathologic, neuroimaging, and/or clinical evidence of permanent injury. Nevertheless, many of the initial studies that illustrated the natural history of this disease, as well as our current standards of practice, predate this updated definition and included only a clinical definition of infarction.

Asymptomatic Patients

In the 1990s, two large randomized controlled trials (RCTs), Asymptomatic Carotid Atherosclerosis Study (ACAS) and the Asymptomatic Carotid Surgery Trial (ACST), showed that carotid endarterectomy (CEA) reduced the incidence of ipsilateral stroke in patients with asymptomatic carotid artery stenosis >60% when compared to medical therapy (eg, aspirin) by 50%. Nevertheless, CEA did not reduce overall stroke and death and did not show any benefit in women or in patients older than 75 years of age. It is important to note that the medical therapy provided in these trials (aspirin) has significantly improved. Currently, the risk of progression of an asymptomatic carotid artery stenosis to occlusion with modern medical therapy is very low. In a cohort of 3681 patients with yearly duplex follow-up, 316 (8.6%) asymptomatic patients had occlusions that occurred during observation. Of these, 80% (254) of the occlusions occurred before the initiation of modern intensive medical therapy[8]. A retrospective community-based cohort study evaluating the effect of contemporary medical therapy (ie, modern lipid lowering, antidiabetic, and antihypertensives) on nonrevascularized asymptomatic patients with carotid artery stenosis (70%-99%) found a mean annual ipsilateral stroke rate of 0.9% (and Kaplan-Meier estimate of 4.7% by 5 years). Over the 4-year period (2008-2012), 21.5% of the cohort had severe (70%-90%) stenosis that progressed to high-grade stenosis (90%-99%), while 8.4% had severe stenosis that progressed to total occlusion. In patients with baseline high-grade stenosis, 28.2% progressed to total occlusion.[9]

Symptomatic Patients

Symptomatic carotid disease is defined as focal neurologic symptoms of sudden onset, in the appropriate carotid artery distribution, within the previous 6 months. The natural history of symptomatic carotid artery stenosis was reflected in the medical arm of the randomized North American Symptomatic Carotid Endarterectomy Trial (NASCET). The 5-year risk of ipsilateral stroke in those medically managed was 18.7% among those with lesions <50% in severity. In those with 50% to 69% stenosis, the risk over the same period was 22.2%. In those with a 70% to 99% stenosis, the 2-year risk of ipsilateral stroke was 26%.[10] Results were similar in the European Carotid Surgery Trial (ECST). The incidence of stroke increased with the severity of stenosis, and the 3-year risk of ipsilateral stroke in symptomatic patients with stenosis greater than 80% was 26.5%. Nevertheless, as the stenosis approaches total occlusion (95%-99%), the risk of ipsilateral stroke goes down to 17.2%.[11]

Clinical Presentation

Symptoms of carotid artery stenosis include the following: ipsilateral transient visual defects (amaurosis fugax) from retinal emboli; contralateral weakness or numbness of an extremity or of the face, or a combination of these; visual field defect; dysarthria; and, in the case of dominant hemisphere involvement, aphasia. The National Institutes of Health Stroke Scale (NIHSS) should be performed in all symptomatic patients to quantify the neurologic deficit, which correlates with outcome. Asymptomatic patients may present with carotid stenosis noted on duplex in the presence of a cervical bruit (class IIA) or carotid screening in the presence of other known or suspected atherosclerotic disease at alternative vascular beds (class IIB for symptomatic peripheral artery disease, coronary artery disease, or ≥2 risk factors such as hypertension [HTN], hyperlipidemia, tobacco use, family history of premature atherosclerosis, or family history of ischemic stroke).[12]

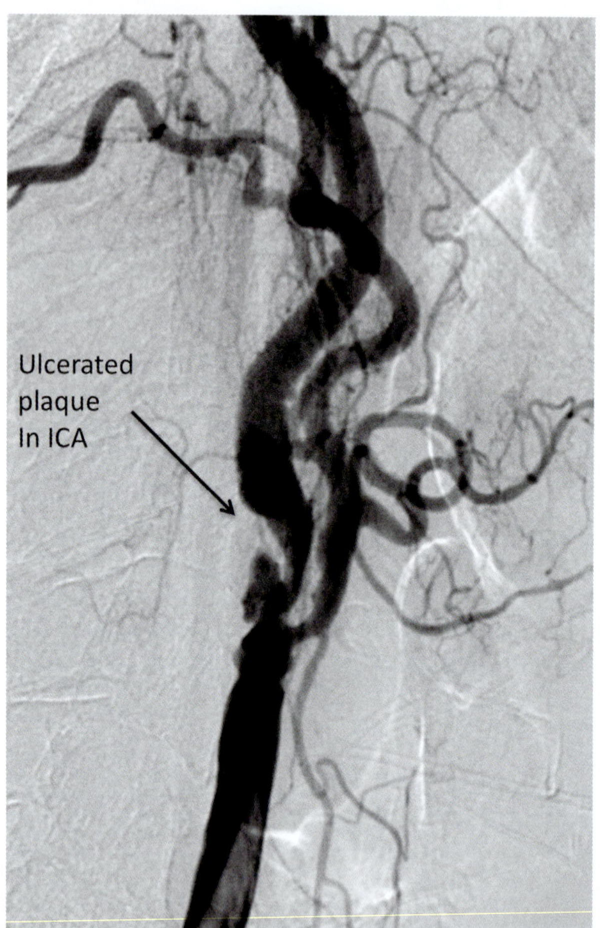

FIGURE 35.1 Catheter angiography of right carotid artery in a patient with recent transient ischemic attack. There is ulcerated plaque at the origin of the internal carotid artery.

Anatomic Imaging

Digital subtraction angiography (DSA) is the gold standard for defining carotid anatomy, with the NASCET method of stenosis measurement, the most widely accepted methodology (**Fig. 35.1**). Invasive cerebral catheter-based angiography carries a risk of iatrogenic cerebral infarction of 0.5% to 1.2%; therefore, noninvasive imaging should be the initial strategy for evaluation. Carotid duplex imaging, transcranial Doppler imaging, computed tomography (CT) angiography (CTA), and magnetic resonance angiography (MRA) are the preferred noninvasive methods of assessment. Duplex imaging represents an optimal choice for initial screening given its safety profile, low cost, and wide availability. Cerebral and cervical imaging should define the aortic arch and the Circle of Willis (**Fig. 35.2**).

Medical Therapy

Current antiatherosclerotic medical therapy has advanced significantly with the development of angiotensin-converting enzyme inhibitors (ACE-Is), angiotensin receptor blockers (ARBs), statin drugs, proprotein convertase subtilisin/kexin type 9 monoclonal antibody/inhibitors (PCSK9s), antidiabetic medications, and newer antiplatelet agents. Medical therapy for carotid atherosclerosis should focus on preventing stroke and stabilizing atherosclerotic lesions to prevent plaque rupture and atheroembolization. Blood pressure control is of paramount importance because it is a primary risk factor for stroke as well as for atrial fibrillation and myocardial infarction (MI), which both increase the likelihood of stroke. ACE-I and ARB are of particular benefit in stroke prevention, particularly in those at higher risk for cardiovascular disease.[12]

Cholesterol lowering with statin drugs in patients treated for atherosclerotic cardiovascular disease (ASCVD) prevention demonstrates a lower risk of stroke. It is possible that statins prevent strokes through pleiotropic effects on endothelial function and plaque stabilization, in addition to their lipid-lowering properties. Current American Heart Association/American Stroke Association (AHA/ASA) stroke guidelines and American College of Cardiology (ACC)/AHA lipid guidelines[6,12] recommend that high-intensity statin therapy be initiated or continued as first-line therapy in patients <75 years of age that have clinical ASCVD unless contraindicated (class I, Level of Evidence [LOE] A) and should be considered in those ≥75 years of age if the benefit outweighs the risk (class IIa, LOE B)[13] (**Table 35.1**). Modern studies (2015-2020) and a meta-analysis evaluating PCSK9 have found, in addition to lowering low-density lipoprotein (LDL) and cardiovascular mortality, an association with lower risk of total and ischemic stroke without increase in hemorrhagic stroke.[15] Consequently, PCSK9i

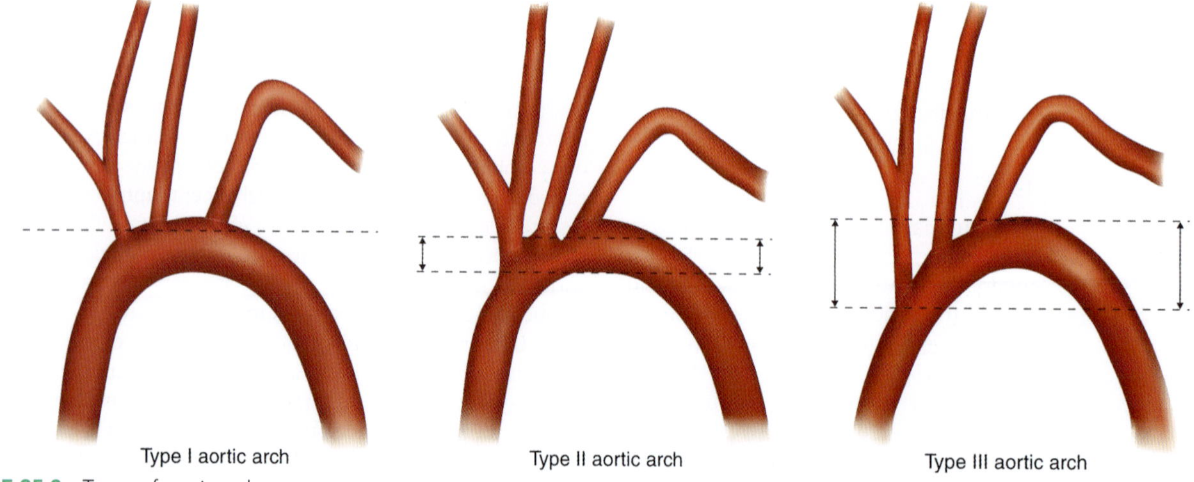

FIGURE 35.2 Types of aortic arch.

TABLE 35.1 AHA/ASA Guidelines for the Primary Prevention of Stroke[7]

Endorsed statin use per 2013 ACC/AHA[14] cholesterol guidelines	ASCVD	Age <75—high-intensity statin Age >75—moderate-intensity statin	Class I LOE A
	LDL > 190	High-intensity statin	
	Age 40-75 with diabetes LDL 70-189	10-y risk >7.5%: high-intensity statin 10-y risk <7.5%: moderate-intensity statin	
	Age 40-75 without ASCVD or diabetes 10-y risk >7.5%	Moderate- to high-intensity statin	
Niacin[a] may be considered for • Low HDL or • Elevated lipoprotein(a)			Class IIb LOE B
Fibric acid derivatives[a] may be considered for • Hypertriglyceridemia			Class IIb LOE C
Nonstatin lipid-lowering therapies[a], such as fibric acid derivatives, bile acid sequestrants, niacin, and ezetimibe may be considered in patients who cannot tolerate statins			Class IIb LOE C

ACC, American College of Cardiology; AHA, American Heart Association; ASA, American Stroke Association; ASCVD, atherosclerotic cardiovascular disease; HDL, high-density lipoprotein; LDL, low-density lipoprotein; LOE, Level of Evidence.
[a]Efficacy in preventing ischemic stroke in patients with these conditions is not established.
From Sacco RL, Kasner SE, Broderick JP, et al. An updated definition of stroke for the 21st century: a statement for healthcare professionals from the American Heart Association/American Stroke Association. *Stroke*. 2013;44(7):2064-2089.

utility for patients with LDL-cholesterol (LDL-C) ≥70 mg/dL while on maximally tolerated statin therapy (with ezetimibe) in setting of known/high-risk ASCVD is highlighted in updates from both the AHA/ASA and ACC.[16,17]

Guidelines also recognize Food and Drug Administration (FDA) approval of statins for stroke prevention in patients with cardiovascular disease and in high-risk hypertensive patients. The Stroke Prevention by Aggressive Reduction in Cholesterol Levels (SPARCL) trial demonstrated that high-dose atorvastatin is effective for secondary stroke prevention in patients with an ischemic stroke or TIA without concomitant coronary heart disease.[18] The Justification for the Use of Statins in Prevention: an Intervention Trial Evaluating Rosuvastatin (JUPITER) study showed that rosuvastatin treatment in patients with normal cholesterol levels but elevated levels of C-reactive protein is effective in reducing the rate of stroke.[19] The Treat Stroke to Target (TST) trial further established that a target LDL-C <70 mg/dL is superior to a higher target (90-110 mg/dL) in preventing major cardiovascular events.[16] Therefore, statins are a cornerstone of stroke treatment and prevention, especially in patients with known ASCVD in any vascular bed.

Antiplatelet medications are a critical component of primary stroke prevention. In the Antithrombotic Trialists' Collaboration meta-analysis of high-risk patients, antiplatelet therapy reduced the occurrence of any vascular event by roughly 25%, nonfatal stroke by about 25%, and death due to vascular cause by about 15%. Aspirin was the most widely used drug with doses of 75 to 150 mg being as beneficial as higher doses. The Women's Health Study found that 100 mg of aspirin every other day resulted in a significant 17% reduction in the risk of stroke over 10 years. High-dose aspirin (160-325 mg daily) provided no more benefit than lower doses but was associated with more side effects. Among patients with symptomatic vascular disease, including stroke, the Clopidogrel versus Aspirin in Patients at Risk of Ischemic Events (CAPRIE) trial demonstrated that clopidogrel 75 mg daily was associated with an 8.7% relative risk reduction in ischemic stroke, MI, or vascular death versus aspirin 325 mg daily (5.32% vs 5.83% P = .043). For the patients who presented with stroke, however, the benefit was not significant. Clopidogrel 75 mg daily plus aspirin 75 mg daily was compared to clopidogrel alone in the Management of Atherothrombosis with Clopidogrel in High-risk Patients (MATCH) trial, which found that among stroke patients, the combination regimen did not improve vascular outcomes but significantly increased major and life-threatening bleeding complications. The Clopidogrel for High Atherothrombotic Risk and Ischemic Stabilization, Management, and Avoidance (CHARISMA) trial included over 4300 patients with a prior TIA or stroke and found that aspirin (75-162 mg daily) was as effective as aspirin plus clopidogrel in preventing future MI, stroke, or cardiovascular death in patients with multiple risk factors or with clinically evident cardiovascular disease. This study also found that 81 mg of aspirin is the optimal dose for safety and efficacy for prevention. The Acute Stroke or Transient Ischemic Attack Treatment with Ticagrelor and Aspirin for Prevention of Stroke and Death (THALES) was a placebo-controlled double-blind RCT of patients with mild-to-moderate acute noncardioembolic ischemic stroke (not undergoing endovascular or intravenous [IV] intervention) wherein patients were assigned in a 1:1 ratio to 30 days of ticagrelor or acetylsalicylic acid (with loading doses). Of the 11,016 patients who underwent randomization, the primary outcome (composite of stroke or death) and secondary outcome of ischemic stroke was lower with ticagrelor-aspirin, but the incidence of disability did not differ significantly and severe bleeding was more frequently seen with ticagrelor + aspirin treatment.[20]

The AHA and ASA guidelines recommend that all patients with carotid atherosclerosis be placed on antiplatelet medications.[6,16] The primary benefit of antiplatelet therapy is in reduction of MI and ischemic cardiovascular events, but complete benefit for prevention of stroke in asymptomatic patients has not been established.[12]

There is uncertainty regarding the best therapy for asymptomatic carotid artery disease. The Carotid Revascularization

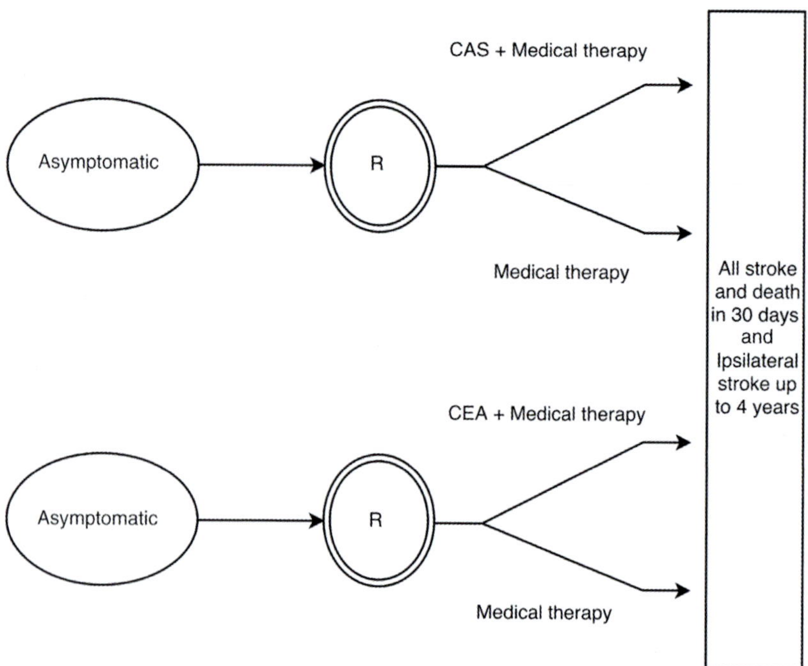

FIGURE 35.3 CREST-2 trial design. CAS, carotid artery stenting; CEA, carotid endarterectomy; CREST, carotid revascularization endarterectomy versus stenting trial.

Endarterectomy versus Stenting Trial (CREST-2) trial is currently enrolling patients and features two parallel arms (**Fig. 35.3**): one compares CEA with contemporary best medical management (BMT) versus BMT alone, and the other arm compares carotid artery stenting (CAS) with BMT versus BMT alone. Comprehensive lifestyle interventions and modern best procedural and medical practices are emphasized in all arms. CREST-2 medical management goals include systolic blood pressure (SBP) <140 mm Hg (<130 mm Hg for diabetes mellitus), LDL <70 mg/dL, hemoglobin A1c <7.0%, smoking cessation, targeted weight management, and more than 30 minutes of moderate exercise three times per week. Two smaller contemporary European trials, the 2nd ECST (n = 429) and Stent-Supported Percutaneous Angioplasty of the Carotid Artery Versus Endarterectomy-2 (SPACE-2, n = 513), completed reduced enrollment with varying degrees of follow-up. Interim 2-year (ECST-2) and 5-year (SPACE-2) have been presented and are concordant. Both trials evaluate revascularization (primarily CEA) with BMT versus BMT alone in asymptomatic patients. Neither trial found a difference in ipsilateral stroke, MI, or death when comparing modern BMT to revascularization with modern BMT. Due to power, recruitment, and execution issues, neither ECST-2 nor SPACE-2 is as robust as CREST-2. Thus, definitive guideline recommendations await the results of CREST-2.[2,21]

Surgical Therapy to Prevent Stroke

Asymptomatic Patients

The purpose of carotid revascularization is to prevent ischemic stroke. There have been three large RCTs comparing CEA to antiplatelet (aspirin) therapy in the treatment of moderate (>50%-60%) carotid stenosis in patients without focal neurologic symptoms, which are all made less relevant by modern medical therapy. The Veterans Affairs Cooperative Study[22] randomized 444 men with asymptomatic carotid stenosis of >50% by angiography to medical therapy plus CEA or medical therapy alone. All patients were assigned aspirin 650 mg twice daily, although many did not tolerate that dose. The 30-day risk of stroke or death in the CEA group was 4.7%. At nearly 4 years of follow-up, the ipsilateral neurologic event rate (including TIA, transient monocular blindness, and fatal and nonfatal stroke) was 8% in the surgical arm and 20.6% in the medical arm (P < .001). The risk of ipsilateral stroke alone was reduced from 9.4% with medical treatment to 4.7% (P < .06) with CEA. Notably, there was no difference between surgery and medical therapy for combined stroke or death.

ACAS randomized 1662 asymptomatic patients with carotid stenosis >60% to medical therapy or medical therapy with CEA.[23] All patients received aspirin 325 mg daily. Angiography was performed only in the CEA group and was associated with a 1.2% risk of stroke. The 30-day risk of stroke or death in the surgical group, including the risk associated with angiography, was 2.7%. The projected 5-year risk of ipsilateral stroke and any perioperative stroke or death was reduced from 11% in the medical arm to 5.1% with CEA. The number of patients needed to treat with surgery to prevent one ipsilateral stroke at 5 years was 19. The benefit for women (17% reduction in events) was less than for men (66% reduction).

ACST evaluated 3120 asymptomatic patients with >60% carotid stenosis by ultrasound. Patients were randomized to CEA with medical management or medical management alone. Drug treatment was left to the discretion of the patients' primary physicians—this usually included antiplatelet medications, antihypertensive therapy, and, in the later years of the study, lipid-lowering agents. The 30-day perioperative risk of stroke or death was 3.1%. The 5-year risk of perioperative death or total stroke was reduced from 11.8% to 6.4% with CEA; roughly, half the strokes were disabling. The benefit of surgery was significant across varying degrees of stenosis (60%-90% stenosis). Nevertheless, CEA did not reduce overall stroke and death and did not show any benefit in women or in patients older than 75 years of age.[23]

Symptomatic Patients

Three, historical, large RCTs have evaluated the benefit of CEA compared to medical therapy in symptomatic patients with moderate to severe carotid artery disease. Medical therapy in these trials is not comparable to contemporary BMT (ie, prestatin). The Veterans Administration 309 trial[24] screened 5000 symptomatic men who presented within 4 months and randomized 189 to either CEA + BMT versus BMT alone. Patients had angiographically defined internal carotid artery (ICA) stenosis ≥50%, but the trial was ended prematurely due to early results from NASCET and ECST. At mean follow-up of almost 1 year, there was a reduction in ipsilateral stroke or TIA (9.4% BMT vs 7.7% in the revascularization arm with an absolute reduction in risk of 11.7%). The benefit of surgery was most profound in patients with stenosis >70% (an absolute risk reduction of 17.7%).

The NASCET trial randomized patients with a TIA or nondisabling stroke within 180 days to CEA + historical BMT (including aspirin) or BMT alone. Patients were originally stratified into three groups based on the degree of carotid stenosis (<50%, 50%-69%, and 70%-99%). About 659 patients with >70% stenosis were randomized to CEA, which demonstrated an absolute risk reduction of 17% (26% CEA vs 9% BMT) of ipsilateral stroke at 2 years.[10] CEA lowered 2-year risk of major or fatal stroke from 13.1% to 2.5%. In patients with <50% stenosis, there was no benefit for stroke prevention with CEA and BMT as compared to BMT alone.[10] The 5-year rate of ipsilateral stroke was 22.2% in those on BMT versus 15.7% for patients who received CEA + BMT (absolute risk reduction of 6.5% for CEA + BMT).

ECST studied 3024 symptomatic patients with carotid stenosis; 60% of patients were randomized to CEA + BMT and 40% to BMT alone. BMT consisted of antihypertensive medications, antiplatelet agents, and antismoking counseling. The 30-day perioperative risk of major stroke or death with revascularization was 7%. There was no benefit to revascularization for stenosis below 70% to 80%. Among patients with a stenosis >80%, the rate of major stroke or death at 3 years was 26.5% with BMT versus 14.9% in the revascularization group (absolute risk reduction of 11.6% with revascularization). There was no benefit for patients who had near occlusion of the carotid artery. Of particular note, ECST criteria for stenosis definition differs from NASCET (eg, 80% stenosis by ECST approximates to 60% by NASCET; **Fig. 35.4**).[25]

A meta-analysis of these three studies found that for lesions <30% (by NASCET criteria), surgery increased the 5-year risk of ipsilateral stroke. CEA provided marginal benefit in patients with 50% to 69% stenosis (absolute risk reduction of 4.6%) but was most beneficial in patients with >70% stenosis (16% absolute risk reduction, $P < .001$). Patients with near occlusion (stenosis causing reduced flow to the distal ICA and/or narrowing of the poststenotic ICA) did not benefit from CEA.[25]

Current AHA/ASA guidelines recommend CEA in symptomatic patients with stenosis of 50% to 99% if the risk of perioperative stroke or death is <6%.[16] The recommended timing for carotid revascularization after a nondisabling stroke or TIA is within the first 2 weeks after the event. In asymptomatic patients, guidelines recommend CEA for stenosis of 60% to 99% if the perioperative risk of stroke is <3% and life expectancy is at least 5 years.[6]

Transcarotid Artery Revascularization

Transcarotid artery revascularization (TCAR) is a distinct stent-based hybrid approach to carotid revascularization that emerged in the mid-2010s. A single manufacturer, Silk Road Medical (Sunnyvale, CA), developed the Enroute system, which consists of an Enhance transcarotid access kit (including a sheath with 10 cm markers), a reverse-flow neuroprotection system (NPS), 4 to 6 mm diameter RX balloons (also a shorter 75 cm working length), a 0.014″ guidewire, and the transcarotid stent system (which itself utilizes the open cell Cordis PRECISE nitinol self-expanding stent on a shorter 57 cm delivery system). The TCAR procedure begins with a surgical cutdown (starting with a 3 cm longitudinal incision) over the proximal ipsilateral common carotid artery (CCA) (immediately cephalad to the clavicle). Stent delivery is directly through this access point, thus avoiding navigation through the aorta and iliofemoral arteries. Standard antiplatelet and anticoagulation practices are observed (including heparin with activated clotting time [ACT] target ≥250 seconds or bivalirudin). After cutdown is performed, a suture is preplaced around the CCA immediately proximal to the puncture site to allow for control of the arteriotomy site at the conclusion of the procedure. The CCA is accessed with standard Seldinger technique. The sheath is introduced, the proximal CCA is clamped, and the CCA flow reversed through the sheath and accompanying NPS (with retrograde flow through the external NPS eventually delivering blood to a common femoral vein). The continuous flow reversal is utilized to provide embolic protection. Thereafter, a guidewire crosses the lesion, and PTA and CAS are performed in similar fashion to transfemoral or transradial CAS, but requiring utilization of the Enroute balloon and stent delivery systems, which have shorter shaft/working lengths (as opposed to transfemoral equipment, which typically has 135 cm shaft length). The Enroute NPS, similar to proximal embolic protection device (EPD), requires contralateral flow crossover through the anterior or posterior circulation. After stenting is completed, the proximal CCA clamp is removed, the sheath is removed, and the previously placed suture deployed to close the arteriotomy site along with resumption of antegrade flow through the CCA. Contraindications for TCAR include any patients not eligible for stent-based revascularization, prior history of radiation therapy, short CCA (<5 cm from arteriotomy to lesion), small CCA (<6 cm), heavily calcified carotid lesion, tracheal stoma, high medical risk, or hostile neck (eg, obesity, immobility, kyphosis).

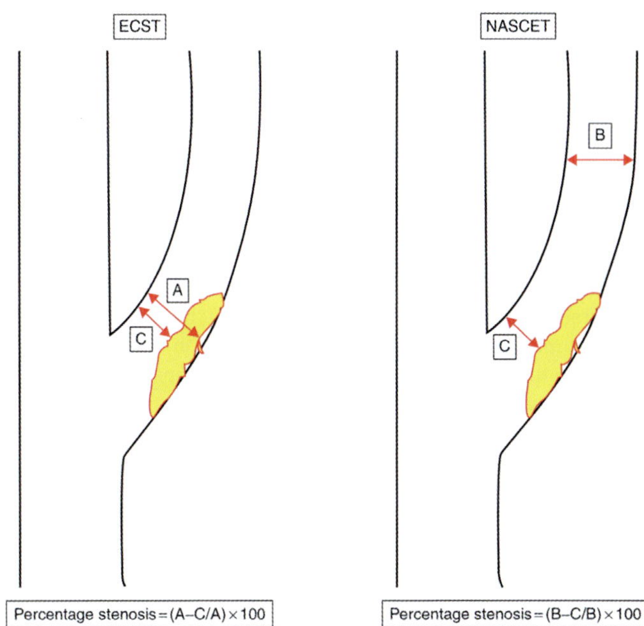

FIGURE 35.4 Angiographic methods for determining carotid stenosis severity. ECST, European Carotid Surgery Trial; NASCET, North American Symptomatic Carotid Endarterectomy Trial.

The Enroute TCAR system has not been evaluated through RCT analysis, but rather clinical data have been obtained solely through registries including the TCAR Surveillance Project (TSP)—an initiative of the Society of Vascular Surgery Patient Safety Organization. TCAR was initially reserved for high surgical risk (HSR) patients, but use has expanded to standard surgical risk patients. Long-term data from the Vascular Quality Initiative-TSP database found that TCAR, as compared to CEA, is associated with a shorter length of stay, lower rates of MI, shorter operative/procedural time, and lower rates of cranial nerve injury with comparable rates of all-cause mortality and ipsilateral stroke.[26] TCAR, similar to CAS and CEA, is an option for appropriate patients while factoring in lesion, anatomic, institutional, and operator experience and other variables. TCAR was included in the Centers for Medicare & Medicaid Services (CMS) 2023 expansion for CAS, and further data will emerge, especially as the procedure moves away from regular proctoring and into real-world use.

Carotid Artery Stenting

Clinical Evidence

Historically, there has been a paucity of high-quality data directly comparing CEA to CAS. However, the second ACST is a multicenter international RCT of CAS versus CEA in asymptomatic severe carotid artery stenosis necessitating revascularization but without a clear superior revascularization strategy (as per the patient and physician). About 3625 patients at 130 centers were randomized to CAS or CEA with follow-up at 1 month postrevascularization and then annually for 5 years. ACST-2 ran from 2008 through 2020 (ie, contemporary practice and medical management), and all operators were anonymized and reviewed for their competency in performing CAS and/or CEA, and intraprocedural modern best practices were observed. Over a mean follow-up duration of 4.9 years, ACST-2 found that serious (disabling or fatal stroke) complications were similarly uncommon after competent CAS or CEA (approximately 1% periprocedural and 0.5% per year long term for both). Nondisabling stroke (modified Rankin score [MRS] of ≤2) was statistically higher with CAS as compared to CEA (2.7% vs 1.9%, *P* = .03), which is consistent with contemporary registry data.[27,28] In totality, ACST-2 offers the highest LOE to date that CAS and CEA are comparable in terms of severe adverse outcomes for asymptomatic patients who are candidates for either procedure and that the overall procedural risk of stroke is low.[25] High-risk features for CEA and CAS are not necessarily interchangeable or equivalent. Features that place a patient at increased risk for complications from CEA and CAS are summarized in **Table 35.2**.

High Surgical Risk Patients

The 2008 Stenting and Angioplasty with Protection in Patients at High Risk for Endarterectomy (SAPPHIRE) trial is an RCT comparing HSR patients treated with CEA to those treated with CAS.[28] About 334 symptomatic patients with stenosis of >50% or an asymptomatic stenosis >80% (~30% were symptomatic) were randomized to CEA or CAS. The primary endpoint of death, stroke, or MI at 30 days along with ipsilateral stroke or death from neurologic cause up to 1 year occurred in 12.2% of the stenting group and 20.1% in the CEA group (*P* = .004 for noninferiority). The 30-day stroke and death rate among the asymptomatic patients was 4.6% for the CAS group and 5.4% for the CEA group. At 3 years, there were no differences between CEA and CAS.

Most contemporary registry data focus on HSR patient (data from over 10,000 HSR patients have been published) . These registries generally include symptomatic patients with >50% stenosis and asymptomatic patients with >70% to 80% stenosis. Data from many of these studies are summarized in **Fig. 35.5**. It is apparent that in HSR patients who require revascularization for stroke prevention, CAS is the preferred procedure in patients who can be treated by an experienced operator and have suitable anatomy for CAS. The current AHA/ASA stroke prevention guidelines regarding carotid revascularization are summarized in **Table 35.3**.

Average or Low Surgical Risk Patients

Five large RCTs in average- or low surgical risk patients have compared CAS to CEA.[30-34] Three of these trials were conducted in Europe, although procedural standards were compromised by allowing very inexperienced CAS operators to participate in the trials and not requiring EPDs to be used. The Endarterectomy Versus Angioplasty in Patients with Symptomatic Severe Carotid Stenosis (EVA-3S) trial randomized symptomatic patients with carotid stenosis of >60% to either CEA or CAS. All patients had to be "suitable candidates" for both procedures and had ipsilateral neurologic symptoms within 120 days of enrollment. The use of EPDs was optional, and many of the investigators were tutored while treating patients. The study was terminated early. The 30-day incidence of stroke or death was 9.6% in the CAS group and 3.9% (*P* = .004) in the CEA group.[33]

The SPACE trial randomized 1214 symptomatic average surgical risk patients to either CEA or CAS.[31] The use of EPDs was

TABLE 35.2 High-Risk Features of CAS and CEA

HIGH-RISK FEATURES FOR CAS		HIGH-RISK FEATURES FOR CEA	
CLINICAL FEATURES	**ANGIOGRAPHIC FEATURES**	**COMORBIDITIES**	**ANATOMIC FEATURES**
Age >75/80	Severe tandem lesions	Age >80	Lesion C2 or higher
Renal failure	>2 acute (90° bends)	Class III/IV CHF or angina	Lesion below clavicle
Multiple lacunar strokes	Circumferential calcification	LM >2-vessel CAD	Prior neck surgery (including ipsilateral CEA)
Dementia	Evidence of thrombus	LVEF <30%	Contralateral carotid occlusion
Bleeding disorder	Poor vascular access	Recent MI (>1 but <30 d)	Contralateral laryngeal nerve palsy
		Severe chronic lung disease	Neck radiation
		Renal failure	Tracheostomy

CAD, coronary artery disease; CAS, carotid artery stenting; CEA, carotid endarterectomy; CHF, congestive heart failure; LM, left main; LVEF, left ventricular ejection fraction; MI, myocardial infarction.

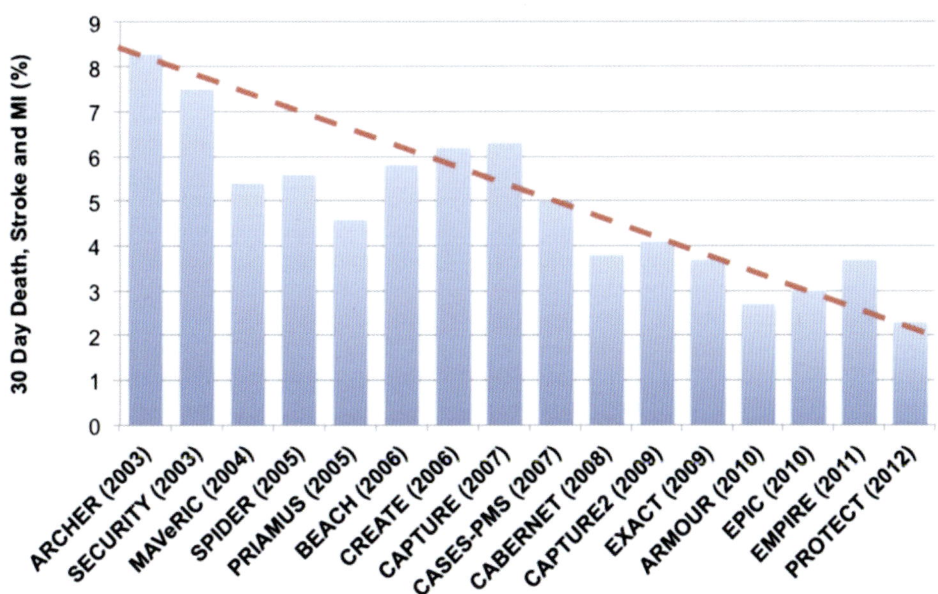

FIGURE 35.5 Trials comparing CAS to CEA in high surgical risk patients. CAS, carotid artery stenting; CEA, carotid endarterectomy; MI, myocardial infarction.

optional, and inexperienced operators were tutored during patient enrollment. The 30-day rate of ipsilateral stroke or death was not different between the two groups (6.8% CAS vs 6.3% CEA, *P* = .09 for noninferiority). Nevertheless, the 2-year outcomes for this trial demonstrated a statistically significant benefit for CAS over CEA in patients <68 years of age.

The International Carotid Stenting Study (ICSS) enrolled over 1700 symptomatic patients and randomized them to either CAS or CEA. Use of EPDs was optional. To qualify as an experienced center, a center had to have a surgeon who had performed 50 CEA procedures and an interventionalist who had performed 10 CAS procedures. If the center was less experienced, they were tutored until considered proficient by their proctor. The center was upgraded to experienced after randomizing 20 patients and if their outcomes were considered acceptable. The patients were assigned to CAS or CEA in a 1:1 fashion and followed up for a median of 4.2 years. The number of fatal or disabling strokes and cumulative 5-year risk did not differ between the CAS and CEA groups (6.4% vs 6.5%). The distribution of mRS scores at 1 year, 5 years, or final follow-up did not differ between treatment groups.[30]

CREST[32] is the largest (*n* = 2502) randomized trial comparing CAS with EPD to CEA in patients at average risk for surgery. It included symptomatic (*n* = 1321) and asymptomatic (*n* = 1181) patients. The primary outcome of periprocedural stroke, death, or MI or follow-up ipsilateral stroke was not significantly different between the two groups (7.2% CAS vs 6.8% CEA). The 30-day risk of all stroke was higher for CAS (4.1% vs 2.3%, *P* = .01), whereas CEA was associated with a higher 30-day risk of MI (2.3% vs 1.1%, *P* = .03). The rate of ipsilateral stroke over a mean follow-up of 4 years was similar between groups. CAS appeared safer than CEA for patients <69 years of age, while CEA yielded better outcomes in those >70 years of age. At 10 years, there continued to be no

TABLE 35.3 Guidelines for Carotid Revascularization[7,29]

	SYMPTOMATIC PATIENTS				ASYMPTOMATIC PATIENTS	
	ESC		AHA/ACCF/SCAI		ESC	AHA/ACCF/SCAI
	50%-69% STENOSIS[a]	70%-99% STENOSIS[a]	50%-69% STENOSIS[b]	70%-99% STENOSIS[b]	>60% STENOSIS[a]	70%-99% STENOSIS[b]
Carotid endarterectomy	Class IIa LOE—A	Class I LOE—A	Class I LOE—B	Class I LOE—A	Class IIa[c] LOE—A	Class IIa LOE—A
Carotid artery stenting	Class IIa[e] Class IIb[f] LOE—B		Class I LOE—B	Class I LOE—B	Class IIb[d] LOE—B	Class IIb LOE—B

ACCF, American College of Cardiology Foundation; AHA, American Heart Association; CTA, computed tomography angiography; ESC, European Society of cardiology; LOE, Level of Evidence; MRA, magnetic resonance angiography; NASCET, North American Symptomatic Carotid Endarterectomy Trial; SCAI, The Society for Cardiovascular Angiography and Interventions.

[a]The severity of stenosis is calculated by duplex ultrasound, CTA, and/or MRA.

[b]The severity of stenosis is defined according to the angiographic criteria by the method used in NASCET but generally corresponds as well to assessment by sonography and other accepted methods of measurement.

[c]Perioperative stroke and death rate <3% and life expectancy >5 y.

[d]In high-volume centers with documented death or stroke rate <3%.

[e]In symptomatic patients at high surgical risk, CAS should be considered an alternative to CEA.

[f]CAS may be considered an alternative to CEA in high-volume centers with a documented death or stroke rate <6%.

From Sacco RL, Kasner SE, Broderick JP, et al. An updated definition of stroke for the 21st century: a statement for healthcare professionals from the American Heart Association/American Stroke Association. *Stroke.* 2013;44(7):2064-2089 and Campbell BC, Mitchell PJ, Kleinig TJ, et al. Endovascular therapy for ischemic stroke with perfusion-imaging selection. *NEJM.* 2015;372(11):1009-1018.

difference for the primary endpoint in symptomatic patients for CAS (13.4%; 95% confidence interval [CI]: 9.7%-17.6%) and in the CEA group (9.8%; 95% CI: 7.2%-12.7%; hazard ratio: 1.17; 95% CI: 0.82-1.66; *P* = .40).

CREST differed from the previous three trials in three significant ways. Most importantly, the European trials, EVA-3S, SPACE, and ICSS, allowed inexperienced operators to treat patients. They allowed interventional operators, but not surgical operators, to be "tutored" during the randomized trial. CREST requirements were more stringent. Many of the "experienced" CAS operators in the first three trials were not very experienced (EVA-3S required that operators perform at least five CAS procedures, ICSS required 10 CAS procedures, and SPACE had no minimum number of carotid stenting procedures required). The frequency of nonculprit carotid circulation neurological events speaks to the critical importance of catheter skills, procedural planning, and training. The value of experience cannot be overstated. Second, CREST mandated the use of EPDs, whereas the other trials did not. Lastly, just over 50% of the patients in CREST were symptomatic, whereas the other trials were entirely for symptomatic patients.

Asymptomatic average surgical risk carotid stenosis patients were enrolled in the Asymptomatic Carotid Trial. CAS was noninferior to CEA with regard to death, stroke, or MI within 30 days after the procedure, or ipsilateral stroke within 1 year (3.8% vs 3.4%). There was no difference for CAS versus CEA for rates of stroke or death within 30 days (2.9% and 1.7% [*P* = .33]). Freedom from ipsilateral stroke from 30 days to 5 years was 97.8% in the CAS group and 97.3% in the CEA group (*P* = .51)[34] (**Fig. 35.6**).

CAS Coverage Expansion

Taken together, the message from these five RCTs is that CAS is a reasonable alternative to CEA in selected average surgical risk patients, when properly performed by experienced operators. Furthermore, in 2022 and early 2023, multiple societies, including the Multispecialty Carotid Alliance (MSCA), American Association of Neurological Surgeons (AANS), and Congress of Neurological Surgeons, urged the CMS to update the National Coverage Determination for Carotid Artery Stenting to include asymptomatic patients as well as standard surgical risk patients given the increasing and concordant data demonstrating equivalent outcomes and long-term stroke prevention between CAS and CEA.[35,36] In late 2023, CMS expanded coverage of CAS (PTA + CAS) to include placement of an FDA-approved carotid stent and FDA-approved or cleared EPD for patients with symptomatic carotid artery stenosis ≥50% or asymptomatic carotid artery stenosis ≥70% provided they also have a neurological assessment by a neurologist or NIHSS-certified health professional before and after CAS. Patients also require a first-line evaluation of stenosis by duplex ultrasonography, a CTA, or MRA (unless contraindicated) to confirm the degree of stenosis (as well as provide additional information about the aortic arch and extracranial and intracranial circulation), and intra-arterial DSA if there is discrepancy between noninvasive imaging results (or in lieu of CTA and/or MRA if there is contraindication to CTA or MRA).[37] CMS expanded coverage of CAS to include standard surgical risk individuals (previously HSR only). And while CMS removed the formal facility approval requirement, they noted that facilities performing CAS must establish and maintain institutional and physician standards to support a dedicated carotid stent program. These standards include clearly delineating a process for granting and maintaining CAS privileges (including monitoring outcomes), having institutional oversight committees for the program to identify minimal case volume (along with risk-adjusted threshold for complications that would require suspension/remediation), ensuring appropriately trained staff are present to fulfill roles and responsibilities for a dedicated carotid stent program, ensuring sufficient appropriate supporting personal and equipment are present for all aspects of uncomplicated and complicated cases, and maintaining an active quality improvement program through assessment of procedural outcomes in order to drive necessary programmatic adjustments to ensure patient safety.[37] CMS also emphasized the need for formal shared decision-making with individuals prior to offering CAS and the need to allow Medicare Administrative Contractors have discretion for coverage of CAS for indications not otherwise covered in the CMS decision memo. The goal is to reduce the significant prior barriers to access to CAS and recognize the increasing data demonstrating safety and efficacy of CAS compared to CEA.[37]

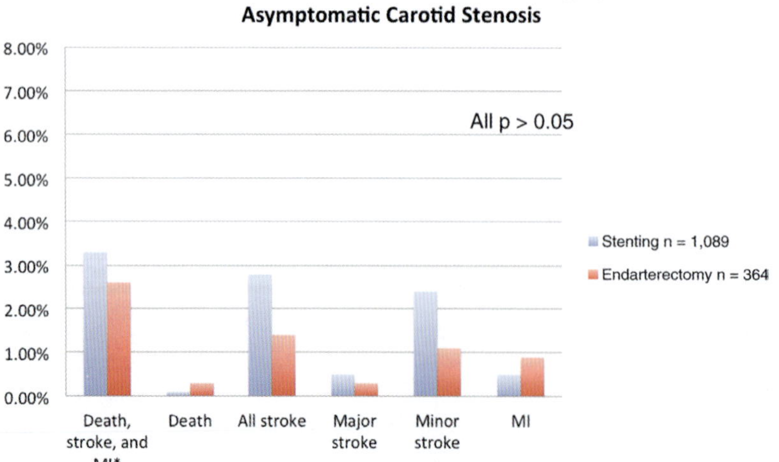

FIGURE 35.6 Results of the Asymptomatic Carotid Trial (ACT-1). MI, myocardial infarction.

Technical Aspects

Baseline Aortography and Cerebral Angiography

Commonly, noninvasive CTA of the aortic arch is performed coincident with CTA visualization of the extracranial and intracranial vessels. This allows identification of high risk or prohibitive proximal anatomy prior to endovascular access. If this noninvasive evaluation is not performed, aortography at the time of endovascular therapy is mandatory both to identify arch type, vertebral origin, and/or congenitally aberrant anatomy. An arch aortogram is performed in the 30° to 45° left anterior oblique (LAO) projection to elongate the arch and optimize identification of the ostia of the cervical vessels. Once the morphology of the aortic arch is determined, catheters are chosen for selective angiography of the cervical arteries supplying the brain (right and left carotid and vertebral arteries [VAs]) and the cerebral vasculature. For a type I arch, Berenstein, angled taper or Judkins Right (JR) catheters are often used. For type II or III arch morphologies, Shepherd's crook-shaped catheters (ie, Simmons or Vitek catheters) may optimize vessel selection though require expertise of use secondary to particular mechanisms of use (**Fig. 35.7**).

Excellent DSA imaging is mandatory for optimal carotid stenting practice. With all catheter injections, meticulous adherence to line preparation to ensure avoidance of air embolization is performed. After an optimal angle is selected to visualize separation of the internal and external carotid arteries, this angle is visualized via sheath injection and a DSA image is utilized to optimize device placement. Simultaneous identification of bony landmarks or the use of prepositioned radiopaque markers or tape can provide confirmation of localization.

Transradial CAS

Historically, transfemoral has been the vascular access approach of choice for most transcatheter interventions, including for CAS. Transradial diagnostic and therapeutic coronary interventions have become increasingly popular and have data to support their efficacy, safety, and outcomes.[38] The transradial approach has become increasingly popular for vascular procedures, and current guidelines recommend it as the primary approach of choice for coronary interventions.[39] Given the benefits of transradial access, especially with regard to vascular access complications, the radial approach has also been introduced in CAS. Transradial CAS should be considered in patients with "bovine" or type III aortic arches as well as in patients with tortuous, severely stenosed, aneurysmal, calcific, or otherwise unfavorable iliofemoral and/or aortic anatomy.[40] Preprocedure planning with CTA or MRA is extremely helpful for planning transradial CAS in order to evaluate for radial size/suitability, arch type (right radial approach for left CCA canulation is technically more difficult in type I aortic arch), atherocalcific disease, and/or unfavorable anatomy such as prohibitive tortuosity.[40] Transradial CAS safety has been evaluated in a subset of the CREST-2 Registry (2868 patients had undergone CAS, of which 213, 3.8%, were transradial) and demonstrated no significant differences between transradial and transfemoral access in regard to major access-related complications or composite of periprocedural stroke or death. Transradial was also associated with lower general anesthesia use and higher use of distal EPD.[41] Transbrachial is also an access option but is associated with higher vascular access complications as compared to the transradial approach. Similar to other transradial interventions, transradial (and transbrachial) should be avoided in the absence of a patent ipsilateral ulnar artery or challenging aortic arch variation (eg, aberrant right subclavian artery).

From the right radial approach, a JR 4, multipurpose, internal mammary, Kimny, or Simmons 2 catheter can be utilized to engage the right CCA (as well as left CCA in patients with bovine type arch). Engaging the left CCA in patients without aberrant anatomy from the right radial approach typically entails looping a 0.035″ guidewire in the sinus of Valsalva (ideally the noncoronary cusp) with the tip of the guidewire extending superiorly toward, or stationed in, the transverse aorta. The catheter is then brought down over the guidewire until it also points superiorly, the guidewire is retracted to allow the catheter to shape, and the entire system then retracted until the catheter engages the ostial left CCA. Thereafter, the guidewire is advanced into the CCA, the catheter advanced over it onto the proximal-to-mid CCA. The guidewire is then removed, and angiography with or without intervention proceeds in a fashion similar to the transfemoral approach. Alternatively, from the right radial approach, the guidewire can be placed in the descending aorta, a Simmons 2 catheter advanced until the tip is in the proximal distal aorta (pointing toward the transverse aorta), and then the guidewire retracted into the Simmons 2 catheter at which point it will be shaped and can be used to directly canulate the left CCA (often with counter clockwise torque of the catheter). LAO angulation aortography as well as roadmap can be helpful in canulating both CCAs via transradial approach and can be performed while the guidewire and guide catheter was in the aortic root. When performing transradial CAS, it is especially important to image the nontarget CCA and ICA first. Of note, the Simmons catheters should be manipulated in a similar fashion as Amplatz curve coronary catheters—pulled back to engage/dive into a vessel and torqued + pushed to disengage from a vessel. Engagement from the left radial artery is similar to the femoral approach, with the use of double-curve catheters (eg, Simmons, Newton) being utilized. Hemostasis after procedural completion is achieved in standard transradial fashion (ie, patent hemostasis).

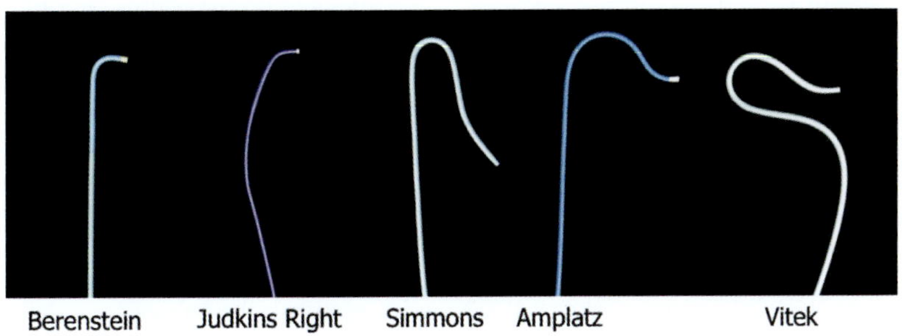

FIGURE 35.7 Catheter shapes most used for engagement of great vessels.

Embolic Protection

Because of the very low incidence of stroke complicating CAS, demonstrating clinical benefit for any EPD in an RCT has been difficult. However the catastrophic potential of iatrogenic embolization coupled with improving outcomes in contemporary CAS trials that utilized EPD, including mandating EPD use for optimal current practice. Two meta-analyses support the use of EPDs.[42,43] Nevertheless, others have failed to demonstrate benefit. Anecdotally, one simply has to retrieve a filter full of debris to realize the empirical benefits relative to the rare complications associated with an EPD.

Proximal protection is an alternative to distal embolic protection. In the United States, only one device remains commercially available: the Mo.Ma system (Medtronic, Minneapolis, MN). The Mo.Ma system consists of a single sheath with two balloons: a proximal balloon to be inflated in the CCA and a distal balloon in the external carotid artery. When the balloons are inflated, blood flow through the ICA is arrested. In order to deploy the system, the external carotid artery is accessed and the sheath and deflated ECA balloon are advanced over the 0.035-in stiff wire into the external carotid artery. The external and common carotid balloons are inflated arresting antegrade flow. Once patient tolerance of balloon occlusion is confirmed, the internal carotid lesion is crossed with a 0.014-in wire, dilated, and stented as described earlier. A distal EPD can be used in conjunction with the Mo.Ma in standard fashion (typically deployed before the Mo.Ma balloons are inflated). Blood is manually aspirated after the stenting procedure to clear the debris distal to the common carotid balloon. Data indicate that proximal embolic protection can provide excellent results. A 1300-patient single-center prospective registry reported 99.7% procedural success with the Mo.Ma device and a 30-day death and stroke rate of 1.38%.[44]

EPDs are standard of care in the United States, and several types exist (**Fig. 35.8**). If the EPD will not cross the lesion, the stenosis may be crossed with a conventional 0.014-in guide wire and subsequently predilated with a small (2.5 mm) balloon. Then, the EPD may be placed. After distal EPD deployment, the lesion is often predilated with an undersized coronary balloon, typically 3 to 4 mm in diameter. A self-expanding stent is then placed across the lesion. The stent covering the origin of the ICA is typically sized to fit the CCA. Though commonly used, there is no demonstrated benefit for using tapered stents. Typically when treating an internal carotid bifurcation lesion, the operator places the stent across the ostium of the external carotid artery.

There are three types of self-expanding stents: closed cell, open cell, and dual layered. Open-cell stents are more flexible and may better navigate tortuous vessels. Closed-cell stents are more rigid but offer better "coverage" of atherosclerotic plaque. While some evidence suggests that the frequency of embolic complications in symptomatic patients is lower with closed-cell stents, other analyses have found no significant correlation between stent design and outcomes. Three leading dual-layered carotid stents have been developed: Scaffold (W.L. Gore and Associates), Roadsaver (Microvention), and CGuard (Inspire-MD). Dual-layered stents are designed with an external self-expanding layer for scaffolding and an internal micromesh layer for plaque coverage, theoretically combining the advantages of an open- and closed-cell stent design. Several studies have demonstrated encouraging results with CAS performed using dual-layered stents.[45-47]

Typical stent sizes are 6 to 10 mm in diameter and 2 to 4 cm in length. Gentle postdilation with a ≤5-mm balloon is often performed to improve stent apposition with the vessel wall. There is no benefit to aggressive postdilation because restenosis and late

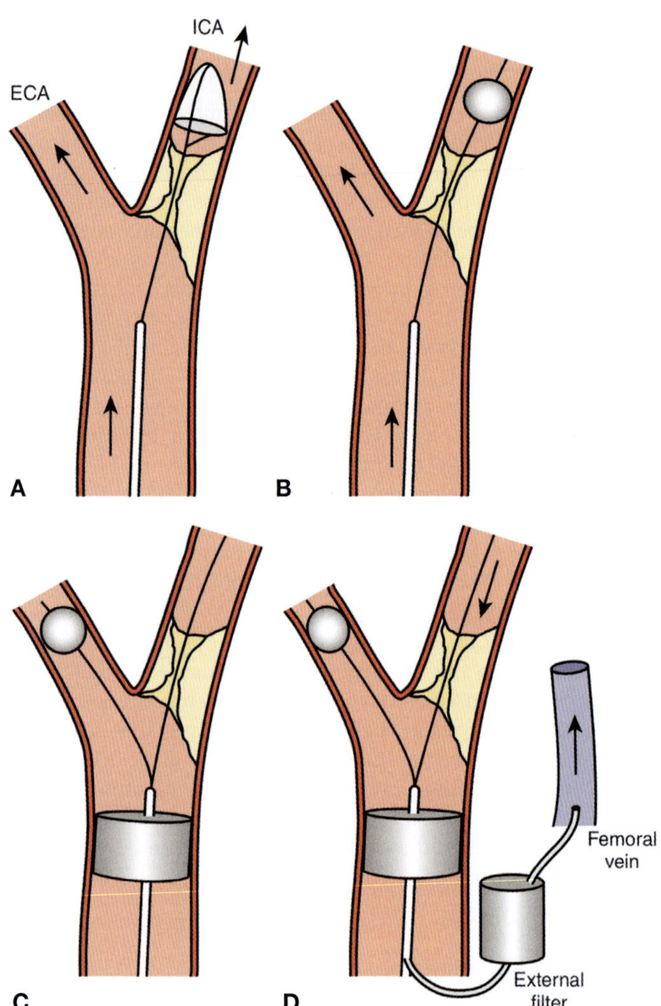

FIGURE 35.8 Embolic protection devices (EPDs). **A,** Filter-type device. **B,** Balloon occlusion of internal carotid artery (ICA). **C and D,** Proximal protection with flow reversal. See text. ECA, external carotid artery.

loss are very low in the carotid artery. Balloons are conservatively sized (<1:1) to minimize vessel trauma/dissection, plaque embolization, and stimulation of the carotid sinus. A poststent carotid diameter stenosis of <50% is an acceptable result. Clinical teams should be prepared for vagal responses including profound hypotension, bradycardia, and heart block when pressure is applied to the carotid bulb. This occurs most frequently at the time of stent postdilatation and can be treated with immediate administration of IV atropine. Other continuous chronotropic therapies or even placement of temporary pacemaker wires can be required to combat this complication in the rare event of persistence.

Following the procedure, if a filter-type EPD is used, the EPD is retrieved. Meticulous caution is required to ensure that the EPD basket is captured sufficiently to allow it to be safely withdrawn through the newly placed stent but without complete collapse, which could result in forced embolization of captured debris. Gentle traction can withdraw the device, but occasionally, manipulation of the sheath or rotation of the neck is required. Final carotid and cerebral angiography is performed after removal. If a proximal protection device is used, aspiration is performed per manufacturer protocol, the balloons are deflated, and then final angiography is performed (**Fig. 35.9**). It is important to confirm that the carotid artery is free of dissection and that the cerebral vasculature

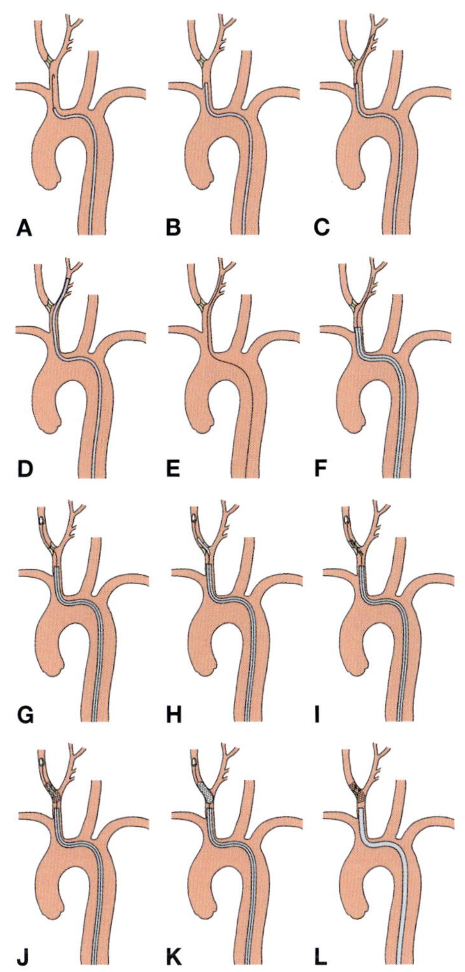

FIGURE 35.9 Stenting of the internal carotid artery (ICA). **A,** The common carotid artery (CCA) is accessed with a diagnostic catheter and standard 0.035-in J wire. **B,** The catheter is advanced over the J wire but remains in the CCA. **C,** The J wire is exchanged for a hydrophilic stiff-angled 0.035″ wire. **D,** The catheter is advanced to the ECA, and the hydrophilic wire is removed. **E,** A stiff Amplatz wire is advanced to the ECA, and the catheter is removed. **F,** A long 6F sheath is advanced over a dilator to the CCA. **G,** After removing the Amplatz wire and dilator, the lesion is crossed with a wire/filter device. **H,** Predilation. **I,** Stent placement. **J,** Stent deployment. The ostium of the ECA is often "jailed". **K,** Postdilation. **L,** Final result.

is intact. Prior to removal of equipment, a neurologic exam assessing speech, movement, and mental status should be performed. If a neurologic deficit is found, a culprit lesion is sought and neurovascular rescue attempted.

It is critical that prior to wiring or manipulation within any supra-aortic vessel that therapeutic anticoagulation (goal ACT >250 seconds) is achieved and maintained throughout the case. Furthermore, meticulous aspiration technique must be utilized, especially since larger equipment (eg, CAS delivery systems) will entrain air within the system while being delivered to the target vessel. Postprocedural care should be standardized across an institution for both CAS and CEA, including regular hemodynamic and neurologic monitoring, especially in the first 24 hours after revascularization.

Aorto-Ostial and Common Carotid Interventions

Coincident or isolated proximal stenotic lesions can be visualized during the workup of carotid artery disease. Revascularization of such lesions can be complicated by the inability to treat within close proximity of an EPD. To treat these lesions, femoral access is obtained with a 6- to 9-French sheath, depending on the diameter of the balloon and stent that will be used.

After anticoagulation and appropriate diagnostic imaging of the target lesion, a 5-French diagnostic catheter is advanced through a guide catheter (ie, a JR 4 or multipurpose guide) to the ostium of the target CCA. The ostial lesion is crossed with a steerable 0.035-in hydrophilic Glidewire (Terumo Interventional Systems, Somerset, NJ). The diagnostic catheter is then advanced across the lesion into the distal vessel. The Glidewire is exchanged for a stiff 0.035-in wire, and the guide catheter is carefully advanced over the diagnostic catheter until it engages the ostium of the CCA. The diagnostic catheter is then slowly removed. An EPD can be placed within the ICA prior to treatment of proximal lesions, but it is often impossible to position the EPD and the proximal lesion within one fluoroscopic plane.

Intravascular ultrasound can be used to allow appropriate visualization and sizing of the lesion. The lesion is predilated with a balloon sized 1:1 with the CCA. As the balloon deflates, the guide is gently advanced or "telescoped" over the balloon and across the lesion. This will facilitate placing the stent across the lesion. The predilation balloon is removed, and a balloon-expandable stent is placed. (In arteries protected by the axial skeleton, balloon-expandable stents are more often used.) After positioning the stent at the target lesion, the guide catheter is withdrawn, uncovering the stent and placing it in contact with the target lesion. The proximal stent should protrude very slightly into the aorta (<1 mm) to ensure lesion coverage. After verifying adequate placement with contrast injections through the guide catheter, the stent is deployed at nominal pressure. As the balloon deflates, the guide is again gently telescoped over the balloon to allow further stents to be delivered distally if needed. A larger semicompliant balloon may be used to flare the protruding portion of the stent in order to facilitate future angiography. Final angiography and neurologic assessment are performed (**Fig. 35.10**).

The access site is managed similarly to other interventional procedures. Sheath removal is performed when the ACT is <170 seconds if a vascular closure device is not used.

Complications and Troubleshooting

Stroke

In a 2009 review of over 54,000 patients, the 30-day risk of stroke during or after CAS was 3.9%.[33] Symptomatic patients were twice as likely to have an adverse event as asymptomatic patients. Most events occur within 24 hours of the procedure. If the patient develops a focal neurologic deficit *during* the procedure, an embolic event is assumed. Immediate cerebral angiography should be performed, and rescue intervention should be attempted. Typically, these emboli are plaque elements not amenable to thrombolysis. Attempts at revascularization with angioplasty and stenting and/or thrombectomy are recommended. Mental status changes *after* the procedure warrant CT evaluation to rule out intracranial bleeding or hyperperfusion syndrome (see the following text). More contemporary data in ACST-2 indicate that with proper patient, technique, and operator selection, the risk of short and long-term complications of CAS is low.[27]

Hemodynamic Instability

Stimulation of the carotid sinus baroreceptor is common during carotid interventions and can cause hypotension and bradycardia.

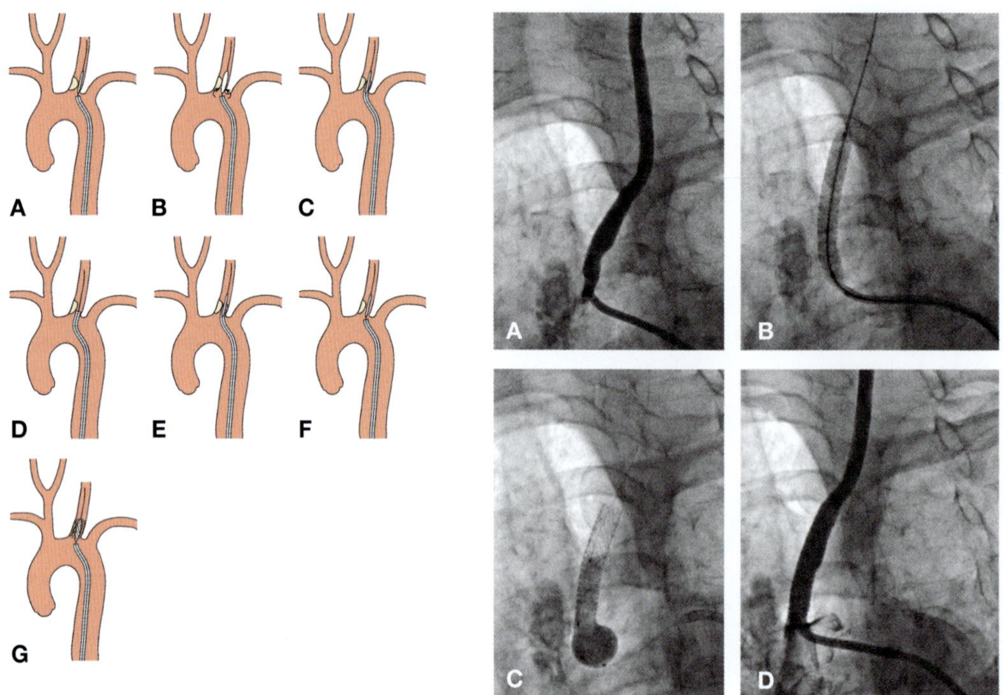

FIGURE 35.10 Dilating and stenting aorto-ostial lesions. Left panel: **A,** The lesion is crossed with a 0.035-in wire and predilation balloon is placed. **B,** The lesion is predilated, and as the balloon deflates, the guide catheter is advanced, thus "swallowing" the balloon. **C,** The guide is now distal to the lesion. **D,**. The balloon is removed. **E,**. A balloon-expandable stent is placed, although a portion of it remains within the guide. **F,** The guide is withdrawn, uncovering the stent and leaving it in contact with the lesion. **G,** The stent is deployed. If a stent is required distally, the stent balloon is "swallowed." Right panel: **A,** Aorto-ostial common carotid stenosis. **B,** Sent inflation with stent partially protruding into the aorta. **C,** Postdilation with Ostial flash balloon. **D,** Final result.

Typically, patients who are most sensitive will react negatively to predilation of the lesion. Acute hypotension can lead to brain hypoperfusion and neurologic symptoms due to impaired cerebral autoregulation. Holding baseline antihypertensive medications on the morning of intervention are prudent to avoid intraprocedural hypotension from baroreceptor activation. Atropine (0.4 to 1 mg) or glycopyrrolate may be used to treat acute bradycardia. A prophylactic dose may be considered before stent deployment if the patient was sensitive to predilation, but there is a risk of urinary retention in men (operator preference and local institutional standards vary in routine utilization of Foley catheter placement) and worsening of acute angle glaucoma. Repeat doses of atropine may can be administered if necessary although alternative parenteral inotropes/vasopressors should be considered if ≥2 mg IV atropine has been administered.

It is reasonable to measure a left ventricular end-diastolic pressure prior to aortography to help guide fluid management, especially in patients with a history of congestive heart failure. Some operators will obtain routine venous access in order to minimized delay when fluid and/or vasopressor administration is needed. Aggressive fluid administration is important in treating hypotension, but vasopressor medications may be needed to maintain an SBP of >100 mm Hg. Repeated boluses, as needed, of 25 to 50 µg of phenylephrine can be utilized. A continuous infusion may be required if hypotension persists. In most patients, however, phenylephrine when required can be weaned within several hours of the procedure, and the patient can ambulate in preparation for discharge the next day. Midodrine 2.5 to 10 mg three times daily (and then titrated downward as tolerated) can be useful to support blood pressure in the setting of prolonged hypotension. Adjusting the patient's antihypertensive regimen will be necessary over the short term. As with many transcatheter procedures, access site bleeding is a common cause of hypotension and should not be overlooked in the setting of postprocedural hypotension.

Hyperperfusion Syndrome and Intracranial Hemorrhage

The opening of a stenotic carotid artery can lead to significant increases in cerebral blood flow, sometimes to levels more than twice that of preprocedure flow. Hyperperfusion syndrome occurs in <1% of carotid stent patients and is defined clinically by the presence of an ipsilateral throbbing headache, a seizure, or a focal neurologic deficit. A chronically stenotic carotid artery can cause the cerebral vasculature to remain in a state of constant maximal vasodilation. When the stenosis is suddenly alleviated, cerebral autoregulatory mechanisms fail to control blood flow, a problem exacerbated by HTN. The resulting elevated cerebral perfusion pressure can lead to cerebral edema or, worse, intracranial hemorrhage (ICH).[48]

Neurologic symptoms from cerebral edema are usually transient but must be addressed. A neurology consultation and head CT should be obtained if this diagnosis is entertained. When diagnosed, strict control of blood pressure is critical, and consideration of mannitol, diuretics, and/or antiepileptic medications (depending on presentation) is warranted. Medications that cause cerebral venous vasodilation (ie, nitroprusside, nitroglycerin) should be avoided. During the procedure, hydralazine IV pushes are preferred if the patient is bradycardic, otherwise labetalol is the preferred choice. When an infusion is required, nicardipine is preferred. Intracranial bleeding is life threatening. If it occurs, antiplatelet medications should be stopped and a neurosurgical team consulted. Strict blood pressure control (goal systolic pressure of 120-140 mm Hg) may decrease the risk of hyperperfusion syndrome and intracranial bleeding.

Follow-Up

Following intervention, patients should be followed to ensure continuation of best medical therapy along, monitoring for focal neurologic symptoms, and Doppler ultrasound (DUS) surveillance. After carotid artery revascularization, it is recommended to obtain DUS studies at baseline (within 1 month of intervention), at 6 months, 12 months, and yearly thereafter.[49] Carotid DUS velocities are altered after stenting, and overestimation of stenosis severity is very common. Thus, the baseline (ie, ≤1 month postintervention) DUS is especially important to serve as a comparator for any changes, which may be especially meaningful compared to standard (ie, nonrevascularized) carotid DUS criteria.[50]

VERTEBRAL ARTERY INTERVENTIONS

The posterior circulation of the brain is supplied by the vertebral arteries (VA). The VAs most commonly originate from the subclavian arteries but can originate directly from the aortic arch in 3% to 5% of individuals.[51] The circle of Willis connects the anterior circulation perfused by the carotid arteries to the posterior circulation but is completely intact in only 20% of patients leading to varied presentation of VA malperfusion.[52]

Classical symptoms of posterior circulation ischemia include dizziness, drop attacks, diplopia, gait disturbance, dysphasia, and bilateral hemianopia. Less frequent symptoms include confusion, global amnesia, syncope, occipital headaches, nausea, vomiting, nystagmus, bilateral facial numbness, cortical blindness, and altered mental status.[53] The natural history of symptomatic vertebral artery stenosis (VAS) is a 5% to 11% incidence of stroke or death at 1 year.[54] Reversible neurologic deficits caused by extracranial VAS carry a 5-year stroke risk of 30%.[55] Symptomatic posterior circulation stenoses that are refractory to medical therapy carry a 5% to 11% incidence of stroke or death at 1 year.[56] Atherosclerotic disease of the VA is most commonly located at the ostium (V0) and proximal segment of the vessel (V1) and typically represents extension of plaque from the subclavian artery. The primary mechanism of stroke in 9% of the cases is artery-to-artery embolism to the distal circulation.

Patients with persistent symptoms and anatomically suitable lesions despite optimal antiatherosclerotic medical therapy should be considered for revascularization. Reasonable candidates for revascularization include patients with symptomatic vertebrobasilar insufficiency and bilateral VAS > 70% or unilateral vertebral stenosis >70% in the presence of an occluded or a hypoplastic contralateral VA.[3] VA revascularization may be considered if vertebral perfusion through the Circle of Willis would increase total cerebral blood flow enough to improve symptomatic patients with diffuse atherosclerotic disease and occlusions of both carotid arteries. VA chronic total occlusions should not be revascularized. Distal embolic debris to V4 and basilar artery perforators supplying the anterior spinal cord and brain stem could potentially be clinically devastating resulting in cerebellar, midbrain, pons, medullary, and brainstem infarctions.

Surgical treatments of proximal vertebral artery occlusive disease are performed rarely and include transsubclavian vertebral endarterectomy and vein patch angioplasty, transposition of the VA to the ipsilateral common carotid or internal artery and reimplantation of the VA with vein graft extension to the subclavian artery. For such proximal VA reconstruction, early complication rates of 2.5% to 25% and perioperative mortality rates of 0% to 4% have been reported.[54,57-59]

Most proximal VA interventions are performed using femoral artery access. A 6-French sheath or guide (including Envoy Multipurpose D or Multipurpose PC) is delivered to the proximal subclavian artery, and the lesion is crossed using a 0.014-inch wire. Predilation with a coronary balloon is optional to facilitate stent delivery but not always necessary in routine cases. Stenting with a balloon-expandable stent is preferred to provide radial strength and reduce restenosis. EPDs are used if the distal vessel is large enough to accommodate the device.[60] With the use of contemporary stenting techniques, procedural success approaches are 100% and periprocedural neurologic complications are rare.

Angioplasty alone carries high rates of restenosis; however, after stenting, the rate of restenosis occurs in 10% or fewer of patients. Lesion length is an independent predictor of restenosis, and this may be considered for the selection of drug-eluting over bare-metal stents for longer lesions. A 2011 meta-analysis of 27 articles and 980 patients undergoing VA stenting reported 1.1% stroke rate (11 patients) and 0.8% TIA (8 patients) at 30 days. Vertebrobasilar infarction (1.3%) and recurrent symptoms (6.5%) remained low at mean follow-up of 21 months.[57] In 2014, a meta-analysis of nine retrospective studies examined 480 lesions treated with 309 bare-metal stents and 175 drug-eluting stents. Drug-eluting stents significantly decreased both angiographic and symptomatic restenosis compared to bare-metal stents: 8.2% versus 23.7% and 4.7% versus 11.7%, respectively.[58]

The Vertebral Artery Stenting Trial enrolled 115 patients with symptomatic VAS and randomized medical therapy versus stenting plus medical therapy. Unfortunately, the trial was prematurely discontinued due to regulatory and funding deficiencies after enrollment of 57 patients in the endovascular arm and 58 patients in the medical therapy arm. There were three strokes and one death (5%) in the stent arm compared to one stroke (2%) in the medical therapy arm at 30 days. At 3-year follow-up, there were more vertebrobasilar strokes with stent therapy compared to medical therapy, 12% (n = 7) versus 7% (n = 4), respectively, but the trial did not show a significant difference in a composite outcome of death, stroke, and MI between the two groups.[59]

In addition to atherosclerotic disease, less common pathologic processes including fibromuscular dysplasia, Takayasu's arteritis, osteophyte compression, dissection, trauma, and other arterial pathologies can result in compromise of VA perfusion. Thoughtful consideration of disease etiology, concordant anatomy, and benefits and risks must always be considered when planning a strategy of therapy for VA disease.

ACUTE STROKE INTERVENTIONS

Rapid reperfusion of cerebral blood flow is extremely important to salvage ischemic brain tissue before infarction. For patients without contraindications, parenteral systemic thrombolytic therapy is a first-line therapy if this therapy is available within 4.5 hours of development of symptoms.[61] In patients presenting with acute ischemic stroke due to the occlusion of a large artery who can be treated with endovascular therapies within 24 hours of the time they were last seen at their neurologic baseline, endovascular therapies for stroke should be considered if clinically available.

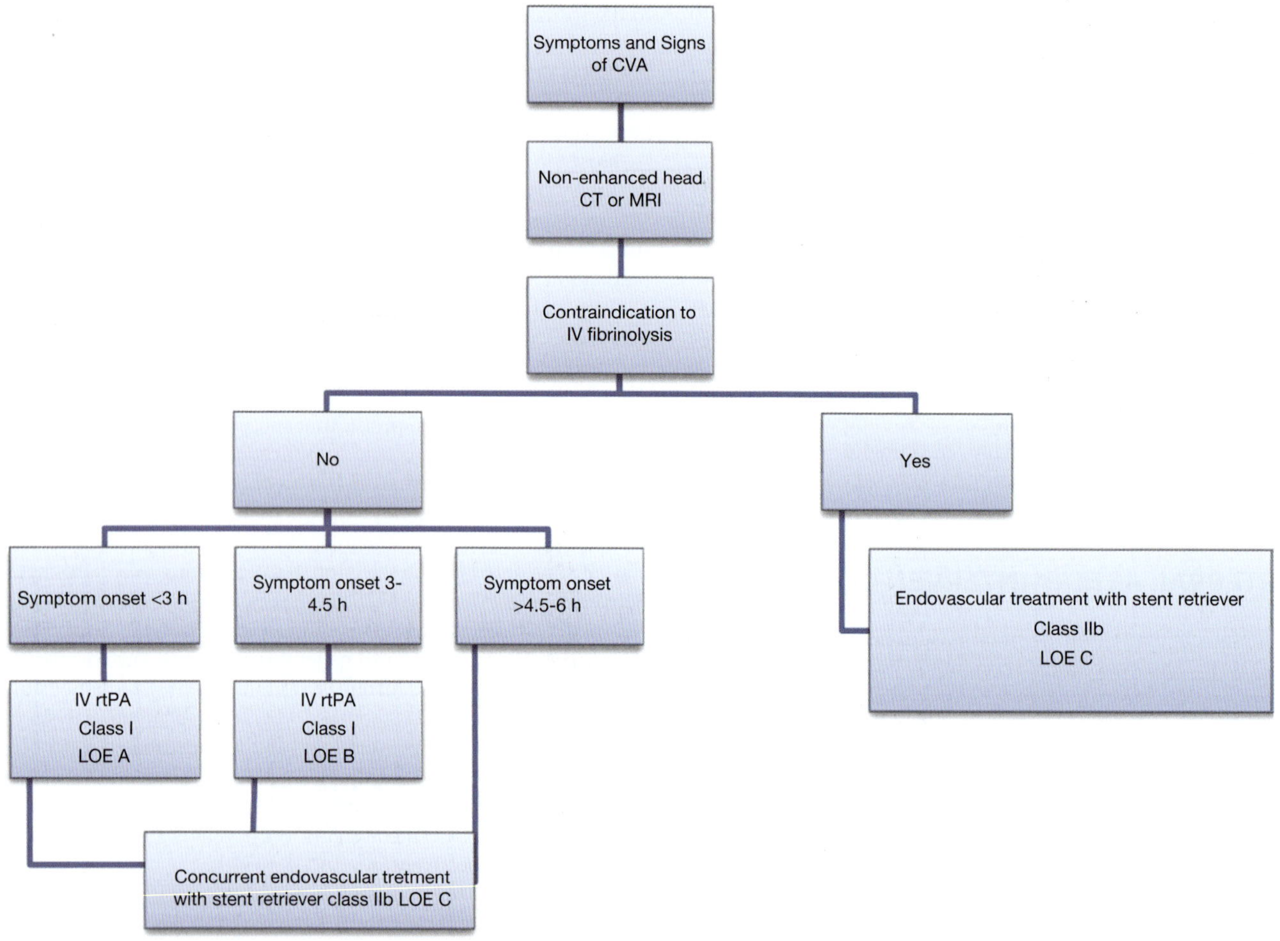

FIGURE 35.11 Algorithm for acute ischemic stroke imaging and treatment. Patients eligible for IV r-tPA should receive IV r-tPA even if endovascular treatments are being considered (class I: LOE A). Observing patients after IV r-tPA to assess for clinical response before pursuing endovascular therapy is not required to achieve beneficial outcomes and is not recommended (class III: LOE B-R). CT, computed tomography; CVA, cerebral vascular accident; IV rtPA, intra-arterial recombinant tissue plasminogen activator; LOE, Level of Evidence; MRI, magnetic resonance imaging.

For the treatment of acute cerebrovascular syndromes, prior trials of endovascular therapy included the intracranial administration of thrombolysis and the use of early generation mechanical thrombectomy devices (Merci and Penumbra with separator devices). These initial trials did not demonstrate conclusive benefit for endovascular therapy but did reveal promising signals toward benefit.[62,63] The benefits of early and effective mechanical reperfusion were balanced against the risks of ICH that was perhaps related to reperfusion of nonviable brain tissue. Newer trials focused on delivering safe and effective reperfusion therapy in stroke patients with viable brain tissue at risk (penumbra), determined by pretreatment brain imaging (**Fig. 35.11**). Treatment paradigms for acute stroke therapy have continued to evolve, driven by the continued introduction of novel endovascular technologies and by improvement in preintervention patient selection driven by radiologic and clinical data.

Advances in Randomized Clinical Trials

Several prospective trials studying mechanical thrombectomy (predating "stent-retriever" devices) for acute ischemic stroke have been negative or inconclusive. The Interventional Management of Stroke III trial, published in 2013, showed no benefit of endovascular therapy following the use of IV thrombolysis over IV thrombolysis alone in the treatment of moderate to severe acute ischemic stroke.[14] Of note, this study did not require CTA prior to enrollment and therefore included patients who did not have intracranial large-vessel occlusion. Newer stent-retriever technology was used only in five patients in this work.

Conversely between December 2014 and April 2015, five multicenter RCTs were published with positive results for endovascular therapy. All these trials included utilization of CTA to select patients with proximal intracranial occlusion and stent retrievers in the performance of thrombectomy in the majority of cases. The Multicenter Randomized Clinical Trial of Endovascular Treatment for Acute Ischemic Stroke in the Netherlands (MR CLEAN), Endovascular Treatment for Small Core and Anterior Circulation Proximal Occlusion With Emphasis on Minimizing CT to Recanalization Times (ESCAPE), Extending the Time for Thrombolysis in Emergency Neurological Deficits-Intra-Arterial (EXTEND-IA), Solitaire With the Intention for Thrombectomy as Primary Endovascular Treatment (SWIFT PRIME), and thrombectomy within 8 hours after Symptom Onset in Ischemic Stroke (REVASCAT) all demonstrated the efficacy of endovascular therapy versus IV intra-arterial recombinant tissue plasminogen activator (tPA) alone in treating patients with acute anterior circulation ischemic stroke. The last three studies were stopped early by their Data Safety Monitoring Boards after the MR CLEAN results were published.[29,64-67]

Inclusion Criteria and Time Window

All five trials utilized CT imaging to select patients. In MR CLEAN, patients were selected based upon plain CT imaging using the Alberta Stroke Program Early CT Score (ASPECTS). In other trials, patients were selected for having a small ischemic core at baseline and either adequate collaterals (using CTA in ESCAPE) or a salvageable brain (using CT perfusion) in EXTEND-IA and SWIFT PRIME trials.[29,64,65] The documentation of a proximal anterior circulation intracranial occlusion with CTA was required in all trials, which is a major difference from the negative endovascular reperfusion trials in the past (**Table 35.4**).

The baseline age and gender characteristics were comparable in all trials. The baseline NIHSS stroke scale was high at about 16. In the EXTEND-IA study, the NIHSS was lower in the conservative group compared to the intervention group (13 vs 16).[29] Patients older than 80 years of age were included in all but SWIFT PRIME trial.[64]

SWIFT PRIME treated patients up to 4.5 hours from the onset of stroke, while MR CLEAN and EXTEND-IA included those up to 6 hours after onset, REVASCAT up to 8 hours, and ESCAPE up to 12 hours. In practice, however, only a few patients who could not have groin puncture by 6 hours were actually included. Therefore, the positive results of the trials mainly apply to patients treated

TABLE 35.4 Summary of Contemporary Trials in Acute Stroke Intervention

PRESTENT RETRIEVER	PATIENTS	STENT-RETRIEVER USE (% AGE)	VASCULAR IMAGING	DEVICE DEPLOYMENT AND/OR IA TPA (TREATMENT ARM)	RECANALIZATION TICI 2B/3 FLOW	PRIMARY ENDPOINT TREATMENT CONTROL COMPARISON
The Interventional Management of Stroke III	656	1.5	No	77%; IA rtPA 41% IA rtPA + device 38% Device only 21% Stent retriever 1.5%	41%	mRS 0-2 at 90 d 40.8% 38.7% 1.5% (−6-9)[a]
MR RESCUE	118	0	CTA, MRA	95% MERCI 58% Penumbra 22% Both 16%	25%	Mean mRS 3.9 3.9 → P = .99
Synthesis expansion	362	14	No	91% IA rtPA alone 66% + device 34%	–	mRS 0-1 at 3 mo → 30.4% 34.8% → 0.71 (0.44-1.14)[a]
Stent-Retriever Era						
MR CLEAN	500	81.5	CTA, MRA, DSA	83.7% Stent retriever 81.5% IAT 21%	58%	Improvement in mRS 1.67 (1.21-2.3)[a] at 90 d
ESCAPE	316	86.1	CTA	91.5% Stent retriever 86.1%	72.4%	Improvement in mRS 3.1 (2.0-4.7)[a] at 90 d
EXTEND-IA	70	100	CTA MRA	77% Stent retriever 100%	86%	Median Reperfusion 100% 37% 4.7 (2.5-9.0)[a] at 24 h ↓ in NIHSS 8 or 80% 37% 6.0 (2.0-18.0)[a] NIHSS 0, 1 at 3 d
SWIFT PRIME	196	100	CTA MRA	88.8% Stent retriever 100%	88%	Rankin shift P < .001 5 and 6 combined
REVASCAT	206	100	CTA MRA, DSA	95% Stent retriever 100%	66%	Improvement in mRS 1.7 (1.05-2.8)[a] at 90 d

CTA, computed tomography angiography; DSA, digital subtraction angiography; IA rtPA, intra-arterial recombinant tissue plasminogen activator; MRA, magnetic resonance angiography; mRS, modified Rankin Scale; NIHSS, National Institutes of Health Stroke Scale; TICI, thrombolysis in cerebral infarction.

[a]95% confidence interval.

within 6 hours from symptom onset. A combined approach with IV thrombolysis and thrombectomy was required in SWIFT PRIME and was used in the majority of patients within the other studies. Most patients in the control groups received IV thrombolysis if they presented within the 4.5-hour time window.

Clinical Outcome

All five recent RCTs demonstrated a benefit with endovascular treatment compared to IV tPA alone with regard to functional outcomes. The percentage of patients achieving a favorable clinical outcome with intra-arterial thrombectomy (IAT) varied between 33% and 71%. There was a consistent positive difference across all studies with a favorable clinical outcome (defined as an mRS of 0-2 at 90 days) between interventional and control arms, favoring IAT by 14% to 31%. The difference between the groups was more pronounced in the trials in which penumbral imaging with CT perfusion was used. Nevertheless, even without imaging selection beyond the unenhanced CT, such as the MR CLEAN study, there was a clear benefit favoring IAT. Importantly, IAT was consistently effective overall among the important prespecified patient subgroups of sex, age, stroke severity, and time of presentation.

Complication and Mortality Rates

In all the studies, IAT added no additional risk of bleeding over standard management with IV tPA. The intracerebral hemorrhage (ICH) risk in both interventional and control arms ranged from 0% to 7%. The fact that in all trials IAT carried no higher bleeding risk compared to IV tPA demonstrates that thrombectomy is safe, and any bleeding risk is caused mainly by thrombolysis. There was an overall trend toward a reduction in mortality with IAT.

Recanalization Rates

Successful recanalization was defined as a thrombolysis in cerebral infarction (TICI) score 2b or 3. The use of stent retrievers in the trials led to recanalization rates between 59% and 88%. The trials also showed that the likelihood of a positive outcome increased with better recanalization. The highest recanalization rates were achieved in SWIFT PRIME (88%) and EXTEND-IA (86%) trials, correlating with the highest rates of favorable clinical outcomes seen in these trials (60% and 71%). The lowest recanalization rate was in MR CLEAN at 59% with a favorable clinical outcome occurring in only 33% of the patients.

Endovascular Technique/Thrombectomy Device

The major difference between these RCTs and earlier mechanical thrombectomy trials was the use of stent retrievers in the majority of the patients (**Table 35.4**). Stent retrievers are self-expandable stent-like devices that are fully retrievable. Therefore, these devices combine the advantages of prompt flow restoration and mechanical thrombectomy (**Fig. 35.12**). The excellent recanalization results with low complication rates of the stent-retriever devices in registries suggested a high rate of favorable clinical outcome.[68,69] This was confirmed in all five RCTs (**Fig. 35.12**).

Meta-Analysis

A large meta-analysis of these trials pooled patient-level data for 1287 subjects.[70] In this work, the rate of functional independence by 90-day mRS score of 0 to 2 was significantly greater for the intervention group compared with the control group (46 vs 27%, odds ratio [OR] 2.35, 95% CI 1.85-2.98). Mechanical thrombectomy was also demonstrated to benefit a wide range of patient subgroups including those with age ≥80 years and those not treated with IV thrombolytic therapy. Of note in this pooled analysis, there was no significant difference between groups in rates of symptomatic ICH or 90-day mortality.

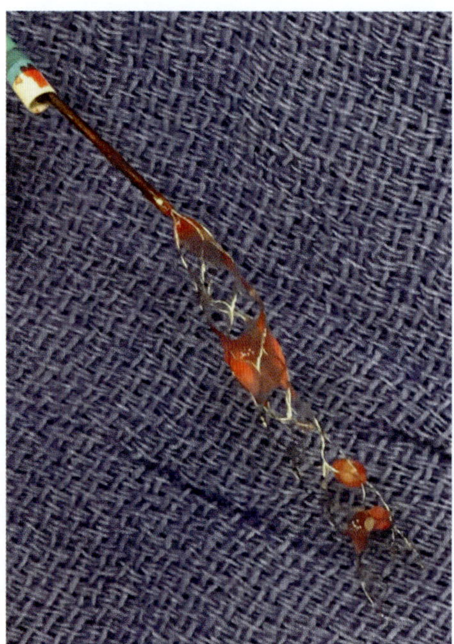

FIGURE 35.12 Stent-retriever device.

Indications and Patient Selection for Endovascular Treatment

Clinical Status

The NIHSS, a quantitative measure of the severity of a stroke, should be performed at the initial examination in all stroke patients, but especially in patients being considered for IV tPA. Patients with significant deficits manifesting as scores between 8 and 20 are more likely to benefit from reperfusion, making them better candidates for treatment.[61] Patients with minor to mild symptoms (NIHSS score <8) and an existing intracranial large-vessel occlusion were not included in the trials. In these patients, the decision to perform additional IAT is based on the operator's experience and the estimated risk of the procedure.

Time of Presentation

IV tPA and IAT reperfusion therapies have both been shown to improve patient outcome. The time window for treatment of both approaches is limited, however. IV thrombolysis can be given up to 4.5 hours after stroke onset. Additional or primary IA therapies can be used up to 12 hours after stroke onset. In anterior circulation strokes, the impact of successful thrombectomy is greater in the first 3 to 4.5 hours after stroke compared to late recanalization after 5 to 8 hours.

In 2018, two RCTs assessed the value of advanced imaging in selecting patients that may benefit from endovascular therapies even when presenting later in the course of stroke. The DAWN (the Clinical Mismatch in the Triage of Wake up and Late Presenting

Strokes Undergoing Neurointervention with Trevo Thrombectomy Procedure) and DEFUSE 3 (Endovascular Therapy Following Imaging Evaluation for Ischaemic Stroke 3) trials implemented CT and magnetic resonance imaging (MRI) in patients with stroke.[71,72] In these trials, patients with large-vessel occlusion and with substantial tissue at risk received benefit from performance of mechanical thrombectomy even when presenting later in their course within 6 to 24 hours after symptom onset.

Imaging of Acute Stroke

Imaging helps identify target intracranial thrombi and measures the extent of salvageable brain tissue. Imaging the brain and the vasculature that supplies it is a vital first step in evaluating patients with acute ischemic stroke. A comprehensive evaluation may be performed with CTA or MRI techniques. The major advantages of CTA compared to MRI are that CTA is widely available, and a stroke imaging protocol that consists of unenhanced CT, CTA, and CT-perfusion imaging can be executed in 5 minutes for the comprehensive evaluation of the extracranial and intracranial circulation, the amount of infarcted brain tissue, and the penumbra.

Computed Tomography

With its widespread availability, short scan time, noninvasiveness nature, and safety, CT has been the traditional first-line imaging modality for the evaluation of acute ischemic stroke. Multimodal CT includes unenhanced CT, CTA, and CT perfusion. Noncontrast CT can identify ICH and detect early signs of acute ischemic stroke. CTA can identify the occlusion site, detect arterial dissection, and grade collateral blood flow, whereas CT perfusion can differentiate between "tissue-at-risk" (the so-called "penumbra") and irreversibly damaged brain tissue.[54] Multimodal CT offers rapid data acquisition and can be performed with modern CT equipment.

Noncontrast CT

In the acute ischemic stroke setting, noncontrast CT has been used to rule out ICH (a contraindication to thrombolysis) or other stroke mimics (eg, tumor, infection, etc.), which preclude the use of thrombolytic therapy, and is also used to measure the extent of early ischemic changes within an ischemic brain. The Alberta Stroke Program Early CT Score (ASPECTS) is a simple and systematic approach evaluating stroke patients.[73] Patients with a high ASPECTS[51,52,71] seem to benefit more from IAT. MR CLEAN, which included patients with ASPECTS of 5 to 7, had an OR of 1.97 for benefit, while those with ASPECTS of 8 to 10 had a beneficial OR of 1.61. Those with ASPECTS of 0 to 4 had no benefit (OR 1.09), suggesting that mechanical thrombectomy has less efficacy in patients with a large ischemic core.

CT Angiography

CTA is widely available, with fast, thin-section, volumetric spiral CT images acquired during the injection of a time-optimized bolus of contrast material for vessel opacification. The entire region from the aortic arch to the circle of Willis can be covered in a single image acquisition. CTA allows a detailed evaluation of the intracranial and extracranial vasculature. Its utility in acute stroke lies in its ability to detect large-vessel occlusion within intracranial vessels and to evaluate the carotid and VAs in the neck. CTA can also depict the leptomeningeal collaterals and can identify large-vessel occlusions with "good" and "poor" collaterals.[74] Good collateral circulation improves the chance of a good neurologic outcome by limiting the extent of brain infarction. The ESCAPE trial used collateral assessment to select patients; the exclusion of participants with a large infarct core and poor collateral circulation was one of the reasons for the high rate of favorable clinical outcome—53%.[75]

CT Perfusion

CT perfusion allows rapid, noninvasive, and quantitative evaluation of cerebral perfusion. CT-perfusion differentiation of the infarct core from the penumbra is based on the concept of cerebral vascular autoregulation. In the penumbra, autoregulation is preserved, mean transit time (MTT) is prolonged, but cerebral blood volume (CBV) is preserved because of vasodilatation and collateral recruitment as part of the autoregulation process. In the infarct core, autoregulation of blood flow is lost, MTT is prolonged, and CBV is reduced. Thus, using appropriate MTT and CBV thresholds, the infarct core and penumbra can be distinguished on CT-perfusion maps. Direct assessment of an individual patient's ischemic penumbra may allow more personalized appropriate selection of candidates for intervention than generalized time criteria because individuals may have different timelines for conversion of penumbra into infarct tissue. CT perfusion was used to select patients for the EXTEND-IA trial, which achieved an impressive rate of good clinical outcome at 71%. Artificial intelligence (AI) is now aiding endovascular stroke physicians by providing perfusion maps and penumbra/core ratio to determine if tissue is viable. AI was used in DAWN and DEFUSE three trials.

Preprocedure Planning

Despite the fact that the efficacy of IV thrombolysis decreases with increased duration of time from the onset of symptoms, less than one-third of stroke patients meet the goal of a "door-to-needle time" of 60 minutes or less due to in-hospital delays.[76] Improvements in prehospital and in-hospital stroke management can translate into faster treatment.[77] Every stroke center should have an optimized stroke management protocol to reduce the "door-to-treatment" time with an on-demand continuously available stroke reperfusion service. When neurointerventional providers are not able to provide interventional stroke coverage, interventional cardiologists with carotid stenting experience have been demonstrated in specific environments to achieve comparable outcomes.[78]

Optimized Stroke Management

Emergency services are instructed to bring patients with a suspected stroke directly to the stroke treatment room, which should be located in close proximity to the CT scanner. After the neurologic examination is performed, the unenhanced CT scan is acquired. If an ICH can be ruled out, CTA and CT perfusion are performed. Within the 4.5-hour time window, patients are treated with IV thrombolytics immediately after exclusion of clinical and neuroradiologic contraindications.

If an occlusion of a large proximal intracranial vessel is identified, the decision to perform endovascular therapy is based on the clinical condition of the patient, the time window (up to 6 hours after stroke onset unless advanced imaging suggests possible benefit), as well as the imaging criteria of the CTA and CT perfusion (the presence of leptomeningeal collaterals and the presence of ischemic penumbra). If the decision to proceed with endovascular therapy is made, the patient is transferred immediately to the angiography suite.

At this point, a decision regarding the need for general anesthesia and ventilation is made, depending on the patient's clinical condition. A subgroup analysis from MR CLEAN indicated that the advantage of IAT may disappear when general anesthesia is performed. One advantage of conscious sedation, compared to general anesthesia is efficiency, in that the procedure begins more quickly. Another major advantage of conscious sedation is the ability to assess clinical status during the procedure and to evaluate the success of treatment. Disadvantages of conscious sedation are the patient's movements, which require experienced operators for a safe and successful procedure.

Using an optimized stroke protocol, with a door-to-device (D2D) time (the time from arrival at the hospital until the thrombectomy device is placed in the target lesion), a D2D time of <100 minutes resulted in a favorable outcome in 66% of patients, compared with 44% of patients with a D2D time of more than 100 minutes.[52] By analogy, the D2D time should play an important role in the outcome of these patients, as it does for the door-to-balloon time in the outcome of patients with ST-segment elevation MI.

Description of the Procedure

From First-Generation Devices to the Flow Restoration Devices (Stent Retriever)

In the last decade, mechanical recanalization devices have been developed to achieve better results than IA thrombolysis alone. The Merci-device and the Penumbra aspiration system were the first devices for which large clinical experiences have been reported.[62,79] Nevertheless, the breakthrough in interventional treatment of acute stroke was achieved by the use of stent-like thrombectomy devices (stent retriever; see **Fig. 35.12**). The stent-retriever devices allow high recanalization rates, with a reduction in the recanalization time and low complication rates.[68,69] In cases with a large thrombus burden, a combination of aspiration through a large lumen reperfusion catheter may be used. In the special groups of patients with extracranial carotid occlusion, arterial dissection, and intracranial stenosis, carotid stenting will be necessary.

Stent-Retriever Technique

Stent retrievers are self-expandable stent-like devices that are fully retrievable. Therefore, these devices combine the advantages of prompt flow restoration and mechanical thrombectomy. The improved clinical outcome with flow restoration devices is due to fast and effective clot removal, and the possibility of temporarily restoring flow. Recanalization rates of TICI 2a/b or 3 flow are high, up to 90%. The results of prospective studies showed high rates of favorable clinical outcomes at 3 months, a low rate of symptomatic ICH, and a low mortality rate. The low mortality rate reflects the low rate of symptomatic ICH and shows the safety of flow-restoration devices compared with reperfusion devices in the past.

Technique of Thrombus Aspiration

Despite the impressive results of the stent-retriever devices with successful recanalization results of up to 95%, there are some vessel occlusions and thrombi that are resistant to this technique, even after repeated recanalization attempts. These vessel occlusions include cases of terminal ICA occlusions. Moreover, "hard" or organized thrombi in other locations, like the middle cerebral artery (MCA), can be resistant to the stent-retriever technique. For these cases, the direct aspiration of the thrombus has been used as an alternative. For direct thrombus aspiration, the most common aspiration catheters used for these purposes are compatible with a 6F neurologic sheath such as Neuron Max 088 (with 0.88″ ID) and Benchmark BMK 096 (0.96″). The current aspiration catheters are extremely trackable. Once in contact with the thrombus, aspiration can be applied through different sizes of catheters depending on the vessel diameter ranging from 0.43″ to 0.72."

Postprocedure Management

The use of vascular closure devices can be routinely used with low complication rates, including in patients that received IV thrombolysis. During intervention, there is no need for any antiplatelet medication. In cases with emergency stent implantation of occlusions at the origin of ICA, antiplatelet therapy is necessary to prevent acute stent thrombosis.[61] In these cases, antiplatelet therapy with IV bridging using GPIIb/IIIa or P2Y12 inhibitor therapy is recommended but should be carefully used in particular if thrombolytics were administered. The overall recommendation after stroke thrombectomy is to start aspirin in the 24- to 48-hour window postprocedure.

Although HTN is common in acute ischemic stroke and is associated with poor outcomes, studies of antihypertensive treatment in this setting have produced conflicting results. A theoretical drawback of blood pressure reduction is that elevated blood pressure may counteract dysfunctional cerebral autoregulation from stroke, but limited evidence suggests that antihypertensive treatment in acute stroke does not change cerebral perfusion. Once IV thrombolytic therapy or thrombectomy are performed, the blood pressure must be maintained below 180/105 mm Hg to limit the risk of ICH.

Potential Complications

Complications that can occur during or after the procedure include distal embolization to the same or other vessel territories, dissection of the arteries, and subarachnoid or ICH. MR CLEAN reported 5.6% incidence of new symptomatic embolism. With distal embolization, the management depends on the relevance of the occluded branch. If the patient is not intubated, a clinical examination can show if a persistent occlusion is relevant or not. If the occluded branch is a relevant one, a stent retriever can be used even in M3 branches of the MCA or in A2 segments of the anterior cerebral artery.

Dissections of the vessels mostly occur in the ICA when a distal access catheter is used. Dissections without flow restriction do not require any therapy. In cases of a flow limiting dissection, stenting of the affected vessel can be performed.

Small subarachnoid hemorrhages are often seen on the control CT and do not require specific therapy. Intracerebral hemorrhage can occur during the procedure due to the intervention or even within 48 hours after the procedure as a result of reperfusion injury. Blood pressure control is a critical element of postprocedure management to limit frequency of this complication. The occurrence of any worsening of neurologic status should be

TABLE 35.5 AHA/ASA[54] Criteria for Endovascular Therapy in Acute Stroke Patients

Criteria for endovascular therapy after acute ischemic stroke (class I; Level of Evidence a)
Prestroke mRS score 0-1
Acute ischemic stroke receiving intravenous r-tPA within 4.5 h of onset according to guidelines from professional medical societies
Causative occlusion of the internal carotid artery or proximal MCA (M1)
Age >18 y
NIHSS score of >6
ASPECTS of >6
Treatment can be initiated (groin puncture) within 6 h of symptom onset

MCA, middle cerebral artery; MI, myocardial infarction; mRS, modified Rankin Scale; NIHSS, National Institutes of Health Stroke Scale; r-tPA, recombinant tissue plasminogen activator.
From Turan TN, Makki AA, Tsappidi S, et al. Risk factors associated with severity and location of intracranial arterial stenosis. *Stroke*. 2010;41(8):1636-1640.

considered a possible sign of ICH, warranting immediate clinical evaluation and an emergency CT scan of the brain. Should ICH be found, reversal of all antithrombotic agents should be performed.

Based on the positive outcomes in RCTs comparing endovascular treatments in suitable patients in conjunction with IV thrombolysis versus thrombolysis alone or in patients in whom IV thrombolysis was contraindicated, the AHA/ASA published a Focused Update in 2015 for the early management of patients with acute ischemic stroke regarding endovascular treatment.[61] Patients should receive endovascular therapy with a stent retriever if they meet the criteria shown in **Table 35.5**.

CONCLUSION

Recently completed RCTs have established mechanical thrombectomy for acute ischemic stroke in patients with large-vessel occlusions and appropriate imaging for brain viability. The current endovascular reperfusion therapies allow high recanalization rates, high rates of favorable clinical outcomes, and low complication rates. Nevertheless, to optimize clinical results, image-guided patient selection and the use of an optimized stroke management protocol are required.

Key Points

- ACCF/ASA/AHA class I Recommendations for Diagnostic Testing in Patients with Symptoms or Signs of Extracranial Carotid Artery Disease:
  1. Initial evaluation of patients with transient retinal or hemispheric neurologic symptoms of possible ischemic origin should include noninvasive imaging for the detection of ECVD (LOE: C).
  2. Duplex ultrasonography is recommended to detect carotid stenosis in patients who develop focal neurologic symptoms corresponding to the territory supplied by the left or right ICA (LOE: C).
  3. In patients with acute focal ischemic neurologic symptoms corresponding to the territory supplied by the left or right ICA, MRA or CTA is indicated to detect carotid stenosis when sonography either cannot be obtained or yields equivocal or otherwise nondiagnostic results (LOE: C).
  4. When extracranial or intracranial cerebrovascular disease is not severe enough to account for neurologic symptoms of suspected ischemic origin, echocardiography should be performed to search for a source of cardiogenic embolism (LOE: C).
- Antihypertensive treatment is recommended for patients with HTN and asymptomatic extracranial carotid or vertebral atherosclerosis to maintain blood pressure below 140/90 mm Hg (class I, LOE: A).
- Patients with extracranial carotid or vertebral atherosclerosis who smoke cigarettes should be advised to quit smoking and be offered smoking cessation interventions to reduce the risks of atherosclerosis progression and stroke (class I, LOE: B).
- Treatment with a statin medication is recommended for all patients with extracranial carotid or vertebral atherosclerosis to reduce LDL-C below 100 mg/dL (class I, LOE: B).
- ACCF/ASA/AHA class I Recommendations for Antiplatelet Therapy in ECVD:
- Antiplatelet therapy with aspirin, 75 to 325 mg daily, is recommended for patients with obstructive or nonobstructive atherosclerosis that involves the extracranial carotid and/or VAs for prevention of MI and other ischemic cardiovascular events. This benefit has not been established for prevention of stroke in asymptomatic patients (class I, LOE: A).
  1. In patients with obstructive or nonobstructive extracranial carotid or vertebral atherosclerosis who have sustained ischemic stroke or TIA, antiplatelet therapy with aspirin alone (75-325 mg daily), clopidogrel alone (75 mg daily), or the combination of aspirin plus extended-release dipyridamole (25 and 200 mg twice daily, respectively) is recommended (class I, LOE: B) and preferred over the combination of aspirin with clopidogrel (class I, LOE: B). Selection of an antiplatelet regimen should be individualized on the basis of patient risk-factor profiles, cost, tolerance, and other clinical characteristics, as well as guidance from regulatory agencies.
  2. Antiplatelet agents are recommended, rather than oral anticoagulation for patients with atherosclerosis of the extracranial carotid or VAs with (LOE: B) or without (LOE: C) ischemic symptoms.
- ACCF/ASA/AHA class I Recommendations for Vascular Imaging in Patients With Vertebral Artery Disease:
  1. CTA or MRA for detection of VA disease should be part of the initial evaluation of patients with neurologic symptoms referable to the posterior circulation and those with subclavian steal syndrome (LOE: C).
  2. Patients with asymptomatic bilateral carotid occlusions or unilateral carotid artery occlusion and incomplete circle of Willis should undergo noninvasive imaging for detection of VA obstructive disease (LOE: C).
  3. In patients whose symptoms suggest posterior cerebral or cerebellar ischemia, MRA or CTA is recommended rather than ultrasound imaging for evaluation of the VAs (LOE: C).

■ ACCF/ASA/AHA Recommendations for Management of Atherosclerotic Risk Factors in Patients With Vertebral Artery Disease:

1. Medical therapy and lifestyle modification to reduce atherosclerotic risk are recommended in patients with vertebral atherosclerosis according to the standards recommended for those with extracranial carotid atherosclerosis (LOE: B).
2. In the absence of contraindications, these patients should also receive antiplatelet therapy with aspirin (75-325 mg daily) to prevent MI and other ischemic events (LOE: B).
3. Antiplatelet drug therapy is recommended as part of the initial management for patients who sustain ischemic stroke or TIA associated with extracranial vertebral atherosclerosis. Aspirin (81-325 mg daily), the combination of aspirin plus extended-release dipyridamole (25 and 200 mg twice daily, respectively), and clopidogrel (75 mg daily) are acceptable options. Selection of an antiplatelet regimen should be individualized (LOE: B).

References

1. Tsao CW, Aday AW, Almarzooq ZI, et al. Heart disease and stroke Statistics-2022 update: a report from the American Heart Association. *Circulation*. 2022;145.8:e153-e639.
2. Reiff T, Eckstein HH, Mansmann U, et al. Carotid endarterectomy or stenting or best medical treatment alone for moderate-to-severe asymptomatic carotid artery stenosis: 5-year results of a multicentre, randomised controlled trial. *Lancet Neurol*. 2022;21(10):877-888.
3. Amarenco P; Steering Committee Investigators of the TIAregistryorg. Risk of stroke after transient ischemic attack or minor stroke. *N Engl J Med*. 2016;375(4):387.
4. Markus HS, King A, Shipley M, et al. Asymptomatic embolisation for prediction of stroke in the Asymptomatic Carotid Emboli Study (ACES): a prospective observational study. *Lancet Neurol*. 2010;9(7):663-671.
5. Jalbert JJ, Nguyen LL, Gerhard-Herman MD, et al. Comparative effectiveness of carotid artery stenting versus carotid endarterectomy among Medicare beneficiaries. *Circ Cardiovasc Qual Outcomes*. 2016;9(3):275-285.
6. Meschia JF, Bushnell C, Boden-Albala B, et al. Guidelines for the primary prevention of stroke: a statement for healthcare professionals from the American Heart Association/American Stroke Association. *Stroke*. 2014;45(12):3754-3832.
7. Sacco RL, Kasner SE, Broderick JP, et al. An updated definition of stroke for the 21st century: a statement for healthcare professionals from the American Heart Association/American Stroke Association. *Stroke*. 2013;44(7):2064-2089.
8. Yang C, Bogiatzi C, Spence JD. Risk of stroke at the time of carotid occlusion. *JAMA Neurol*. 2015;72(11):1261-1267.
9. Chang RW, Tucker L, Rothenberg KA, et al. Incidence of ischemic stroke in patients with asymptomatic severe carotid stenosis without surgical intervention. *JAMA*. 2022;327(20):1974-1982.
10. Barnett HJ, Taylor DW, Eliasziw M, et al. Benefit of carotid endarterectomy in patients with symptomatic moderate or severe stenosis. North American Symptomatic Carotid Endarterectomy Trial Collaborators. *N Engl J Med*. 1998;339(20):1415-1425.
11. Inzitari D, Eliasziw M, Sharpe BL, Fox AJ, Barnett HJ. Risk factors and outcome of patients with carotid artery stenosis presenting with lacunar stroke. North American Symptomatic Carotid Endarterectomy Trial Group. *Neurology*. 2000;54(3):660-666.
12. Brott TG, Halperin JL, Abbara S, et al. 2011 ASA/ACCF/AHA/AANS/ACR/ASNR/CNS/SAIDP/SCAI/SIR/SNIS/SVM/SVS guideline on the management of patients with extracranial carotid and vertebral artery disease: executive summary. *Circulation*. 2011;124:189-532.
13. Stone NJ, Robinson JG, Lichtenstein AH, et al. 2013 ACC/AHA guideline on the treatment of blood cholesterol to reduce atherosclerotic cardiovascular risk in adults: a report of the American College of Cardiology/American Heart Association Task Force on Practice Guidelines. *Circulation*. 2014;129(25 suppl 2):S1-S45.
14. Broderick JP, Palesch YY, Demchuk AM, et al. Endovascular therapy after intravenous t-PA versus t-PA alone for stroke. *NEJM*. 2013;368(10):893-903.
15. Qin J, Liu L, Su XD, et al. The effect of PCSK9 inhibitors on brain stroke prevention: a systematic review and meta-analysis. *Nutr Metab Cardiovasc Dis*. 2021;31(8):2234-2243.
16. Kleindorfer DO, Towfighi A, Chaturvedi S, et al. 2021 guideline for the prevention of stroke in patients with stroke and transient ischemic attack: a guideline from the American Heart Association/American Stroke Association. *Stroke*. 2021;52(7):e364-e467.
17. Lloyd-Jones D, Morris PB, Ballantyne CM, et al. 2022 ACC expert consensus decision pathway on the role of nonstatin therapies for LDL-cholesterol lowering in the management of atherosclerotic cardiovascular disease risk. *J Am Coll Cardiol*. 2022;80(14):1633-1418.
18. Amarenco P, Goldstein LB, Sillesen H, et al. Coronary heart disease risk in patients with stroke or transient ischemic attack and no known coronary heart disease: findings from the Stroke Prevention by Aggressive Reduction in Cholesterol Levels (SPARCL) trial. *Stroke*. 2010;41(3):426-430.
19. Everett BM, Glynn RJ, MacFadyen JG, Ridker PM. Rosuvastatin in the prevention of stroke among men and women with elevated levels of C-reactive protein: justification for the Use of statins in Prevention—an Intervention Trial Evaluating Rosuvastatin (JUPITER). *Circulation*. 2010;121(1):143-150.
20. Johnston SC, Amarenco P, Denison H, et al. Ticagrelor and aspirin or aspirin alone in acute ischemic stroke or TIA. *NEJM*. 2020;383(3):207-217.
21. Nederkoorn PJ. *The 2nd European Carotid Surgery Trial (ECST-2): 2-year interim results*. ESOC; 2023.
22. Hobson RW II, Weiss DG, Fields WS, et al. Efficacy of carotid endarterectomy for asymptomatic carotid stenosis. The Veterans Affairs Cooperative study group. *N Engl J Med*. 1993;328(4):221-227.
23. Endarterectomy for asymptomatic carotid artery stenosis. Executive committee for the asymptomatic carotid atherosclerosis study. *JAMA*. 1995;273:1421-1428.
24. Mayberg MR, Wilson SE, Yatsu F, et al. Carotid endarterectomy and prevention of cerebral ischemia in symptomatic carotid stenosis. Veterans Affairs Cooperative Studies Program 309 Trialist Group. *JAMA*. 1991;266(23):3289-3294.
25. Meschia JF, Brott TG. Lessons from ACST-2. *Stroke*. 2022;53(4):e145-e149.
26. Malas MB, Dakour-Aridi H, Kashyap VS, et al. TransCarotid revascularization with dynamic flow reversal versus carotid endarterectomy in the vascular quality initiative surveillance Project. *Ann Surg*. 2022;276(2):398-403.
27. Halliday A, Bulbulia R, Bonati LH, et al. Second Asymptomatic Carotid Surgery Trial (ACST-2): a randomised comparison of carotid artery stenting versus carotid endarterectomy. *Lancet*. 2021;398(10305):1065-1073.
28. Yadav JS. Carotid stenting in high-risk patients: design and rationale of the SAPPHIRE trial. *Cleve Clin J Med*. 2004;71(suppl 1):S45-S46.
29. Campbell BC, Mitchell PJ, Kleinig TJ, et al. Endovascular therapy for ischemic stroke with perfusion-imaging selection. *NEJM*. 2015;372(11):1009-1018.
30. Bonati LH, Dobson J, Featherstone RL, et al. Long-term outcomes after stenting versus endarterectomy for treatment of symptomatic carotid stenosis: the International Carotid Stenting Study (ICSS) randomised trial. *Lancet*. 2015;385(9967):529-538.
31. SPACE Collaborative Group; Ringleb PA, Allenberg J, Brückmann H, et al. 30 day results from the SPACE trial of stent-protected angioplasty versus carotid endarterectomy in symptomatic patients: a randomised non-inferiority trial. *Lancet*. 2006;368(9543):1239-1247.
32. Mantese VA, Timaran CH, Chiu D, Begg RJ, Brott TG; CREST Investigators. The Carotid Revascularization Endarterectomy versus Stenting Trial (CREST): stenting versus carotid endarterectomy for carotid disease. *Stroke*. 2010;41(10 suppl):S31-S34.
33. Mas JL, Trinquart L, Leys D, et al. Endarterectomy versus angioplasty in patients with symptomatic severe carotid stenosis (EVA-3S) trial: results up to 4 years from a randomised, multicentre trial. *Lancet Neurol*. 2008;7(10):885-892.

34. Rosenfield K, Matsumura JS, Chaturvedi S, et al. Randomized trial of stent versus surgery for asymptomatic carotid stenosis. *N Engl J Med*. 2016;374(11):1011-1020.
35. Stroink AR, Levy EI, Mack WJ. *Letter from American Association of Neurological Surgeons, Congress of Neurological Surgeons, and AANS/CNS Cerebrovascular Section to Coverage and Analysis Group Centers for Medicare & Medicaid Services—Request for Reconsideration of CMS National Coverage Determination (NCD) 20.7*. Percutaneous Transluminal Angioplasty (PTA); 2023.
36. Brott T, for Multispecialty Carotid Alliance (MSCA). et al. *Letter to Centers for Medicare & Medicaid Services Formal Request for Reconsideration of NCD 20.7*; 2022.
37. Centers for Medicare & Medicaid Services (CMS) Decision Memo. *Percutaneous Transluminaimal Angioplasty (PTA) of the Carotid Artery Concurrent with Stenting*; 2023.
38. Thuijs D, Kappetein AP, Serruys PW, et al. Percutaneous coronary intervention versus coronary artery bypass grafting in patients with three-vessel or left main coronary artery disease: 10-year follow-up of the multicentre randomised controlled SYNTAX trial. *Lancet*. 2019;394(10206):1325-1334.
39. Lawton JS, Tamis-Holland JE, Bangalore S, et al. 2021 ACC/AHA/SCAI guideline for coronary artery revascularization: a report of the American College of Cardiology/American Heart Association Joint committee on clinical practice guidelines. *Circulation*. 2022;145(3):e18-e114.
40. Soukas P. Transradial carotid artery stenting. *Vascular Disease Management*. 2017;3:e67-e77.
41. Erben Y, Meschia JF, Heck DV, et al. Safety of the transradial approach to carotid stenting. *Catheter Cardiovasc Interv*. 2022;99(3):814-821.
42. Garg N, Karagiorgos N, Pisimisis GT, et al. Cerebral protection devices reduce periprocedural strokes during carotid angioplasty and stenting: a systematic review of the current literature. *J Endovasc Ther*. 2009;16(4):412-427.
43. Touze E, Trinquart L, Chatellier G, Mas JL. Systematic review of the perioperative risks of stroke or death after carotid angioplasty and stenting. *Stroke*. 2009;40(12):e683-e693.
44. Stabile E, Sannino A, Schiattarella GG, et al. Cerebral embolic lesions detected with diffusion-weighted magnetic resonance imaging following carotid artery stenting: a meta-analysis of 8 studies comparing filter cerebral protection and proximal balloon occlusion. *JACC Cardiovasc Interv*. 2014;7(10):1177-1183.
45. Bosiers M, Deloose K, Torsello G, et al. The CLEAR-ROAD study: evaluation of a new dual layer micromesh stent system for the carotid artery. *EuroIntervention*. 2016;12(5):e671-e676.
46. Giri J, Cox M. Dual-layerd stents: the new standard for carotid stenting? *JACC Cardiovasc Interv*. 2021;14(17):1924-1925.
47. Stabile E, de Donato G, Musialek P, et al. Use of dual-layered stents in endovascular treatment of extracranial stenosis of the internal carotid artery: results of a patient-based meta-analysis of 4 clinical studies. *JACC Cardiovasc Interv*. 2018;11(23):2405-2411.
48. Moulakakis KG, Mylonas SN, Sfyroeras GS, Andrikopoulos V. Hyperperfusion syndrome after carotid revascularization. *J Vasc Surg*. 2009;49(4):1060-1068.
49. American College of Cardiology Foundation, et al. ACCF/ACR/AIUM/ASE/ASN/ICAVL/SCAI/SCCT/SIR/SVM/SVS/SVU [corrected] 2012 appropriate use criteria for peripheral vascular ultrasound and physiological testing part I: arterial ultrasound and physiological testing—a report of the American College of Cardiology Foundation appropriate use criteria task force, American College of Radiology, American Institute of Ultrasound in Medicine, American Society of Echocardiography, American Society of Nephrology, Intersocietal Commission for the Accreditation of Vascular Laboratories, Society for Cardiovascular Angiography and Interventions, Society of Cardiovascular Computed Tomography, Society for Interventional Radiology, Society for Vascular Medicine, Society for Vascular Surgery, [corrected] and Society for Vascular Ultrasound [corrected]. *J Am Coll Cardiol*. 2012;60:242-276.
50. Chi YW, White CJ, Woods TC, Goldman CK. Ultrasound velocity criteria for carotid in-stent restenosis. *Catheter Cardiovasc Interv*. 2007;69(3):349-354.
51. Cavdar S, Arisan E. Variations in the extracranial origin of the human vertebral artery. *Acta Anat*. 1989;135(3):236-238.
52. Fabian TC. Blunt cerebrovascular injuries: anatomic and pathologic heterogeneity create management enigmas. *J Am Coll Surg*. 2013;216(5):873-885.
53. Jenkins JS, White CJ, Ramee SR, et al. Vertebral artery stenting. *Catheter Cardiovasc Interv*. 2001;54:1-5.
54. Turan TN, Makki AA, Tsappidi S, et al. Risk factors associated with severity and location of intracranial arterial stenosis. *Stroke*. 2010;41(8):1636-1640.
55. Crawley F, Brown MM. Percutaneous transluminal angioplasty and stenting for vertebral artery stenosis. *Cochrane Database Syst Rev*. 2000;2000(2):CD000516.
56. Ausman JI, Diaz FG, Sadasivan B, Dujovny M. Intracranial vertebral endarterectomy. *Neurosurgery*. 1990;26(3):465-471.
57. Stayman AN, Nogueira RG, Gupta R. A systematic review of stenting and angioplasty of symptomatic extracranial vertebral artery stenosis. *Stroke*. 2011;42(8):2212-2216.
58. Langwieser N, Prothmann S, Buyer D, et al. Safety and efficacy of different stent types for the endovascular therapy of extracranial vertebral artery disease. *Clin Res Cardiol*. 2014;103(5):353-362.
59. Compter A, van der Worp HB, Schonewille WJ, et al. Stenting versus medical treatment in patients with symptomatic vertebral artery stenosis: a randomised open-label phase 2 trial. *Lancet Neurol*. 2015;14(6):606-614.
60. Jenkins JS, Patel SN, White CJ, et al. Endovascular stenting for vertebral artery stenosis. *J Am Coll Cardiol*. 2010;55(6):538-542.
61. Powers WJ, Derdeyn CP, Biller J, et al. 2015 American Heart Association/American Stroke Association focused update of the 2013 guidelines for the early management of patients with acute ischemic stroke regarding endovascular treatment: a guideline for healthcare professionals from the American Heart Association/American Stroke Association. *Stroke*. 2015;46(10):3020-3035.
62. Smith WS, Sung G, Saver J, et al. Mechanical thrombectomy for acute ischemic stroke: final results of the Multi MERCI trial. *Stroke*. 2008;39(4):1205-1212.
63. Ciccone A, Valvassori L, Nichelatti M, et al. Endovascular treatment for acute ischemic stroke. *NEJM*. 2013;368:901-913.
64. Saver JL, Goyal M, Bonafe A, et al. Stent-retriever thrombectomy after intravenous t-PA vs. t-PA alone in stroke. *NEJM*. 2015;372(24):2285-2295.
65. Berkhemer OA, Fransen PSS, Beumer D, et al. A randomized trial of intraarterial treatment for acute ischemic stroke. *NEJM*. 2015;372(1):11-20.
66. Goyal M, Demchuk AM, Menon BK, et al. Randomized assessment of rapid endovascular treatment of ischemic stroke. *NEJM*. 2015;372(11):1019-1030.
67. Jovin TG, Chamorro A, Cobo E, et al. Thrombectomy within 8 hours after symptom onset in ischemic stroke. *NEJM*. 2015;372(24):2296-2306.
68. Roth C, Reith W, Walter S, et al. Mechanical recanalization with flow restoration in acute ischemic stroke: the ReFlow (mechanical recanalization with flow restoration in acute ischemic stroke) study. *JACC Cardiovasc Interv*. 2013;6(4):386-391.
69. Roth C, Papanagiotou P, Behnke S, et al. Stent-assisted mechanical recanalization for treatment of acute intracerebral artery occlusions. *Stroke*. 2010;41(11):2559-2567.
70. Goyal M, Menon BK, van Zwam WH, et al. Endovascular thrombectomy after large-vessel ischaemic stroke: a meta-analysis of individual patient data from five randomised trials. *Lancet*. 2016;387(10029):1723-1731.
71. Nogueira RG, Jadhav AP, Haussen DC, et al. Thrombectomy 6 to 24 hours after stroke with a Mismatch between deficit and infarct. *NEJM*. 2018;378(1):11-21.
72. Albers GW, Marks MP, Kemp S, et al. Thrombectomy for stroke at 6 to 16 hours with selection by perfusion imaging. *NEJM*. 2018;378(8):708-718.
73. Barber PA, Demchuk AM, Zhang J, Buchan AM. Validity and reliability of a quantitative computed tomography score in predicting outcome of hyperacute stroke before thrombolytic therapy. ASPECTS Study Group. Alberta Stroke Programme early CT score. *Lancet*. 2000;355(9216):1670-1674.
74. Lima FO, Furie KL, Silva GS, et al. The pattern of leptomeningeal collaterals on CT angiography is a strong predictor of long-term functional outcome in stroke patients with large vessel intracranial occlusion. *Stroke*. 2010;41(10):2316-2322.

75. Demchuk AM, Goyal M, Menon BK, et al. Endovascular treatment for Small Core and Anterior circulation Proximal occlusion with Emphasis on minimizing CT to recanalization times (ESCAPE) trial: methodology. *Int J Stroke*. 2015;10(3):429-438.
76. Fonarow GC, Smith EE, Saver JL, et al. Timeliness of tissue-type plasminogen activator therapy in acute ischemic stroke: patient characteristics, hospital factors, and outcomes associated with door-to-needle times within 60 minutes. *Circulation*. 2011;123(7):750-758.
77. Fonarow GC, Smith EE, Saver JL, et al. Improving door-to-needle times in acute ischemic stroke: the design and rationale for the American Heart Association/American Stroke Association's Target—stroke initiative. *Stroke*. 2011;42(10):2983-2989.
78. Htyte N, Parto P, Ragbir S, Jaffe L, White CJ. Predictors of outcomes following catheter-based therapy for acute stroke. *Catheter Cardiovasc Interv*. 2015;85(6):1043-1050.
79. Grunwald IQ, Walter S, Papanagiotou P, et al. Revascularization in acute ischaemic stroke using the penumbra system: the first single center experience. *Eur J Neurol*. 2009;16(11):1210-1216.

Atherosclerotic Renal Artery Disease

Dmitriy Feldman

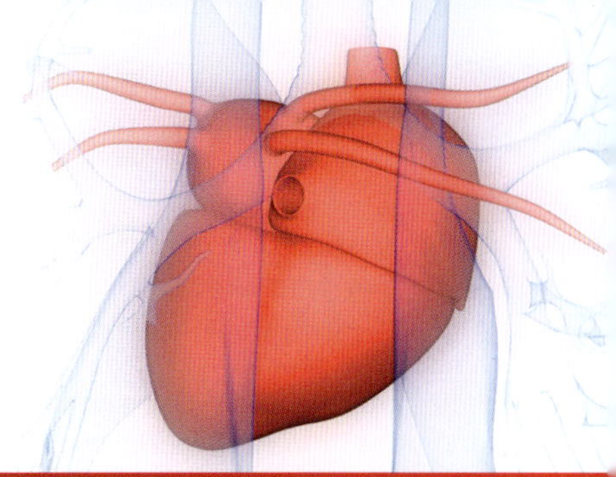

PREVALENCE AND NATURAL HISTORY

Atherosclerotic renal artery stenosis (RAS) is the most common primary disease affecting renal arteries. It is a common cause of secondary hypertension and is found in 0.5% to 5% of all hypertensive patients.[1,2] Renovascular hypertension, pulmonary edema, ischemic nephropathy, and end-stage renal disease (ESRD) are the potential consequences of atherosclerotic RAS.

The prevalence of RAS has been well documented, affecting ~7% of the population aged >65 years.[1] In patients with atherosclerotic coronary and peripheral artery disease (PAD), renal arterial disease has been found to be present in ~30% of patients undergoing screening renal artery angiography at the time of cardiac catheterization. In these patients with underlying coronary artery disease, significant obstructive RAS (>50%) has been reported in 11% to 19% of the patients.[2-4] Prevalence studies have also demonstrated significant RAS in 22% to 59% of the patients with PAD.[5-9] Among the patients with RAS, 44% are found to have bilateral renal artery involvement.[10]

Atherosclerosis accounts for ~90% of cases of stenosis within the renal arterial bed.[11] Common causes of RAS are listed in **Table 36.1**. Atherosclerotic lesions usually involve the origin and proximal third of the main renal artery as well as the perirenal aorta.

TABLE 36.1 Common Causes of RAS

- Atherosclerotic RAS
- FMD
- Renal artery vasculitis
- Diabetic nephropathy (small vessels)
- Thromboangiitis obliterans
- Nephroangiosclerosis (hypertensive injury)
- Dissection of aorta or renal arteries
- Thromboembolic or atheroembolic phenomena
- Transplant RAS
- Extrinsic compression
- Trauma
- Radiation-induced injury
- Scleroderma

RAS, renal artery stenosis.

Fibromuscular dysplasia (FMD) accounts for <10% of cases of RAS and is a group of nonatherosclerotic arterial disease typically involving the distal two-thirds of the main renal artery or its branches. Medial fibroplasia, a subtype of medial FMD, is the histologic finding in 75% to 80% of all cases of FMD. Microscopically, there are alternating areas of thinned media and thickened fibromuscular ridges containing collagen. Some areas of the internal elastic membrane are lost.[12-14] A "string of beads" is used to describe its angiographic appearance, where the "bead" diameter is larger than the proximal vessel. The classification of FMD is demonstrated in **Table 36.2**. Atherosclerosis and FMD are the two most common causes of RAS.

PATHOPHYSIOLOGY OF RAS

RAS leads to kidney hypoperfusion and subsequent activation of the renin-angiotensin-aldosterone pathway. Ischemia triggers the release of renin, and renin leads to the conversion of angiotensin I to angiotensin II. Angiotensin II causes vasoconstriction, which leads to hypertension and enhances the adrenal synthesis of aldosterone. Aldosterone causes sodium and fluid retention, which also promotes the development of hypertension. Together with aldosterone release, the sympathetic nervous system is activated. The totality of these sequences leads to the development of renovascular hypertension, heart failure, and ischemic nephropathy. Early revascularization of atherosclerotic RAS will improve hypertension and associated conditions in these patients. However, this improvement may not be seen in kidneys that have already experienced permanent damage from sustained hypoperfusion.

CLINICAL ENDPOINTS AND PHYSICAL EXAMINATION

Atherosclerotic RAS is a progressive disease. Progression to occlusion is more common in renal arteries with more severe stenosis. Over a 3-year period, Zierler et al found that 48% of patients

TABLE 36.2 Classification of Fibromuscular Dysplasia

TYPE	FREQUENCY	PATHOLOGY
Medial fibroplasias	80%	Alternating areas of thinned media and thickened fibromuscular ridges containing collagen. Internal elastic membrane may be lost in some areas
Perimedial fibroplasias	10%-15%	Extensive collagen deposition in the outer half of the media
Medial hyperplasia	1%-2%	True smooth muscle cell hyperplasia without fibrosis
Intimal fibroplasias	<10%	Circumferential or eccentric deposition of collagen in the intima. No lipid or inflammatory component. Internal elastic lamina fragmented or duplicated
Adventitial (periarterial) fibroplasias	<1%	Dense collagen replaces the fibrous tissue of the adventitia and may extend into the surrounding tissue

had progression of RAS from <60% to >60% stenosis. The renal arteries that progressed to occlusion were each characterized by a stenosis >60% at baseline. Progression of RAS occurred at an average rate of ~7% per year.[15] Although several retrospective studies have indicated that percutaneous renal artery revascularization can improve hypertension, and helps to stabilize or slow the deterioration in renal function, recent randomized prospective trials have not supported the benefit of revascularization procedures. As a result, the relationship between RAS severity and the impact of revascularization on renal function remains poorly understood.

Patients with atherosclerotic RAS who progress to dialysis-dependent ESRD and require dialysis have high mortality rates. The mean life expectancy of individuals older than 65 years with RAS who have ESRD is only ~3 years.[16] This is thought to be due to systemic atherosclerosis and higher rates of cardiovascular and cerebrovascular ischemic events in individuals with atherosclerotic RAS. The severity of renal impairment has also been associated with reduced survival in patients with RAS. In patients with serum creatinine levels <1.4 mg/dL, 3-year survival was 92% (±4%). For serum creatinine levels of between 1.5 and 1.9 mg/dL, 3-year survival was 74% (±8%), and for creatinine >2.0 mg/dL, it was only 51% (±8%) at 3 years.[17]

Individuals with RAS may also experience "flash" pulmonary edema or may manifest a volume-overload state because they lack normal renal function to respond to pressure natriuresis. Also, RAS may play a role in the development of unstable coronary syndromes. It is believed that this may be from an increase in myocardial oxygen demand in patients with underlying coronary disease secondary to peripheral vasoconstriction.

Several clinical features provide relative indications for application of more specific diagnostic testing strategies for RAS (**Table 36.3**). Certain characteristics of hypertension are suggestive of a secondary etiology, including timing of onset, the presence of accelerated, resistant, or malignant hypertension with evidence of end-organ dysfunction, such as new visual or neurologic disturbance, advanced retinopathy, acute decompensated heart failure, and acute renal failure. Classically, hypokalemia associated with such features of hypertension should raise clinical suspicion for RAS. Another indication is the presence of an atrophic kidney (<7-8 cm) or discrepancy in renal sizes >1.5 cm.[18-20] If the renal atrophy is unexplained by a prior history of pyelonephritis, reflux nephropathy, or trauma, then it is an indication for additional renal diagnostic testing to identify the presence of RAS. Cardiac destabilization syndromes that cannot be clearly explained or controlled despite optimal therapy warrant additional diagnostic consideration as well.

TABLE 36.3 Clinical Clues to the Diagnosis of Renal Artery Stenosis

- Onset of hypertension before the age of 30 y or severe hypertension after the age of 55 y
- Accelerated hypertension, defined as a sudden and persistent worsening of previously controlled hypertension
- Resistant hypertension, defined as the failure to achieve goal blood pressure in patients who are adhering to full doses of an appropriate three-drug regimen that includes a diuretic
- Malignant hypertension, which has coexistent evidence of acute end-organ damage
- New azotemia or worsening renal function after the administration of an ACE inhibitor or an ARB agent
- Unexplained atrophic kidney or a discrepancy in size (>1.5 cm) between the two kidneys
- Unexplained renal failure, including individuals starting renal replacement therapy
- Sudden, unexplained pulmonary edema
- Unexplained congestive heart failure or refractory angina
- Multivessel coronary artery disease or PAD

ACE, angiotensin-converting enzyme; ARB, angiotensin II receptor blocker; PAD, peripheral artery disease.

The physical examination of patients with RAS should focus on the assessment of blood pressure because RAS may be associated with sustained or labile hypertension. Assessment for fluid retention, unexplained congestive heart failure, and refractory angina is also useful. The patient should also undergo an evaluation for evidence of atherosclerosis in other vascular territories. The physical exam should include evaluation for a renal abdominal bruit. Epigastric renal bruits that are high pitched with a diastolic component tend to be more hemodynamically significant.

DIAGNOSTIC TESTING

Patients at high risk for RAS should undergo a noninvasive screening test to evaluate for this condition. The American College of Cardiology (ACC) and American Heart Association (AHA) Management Guidelines 2013 gives a class IB recommendation for the use of duplex ultrasound, magnetic resonance angiography (MRA), and computed tomographic angiography (CTA) as diagnostic tests, as well as the gold standard of catheter-based renal artery angiography when noninvasive tests are inconclusive (**Table 36.4**).

RAS is best initially evaluated with a noninvasive imaging modality.[18] Both the main and accessory renal arteries should be assessed to identify the hemodynamic significance of lesions, the site and severity of the stenosis, and associated pathology, including the presence of an abdominal aortic aneurysm or renal or adrenal masses. Imaging modalities such as duplex ultrasound, MRA, and CTA are the most effective diagnostic screening methods. The choice of imaging procedure will depend on patient characteristics, contrast allergy, renal function, and the presence of prior stents or metallic objects. Renal artery duplex ultrasound demonstrates a sensitivity of 84% to 89% and a specificity of 69% to 97% for diagnosing significant RAS depending on the conditions described in **Table 36.4**. Gadolinium-enhanced MRA has been associated with nephrogenic systemic fibrosis, while CTA may cause contrast-induced nephropathy. MRA has the highest sensitivity at 92% to 97% and a specificity of 73% to 93%, while CTA demonstrates the highest specificity range of 82% to 99% and a sensitivity of 59% to 96%.

In contrast, the aforementioned 2013 ACC/AHA Management Guidelines provide a class III recommendation against using captopril renal artery scintigraphy, selective renal vein renin measurements, and plasma renin activity with or without captopril test as screening diagnostic modalities to identify RAS. Captopril renal artery scintigraphy is a relatively specific but insensitive test to demonstrate unilateral RAS; however, the incidence of false negatives is substantial. Measurement of plasma renin levels is discouraged because it is neither a specific nor a sensitive indicator of renovascular hypertension (**Table 36.5**).

TABLE 36.4 Diagnostic Tests for RAS

TEST	ADVANTAGE(S)	DISADVANTAGE(S)
Duplex ultrasound	High sensitivity	Decreased specificity in obese patients
	Surveillance for progression and post-revascularization	Requires patient preparation
		Operator/experience dependent
Magnetic resonance angiogram	Good sensitivity and specificity	Increased false positives
		Not useful if stents are present
Computed tomographic angiography	Good sensitivity and specificity	Ionizing radiation
	Useful to visualize stents	Iodinated contrast
	Provides anatomic information regarding surrounding structures	
Captopril renal artery scintigraphy	Good specificity	Poor sensitivity (~10%-25% false negative)
Renal vein renin	Lateralizing renin predicts treatment response	Poor sensitivity/specificity Invasive
Renal catheter-based angiography	High sensitivity and specificity	Invasive

RAS, renal artery stenosis.

TABLE 36.5 ACC/AHA Recommendations for Diagnostic Methods[18]

Class I

1. Duplex ultrasonography is recommended as a screening test to establish the diagnosis of RAS (level of evidence: B).
2. CTA (in individuals with normal renal function) is recommended as a screening test to establish the diagnosis of RAS (level of evidence: B).
3. MRA is recommended as a screening test to establish the diagnosis of RAS (level of evidence: B).
4. When the clinical index of suspicion is high and the results of noninvasive tests are inconclusive, catheter angiography is recommended as a diagnostic test to establish the diagnosis of RAS (level of evidence: B)

Class III

1. Captopril renal scintigraphy is not recommended as a screening test to establish the diagnosis of RAS (Level of Evidence: C).
2. Selective renal vein renin measurements are not recommended as a useful screening test to establish the diagnosis of RAS (Level of Evidence: B).
3. Plasma renin activity is not recommended as a useful screening test to establish the diagnosis of RAS (Level of Evidence: B).
4. The captopril test (measurement of plasma renin activity after captopril administration) is not recommended as a useful screening test to establish the diagnosis of RAS (Level of Evidence: B).

ACC, American College of Cardiology; AHA, American Heart Association; CTA, computed tomographic angiography; MRA, magnetic resonance angiography; RAS, renal artery stenosis.

RENAL ARTERY ANGIOGRAPHY IN THE CATH LAB

Catheter-based renal angiography remains the gold standard for imaging renal arteries, although the noninvasive testing methods mentioned earlier have superseded it as a screening exam. Angiography is required to establish the diagnosis of RAS in the case of ambiguous noninvasive imaging. It is also indicated in individuals with prespecified clinical conditions in whom concomitant peripheral angiography or coronary angiography is to be performed.

TABLE 36.6 Angiographic and Hemodynamic Significance of RAS[19]

<50% mild stenosis per angiography
50%-70% moderate/indeterminate stenosis per angiography
50%-70% severe/significant when resting mean pressure gradient >10 mm Hg
50%-70% severe/significant when systolic hyperemic pressure gradient >20 mm Hg
50%-70% severe/significant when renal FFR (renal Pd/Pa) <0.80
≥70% severe/significant per angiography

FFR, fractional flow reserve; RAS, renal artery stenosis.

Angiographic stenosis severity can be categorized as:

- mild (<50%),
- moderate/intermediate (50%-70%), and
- severe (>70%).

Such values may not imply the presence of hemodynamically significant stenosis (**Table 36.6**). Angiographic stenoses that are classified as mild (<50%) are not considered hemodynamically significant. Angiographic lesions of >70% are considered to be severe lesions and hemodynamically significant. Moderate/intermediate angiographic stenosis between 50% and 70% may or may not be hemodynamically significant. Data suggest that significant hemodynamic severity is present when there is a resting translesional mean pressure gradient of >10 mm Hg or a translesional peak systolic pressure gradient of >20 mm Hg at rest or during hyperemia, or renal fractional flow reserve (rFFR) of 0.8 or less. Translesional gradients are measured with small catheters, such as a 4-French (F) catheter, or with a 0.014-in pressure wire to obtain P_d/P_a. Caution is advised when using a 4-F or 5-F catheter as it may be occlusive and may artificially raise the gradient. Renal hyperemia for measurement of FFR can be induced with an intrarenal bolus of 32 mg of papaverine or dopamine at 50 µg/kg. Adenosine causes vasoconstriction in the renal circulation and will not induce renal hyperemia.

Intravascular imaging with intravascular ultrasound (IVUS) or optical coherence tomography may provide information regarding minimal luminal area, plaque volume, and stent apposition. Nonetheless, the use of intravascular imaging has not demonstrated improvement in patient outcomes after renal artery stenting.

Catheter-based angiography has a low rate of complications; however, care must be taken to reduce the risks of atheroembolization, vascular complications, bleeding, and contrast-related nephropathy. To avoid these complications, the following is recommended:

- Prehydrate with intravenous fluids prior to the administration of contrast.
- Minimize the use of contrast agents.
- Use iso-osmolar, nonionic contrast agents.
- Obtain as much information as possible from noninvasive studies prior to performing the catheter-based study.

Nonselective angiography using a pigtail or universal catheter (eg, Omni Flush catheter) is performed. Careful catheter manipulation is used to define the status of the aorta and exact locations of the renal ostia in order to facilitate selective cannulation. To reduce contrast volume, aortography can also be performed with diluted contrast and digital subtraction angiography. Alternative angiographic techniques include the use of carbon dioxide angiography or gadolinium as the contrast agent. It is important to make certain that there are no anomalous renal arteries, and that the arterial supply to all portions of the renal parenchyma is visualized.

Selective renal arteriography is used to evaluate the origin of the renal arteries. Selective renal arterial injections provide the most detail and are easily obtained after initially performing screening aortography. When performing aortography, it should be noted that the renal artery origin usually arises at the level of the first lumbar vertebrae (L1). L1 is found just below the T12 ribs. The anteroposterior or ipsilateral (up to 30°) angulations provide the best view of the renal artery ostia in most patients. Acutely angled take-off of the renal artery may require specially shaped catheters, or an upper extremity approach, to achieve coaxial vessel cannulation.

In the majority of cases, retrograde femoral access is used when the renal artery take-off is horizontal, caudal, or mildly cephalad. In some cases, radial access or left brachial is necessary because the take-off of the renal artery is downward angulated. The choice of access is important, given the high rate of concomitant PAD in these patients.

The choice of catheters for selective renal artery angiography is dependent on the anatomy of the renal artery. It is recommended that soft-tipped atraumatic catheters and guide wires be used for these procedures. Commonly used catheters include the internal mammary artery (IMA), JR4, cobra, renal double curve, hockey stick, multipurpose, or SOS Omni. When brachial access is used for a downward angulated renal artery, a 6F or 7F, 90-cm-long vascular sheath (Shuttle, Raabe, Balkan or Ansel sheath, Cook Inc, Bloomington, IN) is advanced over the guide wire and positioned in the suprarenal abdominal aorta. A 4-F to 6-F IMA catheter, multipurpose, or JR4 is then advanced through the long sheath and is used to engage the renal artery with a telescoping technique. Sometimes a catheter is held away from the aorta-renal ostium with a wire in the aorta (0.018-0.035-in) while another (0.014-0.018-in) wire is manipulated into the renal arterial bed using a "no-touch" technique (**Fig. 36.1**). Using such "no-touch" or telescoping techniques will minimize trauma to the perirenal aorta and can help to prevent disruption and embolus of lipid plaque into the distal renal arterial supply.

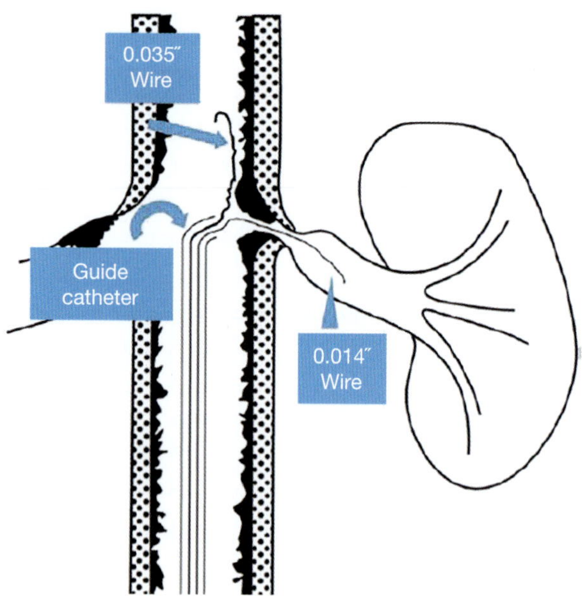

FIGURE 36.1 "No touch" technique. The catheter is held away from the aorta-renal ostium with a 0.018- to 0.035-in wire, while a 0.014- to 0.018-in wire is manipulated into the renal arterial bed. (Reprinted from Rastinehad AR, Siegel DN, Wood BJ, McClure T, ed. *Interventional Urology*. 2nd ed. Springer Cham; 2021, with permission.)

TREATMENT

The goals for medical therapy or revascularization of RAS are as follows:

1. Improve blood pressure control with concomitant reduction in the need for antihypertensive medications.
2. Preserve renal function or delay and prevent the need for renal replacement therapy.
3. Reduce the risk of future cardiovascular events and mortality.

Any intervention, whether medical, endovascular, or surgical, should aim to achieve the relevant clinical goals without significant morbidity or mortality from the intervention.

MEDICAL THERAPY

Angiotensin-converting enzyme (ACE) inhibitors and calcium-channel blockers are effective in the treatment of hypertension in the presence of RAS (**Table 36.7**). They effectively treat hypertension and reduce the risk of progression of renal disease. Treatment with chlorothiazide, hydralazine, and β-blockers are also effective in controlling hypertension in individuals with RAS. In addition, angiotensin II receptor blockers (ARBs) have also shown evidence for controlling blood pressure in individuals with RAS. The use of both ACE inhibitor and ARB for the management of hypertension is safe and is proven to reduce cardiovascular events and slow the progression of renal disease. The remaining aspects of optimal medical therapy for medical management of patients with RAS includes antiplatelet agents, high potency statin ± proprotein convertase subtilisin/kexin type 9 agents, blood glucose control, and lifestyle modifications.

TABLE 36.7 ACC/AHA Guidelines for Medical Treatment for RAS[18]

Class I

1. ACE inhibitors are effective medications for treatment of hypertension associated with unilateral RAS (Level of Evidence: A).
2. Angiotensin receptor blockers are effective medications for treatment of hypertension associated with unilateral RAS (Level of Evidence: B).
3. Calcium-channel blockers are effective medications for treatment of hypertension associated with unilateral RAS (Level of Evidence: A).
4. β-blockers are effective medications for treatment of hypertension associated with RAS (Level of Evidence: A).

ACC, American College of Cardiology; ACE, angiotensin-converting enzyme; AHA, American Heart Association; RAS, renal artery stenosis.

ENDOVASCULAR REVASCULARIZATION

Initial interventional treatment for RAS involved percutaneous transluminal renal angioplasty (PTRA). In the past, several prospective observational trials have indicated that percutaneous PTRA improves blood pressure, with average blood pressure reductions from 10 to 20 mm Hg, and stabilizes or slows the deterioration in renal function. However, recent randomized prospective trials have not supported the benefit of endovascular procedures on clinical outcomes. In 2000, the Dutch RAS Intervention Cooperative (DRASTIC) study was published, where 106 patients were randomly assigned to treatment with PTRA or medical therapy. According to intention-to-treat analysis, at 12 months, there were no significant differences between the angioplasty and drug-therapy groups in systolic and diastolic blood pressures, daily drug doses, or renal function.[21]

With the current use of stent technology and of thienopyridine antiplatelet agents, PTRA with stent deployment has become the gold standard for endovascular RAS intervention. Renal artery stenting overcomes the major complication of elastic recoil with PTRA, which can lead to a restenosis rate of >25% in these vessels. In one of the first trials in 2009 using stent technology, Bax et al in the Stent Placement for Atherosclerotic Stenosis of Renal Artery (STAR) trial randomized 140 patients to stent placement with medical therapy or medical therapy alone to assess for the primary endpoint of worsening renal function. At 2 years of follow-up, there was no statistically significant difference in the primary endpoint, although there was a trend toward benefit in the group with stent placement compared to medical therapy alone (16% vs 22%). Notably, 19% of patients randomized to the intervention arm had <50% stenosis at time of angiography and did not receive stent placement, resulting in only 46 patients who received the intervention treatment compared to 76 patients in the medical therapy arm.[22] Subsequently in the same year, the Angioplasty and Stenting for Renal Artery Lesions (ASTRAL) was published with a much larger study population of 806 patients, who were uniquely identified as a group in which revascularization was deemed to be of unclear benefit by their referring physicians. The study found no difference in outcomes of renal function or events, blood pressure, cardiovascular events, or mortality. However, there was again a trend toward benefit in renal function and blood pressure control in the intervention group. This study highlights the importance of patient selection in revascularization procedures as the patient population specifically excluded those who were considered to likely benefit from intervention, such as patients with flash pulmonary edema, acute renal injury, or rapidly progressive renal disease.[23] The Cardiovascular Outcomes for Renal Atherosclerotic Lesions (CORAL) trial in 2014 enrolled 931 patients to assess whether revascularization in addition to medical therapy would be useful for the prevention of the major adverse clinical events related to hypertension and kidney disease. While renal artery stenting did not show benefit in this trial, a post hoc analysis at 5 years of follow-up did show that individuals with minimal proteinuria who underwent revascularization had better event-free survival from major adverse cardiovascular and renal events and overall survival compared to those on optimal medical therapy alone.[24,25]

In summary, management of patients with atherosclerotic RAS remains controversial. The retrospective and prospective nonrandomized data suggest that endovascular revascularization in addition to optimal medical therapy may be beneficial in select patient populations with specific clinical conditions and criteria.

TABLE 36.8 ACC/AHA Guidelines for Surgical Correction for RAS[18]

Class I

1. Vascular surgical reconstruction is indicated for patients with fibromuscular dysplastic RAS with clinical indications for interventions (same as for percutaneous transluminal angioplasty), especially those exhibiting complex disease that extends into the segmental arteries and those having macroaneurysms (Level of Evidence: B).
2. Vascular surgical reconstruction is indicated for patients with atherosclerotic RAS and clinical indications for intervention, especially those with multiple small renal arteries or early primary branching of the main renal artery (Level of Evidence: B).
3. Vascular surgical reconstruction is indicated for patients with atherosclerotic RAS in combination with pararenal aortic reconstructions (in treatment of aortic aneurysms or severe aortoiliac occlusive disease) (Level of Evidence: C).

ACC, American College of Cardiology, AHA, American Heart Association; RAS, renal artery stenosis.

SURGICAL REVASCULARIZATION

Surgery for atherosclerotic RAS is predominantly limited to patients with concomitant aortic aneurysms, complex renal arterial lesions, or to those who have failed endovascular therapy (**Table 36.8**). When open surgery was compared with endovascular intervention in patients with atherosclerotic RAS, technical procedural success was similar amongst the two groups. The clinical endpoints of hypertension control and renal function preservation were better in the surgical cohort. Major complications occur more in surgical patients, and an excess of 3.1% procedure-related 30-day mortality is observed in the surgical patients. It is therefore suggested that in patients with RAS, who are candidates for either open surgery or endovascular therapy, endovascular intervention should be the first-line therapy unless there are other concomitant indications to undergo open surgery.

INDICATIONS FOR REVASCULARIZATION

The ACC/AHA/Society for Cardiovascular Angiography & Interventions/Society for Interventional Radiology/Society for Vascular Medicine 2018 Appropriate Use Criteria suggest that

TABLE 36.9 Indications for Revascularization for Hemodynamically Significant RAS[19,26]

Appropriate	• In patients with cardiac disturbance syndromes and severe hypertension (sudden-onset flash pulmonary edema or acute coronary syndrome). • In patients with accelerated hypertension, resistant hypertension, malignant hypertension, hypertension with an unexplained unilateral small kidney, and hypertension with intolerance to medications. • In patients with ischemic nephropathy or progressive decline in renal function with bilateral RAS or a solitary viable kidney with RAS (defined as a pole-to-pole kidney length of ≥7 cm).
May be appropriate	• In patients with ischemic nephropathy or progressive decline in renal function with unilateral RAS. • In patients with recurrent congestive heart failure despite optimal medical therapy with unilateral RAS.
Rarely appropriate	• In patients with unilateral, solitary, or bilateral RAS with nonviable small kidneys (pole-to-pole kidney length <7 cm). • In patients with unilateral, solitary, or bilateral RAS with controlled blood pressure and normal renal function. • In patients with unilateral, solitary, or bilateral RAS with chronic ESRD on hemodialysis >3 month • In patients with unilateral, solitary, or bilateral chronic total occlusion of the renal artery.

ESRD, end-stage renal disease; RAS, renal artery stenosis.

hemodynamically significant asymptomatic RAS is defined as RAS in the absence of end-organ dysfunction (eg, idiopathic pulmonary edema, stroke, visual loss, hypertension, or refractory angina) but in the presence of the following[26]:

1. Greater than or equal to 50% to 70% diameter stenosis by visual estimation with a peak translesional gradient (measured with a <5F catheter or pressure wire) of >20 mm Hg or a mean gradient >10 mm Hg, or fractional flow reserve of <0.8;
2. Any stenosis >70% diameter stenosis, or
3. Greater than or equal to 70% diameter stenosis by IVUS measurement.

A number of clinical presentations are indications to consider renal artery intervention in patients with hemodynamically significant RAS (**Table 36.9**). These include individuals with hypertension who cannot tolerate medications, have a unilateral small kidney with RAS, have accelerated hypertension, or have resistant hypertension, defined as requiring more than three antihypertensive medications at maximum tolerated doses. Similarly, intervention should be considered in individuals with progressive renal failure and bilateral RAS, solitary kidney, or unilateral RAS. Cardiac destabilization syndromes in the setting of known significant RAS, such as unexplained or recurrent pulmonary edema, recurrent heart failure despite optimal medical therapy, or unstable angina on maximally tolerated medical therapy, are indications in which intervention may be performed to prevent further events. Comparatively, the ACC/AHA guideline recommendations for revascularization are detailed in **Fig. 36.2**.[27]

PERCUTANEOUS RENAL ARTERY STENTING

Percutaneous transluminal renal balloon angioplasty is the treatment of choice for symptomatic RAS caused by FMD.[12-14] Atherosclerotic aorto-ostial renal artery stenotic lesions are generally not suitable for treatment by balloon angioplasty alone, owing to a high rate of dissections and restenosis, as discussed earlier. Renal artery stent placement has been shown to be superior to balloon angioplasty in the treatment of renal artery atherosclerotic lesions. Larger-diameter renal arteries, and therefore stents, have lower restenosis rates compared to smaller-diameter vessels. Randomized controlled trials have also demonstrated the superiority of renal stents over balloon angioplasty in hypertensive patients with atherosclerotic RAS for procedure success, late patency, and cost-effectiveness.[18,28,29] The potential benefits of renal stent placement include reperfusion of the ischemic kidneys and improvement in the renal hemodynamic parameters.

Patients with a rapid deterioration in renal function derive greater benefit in renal function with stenting than those with stable chronic renal impairment. The lack of any potential benefit in certain patients, and possible deterioration, of renal function may be secondary to hyperperfusion injury, contrast nephropathy, progression of nephrosclerosis, and distal embolization of atherosclerotic material. This potential for embolization of atherothrombotic debris during renal stenting has raised concern that procedure-related renal damage could offset any benefits from improved renal artery blood flow.

Embolic protection devices (EPDs) used during saphenous vein graft angioplasty have been reported to reduce procedural complications and subsequently lead to reduced adverse cardiac events. The use of distal EPDs in renal artery interventions has been advocated as a means of potentially preserving renal function.[30,31] Limited data suggest the use of EPDs to prevent embolization of atheromatous material may lead to improvement in renal function.

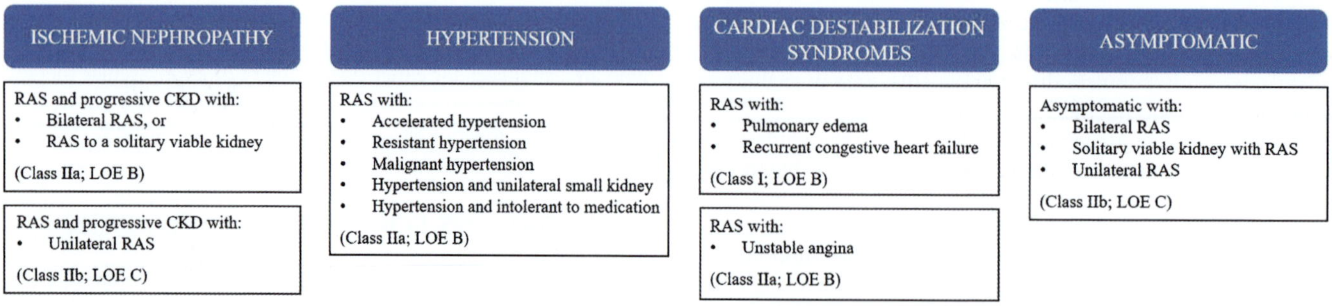

FIGURE 36.2 Summary of the American College of Cardiology/American Heart Association guideline recommendations for revascularization of hemodynamically significant renal artery stenosis.[27]

Other data combining EPDs with abciximab was noted to cause small significant changes in glomerular filtration rate, but no overall improvement in renal function over that existing at baseline prior to renal artery stenting.[32] The evidence supporting the use of EPDs and glycoprotein IIb/IIIa inhibitors has thus far remained unconvincing. The CORAL trial initially mandated the use of EPDs for all randomized to stent treatment; however, soon after trial initiation, this requirement was removed. It was felt that only selective use of EPDs was deemed to be appropriate in patients who were at increased risk for renal dysfunction from potential atheromatous embolization.

The use of intravascular lithotripsy (IVL) for plaque modification in severely calcified coronary and peripheral arterial disease has been demonstrated to be safe and effective in fracturing calcium, achieving luminal gain, and reducing diameter stenosis. The use of IVL in heavily calcified renal arteries has been reported to facilitate lesion preparation as well and promote adequate stent expansion. Prospective trials are needed to further delineate the safety and role of IVL in revascularization of RAS with severe calcification.

TECHNIQUE FOR RA REVASCULARIZATION

Depending on the anatomy seen on initial noninvasive imaging, retrograde common femoral artery (CFA), brachial, or radial artery access is obtained and diagnostic renal arterial angiography is completed, as described in the above section. When retrograde CFA access is chosen, a short 6 to 8F sheath is inserted into the CFA. Also, a 6F or 7F, 55-cm sheath (Ansel, Rabbe, or Shuttle) can be used. Next, a 5F or 6F diagnostic catheter (IMA, cobra, or JR configuration) is advanced to engage the ostium of the renal artery. One approach is to have diagnostic catheters be inserted through a 7 to 8F guiding catheter or 55-cm sheath prior to vessel engagement. This will enable easy exchange and manipulation of the catheters once the wires are in place. Then, a 0.014-in or 0.018-in wire or a soft-tip exchange-length 0.035-in guidewire (eg, Wholey wire) can be used to cross the lesion and positioned in a renal artery branch. A guiding catheter or sheath is positioned in close contact with the renal artery ostium. With this approach, the diagnostic catheter can be removed without losing access to the renal vessel, leaving the guide wire secured in the renal artery, and the guiding catheter or sheath in contact with the ostium of the renal artery.

It is recommended to avoid the use of a hydrophilic Glidewire (Terumo, Somerset, NJ) because this may cause inadvertent vessel perforation and/or dissection. The use of 5F or 6F diagnostic or glide catheters are helpful to locate the ostium of the renal arteries to avoid trauma and potential cholesterol embolization from scraping the aorta, which may occur with larger angioplasty guiding catheters. Using the "no-touch" technique also prevents cholesterol embolization, by avoiding unnecessary scraping of the luminal atherosclerotic aortic plaque through minimizing any manipulation of the guiding catheter during cannulation of the renal artery ostium (**Fig. 36.1**).

After the reference vessel diameter (RVD) is estimated or measured by angiography or intravascular imaging, a peripheral angioplasty balloon (4-8 mm in diameter) is advanced over the guide wire and positioned at the lesion. The lesion is then predilated with a balloon sized 1:1 with the RVD, using the lowest pressure that will fully expand the balloon. Before removal, the balloon is reinflated at a low pressure (1-2 atm) and, while the balloon is deflating, the catheter is advanced across the lesion over the balloon. This maneuver enables the stent to be positioned beyond the lesion site, without risking stent's edges catching on the plaque and reducing the risk of stent embolization. The use of distal vessel protection devices during balloon angioplasty and stenting can reduce and prevent the chance of distal vessel atheroemboli in selected patients, but the data to support their use are very limited.

Balloon-expandable bare metal or drug-eluting stents are used to scaffold the lesion and maximize the angiographic result. The stent is advanced over the guidewire to the lesion site. With gentle contrast injections through the guiding catheter or the sheath, the stent is positioned at the lesion site. When treating ostial lesions, it is important to allow ~1 mm of the stent to protrude into the aorta in order to ensure complete coverage of the diseased ostium of the artery. The stent is deployed at a nominal pressure (6-8 atm), and then the balloon is pulled back and can be used to postdilate and flare the ostial/proximal portion of the stent. Angiography and/or intravascular imaging is then performed and, if inadequate expansion or malapposition of the stent is observed, the operator can repeat dilation of the stent at a higher inflation pressure or with a larger balloon. The goal is to safely reduce the RAS to <30% angiographic stenosis and eliminate the translesional pressure gradient to zero. During angioplasty and stenting, patients may experience abdominal or back discomfort. This may signify stretching of the adventitia and possible vascular rupture. When pain occurs, the balloon should be immediately deflated.

The Szabo technique is another technique used to deploy stents exactly at the aortorenal artery junction, without missing the ostium or protruding too much into the aorta.[33] This technique was initially used in coronary artery ostial lesions but can also be used in guiding and deploying renal stents into position at the aortorenal junction. For the exact deployment, a second 0.014-in wire is inserted through the last cell of a stent for stent deployment. This stent tail wire or anchor technique facilitates precise aorto-ostial stent deployment in cases of atherosclerotic RAS. It also helps to eliminate errors of improper stent positioning at the aortorenal junction and may possibly minimize patient exposure to ionizing radiation and contrast dye (**Figs. 36.3-36.7**).

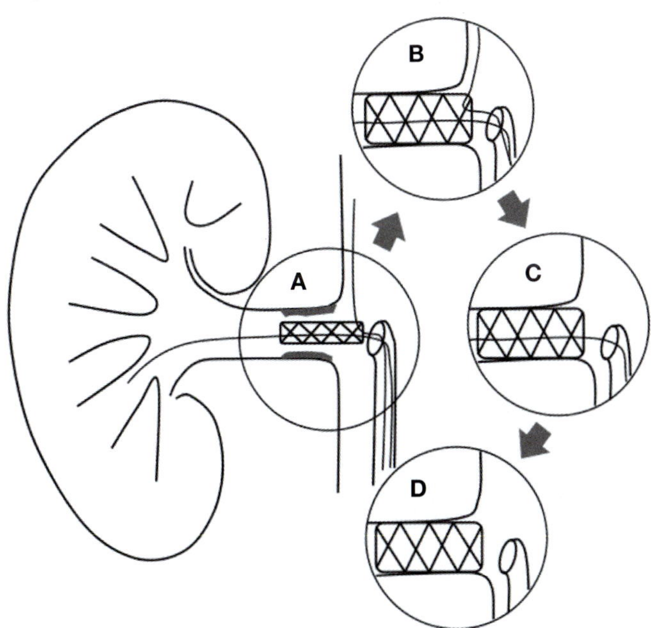

FIGURE 36.3 Szabo technique applied to improve stent deployment in ostial renal artery stenosis. The stent is guided to the lesion with the aid of two wires **(A)**. The aortic wire properly engages the stent at the ostial renal-aorta junction, and the stent is partial deployed **(B)**. The aortic wire is then removed, and the stent is fully deployed **(C)**. Finally, the guide (renal) wire is removed, and the stent remains in the optimal position **(D)**.

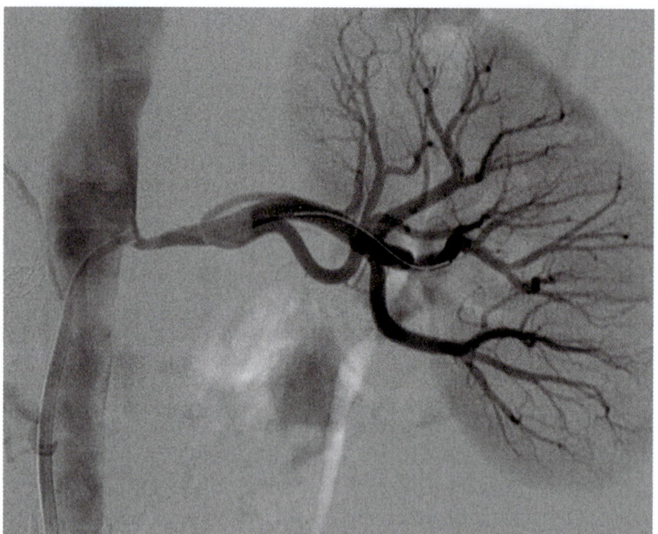

FIGURE 36.4 Angiogram of left renal artery after stenting.

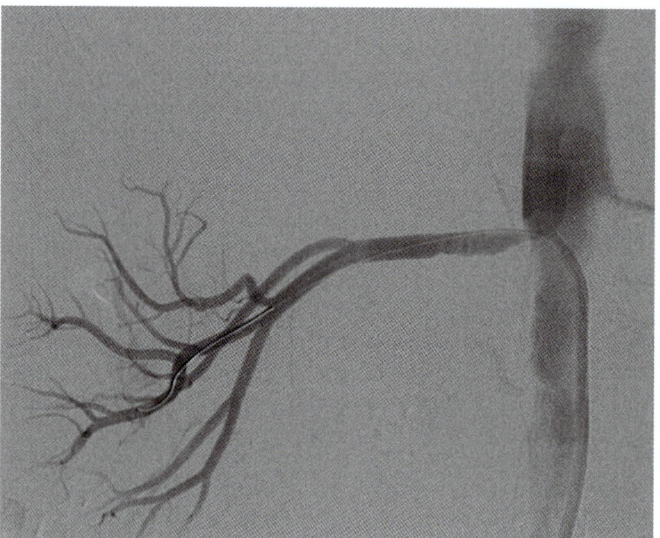

FIGURE 36.6 Angiogram of right renal artery after stenting.

IDENTIFICATION OF PATIENTS WHO MAY BENEFIT FROM REVASCULARIZATION

Baseline mild-to-moderate renal dysfunction appears to be predictive of improved renal function outcomes in patients with RAS who undergo revascularization with stenting. Studies identify a significant and greater renal benefit in patients following revascularization either with a baseline creatinine >1.5 mg/dL or a baseline estimated glomerular filtration rate <60 mL/min/1.73 m^2.[34,35] Minimal proteinuria, suggestive of less kidney damage, has also been associated with improved renal outcomes in these patients.[25] Patients with bilateral renal artery disease and stenting may derive greater benefit compared to those with unilateral disease. Various other clinical parameters have been investigated as predictors of renal outcomes after revascularization, including patient comorbidities, brain natriuretic peptide, and renal resistive index with mixed results.

Clinical predictors for improvement in blood pressure control likely include female sex and higher baseline mean arterial blood pressure or diastolic blood pressure prior to revascularization.[34,36] Some studies suggest that a shorter duration of hypertension (<1-2 years since initial diagnosis) may predict favorable outcomes in terms of improved blood pressure control.

Expert consensus and experimental evidence have suggested that hemodynamic severity of RAS is present when there exists a resting translesional mean pressure gradient of >10 mm Hg, a resting or hyperemic peak systolic gradient of >20 mm Hg, or rFFR ≤0.8. Angiographic stenoses <50% are mild and would not be considered hemodynamically significant or warrant revascularization. The technical aspects of the measurements are described in **Table 36.6**.

Invasive predictors of improved blood pressure after revascularization include measurement of a hyperemic translesional systolic pressure gradient ≥21 mm Hg, using a pressure wire and intra-arterial papaverine to induce renal hyperemia, which has been

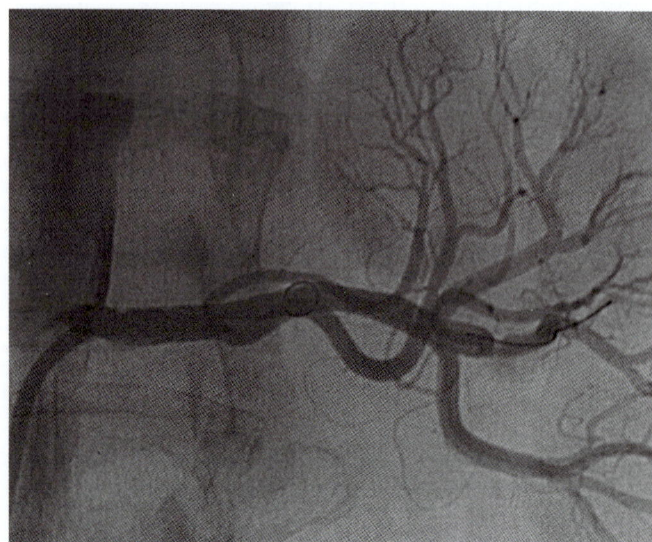

FIGURE 36.5 Right renal artery stenosis.

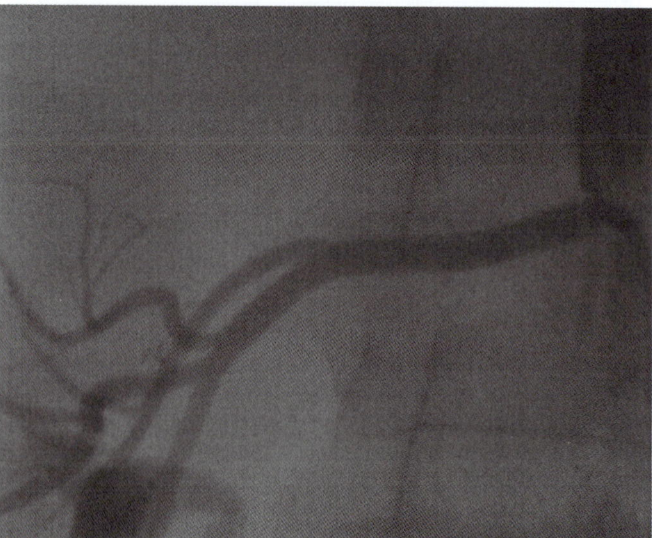

FIGURE 36.7 Szabo technique applied to improve stent deployment in ostial renal artery stenosis. The stent is guided to the lesion with the aid of two wires **(A)**. The aortic wire properly engages the stent at the ostial renal-aorta junction, and the stent is partial deployed **(B)**. The aortic wire is then removed, and the stent is fully deployed **(C)**. Finally, the guide (renal) wire is removed, and the stent remains in the optimal position **(D)**.

shown to identify patients who will develop an improvement in hypertension following revascularization.[37] The lack of a hyperemic response in the kidney may identify patients with intrinsic microvascular or parenchymal disease who will not respond to revascularization. Another trial suggested that a dopamine-induced mean gradient >20 mm Hg was the optimal cutoff point to predict a favorable response to hypertension after renal artery stenting.[38]

Trials investigating resting rFFR, which is the ratio of distal renal pressure to aortic pressure, have suggested that a resting rFFR < 0.9 produced significant elevation in bilateral renal vein renin levels.[39] Therefore, lesions that demonstrated an rFFR < 0.9 may provide reasonable predictive accuracy for blood pressure improvement in patients who have revascularization for RAS. As mentioned previously, an FFR value of <0.8 under hyperemic conditions improved blood pressure control in hypertensive patients as well.[37]

CONCLUSION

Current randomized controlled trials of atherosclerotic renal artery disease comparing renal angioplasty/stenting plus medical therapy versus optimal medical therapy have been mostly negative. These trials should be interpreted with caution given difficulty with enrollment and important selection bias limitations in these trials, which included a heterogeneous population with moderate hypertension, and moderate RAS without systematic examination of hemodynamic significance of renal arterial stenoses. Results from the CORAL trial confirmed that effective medical therapy should be the first line of treatment in patients with presumed renovascular hypertension.[24] In selective patients who fail medical therapy or are unable to tolerate medical therapy, renal artery stenting remains a reasonable option. The CORAL trial also showed that the benefits of medical therapy alone declined over time. At 3 to 5 years of follow-up, the event-free survival declined in this patient group. Clinical evaluation and consideration of renal artery revascularization is needed to ensure patients have access to alternative treatments when medical therapy is not effective. Additional investigations are needed to identify patients who are most likely to benefit from renal artery revascularization compared to medical therapy alone.

At present, aggressive risk factor modification, medical therapy, and blood pressure control remain the mainstay of therapy for renal artery atherosclerosis. Renal artery stenting has been shown to improve outcomes in patients with unstable angina and congestive heart failure. Important indications for revascularization of the renal arteries also include improving blood pressure control and ischemic nephropathy. The ability to perform physiologic lesion assessment using translesional hyperemic pressure gradient and rFFR calculations may aid in identifying patients who will benefit from revascularization. Renal artery stenting is superior to balloon angioplasty in atherosclerotic RAS; nevertheless, balloon angioplasty remains the treatment of choice for FMD.

The main limitation of the randomized control trials for revascularization in atherosclerotic RAS has been patient selection; the trials either included patients without renovascular hypertension or without ischemic nephropathy, with unlikely to be hemodynamically significant RAS lesions, or excluded patients who were most likely to benefit from revascularization as defined by their clinical presentations. Therefore, future prospective randomized trials are still needed to investigate the role of endovascular therapy in carefully selected patients.

Acknowledgments

The authors express our appreciation for the prior version of the chapter published in the third edition of this book by Dr. Pranav M. Patel.

Key Points

- Atherosclerotic RAS is a common cause of secondary hypertension and is a progressive disease associated with high rates of adverse cardiovascular events.
- Activation of the renin-angiotensin-aldosterone pathway from hemodynamically significant RAS leads to development of hypertension, ischemic nephropathy, and cardiac destabilization syndromes.
- Specific clinical features and exam findings should prompt screening with noninvasive imaging. If such testing remains inconclusive, concomitant angiography should be pursued in patients with a high suspicion for RAS; invasive catheter-based renal angiography remains the gold standard for diagnosis.
- Diagnostic renal angiography is ideally performed with a telescoping or "no-touch" technique to minimize complications. Physiologic measurements with resting or hyperemic translesional pressure gradients or FFR may aid in defining hemodynamically significant RAS.
- All patients should be treated with optimal medical therapy, aggressive risk factor modification, and blood pressure control as a first-line management.
- Renal artery angioplasty/stenting with or without EPDs is indicated in certain clinical presentations related to uncontrolled hypertension, progressive renal dysfunction, and recurrent cardiac destabilization syndromes.
- Surgical revascularization is limited to patients with concomitant aortic aneurysms, complex renal arterial lesions, or who have failed endovascular therapy.
- Baseline mild-to-moderate renal dysfunction and lack of significant proteinuria may be predictive of patients who would benefit from revascularization for renal outcomes.
- Predictors for improved blood pressure control may include female sex, higher baseline mean or diastolic blood pressure, new onset hypertension, and invasive physiologic testing suggestive of hemodynamically significant disease.
- To date, randomized controlled trials have not shown clear benefit of renal artery stenting compared to medical therapy alone. However, these studies have been limited by heterogenous patient populations in which intervention was uncertain to be of benefit, highlighting the importance of patient selection for successful revascularization and clinical outcomes.

References

1. Hansen KJ, Edwards MS, Craven TE, et al. Prevalence of renovascular disease in the elderly: a population-based study. *J Vasc Surg*. 2002;36(3):443-451.
2. Harding MB, Smith LR, Himmelstein SI, et al. Renal artery stenosis: prevalence and associated risk factors in patients undergoing routine cardiac catheterization. *J Am Soc Nephrol*. 1992;2(11):1608-1616.

3. Weber-Mzell D, Kotanko P, Schumacher M, Klein W, Skrabal F. Coronary anatomy predicts presence or absence of renal artery stenosis: a prospective study in patients undergoing cardiac catheterization for suspected coronary artery disease. *Eur Heart J*. 2002;23(21):1684-1691.
4. Jean WJ, al-Bitar I, Zwicke DL, Port SC, Schmidt DH, Bajwa TK. High incidence of renal artery stenosis in patients with coronary artery disease. *Cathet Cardiovasc Diagn*. 1994;32(1):8-10.
5. Missouris CG, Buckenham T, Cappuccio FP, MacGregor GA. Renal artery stenosis: a common and important problem in patients with peripheral vascular disease. *Am J Med*. 1994;96(1):10-14.
6. Olin JW, Melia M, Young JR, Graor RA, Risius B. Prevalence of atherosclerotic renal artery stenosis in patients with atherosclerosis elsewhere. *Am J Med*. 1990;88(1N):46N-51N.
7. Rossi GP, Rossi A, Zanin L, et al. Excess prevalence of extracranial carotid artery lesions in renovascular hypertension. *Am J Hypertens*. 1992;5(1):8-15.
8. Metcalfe W, Reid AW, Geddes CC. Prevalence of angiographic atherosclerotic renal artery disease and its relationship to the anatomical extent of peripheral vascular atherosclerosis. *Nephrol Dial Transplant*. 1999;14(1):105-108.
9. Missouris CG, Papavassiliou MB, Khaw K, et al. High prevalence of carotid artery disease in patients with atheromatous renal artery stenosis. *Nephrol Dial Transplant*. 1998;13(4):945-948.
10. Rimmer JM, Gennari FJ. Atherosclerotic renovascular disease and progressive renal failure. *Ann Intern Med*. 1993;118(9):712-719.
11. Safian RD, Textor SC. Renal artery stenosis. *N Engl J Med*. 2001;344(6):431-442.
12. Stanley JC, Wakefield TW. Arterial fibrodysplasia. In: Rutherford RB, ed. *Vascular Surgery*. 6th ed. Saunders; 2004:387-408.
13. Messina LM, Stanley JC. Renal artery fibrodysplasia and renovascular hypertension. In: Rutherford RB, ed. *Vascular Surgery*. 6th ed. Saunders; 2004:1650-1664.
14. Mounier-Vehier C, Haulon S, Devos P, et al. Renal atrophy outcome after revascularization in fibromuscular dysplasia disease. *J Endovasc Ther*. 2002;9(5):605-613.
15. Zierler RE, Bergelin RO, Davidson RC, Cantwell-Gab K, Polissar NL, Strandness DE Jr. A prospective study of disease progression in patients with atherosclerotic renal artery stenosis. *Am J Hypertens*. 1996;9(11):1055-1061.
16. Eggers PW, Connerton R, McMullan M. The Medicare experience with end-stage renal disease: trends in incidence, prevalence, and survival. *Health Care Financ Rev*. 1984;5(3):69-88.
17. Wright JR, Shurrab AE, Cheung C, et al. A prospective study of the determinants of renal functional outcome and mortality in atherosclerotic renovascular disease. *Am J Kidney Dis*. 2002;39(6):1153-1161.
18. Hirsch AT, Haskal ZJ, Hertzer NR, et al. ACC/AHA 2005 guidelines for the management of patients with peripheral arterial disease (lower extremity, renal, mesenteric, and abdominal aortic): executive summary a collaborative report from the American Association for Vascular Surgery/Society for Vascular Surgery, Society for Cardiovascular Angiography and Interventions, Society for Vascular Medicine and Biology, Society of Interventional Radiology, and the ACC/AHA Task Force on Practice Guidelines (Writing Committee to develop guidelines for the management of patients with peripheral arterial disease) endorsed by the American Association of Cardiovascular and Pulmonary Rehabilitation; National Heart, Lung, and Blood Institute; Society for Vascular Nursing; TransAtlantic Inter-Society Consensus; and Vascular Disease Foundation. *J Am Coll Cardiol*. 2006;47(6):1239-1312.
19. Parikh SA, Shishehbor MH, Gray BH, White CJ, Jaff MR. SCAI expert consensus statement for renal artery stenting appropriate use. *Catheter Cardiovasc Interv*. 2014;84(7):1163-1171.
20. Gifford RW Jr, McCormack LJ, Poutasse EF. The atrophic kidney: its role in hypertension. *Mayo Clin Proc*. 1965;40(11):834-852.
21. van Jaarsveld BC, Krijnen P, Pieterman H, et al. The effect of balloon angioplasty on hypertension in atherosclerotic renal-artery stenosis. Dutch Renal Artery Stenosis Intervention Cooperative Study Group. *N Engl J Med*. 2000;342(14):1007-1014.
22. Bax L, Woittiez AJJ, Kouwenberg HJ, et al. Stent placement in patients with atherosclerotic renal artery stenosis and impaired renal function: a randomized trial. *Ann Intern Med*. 2009;150(12):840-848, W150-W151.
23. The ASTRAL Investigators. Revascularization versus medical therapy for renal artery stenosis. *N Engl J Med*. 2009;361:1953-1962.
24. Cooper CJ, Murphy TP, Cutlip DE, et al. Stenting and medical therapy for atherosclerotic renal-artery stenosis. *N Engl J Med*. 2014;370(1):13-22. doi:10.1056/NEJMoa1210753
25. Murphy TP, Cooper CJ, Pencina KM, et al. Relationship of albuminuria and renal artery stent outcomes: results from the CORAL randomized clinical trial (Cardiovascular Outcomes with Renal Artery Lesions). *Hypertension*. 2016;68(5):1145-1152.
26. Bailey SR, Beckman JA, Dao TD, et al. ACC/AHA/SCAI/SIR/SVM 2018 Appropriate use criteria for peripheral artery intervention: a report of the American College of Cardiology appropriate use criteria task force, American Heart Association, Society for Cardiovascular Angiography and Interventions, Society of Interventional Radiology, and Society for Vascular Medicine. *J Am Coll Cardiol*. 2019;73(2):214-237.
27. Anderson JL, Halperin JL, Albert NM, et al. Management of patients with peripheral artery disease (Compilation of 2005 and 2011 ACCF/AHA guideline recommendations): a report of the American College of Cardiology Foundation/American Heart Association Task Force on Practice Guidelines. *Circulation*. 2013;127(13):1425-1443.
28. van de Ven PJ, Kaatee R, Beutler JJ, et al. Arterial stenting and balloon angioplasty in ostial atherosclerotic renovascular disease: a randomised trial. *Lancet*. 1999;353(9149):282-286.
29. Dorros G, Prince C, Mathiak L. Stenting of a renal artery stenosis achieves better relief of the obstructive lesion than balloon angioplasty. *Cathet Cardiovasc Diagn*. 1993;29(3):191-198.
30. Holden A, Hill A. Renal angioplasty and stenting with distal protection of the main renal artery in ischemic nephropathy: early experience. *J Vasc Surg*. 2003;38(5):962-968.
31. Henry M, Klonaris C, Henry I, et al. Protected renal stenting with the PercuSurge GuardWire device: a pilot study. *J Endovasc Ther*. 2001;8(3):227-237.
32. Cooper CJ, Haller ST, Colyer W, et al. Embolic protection and platelet inhibition during renal artery stenting. *Circulation*. 2008;117(21):2752-2760.
33. Salazar M, Kern MJ, Patel PM. Exact deployment of stents in ostial renal artery stenosis using the stent tail wire or Szabo technique. *Catheter Cardiovasc Interv*. 2009;74(6):946-950.
34. Zeller T, Frank U, Müller C, et al. Predictors of improved renal function after percutaneous stent-supported angioplasty of severe atherosclerotic ostial renal artery stenosis. *Circulation*. 2003;108(18):2244-2249.
35. Staub D, Partovi S, Zeller T, et al. Multimarker assessment for the prediction of renal function improvement after percutaneous revascularization for renal artery stenosis. *Cardiovasc Diagn Ther*. 2016;6(3):221-233.
36. Ronden R, Houben AJ, Kessels AG, Stehouwer CD, de Leeuw PW, Kroon AA. Predictors of clinical outcome after stent placement in atherosclerotic renal artery stenosis: a systematic review and meta-analysis of prospective studies. *J Hypertens*. 2010;28(12):2370-2377.
37. Leesar MA, Varma J, Shapira A, et al. Prediction of hypertension improvement after stenting of renal artery stenosis: comparative accuracy of translesional pressure gradients, intravascular ultrasound, and angiography. *J Am Coll Cardiol*. 2009;53(25):2363-2371.
38. Mangiacapra F, Trana C, Sarno G, et al. Translesional pressure gradients to predict blood pressure response after renal artery stenting in patients with renovascular hypertension. *Circ Cardiovasc Interv*. 2010;3(6):537-542.
39. De Bruyne B, Manoharan G, Pijls NHJ, et al. Assessment of renal artery stenosis severity by pressure gradient measurements. *J Am Coll Cardiol*. 2006;48(9):1851-1855.

Deep Venous Thrombosis and Pulmonary Embolism

Andrew J.P. Klein and Prashant Kaul

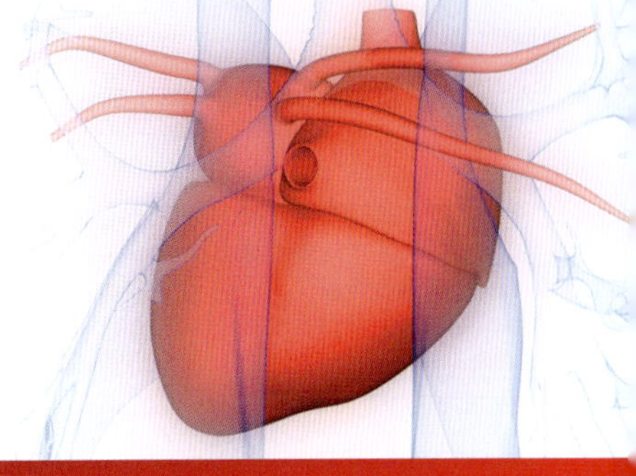

EPIDEMIOLOGY AND DIAGNOSIS

Venous thromboembolism (VTE) represents a source of significant morbidity and mortality and is the third leading cause of cardiovascular death.[1-4] Although most cases are preventable with appropriate pharmacologic and nonpharmacologic prophylaxis, the incidence of VTE appears to be on the rise and is estimated to be one to three cases per 1000 person-years.[2,5] Massive pulmonary embolism (PE), secondary to DVT, causes nearly 300,000 deaths annually in the United States.[6] For those patients who survive their initial PE event, 1% to 5% may develop chronic thromboembolic pulmonary hypertension, which can lead to considerable disability and right-sided heart failure. VTE, even in the absence of PE, can result in a marked decrease in quality of life.[7-9] As many as 20% to 50% of patients with proximal deep venous thrombosis (DVT) may go on to develop some degree of postthrombotic syndrome (PTS) due to valve damage and persistent outflow obstruction despite appropriate anticoagulation.[10,11] Some risk factors for the development of PTS include extensive clot burden, severe symptoms, subtherapeutic anticoagulation, recurrent ipsilateral DVT, obesity, and advanced age.[10,12,13] Interestingly, the total duration of anticoagulation, inherited or acquired thrombophilia, sex, or the circumstances of DVT (provoked, malignancy, or unprovoked) do not seem to influence the risk of developing PTS. Further research is needed to help prevent and treat this limiting condition. Therefore, prevention and early diagnosis with appropriate management are critical.

Diagnosis of acute VTE can be challenging since not all proximal DVTs are clinically apparent. Physical examination, although helpful, is neither sensitive nor specific,[14] and therefore, physicians must take a thorough clinical history and have a high index of suspicion for VTE in the appropriate clinical circumstance. Risk factors for the development of VTE are presented in **Table 37.1** and can be categorized into acquired (some of which may be transient) and genetic factors.[5,15] The diagnostic workup of patients with suspected DVT depends upon the estimated pretest probability (**Fig. 37.1**).[16-18] Importantly, the D-dimer test is highly sensitive but cannot rule out VTE in those with high pretest probability. Such patients should proceed to imaging without D-dimer testing with whole leg compression duplex ultrasonography for suspected DVT and computed tomography angiography or ventilation-perfusion scan for suspected PE.[17]

It is important to assess the severity of illness, identify important comorbid conditions (eg, pregnancy, cancer), and recognize contraindications to anticoagulation at the time of diagnosis since this will often alter management. For patients with DVT, signs of blanching, cyanosis, edema, compartment syndrome, or even venous gangrene are suggestive of phlegmasia cerulea dolens, which is associated with significantly higher morbidity and mortality.[19-21] Furthermore, all proximal DVTs should not be considered the same. Those with iliofemoral DVT have low rates of recanalization and higher rates of recurrent thrombosis.[22] For those with PE, risk stratification should be performed using a validated prognostic model such as the PE severity index (**Table 37.2**).[23-26]

TABLE 37.1 Risk Factors for the Development of VTE

Acquired

- Acute medical illness
- Inflammatory bowel disease
- Nephrotic syndrome
- Age >60 y
- Previous VTE
- Cancer or chemotherapy
- Surgery
- Trauma
- Immobility
- Pregnancy
- Estrogen therapy
- Obesity
- Antiphospholipid antibody syndrome
- May-Thurner syndrome

Genetic

- Antithrombin deficiency
- Protein C deficiency
- Protein S deficiency
- Hyperhomocysteinemia
- Prothrombin gene mutation
- Factor V Leiden mutation
- Elevated factor VIII levels

VTE, venous thromboembolism.

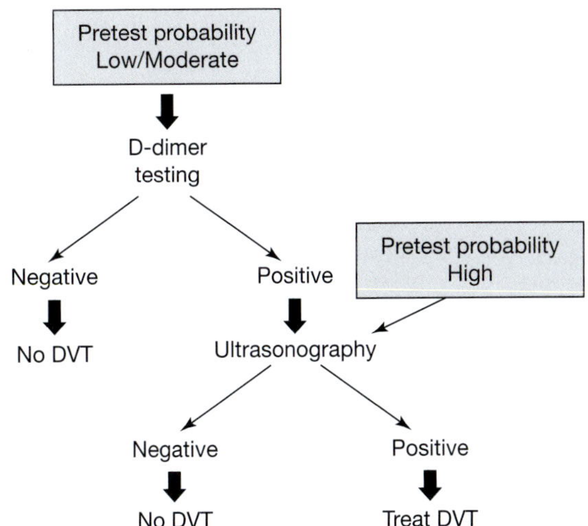

FIGURE 37.1 Diagnostic algorithm for suspected deep venous thrombosis (DVT).

TABLE 37.2 Simplified Pulmonary Embolism Severity Index Score

PREDICTOR	POINTS
Age >80 y	1
History of cancer	1
COPD	1
Pulse > 100 bpm	1
SBP < 100 mm Hg	1
SaO_2 < 90%	1
Score >1 = high risk	

COPD, chronic obstructive pulmonary disease; SBP, systolic blood pressure.

MEDICAL MANAGEMENT

Prompt initiation of therapeutic anticoagulation remains the cornerstone of treatment of patients with suspected and confirmed VTE. Treatment should not be delayed for imaging results, especially if the pretest probability is high. Anticoagulation prevents thrombus propagation, recurrence, and the development of new thrombi but does not dissolve thrombi that already exist. Currently available direct-acting oral anticoagulant (DOAC) options are shown in **Table 37.3**, and recent guidelines give a weak recommendation for their use as first-line treatment of patients without cancer.[27] For those with cancer, low-molecular-weight heparin (LMWH) is the preferred agent.[27] DOACs and LMWH offer fairly predictable pharmacomechanics when compared with unfractionated heparin, with a rapid onset of action and short time to achieving therapeutic anticoagulation. Rivaroxaban and apixaban can be given as monotherapy without parenteral anticoagulation and are therefore the most commonly used. Dabigatran and edoxaban were studied in patients who initially received 5 to 10 days of parenteral anticoagulation. Of note, for those patients with DVT and swelling, the routine use of compression stockings during the acute phase to prevent PTS is not recommended based on the negative randomized controlled SOX (Compression Stockings to Prevent the Post-Thrombotic Limb Syndrome) trial.[27,28]

A minimum of 3 months of therapeutic anticoagulation should be administered to all patients with acute VTE regardless of whether reversible or transient risk factors (provoked) are identified.[27] Anticoagulation may be discontinued in patients with transient risk factors, but it should be continued indefinitely (potentially at reduced doses) in those patients with a second event, with cancer, and perhaps in those with unprovoked DVT. If anticoagulation needs to be discontinued for patients with unprovoked cases due to intolerance, then aspirin should be prescribed indefinitely.[29,30]

CATHETER-DIRECTED MANAGEMENT OF ACUTE DVT

As discussed previously, the purpose of conventional therapy with anticoagulation for DVT is to prevent propagation of the clot and the development of new clots and to reduce the risk for PE. Anticoagulation does not resolve the existing clot, reduce the risk of developing venous valvular damage, prevent venous hypertension, or rapidly resolve symptoms, leaving patients with proximal iliofemoral DVT with large thrombus burden vulnerable to the development of venous stasis ulcers, PTS, and potentially even PE. In such patients, early catheter-directed therapy may prevent PTS and provide faster symptom relief compared with anticoagulation alone.[31-38] In the National Venous Thrombolysis Registry, 66% of patients had acute DVT and 19% had acute-on-chronic DVT, most (75%) of which involved the iliofemoral system.[35] This study reported a success rate of 65% with a 1-year patency rate of 96% in those who had initial procedural success.[35,39] Importantly, incomplete clot lysis was associated with venous valvular incompetence, whereas optimal clot lysis was associated with improved valvular function. The rate of bleeding associated with catheter-directed thrombolysis (CDT) appears to be low (<10%), and most bleeding is related to the access site with intracranial events limited to <1%.[34,35,40] Despite initial studies suggesting that catheter-based therapies may be the optimal approach for patients with DVT, the multicenter randomized ATTRACT (Acute Venous Thrombosis: Thrombus Removal with Adjunctive Catheter-Directed Thrombolysis) trial did not meet its primary endpoint to reduce PTS. This randomized controlled trial involved 692 patients with acute proximal deep vein thrombosis randomized to receive either anticoagulation alone (control group) or anticoagulation plus pharmacomechanical thrombolysis (catheter-mediated or device-mediated intrathrombus delivery of recombinant tissue plasminogen activator and thrombus aspiration or maceration, with or without stenting). The primary endpoint was development of the PTS between 6 and 24 months of follow-up. There was no significant between-group difference in the percentage of patients with the PTS (47% in the pharmacomechanical-thrombolysis

TABLE 37.3 Direct-Acting Oral Anticoagulant Options

	DABIGATRAN	RIVAROXABAN	APIXABAN	EDOXABAN
Target	Thrombin (IIa)	Xa	Xa	Xa
Time to peak (h)	1.5-3	2-3	3-4	1-2
Half-life (h)	14-17	5-9	8-15	10-14
Renal excretion %	>80	66	25	50
Antidote	Idarucizumab	None	None	None
Dosing	Oral, once or twice daily	Oral, once or twice daily	Oral, twice daily	Oral, once daily
FDA-labeled indications	• NVAF • VTE ppx THA • VTE tx	• NVAF • VTE ppx THA, TKA • VTE tx	• NVAF • VTE ppx THA, TKA • VTE tx	• NVAF • VTE tx

FDA, US Food and Drug Administration; NVAF, nonvalvular atrial fibrillation; THA, total hip arthroplasty; TKA, total knee arthroplasty; VTE, venous thromboembolism.

group and 48% in the control group; risk ratio, 0.96; 95% confidence interval [CI], 0.82-1.11; $P = .56$). In fact, pharmacomechanical thrombolysis led to more major bleeding events within 10 days (1.7% vs 0.3% of patients, $P = .049$) with no significant difference in recurrent VTE at 24 months. Moderate to severe PTS occurred in 18% of patients in the pharmacomechanical-thrombolysis group versus 24% of those in the control group (risk ratio, 0.73; 95% CI, 0.54-0.98; $P = .04$). Severity scores for the PTS were also lower in the pharmacomechanical-thrombolysis group at 6, 12, 18, and 24 months of follow-up ($P < .01$ for the comparison of the Villalta scores at each time point), although the improvement in quality of life from baseline to 24 months did not differ significantly between the treatment groups.[41]

While routine use of catheter-directed treatment is not encouraged by current guidelines, young patients with acute symptomatic phlegmasia cerulea dolens (especially with a threatened limb), large thrombus burden within the inferior vena cava (IVC), or symptomatic massive iliofemoral and femoral vein thrombosis should be considered for catheter-based treatment as an adjunct to anticoagulation, since these are the patients at highest risk for PTS.[11,27] Until further data are available from randomized trials, isolated femoropopliteal DVT should most likely be treated with medical therapy alone; however, this decision should be personalized. In all cases, the risk of bleeding must be relatively low and the thrombus must be fairly acute (within 2-4 weeks) in order to have the highest chance of clot dissolution.[42] Additional contraindications include recent stroke, gastrointestinal bleed, surgery, trauma, and presence of malignancy or pregnancy.

Catheter-based therapies can be divided into three major categories: catheter-based lysis alone, mechanical thrombectomy without lysis, and pharmacomechanical thrombolysis plus/minus thrombectomy (eg, PMCT, pharmacomechanical catheter thrombectomy/thrombolysis). Nevertheless, a combination of these therapies is often needed. Options for catheter-based lysis include administration of a thrombolytic agent directly into the thrombus for 48 to 72 hours via an infusion catheter with multiple sideholes. Mechanically enhanced thrombolysis can be achieved by rheolytic thrombectomy. Pharmacomechanical thrombolysis can be achieved by pulse spray via the AngioJet device or by ultrasound-based methods such as EKOS. Any combination of these therapies may be used, and one approach is shown in **Figure 37.2**. The latter two strategies (often referred to as PMCT) are preferred and have been shown to reduce the total thrombolytic dose, the duration of exposure to thrombolytic drugs, cost, and hospital days and may result in more effective clot dissolution.[43-48]

For iliofemoral DVT, the ipsilateral popliteal vein is typically accessed, ideally with a single puncture using ultrasound guidance. The thrombus is crossed with a 0.035-in hydrophilic guide wire, and the thrombolytic delivery system is advanced over the wire into position. With the 5.2-French ultrasound-enhanced system (EkoSonic Endovascular System, **Fig. 37.3**), the thrombolytic agent is continuously infused into the catheter and ultrasound waves accelerate thrombolysis by mechanically disturbing the fibrin matrix and exposing more binding sites for the agent to work. The ultrasound waves also serve to push the thrombolytic drug deeper into the clot. After 12 to 24 hours, repeat venography is performed to assess the clot burden and determine the need for further treatment with either additional thrombolytic infusion or percutaneous thrombectomy. Close monitoring in an intensive care unit for complications such as bleeding or PE is required. Partial thromboplastin time and fibrinogen levels are obtained every 4 to 6 hours. If the fibrinogen level drops to <100 mg/dL, the thrombolytic infusion is reduced or stopped. Intravenous fluids should be administered if possible, because hemolysis may result in renal insufficiency. The AngioJet rheolytic thrombectomy system (**Fig. 37.4**) involves spraying the thrombolytic agent into the thrombus and allowing it to percolate for 15 to 30 minutes followed by thrombectomy with high-pressure pulsatile saline jets that macerate and fragment the thrombus. For large thrombus burden in the IVC, suction thrombectomy using the AngioVac venovenous bypass system can be considered. This device, which requires a perfusionist, uses suction through a 22-Fr central venous cannula via a centrifugal pump, filtration via an external filtering system, and then reinfusion via a 17-Fr central venous cannula.

Residual stenosis due to a fibrotic organized thrombus or webs may be present after PMCT and is associated with recurrent thrombosis and PTS.[49-51] Balloon angioplasty with or without stenting is commonly performed in such cases to relieve outflow obstruction and has been shown to reduce recurrent thrombosis, improve quality of life, and reduce PTS.[52,53] Wall stents are typically used for IVC stenosis and are usually safe to balloon across an occluded IVC filter.[54] Intravascular ultrasound imaging can assist with accurate placement and is essential for accurate sizing of these devices. For infrainguinal stenoses, self-expanding stents are preferred, given their resistance to extrinsic compression. Postprocedural duplex ultrasonography is typically performed at 6- to 12-month intervals to assess for patency or restenosis.

PULMONARY EMBOLISM

Pathophysiology

When embolization of a DVT occurs, the pathology of this disease expands to include the right side of the heart. The right ventricle (RV) is a thin-walled structure compared with its left-sided counterpart and normally operates under a low-pressure system. The obstruction that occurs with a PE may trigger a spiral of events leading to RV failure and ultimately death. Once >30% of the pulmonary circulation is obstructed, the pulmonary artery pressure rises leading to RV dilatation, which causes tachycardia and an increase in contractility and activation of the sympathetic nervous system. As RV dilation increases, so does the intramural pressure, which in turn reduces coronary blood flow and the contractility of the left and right ventricles. This can lead to an inability to get blood into the lungs and then back to the left side of heart, which leads to systemic hypotension. Hypotension may also occur as a result of bowing of the intraventricular septum into the left ventricle, leading to decreased filling of the left ventricle.[55,56]

RISK STRATIFICATION

Prompt diagnosis is critical for the survival of patients with PE. As noted previously, these patients should receive immediate Anticoagulation (AC) preferably with LMWH over unfractionated heparin (UFH) if the pretest probability is high enough. Risk classification via the European Guidelines is recommended at this time.[57] This stratification involves the hemodynamic stability of the patient and the absence or presence of right ventricular strain as noted by biomarkers (troponin and B-type natriuretic peptide) and by imaging (computed tomography or echo) (**Table 37.4**). Patients may be classified as (1) high risk (formerly called massive) when hypotension and/or cardiac arrest is present, (2) intermediate

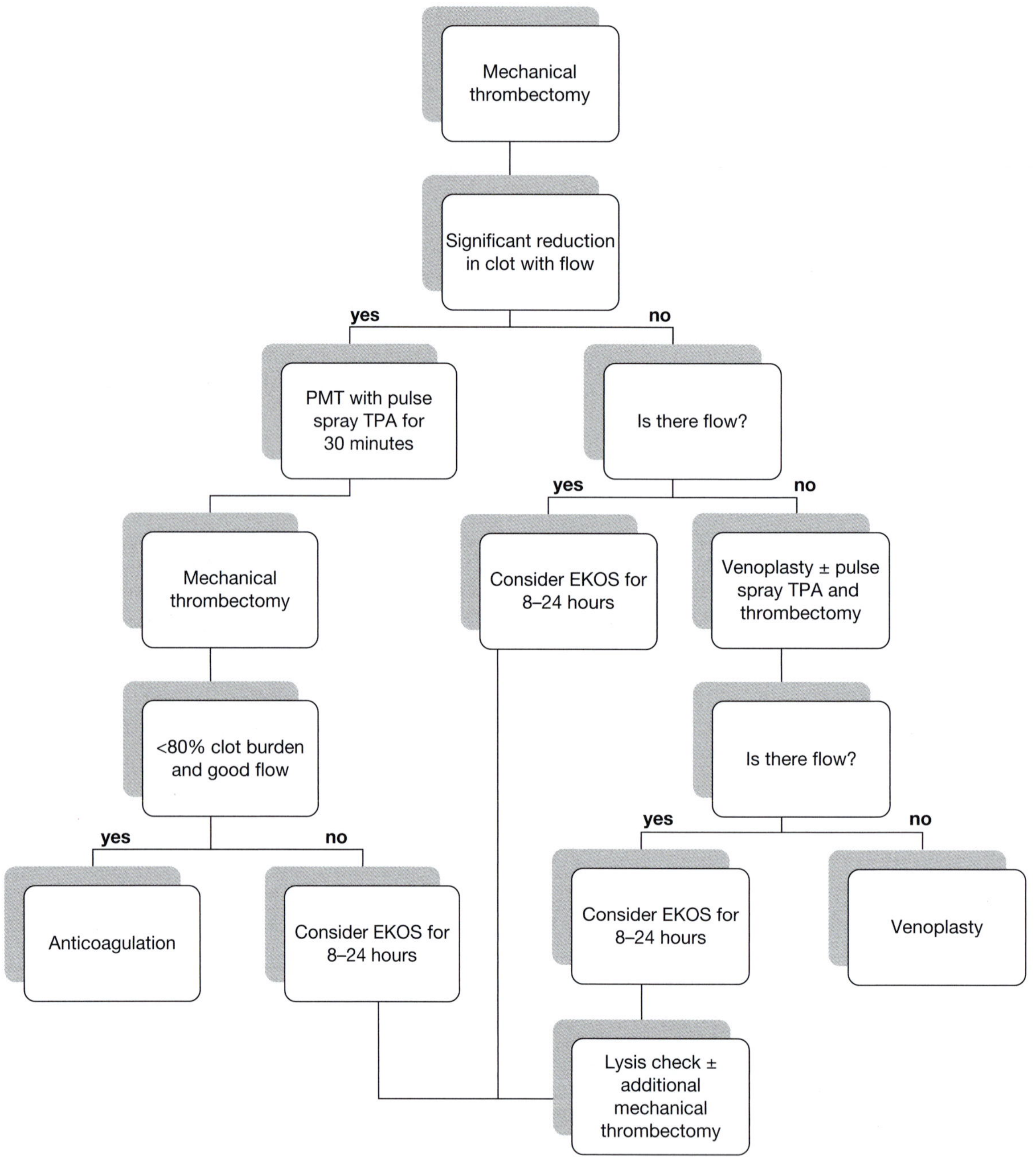

FIGURE 37.2 Approach to catheter-based treatment of acute iliofemoral deep venous thrombosis. PMT, pharmacomechanical thrombectomy; TPA, tissue plasminogen activator.

risk (formerly called submassive) when the blood pressure is normal but there is either a high degree of RV strain (intermediate high risk) or a small amount of RV strain (intermediate low risk), or (3) low-risk patients who have no evidence of RV strain and are normotensive. The intermediate high risk category involves positive biomarkers and imaging while the intermediate low risk category may include either imaging criteria or biomarkers but not both.

Treatment

The first-line therapy for all patients with PE is rapid administration of anticoagulation with either LMWH or UFH. LMWH given its rapid time to full AC is recommended. For patients with low-risk PE, AC alone is sufficient given that these patients have a low mortality rate. Whether these patients need to be hospitalized is currently being evaluated. Ongoing studies evaluating the immediate use of DOACs and discharge from the hospital are ongoing.[58] The low mortality rate associated with this type of PE is reassuring.

Patients with an intermediate-risk PE may be considered for advanced therapies in addition to anticoagulation. Similar to the management of DVT, options for endovascular therapies include catheter-based lysis alone, mechanical thrombectomy without lysis, and mechanical thrombectomy with lysis. There are no current studies favoring one treatment over the other, and the ongoing HI-PEITHO study is comparing AC versus EKOS for those patients presenting with intermediate high-risk PE. Catheter-based thrombolysis (also known as CDT) is exactly as described for DVT and may involve an end-hole catheter such as a Craig-MacNamara or ultrasound-assisted CDT such as the EKOS catheter. One small study (SUNSET trial) failed to show any difference between these

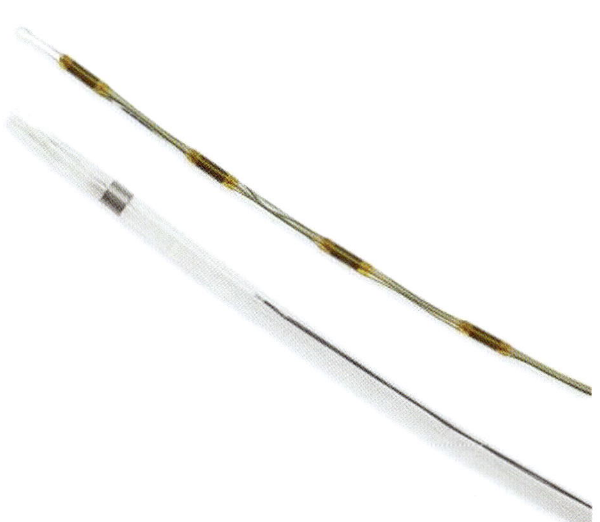

FIGURE 37.3 EkoSonic endovascular system.

two catheters, although larger studies are needed given the cost differential present. Typically these catheters are placed into the clot and the administration of thrombolytics may occur over 6 to 48 hours with operator-chosen rates of tissue plasminogen activator (typically 0.5-2 mg/h). Given the low systemic amounts of thrombolytics being administered locally, the risk of intracranial hemorrhage has been very low in all of the studies to date. Often, these patients are watched carefully in an intensive care unit setting to monitor for any bleeding and typically, in contrast to DVT management, repeat angiography is not performed after thrombolysis.

Mechanical thrombectomy of pulmonary emboli is performed via large-bore sheaths (22-26 Fr) and large devices (18-24 Fr), which must be advanced across the right side of the heart. Operators must ensure that the wires are not entangled in tricuspid valve chordae, or valvular damage may ensue. One technique to prevent this is to advance a standard pulmonary artery catheter through the right side of the heart and use an exchange length wire to then advance a catheter that will accommodate a 0.035-in wire, such as a pigtail catheter, through the right side of the heart to perform angiography and ultimately exchange for a stiff wire (typically a 1-cm tip stiff Amplatz wire), which will then allow for safer transit of the large catheter through the right side of the heart. All these devices use a variation of a suction mechanism to remove the thrombus and thus unload the RV. These devices may be used with or without the intrapulmonary artery administration of tPA, which can be used to treat more distal thrombus and soften the larger clot that may present. There are no current studies favoring one device over another. Currently available devices include the Inari FlowTriever, the Penumbra (available in numerous sizes), and the AngioDynamics AlphaVac. The number of devices in this market is rapidly expanding despite the lack of data supporting any superiority of thrombectomy over CDT or medical therapy alone.

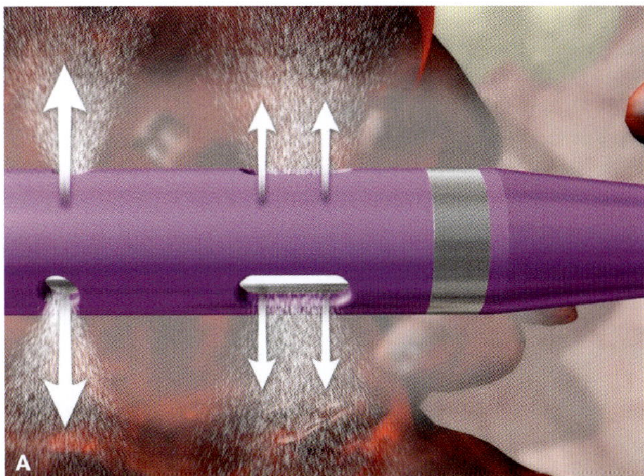

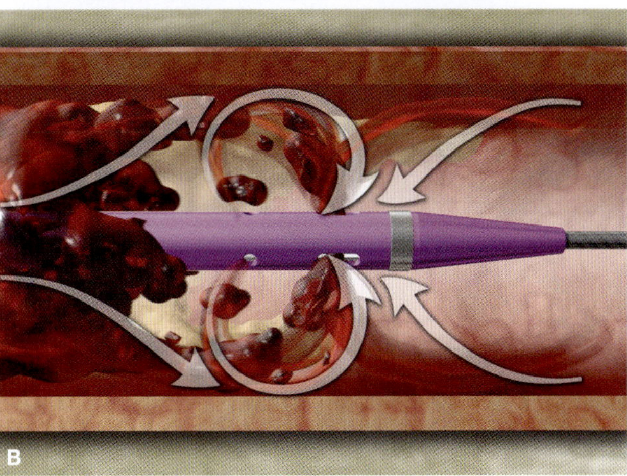

FIGURE 37.4 AngioJet rheolytic thrombectomy system. **A:** Top panel demonstrates power pulse feature where tPA is sprayed into the thrombus. **B:** Bottom panel demonstrates the mechanism of thrombus removal, where high-velocity flow creates a low-pressure zone within and surrounding the catheter tip. The thrombus is subsequently pulled into the catheter. tPA, tissue plasminogen activator.

Patients presenting with high-risk (formerly known as massive) PE are at the highest risk for mortality. These patients are critically ill

TABLE 37.4 Risk Stratification of Pulmonary Embolism

CATEGORY	HEMODYNAMICS	BIOMARKERSTROPONIN BNP	IMAGING OF RV STRAIN (CT OR ECHO)
High	Unstable	+++	+++
Intermediate-high	Stable	++	++
Intermediate-low[a]	Stable	±	±
Low	Stable	None	None

Risk stratification of pulmonary embolism based on European Guidelines.
[a]Intermediate-low risk includes RV strain by imaging or biomarkers but not both.
BNP, B-type natriuretic peptide; CT, computed tomography; RV, right ventricle.
Adopted from Konstantinides SV, Meyer G, Becattini C, et al. 2019 ESC Guidelines for the diagnosis and management of acute pulmonary embolism developed in collaboration with the European Respiratory Society (ERS): the Task Force for the diagnosis and management of acute pulmonary embolism of the European Society of Cardiology (ESC). *Eur Respir J.* 2019;54(3):1901647.

and require immediate intervention as well as stabilization of their shock state. There are data suggesting that immediate cannulation of these patients with venous arterial extracorporeal membrane oxygenation (VA ECMO) is the best option when it is available. For patients who are unstable and ECMO is not an option, systemic thrombolysis is the preferred therapy given its ease of administration and availability. ECMO cannulation permits stabilization of the shock state and rests the RV, thereby allowing for more time to decide on a more advanced strategy, such as lysis, catheter-based or surgical. Although single center and retrospective, one study has highlighted the safety and efficacy of an ECMO and then surgical approach for these patients.[59] Catheter-based intervention for high-risk PE with or without ECMO support is also a valid approach depending on local expertise and availability of an angiography suite. There are also other catheter-based support devices such as the ProtekDuo and the Impella RP, which also may be used to support RV function. Catheter-based intervention for high-risk PE includes CDT as well as thrombectomy. Given the ability of thrombectomy to rapidly remove thrombus, which in turn can stabilize hemodynamics, it is often considered in this patient subset primarily over CDT alone. Combination therapy with upfront thrombectomy to treat central clot followed by the placement of CDT to treat thrombus in the smaller vascular beds is another potential technique.

In addition to catheter-based therapy, pulmonary embolectomy is also a therapeutic option for these patients. There has been a recent resurgence of surgical embolectomy, and in experienced hands this technique is very safe and effective, albeit morbid given the need for sternotomy.[60] Surgical intervention for PE and the use of ECMO was recently reviewed and published by the American Heart Association.[61] This document underscores the utility of this approach, validating it as an option for patients with intermediate- and high-risk PE.

The duration of anticoagulation for PE is the same as for DVT and is recommended for 3 months after the initial event. Current CHEST guidelines[62] note that some patients should be considered for "extended" therapy anticoagulation (up to 4 years) based on the nature of the risk factor that caused the initial event and each case should be evaluated on an individual basis. The guidelines are divided into the following four categories:

A) VTE provoked by a major transient risk factor (present within the 3 months before VTE diagnosis), eg, surgery with general anesthesia for greater than 30 minutes, confinement to bed in hospital (only "bathroom privileges") for at least 3 days with an acute illness, cesarean section, major trauma.
B) VTE provoked by a minor transient risk factor (present within the 2 months before VTE diagnosis), eg, surgery with general anesthesia for less than 30 minutes, admission to hospital for less than 3 days with an acute illness, estrogen therapy, pregnancy, or puerperium, confinement to bed out of hospital for at least 3 days with an acute illness, leg injury associated with reduced mobility for at least 3 days, prolonged car or air travel.
C) VTE provoked by a persistent risk factor, eg, active cancer, antiphospholipid syndrome.
D) Unprovoked PE.

Notwithstanding the paucity of data for the superiority of any individual therapy, our recommendation is that, given the prevalence of the disease, its mortality impact, and the multiple various therapeutic options, a PERT (pulmonary embolism response team)[63] should be formulated at every hospital and should consist of a multidisciplinary team of physicians who treat these patients. These include members of the emergency response team, hematology/oncology, vascular endovascular medicine, interventional cardiology, interventional radiology, vascular surgery, cardiothoracic surgery, pulmonary and critical care medicine, surgical critical care, anesthesia, as well as hospitalist medicine. VTE/PE is a pervasive and deadly disease that is best managed by a multidisciplinary team dedicated to optimizing patient outcomes while minimizing morbidity and mortality.

Key Points

- Risk factors for VTE can be categorized into acquired and genetic factors.
- The diagnostic workup of suspected DVT depends upon the estimated pretest probability.
- The D-dimer test is highly sensitive but cannot rule out VTE in those with high pretest probability. High-probability patients should proceed to imaging without D-dimer testing (ie, whole leg compression duplex ultrasonography for suspected DVT and computed tomography angiography or ventilation-perfusion scan for suspected PE).
- A minimum of 3 months of therapeutic anticoagulation should be administered to all patients with acute VTE regardless of whether reversible or transient risk factors are identified.
- PMCT has not been shown to reduce PTS, although in patients with large iliofemoral or IVC thrombus or those with phlegmasia ceruleans dolens, it should be considered.
- Patients with PE should be rapidly anticoagulated and then risk stratified per the European Society of Cardiology guidelines.
- Patients with intermediate- or high-risk PE may be candidates for catheter- or surgical-based therapies including catheter-directed thrombolysis/thrombectomy or surgical embolectomy.
- Patients with low-risk PE can be treated with AC alone.
- There is a marked risk of reoccurrence with PE and this risk can be mitigated by longer AC, perhaps at lower dosing depending on whether the initial event was provoked or unprovoked.
- Each hospital/hospital system should consider the formation of a Pulmonary Embolism Response Team (PERT) to permit the rapid identification, triage, and treatment of patients with pulmonary embolism.

References

1. Heit JA. The epidemiology of venous thromboembolism in the community. *Arterioscler Thromb Vasc Biol*. 2008;28(3):370-372.
2. Huang W, Goldberg RJ, Anderson FA, Kiefe CI, Spencer FA. Secular trends in occurrence of acute venous thromboembolism: the Worcester VTE study (1985-2009). *Am J Med*. 2014;127(9):829-839.e5.
3. Kahn SR, Lim W, Dunn AS, et al. Prevention of VTE in nonsurgical patients: antithrombotic therapy and prevention of thrombosis, 9th ed—American College of chest physicians evidence-based clinical practice guidelines. *Chest*. 2012;141(2 suppl):e195S-e226S.
4. Lindblad B, Sternby NH, Bergqvist D. Incidence of venous thromboembolism verified by necropsy over 30 years. *BMJ*. 1991;302(6778):709-711.

5. Dobromirski M, Cohen AT. How I manage venous thromboembolism risk in hospitalized medical patients. *Blood*. 2012;120(8):1562-1569.
6. Tapson VF. Acute pulmonary embolism. *N Engl J Med*. 2008;358(10):1037-1052.
7. Guanella R, Ducruet T, Johri M, et al. Economic burden and cost determinants of deep vein thrombosis during 2 years following diagnosis: a prospective evaluation. *J Thromb Haemost*. 2011;9(12):2397-2405.
8. Kahn SR, Shbaklo H, Lamping DL, et al. Determinants of health-related quality of life during the 2 years following deep vein thrombosis. *J Thromb Haemost*. 2008;6(7):1105-1112.
9. Page RL II, Ghushchyan V, Gifford B, et al. Hidden costs associated with venous thromboembolism: impact of lost productivity on employers and employees. *J Occup Environ Med*. 2014;56(9):979-985.
10. van Dongen CJ, Prandoni P, Frulla M, Marchiori A, Prins MH, Hutten BA. Relation between quality of anticoagulant treatment and the development of the postthrombotic syndrome. *J Thromb Haemost*. 2005;3(5):939-942.
11. Kahn SR, Comerota AJ, Cushman M, et al. The postthrombotic syndrome: evidence based prevention, diagnosis, and treatment strategies—a scientific statement from the American Heart Association. *Circulation*. 2014;130(18):1636-1661.
12. Ageno W, Piantanida E, Dentali F, et al. Body mass index is associated with the development of the post-thrombotic syndrome. *Thromb Haemost*. 2003;89(2):305-309.
13. Chitsike RS, Rodger MA, Kovacs MJ, et al. Risk of post-thrombotic syndrome after subtherapeutic warfarin anticoagulation for a first unprovoked deep vein thrombosis: results from the REVERSE study. *J Thromb Haemost*. 2012;10:2039-2044.
14. Goodacre S, Sutton AJ, Sampson FC. Meta-analysis: the value of clinical assessment in the diagnosis of deep venous thrombosis. *Ann Intern Med*. 2005;143(2):129-139.
15. Bauer KA. The thrombophilias: well-defined risk factors with uncertain therapeutic implications. *Ann Intern Med*. 2001;135(5):367-373.
16. Wells PS, Anderson DR, Bormanis J, et al. Value of assessment of pretest probability of deep-vein thrombosis in clinical management. *Lancet*. 1997;350(9094):1795-1798.
17. Bates SM, Jaeschke R, Stevens SM, et al. Diagnosis of DVT: antithrombotic therapy and prevention of thrombosis, 9th ed—American College of chest physicians evidence-based clinical practice guidelines. *Chest*. 2012;141(2 suppl):e351S-e418S.
18. Wells PS, Anderson DR, Rodger M, et al. Derivation of a simple clinical model to categorize patients probability of pulmonary embolism: increasing the models utility with the SimpliRED D-dimer. *Thromb Haemost*. 2000;83(3):416-420.
19. Sarwar S, Narra S, Munir A. Phlegmasia cerulea dolens. *Tex Heart Inst J*. 2009;36(1):76-77.
20. Haimovici H. The ischemic forms of venous thrombosis. 1. Phlegmasia cerulea dolens. 2. Venous gangrene. *J Cardiovasc Surg*. 1965;5(6):164-173.
21. Jaff MR, McMurtry MS, Archer SL, et al. Management of massive and submassive pulmonary embolism, iliofemoral deep vein thrombosis, and chronic thromboembolic pulmonary hypertension: a scientific statement from the American Heart Association. *Circulation*. 2011;123(16):1788-1830.
22. Douketis JD, Crowther MA, Foster GA, Ginsberg JS. Does the location of thrombosis determine the risk of disease recurrence in patients with proximal deep vein thrombosis? *Am J Med*. 2001;110(7):515-519.
23. Jimenez D, Lobo JL, Fernandez-Golfin C, et al. Effectiveness of prognosticating pulmonary embolism using the ESC algorithm and the Bova score. *Thromb Haemost*. 2016;115(4):827-834.
24. Jimenez D, Kopecna D, Tapson V, et al. Derivation and validation of multimarker prognostication for normotensive patients with acute symptomatic pulmonary embolism. *Am J Respir Crit Care Med*. 2014;189(6):718-726.
25. Wicki J, Perrier A, Perneger TV, Bounameaux H, Junod AF. Predicting adverse outcome in patients with acute pulmonary embolism: a risk score. *Thromb Haemost*. 2000;84(4):548-552.
26. Aujesky D, Obrosky DS, Stone RA, et al. Derivation and validation of a prognostic model for pulmonary embolism. *Am J Respir Crit Care Med*. 2005;172(8):1041-1046.
27. Kearon C, Akl EA, Ornelas J, et al. Antithrombotic therapy for VTE disease: CHEST guideline and expert panel report. *Chest*. 2016;149(2):315-352.
28. Kahn SR, Shapiro S, Wells PS, et al. Compression stockings to prevent post-thrombotic syndrome: a randomised placebo-controlled trial. *Lancet*. 2014;383(9920):880-888.
29. Becattini C, Agnelli G, Schenone A, et al. Aspirin for preventing the recurrence of venous thromboembolism. *N Engl J Med*. 2012;366(21):1959-1967.
30. Brighton TA, Eikelboom JW, Mann K, et al. Low-dose aspirin for preventing recurrent venous thromboembolism. *N Engl J Med*. 2012;367(21):1979-1987.
31. Comerota AJ, Throm RC, Mathias SD, Haughton S, Mewissen M. Catheter-directed thrombolysis for iliofemoral deep venous thrombosis improves health-related quality of life. *J Vasc Surg*. 2000;32(1):130-137.
32. Elsharawy M, Elzayat E. Early results of thrombolysis vs anticoagulation in iliofemoral venous thrombosis. A randomised clinical trial. *Eur J Vasc Endovasc Surg*. 2002;24(3):209-214.
33. AbuRahma AF, Perkins SE, Wulu JT, Ng HK. Iliofemoral deep vein thrombosis: conventional therapy versus lysis and percutaneous transluminal angioplasty and stenting. *Ann Surg*. 2001;233(6):752-760.
34. Vedantham S, Thorpe PE, Cardella JF, et al. Quality improvement guidelines for the treatment of lower extremity deep vein thrombosis with use of endovascular thrombus removal. *J Vasc Interv Radiol*. 2006;17(3):435-448. quiz 48.
35. Mewissen MW, Seabrook GR, Meissner MH, Cynamon J, Labropoulos N, Haughton SH. Catheter-directed thrombolysis for lower extremity deep venous thrombosis: report of a national multicenter registry. *Radiology*. 1999;211(1):39-49.
36. Meissner MH, Manzo RA, Bergelin RO, Markel A, Strandness DE Jr. Deep venous insufficiency: the relationship between lysis and subsequent reflux. *J Vasc Surg*. 1993;18(4):596-608. discussion 6-8.
37. Watson L, Broderick C, Armon MP. Thrombolysis for acute deep vein thrombosis. *Cochrane Database Syst Rev*. 2016;11:CD002783.
38. Enden T, Haig Y, Kløw NE, et al. Long-term outcome after additional catheter-directed thrombolysis versus standard treatment for acute iliofemoral deep vein thrombosis (the CaVenT study): a randomised controlled trial. *Lancet*. 2012;379(9810):31-38.
39. Bjarnason H, Kruse JR, Asinger DA, et al. Iliofemoral deep venous thrombosis: safety and efficacy outcome during 5 years of catheter-directed thrombolytic therapy. *J Vasc Interv Radiol*. 1997;8(3):405-418.
40. Patel N, Sacks D, Patel RI, et al. SIR reporting standards for the treatment of acute limb ischemia with use of transluminal removal of arterial thrombus. *J Vasc Interv Radiol*. 2003;14(9 pt 2):S453-S465.
41. Vedantham S, Goldhaber SZ, Julian JA, et al. Pharmacomechanical catheter-directed thrombolysis for deep-vein thrombosis. *N Engl J Med*. 2017;377(23):2240-2252. doi:10.1056/NEJMoa1615066
42. Theiss W, Wirtzfeld A, Fink U, Maubach P. The success rate of fibrinolytic therapy in fresh and old thrombosis of the iliac and femoral veins. *Angiology*. 1983;34(1):61-69.
43. Martinez Trabal JL, Comerota AJ, LaPorte FB, Kazanjian S, DiSalle R, Sepanski DM. The quantitative benefit of Isolated, Segmental, Pharmacomechanical Thrombolysis (ISPMT) for iliofemoral venous thrombosis. *J Vasc Surg*. 2008;48(6):1532-1537.
44. Parikh S, Motarjeme A, McNamara T, et al. Ultrasound-accelerated thrombolysis for the treatment of deep vein thrombosis: initial clinical experience. *J Vasc Interv Radiol*. 2008;19(4):521-528.
45. O'Sullivan GJ, Lohan DG, Gough N, Cronin CG, Kee ST. Pharmacomechanical thrombectomy of acute deep vein thrombosis with the Trellis-8 isolated thrombolysis catheter. *J Vasc Interv Radiol*. 2007;18(6):715-724.
46. Hartung O, Loundou AD, Barthelemy P, Arnoux D, Boufi M, Alimi YS. Endovascular management of chronic disabling ilio-caval obstructive lesions: long-term results. *Eur J Vasc Endovasc Surg*. 2009;38(1):118-124.
47. Latchana N, Dowell JD, Al Taani J, Michaels A, Elkhammas E, Black SM. Ultrasound-accelerated, catheter-directed thrombolysis for inferior vena cava thrombosis after an orthotopic liver transplant. *Exp Clin Transplant*. 2015;13(1):96-99.
48. Lin PH, Zhou W, Dardik A, et al. Catheter-direct thrombolysis versus pharmacomechanical thrombectomy for treatment of symptomatic lower extremity deep venous thrombosis. *Am J Surg*. 2006;192(6):782-788.
49. Hartung O, Benmiloud F, Barthelemy P, Dubuc M, Boufi M, Alimi YS. Late results of surgical venous thrombectomy with iliocaval stenting. *J Vasc Surg*. 2008;47(2):381-387.

50. Neglen P. Stenting is the "Method-of-Choice" to treat iliofemoral venous outflow obstruction. *J Endovasc Ther*. 2009;16(4):492-493.
51. George R, Verma H, Ram B, Tripathi R. The effect of deep venous stenting on healing of lower limb venous ulcers. *Eur J Vasc Endovasc Surg*. 2014;48(3):330-336.
52. Alkhouli M, Zack CJ, Zhao H, Shafi I, Bashir R. Comparative outcomes of catheter-directed thrombolysis plus anticoagulation versus anticoagulation alone in the treatment of inferior vena caval thrombosis. *Circ Cardiovasc Interv*. 2015;8(2):e001882.
53. Delis KT, Bountouroglou D, Mansfield AO. Venous claudication in iliofemoral thrombosis: long-term effects on venous hemodynamics, clinical status, and quality of life. *Ann Surg*. 2004;239(1):118-126.
54. Neglen P, Oglesbee M, Olivier J, Raju S. Stenting of chronically obstructed inferior vena cava filters. *J Vasc Surg*. 2011;54(1):153-161.
55. McIntyre KM, Sasahara AA. The hemodynamic response to pulmonary embolism in patients without prior cardiopulmonary disease. *Am J Cardiol*. 1971;28(3):288-294.
56. Piazza G, Goldhaber SZ. Management of submassive pulmonary embolism. *Circulation*. 2010;122(11):1124-1129.
57. Konstantinides SV, Meyer G, Becattini C, et al. 2019 ESC Guidelines for the diagnosis and management of acute pulmonary embolism developed in collaboration with the European Respiratory Society (ERS): the Task Force for the diagnosis and management of acute pulmonary embolism of the European Society of Cardiology (ESC). *Eur Respir J*. 2019;54(3):1901647.
58. Singer AJ, Xiang J, Kabrhel C, et al. Multicenter trial of rivaroxaban for early discharge of pulmonary embolism from the emergency department (MERCURY PE): rationale and design. *Acad Emerg Med*. 2016;23(11):1280-1286.
59. Goldberg JB, Spevack DM, Ahsan S, et al. Comparison of surgical embolectomy and veno-arterial extracorporeal membrane oxygenation for massive pulmonary embolism. *Semin Thorac Cardiovasc Surg*. 2022;34(3):934-942.
60. Goldberg JB, Spevack DM, Ahsan S, et al. Survival and right ventricular function after surgical management of acute pulmonary embolism. *J Am Coll Cardiol*. 2020;76(8):903-911.
61. Goldberg JB, Giri J, Kobayashi T, et al. Surgical management and mechanical circulatory support in high-risk pulmonary embolisms: historical context, current status, and future directions—a scientific statement from the American Heart Association. *Circulation*. 2023;147(9):e628-e647.
62. Stevens SM, Woller SC, Kreuziger LB, et al. Antithrombotic therapy for VTE disease: second update of the CHEST guideline and expert panel report. *Chest*. 2021;160(6):e545-e608.
63. Provias T, Dudzinski DM, Jaff MR, et al. The Massachusetts General Hospital Pulmonary Embolism Response Team (MGH PERT): creation of a multidisciplinary program to improve care of patients with massive and submassive pulmonary embolism. *Hosp Pract (1995)*. 2014;42(1):31-37. doi:10.3810/hp.2014.02.1089

Introduction to Structural Imaging

Daniel Shpilsky and Dee Dee Wang

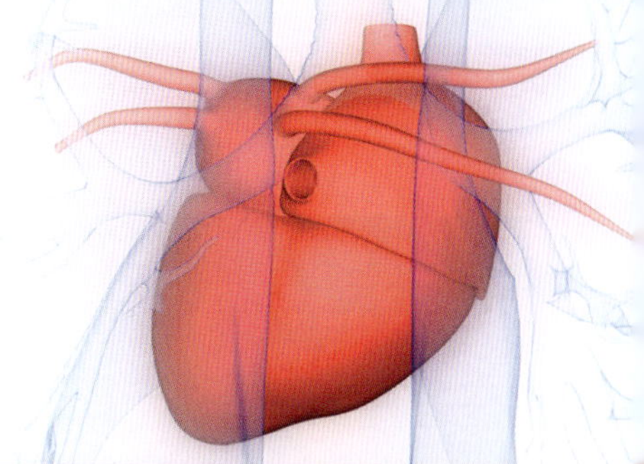

INTRODUCTION

Structural imaging is a new subspecialty within the field of cardiovascular medicine. Training in structural imaging requires horizontal integration of knowledge and understanding between multidisciplinary heart teams, multiple different imaging technology interfaces, and device-specific technology understanding. In this chapter, introduction to structural imaging is less about imaging as a modality, but an introduction to the concept of utilizing imaging to create protocols to understand the engineering of commonly encountered transcatheter devices.

LEFT ATRIAL APPENDAGE OCCLUSION

Preprocedural Planning: Transesophageal Echocardiogram

Preprocedural transesophageal echocardiogram (TEE) evaluation must include left atrial appendage (LAA) size and morphology in addition to a full assessment of the presence/size/location of any pericardial effusion, biventricular function, concomitant valvular disease, and ruling out LAA thrombus.

Watchman (Boston Scientific)

With regard to device size planning, the LAA is measured at the level of the left circumflex artery to ~10 to 20 mm from the tip of the coumadin ridge to create a virtual landing zone plane of where the device will sit once deployed.[1] The appendage landing zone diameter is measured at midend systole when orifice size is largest at 0°, 45°, 90°, and 135° views (**Fig. 38.1**). A line perpendicular to the landing zone dimension is measured to the distal portion of the appendage tip to evaluate depth. To ensure the maximum dimensions have been obtained, a 3D data set of the LAA should be acquired and 3D multiplanar reconstruction (MPR) can then be analyzed to assess landing zone area and maximize dimension to further guide device sizing (**Fig. 38.2**). A description of LAA morphology is also helpful in procedural planning and includes appendage shape, number/location of lobes, and the presence of prominent trabeculations/pectinate ridges, which can all influence device selection and implantation strategy. Appendage axis/trajectory (ie, superior-anterior, inferior-anterior) relative to the interatrial fossa helps further delineate optimal sheath selection and trans-septal puncture location.

Amulet (Abbott)

Preprocedural TEE planning for Amulet device is similar. Given the presence of both a lobe and cover sealing mechanism, notation should also be made about proximity to nearby structures including mitral annulus and left upper pulmonary vein (LUPV) to avoid device interaction. The Amulet landing zone, ie, where the lobe sits, is measured 10 to 12 mm from the appendage Os. The distinction between 10 and 12 mm from the Os is dependent on the Amulet device size that will be chosen. Measurements are again made at midend systole at angles 0°, 45°, 90°, and 135° views in addition to 3D MPR.

Preprocedural Planning: Computed Tomography

Cardiac computed tomography (CT) for preprocedural planning of LAA intervention may offer several advantages over TEE including a noninvasive evaluation without requirement for procedural sedation, increased spatial resolution, and a more accurate evaluation of LAA morphology, sizing, and distance to adjacent structures (ie, LUPV, mitral valve [MV] annulus). The LAA is a highly complex and heterogeneous structure with variations in shape, number of lobes, trabeculations, and pectinate muscle such that CT planning may offer advantages in planning device selection and sizing given superior spatial resolution. CT can also be used to rule out LAA thrombus with the use of delayed acquisition imaging. CT acquisition for LAA evaluation involves contrast-enhanced, retrospective electrocardiogram (ECG)-gated imaging with further specifications based on scanner and institutional preferences.[2,3] Measurements of LAA area/dimensions should be made at end systole (late atrial diastole) when the left atrium (LA)/appendage is largest (typically corresponding to 30%-40% of the RR interval). On axial slices, the appendage can be found at the level of the circumflex artery. For Watchman planning, orthogonal cross-sections across the LAA landing zone can then be created from the prior coronal and sagittal planes and the resultant "enface" view is used to measure area and maximum/minimum dimensions (**Fig. 38.3**). Depth from the landing zone to appendage tip is also measured. A 3D volume-rendered projection of the LA and LAA can be created to help demonstrate optimal trans-septal crossing, orifice angulation, and LAA morphology. A simulated C-arm fluoroscopy angle can also be created to help predict optimal C-arm implantation angle for the implanter (**Fig. 38.4**).

For Amulet devices, a measurement is done at the LAA ostium and again at the LAA device landing zone defined by the circumflex artery (**Figs. 38.5** and **38.6**). Landing zone dimensions, area, and distance of the pulmonary vein to MV annulus are included in the final report (**Figs. 38.5** and **38.6**).

INTRAPROCEDURAL GUIDANCE

Watchman

The Watchman device consists of a self-expanding nitinol frame covered by a thin polyester membrane.[1] Hooks around the mid-perimeter secure the device to the LAA wall. Current-generation Watchman FLX devices are used to treat LAA ostia ranging from 14 to 31.5 mm and come in five sizes.[4] Recommendations for device selection specify that the device should be 10% to 30% larger than the LAA body to have sufficient compression for stable

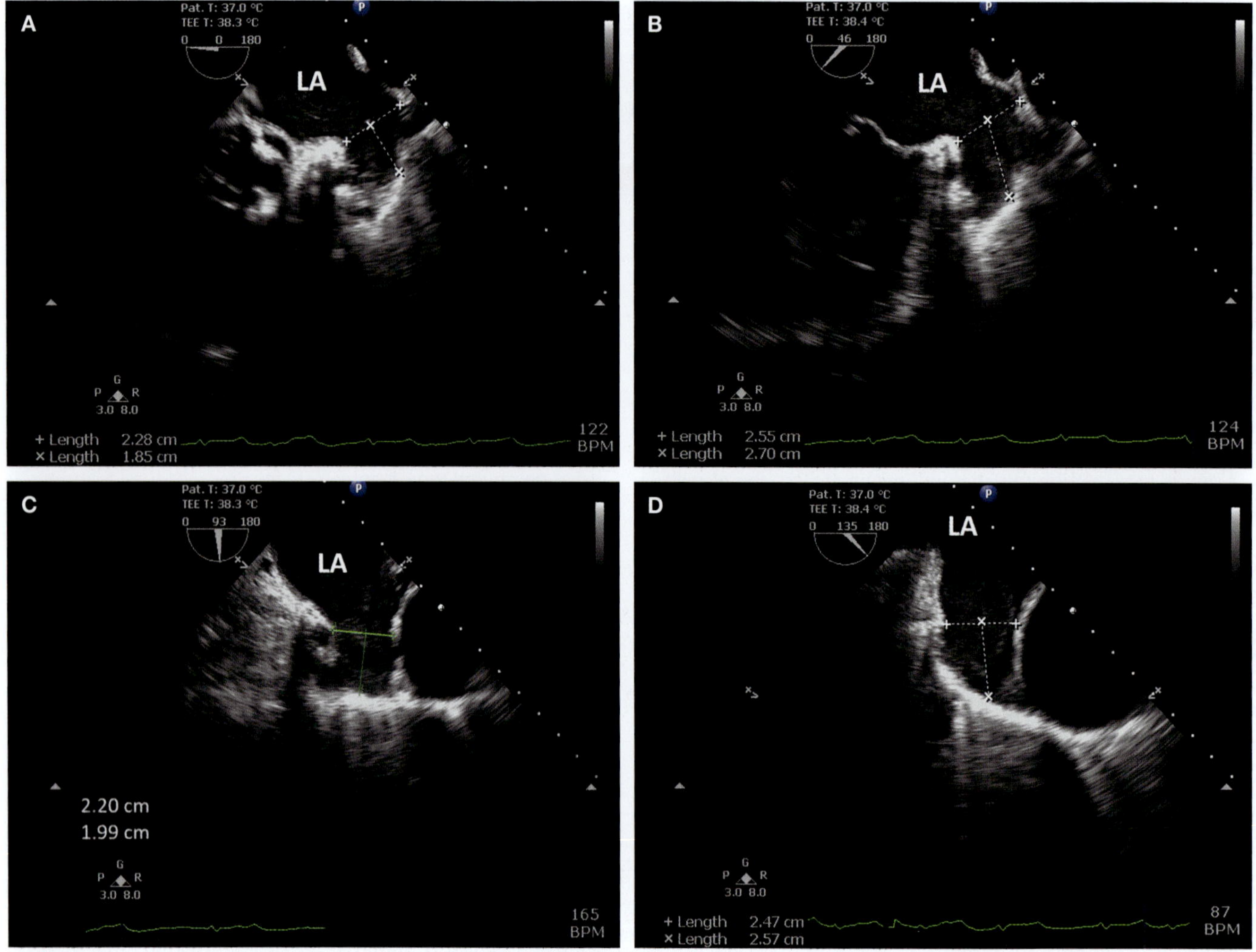

FIGURE 38.1 2D sizing for Watchman FLX device at **(A)** 0°, **(B)** 45°, **(C)** 90°, and **(D)** 135°. Measurements of LAA diameter taken at level of circumflex artery to ~10 to 20 mm from tip of the coumadin ridge. Implantation depth measured perpendicular to diameter axis. Largest diameter visualized in 45° view (2.55 × 2.70 cm) and favors implantation of 31 mm device. LA, left atrium; LAA, left atrial appendage.

positioning.[1] Additionally, adequate depth is necessary such that the minimum depth required is 50% of the device size (ie, for a 24-mm Watchman FLX, the LAA should be at least 12 mm in depth). Intraprocedural guidance initially involves trans-septal crossing using biplane imaging of the fossa with both the short axis (anterior-posterior dimension) and bicaval views (superior-inferior dimension). The ideal crossing spot is at a midinferior and mid-posterior location on the fossa, which allows for optimal coaxiality with the appendage and the catheter to most easily engage the LAA ostium (**Figs. 38.7** and **38.8**).[4] Once trans-septal access is obtained, TEE and fluoroscopy are used to guide the delivery catheter into the anterior lobe of the LAA (**Fig. 38.9**). The device flex ball is formed under fluoroscopic and echocardiographic guidance and ultimately deployed. While the Watchman device is still attached to the delivery catheter, the interventional imaging physician can perform device assessment using the Boston Scientific PASS criteria (position, anchoring, size, and seal). For positioning, the device should be at or just distal to the appendage orifice without any tilt or protruding shoulder. A device too distal may result in uncovered lobes, incomplete seal, or residual flow into the LAA. A device too proximal may result in protrusion into the LA or low compression/unstable device. The implanter can assess anchoring by a "tug test" in which a gentle pullback on the catheter ensures the device is stable. Device size is assessed by percentage compression at 0°, 45°, 90°, and 135° with a target of 10% to 30% and is calculated by (device width − compressed width)/(device width) (**Fig. 38.10**). Finally, device seal is assessed by evaluating for peridevice leak (PDL) at the aforementioned angles at a reduced Nyquist limit to help identify color jets between the device and appendage walls. At completion of the procedure, final assessment should note the presence or change in pericardial effusion size/location and direction of flow across the iatrogenic atrial septal defect.

Amulet

The Amulet device is a dual-seal device comprised of an inner Nitinol mesh lobe with an outer cover. Intraprocedural guidance is similar to that of the Watchman FLX device. Current generation devices come in eight sizes. A minimum LAA depth of 10 to 12 mm (depending on device size chosen) is required for successful implantation. Prior to device release, verification of stability is assessed with the Abbott "CLOSE" criteria. The lobe should be at least 2/3 distal to the Circumflex artery. Adequate Lobe compression is evaluated by fluoroscopic and TEE imaging. The Orientation of the lobe should align with the axis of the LAA neck. There should be Separation between the device lobe and disc. Finally, the disc should be Elliptical in

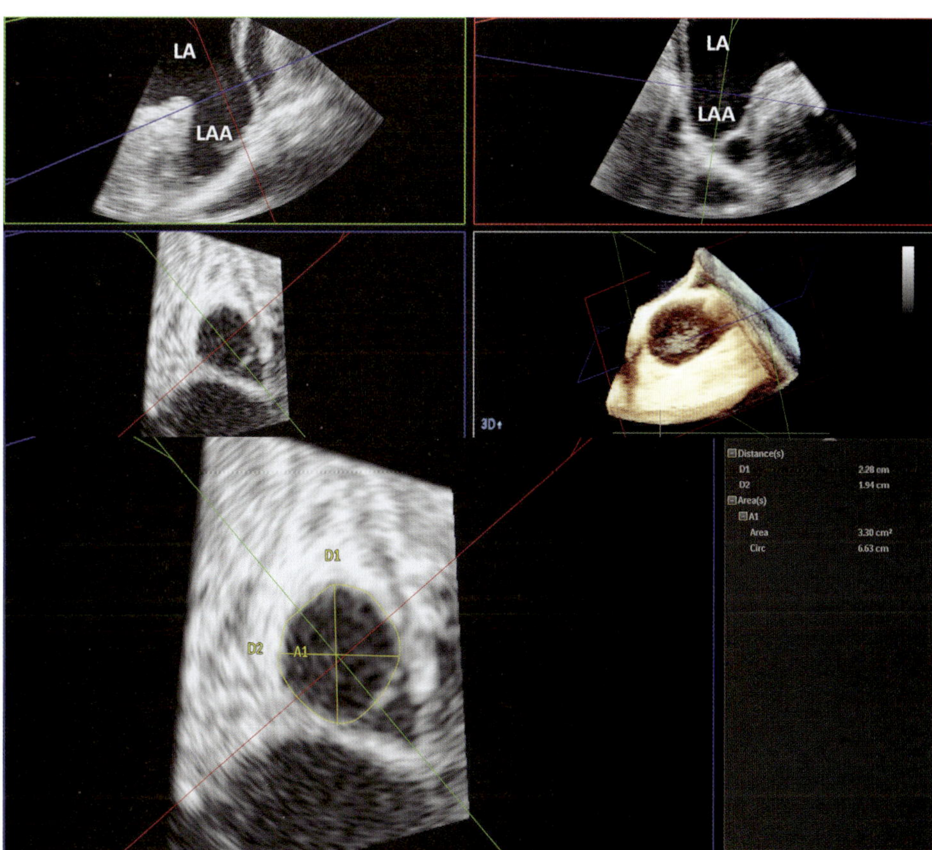

FIGURE 38.2 3D MPR of LAA measuring 2.28 × 1.94 cm in dimension and area of 3.30 cm^2. LA, left atrium; LAA, left atrial appendage; MPR, multiplanar reconstruction.

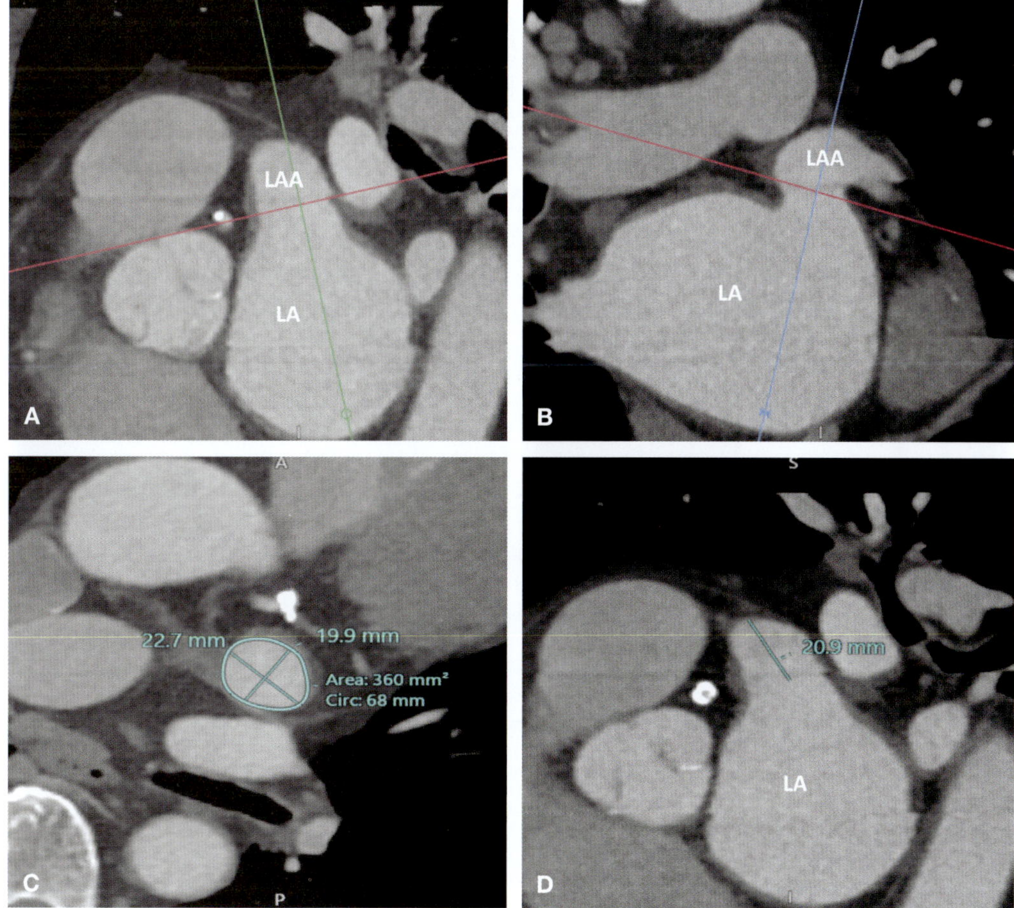

FIGURE 38.3 CT sizing for Watchman device via multiplanar reconstruction. **A,** Former sagittal plane. **B,** Former coronal plane. **C,** En face short axis where dimensions and area are measured. **D,** Depth to appendage tip. CT, computed tomography; LA, left atrium; LAA, left atrial appendage.

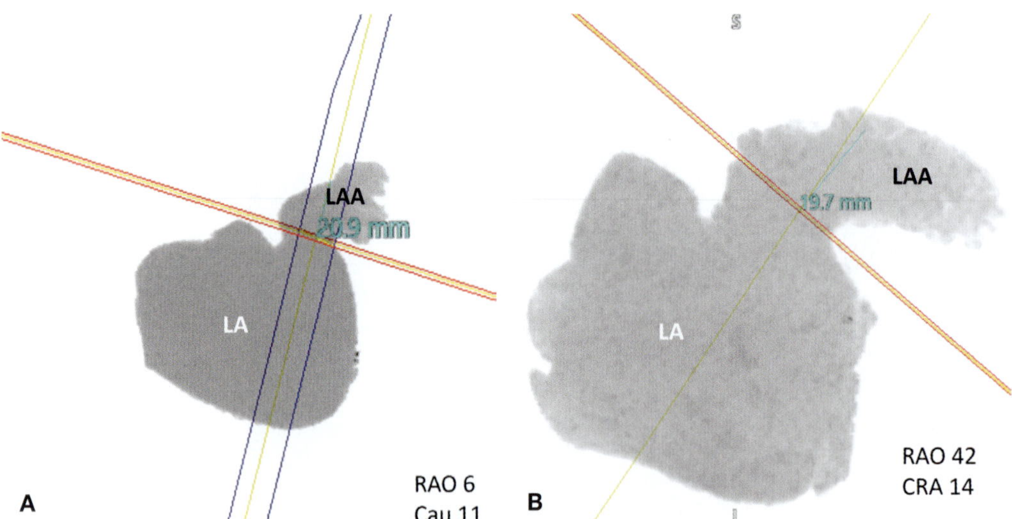

FIGURE 38.4 **A,** Simulated C-arm fluoroscopy angle for optimal catheter coaxiality for Watchman device. **B,** Simulated C-arm fluoroscopy angle for optimal catheter coaxiality for Amulet device. LA, left atrium; LAA, left atrial appendage.

shape, ie, as a concave disc. **Figure 38.11** demonstrates well-seated Watchman and Amulet devices by both TEE and CT.

Postprocedural Evaluation: TEE and CT

About 45 days post-LAA occlusion, the device should be evaluated by TEE or cardiac CT to evaluate for device stability and the absence of complications including PDL (**Fig. 38.12A and D**), device-related thrombus (DRT) (**Fig. 38.12B-D**), and less commonly device embolization. By TEE, the device is evaluated at the similar implantation angles of 0°, 45°, 90°, and 135° looking for PDL at a reduced Nyquist limit and ensuring the threaded insert portion at the tip of the device is clearly seen and there are no attached mobile echogenic structures to suggest DRT. PDL width

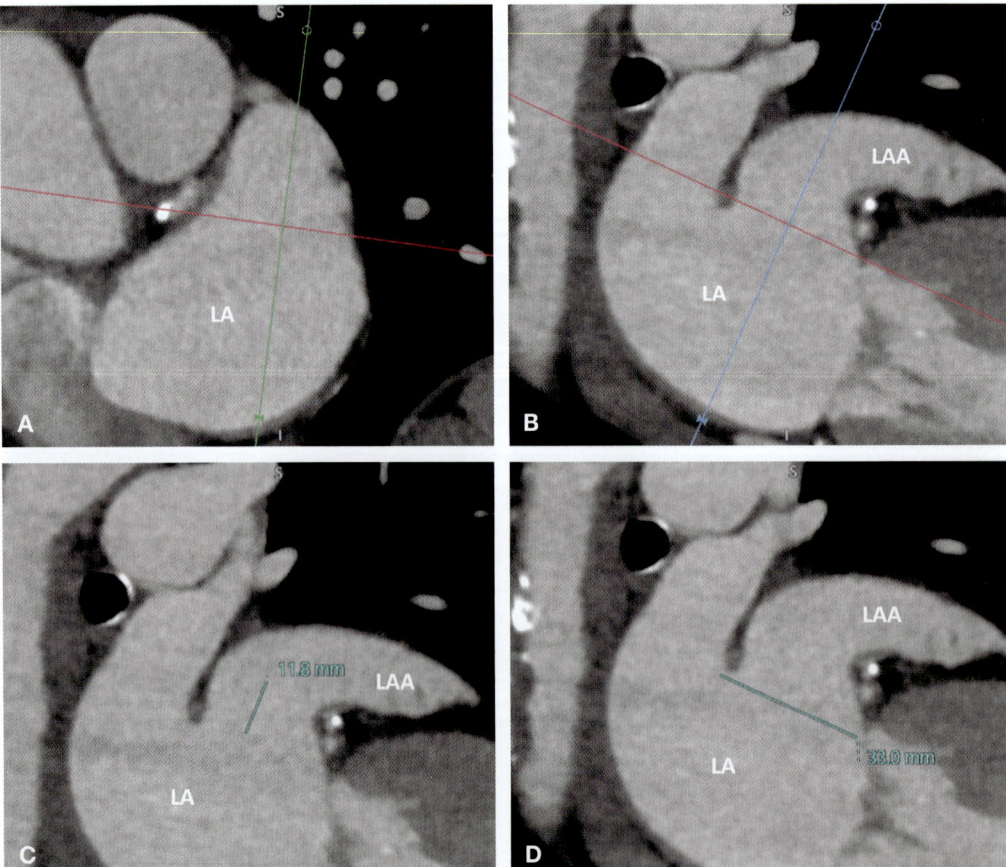

FIGURE 38.5 Multiplanar reconstruction of left atrial appendage ostium. **A,** LAA ostium dimension former sagittal plane. **B,** LAA ostium former coronal plane. **C,** 12 mm from appendage ostium to virtual landing zone for Amulet device. **D,** Distance of left upper pulmonary vein to mitral valve annulus. LA, left atrium; LAA, left atrial appendage.

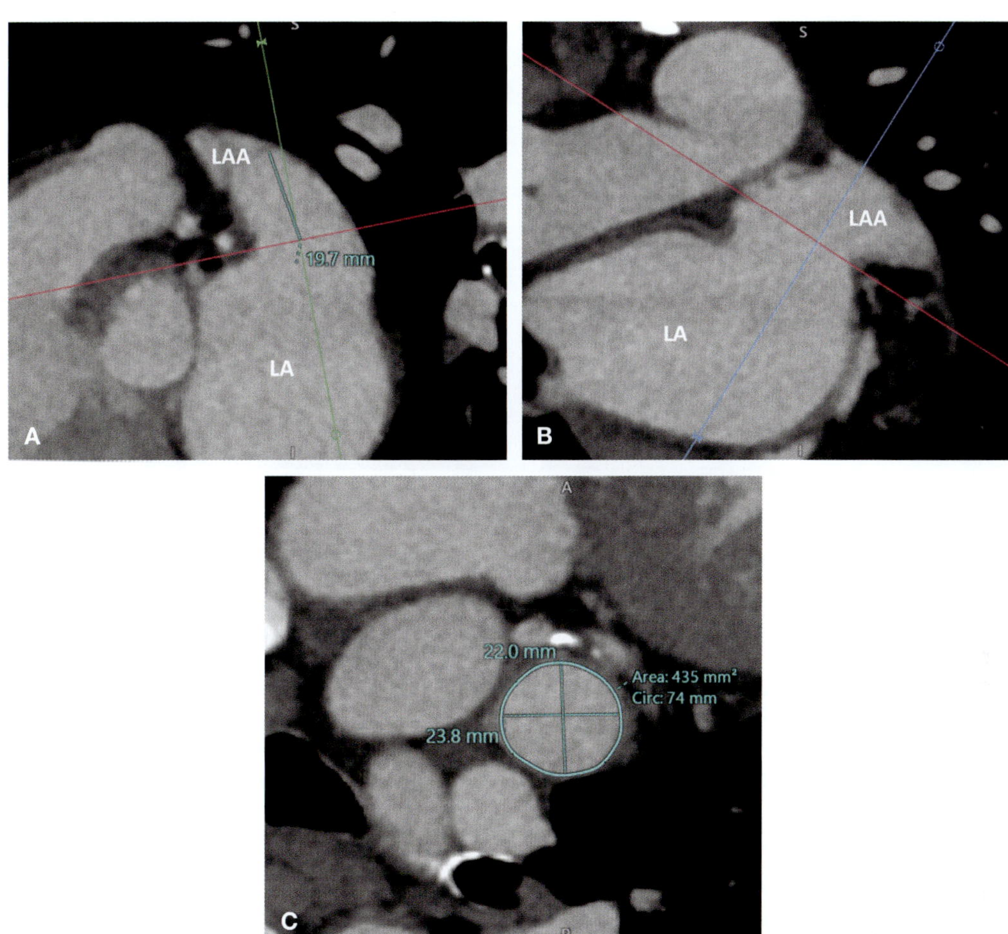

FIGURE 38.6 Amulet plug landing zone. **A,** Former sagittal plane and distance of landing zone to LAA tip. **B,** Former coronal plane. **C,** En face short axis landing zone dimensions and area. LAA, left atrial appendage.

by TEE can be determined by measuring the width of the color jet at its neck. Similarly, postprocedure CT can evaluate for the presence of PDL (contrast filling the distal LAA, ie, similar Hounsfield unit as compared to proximal LA) and size of PDL gap as well as for DRT. **Figure 38.13** additionally shows PDL from an uncovered accessory lobe due to a suboptimally positioned Watchman device.

MV TRANSCATHETER EDGE-TO-EDGE REPAIR

Preprocedural Echocardiographic Imaging

Initial evaluation for MV transcatheter edge-to-edge repair (TEER) candidacy begins with a screening echocardiogram (transthoracic

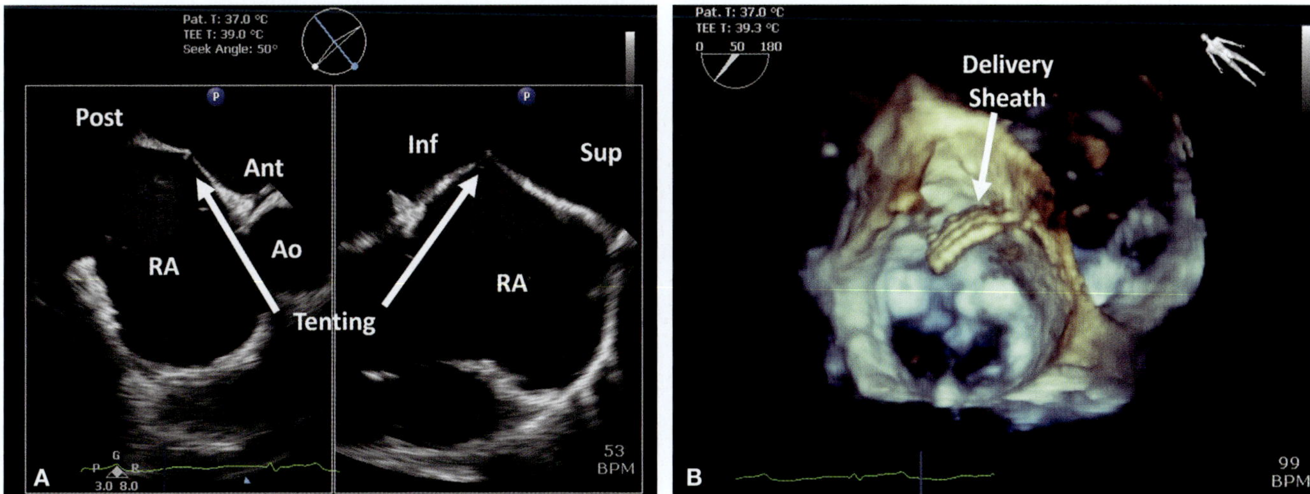

FIGURE 38.7 **A,** Tenting of interatrial septum using biplane imaging. Positioning of catheter is midseptum along anterior-posterior short axis and mid/inferior septum along superior-inferior axis. **B,** Delivery sheath across interatrial septum. Ant, anterior; Ao, aorta; Inf, inferior; Post, posterior; RA, right atrium; Sup, superior.

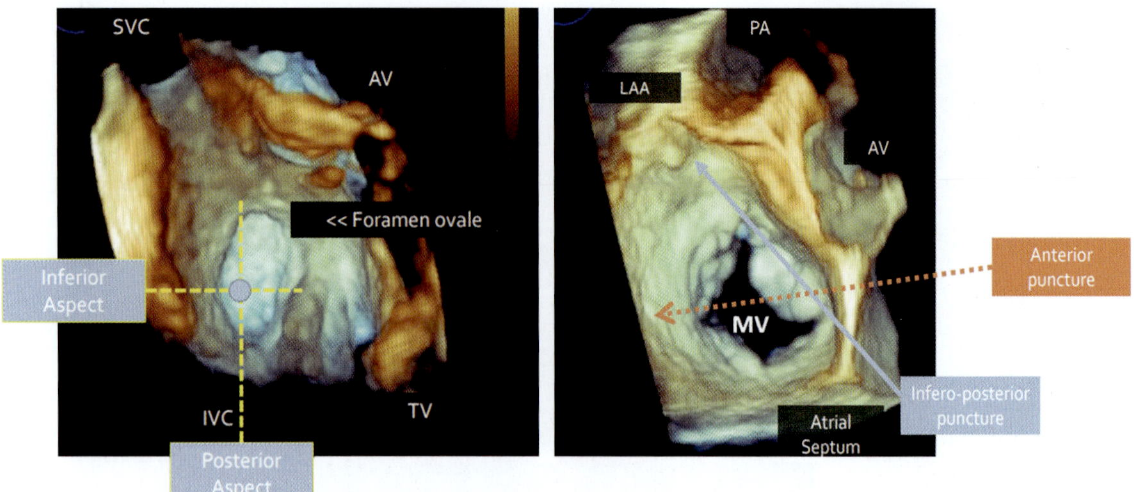

FIGURE 38.8 *Left Image*: 3D representation of optimal inferior-posterior trans-septal crossing site on the fossa. *Right image*: 3D representation of optimal coaxiality of inferior-posterior puncture site to the LAA ostium. LAA, left atrial appendage.

echocardiogram [TTE] and TEE) to delineate mitral regurgitation severity, pathologic mechanism, jet origin, biventricular size and function, the presence of pericardial effusion or LAA thrombus, concomitant valvular disease, and procedural feasibility. Important procedural characteristics include leaflet length/calcification, leaflet tip orifice area, mean diastolic mitral gradient, flail width/gap, and potential subvalvular interactions.

Evaluating MR Severity

Evaluating MR severity should include both qualitative but more importantly quantitative parameters.[5,6] Severe MR can be qualitatively visualized by a large jet area and a dense, holosystolic (sometimes triangular), continuous wave Doppler profile. On transthoracic imaging, very eccentric jets may be underestimated and suboptimally visualized, and Doppler alignment is further challenging. TEE imaging will help better characterize eccentric jet severity and pathology (**Fig. 38.14**). The semiquantitative parameter of vena contracta (VC) width is useful but can be limited by multiple jets, color gain, and arrhythmias such as atrial fibrillation. Pulmonary vein flow, specifically systolic flow reversal, is a specific sign but less sensitive parameter. Quantitative parameters include 2D PISA (proximal isovelocity surface area) for effective regurgitant orifice area and regurgitant volume (RV) calculation, MV RV by continuity equation, and 3D VC. Although quantitation of MR severity should be routinely performed, understanding limitations is important. The 2D PISA method assumes a circular orifice, but functional (secondary) mitral regurgitation typically

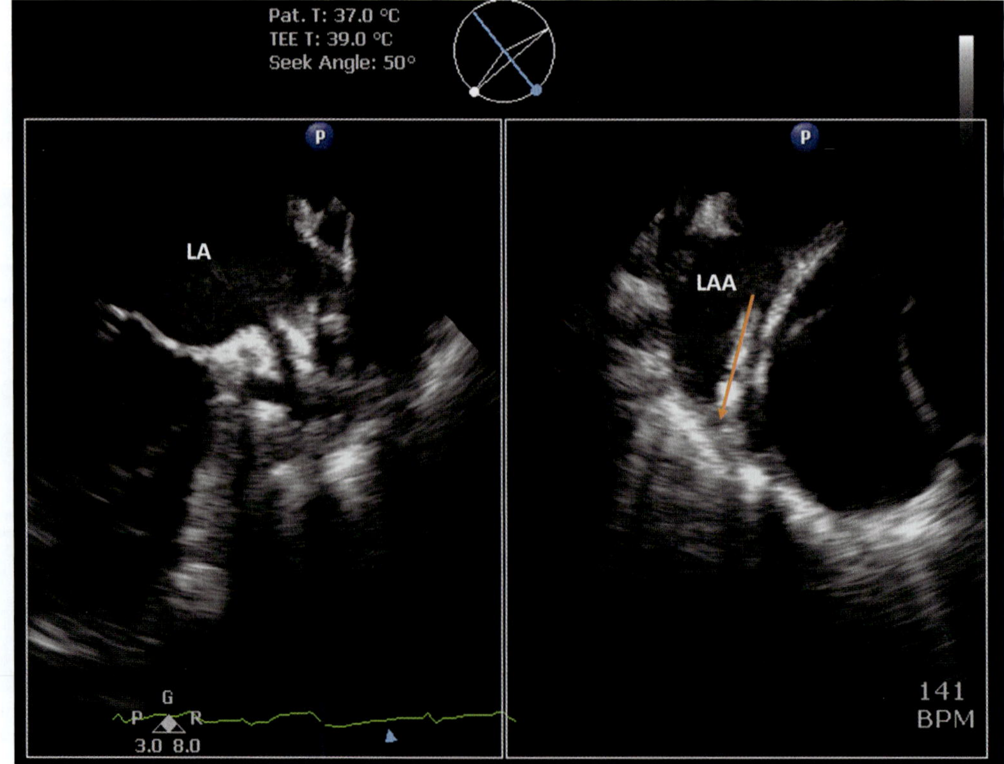

FIGURE 38.9 Biplane image of LAA from 50° and 140° angles. In 140° view, catheter trajectory (red arrow) is optimally placed anteriorly within the appendage. LA, left atrium; LAA, left atrial appendage.

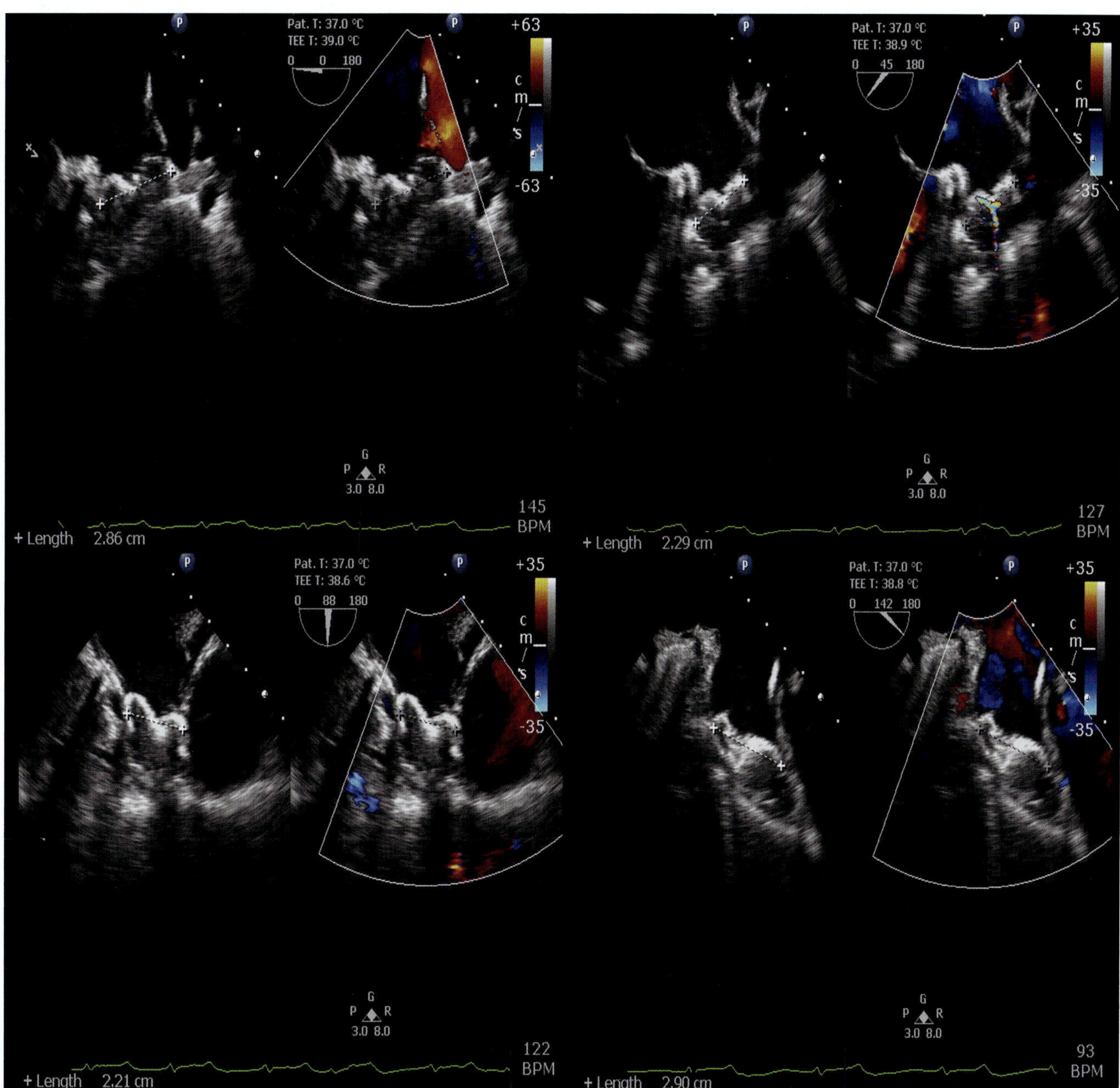

FIGURE 38.10 TEE color compare post 35 mm Watchman implantation at 0°, 45°, 90°, and 135° views. Left-sided images show Watchman dimension at ""shoulder" of device for compression assessment (ranging 17%-37%). Right-sided images show no evidence of peridevice leak with color Doppler at aliasing velocity 35 cm/s. TEE, transesophageal echocardiogram.

produces a more elliptical orifice such that MR severity may be underestimated. Furthermore, the presence of multiple jets can again underestimate regurgitation severity if PISA is only used to quantify a single jet. Additionally, MR can be dynamic throughout systole with a classic example being late systolic MR due to MV prolapse. Quantitation by continuity method relies on accurate measurement of left ventricular outflow tract (LVOT) and mitral annular diameters and assumes a circular orifice. These assumptions can be somewhat overcome by sizing using 3D MPR to measure mitral annulus area ± LVOT area. Concomitant valvular disease, shunting, or outflow tract obstruction may result in over- or underestimation of MR severity and arrhythmias such as atrial fibrillation can result in beat-to-beat variability in stroke volumes. 3D VC may help overcome some of the above challenges but requires technical precision, is technically challenging in the presence of multiple jets, and VC area may vary throughout systole. Quantitative analysis is also affected by loading and hemodynamic conditions such as volume status and blood pressure especially for functional mitral regurgitation. Loading conditions and qualitative/quantitative parameters should be taken into context of the underlying pathology to form a formal assessment of MR severity. When generating the valvular heart disease echo final report, it is imperative that serial echocardiographic/imaging studies be reviewed to generate comparison reads to help multidisciplinary heart teams understand the presence or the absence of any signs of disease progression. Multimodality imaging with cardiac CT and MRI should be considered in the appropriate context to for better spatial resolution and volumetric assessment respectively.

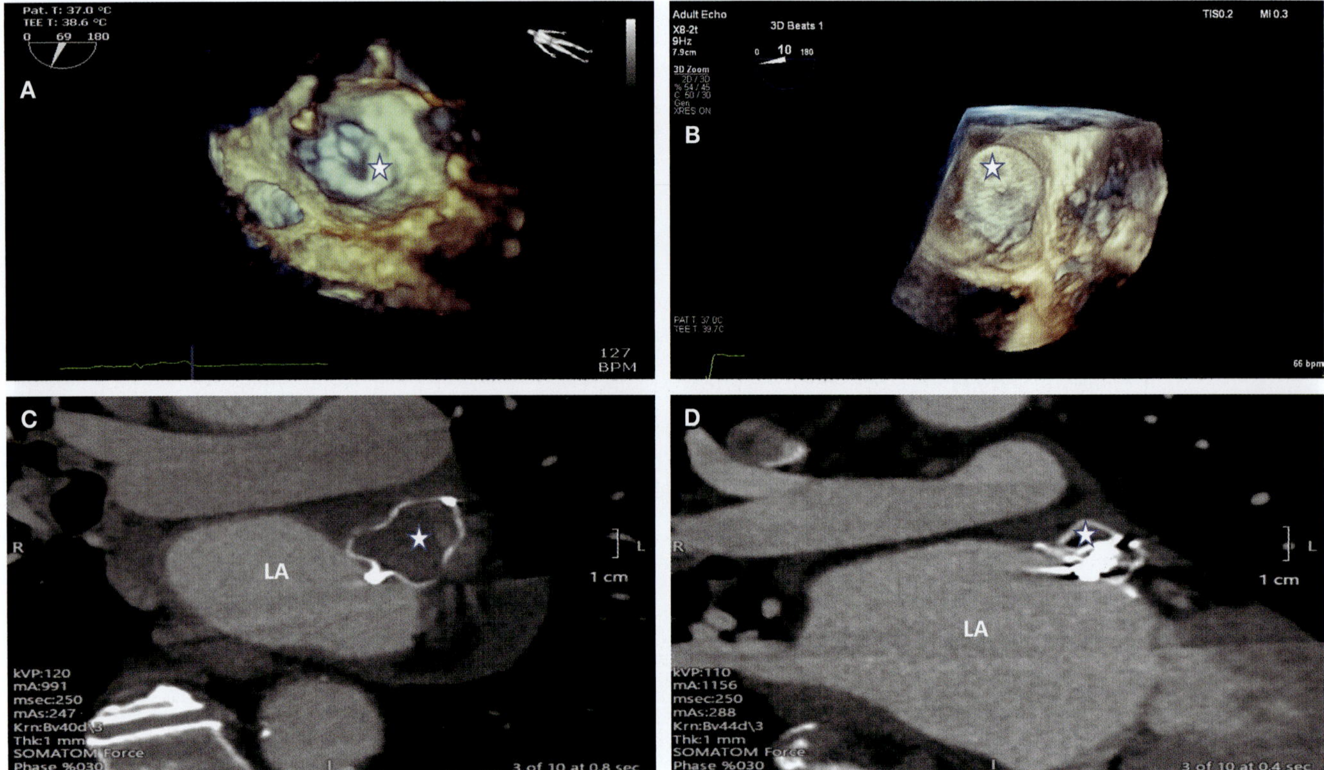

FIGURE 38.11 **A,** TEE 3D zoom of well-seated Watchman device in LAA. **B,** TEE 3D zoom of well-seated Amulet device. **C,** CT post-Watchman device. **D,** CT post-Amulet device. *Left atrial appendage occluder device. CT, computed tomography; LA, left atrium; LAA, left atrial appendage; TEE, transesophageal echocardiogram.

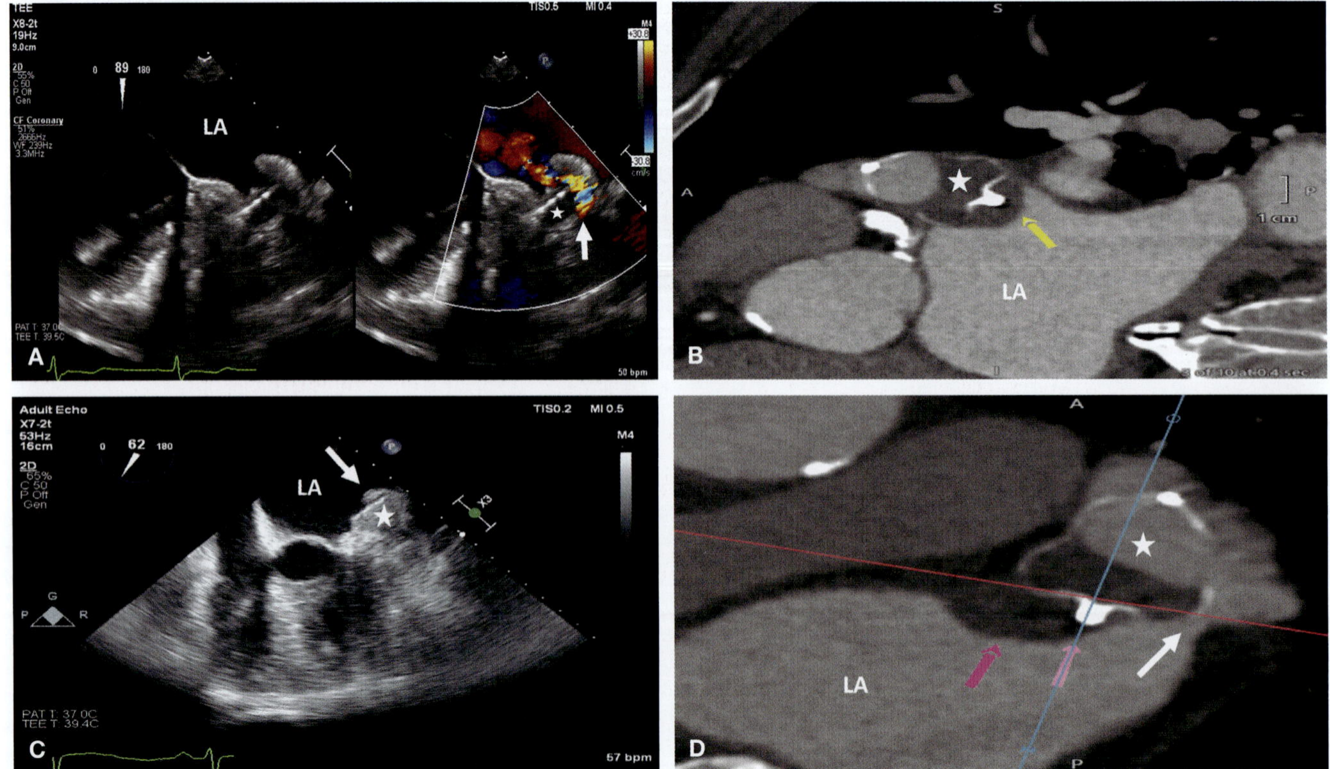

FIGURE 38.12 **A,** Post-Watchman TEE with significant peridevice leak (*white arrow*). **B,** Post-Watchman CT with device-related thrombus (*yellow arrow*). **C,** Post-Watchman TEE device-related thrombus (*white arrow*). **D,** Post-Watchman TEE showing device-related thrombus (*pink arrows*) and peridevice leak (*white arrow*). *Left atrial appendage occluder device. LA, left atrium; TEE, transesophageal echocardiogram.

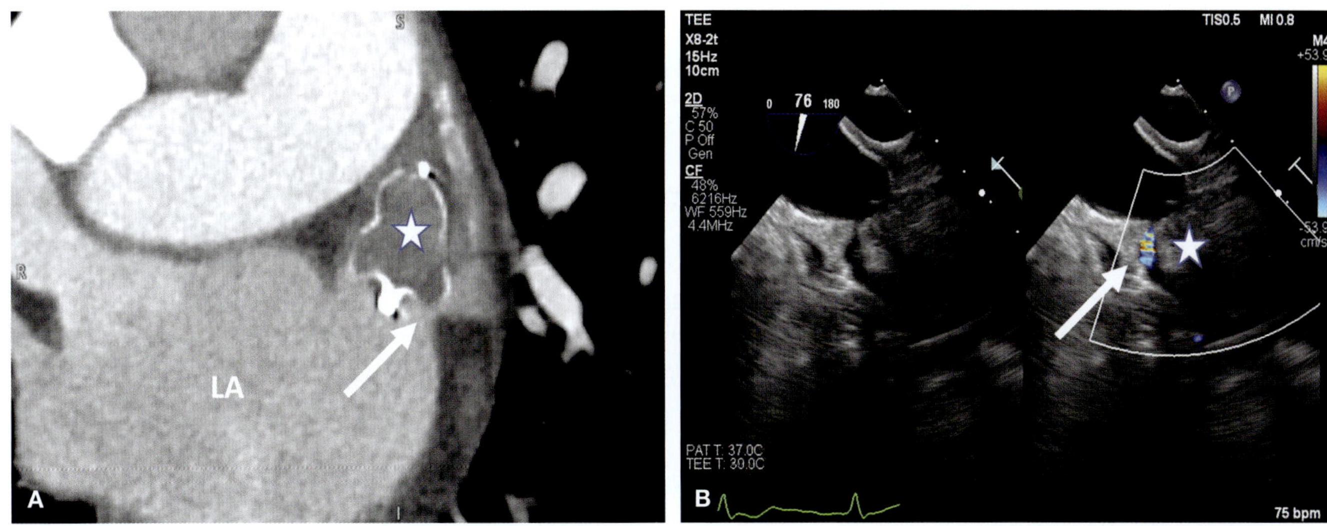

FIGURE 38.13 **A,** Post-Watchman CT with peridevice leak due to uncovered accessory lobe (*white arrow*). **B,** Post-Watchman TEE with peridevice leak due to uncovered accessory lobe (*white arrow*). *Left atrial appendage occluder device. LA, left atrium; TEE, transesophageal echocardiogram.

MV TEER Feasibility

Appropriate patient selection and the identification of challenging anatomy preprocedurally can assist with appropriate planning and optimizing intraprocedural success. **Table 38.1** demonstrates criteria for optimal, challenging, and unsuitable candidates for MV TEER and can be assessed during screening echocardiograms.[7,8] Current commercially available G4 MitraClip (Abbott) devices include the XT, NT, XTw, and NTw models.[7] XT devices have arm dimensions of 12 mm and are favorable in primary/degenerative pathologies where longer leaflet lengths and larger coaptation gaps exist whilst the NT devices are more suitable to shorter/more restricted MV leaflets and have an arm length of 9 mm. The "w" designation indicates wider grasp of 6 mm versus standard grasp of 4 mm. Wider MitraClip models favor wider/elongated jets.

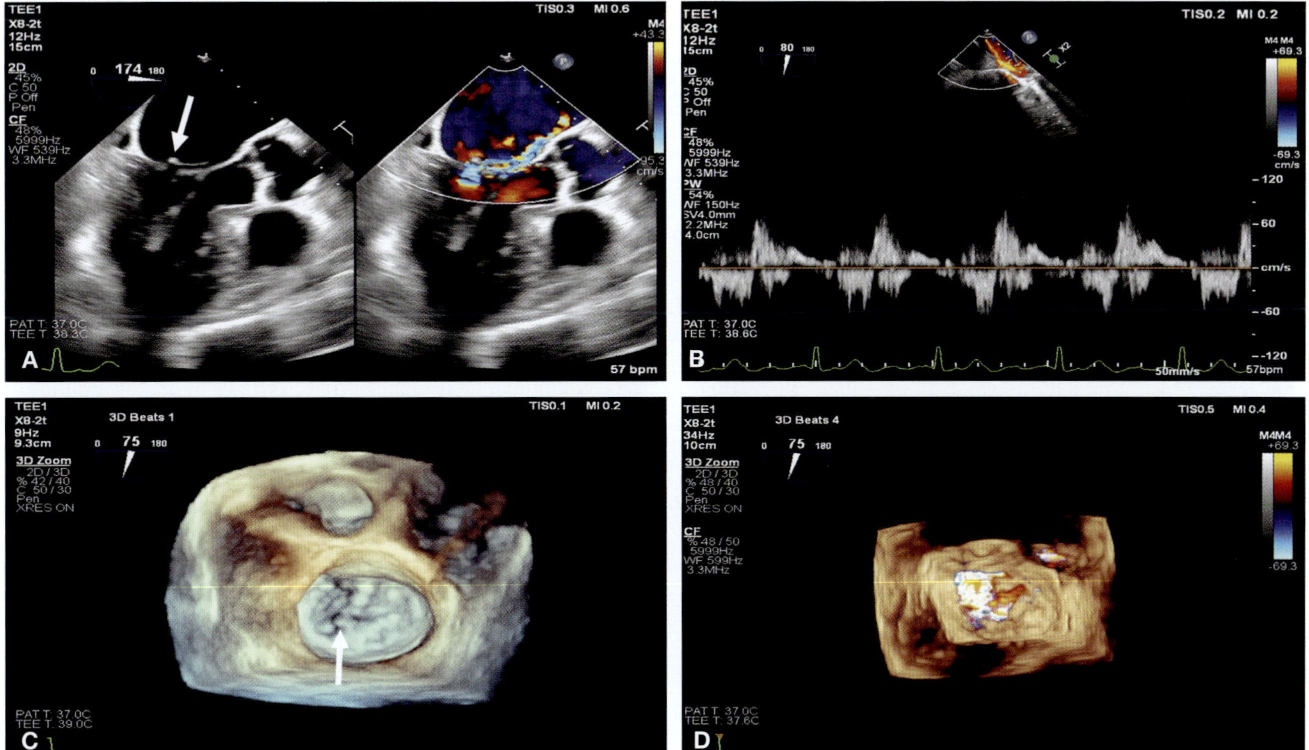

FIGURE 38.14 **A,** TEE long-axis color compare image with reduced aliasing velocity demonstrating PISA shell of eccentric and anteriorly directed mitral regurgitant jet due to flail of P2 scallop (*white arrow*). **B,** Pulmonary vein systolic flow reversal. **C,** 3D zoom surgeon's view of mitral valve with flail of lateral aspect of P2 scallop (*white arrow*). **D,** 3D color zoom with anteriorly directed eccentric mitral regurgitation. PISA, proximal isovelocity surface area; TEE, transesophageal echocardiogram.

TABLE 38.1 MV TEER Feasibility

OPTIMAL	ANATOMICALLY CHALLENGING	LOWER LIKELIHOOD OF PROCEDURAL SUCCESS
Central A2-P2 pathology	Commissural pathology (A1-P1, A3-P3); multiple segments	Cleft, perforation
No calcification or MV chordae in grasping zone	Calcification or chordae adjacent to grasping zone	Heavy calcification at grasping zone
MVA > 4 cm^2	MVA 3-4 cm^2	MVA ≤ 3 cm^2
Transmitral gradient <5 mm Hg	Transmitral gradient >5 mm Hg	
Posterior leaflet length >10 mm	Posterior leaflet length 6-10 mm	Posterior leaflet length <6 mm
Normal leaflet mobility and thickness	Excessive leaflet mobility, restricted leaflet, Barlow's disease	Rheumatic MV leaflets, friable leaflets
Tenting height <11 mm	Tenting height ≥11 mm	
Flail width <15 mm Flail gap <10 mm	Flail width ≥15 mm Flail gap ≥10 mm	
		LVEDD > 70 mm LVEF < 20%

LVEDD, left ventricular end-diastolic diameter; LVEF, left ventricular ejection fraction.

INTRAPROCEDURAL GUIDANCE

Trans-Septal Puncture

The guiding of trans-septal access to attain adequate height is of the utmost importance to optimize catheter trajectory and device delivery. It becomes even more crucial when additional height is needed for medial commissural jets. Identification of the thin portion of the interatrial septum (IAS) by both 2D and 3D TEE can be utilized. 3D TEE is helpful to demonstrate the location of the fossa relative to MV leaflet pathology to help determine ideal trans-septal crossing location (**Fig. 38.15**). Once the catheter has been advanced into the superior vena cava (SVC), the interventionalist should let the interventional imaging physician know they are ready to bring the catheter down to the IAS. The interventional imaging physician should obtain a biplane view of the IAS from the midesophageal short axis (~20°-55°) representing anterior and posterior trajectory and the orthogonal bicaval view representing superior and inferior trajectory (**Figure 38.15A**). As the catheter is brought into view adjacent to the septum, the interventional imaging physician can begin to guide the catheter to a more ideal crossing location, typically on the superior-posterior aspect of the fossa. Once a suitable position is identified, the catheter should be tenting the fossa from the right atrium into the LA to help determine a tenting height. Tenting height can be assessed in a traditional 2D midesophageal 4-chamber view or with a 3D view (**Fig. 38.15B and C**). Ideal trans-septal height of 4.5 to 5.0 cm but at least 4.0 cm should be obtained. If an adequate tenting height has been achieved, trans-septal crossing can be visualized under 3D guidance to determine wire, sheath, and steerable guide catheter (SGC) crossing and the relative position to the atrial walls, LAA, and LUPV (**Fig. 38.15D**). Once trans-septal access has been obtained, evaluation for new or changing pericardial effusion should take place and subsequently at any time hypotension is present.

Initially, a wire is advanced into the LA and anchored in the LUPV. The SGC with its dilator is then advanced over the wire across the septum with the SGC appearing as a double orifice tubular catheter and the dilator tip appearing conical at its tip. Once the SGC is within the LA, the distance to the septum can be measured to ensure an adequate and safe length has been achieved.

Device Orientation, Positioning/Trajectory, and Gripper Identification

While the clip delivery system (CDS) is being prepared, the interventional imaging physician can optimize a 3D zoom "surgeon's view" of the MV with the lateral and medial commissures at 10 and 2 on the clock face. If feasible, ideal 3D imaging should not only show the MV enface but should also depict the guide catheter across the septum and left atrial walls (**Fig. 38.16A**). Once the clip is loaded into the SGC, the interventional imaging physician can assist in visualization of the clip as it makes its way out of the catheter and into the LA. Visualization of the clip should take place the entire time as it is steered toward the MV annulus making sure it is clear of LA walls, LAA, and LUPV. Clip trajectory can be checked in a traditional 2D biplane view encompassing the midesophageal commissural and orthogonal long axis views (**Fig. 38.17A**). The interventionalist can advance the CDS as if to cross the mitral annular plane simulating the expected trajectory and ensuring the CDS is being directed over the primary jet location. Maneuvers can be undertaken to correct suboptimal medial/lateral trajectories or tilting toward the aorta known as an "aorta hugger." This can also be shown in the 3D view by tilting the trackball to show catheter trajectory across the fossa relative to MV annulus (**Fig. 38.16B**). Once optimal positioning and trajectory have been obtained, clip orientation can take place. With A2-P2 leaflet pathology, the clip is typically oriented at a 12-6 position on the clock face perpendicular to the line of coaptation; while lateral and medial commissural jet pathologies may require a clocking and counterclocking of the clip respectively to again be perpendicular to the plane of coaptation (~1 and 7 for lateral grasp; ~11 and 5 for medial grasp). Once completed, gripper identification can take place. The grippers are the part of the clip used to grasp opposing anterior/posterior leaflets. With the clip open, the interventional imaging physician can assist in identification of which gripper corresponds to anterior versus posterior. All these checks and maneuvers can be performed again as needed to ensure ideal positioning and trajectory are in place prior to crossing the MV annulus.

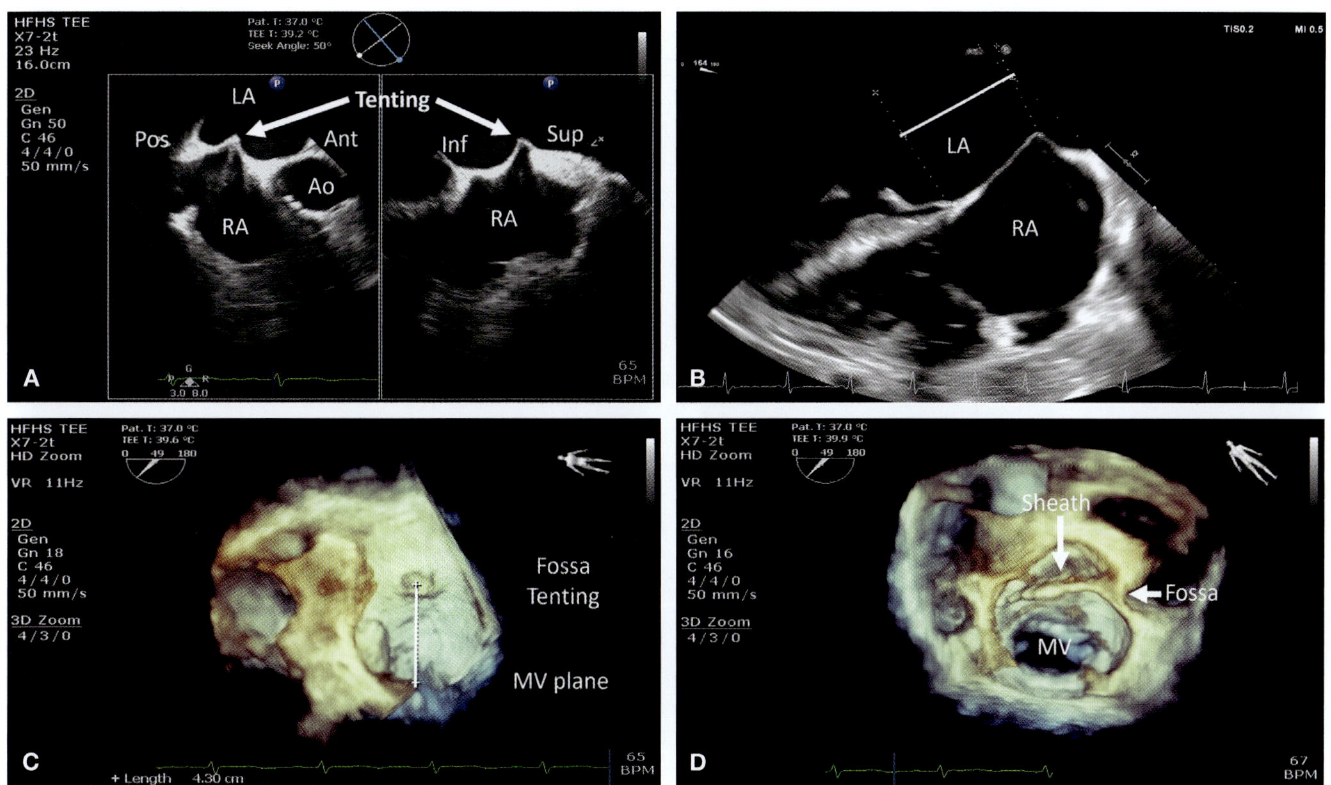

FIGURE 38.15 **A,** Tenting of interatrial septum visualized by biplane imaging (short axis on left and modified bicaval view on right). Positioning of catheter is midseptum along anterior-posterior short axis and superior along superior-inferior axis. **B,** 2D tenting height (*white line*) measured from tenting location to mitral valve annular plane. **C,** 3D tenting height (*white line*) from tenting location on fossa to mitral valve annular plane. **D,** 3D trans-septal crossing site with sheath across the septum into the left atrium. Ant, anterior; Ao, aorta; Inf, inferior; LA, left atrium; MV, mitral valve; Pos, posterior; RA, right atrium; Sup, superior.

Crossing the MV Annulus and Leaflet Grasping

With the above steps completed, the clip device can be advanced across the MV annulus into the left ventricle (LV) using 2D biplane imaging of the commissural and long-axis views (**Fig. 38.17A**). Nonstandard and off-axis views may be necessary to visualize the clip away from the shadow of the shaft/CDS. Once in the LV, clip orientation relative to the clock face may need to be checked again if the clip has rotated. With the clip in the LV, the interventional imaging physician can obtain a long-axis "grasping" view as the interventionalist opens the clip arms and begins to retract the CDS toward the MV leaflets. Color compare mode can be used to ensure the device is over the most significant jet pathology (**Fig. 38.17B**). Once both leaflets are adequately captured (at least 9 mm of leaflet using XT clip and 6 mm of leaflet using NT clip), the interventionalist will lower the grippers and begin to close the clip. With grippers lowered, a quick assessment for the "gripper sign" can

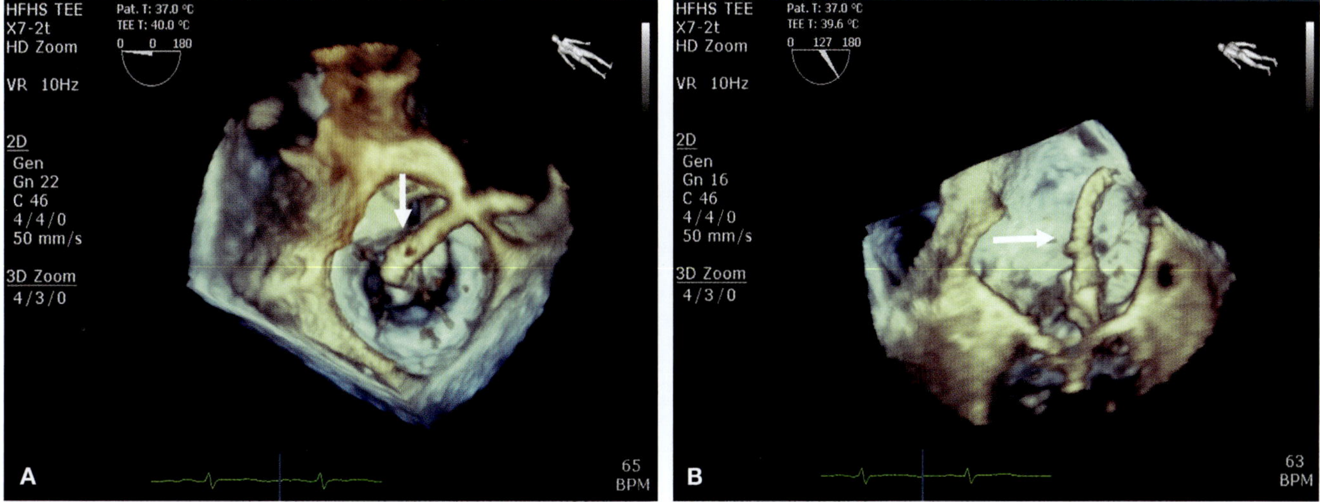

FIGURE 38.16 **A,** 3D TEE orientation of clip delivery system (*white arrow*) in left atrium. **B,** 3D TEE trajectory of clip-delivery system (*white arrow*). TEE, transesophageal echocardiogram.

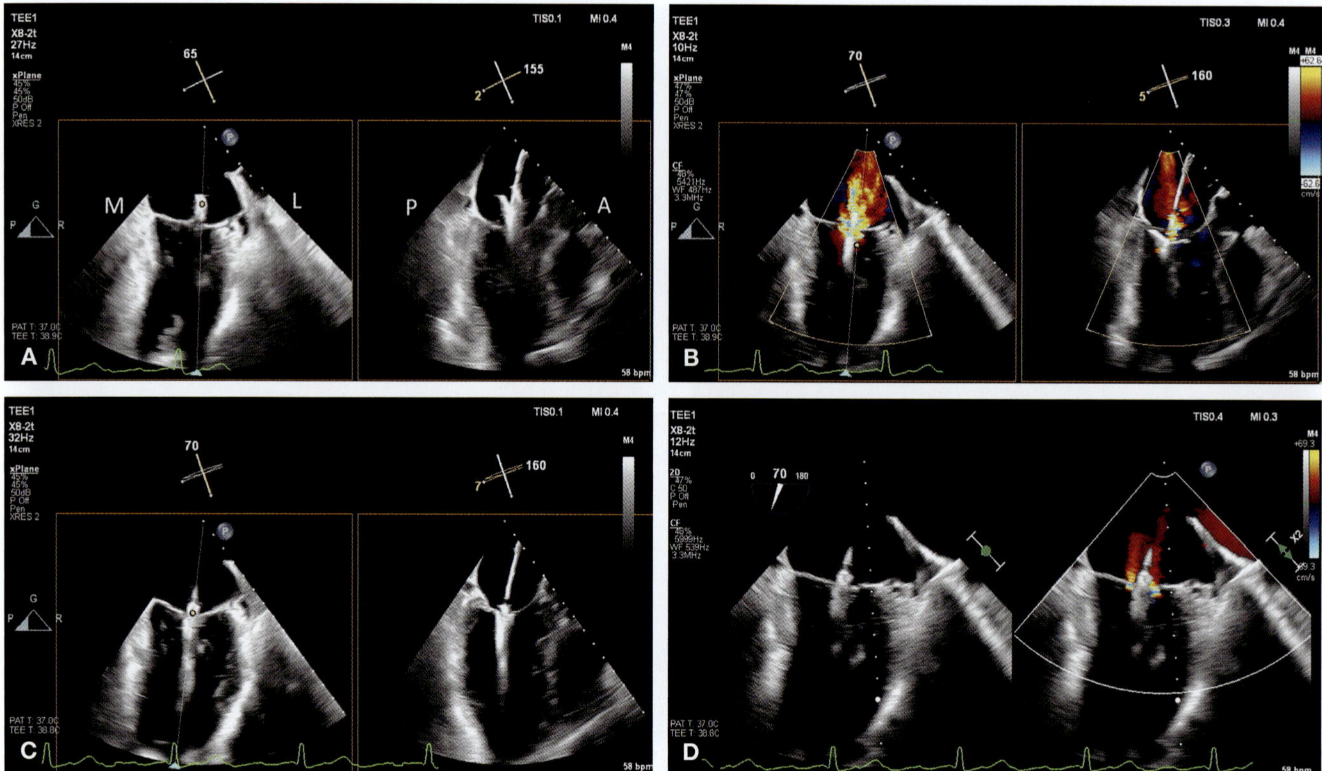

FIGURE 38.17 TEE guidance of leaflet grasp using MitraClip device as demonstrated by 2D biplane imaging of commissural and long axis views (**A-C**). **A,** Clip trajectory along lateral/medial and anterior/posterior axis. **B,** Color Doppler demonstrating open MitraClip device over most significant regurgitant jet. **C,** MitraClip device after lowering of grippers and device closure demonstrating adequate leaflet grasps of both anterior and posterior leaflets. **D,** MitraClip in closed and locked position in commissural view demonstrating trace residual mitral regurgitation medial and lateral to the clip. A, anterior; L, lateral; M, medial; P, posterior; TEE, transesophageal echocardiogram.

be visualized and is defined by slight lifting of the gripper arms during systolic motion of the MV ensuring leaflets have adequate insertion.

Evaluation of the Grasp

Assessment should now include visualization of optimal leaflet grasping and insertion into the clip device at grasping and 0° views. These views in addition to commissural and 90° can be used with color compare to evaluate reduction in MR severity and any residual jets of significance (**Fig. 38.17C and D**) and help determine the need for additional clips. Evaluation at multiple angles can help identify any remaining eccentric jets. In the commissural view, diastolic mitral gradients lateral and medial to the clip should be measured to identify an average acceptable gradient (ideally averaging to <5 mm Hg). Pulmonary vein flow can be checked in all veins as feasible to assess for improvement from baseline. A 3D zoom surgeon's view should be obtained to evaluate for clip orientation and adequate tissue bridge (**Fig. 38.18**). 3D color can also be utilized to further demonstrate MR reduction and any residual jets. After full closure of the clip and release from the CDS, the interventional imaging physician should ensure clip stability and no change in MR severity. The residual distal tip of the CDS must be visualized at all times as it is guided back into the SGC and can be done under 3D zoom surgeon's view. Final assessment of the clip, mitral gradients, degree of residual MR, and 3D orientation/tissue bridge can again be assessed at this time prior to removal of the SGC into the right atrium. If satisfactory results have been achieved, evaluation for change in biventricular function, pericardial effusion, and color/spectral Doppler flow across the iatrogenic atrial septal defect should take place.

TRANSCATHETER MV REPLACEMENT

Overview

In select patients with severe mitral stenosis or severe mitral regurgitation who are not candidates for MV TEER, transcatheter MV replacement may be a feasible option. Although the technology is

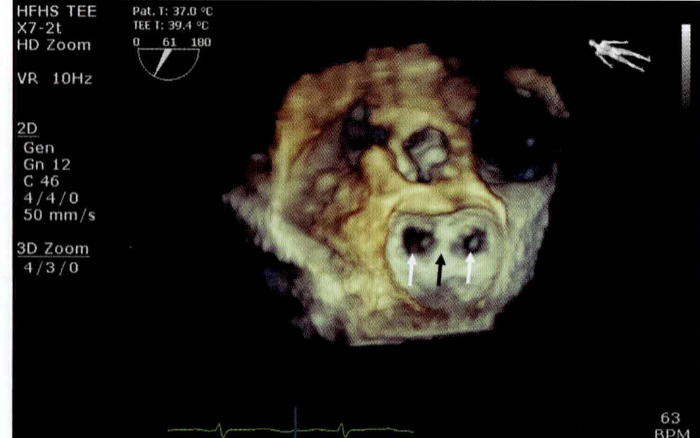

FIGURE 38.18 3D zoom Surgeon's view post-MitraClip deployment demonstrating adequate tissue bridge (*black arrow*) and residual double orifice valve (*white arrows*).

still growing, clinical trials and off-label use of commercial valves used for transcutaneous aortic valve replacement (TAVR) are becoming increasingly utilized with successful results. The most challenging component to this procedure has been evaluating transcatheter device fit in relation to the asymmetric saddle-shaped annulus, complex subvalvular apparatus, and to the LVOT.[9] Additionally, anchoring the transcatheter device in various annuli such as valve-in-valve (ViV), valve-in-ring (ViR), and valve-in-mitral annular calcification (ViMAC) pose unique considerations. Given MV proximity to the aortic valve and LVOT, left ventricular outflow tract obstruction (LVOTO) is the most feared complication given the potentially fatal outcome.[10]

CT Planning

CT planning for transcatheter mitral valve replacement (TMVR) initially involves evaluation of MV annular area and dimensions. Mitral annulus sizing measurements are typically obtained in end diastole when the annulus is largest in size. This can be done by creating a 3-chamber projection and orthogonal commissural projection with crosshairs lined up at the MV annulus (**Fig. 38.19A and B**). This results in a short axis en face view traditionally demonstrating a saddle- or D-shaped MV annulus in which area, lateral-medial dimension (commissural), and anterior-posterior dimension can all be measured (**Fig. 38.19C**). **Figure 38.19** demonstrates a baseline bioprosthetic MV replacement in which the annulus has conformed to the circular nature of the prosthesis. Oversizing is often more critical in TMVR as compared to TAVR to prevent device migration and embolization. For ViV TMVR, CT sizing can be compared to true inner diameter ID of the existing surgical prosthesis proposed by Bapat.[11] CT can also be utilized to predict optimal fluoroscopic C-arm angle for TMVR deployment (**Fig. 38.19D**). Transapical access can also be planned as needed by identifying degree of LV apical muscle thickness, distance from important landmarks such as left anterior descending artery, distance of skin to LV apex, and optimal access site using 3D volume rendering.

Special Considerations[12-14]: In cases of ViMAC planning, the degree and distribution of calcification in addition to calcium protrusion into MV orifice should be identified to ensure adequate anchoring is feasible and minimal deformation will occur to an

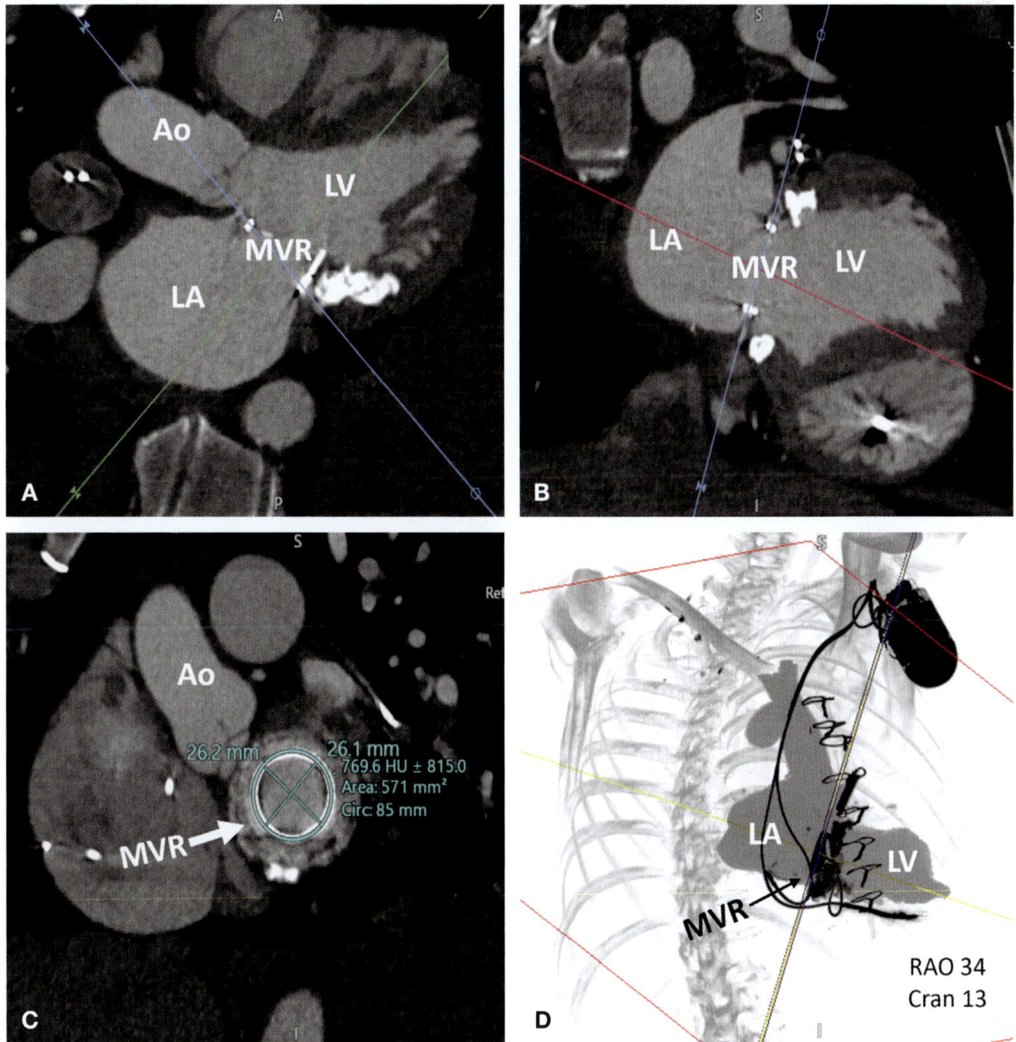

FIGURE 38.19 **A,** Former sagittal plane with blue axis lined up on struts of prior bioprosthetic surgical mitral valve replacement. **B,** Former coronal plane with blue axis lined up on struts of prior bioprosthetic surgical mitral valve replacement. **C,** Resultant en face short axis of bioprosthetic surgical MVR with dimensions, area, and perimeter outlined. **D,** Simulated C-arm fluoroscopy angle for coplanar alignment along mitral annulus for anticipated TMVR deployment. Markers such as pacemaker leads and sternotomy wires included as helpful landmarks transcatheter heart valve alignment. Ao, aorta; LA, left atrium; LV, left ventricle; MVR, mitral valve replacement; TMVR, transcatheter mitral valve replacement.

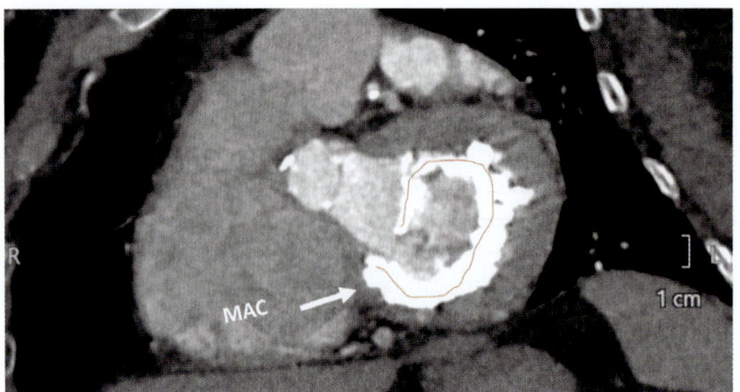

FIGURE 38.20 CT analysis of mitral valve in short axis demonstrating near-circumferential MAC involving both lateral and medial trigones (*outlined by red line*). CT, computed tomography; MAC, mitral annular calcification.

implanted prosthesis (**Fig. 38.20**). Circumferential calcification involving the commissures is preferred for optimal anchoring success. In cases of ViR, annuloplasty ring shape and size must be known to determine suitability for TMVR. Circular rings are most ideal, but if not present, oval rings that are complete and deformable (semirigid) are preferred. An additional key measurement for ViR and ViMAC case planning may also include MV anterior leaflet length given interaction with LVOT after TMVR deployment.

Risk assessment for LVOTO is challenging given multiple influencing factors including aortomitral angle, size/shape of the LV, hyperdynamic LV function, septal hypertrophy, anterior MV leaflet length, and prosthesis choice/positioning.[12-16] Specialized 3D postprocessing software can be utilized to predict the neo-LVOT area based on specified device size and depth of implantation (**Fig. 38.21**). This is done by simulating a virtually implanted TMVR prosthesis at the specified depth during systole within the pre-existing surgical prosthesis, annuloplasty ring, or MAC. The virtual area of the neo-LVOT can then be measured at the narrowest location with borders encompassing the basal interventricular septum, TMVR device strut, and the displaced anterior MV leaflet. Predicted neo-LVOT area ≤189.4 mm^2 has been validated to have high sensitivity and specificity for detecting post-TMVR LVOTO.[17] This cutoff is most predictive in ViV TMVR and progressively less predictive in ViR and ViMAC cases. Additionally, an elongated anterior MV leaflet (>25 mm in length or larger than the LVOT diameter) increases risk for LVOTO. Consideration may be given to alcohol septal ablation (ASA) in patients deemed high risk for LVOTO. If ASA is not feasible, anterior MV leaflet laceration may also be an option.

INTRAPROCEDURAL ECHOCARDIOGRAPHIC GUIDANCE

Intraprocedurally, TMVR guidance relies on transesophageal echocardiography for trans-septal or apical access, guidance across the MV annulus, possible pre/postdeployment balloon dilation, and valve positioning prior to deployment as needed. Baseline assessment should include evaluation for pericardial effusion, LAA thrombus, biventricular function, concomitant valve disease, LVOT gradient, and baseline MV assessment including degree of regurgitation/stenosis and mitral diastolic mean gradient (**Fig. 38.22A-C**). For transapical access, TEE can help demonstrate apical puncture by visualizing the cardiac surgeon's finger poking at the apex. For trans-septal access, a short axis (anterior-posterior dimension) and orthogonal bicaval view (superior-inferior dimension) should be shown. Optimal access site is posterior in the short axis and midfossa in the bicaval window or as best predicted by preprocedural CT analysis. As mentioned, TEE can be used to guide pre- or postdeployment balloon dilation (**Fig. 38.23**). Prior to device deployment, TEE can be used to help confirm ideal positioning and device trajectory/coaxiality utilizing 2D biplane imaging (commissural/long axis views), live

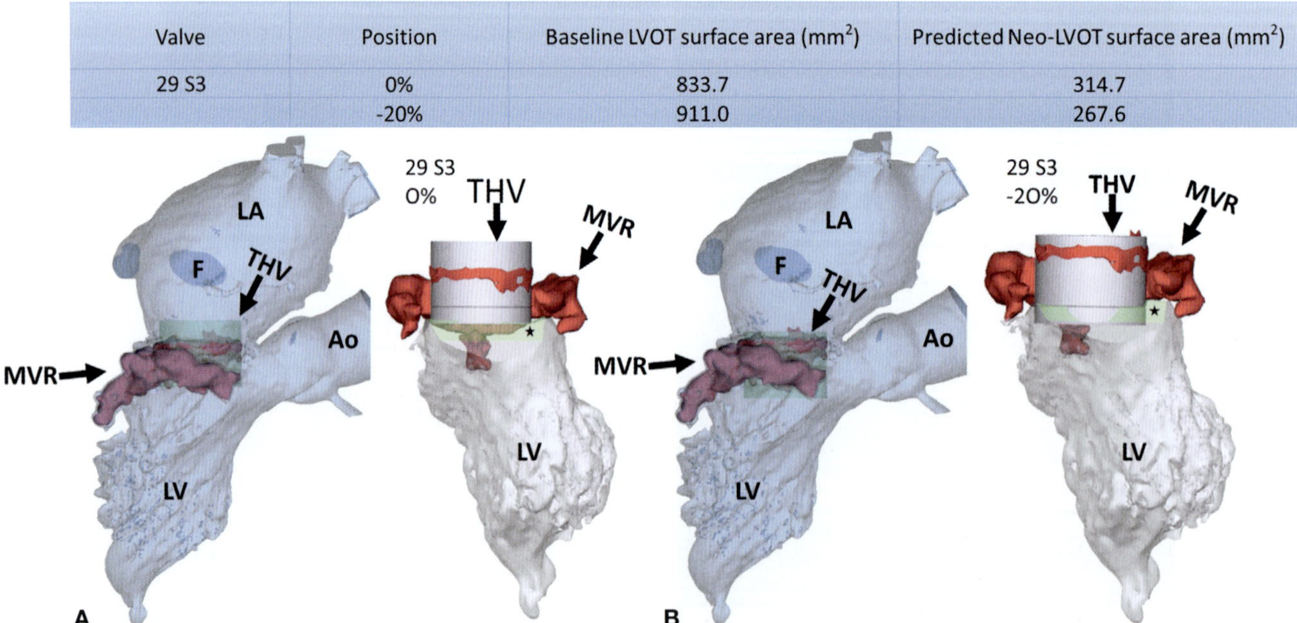

Valve	Position	Baseline LVOT surface area (mm^2)	Predicted Neo-LVOT surface area (mm^2)
29 S3	0%	833.7	314.7
	-20%	911.0	267.6

FIGURE 38.21 3D postprocessing software modeling Edwards 29 Sapien 3 balloon-expandable valve in prior bioprosthetic surgical MVR at (**A**) 0% or THV aligned completely within the LA and (**B**) −20% or THC aligned 20% into LV and 80% into LA. Neo-LVOT surface area modeling in this case demonstrates low risk of LVOT obstruction. *Simulated neo-LVOT. Ao, aorta; F, interatrial fossa; LA, left atrium; LV, left ventricle; LVOT, left ventricular outflow tract; MVR, mitral valve replacement; THV, simulated transcatheter heart valve.

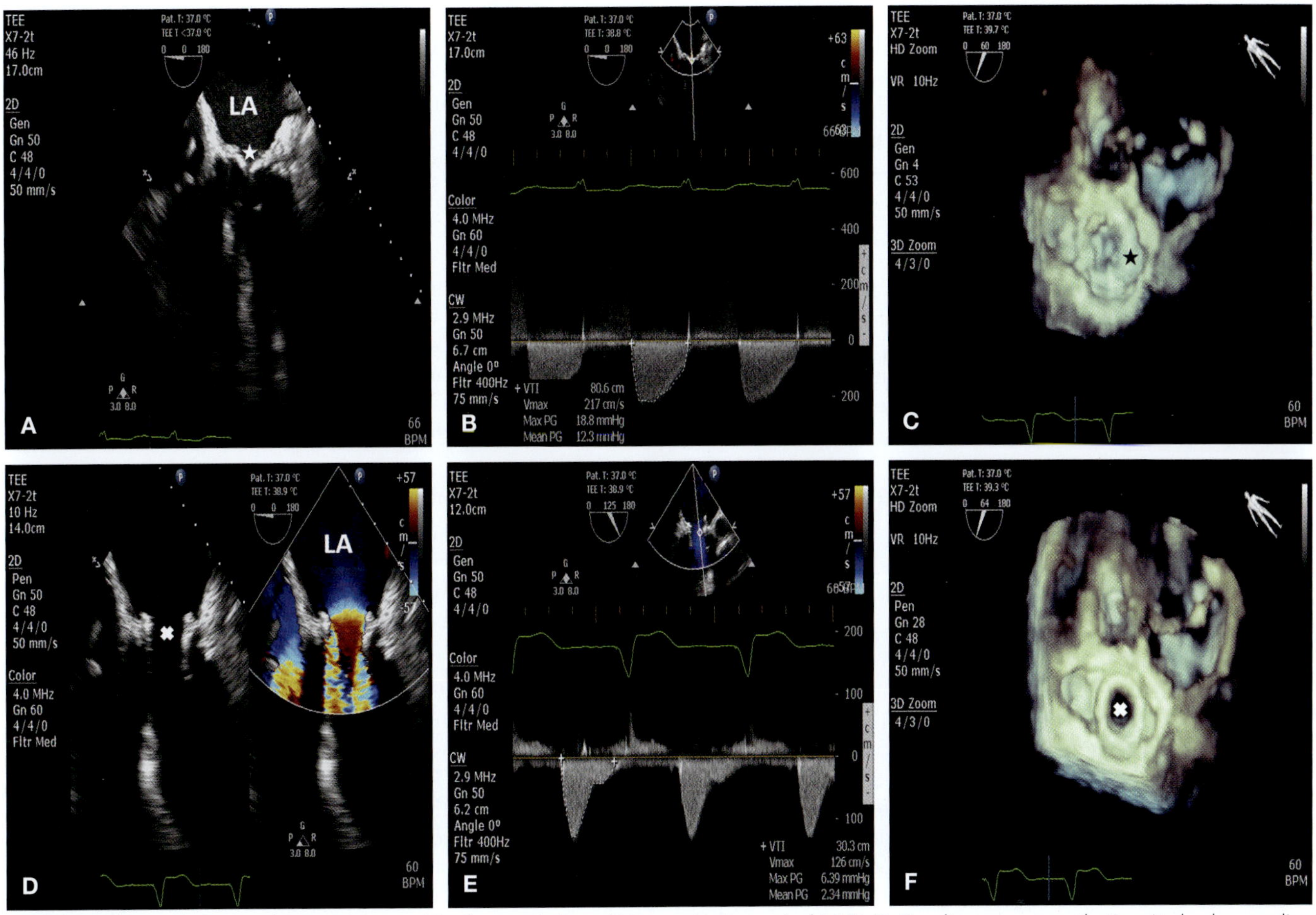

FIGURE 38.22 **A,** Severe degeneration and leaflet restriction of bioprosthetic surgical MVR. **B,** Baseline mean prosthetic mitral valve gradient 12.3 mm Hg. **C,** 3D zoom of bioprosthetic surgical MVR with leaflet restriction demonstrated in diastole. **D,** Post TMVR with complete leaflet opening/flattening against valve frame. **E,** Post TMVR mean mitral valve gradient 2.3 mm Hg. **F,** 3D zoom post TMVR showing leaflet opening in diastole. *Bioprosthetic surgical AVR. X (TMVR). LA, left atrium; MVR, mitral valve replacement; TMVR, transcatheter mitral valve replacement.

3D, or 3D MPR. During deployment, balloon-expandable valves shorten almost exclusively from the atrial side such that the landing zone can be assessed by the ventricular portion of the stent. Positioning of the device too atrial can increase risk of skirt leak and worst case scenario device embolization; while too ventricular of a position can increase risk of LVOTO. For ViR or ViMAC cases utilizing balloon-expandable transcatheter valves, unless otherwise predicted by CT, the most desirable position is ~80% of valve stent in the LV and 20% in the LA.[12-14] For ViV TMVR, the stent frame is typically aligned with the ventricular edge of the existing bioprosthesis, which is often assessed by fluoroscopic markers. Immediately after TMVR deployment, assessment of anchoring,

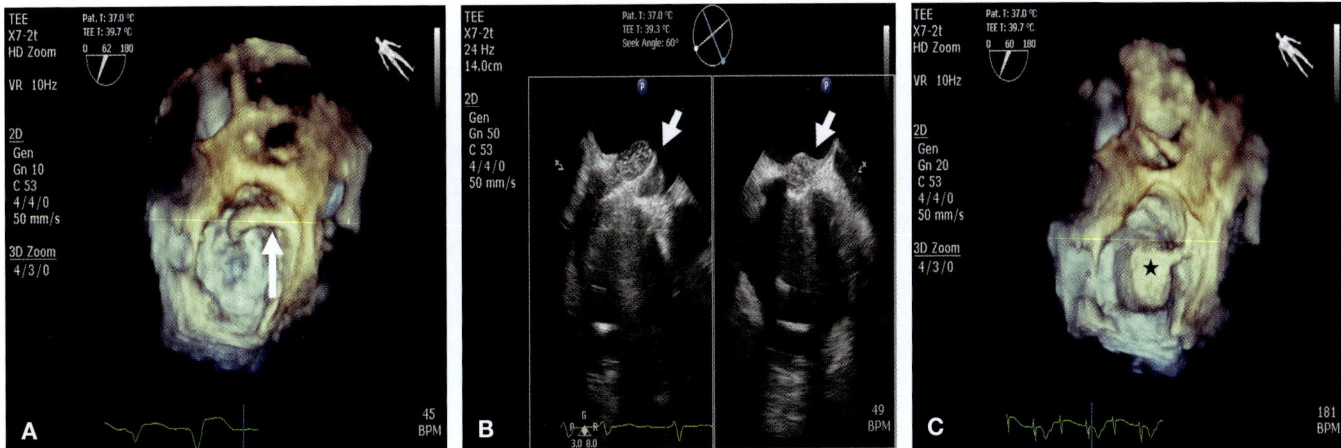

FIGURE 38.23 **A,** Trans-septal sheath (*white arrow*) across interatrial septum and across surgical mitral valve prosthesis. **B,** 2D biplane view (commissural/long axis angles) of pre-TMVR balloon dilation (*white arrows*). **C,** 3D zoom of pre-TMVR balloon dilation (*black star*). TMVR, transcatheter mitral valve replacement.

position, seal, valve function, and LVOT flow/gradients must be performed. Final assessment should include 2D/3D leaflet motion, ruling out central/paravalvular regurgitation, final MV diastolic gradient, biventricular function, wall motion, flow direction across the iatrogenic atrial septal defect, and development of pericardial effusion (**Fig. 38.22D-F**).

Postprocedural Evaluation

Routine follow-up with TTE prior to discharge and at 3 to 6 month and 1-year follow-up should be obtained. If any evidence of morphologic valve deterioration is present along with prosthetic valve dysfunction (increase in mean diastolic gradient at similar heart rate or new/worsening regurgitation), the patient should be referred for TEE and possible cardiac CT as deemed necessary.

TRANSCUTANEOUS AORTIC VALVE REPLACEMENT

CT Planning

TAVR CT has significantly advanced the field and improved clinical outcomes allowing for assessment of everything from vascular access planning to valve sizing to identifying high-risk features and finally assessment of postprocedural complications such as hypoattenuating leaflet thickening (HALT).

CT data acquisition and scanning protocols vary institution to institution and based on scanner manufacturer. Acquisition typically involves ECG-gated scanning of the aortic root, valvular, and subvalvular structures and nongated scanning of the aorta, carotid, subclavian, iliac, and femoral vessels.[18] ECG-gated data of thoracic structures are acquired covering the entire cardiac cycle to ensure both systolic and diastolic measurements can be obtained. This is typically done with retrospective ECG gating as prospective triggering is more susceptible to heart rate variability such as ectopic beats and variable R-R intervals in atrial fibrillation.

After scanning is complete, ECG-gated CT data can be reconstructed in an axial data set with <1 mm slice thickness. MPRs of coronal and sagittal planes can then be generated from the primary axial data set. Primary data should be reviewed to ensure anatomic structures of interest appear without any artifacts traversing the field that could affect visualization and accurate measurements. The data set is then typically reconstructed in 10% intervals of the cardiac cycle to identify systolic versus diastolic phases with 0% to 40% corresponding to systole and 50% to 100% corresponding to diastole. Non-ECG gated data of the aorta and additional vasculature are reconstructed into an axial data set with ≤1.5 mm slice thickness.

Aortic Valve Annulus and LVOT Area

For TAVR planning, the aortic valve annulus is a virtual plane defined by the most basal attachment points of the aortic valve cusps. Identification of the basal attachment points and construction of the virtual anulus plane is done in both systolic and diastolic phases to identify the largest and smallest annulus possible. The process of creating the virtual plane is software dependent. Once identified, this plane can be traced to identify key measurements, including annular area, perimeter, and maximum/minimum dimensions (**Fig. 38.24**). Ideal imaging should encompass sharp annular contours separating contrasted blood pool from the aortic annulus and exclude image artifacts and noise.

After the virtual annular plane has been created and measured, a line perpendicular to this plane can be measured 5 mm into the LV to identify the LVOT plane. A similar area and maximum/minimum dimension should be measured.

Device Sizing

The device landing zone comprises the aortic valve cusps, aortic annulus, and the LVOT. Device sizing is based on manufacturer-specific measurements of individual TAVR valves relative to either annulus area or circumference. If sizing is based on annular area such as for Sapien 3 Ultra devices (Edwards), the current recommendation is to use a device that ranges between 5% undersized to up to 20% oversized relative to the annulus. The % over/undersizing can be calculated by ([TAVR nominal area measurement − CT annulus area]/[CT annulus area]) × 100.

Special Considerations

Attention should be made to the degree of annular and subannular calcification given increased risk of paravalvular leak (PVL) or root injury with aggressive oversizing (specifically with large, spiculated, and protruding nodules).

Coronary Heights

Left and right coronary heights should be measured from the virtual annulus to the ostium of the coronary artery in both systolic and diastolic phases (**Fig. 38.25**). Coronary ostial height <10 mm may be associated with increased risk of coronary occlusion. If coronary heights are borderline or less than the recommended height for TAVR implantation in either native valves or surgical protheses, measurement of coronary ostium to opposing wall or coronary ostium to prosthesis frame can be done to further assess the risk of coronary occlusion (**Fig. 38.26**).

Additional Measurements

Additional diastolic measurements should include sinotubular junction (STJ) dimensions, STJ height, sinus of Valsalva (SOV) dimensions, aortic root angle, commissure heights, and maximum ascending aorta dimensions (**Fig. 38.27**). SOV mean diameter <30 mm may be associated with increased risk of coronary occlusion.[19] STJ diameter and height are important when considering anticipated TAVR device and size to help predict any possible risk of STJ injury. Ascending aorta measurements are conducted to evaluate for aortopathy that may favor surgery if intervention to both valve and aorta are indicated. A root angle >50° should be flagged to the interventional team given associated risks and challenges for optimal catheter trajectory and TAVR delivery.

A C-arm projection (**Fig. 38.28**) should be provided to simulate fluoroscopic C-arm angulation in which the aortic valve cusps overlap for optimal TAVR valve alignment and deployment.

Vasculature Analysis

Sizing analysis of the abdominal aorta, iliac, and femoral vessels is standard and should always be included given that the femoral vessels are the preferred access site for the TAVR procedure. Minimum dimensions via coronal overlay in each segment of the femoral, external iliac, and common iliac artery can be provided to demonstrate sizing, vessel tortuosity, and calcium distribution (**Fig. 38.29**). Corresponding axial cross-sections demonstrate luminal dimension, plaque morphology, calcium distribution, and other important characteristics such as dissection flaps.

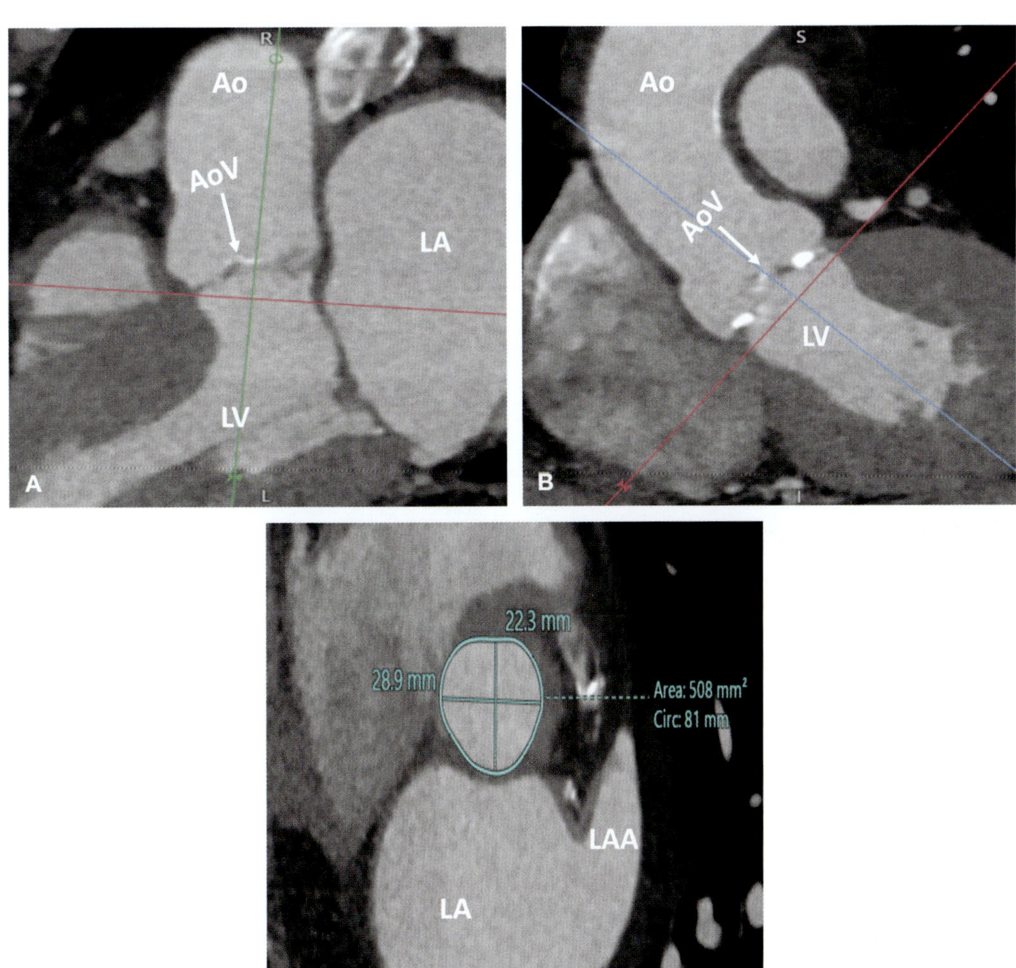

FIGURE 38.24 **A,** Former sagittal plane aligned at base of right coronary cusp of aortic valve for virtual annular plane. **B,** Former coronal plane aligned at base of left and noncoronary cusps of aortic valve to define virtual annulus plane. **C,** En face view of virtual annulus with dimensions, area, and perimeter reported. Ao, aorta; AoV, aortic valve; LA, left atrium; LAA, left atrial appendage; LV, left ventricle.

In cases in which femoral access is not feasible, alternative access can be planned to include carotid, subclavian, and transcaval access. Carotid sizing should also be routinely provided for cerebral embolic protection planning as deemed appropriate.

Post TAVR Echocardiographic Assessment

Post-TAVR Echocardiography is important for obtaining baseline gradients and effective orifice area and for evaluating for PVL. Measurements should include peak and mean gradients across the TAVR prosthesis using continuous wave Doppler. Neo-LVOT diameter can be acquired using a zoomed systolic frame in which the outer-to-outer stent diameter is ideally measured.[20,21] A corresponding pulsed wave Doppler of the LVOT velocity should be acquired with the sample volume just apical to the transcatheter valve.

Follow-up routine echocardiograms should be obtained, and any clinical change should also prompt further evaluation for prosthetic valve dysfunction. According to VARC3 criteria,[22] prosthetic valve dysfunction may include structural valve deterioration inherent to the prosthesis itself, nonstructural dysfunction including PVL and patient-prosthesis mismatch, leaflet thrombosis, and endocarditis. Significant hemodynamic changes should be noted including a change in mean gradient in the context of the patients' prior and current left ventricular ejection fraction and blood pressure hemodynamics (**Table 38.2**). Additional morphologic changes, such as leaflet thickening, decreased mobility, calcification, and pannus, should be compared to baseline morphology performed 1 to 3 months postintervention.

New or worsening TAVR regurgitation must be thoroughly investigated.[23,24] By TTE, PVL should be evaluated in parasternal long and short axis views and may require sweeping the probe back and forth from aorta through LVOT to best evaluate for any eccentric jets or jets obscured by acoustic shadowing. The circumferential extent on short axis imaging is helpful in assessing severity but can also over- or underestimate severity depending on jet origin location and jet splay as it expands in the LVOT. Low or high stent position, noncircular/irregular shape, and free space between stent frame and native annulus are all red flags for significant PVL. Apical 3- and 5-chamber views should also be acquired with lateral-medial, anterior-posterior, and rotational sweeps to identify the largest jet origin. The width of the jet at its origin in parasternal and apical views in relation to LVOT diameter may be the most helpful in characterizing regurgitant lesion severity. Further comprehensive evaluation includes pressure half-time, RV estimation by difference in right and left ventricular stroke volumes, and pulse wave Doppler of the abdominal and thoracic aorta demonstrating holodiastolic flow reversal. Other echocardiographic clues include

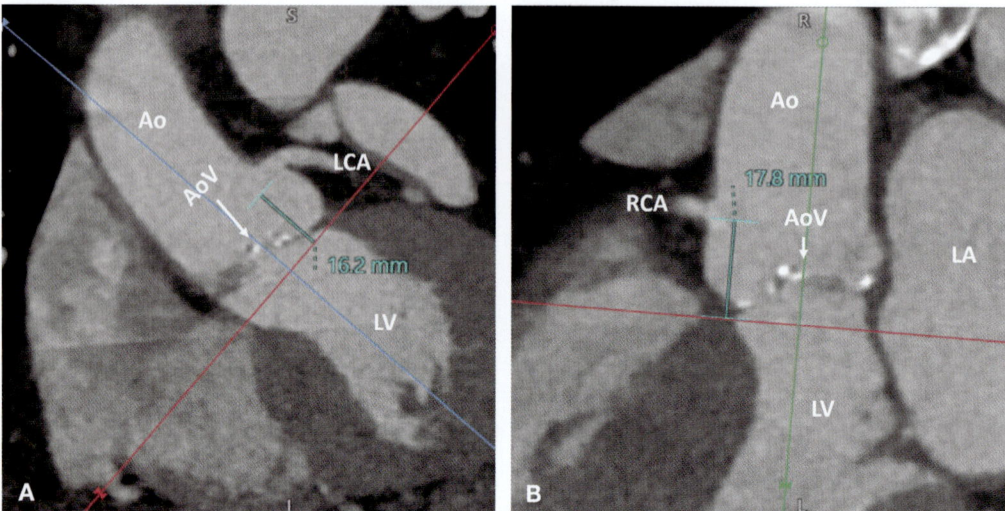

FIGURE 38.25 **A,** Left coronary height from aortic valve annulus to left main coronary artery ostium. **B,** Right coronary height from aortic valve annulus to right coronary artery ostium. Ao, aorta; AoV, aortic valve; LA, left atrium; LAA, left atrial appendage; LCA, left coronary artery; LV, left ventricle; RCA, right coronary artery.

increase in LV size or worsening of LV ejection fraction, but this may take some time to develop.

If any suspicion is raised about the severity of central or paravalvular regurgitation, additional imaging modalities such as TEE, cardiovascular magnetic resonance, or fluoroscopy/hemodynamic assessment should be considered. **Figure 38.30** demonstrates a case of paravalvular regurgitation detected on routine TTE with severe PVL confirmed on supplemental TEE images. CT imaging was utilized to characterize PVL size for transcatheter closure planning (**Fig. 38.31**).

Post-TAVR CT Assessment

Post-TAVR CT assessment may be indicated in patients who have developed new or worsening heart failure symptoms, a new murmur picked up on physical examination, or significant increase in gradients from baseline identified by echocardiogram.[18] CT can assist in the identification of post-TAVR complications, such as HALT, valve thrombosis, and infective endocarditis. **Figure 38.32** demonstrates HALT in a patient referred for CT due to a significant increase in transvalvular gradients from baseline.

TRICUSPID VALVE IMAGING

Tricuspid regurgitation (TR) in the setting of right heart failure is an independent predictor of morbidity and mortality. As transcatheter technologies have developed, intervention for TR has become more feasible.[25] Multiple clinical trials are ongoing to evaluate effectiveness and clinical outcomes in TR intervention and currently include devices for tricuspid valve edge-to-edge repair (TV TEER), transcatheter tricuspid valve replacement, and caval valve implantation (CAVI).

Preprocedural TEE

Screening for TR severity by echocardiography includes a thorough qualitative and quantitative evaluation similar to that of MR.[26-28]

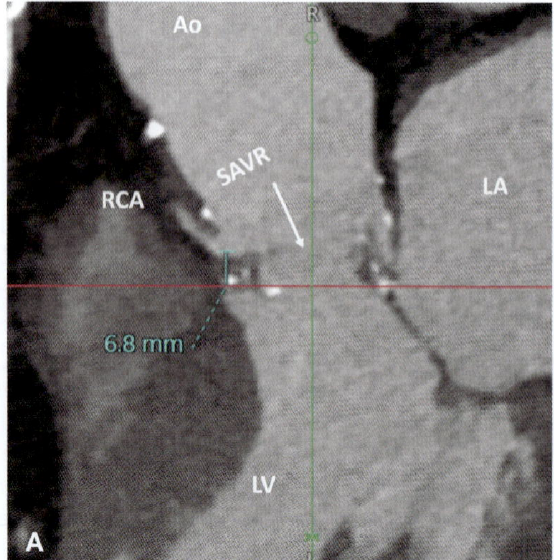

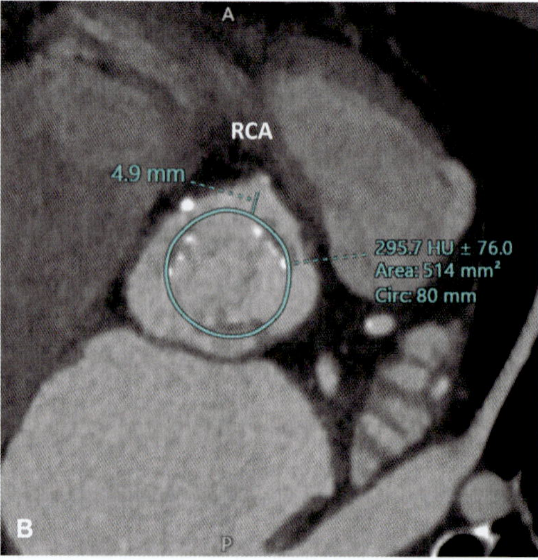

FIGURE 38.26 **A,** Surgical aortic valve annulus to right coronary artery ostium height (6.8 mm) indicating at risk coronary artery. **B,** Surgical aortic valve frame to right coronary ostium distance (4.9 mm). Ao, aorta; AVR, aortic valve replacement; LA, left atrium; LV, left ventricle; RCA, right coronary artery.

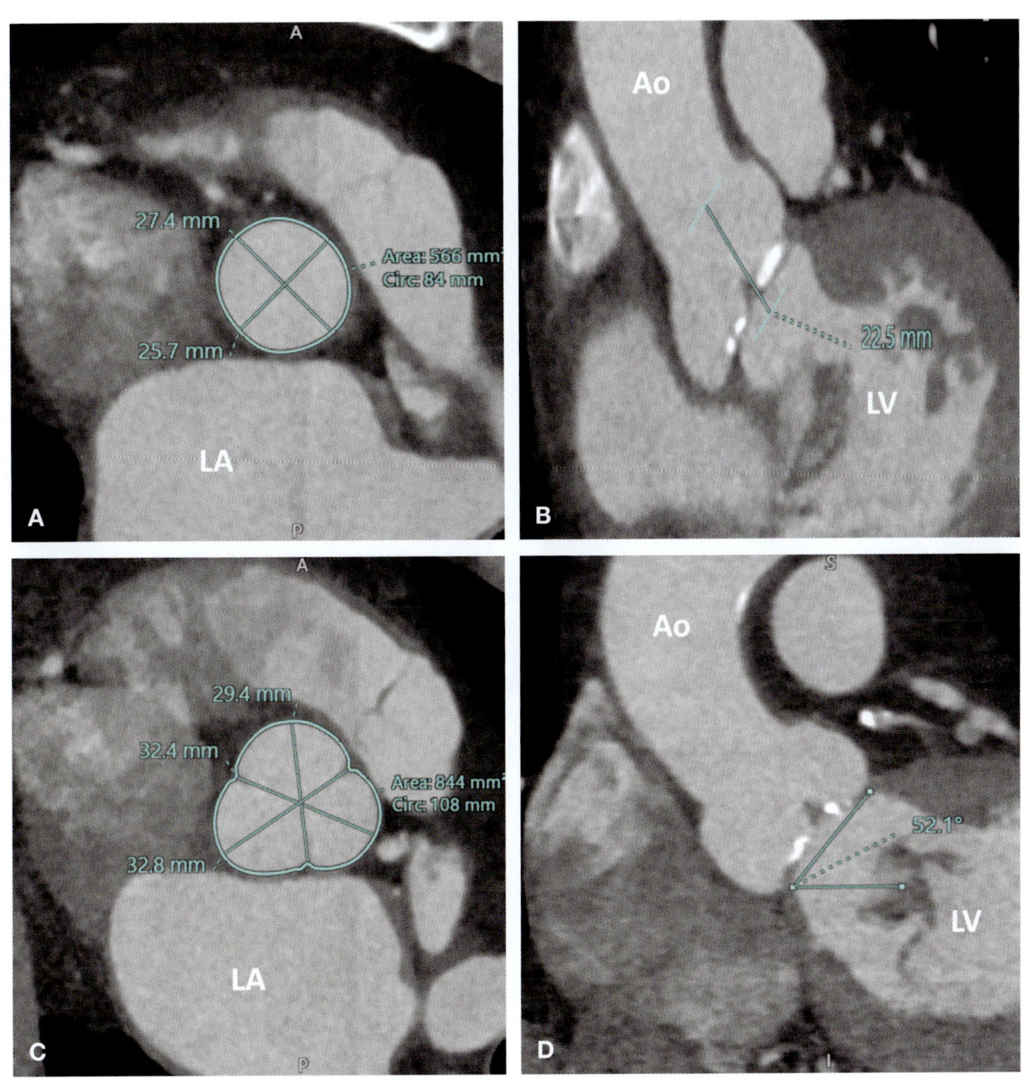

FIGURE 38.27 **A,** Sinotubular junction area and dimensions. **B,** Sinotubular junction height. **C,** Sinus of Valsalva area and dimensions. **D,** Aorta root angle. Ao, aorta; LA, left atrium; LV, left ventricle.

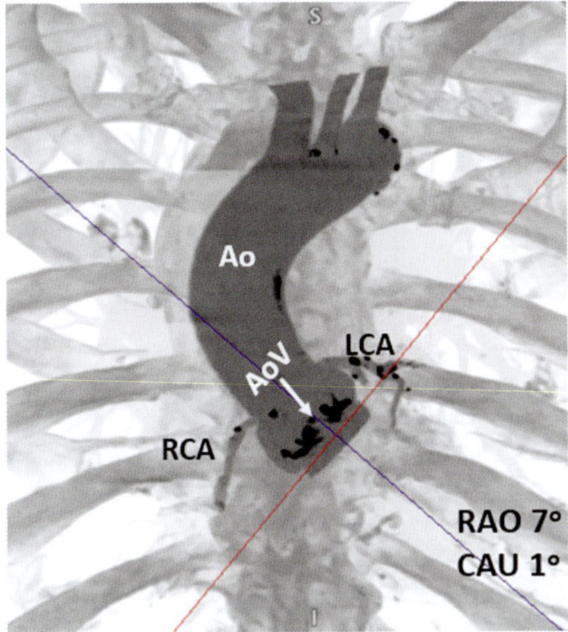

FIGURE 38.28 Simulated fluoroscopic C-arm angulation for optimal cusp overlap for TAVR implantation. Ao, aorta; AoV, aortic valve; LCA, left coronary artery; LV, left ventricle; RCA, right coronary artery; TAVR, transcutaneous aortic valve replacement.

Understanding leaflet anatomy, mechanism of TR (primary/secondary/pacemaker-lead related), and the geography of nearby native or implanted intracardiac structures are important for potential device selection and intervention.

Screening echocardiogram should include evaluation of right atrial (RA) size and right ventricular (RV) size/function by 2D and 3D methods and potentially RV strain as applicable. With TEE, identifying the TR mechanism should be undertaken by full visualization of TV leaflets at multiple angles and levels including midesophageal, deep esophageal, and transgastric windows (**Fig. 38.33**). Color Doppler, biplane imaging, and color compare mode can be utilized to help define TR jet origin and direction. As part of this assessment, VC width should be measured and 2D PISA should be used to calculate regurgitant orifice area and RV. An additional quantitative parameter for TR severity includes RV calculation by continuity method comparing stroke volume across the TV and pulmonic valves (assuming no significant pulmonic valve disease is present). This requires accurate right ventricular outflow tract (RVOT) diameter and tricuspid annular diameter (or preferably area acquired by 3D MPR) in addition to pulse wave Doppler at the tricuspid annulus and RVOT. Each parameter has its own limitations and may be prone to measurement error depending on method of quantification used and TR characteristics. Issues include noncircular regurgitant orifice area, eccentric jets, multiple jets, etc. Hepatic vein systolic flow reversal is also a specific marker

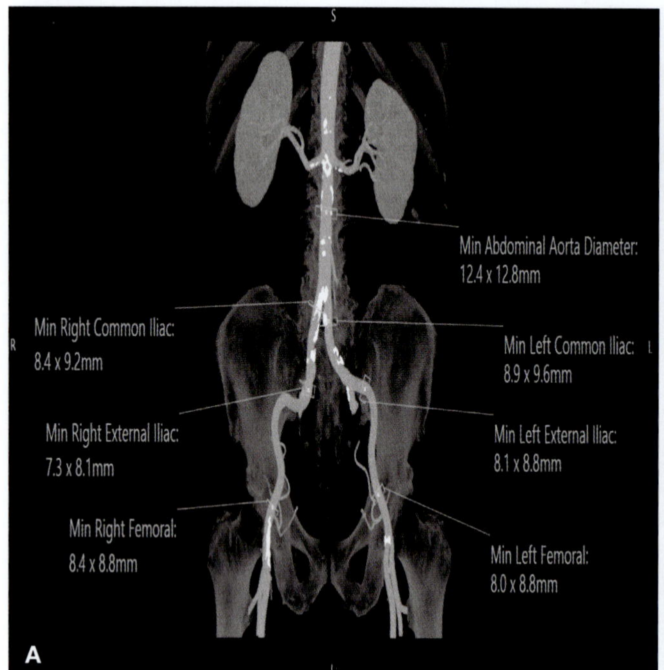

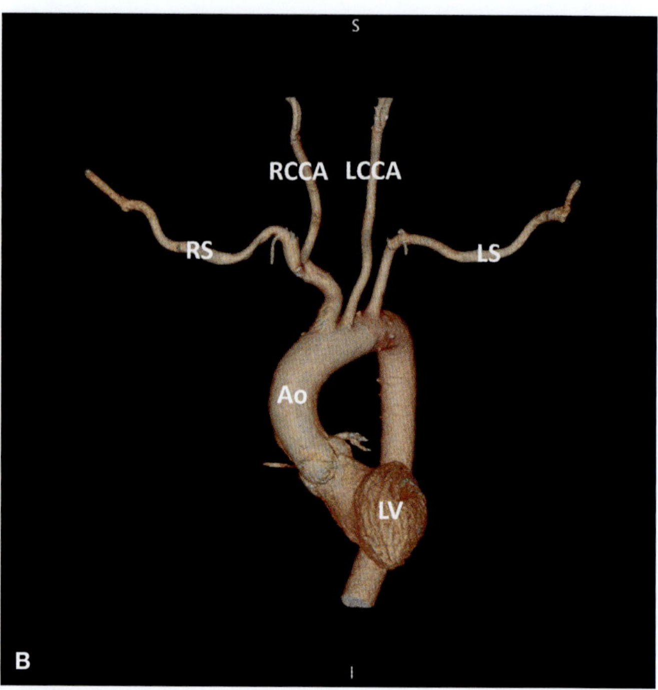

FIGURE 38.29 **A,** Coronal overlay demonstrating minimum dimensions of femoral, external iliac, common iliac arteries, and aorta. **B,** 3D volume rendering of aorta, subclavian, and carotid vessels. Ao, aorta; LCCA, left common carotid artery; LS, left subclavian artery; LV, left ventricle; RCCA, right common carotid artery; RS, right subclavian artery.

for TR severity but may be impacted by RA size/compliance and RV function.[26] Visualization of TV leaflets in 3D from mid/deep-esophageal and transgastric windows assists greatly in understanding TR mechanism including leaflet malcoaptation, interaction with pacemaker/defibrillator leads, or flail/prolapsing segments. It is also beneficial in defining the number of TV leaflets present. Additionally, 3D VC may further help delineate severity by a quantitative approach given the inherent noncircular regurgitant orifice area of TR (**Fig. 38.34**). If discordant findings of TR severity with patient symptoms/exam exist, invasive hemodynamics from right heart catheterization may be utilized to evaluate for findings such as elevated RA pressure and ventricularization of RA wave forms. Additionally, cardiac MRI may also be considered in appropriate patients to help quantify TR RV/regurgitant fraction and to assess RV size and function.

Preprocedural CT

Cardiac CT is important for device planning and sizing.[27-29] TV CT scanning is done via ECG-gated retrospective acquisition covering the entire cardiac cycle. The contrast bolus is timed for optimal opacification of right heart structures. Once completed, MPR allows for measurement of the tricuspid annulus at its largest area/dimensions in end diastole (**Fig. 38.35A-C**). Additional measurements can be made to nearby structures of significance such as annulus to papillary muscle distance for transcatheter TV replacement planning (**Fig. 38.35D**) and RA/IVC junction distance to hepatic vein distance for CAVI. Cardiac CT is also helpful for identifying the best fluoroscopic angle for coplanar alignment along the tricuspid annulus (**Fig. 38.35E**). With retrospective acquisition, a full cardiac cycle data set can be reconstructed to demonstrate contrast reflux into the IVC and hepatic veins (**Fig. 38.35F**).

TABLE 38.2 Bioprosthetic Valve Deterioration Classification

	MODERATE HEMODYNAMIC VALVE DETERIORATION	SEVERE HEMODYNAMIC VALVE DETERIORATION
Hemodynamic changes	Compared to baseline: • Increase in mean gradient ≥10 mm Hg resulting in mean gradient ≥20 mm Hg And • Concomitant decrease in EOA ≥0.3 cm^2 or ≥25% And/Or • Decrease in Doppler velocity index ≥0.1 or ≥20%	Compared to baseline: • Increase in mean gradient ≥20 mm Hg resulting in mean gradient ≥30 mm Hg And • Concomitant decrease in EOA ≥0.6 cm^2 or ≥50% And/Or • Decrease in Doppler velocity index ≥0.2 or ≥40%
Change in AR severity	New occurrence or increase of ≥1 grade of intraprosthetic AR resulting in ≥ moderate AR	New occurrence or increase of ≥2 grade of intraprosthetic AR resulting in severe AR

AR, aortic regurgitation.

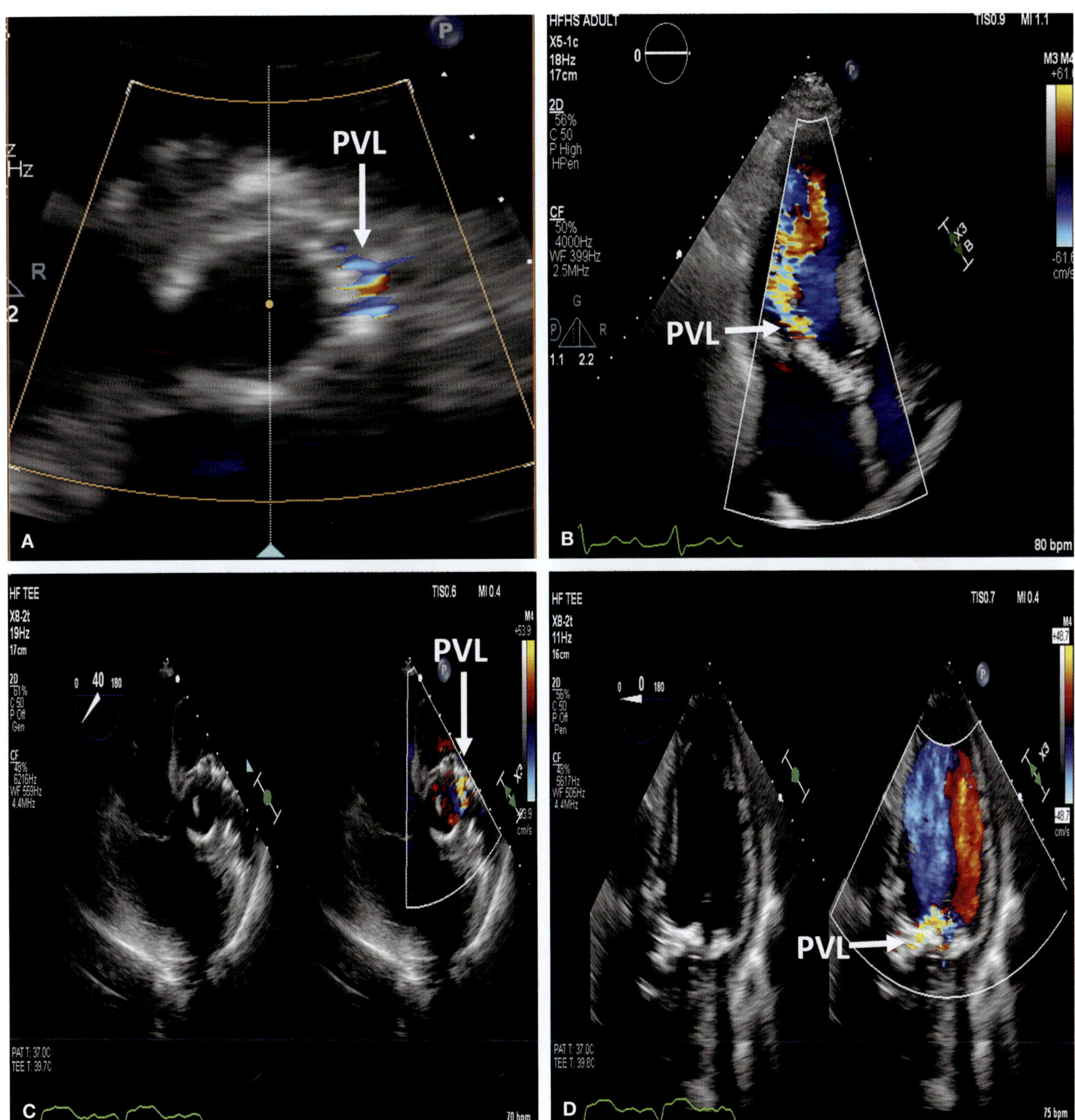

FIGURE 38.30 **A,** TTE short axis of TAVR valve with PVL adjacent to left coronary cusp. **B,** TTE Apical 3-chamber demonstrating severe posterior PVL. **C,** TEE short axis of TAVR valve with PVL adjacent to left coronary cusp. **D,** Deep transgastric view of posteriorly directed PVL. PVL, paravalvular leak; TAVR, transcutaneous aortic valve replacement; TEE, transesophageal echocardiogram; TTE, transthoracic echocardiogram.

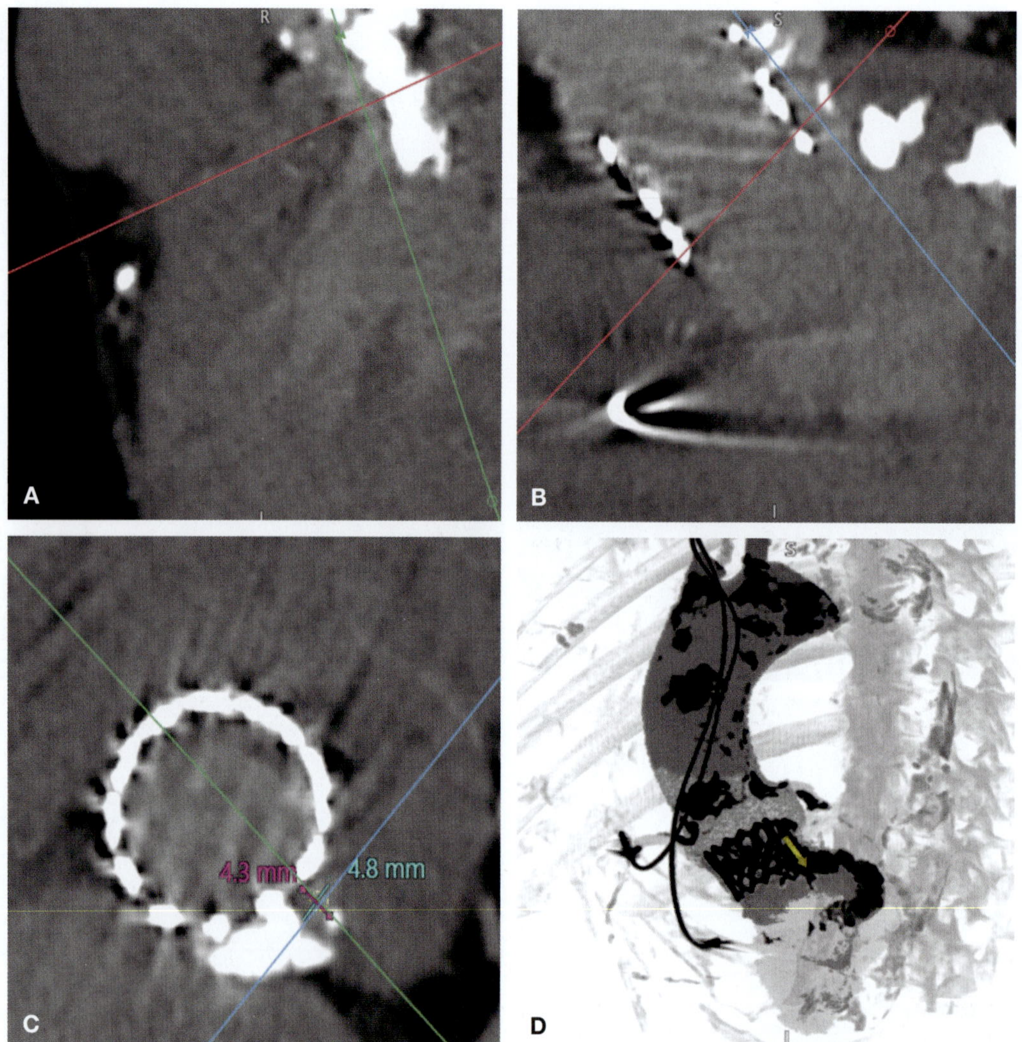

FIGURE 38.31 **A,** Former sagittal plane with red plane through PVL neck. **B,** Former coronal plane with red plane through PVL neck. **C,** En face view of PVL neck with dimensions measuring 4.3 × 4.8 mm. **D,** Simulated C-arm fluoroscopy angle for transcatheter engagement of PVL for closure via retro-aortic approach. PVL, paravalvular leak.

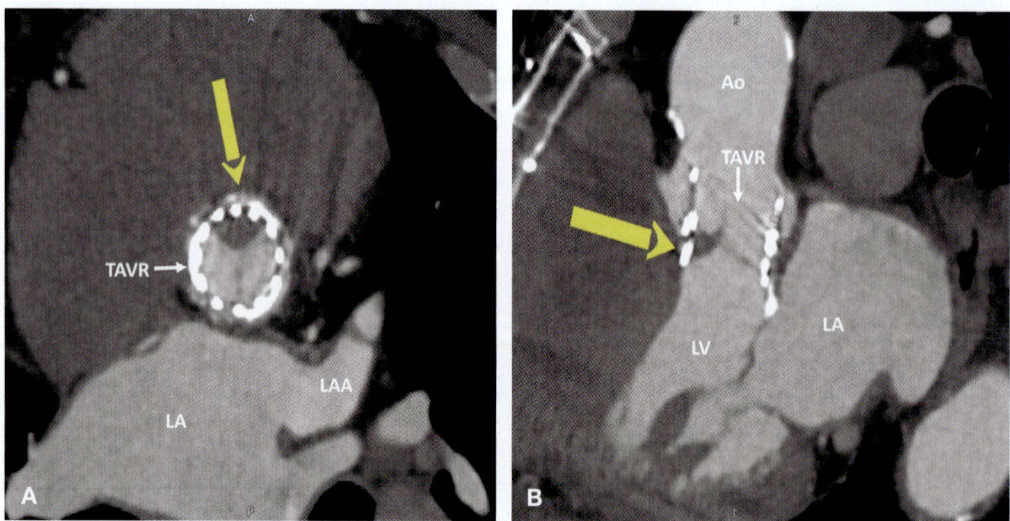

FIGURE 38.32 HALT (hypoattenuating leaflet thickening) of right coronary cusp of TAVR valve (*yellow arrow*). Ao, aorta; LA, left atrium; LAA, left atrial appendage; LV, left ventricle; TAVR, transcutaneous aortic valve replacement.

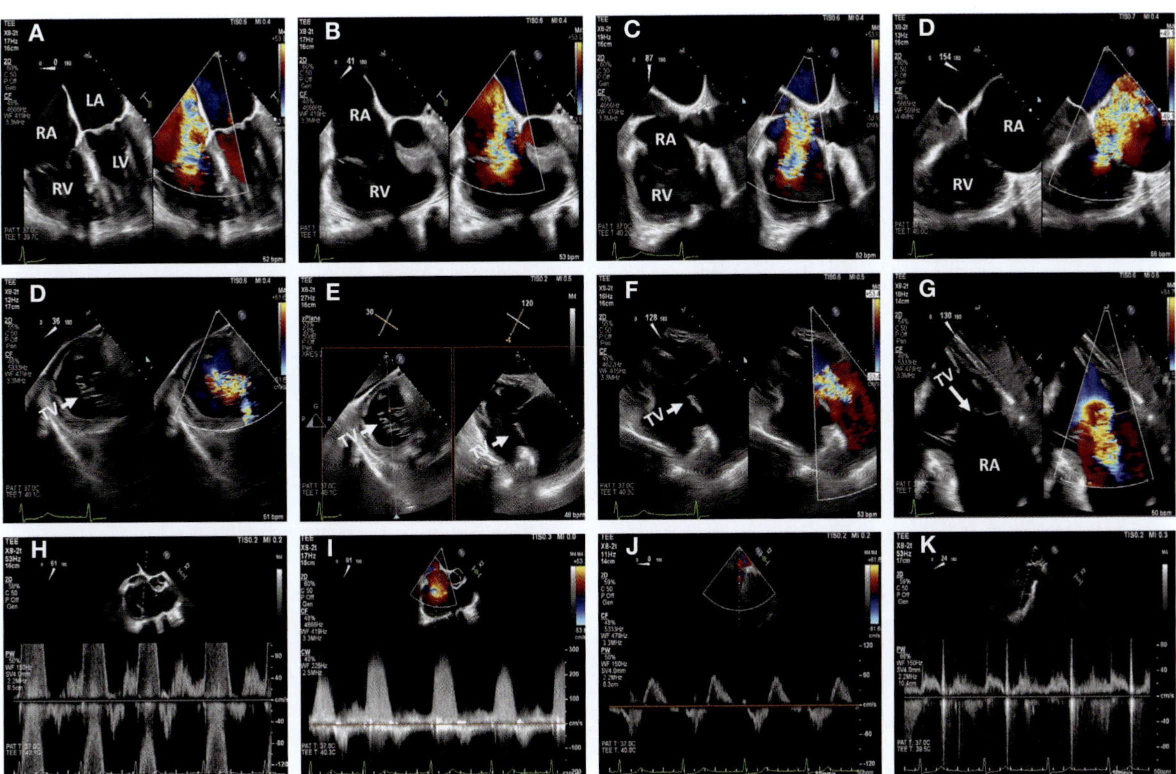

FIGURE 38.33 **A,** Severe TR 0° view. **B,** Severe TR ~45° view (inflow-outflow). **C,** Severe TR ~90° view. **D,** Severe TR 154° view. **D,** Transgastric view of tricuspid valve. **E,** Biplane transgastric short and long axis tricuspid valve. **F,** Transgastric long axis view tricuspid valve. **G,** Deep transgastric view of tricuspid valve. **H,** Pulse wave Doppler at tricuspid valve annulus. **I,** Continuous wave Doppler of tricuspid regurgitant jet. **J,** Pulse wave Doppler demonstrating hepatic vein systolic flow reversal. **K,** Pulse wave Doppler of right ventricular outflow tract from upper esophageal window. LA, left atrium; RA, right atrium; RV, right ventricle; TV, tricuspid valve.

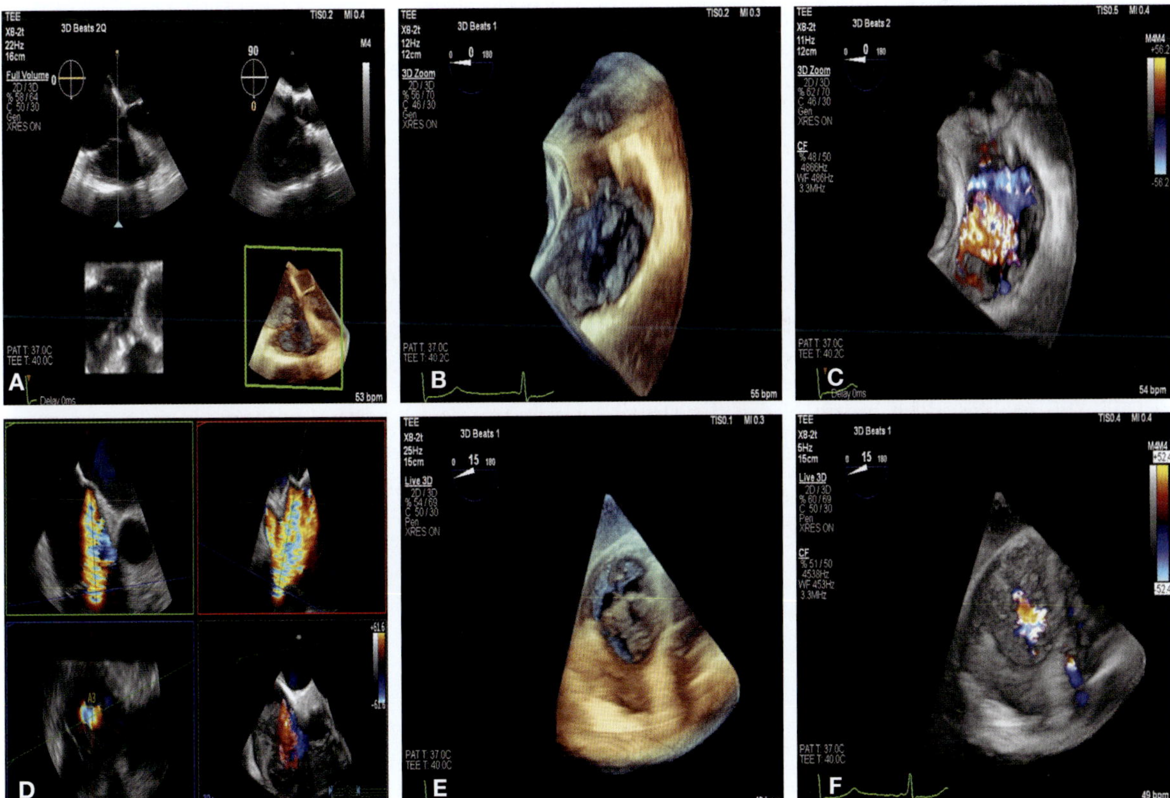

FIGURE 38.34 **A,** Full volume of right ventricle for 3D right ventricular ejection fraction estimation. **B,** 3D zoom of tricuspid valve in midesophageal window. **C,** 3D color of tricuspid regurgitation in midesophageal window. **D,** 3D vena contracta area of tricuspid regurgitation. **E,** Live 3D of tricuspid valve in transgastric window. **F,** 3D color of tricuspid regurgitation in transgastric window.

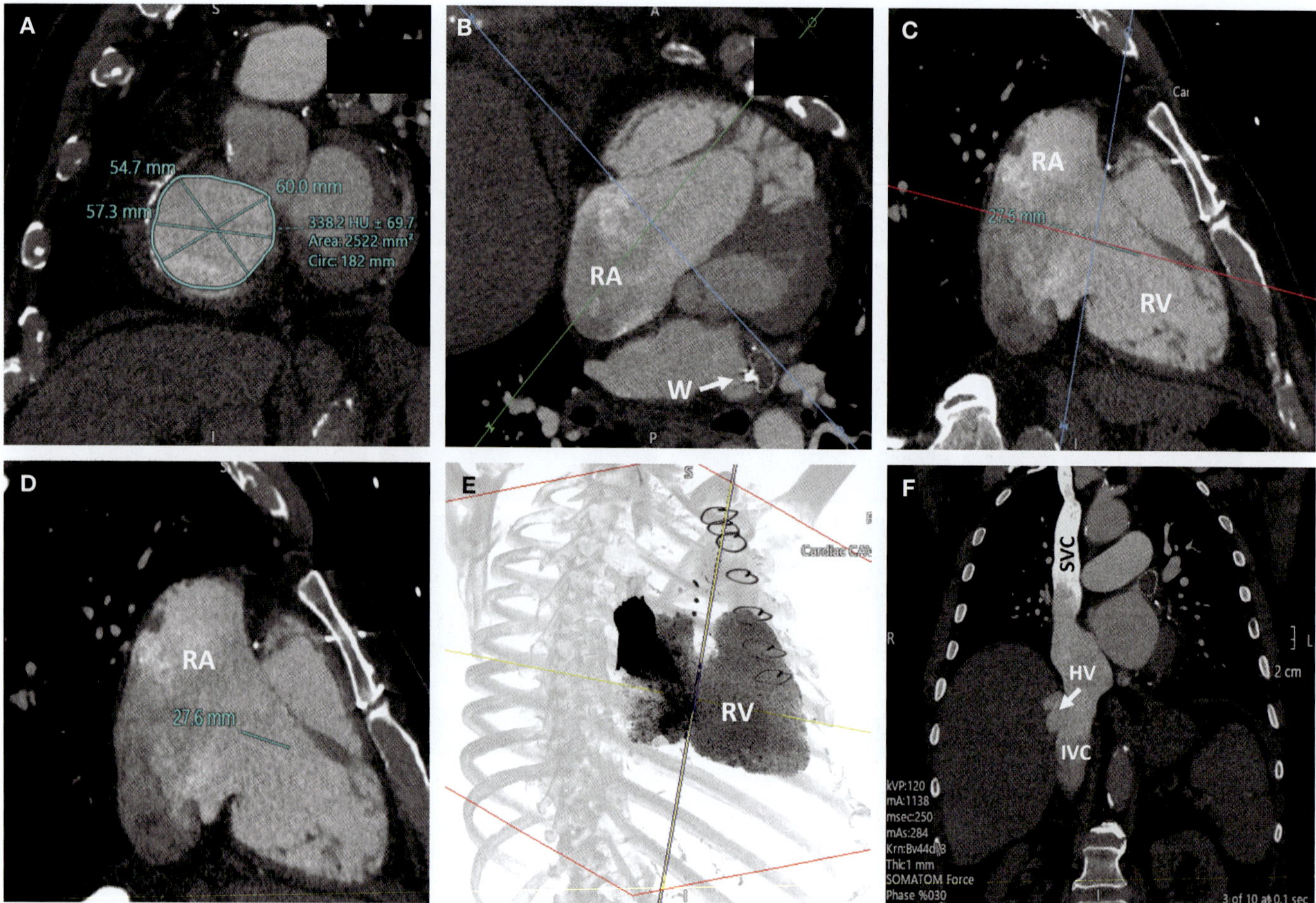

FIGURE 38.35 **A,** En face tricuspid valve annulus with measurements of dimensions, area, and circumference. **B,** Former sagittal plane with blue axis across tricuspid valve annulus. **C,** Former coronal plane with blue axis across tricuspid valve annulus. **D,** Measurement of distance from tricuspid annulus to RV papillary muscle. **E,** Simulated C-arm angle demonstrating best fluoroscopic view for coplanar alignment along tricuspid annulus. **F,** Contrast reflux into IVC and hepatic veins. IVC, inferior vena cava; RA, right atrium; RV, right ventricle; SVC, superior vena cava; W, Watchman device.

PATENT FORAMEN OVALE/ATRIAL SEPTAL DEFECT CLOSURE

In patients who have an indication for patent foramen ovale (PFO) or atrial septal defect (ASD) closure, transcatheter approach has been successfully guided by both intracardiac echocardiography (ICE) and TEE. TEE has the added benefit of superior spatial and temporal resolution compared to current generation ICE catheters. Proper defect sizing is important for device selection. Additionally, for native PFOs/ASDs, identification of sufficient anterior/posterior and SVC/IVC rims is important for device anchoring.

In cases requiring trans-septal access for left heart procedures, occasional closure of iatrogenic ASDs is required in patients with severely elevated right heart pressures such as those with severe pulmonary hypertension or severe TR due to consequential right-to-left or bidirectional shunting. This should be demonstrated by color and pulse wave Doppler prior to removal of left atrial access (**Fig. 38.36A**). A 3D MPR of the defect can be obtained to assist with device sizing (**Fig. 38.36B**). Typically, a midesophageal biplane view of the IAS from both the short axis (anterior-posterior trajectory) and bicaval planes (superior-inferior trajectory) is most helpful to help guide closure (**Fig. 38.36C**). Additionally, 3D imaging can be used for device alignment and identification of disc apposition from both the LA and RA sides (**Fig. 38.36D**).

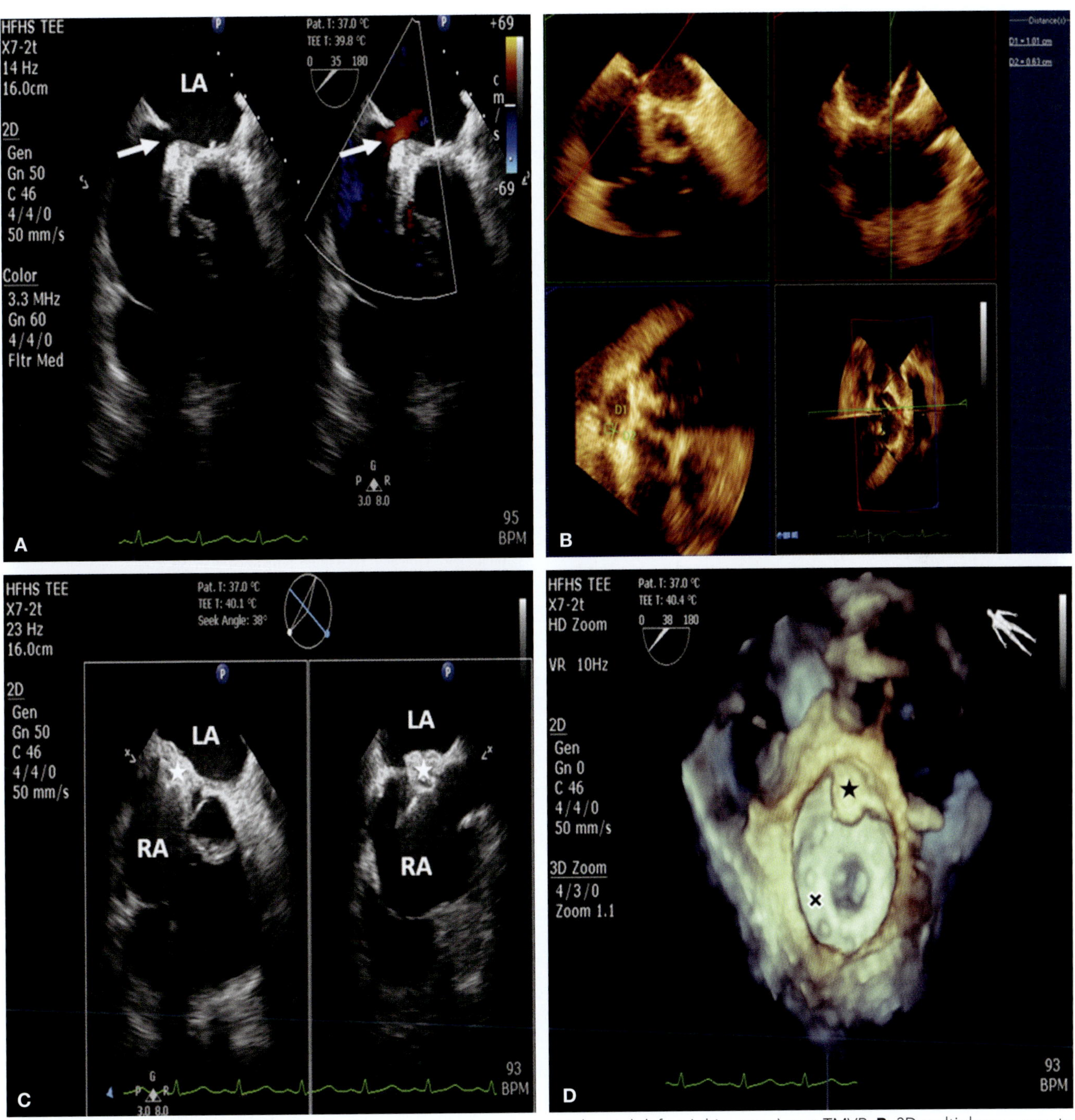

FIGURE 38.36 **A,** Right to left flow by color Doppler across iatrogenic atrial septal defect (white arrow) post TMVR. **B,** 3D multiplanar reconstruction for sizing of iatrogenic atrial septal defect. **C,** Amplatzer septal occluder device (Abbott) sealing iatrogenic atrial septal defect visualized in 2D biplane imaging (short axis on left; bicaval view on right). **D,** 3D zoom of catheter across iatrogenic septal defect with Amplatzer septal occluder device (Abbott). *Amplatzer septal occlude device); × (TMVR). LA, left atrium; RA, right atrium; TMVR, transcatheter mitral valve replacement.

SUMMARY

In summary, there is significant value to pre-, post-, and intra-procedural imaging for transcatheter interventions. The field of structural heart imaging has grown immensely with the integration of multiple imaging modalities for procedural planning/guidance in conjunction with the expertise of the interventional imaging physician and the development of transcatheter technologies. Structural imaging is a tool utilized by interventional imaging physicians to understand the engineering behind each type of transcatheter device in order to guide multidisciplinary heart team discussions on optimal patient-specific anatomical treatment pathways. Structural imaging is not just about providing images but about the physician know-how required to integrate patient-specific pathology and anatomy to novel device-specific technologies.

References

1. Faletra FF, Saric M, Saw J, et al. Imaging for patient's selection and guidance of LAA and ASD percutaneous and surgical closure. *JACC Cardiovasc Imaging*. 14(1):3-21.
2. Korsholm K, Berti S, Iriart X, et al. Expert recommendations on cardiac computed tomography for planning transcatheter left atrial appendage occlusion. *JACC Cardiovasc Interv*. 2020;13(3):277-292.
3. Kaafarani M, Saw J, Daniels M, et al. Role of CT imaging in left atrial appendage occlusion for the Watchman device. *Cardiovasc Diagn Ther*. 2020;10(1):45-58.
4. Vainrib AF, Harb SC, Jaber W, et al. Left arial appendage occlusion/exclusion: procedural image guidance with transesophageal echocardiography. *J Am Soc Echocardiogr*. 2017;31(4):454-474.
5. Grayburn P, Thomas JD. Basic Principles of the echocardiographic evaluation of mitral regurgitation. *JACC Cardiovasc Imaging*. 2021;14(4):843-853.
6. Zoghbi WA, Adams D, Bonow RO, et al. Recommendations for noninvasive evaluation of native valvular regurgitation. *J Am Soc Echocardiogr*. 2017;30(4):303-371.
7. Mackenson GB, Garcia-Sayan E. *Patient selection for transcatheter mitral leaflet repair. Transcatheter Edge-to-Edge Repair*. Asgar AW, Rogers JH. 2022.
8. Flint N, Price MJ, Little SH, et al. State of the art: transcatheter edge-to-edge repair for complex mitral regurgitation. *J Am Soc Echocardiogr*. 2021;34(10):1025-1037.
9. Hensey M, Brown RA, Lal S, et al. Transcatheter mitral valve replacement: an update on current techniques, technologies, and future directions. *JACC Cardiovasc Interv*. 2021;14(5):489-500.
10. Reid A, Ben Zekry S, Turaga M, et al. Neo-LVOT and transcatheter mitral valve replacement: expert recommendations. *JACC Cardiovasc Imaging*. 2021;14(4):854-866.
11. Bapat V. Valve-in-valve apps: why and how they were developed and how to use them. *Eurointervention*. 2014;10(suppl U):U44-U51.
12. Little SH, Bapat V, Blanke P, Guerrero M, Rajagopal V, Siegel R. Imaging guidance for transcatheter mitral valve intervention on prosthetic valves, rings, and annular calcification. *JACC Cardiovasc Imaging*. 2021;14(1):22-40.
13. Garcia-Sayan E, Chen T, Khalique OK. Multimodality cardiac imaging for procedural planning and guidance of transcatheter mitral valve replacement and mitral paravalvular leak closure. *Front Cardiovasc Med*. 2021;8:582925.
14. Blanke P, Naoum C, Webb J, et al. Multimodality imaging in the context of transcatheter mitral valve replacement: establishing consensus among modalities and disciplines. *JACC Cardiovasc Imaging*. 2015;8(10):1191-1208.
15. Hashimoto G, Lopes BBC, Sato H, et al. Computed tomography planning for transcatheter mitral valve replacement. *Struct Heart*. 2022;6(1):100012.
16. Ge Y, Gupta S, Fentanes E, et al. Role of cardiac CT in pre-procedure planning for transcatheter mitral valve replacement. *JACC Cardiovasc Imaging*. 2021;14(8):1571-1580.
17. Wang DD, Eng MH, Greenbaum AB, et al. Validating a prediction modeling tool for left ventricular outflow tract (LVOT) obstruction after transcatheter mitral valve replacement (TMVR). *Catheter Cardiovasc Interv*. 2018;92(2):379-387.
18. Blanke P, Weir-McCall JR, Achenbach S, et al. Computed tomography imaging in the context of transcatheter aortic valve implantation (TAVI)/transcatheter aortic valve replacement (TAVR): an expert consensus document of the Society of Cardiovascular Computed Tomography. *J Cardiovasc Comput Tomogr*. 2019;13:1-20.
19. Ribeiro HB, Webb JG, Makkar RR, et al. Predictive factors, management, and clinical outcomes of coronary obstruction following transcatheter aortic valve implantation: insights from a large multicenter registry. *JACC (J Am Coll Cardiol)*. 2013;62(17):1552-1562.
20. Hahn RT, Nicoara A, Kapadia S, Svensson L, Martin R. Echocardiographic imaging for transcatheter aortic valve replacement. *J Am Soc Echocardiogr*. 2018;31(4):405-433.
21. Hahn RT, Leipsic J, Douglas PS, et al. Comprehensive echocardiographic assessment of normal transcatheter valve function. *JACC Cardiovasc Imaging*. 2019;12(1):25-34.
22. Genereux P, Généreux P, Piazza N, et al. Valve academic research consortium 3: updated endpoint definitions for aortic valve clinical research. *J Am Coll Cardiol*. 2021;77(21):2717-2746.
23. Pibarot P, Hahn RT, Weissman NJ, Monaghan MJ. Assessment of paravalvular regurgitation following TAVR: a proposal of unifying grading scheme. *JACC Cardiovasc Imaging*. 2015;8(3):340-360.
24. Zoghbi WA, Asch FM, Bruce C, et al. Guideilnes for the evaluation of valvular regurgitation after percutaneous valve repair or replacement. *J Am Soc Echocardiogr*. 2019;32(7):914-917.
25. Hahn RT, Nabauer M, Zuber M, et al. Intraprocedural imaging of transcatheter tricuspid valve interventions. *JACC Cardiovasc Imaging*. 2019;12(3):532-553.
26. Hahn RT, Mahmood F, Kodali S, et al. Core competencies in Echocardiography for imaging Structural Heart disease interventions: an expert consensus statement. *JACC Cardiovasc Imaging*. 2019;12(12):2560-2570.
27. Khalique OK, Cavalcante JL, Shah D, et al. Multimodality imaging of the tricuspid valve and right heart anatomy. *JACC Cardiovasc Imaging*. 2019;12(3):516-531.
28. Singulane CC, Singh A, Addetia K, Yamat M, Lang RM. Developing insights regarding tricuspid valve regurgitation: morphology, assessment of severity, and the need for a novel grading scheme. *Struct Heart*. 2022;6(1):100026.
29. Agricola E, Asmarats L, Maisano F, et al. Imaging for tricuspid valve repair and replacement. *JACC Cardiovasc Imaging*. 2021;14(1):61-111.

Atrial Septal Defect and Patent Foramen Ovale

Fareed Moses S. Collado and Clifford J. Kavinsky

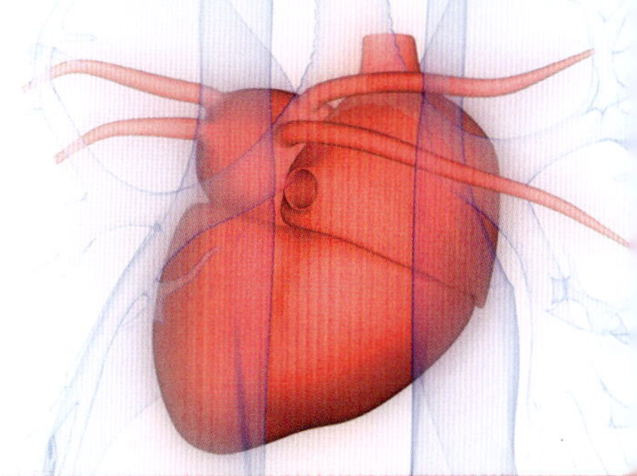

EMBRYOLOGY OF THE ATRIAL SEPTUM

The interatrial septum is developed by a series of embryological events formed by the septum primum, the anterosuperior and the posteroinferior cushions of the atrioventricular (AV) canal, the septum secundum, the left sinus valve, and the "spina vestibuli."[1] In the sixth week of development, the primary atrium is formed by several embryological changes forming a single cavity. Once the formation of the primary atrium is complete, atrial septation begins.

The first indication of atrial septation is the formation of the primary atrial septum or the ***septum primum***. It begins with a muscular crescent growing in the atrial cavity with a mesenchymal cap on its leading edge. Simultaneously, AV endocardial cushions are dividing the AV canal. The space of the leading edge of the ***septum primum*** as it approaches the endocardial cushion forms the primary atrial foramen or the ***ostium primum***. The complete union of the ***septum primum*** and the AV endocardial cushion closes the ***ostium primum***. Prior to closure of the ***ostium primum***, multiple perforations appear in the septum primum to form ***the ostium secundum***. At the anterosuperior rim, a second septum (***septum secundum)*** is formed. It is an in-folding between the junction of the superior caval vein to the right atrium and the right pulmonary veins to the left atrium. The tunneled structure formed by the lower rim of the septum secundum and the ostium secundum is called the foramen ovale (FO).

After completion of septation, the two formed atria each possess a part of the body of the primary atrium, an appendage, a vestibule, and a venous component (pulmonary veins and vena cavae). The two chambers remain in continuity through a tunneled structure formed by the lower rim of the septum secundum and the ostium secundum (part of the septum primum) and form the FO.

During fetal development, placental blood flows from a higher-pressure right atrium to the left atrium through the FO. After birth, lung function and circulation commence, thus increasing left atrial pressure. When the septum primum and septum secundum fuses, the FO closes and the oval depression now becomes the fossa ovalis.

Atrial Septal Defect

Secundum Atrial Septal Defect

The most common atrial septal defect (ASD) is a secundum ASD (**Fig. 39.1B**), accounting for ~75% of all ASDs. The secundum-type defect results from either deficient growth of the septum secundum or excessive resorption of the septum primum. Both scenarios result in a centrally located septal defect (near the area of the fossa ovalis in normal hearts) of varying size, shape, and degree of shunting.

With the exception of very large secundum ASDs (>35 mm), and those defects with insufficient rim tissue to accommodate a closure device, transcatheter closure is recommended over surgery as first-line therapy for ASD closure.[2]

Primum ASD

Primum ASDs (**Fig. 39.1D**) (also referred to as AV septal defects, AV canal defects, and endocardial cushion defects) are less common than the secundum type (15%-20% of all ASDs). Partial primum ASDs consist of an absence of the inferior portion of the interatrial septum and frequently associated with a cleft mitral valve. Complete primum ASDs are marked by an inlet ventricular septal defect (VSD) and a single AV valve.

Sinus Venosus ASD and Unroofed Coronary Sinus

The least common type of ASDs are sinus venosus (~5%) and unroofed coronary sinus (<1%) defects. Sinus venosus defects most commonly result from deficiency of the common wall between the superior vena cava (SVC) and left atrium (**Fig. 39.1A**), involving the superior and posterior portion of the septum, and are invariably associated with an anomalous right upper pulmonary vein draining into the right atrium. Less frequently, the defect is in the inferior-posterior septum, associated with the inferior vena cava (IVC) and an anomalous right lower pulmonary vein draining into the right atrium (**Fig. 39.1C**). The unroofed coronary sinus is an

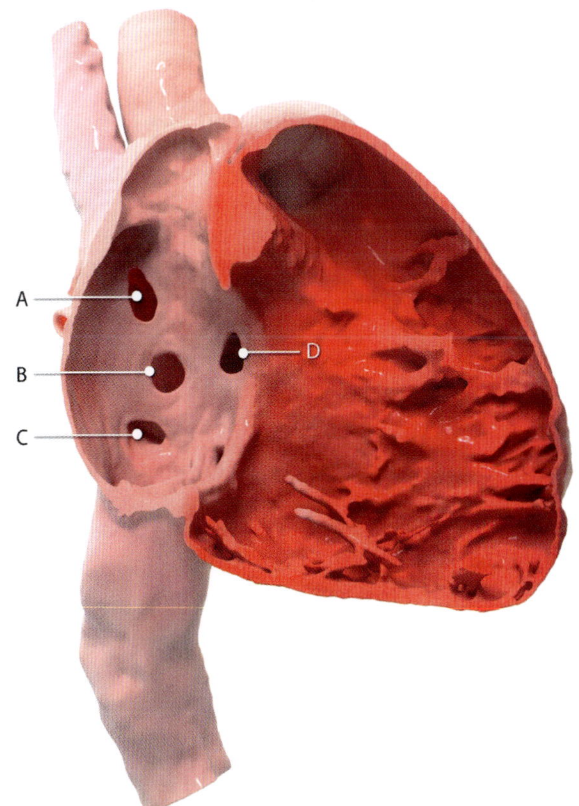

FIGURE 39.1 Atrial septal defect morphologies: superior sinus venosus **(A)**, secundum **(B)**, inferior sinus venosus **(C)**, and primum **(D)**. (Courtesy of Adam Hansgen.)

open communication between the left atrium and the coronary sinus, allowing left-to-right shunting through the intact coronary sinus inlet into the right atrium.

Current available ASD closure devices are approved for closure of secundum-type ASDs. However, primum ASDs, sinus venosus, and coronary sinus defects should be generally closed surgically due to the following: (1) the absence of appropriate rims, (2) the proximity of the AV valves and conduction system to the closure device, (3) and the presence of other congenital heart defects that may require surgical correction.

Indications for ASD Closure

Table 39.1 lists the summary of current recommendations for ASD closure from the 2018 American Heart Association/American College of Cardiology Guidelines for Management of Adults with Congenital Heart Disease.[2]

Transcatheter Closure of ASDs

The first percutaneous closure of an ASD was done in 1975 on a 17-year-old girl using a 35 mm King and Mills Cardiac Umbrella. The device was composed of six stainless steel struts with fixation barbs and Dacron covering for each opposing umbrella.[3] Contemporary iterations of ASD closure devices use the same design as the King and Mills Cardiac umbrella with two opposing discs connected by a waist. The current ASD devices available for commercial use in the United States include the Gore Cardioform ASD Occluder (**Fig. 39.2A**), Gore Cardioform Septal occluder (also used for patent foramen ovale [PFO] closures) (**Fig. 39.2B**), Amplatzer Septal Occluder (**Fig. 39.3B**), and Amplatzer Cribriform Occluder (**Fig. 39.3C**). Other devices are CE marked and are also commercially available outside the United States such as the Occlutech Figulla Flex II device. **Fig. 39.4** shows the fluoroscopic profile of the Amplatzer Septal Occluder (A) and the Gore Cardioform Septal Occluder (B).

The current device designs can be categorized into self-centering and non-self-centering devices. Self-centering devices (Gore Cardioform ASD Occluder and Amplatzer Septal Occluder) have wide waists that completely straddles the defect (**Fig. 39.5**). On the other hand, non-self-centering devices (Gore Cardioform Septal Occluder and Amplatzer Cribriform Occluder) have thin waists connecting the right and left atrial discs.

Procedural preparation and planning are integral steps in transcatheter closure of ASDs. Preprocedural cardiac catheterization is not required for all patients undergoing ASD closure. However, it may be necessary for decision making or to clarify discrepant or inconclusive noninvasive imaging data.[2] Preprocedure hemodynamic assessment with right heart catheterization may also provide valuable information including shunt size (ratio of pulmonary flow: systemic flow or Qp:Qs) and the presence of significant pulmonary hypertension. Cardiac computed tomography may provide further anatomical detail such as deficient rims, the shape of the defect, and the presence of other congenital heart defects (ie, anomalous pulmonary venous connections) that may influence decision making.

TABLE 39.1 Summary of Recommendations for ASD Closure From the 2018 AHA/ACC Guideline for the Management of Adults With Congenital Heart Disease

RECOMMENDATION	CLASS	LOE
Transcatheter or surgical closure is recommended in adults with isolated secundum ASD causing impaired functional capacity, right atrial and/or RV enlargement, and net left to-right shunt sufficiently large to cause physiological sequelae ([Qp:Qs] ≥1.5:1) without cyanosis at rest or during exercise. Systolic PA pressure should be <1/2 of systolic systemic pressure and PVR is <1/3 of the SVR	I	B-NR
Surgical closure is recommended in adults with primum ASD, sinus venosus defect, or coronary sinus defect causing impaired functional capacity, right atrial and/or RV enlargement, and net left-to-right shunt sufficiently large to cause physiological sequelae ([Qp:Qs] ≥1.5:1) without cyanosis at rest or during exercise. Systolic PA pressure should be <1/2 of systolic systemic pressure and PVR is <1/3 of the SVR	I	B-NR
Transcatheter or surgical closure is reasonable in asymptomatic adults with isolated secundum ASD, right atrial and RV enlargement, and net left-to-right shunt sufficiently large to cause physiological sequelae ([Qp:Qs] ≥1.5:1), without cyanosis at rest or during exercise. Systolic PA pressure <1/2 of systolic systemic pressure and PVR is <1/3 of the SVR	IIa	C-LD
Surgical closure of a secundum ASD in adults is reasonable when a concomitant surgical procedure is being performed, and there is a net left-to-right shunt sufficiently large to cause physiological sequelae ([Qp:Qs] ≥1.5:1) and RA and RV enlargement without cyanosis at rest or during exercise	IIa	C-LD
Transcatheter or surgical closure may be considered for adults with ASD when net left-to-right shunt ([Qp:Qs] ≥1.5:1), PA systolic pressure is ≥1/2 systemic systolic pressure, and/or PVR is >1/3 of the SVR	IIb	B-NR
ASD closure should not be performed in adults with PA systolic pressure >2/3 of systemic systolic pressure, PVR >2/3 of the SVR, and/or a net right-to-left shunt	III—Harm	C-LD

ACC, American College of Cardiology; AHA, American Heart Association; ASD, atrial septal defect; B-NR, nonrandomized study; Class I, strong recommendation; Class IIa, moderate recommendation; Class IIb, weak recommendation; Class III, harm; Class III, no benefit; C-LD, limited data; LOE, Level of Evidence; PA, pulmonary artery; PVR, pulmonary vascular resistance; Qp:Qs, pulmonary-systemic blood flow ratio; RA, right atrium; RV, right ventricle; SVR, systemic vascular resistance.

Balloon Sizing Using Stop-Flow Technique

Balloon sizing is an important step in percutaneous ASD closure, while in PFO closure, balloon sizing is not necessary but may occasionally be used to assess tunnel length and compliance. There are several sizing balloons commercially available. The Amplatzer sizing balloon II is commonly used. It is a triple-lumen compliant balloon with three radio-opaque marker bands to aid in fluoroscopic calibration and measurement. The center of the balloon has two radio-opaque marker bands that are 0.4 mm apart. These two central marker bands are used to profile the balloon in an

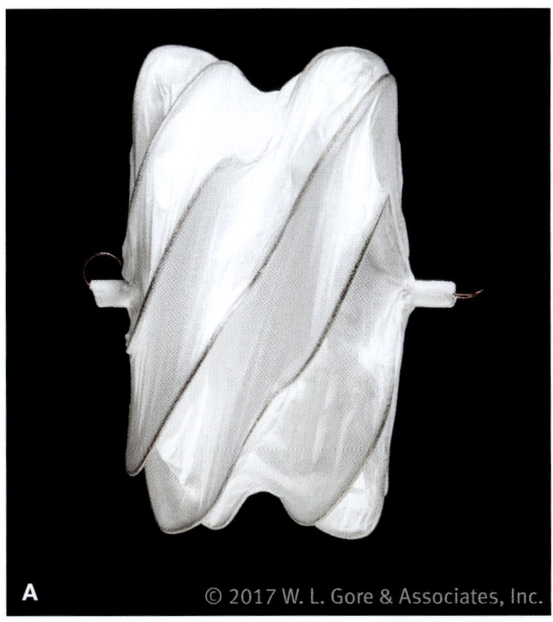

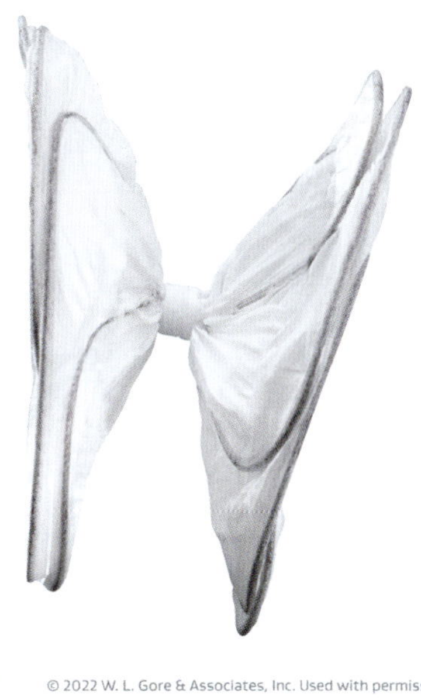

FIGURE 39.2 **A:** Gore Cardioform ASD Occluder and **(B)** Gore Cardioform Septal Occluder. ASD, atrial septal defect.

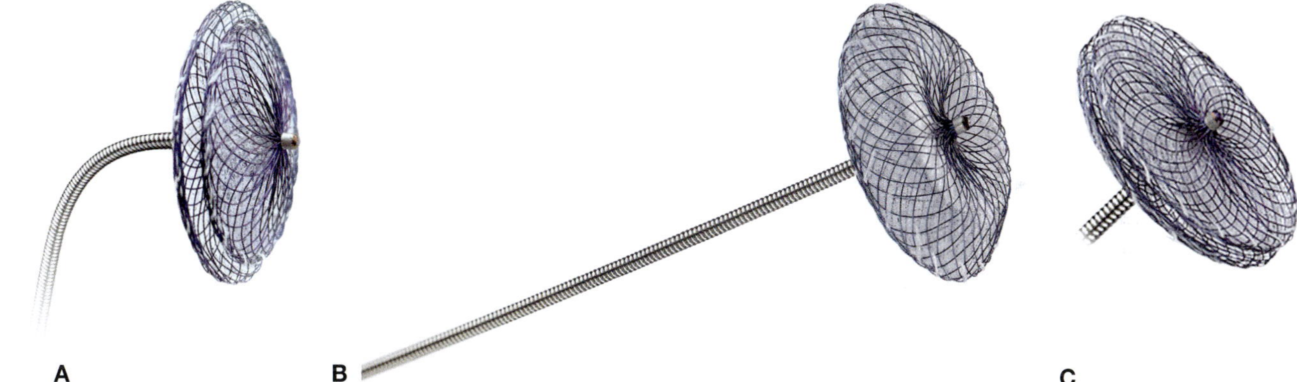

FIGURE 39.3 **A:** Amplatzer PFO Occluder, **(B)** Amplatzer Septal Occluder, and **(C)** Amplatzer Cribriform Occluder. PFO, patent foramen ovale.

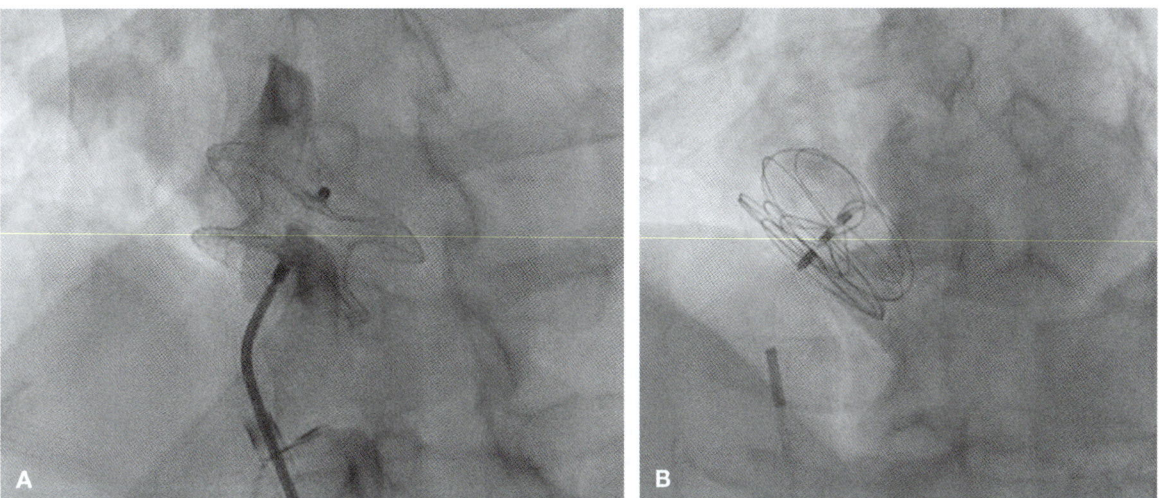

FIGURE 39.4 **A:** Amplatzer Septal Occluder and **(B)** Gore Cardioform Septal Occluder device in situ.

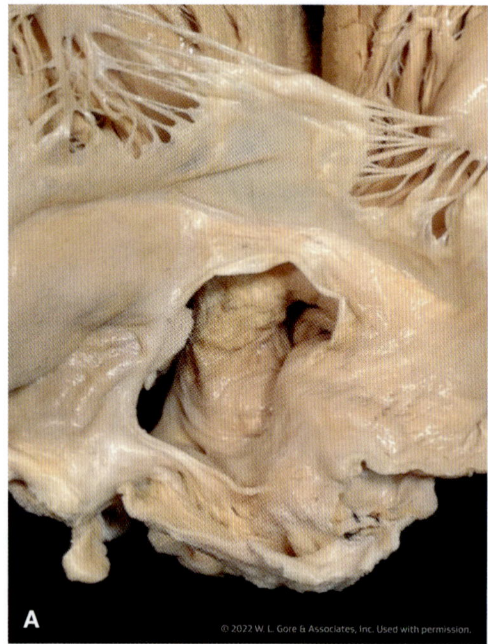

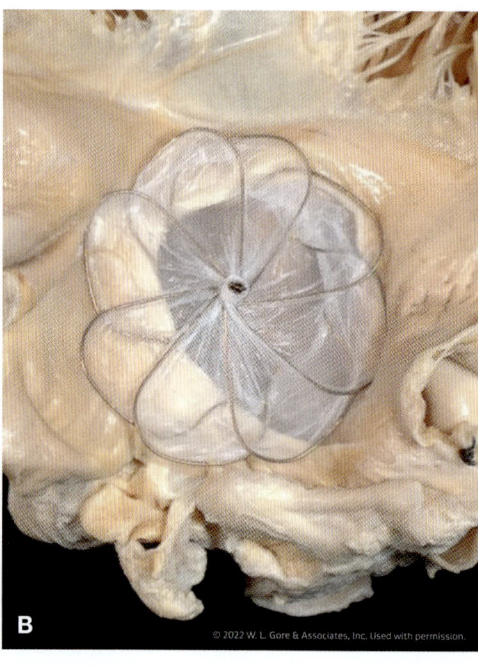

FIGURE 39.5 Large atrial septal defect **(A)** as seen in the left atrial side. Gore Cardioform ASD Occluder in situ **(B)**. ASD, atrial septal defect.

optimal fluoroscopic view (usually shallow left anterior oblique) to avoid inaccurate measurements due to balloon foreshortening. The most proximal marker band is 15 mm from the first central marker band. Fluoroscopic measurement of the balloon is calibrated from this distance (**Fig. 39.6A**). The balloon is advanced over a stiff 0.035 in guidewire under fluoroscopic and echocardiographic guidance and slowly inflated until color flow across the defect ceases (stop-flow technique) (**Fig. 39.6B**). Once balloon sizing is completed, four sets of defect size criteria are considered: (1) unstretched diameter by echocardiogram (either transesophageal echocardiogram [TEE] or intracardiac echocardiogram [ICE]), (2) the diameter as determined by the width of the color Doppler signal across the defect, (3) the fluoroscopic measurement of the stretched diameter obtained by measuring the waist of the inflated balloon, and (4) stretched diameter by stop-flow technique. The stretched diameter will always be larger than the unstretched diameter. Once the size of the defect is measured, device type and size are chosen. In self-centering devices, the recommended device size is equal to or slightly larger (~2 mm) than the stop-flow diameter. If balloon sizing is not done, then a self-centering device approximately 25% larger than the diameter of the defect should be chosen. However, if a non-self-centering device is chosen, a device twice the size of the defect is recommended under the instructions for use of the selected device.

PATENT FO

A PFO is formed when there is an incomplete postnatal fusion of the ***septum secundum*** and ***septum primum***.[4] A PFO with a right-to-left shunt is a potential conduit for venous thrombi to reach the arterial circulation causing paradoxical embolism including stroke (**Fig. 39.7**). An ischemic stroke is deemed cryptogenic when it is not attributed to definite large-vessel atherosclerosis, small artery disease, or embolism despite extensive vascular, serologic, and cardiac evaluation.[5] PFO is common and found in approximately 25% of the adult population. Having a PFO has not been shown to increase the risk of ischemic stroke.[6,7] However, studies have shown that approximately 40% of cryptogenic strokes have a PFO.[7] This suggests that paradoxical embolism may be the culprit for a fraction of cryptogenic strokes. An atrial septal aneurysm (which is an outpouching of redundant atrial septal tissue caused by a primary defect of the fossa ovalis or by sustained interatrial pressure difference) in combination with a PFO can increase the likelihood that a given cryptogenic stroke event may be due to a paradoxical embolism.[8] Similarly, the finding of a large right-to-left shunt through a PFO in a young (<60) cryptogenic stroke patient increases the likelihood that the stroke was due to a paradoxical embolism.[9]

Indications for PFO Closure

Percutaneous closure of PFO for the prevention of recurrent ischemic stroke has historically been controversial. This is mainly due to the negative results of the early randomized clinical trials comparing PFO closure device to medical therapy. The CLOSURE I (STARFlex Septal Occluder) and PC (Amplatzer PFO Occluder) trials did not achieve the prespecified clinical endpoint for efficacy.[10,11] These two negative trials created such an impact in the field of neurology and cardiology such that in the 2016 guidelines of the American Academy of Neurology, the use of PFO closure for cryptogenic stroke was discouraged.[12]

The results of the more recent landmark trials, RESPECT (long-term follow up) and REDUCE resurrected the use of PFO closure for stroke prevention (**Table 39.2**). The RESPECT trial (Amplatzer PFO Occluder) and the REDUCE Trial (Gore Cardioform Septal Occluder) demonstrated superiority of PFO closure device over medical therapy for secondary prevention of stroke.[13,14] Subsequently, the Food and Drug Administration (FDA) approved the Amplatzer PFO Occluder (Abbott Structural, Santa Clara, CA) and the Gore Cardioform Septal Occluder (W. L. Gore and Associates, Inc, Newark, DE) in 2016 and 2018, respectively. The US FDA approval states, PFO closure is indicated *"to reduce the risk of recurrent ischemic stroke in patients, predominantly between the ages of 18 and 60 years, who have had a cryptogenic stroke due to a presumed paradoxical embolism, as determined by a neurologist*

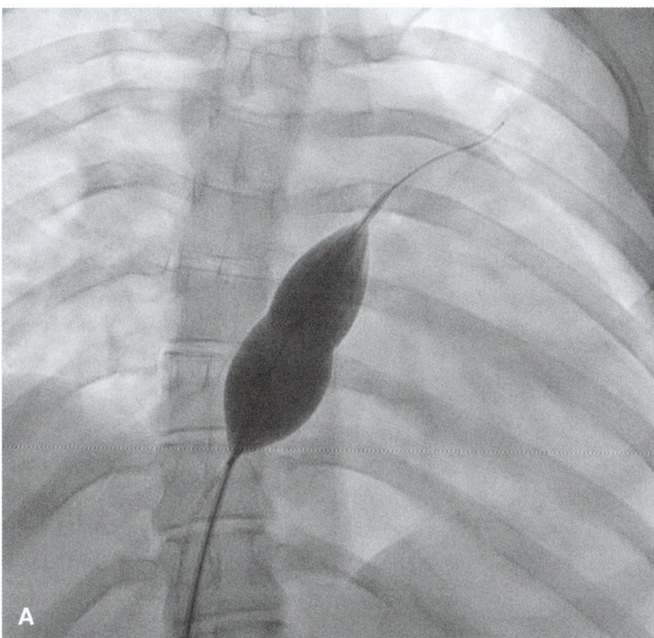

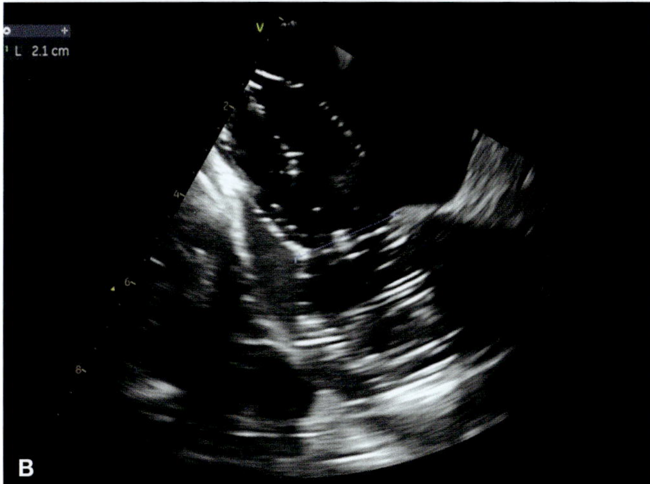

FIGURE 39.6 **A:** Fluoroscopic and **(B)** ICE image of sizing balloon using stop-flow technique (color Doppler not shown). ICE, intracardiac echocardiogram.

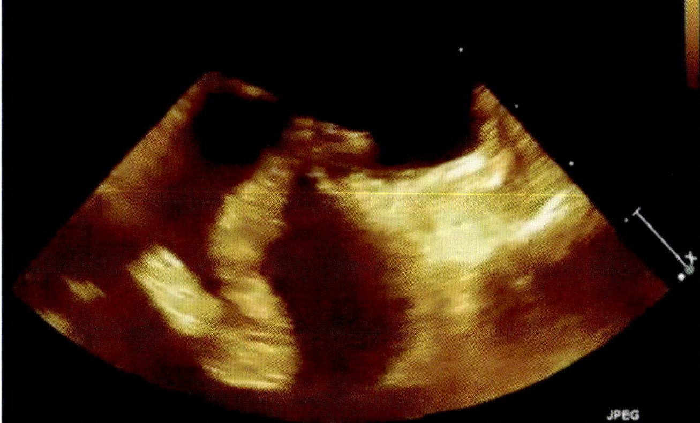

FIGURE 39.7 Transesophageal echocardiogram image of a thrombus in transit across a PFO. LA, left atrium; PFO, patent foramen ovale; RA, right atrium.

and cardiologist following an evaluation to exclude known causes of ischemic stroke."

In 2020, the American Academy of Neurology updated their practice advisory on PFO closure for secondary stroke prevention. The advisory states "*In patients younger than 60 years with a PFO and embolic-appearing infarct and no other mechanism of stroke identified, clinicians may recommend closure following a discussion of potential benefits (absolute recurrent stroke risk reduction of 3.4% at 5 years) and risks (periprocedural complication rate of 3.9% and increased absolute rate of non-periprocedural atrial fibrillation of 0.33% per year).*"[15]

PFO Closure in PFO-Associated Stroke

The heart-brain team, composed of a cardiologist and a stroke neurologist, should rule out other causes of stroke through an extensive evaluation. Atrial fibrillation (AF) should be ruled out with noninvasive electrocardiographic monitoring. The ideal duration of monitoring is unclear; however, monitoring for 30 days is suggested.[16]

Table 39.3 outlines the current Society for Cardiovascular Angiography and Interventions (SCAI) guideline recommendations for PFO closure with prior PFO-associated stroke.[17]

The Risk of Paradoxical Embolism (RoPE) score is a useful assessment tool to determine the probability that a PFO is the culprit for a cryptogenic stroke (**Table 39.4**). A high RoPE score directly correlates with an increased likelihood that a PFO is the culprit for the index stroke. A RoPE score of 7 or more helps identify patients who may benefit from PFO closure. On the other hand, the risk-benefit ratio of performing PFO closure in patients with a RoPE score less than 7 should be evaluated carefully.[18] The RoPE score, however, does not take into consideration the structural features of a PFO. The PFO-Associated Stroke Causal Likelihood (PASCAL) classification system combines the RoPE score with high-risk PFO features, including a large right-to-left shunt or an atrial septal aneurysm. The PASCAL classification algorithmically assigns a likely causal relationship between PFO and stroke into three categories: unlikely, possible, and probable.[19] The operator should keep in mind that both scoring systems are used as a guide and not used to determine indication for PFO closure.

PFO Closure in Other Conditions

Indications for PFO closure in conditions other than a PFO-associated stroke are uncertain due to a paucity of prospective clinical trial data. **Table 39.5** summarizes the SCAI recommendations for PFO closure in other conditions. PFO closure is not recommended in the following conditions: debilitating migraines refractory to conventional medical therapy, atrial septal aneurysm, or deep vein thrombosis without a prior stroke, transient ischemic attack, SCUBA diving to prevent decompression sickness, and thrombophilia. In patients with a PFO and platypnea-orthodeoxia syndrome or systemic embolism without a prior stroke, PFO closure is recommended over medical therapy alone. However, patients may decline PFO closure in these conditions if the risks outweigh the benefits of the procedure.[17]

Heart-Brain Team Evaluation

A patient-centered multidisciplinary team evaluation should be implemented to help identify stroke patients who will benefit from PFO closure. The FDA approval of the two PFO closure devices clearly mandates that patients be evaluated by both a cardiologist and a neurologist prior to consideration of PFO closure and

TABLE 39.2 Contemporary Randomized Trials on PFO

TRIAL	YEAR PUBLISHED	PFO CLOSURE DEVICE USED	CONTROL ARM(S)	PRIMARY ENDPOINT	CONCLUSIONS
CLOSURE I	2012	STARFlex	Aspirin and/or warfarin (INR 2-3)	Composite of stroke/TIA, all-cause mortality, death from neurologic causes	Closure is not superior to medical therapy
PC Trial	2013	Amplatzer PFO Occluder	Antiplatelet therapy or oral anticoagulation	Composite of death, nonfatal stroke, TIA, or peripheral embolism	Closure is not superior to medical therapy
RESPECT	2013	Amplatzer PFO Occluder	Aspirin or warfarin or clopidogrel, or aspirin with extended-release dipyridamole	Composite of recurrent nonfatal ischemic stroke, fatal ischemic stroke, or early death after randomization	No significant benefit for closure (intention-to treat analysis) Closure is superior to medical therapy (as-treated analysis)
RESPECT (long-term follow-up)	2017	Amplatzer PFO Occluder	Aspirin or warfarin or clopidogrel, oraspirin with extended-release dipyridamole	Composite of recurrent nonfatal ischemic stroke, fatal ischemic stroke, or early death after randomization	Closure is superior to medical therapy on extended follow-up in intention-to-treat analysis
CLOSE	2017	Any CE marked PFO device	1. .*Antiplatelet arm*: Aspirin or clopidogrel or aspirin with extended-release dipyridamole 2. .*Oral anticoagulant arm*: Vitamin K antagonists or NOACs	Recurrent fatal or nonfatal stroke	Closure is superior to antiplatelet in patients with ASA or PFO with large shunt Anticoagulant is equivalent to antiplatelet therapy
REDUCE	2017	Helex Septal Occluder and Cardioform Septal Occluder	Aspirin or clopidogrel or aspirin with dipyridamole	1. .Recurrent stroke 2. .New brain infarct inclusive of silent brain infarct (SBI)	Closure is superior to antiplatelet therapy
DEFENSE-PFO	2018	Amplatzer PFO Occluder	Aspirin or aspirin and clopidogrel, or aspirin and cilostazol, or warfarin	Stroke, vascular death, or TIMI-defined major bleeding	Closure in patients with high-risk PFO characteristics resulted in lower rate of ischemic stroke vs medical therapy

ASA, atrial septal aneurysm; CLOSE, closure of patent foramen ovale or anticoagulants versus antiplatelet therapy to prevent stroke recurrence; CLOSURE I, evaluation of the STARFlex septal closure system in patients with a stroke and/or transient ischemic attack due to presumed paradoxical embolism through a patent foramen ovale; DEFENSE-PFO, device closure versus medical therapy for cryptogenic stroke patients with high-risk patent foramen ovale; INR, International normalized ratio; NOAC, novel oral anticoagulant; PC, percutaneous closure of patent foramen ovale using the AMPLATZER PFO occluder with medical treatment in patients with cryptogenic embolism; PFO, patent foramen ovale; REDUCE, GORE HELEX septal occluder/GORE CARDIOFORM septal occluder and antiplatelet medical management for reduction of recurrent stroke or imaging-confirmed TIA in patients with patent foramen ovale; RESPECT, randomized evaluation of recurrent stroke comparing PFO closure to established current standard of care treatment; TIA, transient ischemic attack; TIMI, thrombolysis in myocardial infarction.

that patients treated with these devices be followed prospectively as part of a postapproval study. The heart-brain team promotes a shared decision making process, ensures proper patient selection, serves to prevent inappropriate PFO closure, and mitigates unnecessary risks.[12]

Amplatzer PFO Occluder

After the RESPECT (long-term follow-up) trial results, the FDA approved the Amplatzer PFO Occluder. It is the first device to be FDA approved in the United States for PFO closure. The device has two self-expanding discs composed of a nickel-titanium (Nitinol) wire mesh with a wire diameter of 0.005 to 0.006 in. The current iteration of the device (Amplatzer Talisman PFO occluder) is available in four sizes (18, 25, 30, and 35 mm) (**Fig. 39.8**). The sizes of the asymmetric disc design are based on the right atrial disc diameter. The device is preattached to the delivery cable and goes through a proprietary 8 or 9F introducer sheath. After crossing the PFO with a 0.035 in guide wire, the delivery sheath and dilator ensemble is advanced into the left atrium. The wire and dilator are removed, and the loaded device is inserted. The device is then unsheathed in the left atrium. The left atrial disc is deployed and is pulled back and held against the atrial septum while the right atrial disc is deployed. The device is released by counterclockwise rotation of the delivery cable using the included vise.

Gore Cardioform Septal Occluder

After the REDUCE study, the FDA approved the Gore Cardioform Septal Occluder for PFO closure. The device is composed of two symmetrical discs formed by platinum-filled nitinol wire frames (**Figs. 39.2B** and **39.4B**). The device is covered by a proprietary thromboresistant expanded polytetrafluoroethylene material, which also allows tissue ingrowth and endothelialization

TABLE 39.3 Summary of SCAI Guideline Recommendations for PFO Closure With Prior PFO-Associated Stroke

CONDITION	RECOMMENDATION BY SCAI GUIDELINE PANEL	STRENGTH OF RECOMMENDATION	CERTAINTY OF EVIDENCE	REMARKS
Patients between ages of 18 and 60 y with a prior PFO-associated stroke and no other indications for treatment with anticoagulation	Suggests PFO closure plus antiplatelet therapy rather than anticoagulation therapy alone	Conditional	Low	This recommendation is independent of patient anatomy (ie, presence of ASA, size of shunt) due to limited clinical data on these subpopulations. A RoPE score ≥7 may identify patients who are likely to receive greater benefit from PFO closure
Patients 60 y or older with a prior PFO-associated stroke and no other indications for treatment with anticoagulation	Suggests PFO closure plus antiplatelet therapy rather than long-term anticoagulation therapy alone	Conditional	Very low	Patients in this age group who place a lower value on the uncertain benefits of PFO closure and a higher value on the possible procedure-related risks may reasonably decline PFO closure

ASA, atrial septal aneurysm; PFO, patent foramen ovale; RoPE, Risk of Paradoxical Embolism score; SCAI, Society of Cardiovascular Angiography and Interventions.

(**Fig. 39.9A and B**). A 0.035 or 0.018 in guidewire may be used to advance the delivery system into the left atrium. An 11 or 12F introducer sheath may be used if an 0.018 or 0.035 in guidewire is chosen, respectively. The device was designed to be soft and conformable to surrounding anatomy of the atrial septum with minimal injury and risk of erosion. It is available in a variety of sizes (20, 25, and 30 mm) and preloaded in its own delivery system (**Fig. 39.10A**). After crossing the PFO with the chosen guidewire, the preloaded device in the delivery catheter is inserted through a "rapid exchange" wire port. When the tip of the delivery catheter is in the middle left atrium, the guidewire is removed. The device is then deployed using the slider in the handle to unsheath and deploy the discs (**Fig. 39.11E**). The device is then locked. Finally, the device is fully released by gently pulling the cord in the handle.

Several key assessments should be done to ensure successful deployment before the device is released (**Fig. 39.11**). The device should be evaluated in the long axis (SVC rim) and short axis (aortic rim) using ICE or TEE (**Fig. 39.11F and G**). Device stability can be challenged using a "tug test" by gently pulling on the delivery system while watching under fluoroscopy and echocardiography. Any residual shunt should be carefully assessed by color Doppler. Both devices are recapturable if the initial deployment is unsatisfactory. After the device is released, residual shunting and final device position is once again reassessed using color Doppler and injection of agitated saline (**Fig. 39.11H**).

TABLE 39.4 Risk of Paradoxical Embolism (RoPE) Score

CRITERIA	POINT(S)
No history of hypertension	1
No history of diabetes	1
No history of TIA or stroke	1
Nonsmoker	1
Cortical infarct on imaging	1
Age	
18-29	5
30-39	4
40-49	3
50-59	2
60-69	1
>70	0

TIA, transient ischemic attack.

Intraprocedural Imaging

Intraprocedural echocardiographic imaging is mandatory during ASD and PFO closure and is considered standard of care. The atrial septum and its surrounding structures should be carefully evaluated prior to device deployment. TEE and ICE are equally acceptable modes of imaging with each offering advantages and disadvantages. A second venous access is needed if ICE is chosen. The use of ICE avoids the use of general anesthesia and a second operator during the procedure. ICE can be used for assessment of shunt via color Doppler and provides optimal visualization of the septal rims and the ASD or PFO device (**Fig. 39.12**). Currently available 3D/4D ICE catheters (NuVision by Biosense Webster, Inc, AcuNav by Siemens, and VeriSight Pro by Philips) may provide better anatomic detail compared to the traditional 2D ICE imaging.

A detailed evaluation of the interatrial septum and its surrounding structures should be performed. The presence of atrial septal aneurysm, long tunnel (more than 12 mm), and thick septum secundum increase the difficulty of PFO closure and may require larger PFO devices. In ASD closures, the operator should also be familiar with the atrial septal rims: aortic rim, SVC rim, superior rim (between the SVC rim and the aortic rim), the posterior rim (opposite the aortic rim), IVC rim, and the AV rim (**Fig. 39.13**).[20] Regardless of imaging modality, a complete evaluation of the interatrial septum and its surrounding structures is mandatory in order to deploy an ASD or PFO device safely and effectively.

Perioperative Care

Anticoagulation with intravenous unfractionated heparin at a dose of 70 to 100 IU/kg to maintain an activated clotting time of more than 250 seconds is recommended in both PFO and ASD closures. Heparin is given once vascular access is obtained.

TABLE 39.5 Summary of SCAI Guideline Recommendations for PFO Closure Without a PFO-Associated Stroke

CONDITION	RECOMMENDATION BY SCAI GUIDELINE PANEL	STRENGTH OF RECOMMENDATION	CERTAINTY OF EVIDENCE	REMARKS
Migraines and without a prior PFO-associated stroke	Suggests against routine use of PFO closure for the treatment of migraine	Conditional	Moderate	Patients, particularly those with debilitating migraines, who have failed to benefit from conventional medical therapy, and who place a high value on the uncertain benefits of having their PFO closed and a lower value on the uncertain harms, may reasonably choose PFO closure
SCUBA divers with prior decompression illness and without a prior PFO-associated stroke	Suggests against the routine use of PFO closure to prevent decompression illness	Conditional	Very low	Patients who place a high value on the potential, but uncertain, benefits of having their PFO closed and a lower value on risks may reasonably choose PFO closure
Platypnea-orthodeoxia syndrome (POS) and without a prior PFO-associated stroke, in whom other causes of hypoxia have been excluded	Suggests PFO closure rather than no PFO closure	Conditional	Very low	Patients who place a higher value on the risks of closure and a lower value on the uncertain benefits may reasonably decline PFO closure
Thrombophilia and without a prior PFO-associated stroke	Suggests against the use of PFO closure in addition to antithrombotic therapy	Conditional	Very low	
The presence of an atrial septal aneurysm without a prior PFO-associated stroke	Suggests against the use of PFO closure	Conditional	Very low	
Systemic embolism without a prior PFO-associated stroke, in whom other embolic etiologies have been excluded	Suggests PFO closure rather than medical therapy alone	Conditional	Very low	Patients who place a high value on the risks and a lower value on the uncertain benefits may reasonably decline PFO closure
History of TIA and without a prior PFO-associated stroke	Suggests against PFO closure	Conditional	Very low	Patients, particularly those with recurrent high-probability TIAs, who place a high value on the uncertain benefits and a low value on procedural risks would reasonably choose PFO closure
History of deep vein thrombosis and without a prior PFO-associated stroke	Suggests against PFO closure	Conditional	Very low	

PFO, patent foramen ovale; SCAI, Society for Cardiovascular Angiography and Interventions; TIA, transient ischemic attack.

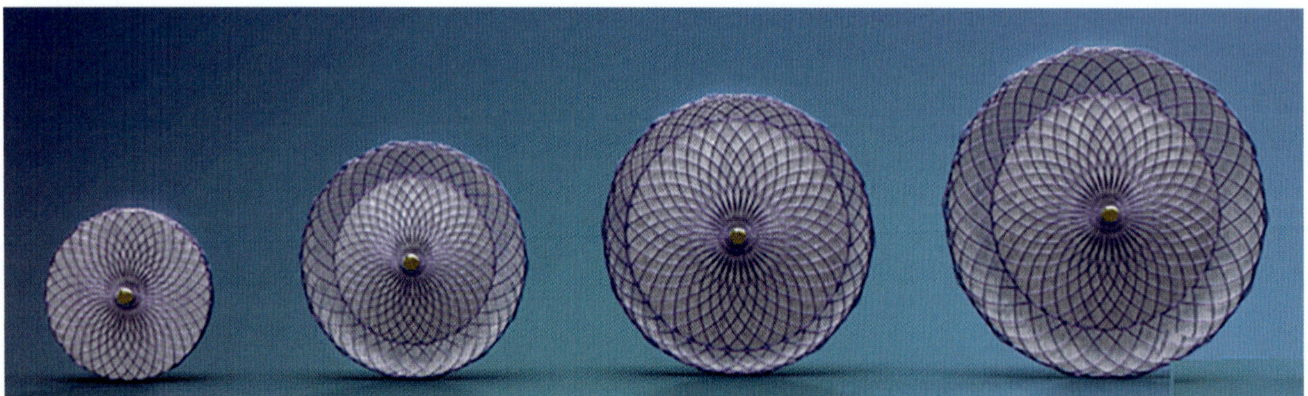

FIGURE 39.8 Amplatzer PFO Occluder sizes. Note the larger right atrial disc compared to the left atrial disc except on the smallest size (18 mm). PFO, patent foramen ovale.

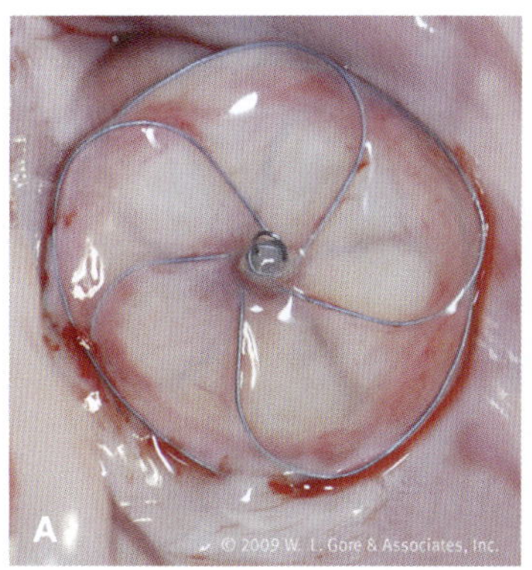

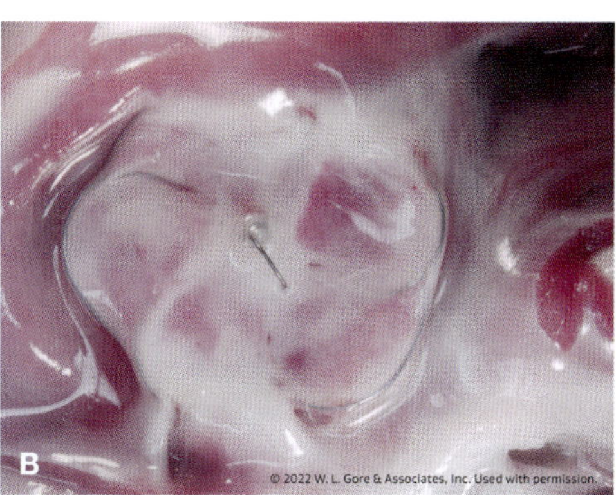

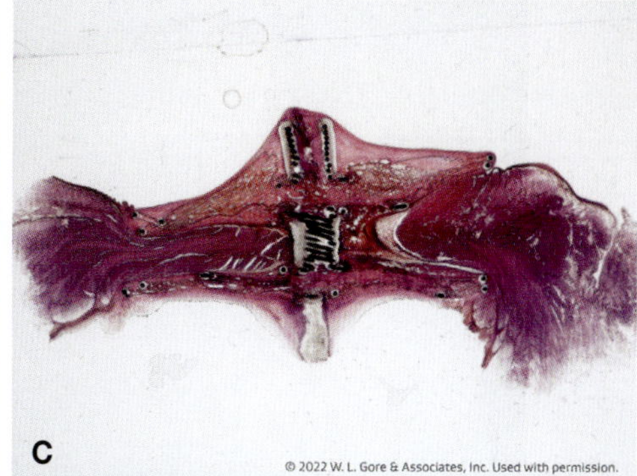

FIGURE 39.9 Gross and histopathology **(C)** of a Gore Cardioform Septal Occluder at **(A)** 30 days and **(B)** 90 days in a canine model.

Postoperatively, patients generally receive dual antiplatelet therapy with aspirin and clopidogrel, although this is not a data-driven recommendation. The optimal duration for postprocedural antiplatelet therapy is also unclear. Based on the PFO landmark trials, dual antiplatelet therapy is given for 1 to 3 months and then followed by aspirin monotherapy. Postprocedure, transthoracic echocardiogram prior to discharge is done to evaluate device stability, residual shunts, and assessing for pericardial effusion. Serial echocardiograms may be done in 1 and 6 months postprocedure. The optimal duration and frequency of follow-up echocardiograms post-PFO and ASD closure remains unclear. Infective endocarditis prophylaxis prior to dental procedures is indicated for the first 6 months.[21] Antibiotic prophylaxis is not required for nondental procedures (ie, colonoscopy, cystoscopy, and TEE).

Complications of Transcatheter ASD and PFO Closure

Percutaneous ASD and PFO closure are generally safe when performed by experienced operators with excellent imaging guidance. Most complications may be avoided with proper patient selection, preprocedural planning, optimal imaging guidance, and thoughtful device selection and sizing.

Both procedures are associated with all the usual risks that are inherent in any transcatheter cardiac procedure. These include vascular injury, vessel or cardiac perforation, stroke, infection, and complications related to anesthesia. Although serious complications are exceedingly rare, specific complications related to both procedures are notable. Device embolization following PFO closure may occur as low as 0.7% although none occurred during the landmark PFO trials. Residual shunt was relatively common with the early generation PFO devices. Fortunately, embolic event rate remained low despite the high incidence of residual shunt postimplant. Data from the RESPECT (0.4%) and CLOSE (0.8%) trials showed low incidence of significant residual shunts using the contemporary devices.[14,22] AF is an important postprocedure complication especially for PFO closures because it may be the culprit for future embolic strokes. The incidence of AF in PFO closures is as low as 0.3%. The mechanism of AF postprocedure is not clearly known but may be related to device irritation, local stretch, or formation of reentry circuits.

Other rare but significant complications related to both procedures include device-related thrombus, nickel allergy, and pacemaker lead entrapment within the device.

Device erosion and cardiac perforation is one of the most feared complications of both transcatheter PFO and ASD closure but mostly reported in ASD closures. The incidence of device erosion from the Amplatzer PFO occluder and Amplatzer Septal Occluder was 0.018% and 0.1%, respectively.[23] Deficient rims (specifically the aortic rim) and device oversizing were identified as potential risks for device erosion. Patients usually present with cardiac tamponade from hemopericardium or sudden death. Interestingly, no reported erosions were seen in the Gore devices. However, in the Gore Helex Device (predecessor of the Gore Cardioform Septal Occluder), wire frame fractures and perforations leading to hemopericardium were reported.[24]

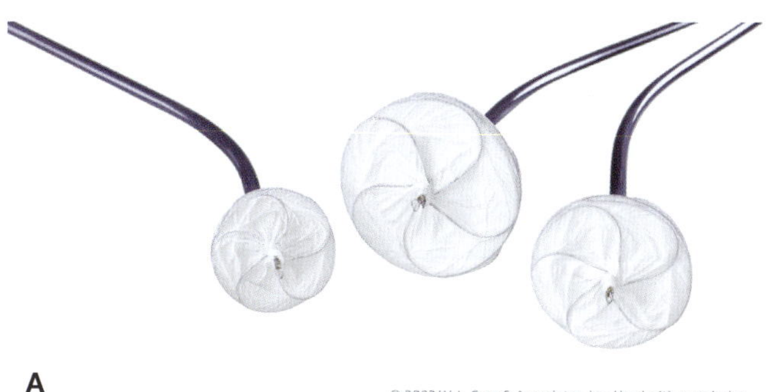

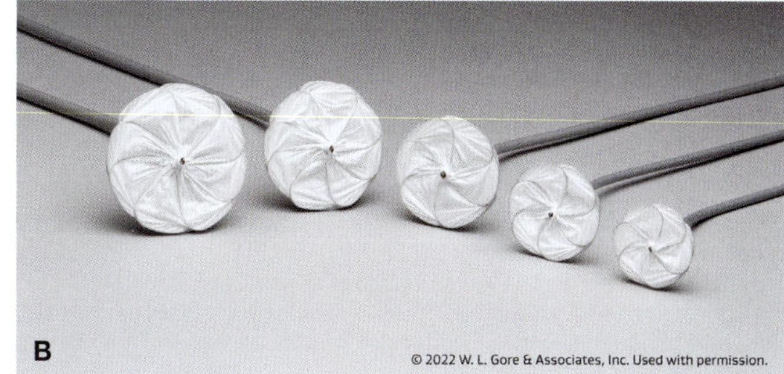

FIGURE 39.10 Available sizes of the **(A)** Gore Cardioform Septal Occloder and the **(B)** Gore Cardioform ASD Occluder. ASD, atrial septal defect.

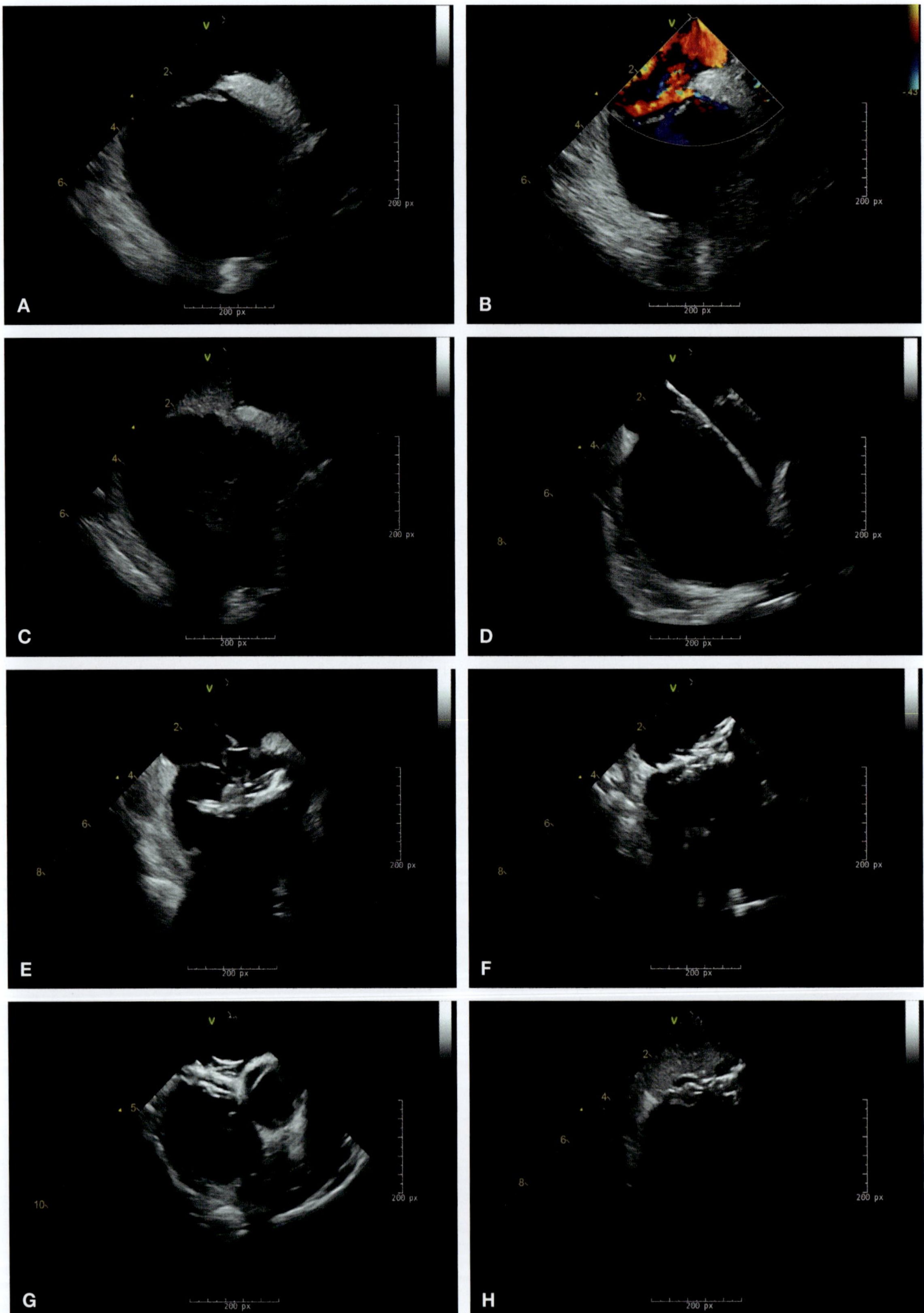

FIGURE 39.11 ICE images of a **(A)** PFO demonstrating a right to left shunt by **(B)** color Doppler and **(C)** agitated saline. **D:** An 0. 035 in wire is shown across the PFO. **E:** The left atrial disc of a Gore Cardioform Septal Occluder is initially deployed in the left atrium and then the right atrial disc in the right atrium. A fully deployed device is seen here in the **(F)** long-axis and **(G)** short-axis view. **H:** Agitated saline study after deployment showed no further right to left shunt. ICE, intracardiac echocardiogram; PFO, patent foramen ovale.

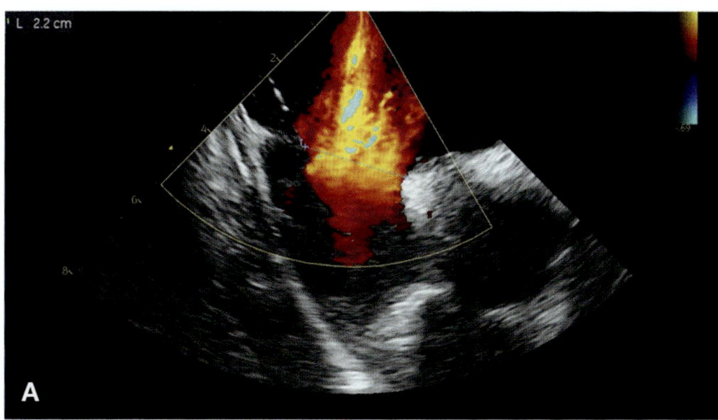

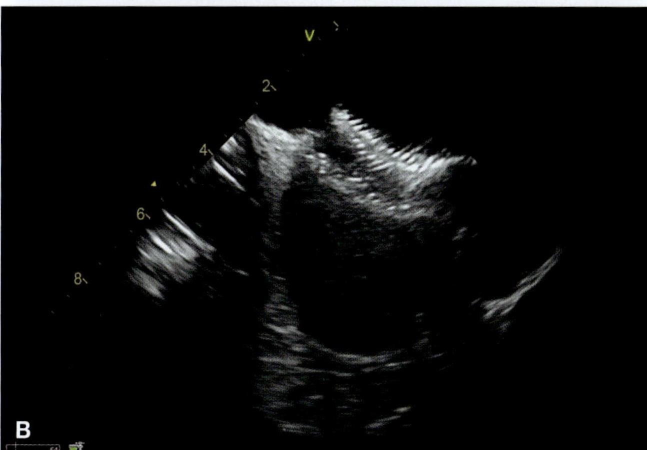

FIGURE 39.12 **A:** ICE image of a large secundum ASD with left-to-right shunt by **(B)** color Doppler and after Amplatzer Septal Occluder implant. Ao, aorta; ASD, atrial septal defect; ICE, intracardiac echocardiogram; LA, left atrium; RA, right atrium.

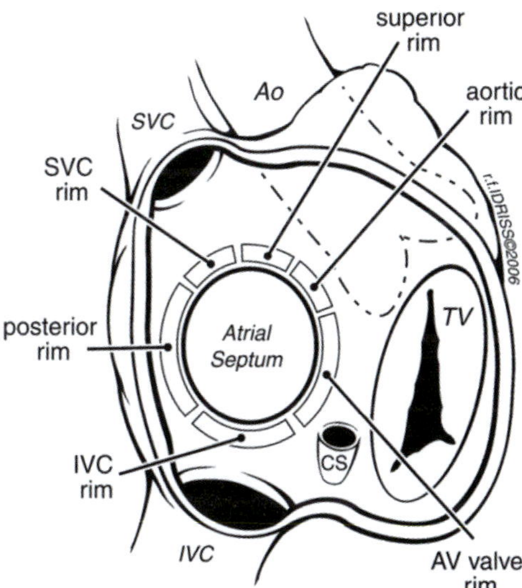

FIGURE 39.13 Atrial septum rims and surrounding structures as seen from the right atrium. Ao, aorta; IVC, inferior vena cava; SVC, superior vena cava; TV, tricuspid valve. (Reprinted from Amin Z. Transcatheter closure of secundum atrial septal defects. *Catheter Cardiovasc Interv.* 2006;68(5):778-787.)

Key Points

- Transcatheter or surgical closure is recommended in isolated secundum ASDs with suitable anatomy, while surgical closure is recommended in primum ASDs, sinus venosus, and unroofed coronary sinus defects.
- Knowledge and identification of the atrial septal rims prior to ASD and PFO closure are critical.
- PFO closure is indicated to prevent recurrent ischemic stroke in patients who had a cryptogenic stroke presumed to be embolic after thorough evaluation by the heart-brain team.
- The RoPE score and the PASCAL classification system are helpful tools in assessing patients who may benefit from PFO closure.
- The Gore Cardioform Septal Occluder and the Amplatzer PFO Occluder are currently the only FDA-approved devices for PFO closure in the United States.
- ASD closure devices available in the United States include the self-centering devices (Gore Cardioform ASD Occluder and Amplatzer Septal Occluder) and non-self-centering devices (Gore Cardioform Septal Occluder and Amplatzer Cribriform Occluder).

References

1. Anderson RH, Brown NA, Webb S. Development and structure of the atrial septum. *Heart*. 2002;88(1):104-110.
2. Stout KK, Daniels CJ, Aboulhosn JA, et al. 2018 AHA/ACC guideline for the management of adults with congenital heart disease: a report of the American College of Cardiology/American Heart Association Task Force on Clinical Practice Guidelines. *Circulation*. 2019;139(14):e698-e800.
3. King TD, Mills NL. Nonoperative closure of atrial septal defects. *Surgery*. 1974;75(3):383-388.
4. Collado FMS, Poulin MF, Murphy JJ, Jneid H, Kavinsky CJ. Patent foramen ovale closure for stroke prevention and other disorders. *J Am Heart Assoc*. 2018;7(12):e007146.
5. Adams HP Jr, Bendixen BH, Kappelle LJ, et al. Classification of subtype of acute ischemic stroke. Definitions for use in a multicenter clinical trial. TOAST. Trial of Org 10172 in Acute Stroke Treatment. *Stroke*. 1993;24(1):35-41.
6. Overell JR, Bone I, Lees KR. Interatrial septal abnormalities and stroke: a meta-analysis of case-control studies. *Neurology*. 2000;55(8):1172-1179.
7. Lechat P, Mas JL, Lascault G, et al. Prevalence of patent foramen ovale in patients with stroke. *N Engl J Med*. 1988;318(18):1148-1152.
8. Mas JL, Arquizan C, Lamy C, et al. Recurrent cerebrovascular events associated with patent foramen ovale, atrial septal aneurysm, or both. *N Engl J Med*. 2001;345(24):1740-1746.
9. Wahl A, Krumsdorf U, Meier B, et al. Transcatheter treatment of atrial septal aneurysm associated with patent foramen ovale for prevention of recurrent paradoxical embolism in high-risk patients. *J Am Coll Cardiol*. 2005;45(3):377-380.
10. Meier B, Kalesan B, Mattle HP, et al. Percutaneous closure of patent foramen ovale in cryptogenic embolism. *N Engl J Med*. 2013;368(12):1083-1091.
11. Furlan AJ, Reisman M, Massaro J, et al. Closure or medical therapy for cryptogenic stroke with patent foramen ovale. *N Engl J Med*. 2012;366(11):991-999.
12. Collado FMS, Kavinsky CJ. The heart-brain team approach in patent foramen ovale closure. *Front Neurol*. 2020;11:561938.

13. Søndergaard L, Kasner SE, Rhodes JF, et al. Patent foramen ovale closure or antiplatelet therapy for cryptogenic stroke. *N Engl J Med*. 2017;377(11):1033-1042.
14. Saver JL, Carroll JD, Thaler DE, et al. Long-term outcomes of patent foramen ovale closure or medical therapy after stroke. *N Engl J Med*. 2017;377(11):1022-1032.
15. Messe SR, Gronseth GS, Kent DM, et al. Practice advisory update summary: patent foramen ovale and secondary stroke prevention—report of the Guideline Subcommittee of the American Academy of Neurology. *Neurology*. 2020;94(20):876-885.
16. Gladstone DJ, Spring M, Dorian P, et al. Atrial fibrillation in patients with cryptogenic stroke. *N Engl J Med*. 2014;370(26):2467-2477.
17. Kavinsky CJ, Szerlip M, Goldsweig AM, et al. SCAI guidelines for the management of patent foramen ovale. *J Soc Cardiovasc Angiogr Interv*. 2022;1(4):100039.
18. Kent DM, Ruthazer R, Weimar C, et al. An index to identify stroke-related vs incidental patent foramen ovale in cryptogenic stroke. *Neurology*. 2013;81(7):619-625.
19. Kent DM, Saver JL, Kasner SE, et al. Heterogeneity of treatment effects in an analysis of pooled individual patient data from randomized trials of device closure of patent foramen ovale after stroke. *JAMA*. 2021;326(22):2277-2286.
20. Amin Z. Transcatheter closure of secundum atrial septal defects. *Catheter Cardiovasc Interv*. 2006;68(5):778-787.
21. Nishimura RA, Otto CM, Bonow RO, et al. 2014 AHA/ACC guideline for the management of patients with valvular heart disease: a report of the American College of Cardiology/American Heart Association Task Force on Practice Guidelines. *Circulation*. 2014;129(23):e521-e643.
22. Mas JL, Derumeaux G, Guillon B, et al. Patent foramen ovale closure or anticoagulation vs. antiplatelets after stroke. *N Engl J Med*. 2017;377(11): 1011-1021.
23. Amin Z, Hijazi ZM, Bass JL, Cheatham JP, Hellenbrand WE, Kleinman CS. Erosion of Amplatzer septal occluder device after closure of secundum atrial septal defects: review of registry of complications and recommendations to minimize future risk. *Catheter Cardiovasc Interv*. 2004;63(4):496-502.
24. Fagan T, Dreher D, Cutright W, Jacobson J, Latson L; GORE HELEX Septal Occluder Working Group. Fracture of the GORE HELEX septal occluder: associated factors and clinical outcomes. *Catheter Cardiovasc Interv*. 2009;73(7):941-948.

Left Atrial Appendage Occlusion

Rony Lahoud and Andrew Goldsweig

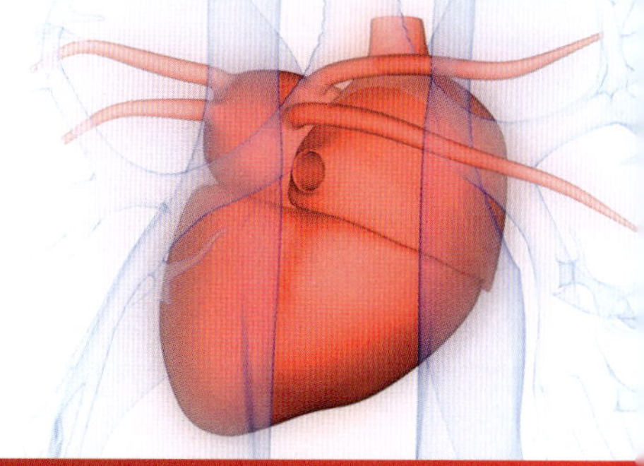

ATRIAL FIBRILLATION AND THE LEFT ATRIAL APPENDAGE

Atrial Fibrillation and Stroke Risk

Atrial fibrillation (AF) is the most common sustained arrhythmia globally. AF is projected to continue increasing in prevalence with the aging population as increasing age is a major risk factor for AF. AF is associated with a 4-5-fold increase in the risk of stroke and is estimated to account for nearly 25% of all strokes in the United States.[1] AF-related ischemic strokes appear to be more severe and confer a worse overall prognosis than non-AF-related strokes. The frequency or individual burden of AF does not appear to temper the risk, as paroxysmal, persistent, and permanent AF seem to confer similar risk of stroke.

Stroke prevention is therefore a central tenet of AF management.[2] The increased risk of thromboembolic stroke with AF is not uniform across patients and may be estimated using two well-validated scores: the CHA2DS$_2$ and the CHA2DS$_2$-VASc scores (**Table 40.1**). These scores use simple individual-level variables to estimate the yearly stroke risk and guide management.

Anticoagulation and Bleeding Risk

Historically, oral anticoagulants (OACs) have been the first line of therapy to reduce the risk of ischemic stroke in patients with AF. Warfarin, a vitamin K-dependent OAC, was the standard of care for decades but is limited by numerous drug-drug and food-drug interactions requiring dietary restriction, frequent blood testing to monitor its relatively narrow therapeutic range, and resultant nonadherence.[3] Newer non-vitamin K-dependent anticoagulants are safer and easier to use but are still limited by bleeding risk and high lifetime cost leading to poor adherence.[4] Elevated bleeding risk is especially concerning in elderly patients, who frequently have comorbidities and gait instability that increase their risks. Bleeding risks, fall risks, cognitive issues, drug interactions, and allergies make many physicians reluctant to prescribe OACs and patients less willing to adhere to them. In fact, anticoagulants are not used by >50% of eligible patients due to bleeding concerns, intolerance, or noncompliance.[5] The HAS-BLED (**Table 40.2**) score is a well-validated score aimed to predict the risk of bleeding events. When considering alternatives to anticoagulation for stroke prevention in AF, determination of the bleeding risk is an integral part of the assessment.

Rationale for Left Atrial Appendage Occlusion

The left atrial appendage (LAA) is the predominant source of thromboembolism in AF, accounting for 91% of strokes.[6] LAA occlusion (LAAO) eliminates the nidus for thrombus formation, thereby reducing the thromboembolic risk in AF while abrogating the need for long-term anticoagulation and its associated bleeding risk. Transcatheter LAAO thus provides a nonpharmacologic approach to stroke prevention for AF patients, meeting a large unmet need for prevention of AF-associated ischemic strokes.

TABLE 40.1 Thromboembolic Risk Scores for Patients With Atrial Fibrillation

CHADS$_2$	
Characteristic	**Points**
Congestive heart failure	1
Hypertension	1
Age ≥75 years	1
Diabetes mellitus	1
Stroke, transient ischemic attack, or thromboembolism	2
Maximum score	6
CHA$_2$DS$_2$-VASC	
Characteristic	**Points**
Congestive heart failure	1
Hypertension	1
Age ≥75 years	2
Diabetes mellitus	1
Stroke, transient ischemic attack, or thromboembolism	2
Vascular disease (prior MI, PAD, or aortic plaque)	1
Age 65-74 years	1
Sex category = female	1
Maximum score	9

MI, myocardial infarction; PAD, peripheral arterial disease.

Adapted from January CT, Wann LS, Alpert JS, et al. 2014 AHA/ACC/HRS guideline for the management of patients with atrial fibrillation: a report of the American College of Cardiology/ American Heart Association Task Force on Practice Guidelines and the Heart Rhythm Society. *J Am Coll Cardiol.* 2014;64:e1-e76.

The concept of LAA intervention for stroke prevention was first described in 1949 with a reported surgical excision of the LAA for the "prophylaxis of recurrent thrombi,"[6] but surgical LAA intervention only became more mainstream in the late 1990s.[6] Percutaneous LAAO devices emerged in the early 2000s and first received approval in the United States in 2015.

LAA Anatomy

The LAA is a multilobed trabeculated structure with a narrow neck, predisposing to stagnation of blood and thrombosis. The LAA arises anteriorly and superiorly from the left atrium. The LAA ostium is formed *superiorly* by the limbus of the left upper pulmonary vein (LUPV) and *inferiorly* by the mitral valve annulus and the left atrioventricular groove, which contains the left circumflex coronary artery (**Fig. 40.1**). The morphology of the LAA is variable and can be generally classified into one of the following categories:

TABLE 40.2 HAS-BLED Bleeding Risk Score

CHARACTERISTIC	POINTS
Hypertension (uncontrolled systolic blood pressure >160 mm Hg)	1
Abnormal liver or renal function[a]	1 each, maximum 2
Stroke (previous history)	1
Bleeding history or disposition (eg, anemia)	1
Labile INR (ie, time in therapeutic range <60%)	1
Elderly age (>65 y)	1
Drugs that promote bleeding or excess alcohol consumption (>7 U/wk)	1 each, maximum 2
Maximum score	9

INR, international normalized ratio.

[a]Abnormal liver function was defined as cirrhosis or biochemical evidence of significant hepatic derangement; abnormal renal function was defined as serum creatinine >200 µmol/L (2.26 mg/dL).

Adapted from Pisters R, Lane DA, Nieuwlaat R, de Vos CB, Crijns HJGM, Lip GYH. A novel user-friendly score (HAS-BLED) to assess 1-year risk of major bleeding in patients with atrial fibrillation: the Euro Heart Survey. *Chest*. 2010;138:1093-1100.

windsock, chicken wing cactus, and cauliflower (**Fig. 40.2**). The chicken wing-type anatomy may be particularly challenging for successful transcatheter closure.

Transthoracic echocardiography (TTE) is insufficient to evaluate LAA anatomy because the LAA is located close to the sternum and cannot be well visualized via surface ultrasound windows. A thorough evaluation of the LAA by transesophageal echocardiography (TEE) includes an assessment for LAA thrombus, the presence of baseline pericardial effusion, and the interrogation of the appendage from the midesophageal view in four planes (0°, 45°, 90°, and 135°) to determine the overall shape, depth, and number of lobes and the maximal width and depth of the LAA ostium. For the purpose of LAA closure, the ostial diameter is defined as the distance from a point just distal to the left circumflex artery to approximately 1 to 2 cm from the tip of the LUPV limbus. Cardiac computed tomography (CT) can be an excellent imaging tool for LAAO planning and is increasingly used given its superior spatial resolution to TEE. While not incorporated in the initial clinical studies for LAAO, CT can be very useful in cases where the LAA anatomy is unclear or TEE is contraindicated.

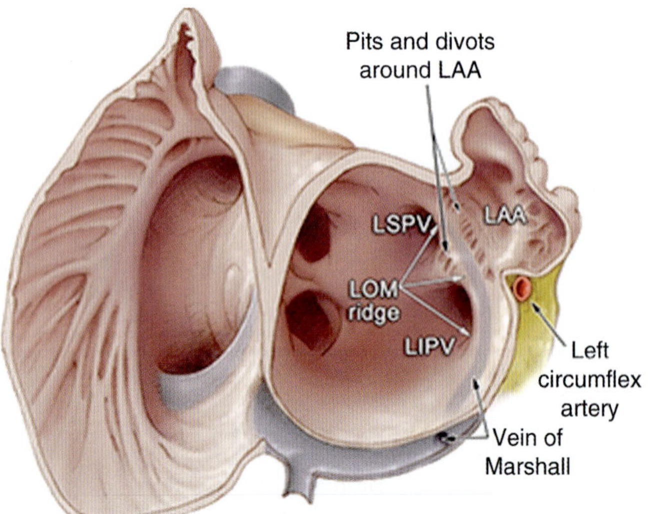

FIGURE 40.1 Anatomy of the left atrial appendage and surrounding structures.

LAA OCCLUSION

Indications

Assessments of thromboembolic and bleeding risks as outlined above are essential components for patient selection for LAAO because the procedure is specifically indicated for patients with an elevated stroke risk and who have a rationale to seek a nonpharmacologic approach to stroke reduction (Box 40.1). The 2019 American Heart Association/American College of Cardiology/Heart Rhythm Society Guideline for the Management of Patients with Atrial Fibrillation[7] recommends that treatment with an OAC or aspirin be considered in nonvalvular AF and a CHA2DS$_2$-VASc score of 1 (class IIB, Level of Evidence: C) and recommends the use of OACs in patients with CHA2DS$_2$-VASc score ≥2 (class I, Level of Evidence: A). Percutaneous LAAO for patients with increased stroke risk and contraindications to long-term anticoagulation received a class IIb recommendation with Level of Evidence B – nonrandomized (**Table 40.3**).

Several devices have been developed to close the LAA. At present, two devices have been approved by the Food and Drug Administration (FDA) for clinical use in the United States: the WATCHMAN device (Boston Scientific, Marlborough, MA) in 2015 and the Amulet device (Abbott, Chicago, IL) in 2021 (**Fig. 40.3**).

LAAO Versus Anticoagulation

The safety and clinical efficacy of WATCHMAN LAA closure have been evaluated in three randomized controlled trials that tested whether LAAO was noninferior to anticoagulation for the primary efficacy endpoint of stroke, systemic embolism, and cardiovascular/unexplained death in AF patients who were eligible for long-term OAC.

PROTECT-AF

The PROTECT-AF (WATCHMAN Left Atrial Appendage System for Embolic Protection in Patients with Atrial Fibrillation) trial randomly assigned 707 AF patients with a CHADS$_2$ score ≥1 who were eligible for long-term OAC to either WATCHMAN LAA closure or warfarin in a 2:1 ratio.[8] LAAO was both noninferior and superior to warfarin for the primary efficacy endpoint at a mean follow-up of 3.8 ± 1.7 years (2625 patient-years) (rate ratio, 0.60 [95% credible interval [CrI], 0.41-1.05, posterior probability of noninferiority >99.9%, and posterior probability for superiority = 96%) (**Fig. 40.4**). Cardiovascular and all-cause mortality were reduced with LAAO (hazard ratio [HR], 0.40 [95% confidence interval [CI], 0.21-0.75], *P* = .005 and HR 0.66 [95% CI, 0.45-0.98], *P* = .04, respectively). Safety events were initially greater in the LAAO group, driven by procedural complications, although by the end of the follow-up, the overall rate of safety events in both arms was similar due to bleeding events in the warfarin group[9] (**Fig. 40.4**). Peridevice leak (PDL) on follow-up TEE was frequent (41% and 32% of patients at 6 weeks and 1-year postprocedure, respectively), was mostly <3 mm in diameter, and did not appear to be associated with thromboembolic events.[10]

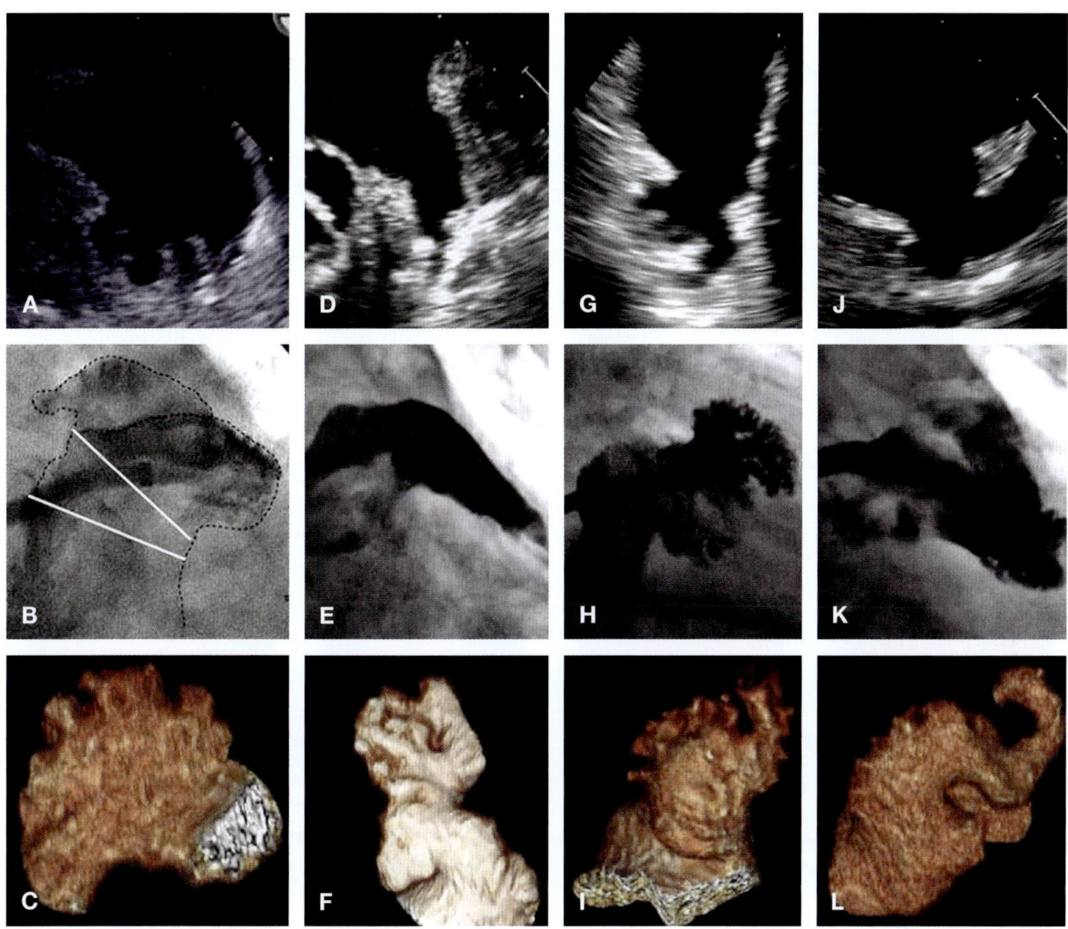

FIGURE 40.2 Various morphologies of the left atrial appendage. The four proposed classifications of LAA morphologies as shown by transesophageal echocardiography (**top**), cineangiography (**middle**), and 3D-computed tomography (**bottom**). **A-C:** Cauliflower; **D-F:** windsock; **G-I:** cactus; **J-L:** chicken wing. (Adapted from Beigel R, Wunderlich NC, Ho SY, Arsanjani R, Siegel RJ. The left atrial appendage: anatomy, function, and noninvasive evaluation. *J Am Coll Cardiol Img.* 2014;7(12):1251-1265.)

Box 40.1 Indications Left Atrial Appendage Occlusion

Left atrial appendage occlusion (LAAO) is indicated to reduce the risk of thromboembolism from the LAA in patients with nonvalvular AF who

- Are at increased risk for stroke and systemic embolism based on CHA2DS$_2$-VASc score (≥2 [men] or ≥3 [women] as per the ESC 2020 and ACC/AHA 2019 updates)
- Have a minimum of 1 year of life expectancy with a quality of life to benefit from LAAO
- Have an appropriate rationale to seek a nonpharmacologic alternative to anticoagulation therapy, taking into account the safety and effectiveness of the device compared to anticoagulation therapy. This includes patients with increased bleeding risks (eg, HAS-BLED score ≥3) or OAC intolerance, including prior bleeding, fall risk, uncontrolled hypertension, renal or liver failure, alcohol use, concomitant antiplatelet or nonsteroidal agents, high-risk occupations, noncompliance, labile international normalized ratio (INR), OAC intolerance/allergy, and drug interactions
- Had a patient-provider discussion for shared decision making

PREVAIL

The aim of the smaller PREVAIL (Prospective Randomized Evaluation of the WATCHMAN Left Atrial Appendage Closure Device In Patients with Atrial Fibrillation vs Long Term Warfarin Therapy) trial was to confirm procedural safety, particularly among newer operators, and to explore further the clinical efficacy of LAAO compared with warfarin.[11] A total of 407 AF patients with CHADS$_2$ ≥ 2 were randomly assigned to either WATCHMAN LAA closure or warfarin in a 2:1 ratio. The WATCHMAN device met the performance goal for procedural and device safety prespecified by the sponsor and the FDA, with safety events occurring in 2.2% of patients. Implantation by new operators was not associated with reduced rates of implant success or an increased risk of major adverse events. The rate of procedural complications, including stroke and pericardial effusions requiring intervention, was significantly reduced in PREVAIL compared to PROTECT-AF. At a mean follow-up of 11.8 ± 5.8 months, the primary efficacy endpoint of stroke, systemic embolism, or cardiovascular death was similar between study arms, but LAAO did not achieve noninferiority (device event rate, 0.064 vs warfarin event rate, 0.064; rate ratio, 1.07 [95% CrI, 0.57-1.89], rate ratio for noninferiority criterion: upper bound of 95% CrI < 1.75).

A pooled patient-level meta-analysis of PROTECT-AF and PREVAIL demonstrated that the rate of the primary efficacy

TABLE 40.3 2019 AHA/ACC/HRS Focused Update of the 2014 AHA/ACC/HRS Guideline for the Management of Patients With AF

RECOMMENDATIONS	CLASS	LEVEL	REF
After surgical occlusion or exclusion of the LAA, it is recommended to continue anticoagulation in at-risk patients with AF for stroke prevention	I	B	461, 462
LAA occlusion may be considered for stroke prevention in patients with AF and contraindications for long-term anticoagulant treatment (eg, those with a previous life-threatening bleed without a reversible cause)	IIb	B	449, 453, 454
Surgical occlusion or exclusion of the LAA may be considered for stroke prevention in patients with AF undergoing cardiac surgery	IIb	B	463
Surgical occlusion or exclusion of the LAA may be considered for stroke prevention in patients undergoing thoracoscopic AF surgery	IIb	B	468

ACC, American College of Cardiology; AF, atrial fibrillation; AHA, American Heart Association; HRS, Heart Rhythm Society; LAA, left atrial appendage.

endpoint was similar with LAAO compared with chronic warfarin therapy (HR, 0.79; 95% CI, 0.53-1.2, P = .22).[12] All-cause stroke and systemic embolism were similar between LAAO and warfarin; there were numerically more ischemic strokes in the device group, significantly more hemorrhagic strokes in the warfarin group, and significantly fewer cardiovascular deaths in the device group. Another pooled analysis demonstrated a significant reduction in major bleeding with LAAO once the 6-month period of postprocedure pharmacotherapy was completed.[12]

PRAGUE-17

The PRAGUE-17 (Left Atrial Appendage Closure vs Novel Anticoagulation Agents in Atrial Fibrillation) study is the only completed randomized controlled trial to date comparing LAAO with direct oral anticoagulants (DOACs). The study, which enrolled 402 patients randomized 1:1 to WATCHMAN or DOAC, showed noninferiority of LAAO compared with DOAC for a composite endpoint that combined ischemic and bleeding events with 4 years of follow-up.[13,14] The study was underpowered to assess the specific impact of LAAO on lowering ischemic events alone.

Amulet Versus WATCHMAN

The Amulet device has been compared to the WATCHMAN device in two clinical trials, resulting in approval of Amulet in the United States.

SWISS-APERO

The SWISS-APERO (Comparison of Amplatzer Amulet and Watchman Device in Patients Undergoing Left Atrial Appendage Closure) trial randomized 221 patients to receive the Amulet versus WATCHMAN device and noted similar rates of residual LAA flow in both the devices at 45-day postimplant on CT angiography (CTA; 67.6% vs 70%, respectively, P = .001). Intradevice leaks were more common with the Amulet device (44.8% vs 23%, P = .001), while TEE-defined PDL of >5 mm were more common with the WATCHMAN device (13.7% vs 27.5%, P = .02). Use of the Amulet device was associated with higher procedure-related major complications (9.0% vs 2.7%,

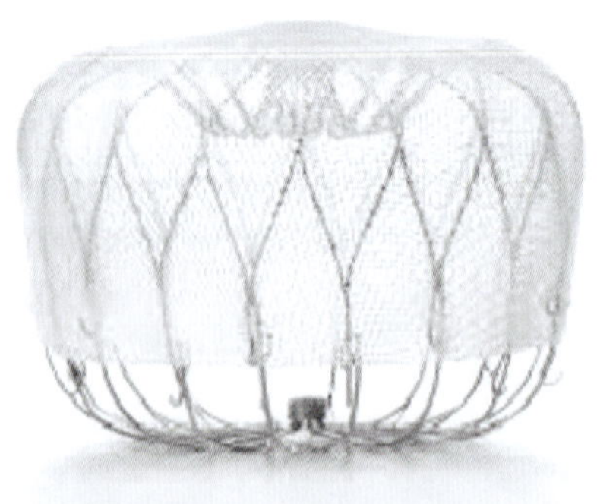

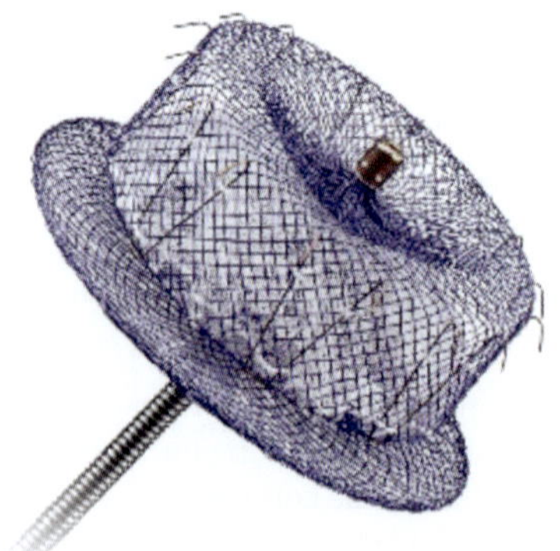

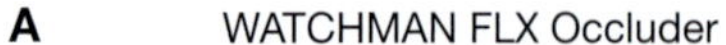

FIGURE 40.3 Long-term clinical and safety outcomes in the PROTECT-AF randomized trial of WATCHMAN LAA closure compared with warfarin therapy. **A:** Primary efficacy outcome of cardiovascular death, stroke, or systemic embolism. At a mean of 3.8 years (2621 patient-years) of follow-up, transcatheter LAA occlusion with the WATCHMAN met prespecified criteria for noninferiority and superiority compared with warfarin. **B:** Primary safety outcomes, a composite of major bleeding events and procedure-related complications. While an early hazard was apparent around the periprocedural period with device therapy, the overall rate of safety events was similar in both groups, primarily due to ongoing bleeding events in the warfarin group. LAA, left atrial appendage; PROTECT-AF, WATCHMAN Left Atrial Appendage System for Embolic Protection in Patients with Atrial Fibrillation. (Adapted from Reddy VY, Sievert H, Halperin J, et al. Percutaneous left atrial appendage closure vs warfarin for atrial fibrillation: a randomized clinical trial. *JAMA.* 2014;312:1988-1998.)

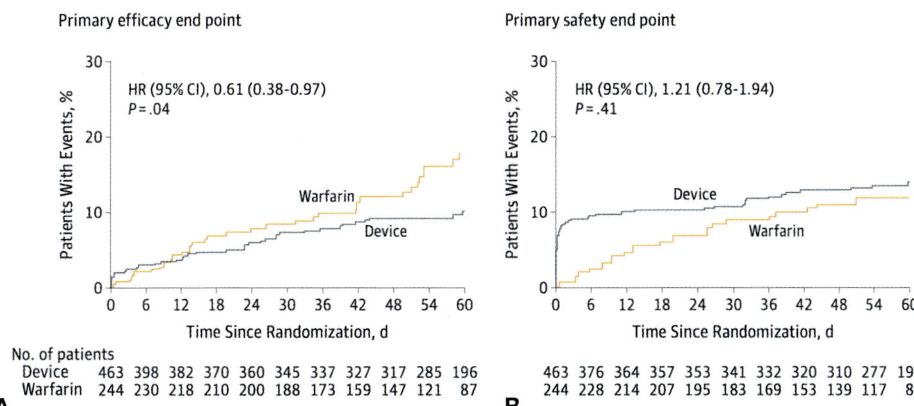

FIGURE 40.4 WATCHMAN FLX and Amulet devices.

P = .047) due to higher rates of major bleeding and pericardial effusions.[15]

AMULET US-IDE

The AMULET US-IDE (Investigational Device Exemption) trial was the largest LAAO trial to date, randomizing 1878 patients with nonvalvular AF to receive the Amulet versus WATCHMAN device in 1:1 fashion.[16]Amulet was noninferior to WATCHMAN with regard to safety, using a composite of all-cause mortality, procedure-related complications, or major bleeding at 12 months (14.5% with Amulet vs 14.7% with WATCHMAN). Efficacy, a composite of ischemic stroke or systemic embolism at 18 months, was similar between the two devices (2.8% for both devices). Procedure-related complications (device embolization or pericardial effusion) were higher in the Amulet group (4.5% vs 2.5%, P = .02), while moderate-to-severe PDL at 12 months was lower in the Amulet group (10% vs 22%, P < .001).

Trials in Progress

As reflected in the societal guidelines above (Level of Evidence: B), more randomized data are needed to support the efficacy of LAAO.[17,18] The two largest trials in progress are the CHAMPION-AF (NCT04394546, n = 3000) and CATALYST (NCT04226547, n = 2650) trials, randomizing AF patients who are eligible for long-term DOAC to LAAO with WATCHMAN FLX or Amulet, respectively, versus long-term DOAC. The outcomes assessed are ischemic stroke, systemic embolization, cardiovascular death, and nonprocedural major bleeding at 2 to 3 years.

Finally, there is rising interest in the concept of using LAAO *in combination* with DOAC to reduce ischemic risk even further. This concept was fueled by the recent LAAOS III trial, which showed a 33% relative risk reduction in ischemic stroke or systemic embolization in patients undergoing surgical LAA closure with chronic anticoagulation versus anticoagulation alone.[19,20]

Postprocedure Antithrombotic Regimens

For the WATCHMAN device, there are two FDA-approved options for postprocedure antithrombotic therapy. Discharge on aspirin plus anticoagulant is well established based upon the PROTECT-AF and PREVAIL trials; or discharge on dual antiplatelet therapy (DAPT) with aspirin and clopidogrel appears equivalent based upon recent trial and registry results.[21,22] If patients receive aspirin plus anticoagulation at discharge, they are transitioned to DAPT at 45 days postprocedure if no device-related thrombus (DRT) or PDL > 5 mm is observed on imaging. All patients are transitioned to aspirin monotherapy at 6 months postprocedure. For the Amulet device, discharge on DAPT for 6 months followed by aspirin monotherapy is well established based on the Amulet IDE study and was approved by the FDA with device approval in 2021.

LAAO DEVICES AND PROCEDURES

WATCHMAN FLX

The WATCHMAN FLX device is composed of a self-expanding nitinol frame with a polyethylene terephthalate fabric 160 mm pore mesh cap (**Fig. 40.3A**). Two rows of distal fixation anchors and radial force at the device shoulders secure the device within the LAA trabeculae. The device attaches to a delivery cable at a central threaded insert. The device size corresponds to the width of the device at its proximal shoulders. The length of the device is roughly half its width when compressed 10% to 15%, a change from the prior version of the device to allow for implantation in shallower appendages.

Amulet

The Amulet device is made of a self-expanding nitinol mesh and consists of a lobe and a disc connected by a central waist, with polyester patches sewn into both the lobe and disc to facilitate occlusion (**Fig. 40.3B**). The lobe has stabilizing wires that anchor the device within the LAA trabeculae. The device has a threaded screw attachment at the proximal end for connection to the delivery cable and radiopaque markers at each end.

LAAO PROCEDURE

The LAAO procedure (**Fig. 40.5**) is performed via femoral venous access (right-sided whenever possible) with recommended ultrasound guidance. Commonly, radial arterial access is obtained for blood pressure monitoring. From the femoral vein, trans-septal puncture is performed using standard techniques and TEE or intracardiac echocardiography (ICE) and fluoroscopy guidance. Since the trans-septal puncture should be perpendicular to the ostium of the LAA, an inferior and posterior location along the fossa ovalis is usually desired. The 90° TEE view is especially helpful in gaging

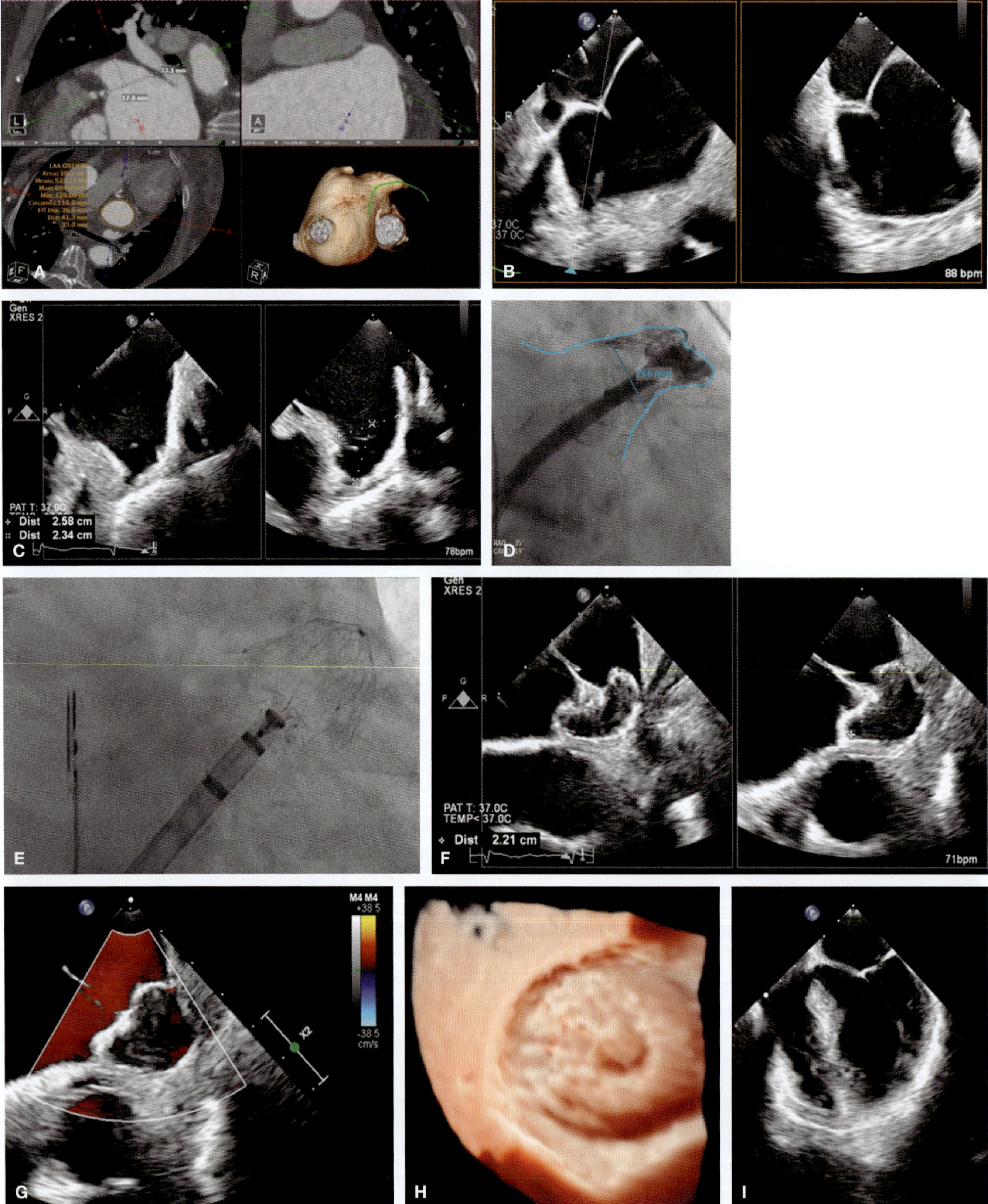

FIGURE 40.5 Step-by-step description of the LAAO procedure including computed tomography, fluoroscopy, and echocardiography images. **A.** Pre-procedure CT for procedure planning. **B.** Echocardiography-guided transseptal puncture. **C.** Echocardiographic LAA measurement. **D.** Fluoroscopic LAA measurement. **E.** Device implantation. **F.** Measurement of device compression. **G.** Assessment for peri-device leak with color Doppler. **H.** Device release. **I.** Echocardiographic assessment for pericardial effusion. LAAO, left atrial appendage occlusion.

TABLE 40.4 TEE Versus ICE for Intraprocedural Imaging

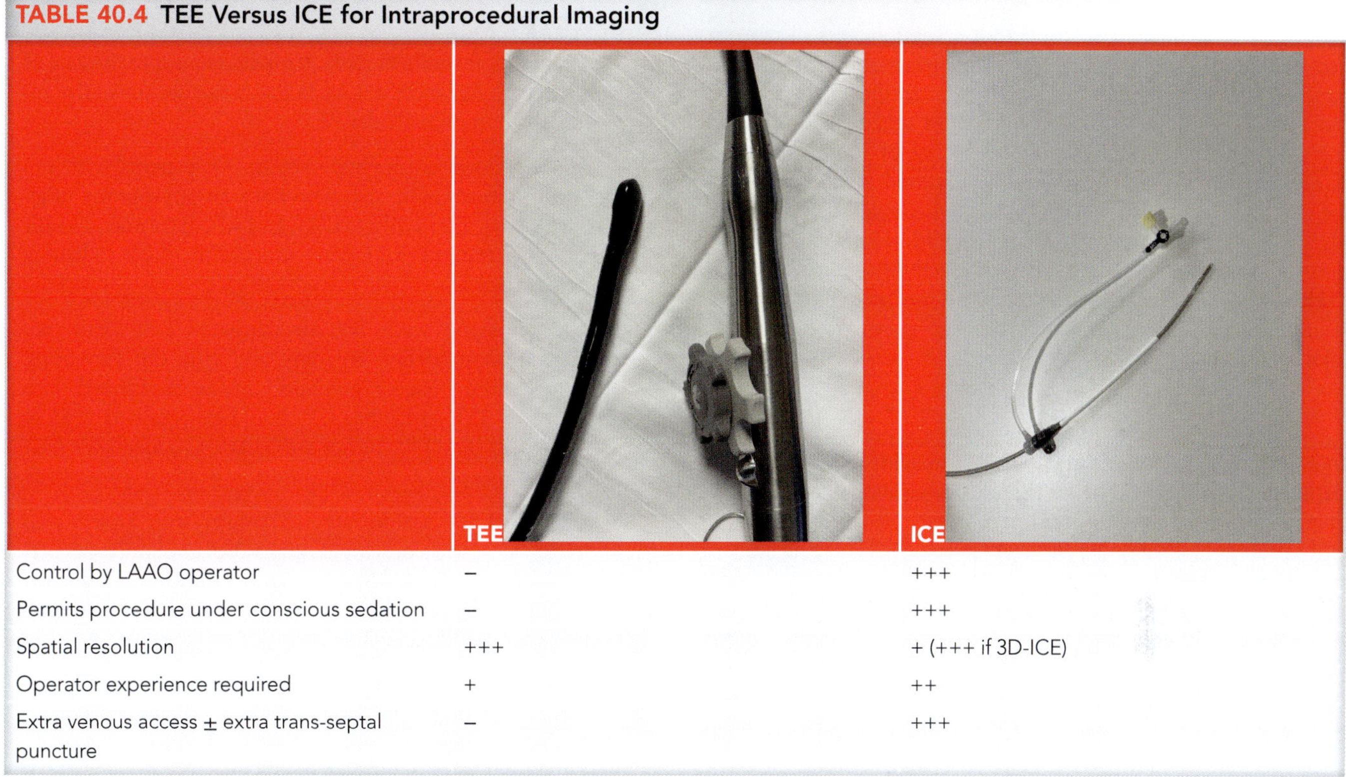

Control by LAAO operator	–	+++
Permits procedure under conscious sedation	–	+++
Spatial resolution	+++	+ (+++ if 3D-ICE)
Operator experience required	+	++
Extra venous access ± extra trans-septal puncture	–	+++

ICE, intracardiac echocardiography; LAAO, left atrial appendage occlusion; TEE, transesophageal echocardiography.

the direction of the LAA, with most appendages oriented anteriorly and superiorly. Following trans-septal puncture, a device-specific delivery sheath is delivered to the left atrium, over either a stiff wire anchored in the left superior pulmonary vein or a pigtail-shaped wire placed in the left atrium. The WATCHMAN device is delivered through a 14-Fr sheath with one of the three shapes corresponding to LAA morphology. The Amulet device can be delivered through either a 12- or 14-Fr TorqueVue sheath depending upon device size or through a 19-Fr steerable sheath.

The device delivery sheath is then advanced over a pigtail catheter, which is positioned in the LAA. The pigtail catheter allows for contrast angiography of the appendage.

Device deployment is visualized using both echocardiography (TEE or ICE) and fluoroscopy. Echocardiography and contrast angiography should be used after deployment to verify placement.

WATCHMAN device implantation is assessed using the PASS criteria:

P: Position (plane of maximal device diameter at the LAA ostium),
A: Anchor (gently pull back and release to ensure no device movement on a "tug test"),
S: Size (10%-30% compression on TEE/ICE) and
S: Seal (no PDL > 5 mm and all lobes covered).

Amulet device implantation is assessed using the CLOSE criteria:

C: A minimum of the 2/3 of the device lobe distal to the left circumflex coronary artery
L: Lobe of the device slightly compressed with good apposition to the LAA wall
O: Orientation of the lobe is coaxial with the landing zone
S: Separation of the disc from the lobe
E: Elliptical concave shape of the disc

After device deployment, hemostasis at the femoral venous access site is achieved by device-mediated closure, external figure-of-eight suture, or manual compression.

PERIPROCEDURAL IMAGING

Preprocedural Imaging

Baseline preprocedural imaging with TEE or cardiac CTA is recommended prior to starting the procedure to define LAA anatomy and to rule out the presence of thrombus.

With TEE, multiple two-dimensional images of the LAA should be obtained at multiple angles (0°, 45°, 90°, and 135°) to identify the maximal width of the LAA ostium along with straight-line depth dimensions obtained from the center of the planned landing zone to the LAA wall. Adequate hydration (ideally left atrial pressure >12 mm Hg) should be ensured at the time of measurement, and all measurements should be obtained during ventricular systole to ensure maximal filling of the LAA. Three-dimensional (3D) TEE imaging of the LAA can provide improved accuracy for sizing measurements.

With gated cardiac CT, measurements of the LAA ostium should be performed utilizing 3D multiplanar reformatted images during midlate ventricular systole. As mentioned above, CT is an increasingly used technology, partially due to its noninvasive nature and superior spatial resolution to TEE.[23]

Intraprocedural Imaging

Intraprocedural imaging is critical for several aspects of the procedure including ruling out LAA thrombus, monitoring for pericardial effusion, guidance of trans-septal puncture, visualization of device implantation, stability, compression, and PDL, and assessment of iatrogenic ASD.[24] Therefore, the use of fluoroscopy alone is not recommended.[23] TEE was the required imaging modality for the trials leading to WATCHMAN and Amulet device approvals and remains the mainstay of intraprocedural imaging, offering generally superior resolution and reproducibility compared to ICE (**Table 40.4**). ICE can nonetheless be a powerful tool in the hands of an experienced operator and has been shown to be safe and effective in small studies.[25]

Postprocedural Imaging

In addition to intraprocedural TEE/ICE imaging following device deployment to assess for immediate complications and a predischarge TTE to assess for delayed pericardial effusion or rare device embolization, a 45-day (45-90 days) post-LAAO imaging study is important in guiding management. The 45-day post-LAAO study should assess for both DRT and PDL. The most commonly used modality is TEE, allowing for visualization of both complications. Cardiac CTA is an increasingly popular modality, offering a less invasive approach, a comparable rate of detection of DRT, and possibly a greater rate of detection of PDL compared to TEE.[26] Based upon the PROTECT-AF and PREVAL trial protocols, the presence of PDL >5 mm should be treated with continued anticoagulation and serial LAA imaging to assess for reduction in PDL size.

COMPLICATIONS

Major complications associated with LAAO include pericardial effusion and cardiac tamponade, procedural stroke, device embolization, and vascular injury or bleeding.[27] In PROTECT-AF trial, serious pericardial effusion (requiring drainage or surgical intervention) occurred in 4.8% of patients.[9] However, procedural outcomes have improved since this initial experience, with pericardial effusions occurring in 1% to 3% of commercial cases.[22] Nonetheless, pericardial effusion remains the most common adverse event associated with LAAO, and operators should have pericardiocentesis equipment easily accessible while performing the procedure. The second major procedural complication identified in the PROTECT-AF trial was periprocedural cerebrovascular accident, occurring in 0.9% of patients. More recent data from the National Cardiovascular Data Registry show the occurrence of ischemic stroke down to 0.12% of cases, and hemorrhagic strokes down to 0.01%.[22] Device embolization remains an uncommon complication, occurring in 0.07% of patients.[22]

Late adverse events consist primarily of DRT and PDL, noted on follow-up imaging. DRT is observed in approximately 3% to 4% of cases. The significance of DRT is still emerging, but there is a well-established association with thromboembolic events.[28] While patients are commonly treated with extended anticoagulant therapy when DRT is noted, the appropriate treatment regimen remains unknown. PDL > 5 mm is noted in ~1% to 3% of cases on TEE at 45 to 90 days postprocedure. The exact significance of PDL remains unclear, given the heterogeneous nature of leaks and varying definitions associated with it. Recent studies suggest increased rates of strokes but offer no insights on ideal management strategies for PDL.[29,30]

Key Points

- Prevention of thromboembolic stroke is central to the care of patients with AF, and the LAA is the major source of thromboembolism in nonvalvular AF.
- LAAO is appropriate for nonvalvular AF patients with elevated thromboembolic risk who have an appropriate rationale to seek an alternative to OAC and who have adequate life expectancy (minimum >1 year) and quality of life to benefit from LAAO.
- Baseline imaging with TEE or cardiac CT is important before LAAO to define anatomy and rule out thrombus. Intraprocedural imaging guidance can be performed with TEE or ICE. TEE or cardiac CT should be obtained at 45 to 90 days post-LAAO for device surveillance to assess for DRT and PDL.
- Following LAAO, antithrombotic therapy with aspirin plus warfarin, a DOAC, or clopidogrel (DAPT) should be prescribed for up to 6 months followed by aspirin monotherapy according to the studied regimen for each device and with consideration of the bleeding risks of each patient.
- The most common procedural complications of LAAO are pericardial effusion and periprocedural stroke. Both have decreased in frequency with improving operator experience and iterative device improvements. Long-term issues associated with LAAO include DRT and PDL, which remain the focus of ongoing studies to understand their significance and optimal treatment strategies.

Acknowledgments

The authors thank Matthew Price, MD, FSCAI whose chapter in the previous edition of this book served as an excellent guide.

For further review and interactivities, please see the chapter-based multiple choice questions and videos accessible in the complimentary eBook bundled with this text. Access instructions are located in the inside front cover.

References

1. Benjamin EJ, Muntner P, Alonso A, et al. Heart disease and stroke statistics-2019 update: a report from the American Heart Association. *Circulation*. 2019;139(10):e56-e528.
2. Reddy VY, Doshi SK, Kar S, et al. 5-Year outcomes after left atrial appendage closure: from the PREVAIL and PROTECT AF trials. *J Am Coll Cardiol*. 2017;70(24):2964-2975.
3. Price MJ, Valderrabano M. Left atrial appendage closure to prevent stroke in patients with atrial fibrillation. *Circulation*. 2014;130(2):202-212.
4. Marzec LN, Wang J, Shah ND, et al. Influence of direct oral anticoagulants on rates of oral anticoagulation for atrial fibrillation. *J Am Coll Cardiol*. 2017;69(20):2475-2484.
5. Holmes DR Jr, Alkhouli M, Reddy V. Left atrial appendage occlusion for the unmet clinical needs of stroke prevention in nonvalvular atrial fibrillation. *Mayo Clin Proc*. 2019;94(5):864-874.
6. Blackshear JL, Odell JA. Appendage obliteration to reduce stroke in cardiac surgical patients with atrial fibrillation. *Ann Thorac Surg*. 1996;61(2):755-759.

7. January CT, Wann LS, Calkins H, et al. 2019 AHA/ACC/HRS focused update of the 2014 AHA/ACC/HRS guideline for the management of patients with atrial fibrillation: a report of the American College of Cardiology/American Heart Association Task force on clinical practice guidelines and the heart rhythm society. *J Am Coll Cardiol*. 2019;74(1):104-132.
8. Holmes DR, Reddy VY, Turi ZG, et al. Percutaneous closure of the left atrial appendage versus warfarin therapy for prevention of stroke in patients with atrial fibrillation: a randomised non-inferiority trial. *Lancet*. 2009;374(9689):534-542.
9. Reddy VY, Sievert H, Halperin J, et al. Percutaneous left atrial appendage closure vs warfarin for atrial fibrillation: a randomized clinical trial. *JAMA*. 2014;312(19):1988-1998.
10. Viles-Gonzalez JF, Kar S, Douglas P, et al. The clinical impact of incomplete left atrial appendage closure with the watchman device in patients with atrial fibrillation: a PROTECT AF (percutaneous closure of the left atrial appendage versus warfarin therapy for prevention of stroke in patients with atrial fibrillation) substudy. *J Am Coll Cardiol*. 2012;59(10):923-929.
11. Holmes DR Jr, Kar S, Price MJ, et al. Prospective randomized evaluation of the watchman left atrial appendage closure device in patients with atrial fibrillation versus long-term warfarin therapy: the PREVAIL trial. *J Am Coll Cardiol*. 2014;64(1):1-12.
12. Holmes DR Jr, Doshi SK, Kar S, et al. Left atrial appendage closure as an alternative to warfarin for stroke prevention in atrial fibrillation: a patient-level meta-analysis. *J Am Coll Cardiol*. 2015;65(24):2614-2623.
13. Osmancik P, Herman D, Neuzil P, et al. Left atrial appendage closure versus direct oral anticoagulants in high-risk patients with atrial fibrillation. *J Am Coll Cardiol*. 2020;75(25):3122-3135.
14. Osmancik P, Herman D, Neuzil P, et al. 4-Year outcomes after left atrial appendage closure versus nonwarfarin oral anticoagulation for atrial fibrillation. *J Am Coll Cardiol*. 2022;79(1):1-14.
15. Galea R, De Marco F, Meneveau N, et al. Amulet or watchman device for percutaneous left atrial appendage closure: primary results of the SWISS-APERO randomized clinical trial. *Circulation*. 2022;145(10):724-738.
16. Lakkireddy D, Thaler D, Ellis CR, et al. Amplatzer amulet left atrial appendage occluder versus watchman device for stroke prophylaxis (Amulet IDE): a randomized, controlled trial. *Circulation*. 2021;144(19):1543-1552.
17. Khan MS, Ochani RK, Shaikh A, et al. Fragility Index in cardiovascular randomized controlled trials. *Circ Cardiovasc Qual Outcomes*. 2019;12(12):e005755.
18. Alkhouli M, Ellis CR, Daniels M, et al. Left atrial appendage occlusion. *JACC (J Am Coll Cardiol)*. 2022;1(5):100136.
19. Whitlock R, Healey J, Vincent J, et al. Rationale and design of the left atrial appendage occlusion study (LAAOS) III. *Ann Cardiothorac Surg*. 2014;3(1):45-54.
20. Verma S, Bhatt DL, Tseng EE. Time to remove the left atrial appendage at surgery: LAAOS III in perspective. *Circulation*. 2021;144(14):1088-1090.
21. Osman M, Busu T, Osman K, et al. Short-term antiplatelet versus anticoagulant therapy after left atrial appendage occlusion: a systematic review and meta-analysis. *JACC Clin Electrophysiol*. 2020;6(5):494-506.
22. Freeman JV, Varosy P, Price MJ, et al. The NCDR left atrial appendage occlusion registry. *J Am Coll Cardiol*. 2020;75(13):1503-1518.
23. Saw J, Holmes DR, Cavalcante JL, et al. SCAI/HRS expert consensus statement on transcatheter Left Atrial Appendage Closure (LAAC). *Journal of the Society for Cardiovascular Angiography & Interventions*. 2023;16(11):1384-1400.
24. Alkhouli M, Chaker Z, Alqahtani F, Raslan S, Raybuck B. Outcomes of routine intracardiac echocardiography to guide left atrial appendage occlusion. *JACC Clin Electrophysiol*. 2020;6(4):393-400.
25. Berti S, Pastormerlo LE, Santoro G, et al. Intracardiac versus transesophageal echocardiographic guidance for left atrial appendage occlusion: the LAAO Italian multicenter registry. *JACC Cardiovasc Interv*. 2018;11(11):1086-1092.
26. Qamar SR, Jalal S, Nicolaou S, Tsang M, Gilhofer T, Saw J. Comparison of cardiac computed tomography angiography and transoesophageal echocardiography for device surveillance after left atrial appendage closure. *EuroIntervention*. 2019;15(8):663-670.
27. Price MJ. Prevention and management of complications of left atrial appendage closure devices. *Interv Cardiol Clin*. 2014;3(2):301-311.
28. Alkhouli M, Busu T, Shah K, Osman M, Alqahtani F, Raybuck B. Incidence and clinical impact of device-related thrombus following Percutaneous left atrial appendage occlusion: a meta-analysis. *JACC Clin Electrophysiol*. 2018;4(12):1629-1637.
29. Dukkipati SR, Holmes DR Jr, Doshi SK, et al. Impact of peridevice leak on 5-year outcomes after left atrial appendage closure. *J Am Coll Cardiol*. 2022;80(5):469-483.
30. Alkhouli M, Du C, Killu A, et al. Clinical impact of residual leaks following left atrial appendage occlusion: insights from the NCDR LAAO registry. *JACC Clin Electrophysiol*. 2022;8(6):766-778.
31. Lip GY, Nieuwlaat R, Pisters R, Lane DA, Crijns HJGM. Refining clinical risk stratification for predicting stroke and thromboembolism in atrial fibrillation using a novel risk factor-based approach: the euro heart survey on atrial fibrillation. *Chest*. 2010;137(2):263-272.
32. Price MJ, Valderrábano M, Zimmerman S, et al. Periprocedural pericardial effusion complicating transcatheter left atrial appendage occlusion: a report from the NCDR LAAO registry. *Circ Cardiovasc Interv*. 2022;15(5):e011718.

Transcatheter Mitral Valve Repair and Replacement

Abdullah Al-Abcha, Teodora Donisan, Emily Cendrowski, Trevor Simard, and Mayra Elizabeth Guerrero

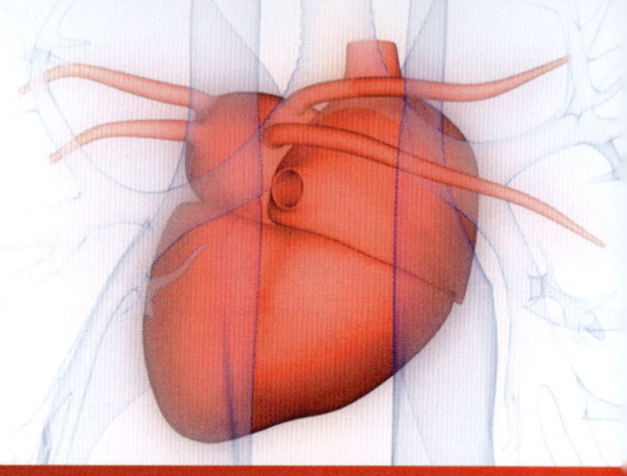

INTRODUCTION

Transcatheter mitral valve (MV) interventions are evolving into a viable treatment option for several mitral pathologies ranging from rheumatic mitral valve stenosis (MS), primary or secondary mitral regurgitation (MR), failed surgical bioprostheses or annuloplasty rings, and degenerative calcific MS or MR in the setting of mitral annulus calcification (MAC). Many advances have occurred in the last 4 decades since mitral valvuloplasty was first described by Inoue in 1982 and his first series of cases published in 1984.[1] Transcatheter edge-to-edge repair (TEER) with the MitraClip device (Abbott Vascular, Santa Clara, CA) proved to be a safe procedure with efficacy noninferior to surgical repair in primary MR[2] and superior to medical treatment in secondary MR[3] leading to approval and inclusion in guideline recommendations for high-surgical risk patients with primary MR as well as secondary MR irrespective of surgical risk.[4] Transcatheter mitral valve replacement (TMVR) has emerged as an alternative approach for patients who are not candidates for transcatheter repair. The TMVR era first started with the use of aortic balloon-expandable transcatheter valves for mitral valve-in-valve (MViV), mitral valve-in-ring (MViR), or valve-in-MAC (ViMAC) procedures. Since then, the field has rapidly evolved generating numerous transcatheter heart valves (THVs) specifically designed for the MV, with several already being evaluated in pivotal trials. This chapter reviews both transcatheter MV repair and TMVR therapies approved for commercial use as well as TMVR technology being evaluated in pivotal clinical trials.

TRANSCATHETER MV REPAIR

The two main types of transcatheter MV repair are balloon commissurotomy or valvuloplasty and edge-to-edge repair. Newer technologies are being developed utilizing a variety of mechanisms, including direct or indirect annuloplasty, chordal repair, ventricular remodeling, and enhanced coaptation though leaflet extensions. Most remain in early stages of evaluation and are not commercially available. Therefore, we consider those are outside the scope of this chapter. The main focus will be on technologies available and needed in the daily practice of contemporary interventional cardiology practices.

Transcatheter MV Repair for MS

MS: Causes, Symptoms, and Complications

MS is a complex valve disease caused by structural changes of the MV apparatus leading to increased resistance to transmitral flow as well as increased left atrial (LA) and pulmonary arterial systolic pressure.[5] In developing countries, MS is predominantly caused by rheumatic fever; however, in industrialized countries, degenerative MS is increasingly prevalent given ever-increasing life expectancy.[6] Rheumatic fever is an autoimmune reaction to streptococcal infections, leading to rheumatic heart disease (RHD) characterized by both valvular and myocardial inflammation and damage. Despite decreasing prevalence, rheumatic fever remains an important clinical concern worldwide including in developed areas, most frequently in immigrants or the elderly.[7] Degenerative MS can arise from MAC and/or mitral leaflets, especially in the elderly or in patients undergoing renal replacement therapy.[8] Mitral bioprosthetic valve stenosis is an increasingly common cause of MS with dedicated criteria being developed.[9] Other less frequent causes of MS include congenital heart disease, endocarditis, carcinoid heart disease, infiltrative disease, systemic inflammatory diseases, or cancer treatment related.[10] The hallmark symptom of MS is exertional dyspnea, which usually occurs when the mitral valve area (MVA) is ≤1.5 cm^2.[11] Other symptoms of MS include chest discomfort, hemoptysis, and pressure effects on surrounding structures (ie, dysphagia from LA compression of the esophagus). MS can be complicated by a higher thromboembolic risk, given the association with LA enlargement, stasis, and atrial fibrillation.[12]

Morphologic Features of MS

Morphologically, rheumatic mitral disease leads to a funnel-shaped geometry, with diffuse fibrous thickening of the margins of closure and leaflets, commissural fusion, and shortening, thickening, and fusion of the chordae (**Fig. 41.1**). While RHD typically spares the annulus, in degenerative MS due to MAC, this is primary driving pathology, particularly of the posterior annulus. Degenerative MS may also extend into the base of the leaflets leading to leaflet thickening and calcified nodules. Accordingly, the mechanism of stenosis due to MAC likely arises from both impairments in physiologic annular dilation during diastole and restricted leaflet motion.[13]

Diagnostic Findings and Evaluation of MS

Transthoracic echocardiography (TTE) is essential in establishing the diagnosis and severity of MS, while also evaluating associated valvular pathologies.[14] Hemodynamic severity is reflected by MVA, with severe MS typically represented by an MVA ≤1.5 cm^2, typically translating to a transmitral mean gradient of >5 to 10 mm Hg or diastolic pressure half time of ≥150 ms. If there are discordances between symptoms and imaging findings, exercise testing or cardiac catheterization are recommended and will also enable diagnosis of the underlying pathology of MS, which has important management implications.[15]

Treatment of MS

In patients with MS, medical therapy with diuretics, beta blockers, calcium channel blockers, or ivabradine to optimize heart rate control can improve valvular hemodynamics, translating to symptomatic improvement.[11] Concomitant atrial fibrillation or flutter are often present and warrant anticoagulation with vitamin K antagonists.[11] Transcatheter interventions for MS are based largely upon the underlying pathology, highlighting the importance of detailed anatomic assessment prior to discerning an interventional strategy.

	Rheumatic mitral stenosis	Degenerative mitral stenosis
Leaflets	• Thick and retracted • Commissural fusion • Reduced orifice -> "fishmouth" opening	• Leaflet base calcification • No commissural fusion • Leaflet tips are unaffected
Annulus	• Spared	• Calcified (posteriorly most prominent) • Tunnel-like stenosis leading to apical displacement of the leaflet hinge point
Transthoracic echocardiogram	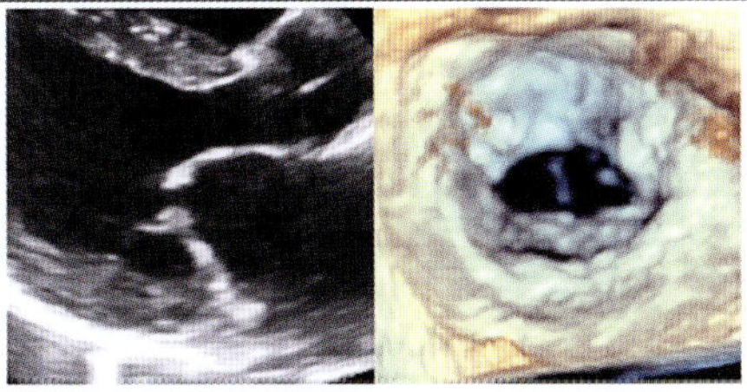	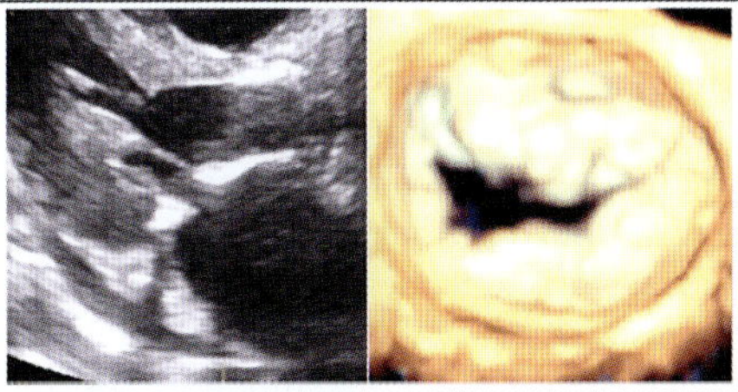

FIGURE 41.1 Transthoracic and transesophageal echocardiogram images of rheumatic (*Left*) or degenerative mitral stenosis (*Right*).

Percutaneous mitral balloon valvuloplasty or commissurotomy (PMBC) is often the first-line intervention for patients with severe rheumatic MS who have favorable anatomy, with a goal of preventing or delaying eventual surgical MV replacement, though upfront surgical intervention can also be considered particularly if anatomy is not favorable for PMBC (**Table 41.1**).[11,15] Indeed, of patients undergoing PMBC for rheumatic MS, 70% to 80% were asymptomatic at 10 years and 30% to 40% at 20 years.[16,17] PMBC should be performed in specialized heart valve centers, with the ultimate choice between PMBC and surgical approach being driven by patient and anatomic considerations in combination with local expertise.[15] PMBC remains underused worldwide given cost and availability concerns.[18]

Patients with calcific MS have worse prognoses, with a 5-year survival rate of <50%.[19] Surgical commissurotomy has been reported to relieve stenosis, though it should be performed in centers with a high level of expertise and requires further study. TMVR represents a promising alternative approach although this is an area of ongoing study and technical development—an area we expand on later in this chapter.[13]

Percutaneous Balloon Commissurotomy

Indications

When PMBC is considered, TTE often provides sufficient morphologic evaluation to determine candidacy, though transesophageal echocardiography (TEE) affords additional insights into

TABLE 41.1 2020 AHA/ACC Guideline Recommendations for Mitral Stenosis Intervention[4]

Recommendations for Patients With Rheumatic MS
Class 1 recommendations
PMBC = recommended—if symptomatic, severe rheumatic MS (MVA ≤1.5 cm²), favorable valve morphology, <moderate MR, and the absence of LA thrombus
Mitral surgery = recommended—if severely symptomatic, severe rheumatic MS (MVA ≤1.5 cm²), not candidates for/have failed prior PMBC, require other cardiac procedures, no access to PMBC
Class 2a recommendations
PMBC = reasonable—if asymptomatic, severe rheumatic MS (MVA ≤1.5 cm²), favorable valve morphology, <moderate MR, the absence of LA thrombus, PA systolic pressures >50 mm Hg
Class 2b recommendations
PMBC = may be considered—if asymptomatic, severe rheumatic MS (MVA ≤1.5 cm²), favorable valve morphology, <moderate MR, the absence of LA thrombus, new onset AF
PMBC = may be considered—if symptomatic, rheumatic MS and MVA >1.5 cm², hemodynamic evidence of significant MS (PCWP >15 mm Hg or a mean MV gradient >15 mm Hg during exercise)
PMBC = may be considered—if severely symptomatic, severe rheumatic MS (MVA ≤1.5 cm²), suboptimal valve anatomy, not candidates for surgery
Recommendations for Patients With Degenerative MS
Class 2b recommendations
PMBC = may be considered—if severely symptomatic, severe degenerative MS, only after discussion of the high procedural risk and the individual patient's preferences and values

LA, left atrium; MR, mitral regurgitation; MS, mitral stenosis; MV, mitral valve; PA, pulmonary artery; PCWP, postcapillary wedge pressure; PMBC, percutaneous mitral balloon commissurotomy.

From Otto CM, Nishimura RA, Bonow RO, et al. 2020 ACC/AHA guideline for the management of patients with valvular heart disease: a report of the American college of cardiology/American heart association joint committee on clinical practice guidelines. *Circulation.* 2021;143:e72-e227.

morphology, concomitant MR, and to ensure the absence of LA thrombus.[15] MV morphology, suitability for PMBC, and prediction of outcomes after PMBC can be obtained using multiple score calculators (**Table 41.2**).[10,20-23] These scores grade the severity of valve thickening, mobility, fusion, and subvalvular calcification assist with PMBC suitability assessment. The short axis transthoracic echo view can be used to assess the symmetry of commissural fusion (**Fig. 41.2**). Symmetric commissural fusion and the absence of leaflet calcification are associated with the best balloon dilatation results. Asymmetric fusion and/or calcification of the commissures typically yield less optimal results from balloon dilatation because of the reduced ability of the balloon to split the commissures in a controlled predictable fashion.

Based on the current guidelines, PMBC is recommended in symptomatic patients with an MVA of ≤1.5 cm^2, favorable valve morphology, without significant MR or LA thrombus (**Table 41.1**).[15] PMBC can be a reasonable option for asymptomatic patients with severe rheumatic MS as well, if no significant MR or LA thrombus is present and if PA systolic pressure is >50 mm Hg. PMBC may be considered even in patients who are symptomatic but have rheumatic MS with MVA >1.5 cm,^{2} if there are hemodynamic markers of significant MS, including a PCWP >15 mm Hg or a mean MS gradient >15 mm Hg during exercise.

Prior to intervention, invasive coronary angiography is recommended in patients with chest pain and signs of ischemia, decreased left ventricle (LV) systolic function, history of coronary artery disease, men >40 years of age, and postmenopausal women to ensure there is no concomitant coronary artery disease, which could alter management strategies.

Technique

PMBC can be performed utilizing single balloons, double balloons, and the commonly used Inoue balloon (Toray Medical Co, Ltd) (**Fig. 41.3**). The Inoue balloon is an established approach, with a >95% procedural success rate (symptomatic improvement and an average increase in MVA to 1.9 ± 0.3 cm^2), and with a very low in-hospital mortality.[24] PMBC is performed in the cardiac catheterization laboratory under conscious sedation or general anesthesia.

LA thrombus is a relative contraindication for PMBC, given the need for trans-septal (TS) puncture (TSP) and LA access. Accordingly, TEE should be performed prior to PMBC to assess for the presence of intracardiac thrombi. If thrombus is present, typically a trial of anticoagulation and reassessment for thrombus resolution would be pursued or surgery may be considered as an alternative. It is not uniformly agreed upon whether PMBC can be performed in the presence of thrombi. Some interventionalists suggest performing PMBC using a modified Inoue technique for selected patients with laminar thrombus confined to the left atrial appendage (LAA), while others prefer to trial anticoagulation and reassess for resolution.[25]

TABLE 41.2 Main Scoring Systems Used to Assess Suitability and Prognosis of Percutaneous Mitral Balloon Commissurotomy

REFERENCE	CHARACTERISTICS	SCORING SYSTEM

Wilkins score[20]	• 2D TTE;
	• Semiquantitative assessment:
	  • Mobility (1-4)
	  • Thickening (1-4)
	  • Calcification (1-4)
	  • Subvalvular fusion (1-4)
		• Maximal score = 16;
		• Score ≤8:
		  • Pliable, noncalcified valve, little subvalvular fusion;
		  • Predictive of immediate success, low rate of restenosis.
		• Score >8:
		  • More calcified, immobile, and thickened valve leaflets, subvalvular fusion;
		  • Associated with less optimal results and a higher rate of restenosis.

Cormier score[21]	• 2D TTE & fluoroscopic (calcification) assessment:
	  • Mobility
	  • Subvalvular fusion
	  • Leaflet calcification
		• Group 1 correlates with Wilkins score 7-9:
		  • Pliable noncalcified anterior mitral leaflet, mild subvalvular disease;
		• Group 2 correlates with Wilkins score 8-12:
		  • Pliable noncalcified anterior mitral leaflet, severe subvalvular disease;
		• Group 3 correlates with Wilkins score 10-15:
		  • Any calcification of mitral valve as assessed by fluoroscopy.

Assessment of commissural calcium[22]	• 2D TTE; • Detection of high-intensity bright echoes => amount of calcification in each half of the medial and lateral commissures (0-4).	• Grade of intercomissural calcium = predictor of achieving an MV area post-PMBC >1.5 cm^2 without creating significant MR;

RT3DE score[23]	• Real-time 3D TTE;
	• Divide each mitral valve leaflet into 3 scallops;
	• Composed of 31 points:
	  • Thickness (6 points)
	  • Mobility (6 points)
	  • Calcification (10 points)
	  • Subvalvular apparatus involvement (9 points)
		• Mild (<8);
		• Moderate (8-13);
		• Severe (≥14).

MR, mitral regurgitation; MV, mitral valve; PMBC, percutaneous mitral balloon valvuloplasty or commissurotomy; TTE, transthoracic echocardiography.
Adapted from Giannini C, Mazzola M, Pugliese NR, Petronio AS. Mitral valve stenosis in the current era: a changing landscape. *J Cardiovasc Med.* 2022;23(11):701-709. doi:10.2459/jcm.0000000000001384

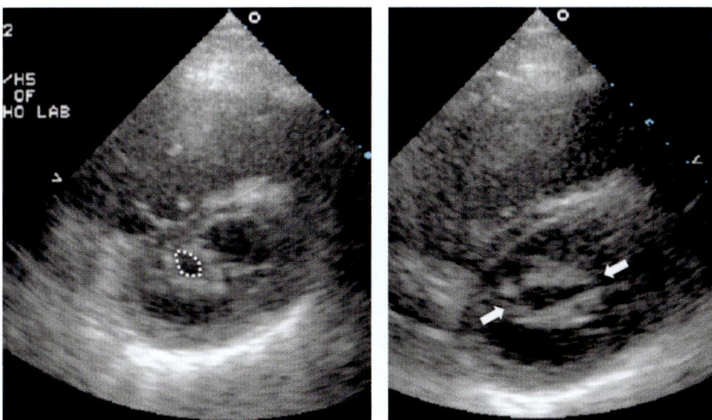

FIGURE 41.2 The left panel shows a short-axis transthoracic echocardiographic image at the level of the mitral valve orifice. Planimetry of the orifice shows the typical fishmouth appearance (*dotted circle*). The interventricular septum is flattened due to chronic pulmonary hypertension. There is dense and symmetrical commissural fusion. On the right, after balloon mitral commissurotomy, there is bilateral commissural splitting, shown by the *white arrows*. The interventricular septum is now more round, consistent with immediate diminution of the pulmonary artery pressure.

In most cases, PMBC is performed using an antegrade transvenous approach, with access to the LA obtained through TSP with a dedicated apparatus. The puncture site is typically located slightly posterior and inferior to the midfossa, and heparin is administered to maintain therapeutic acceptance and commitment therapy (ACT) throughout left-sided access.

Appropriate balloon sizing is crucial to avoid injury to the MV leaflets and apparatus during balloon inflation and resultant MR. Various methods for sizing have been suggested, including patient height, body surface area, or measuring the maximal intercommissural diameter.[26,27] Once access to the LA is achieved, the selected balloon is inserted and directed toward the LV across the MV with fluoroscopic and echocardiographic guidance. TEE helps direct the catheters and wires away from the LAA, position the balloon correctly, and determine the optimal position between the mitral leaflets. If resistance crossing the valve with the deflated Inoue balloon is encountered, described as the "balloon impasse" sign, balloon downsizing should be considered.[28] Care must be taken not to inflate the balloon in the subvalvular region to reduce the risk of chordal rupture, leaflet tearing, or damage to the papillary muscle.

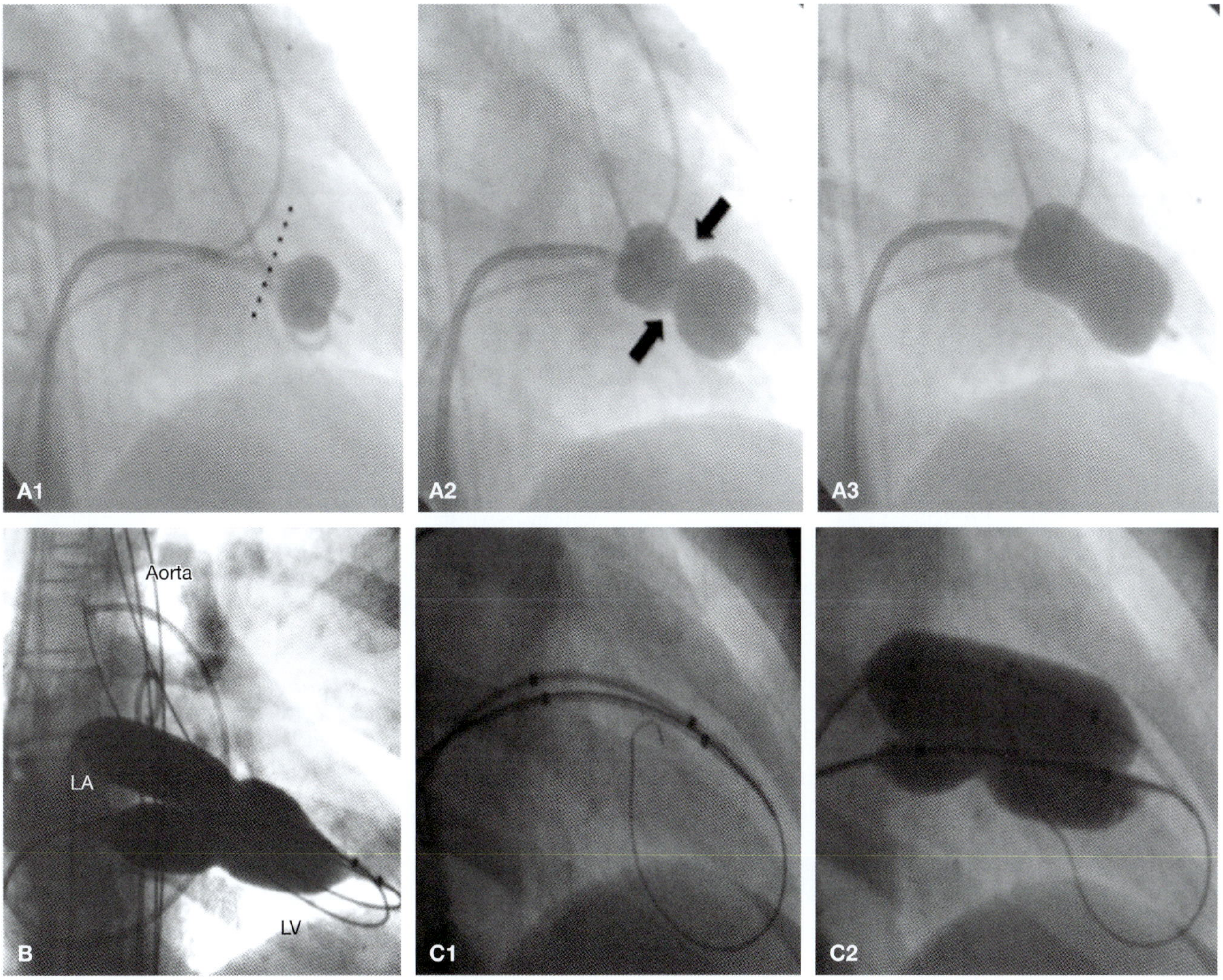

FIGURE 41.3 *Panels A1-A3* show the Inoue-balloon catheter in a partially inflated state and pulled back to the mitral valve plane (A1, *dotted line*), followed by continued inflation, when the waist of the balloon engages the mitral orifice (A2, *black arrows*), to the final appearance of the fully inflated balloon (A3). *Panel B* illustrates the double balloon technique, where 2 conventional balloons are shown positioned across the mitral orifice. Double wires can be seen from the left atrium (LA), across the mitral valve, through the left ventricle (LV), into the aorta. *Panels C1-C2* show the multitrack system. A single wire looped in the LV apex can be seen in panel C1. The superior balloon is delivered via a short monorail, and the over-the-wire balloon is below it, with a single wire used for a double balloon approach (C1-C2).

Special attention is required during PMBC in high-risk patients, such as the elderly, pregnant women, very severe MS, extensive subvalvular involvement, severe calcification in commissural areas, severe pulmonary arterial hypertension, and patients with asymmetric MV opening. Hemodynamic parameters should be closely monitored during each balloon inflation to detect any transient hemodynamic deterioration. Commissures can be seen to open fluoroscopically, as the constriction at the level of the balloon disappears. Hemodynamic changes should also occur immediately (**Fig. 41.4**).

Criteria for discontinuing a PMBC procedure include an MVA >1 cm^2/m^2 body surface area, complete commissural opening in at least one commissure, and the occurrence or worsening of MR >grade 1. The success of PMBC is defined as an increase in MVA of at least 1.5 cm^2 without complications and particularly MR grade <2.[15] If the result is unsatisfactory, balloon inflation can be repeated by increasing the size incrementally until the desired MV opening is achieved or a worsening of MR occurs.

The prediction of outcomes following PMBC involves multiple factors, including clinical, anatomical, and hemodynamic parameters, including older age, previous commissurotomy, the presence of atrial fibrillation, baseline MR, elevated pulmonary artery pressure and pulmonary vascular resistance, higher echocardiographic grouping (≥2) or Wilkins score (≥8), commissural grade ≥2, severe subvalvular involvement, lower MVA after PMBC, and MR grade ≥2+ after PMBC.[29,30]

Periprocedural Complications

During a PMBC procedure, it is crucial to promptly detect any complications that may arise. These complications include[31]:

- Cardiac tamponade: Occurring in 0% to 2% of cases, it can be caused by inadvertent puncture of the aorta or cardiac walls. Prompt recognition followed by either anticoagulation reversal and monitoring, pericardiocentesis or even surgery may be required.

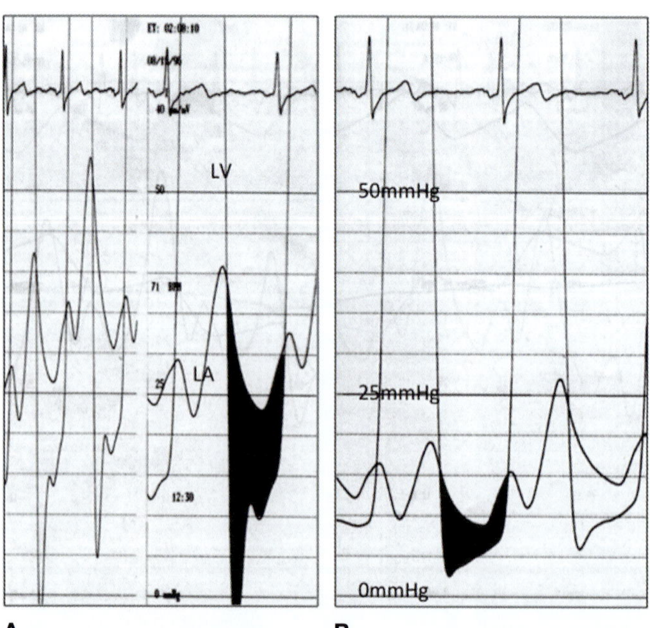

FIGURE 41.4 **Panel A** and its shaded area show a large transmitral pressure gradient. **Panel B** is immediately after PMBC, the shaded area is significantly smaller, signifying a reduced transmitral gradient. The left atrial waveforms do not show increases in V waves, reassuring us that no significant mitral regurgitation has occurred. PMBC, percutaneous mitral balloon valvuloplasty or commissurotomy.

- Embolic events: Air or thromboembolism can occur in 0% to 4% of cases. Careful deairing of the balloon, aspiration and flushing of catheters, and keeping the catheter hub below the heart level during insertion or removal can prevent air embolic events. Thromboembolism may result from dislodged intracardiac thrombotic material or acute thrombus formation on the apparatus. Thorough intracardiac thrombus assessment preprocedurally and maintaining the activated clotting time between 250 and 300 seconds during the procedure can minimize the risk.
- Significant MR: Incidence ranges from 1.4% to 9.1%. MR may increase or develop due to commissural tearing, rupture in noncommissural regions of the leaflets, or inadequate leaflet coaptation caused by severe calcification or rupture of the subvalvular mitral apparatus. Choosing an appropriate balloon size, proper balloon positioning during inflation, and careful step-by-step balloon inflation with close echocardiographic monitoring can help reduce this complication. If severe MR is encountered, surgical MV replacement will often be required.
- Iatrogenic atrial septal defects (ASDs) after TSP: These ASDs are typically small, clinically insignificant, and do not appear to worsen long-term outcomes. In fact, ASDs may provide further symptomatic relief via decompression of elevated LA pressures as observed in Lutembacher syndrome with congenital ASDs and concomitant MS.[32] Indeed, LA decompression via left-to-right shunting is being explored as a therapeutic approach for patients with LA hypertension.[33,34]

Special Considerations

Mixed Valvular Disease

The assessment and management of multivalvular disease is complex and may require invasive hemodynamic testing.[35] In cases with concurrent MS and tricuspid regurgitation (TR), surgical intervention on both valves is advised.[11,15] PMBC alone can be considered if TR is thought to be functional, in the setting of moderate atrial enlargement and pulmonary hypertension.[11] In patients with concurrent MS and aortic disease, PMBC can be considered to manage MS and postpone the need for surgical treatment of both valves.[11,15]

Mitral Restenosis After PMBC

Restenosis can occur after PMBC with time, and it can be associated with increased incidence of major adverse cardiovascular events.[36] For patients with restenosis following mitral commissurotomy, PMBC has demonstrated effectiveness and provides satisfactory immediate outcomes, regardless of the type of previous commissurotomy procedures performed.[37] While Australian guidelines suggest redo-PMBC,[38] European and Japanese guidelines recommend a surgical approach, with redo-PMBC saved only for patients with high surgical risks and anatomy suitable for PMBC.[39,40] The American College of Cardiology/American Heart Association guidelines do not have recommendations in this regard. Accordingly, assessment of both patient and anatomic characteristics should guide the patient discussion as to whether to proceed with repeat PMBC versus surgical evaluation.

MS During Pregnancy

Women with MS should ideally undergo cardiology or cardio-obstetrics evaluation prior to pregnancy to discuss risks and best ways to mitigate them before exposure to hemodynamic changes that occur with pregnancy.[11,38] Exercise stress testing can be considered in asymptomatic patients with severe MS who are planning to become pregnant, to identify whether symptoms or increases in pulmonary artery pressures occur.[15] Stroke volume and transvalvular gradients can increase during pregnancy, and this can precipitate heart failure (HF), arrhythmias, or pulmonary hypertension.[41]

In fact, more than 50% of asymptomatic patients will develop HF symptoms during pregnancy.[42] Fetal health can be endangered by MS, which can lead to intrauterine growth restriction, low birth weights, and fetal death.[43] Guidelines recommend treatment of severe asymptomatic MS prior to pregnancy.[11,15,38]

In pregnant women with MS, a multidisciplinary approach is recommended, with a team including obstetricians, cardiologists (or cardio-obstetrics specialists), and anesthetists. Medical management should be optimized with pregnancy-appropriate beta blockers for heart rate control and diuretics to prevent volume overload. Pregnant patients with symptomatic severe MS despite medical therapy should be considered for PMBC.[11,15,38] MV surgery should only be considered in select cases, as it can carry significant risks to both the mother and the fetus.[44]

Transcatheter Edge-to-Edge Repair

Overview

MR is the most common valvular heart disease in the United States and is associated with increased morbidity and mortality.[45] The normal function of the MV depends on the interplay of all its components, including the annulus, leaflets, chordae, and papillary muscles, as well as the LA and LV size and function. Morphological, geometrical, and functional distortion of these components results in MV dysfunction. MR can be broadly classified into two distinct categories: primary or degenerative MR and secondary or functional MR. Primary or secondary are considered more appropriate descriptions than degenerative or functional. Primary MR occurs due to intrinsic distortion of the valve itself, such as leaflet prolapse or flail, as well as abnormalities in the chordae. On the other hand, secondary MR occurs secondary to LA or LV abnormalities. The mechanism of secondary MR is due to imbalance between closing and tethering forces of the MV in the presence of a structurally normal valve resulting in a coaptation defect. Secondary MR is further stratified into atrial and ventricular secondary MR.[46] Ventricular secondary MR is due to global or regional left ventricular abnormalities that result in tethering of the leaflets. Less commonly, secondary MR can occur in patients with normal LV geometry and is primarily due to mitral annular enlargement with poor coaptation secondary to LA enlargement. This mechanism is referred to as atrial secondary MR. Another classification of MR is the Carpentier classification and is primarily based on leaflet motion (**Fig. 41.5**).[47]

Surgical interventions are the first-line therapy for patients with severe primary MR. However, given the aging population and the growing number of patients with severe symptomatic MR who are at high surgical risk, TEER has emerged as a paradigm shift in the management of this patient population. The underlying principle of TEER, similar to the surgical Alfieri stitch, relies on the approximation of the anterior and posterior leaflets of the MV to restore valvular competency and reduce the extent of regurgitant blood. Randomized clinical trials (RCTs) have demonstrated its safety and efficacy in the management of primary and secondary MR.[2,3] Current guidelines recommend TEER in high-surgical risk patients with severe symptomatic primary MR and favorable anatomy for TEER (class IIa recommendation) as well as patients with severe secondary MR and left ventricular ejection fraction (LVEF) <50% who remain symptomatic despite guideline-directed medical therapy (GDMT) and have favorable anatomy for TEER (class IIa recommendation).[4]

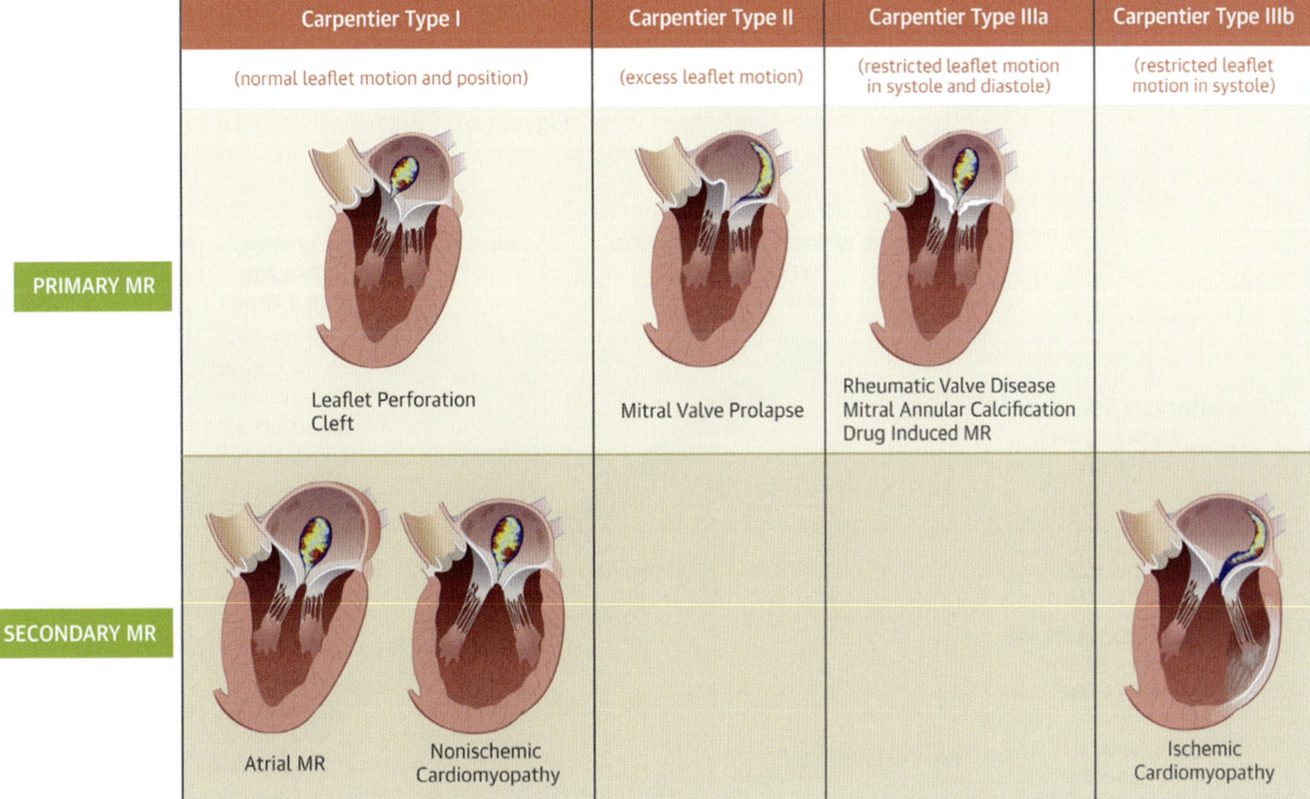

FIGURE 41.5 Carpentier classification of mitral regurgitation. MR, mitral regurgitation. (Adapted from El Sabbagh A, Reddy YNV, Nishimura RA. Mitral valve regurgitation in the contemporary era: insights into diagnosis, management, and future directions. *JACC Cardiovasc Imaging*. 2018;11(4):628-643. doi:10.1016/j.jcmg.2018.01.009)

The Role of TEER in Specific Patient Populations

Primary MR

The EVEREST (Endovascular Valve Edge-to-Edge Repair Study) feasibility trial demonstrated the safety of TEER in 107 patients with severe primary and/or secondary MR.[48] The EVEREST II trial was the first large-scale RCT that assessed the safety and efficacy of TEER in patients with severe MR compared to conventional surgical repair or replacement.[2] TEER was performed with the MitraClip (Abbott Vascular, Santa Clara, CA) device. Eligibility criteria included symptomatic patients with severe MR, and asymptomatic patients were required to have one of the following: an LVEF of 25% to 60%, LV end-systolic diameter of 40 to 55 mm, pulmonary hypertension, or new onset atrial fibrillation. A total of 279 patients were included, 73% of whom had primary MR. At 30 days, major adverse events were significantly lower in the TEER arm (15% vs 48%, $P < .001$) with similar rate of mortality at 1 year. Subsequently, in March 2013, the US Food and Drug Administration (FDA) approved the use of the MitraClip for high-surgical risk patients with symptomatic primary MR.[49] Subsequently, two ongoing clinical trials investigate the efficacy of TEER versus surgical repair in patients with degenerative MR.[50-52] The REPAIR MR (Percutaneous MitraClip Device or Surgical Mitral Valve REpair in PAtients With PrImaRy MItral Regurgitation) trial (NCT: NCT04198870) evaluates outcomes of TEER versus mitral surgery in patients who are candidates for surgery.[51] Similarly, the PRIMARY (PeRcutanoeus of surgIcal MitrAl Valve RepaIr) trial (NCT05051033) compares outcomes of TEER in primary MR versus mitral surgery.[52] These trials will provide insights to further optimize contemporary interventional strategies.

In addition to the MitraClip device, the PASCAL (Edwards Lifesciences) device has been developed for the treatment of MR. Early single-arm studies demonstrated the safety in terms of complications and survival as well as efficacy of the device in terms of durable MR reduction.[53-55] There are no RCTs evaluating its efficacy against surgical repair; however, the CLASP IID trial evaluated the safety and efficacy of the PASCAL device compared with the MitraClip device in patients with severe symptomatic primary MR who are at a prohibitive surgical risk.[56] A total of 180 patients were included, and the primary efficacy endpoint of MR ≤2 at 6 months was met with noninferiority of the PASCAL device (PASCAL 96.5% vs MitraClip 96.8%). Additionally, the primary safety point as a composite of major adverse events was similar between the two systems (PASCAL 3.4% vs MitraClip 4.8%). Subsequently, the FDA approved the PASCAL device for the treatment of patients with severe symptomatic primary MR.[57]

Secondary MR

Two RCTs assessed the benefit of TEER in patients with secondary MR. The MITRA-FR trial (Percutaneous Repair with the MitraClip Device for Severe Functional/Secondary Mitral Regurgitation) included 304 patients with severe secondary MR who were randomized to either undergo MitraClip in addition to medical therapy or to receive medical therapy alone.[58] Severe MR was defined as an effective regurgitant orifice area (EROA) >0.2 cm^2 and/or regurgitant volume (RV) >30 mL and LVEF between 15% and 40%. At 12 months, all-cause mortality (MitraClip 24.3% vs control 22.4%), as well as the rate of HF hospitalization (MitraClip 48.7% vs control 47.4%), did not differ between the two groups. On the other hand, the COAPT trial included 614 patients with moderate-to-severe or severe secondary MR who were randomized to either undergo MitraClip in addition to medial therapy or to receive medical therapy alone.[3] Moderate-to-severe MR was defined as an EROA >0.3 cm^2 and/or RV 45 mL and LVEF ≥20%. At 24 months, all-cause mortality (MitraClip 21.1% vs control 46.1%) and HF hospitalization (MitraClip 35.8% vs control 67.9%) were significantly lower in the MitraClip arm.

There are several possible explanations for the differences in the results of the trials.[59-61] The concept of disproportionate MR has been proposed as patients in the COAPT trial had an EROA almost 30% higher with LV volumes that were almost 30% smaller than patients in the MITRA-FR trial. This is suggestive that the MR is the primary driver of symptoms, not the LV dysfunction as the degree of MR is disproportionate to the degree of LV enlargement (**Fig. 41.6**).[59] Additionally, GDMT for HF was optimized prior to randomization in the COAPT trial; however, GDMT was

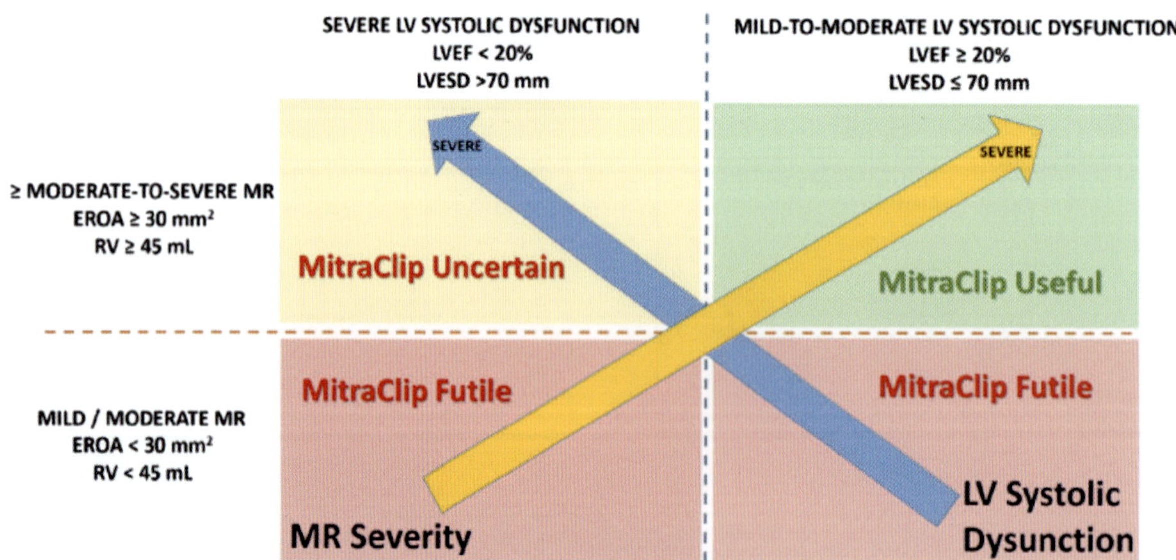

FIGURE 41.6 Utility of mitral transcatheter edge-to-edge repair according to the degree of mitral regurgitation and left ventricular size and systolic function. EROA, effective regurgitant orifice area, LV, left ventricle; LVEF, left ventricular ejection fraction; LVESD, left ventricular end-systolic diameter; MR, mitral regurgitation; RV, regurgitant volume. (From Pibarot P, Delgado V, Bax JJ. MITRA-FR vs. COAPT: lessons from two trials with diametrically opposed results. *Eur Heart J Cardiovasc Imaging.* 2019;20(6):620-624. doi:10.1093/ehjci/jez073)

not optimized at baseline in the MITRA-FR trial. Furthermore, the COAPT trial had a more aggressive strategy for MR correction with more clips placed per patient and had a higher rate of sustained MR reduction compared to the MITRA-FR trial. As a result, the FDA approved the use of MitraClip in patients with moderate-to-severe or severe secondary MR and LVEF 20% to 50% who remained symptomatic despite maximally tolerated GDMT.[62]

The role of TEER in atrial secondary MR has not been assessed in RCTs. However, several retrospective studies examined the efficacy of TEER in this subset of patients (**Table 41.3**).[63-69] Notably, the definition of atrial secondary MR varied across the studies. All studies required patients with atrial secondary MR to have normal LVEF; however, some studies required the presence of atrial fibrillation, some required LA enlargement, and others required both. Yoon et al[65] reported the results of TEER in 1044 patients, 11.1% of whom had atrial secondary MR and 48.4% had ventricular secondary MR. At 2-year follow-up, the composite outcome of all-cause mortality and HF hospitalization was significantly higher in patients with ventricular secondary MR compared to atrial secondary MR (42.3% vs 31.5%, *P* = .022, respectively). Doldi et al reported the outcomes of TEER in 1608 patients, 7.8% of whom had atrial MR. Procedural success, defined as MR ≤2, was significantly higher in ventricular MR (94%) compared to atrial MR (87%, *P* = .003).[64] However, the rate of all-cause mortality and

TABLE 41.3 Characteristics and Outcomes of Studies That Evaluated Transcatheter Edge-to-Edge Repair in Patients With Atrial Functional Mitral Regurgitation

STUDY	DEFINITION OF AFMR	STUDY DESIGN	POPULATION	PRIMARY OUTCOME	SECONDARY OUTCOMES
Simard 2022[64]	• Structurally normal mitral valve • LVEF ≥50% and no RWMAs • No LV dilatation • LA enlargement (>48 mL/m²)	Observational, retrospective, single center (*n* = 306)	vFMR in 12.1% aFMR in 6.9%	Device success was similar with aFMR (57%) vs vFMR (73%) vs DMR (64%) LAP decreased after TEER for DMR and vFMR but not after TEER for Afmr	No difference in MR grade or major adverse events at 1 y
Doldi 2022[65]	• Structurally normal mitral valve • LVEF ≥50% and no RWMAs • Dilated LA	Observational, retrospective, international registry (*n* = 1608)	aFMR in 7.8% vFMR in 84%	Procedural success defined as MR ≤2 was significantly higher in vFMR (94%) compared to aFMR (87%, *P* = .003)	The estimated 2-y survival rate in aFMR was 70.4% 2-y survival was similar between aFMR and vFMR patients
Yoon 2022[66]	• Structurally normal mitral valve • No or mild LV remodeling • Moderate/severe LA dilatation	Observational, retrospective, single center (*n* = 1044)	vFMR in 48.4% aFMR in 11.1%	2-year rate of death or HF hospitalization higher for vFMR (42.3%) and aFMR (31.5%) compared to DMR (21.6%) (*P* < .001)	No difference in residual MR ≥3 at discharge or at 1 mo
Sodhi 2022[67]	• Structurally normal mitral valve • LVEF ≥45% and no RWMAs • History of AF • LA enlargement	Observational, prospective, multicenter (*n* = 835)	vFMR in 43.1% aFMR in 6.3%	1-y reduction of MR to ≤2 was 100% in aFMR and 99.5% in vFMR	No difference in 30-d major adverse events, 1-y death, or 1-y HF hospitalization
Tanaka 2022[68]	• Structurally normal mitral valve • LVEF >50% and no RWMAs • No LV enlargement	Observational, retrospective, single center (*n* = 415)	aFMR in 24.8% of all FMRs	Rate of MR reduction to ≤1 at discharge in patients with aFMR (79.7%)	MitraClip NTR/XTR or G4 was associated more patients with residual MR ≤1+
Popolo et al, 2022[69]	• Structurally normal MV • LVEF ≥50% and LVEDD <55 mm • History of AF	Observational, retrospective, multicenter (*n* = 1153)	vFMR in 58.1% aFMR in 7.5%	Rates of technical (97%), device (83%), and procedural (80%) success in aFMR cohort MR ≤2 was sustained in 89%	TEER for aFMR resulted in positive LA and annular remodelling
Benito-González 2021[70]	Structurally normal MV LVEF >50% and no RWMA history of AF	Observational, retrospective, multicenter (*n* = 1074)	vFMR in 58.1% aFMR in 4.5%	Procedural success was 91.7% with aFMR vs 88.9% with vFMR and 87.6% with DMR No difference in MR grade at 1 y	No difference in 1-y incidence of death or HF hospitalization

AF, atrial fibrillation; aFMR, atrial functional mitral regurgitation; DMR, degenerative mitral regurgitation; HF, heart failure; LA, left atrium; LAP, left atrial pressure; LVEDD, left ventricular end-diastolic diameter; LVEF, left ventricular ejection fraction; MR, mitral regurgitation; MV, mitral valve; RWMA, regional wall motion abnormality; TEER, transcatheter edge-to-edge repair; vFMR, ventricular mitral regurgitation.

HF hospitalization was similar between the two arms at 2 years. Despite the knowledge gap in this patient population, the results from retrospective data provide reassurance, and TEER appears to be a promising treatment for these patients. However, RCTs are needed to confirm its efficacy.

Cardiogenic Shock

Cardiogenic shock (CS) continues to have a persistently high mortality, with few interventions that improve prognosis. Multiple studies have demonstrated that moderate-severe MR is prevalent in up to 20% of patients admitted with CS and increases the risk of mortality by up to 60%.[70,71] TEER has emerged as an effective treatment for high-risk patients with severe symptomatic MR. The clinical benefit of TEER has been investigated in patients with CS and moderate to severe or severe MR who were not surgical candidates and were treated with TEER.[70] A patient-level analysis including 141 patients across 14 institutions demonstrated an in-hospital mortality of 15.6% and 42.6% at 1 year.[72] A comprehensive analysis of the transcatheter valve therapy (TVT) registry included 3797 patients with CS and MR.[73] MR etiology was primary in 53.4% and secondary in 27.5% (mixed or other in 19%). At 1 year, device success was associated with significantly lower all-cause mortality (34.6% vs 55.5%; $P < .001$) and a lower composite of mortality or HF hospitalization (29.6% vs 45.2%; $P < .001$). Currently, the CAPITAL MINOS (transcatheter Mitral valve repair for INOtrope dependent cardiogenic Shock) trial (NCT 05298124) is an ongoing open-label and multicenter RCT comparing TEER to medical therapy in patients with CS and MR.[74]

TEER Devices

MitraClip

The MitraClip device is the first TEER system that was approved for the management of severe MR (**Figs. 41.7** and **41.8**). The first-in-human implantation of the MitraClip was in 2003, and since then, the MitraClip system has undergone multiple technical iterations to improve device handling (**Fig. 41.9**).[75] The third generation of the MitraClip (XTR and NTR) was commercially available in 2018. The MitraClip XTR had longer clip arms compared to the previous generation and to the NTR system, which adds an additional 3 mm in length and 2 frictional elements to each clip arm.[76] These features resulted in increased coaptation surface area and potentially improved leaflet grasping especially in complex anatomy with larger coaptation gap. Additionally, the third-generation XTR and NTR devices had a new clip delivery shaft that was longer and stiffer to maintain clip orientation when crossing the MV into the ventricle. The additional 1.5 cm in the length of the shaft allows for greater height of the TSP. This allows for a greater range of motion of the guiding catheter and the clip in the LA. However, the third-generation MitraClips had a few limitations. The two

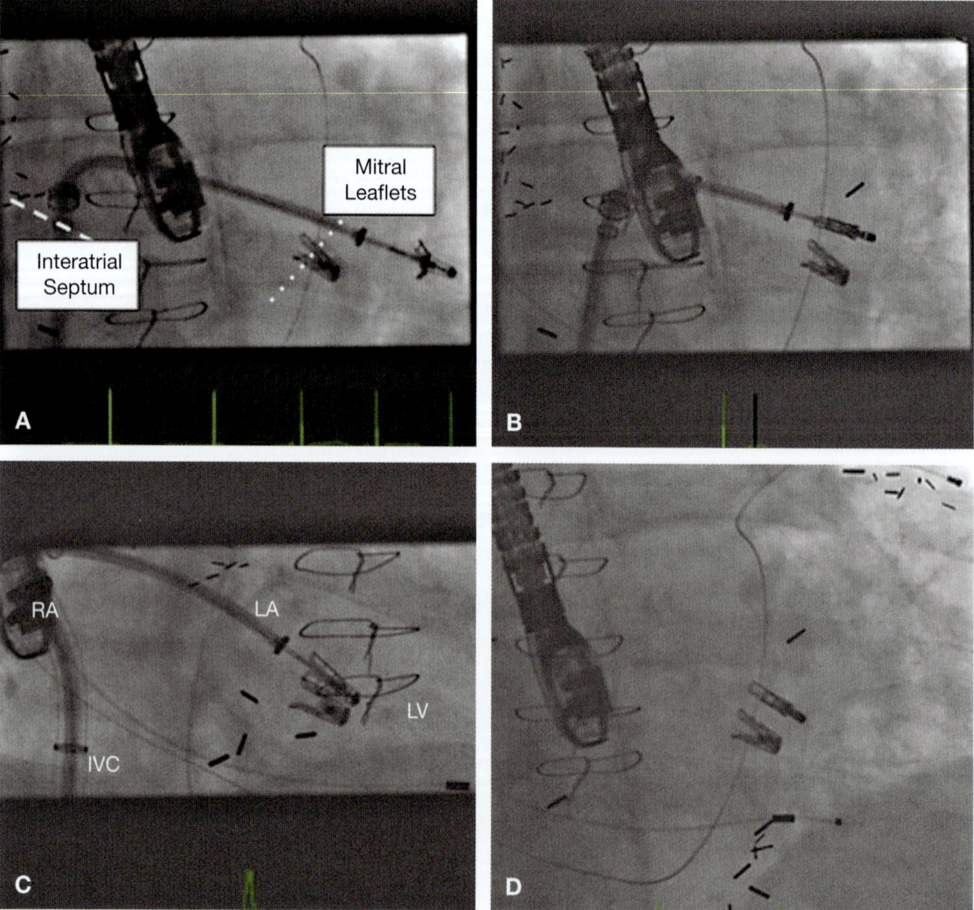

FIGURE 41.7 **Panel A,** shows the MitraClip device already implanted and a second MitraClip device inserted through the guide catheter and passed across the mitral valve into the left ventricle. A transesophageal echo probe is noted in the picture. **Panel B,** shows the clip having been pulled back and closed to capture the mitral leaflets next to the first device. **Panel C,** shows the clip ready to be released. **Panel D,** shows the clip released. IVC, inferior vena cava; LA, left atrium; LV, left ventricle; RA, right atrium.

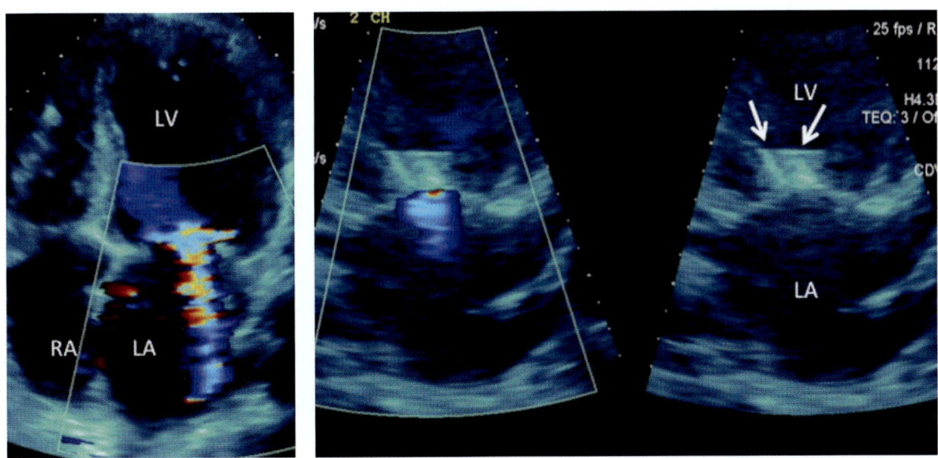

FIGURE 41.8 On the *left* is a transthoracic echocardiogram from the MitraClip patient in Figure 7, taken before the MitraClip procedure. Severe mitral regurgitation is easily seen. On the *right*, two clips can be seen, denoted by the *arrows*. The mitral regurgitation has been reduced to a trivial grade. LA, left atrium; LV, left ventricle.

graspers of the MitraClip XTR and NTR did not move independently, preventing independent grasping of the anterior and posterior mitral leaflets. Early clinical experience demonstrated that the MitraClip XTR might be associated with a relatively higher risk of leaflet tear.[77] However, results from the EXPAND registry in 1041 who underwent TEER with the third-generation MitraClip did not show higher rate of adverse leaflet events of the XTR system compared to the NTR system.[78]

The newest MitraClip "Generation 4" or "G4" was launched in 2019 to overcome these limitations.[79] The MitraClip G4 system is composed of two rigid arms of cobalt-chromium alloy with flexible nitinol-based grippers (**Fig. 41.10**). These grippers are equipped with either four or six small hooks that provide the frictional element. There are four available sizes compared to the two sizes of the third generation (**Table 41.4**). Similar to the third-generation XTR system, the XT/XTW systems have longer clip arms that allow the treatment of a larger coaptation gap. Additionally, MitraClip G4 can grasp each leaflet independently and has the ability to continuously monitor the LA pressure, which was not possible with the previous generation. Early clinical experience with the MitraClip G4 demonstrated excellent procedural results with MR reduction to ≤2+ in 96.6% of patients at 30 days.[79]

PASCAL

The PASCAL TEER system was first implanted in 2016 and was reported in a compassionate use framework in 23 patients with complex anatomy.[80] The currently available second generation of the PASCAL system was launched in August 2022 and consists of 3 embedded catheters that allow high range of motion in the LA (**Fig. 41.11**). The PASCAL systems are nitinol-based implants composed of two spring-loaded paddles with 26 mm grasping length, two clasps, and a central spacer. The central spacer's role is to fill part of the coaptation gap. Additionally, the nitinol claps can be controlled and maneuvered independently enabling leaflet optimization and staged capture of the leaflets. There are two available implants, the PASCAL P10 and the PASCAL ACE system. The PASCAL P10 system has 10 mm clasps, while the PASCAL ACE has clasps that are 6 mm wide to accommodate smaller anatomy.[81]

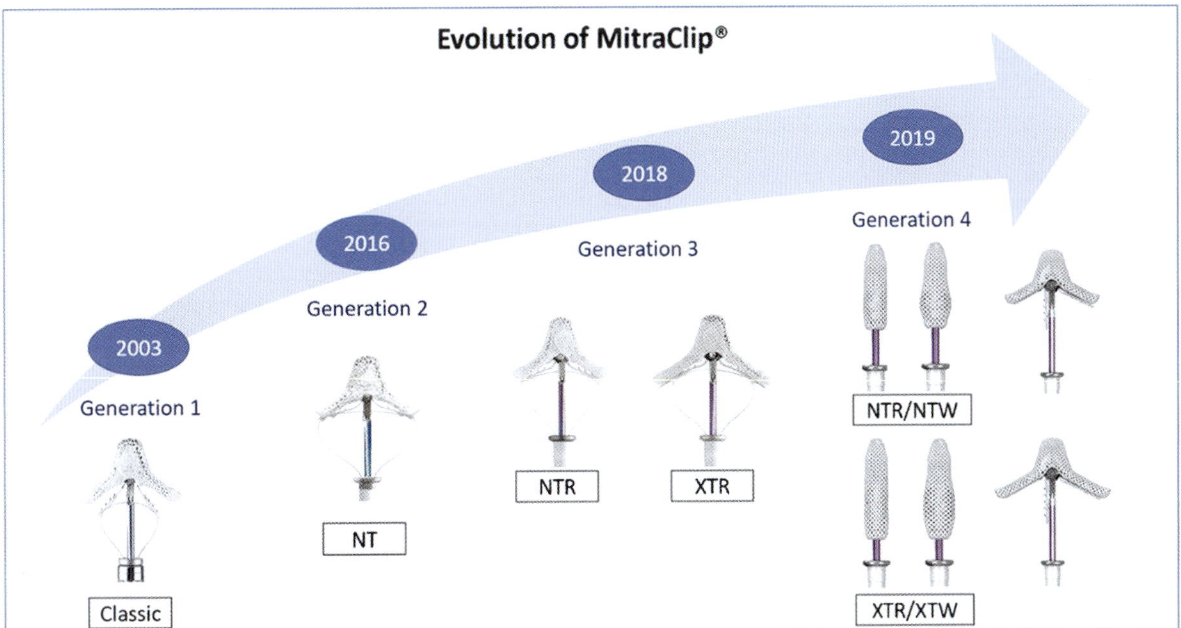

FIGURE 41.9 Evolution of the MitraClip. (From Schnitzler K, Hell M, Geyer M, Kreidel F, Münzel T, von Bardeleben RS. Complications following MitraClip implantation. *Curr Cardiol Rep*. 2021;23(9):131. doi:10.1007/s11886-021-01553-9

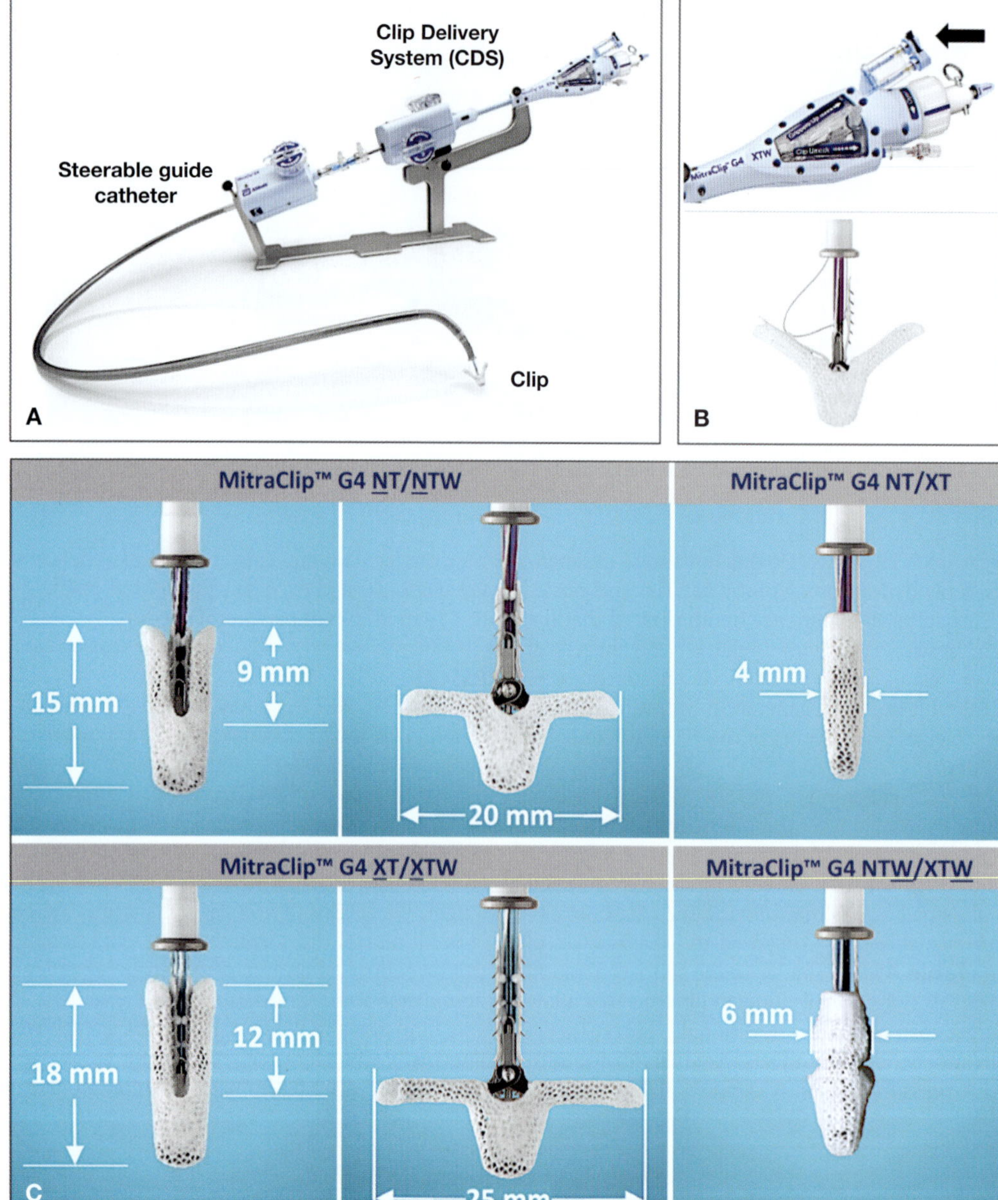

FIGURE 41.10 **A,** All components of the G4 System. **B,** Two independent gripper levers. **C,** The MitraClip G4 includes four clip sizes (NT, XT, NTW, and XTW) offering more options for patient-tailored mitral valve repair. (Reproduced from De Backer O, Wong I, Taramasso M, Maisano F, Franzen O, Søndergaard L. Transcatheter mitral valve repair: an overview of current and future devices [published correction appears in *Open Heart*. 2021;8(1)]. *Open Heart*. 2021;8(1):e001564, with permission from BMJ Publishing Group Ltd.)

The Role of Echocardiography and Anatomical Consideration in TEER

TTE is the initial modality utilized to quantify the severity of MR and to discern the etiology of the MV dysfunction. Thereafter, TEE plays a crucial role in preprocedural analysis of the morphology and function of the leaflets as well as intraprocedural guidance.[82] Recent advances in TEE including x-plane imaging, 3D multiplanar reconstruction (MPR), and transillumination imaging have further enhanced the role of TEE in TEER (**Fig. 41.12**).[83] X-plane imaging allows the visualization of structures in two imaging planes at

TABLE 41.4 Characteristics of the Different MitraClip Generation 4 Systems

	MITRACLIP G4 NT	MITRACLIP G4 NTW	MITRACLIP G4 XT	MITRACLIP G4 XTW
Clip arm length	9 mm	9 mm	12 mm	12 mm
Clip width	4 mm	6 mm	4 mm	6 mm
Number of hooks	4	4	6	6

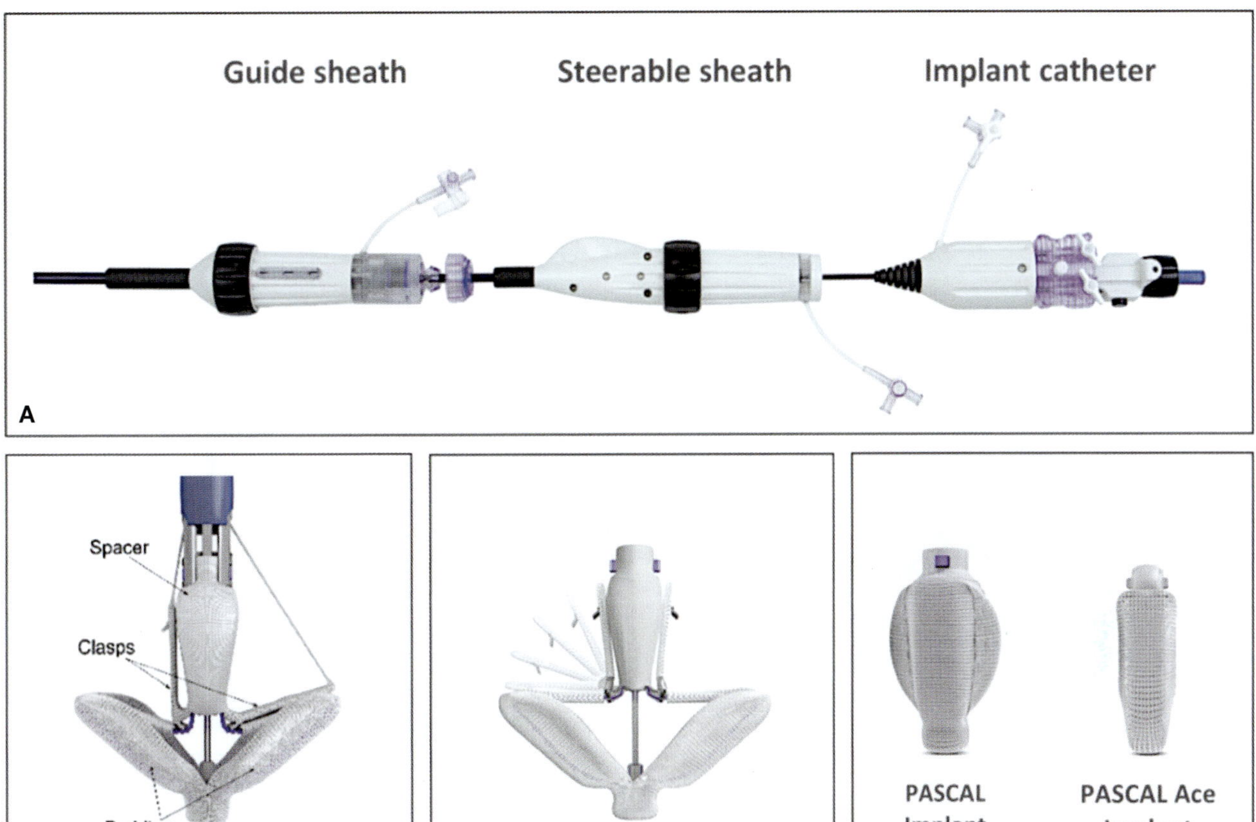

FIGURE 41.11 **A,** The three components of the PASCAL delivery system. **B,** The PASCAL implant consists of two paddles, two clasps, and a central spacer. **C,** Independent leaflet capture. **D,** The newest generation PASCAL Ace implant. (Reproduced from De Backer O, Wong I, Taramasso M, Maisano F, Franzen O, Søndergaard L. Transcatheter mitral valve repair: an overview of current and future devices [published correction appears in *Open Heart*. 2021;8(1)]. *Open Heart*. 2021;8(1):e001564. doi:10.1136/openhrt-2020 to 001564)

the same time that are usually orthogonal to each other, while live 3D MPR technique allows the display of multiple planes as well as a 3D en-face view of the MV while the transillumination imaging technique adds a virtual light source to highlight structures and enhance depth perception compared to conventional 3D images.[83]

There are multiple factors that play a role in achieving optimal results in patients undergoing TEER. This includes anatomical, patient related, and clinical factors. The optimal anatomic candidates for TEER are patients who meet the eligibility criteria for EVEREST II trial with primarily A2/P2 pathology, minimal calcium at grasping area and an MVA >4 cm^2 [58] and COAPT with A2/P2 pathology, and adequate posterior leaflet length.[3] TEE plays an important role in identifying these anatomical factors for optimum patient selection as well as the detection of unsuitable anatomy for TEER.[84]

An expert consensus document has addressed the unsuitability factors for TEER (**Fig. 41.13**).[84] There are two main categories in terms of anatomical considerations in patients undergoing TEER: (i) anatomical factors associated with MS after TEER and (ii) anatomical factors associated with inadequate reduction in MR. Patients with Carpentier IIIa and MAC are at high risk of developing MS after TEER. Frequently, there is leaflet thickening and/or subvalvular disease that precipitate these patients to develop MS. The mechanism of MR in patients with MAC is either due to the extension of the calcium onto the leaflets or the retraction of the posterior leaflet from MAC. Either way, TEER in this subset of patients might result in high inflow gradients immediately postprocedure or in subsequent months or years if/when MAC severity progresses.

Another subset of patients at risk of MS are those with small MVA at baseline, especially those with MR after a previous surgical repair with annuloplasty ring or band. An MVA less than 3.5 cm^2 has been associated with high risk of MS after TEER. Additionally, patients with residual or recurrent MR after TEER have lower long-term survival.[85,86] Thus, it is important to identify anatomical factors associated with inadequate reduction of MR as these patients can be evaluated for MV therapies other than TEER such as TMVR. A short posterior leaflet makes the procedure more challenging. A cutoff of less than 5 mm posterior leaflet length has been deemed unsuitable for TEER due to lack of tissue available for adequate grasping of leaflet into the device. Additionally, patients with Barlow disease often have calcification, multiple regurgitant jets, and redundancy that can limit the ability to reduce MR with TEER.

TEER is usually performed under TEE guidance. This includes guiding TSP, clip steering and positioning, leaflet grasping, and pre- as well as post-deployment evaluation.[83] Intracardiac echocardiography (ICE) has emerged as an alternative to TEE in cases when TEE cannot be performed or when general anesthesia needs to be avoided. The efficacy and safety of ICE-guided TEER has been reported in several case reports.[87]

Future Directions and Transcatheter MV Repair Systems

In addition to TEER, multiple transcatheter systems have been developed as therapeutic interventions that targets the mitral annulus and chordae. This includes transcatheter mitral annuloplasty and transcatheter MV chordal repair. Transcatheter mitral

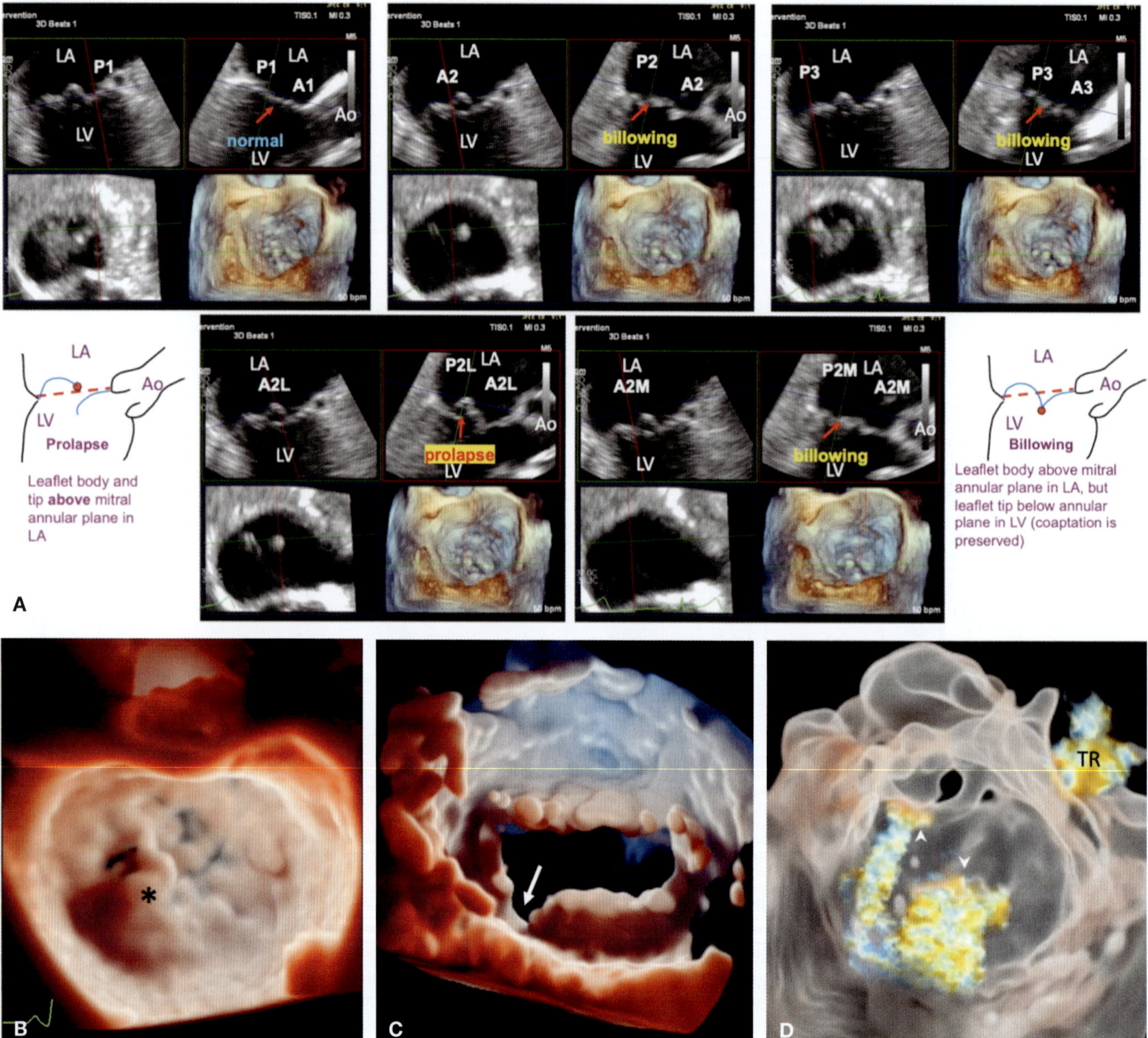

FIGURE 41.12 **A,** Segmental analysis of leaflet edge anatomy using live 3D MPR on 3D TEE data set of a patient with diffuse myxomatous MV disease. Prolapse is seen in the lateral part of the A2 segment (A2L); other segments show either leaflet billowing or normal leaflet motion. **B,** Transillumination imaging in a patient with a flail P2 segment (*). **C,** Transillumination imaging of the MV viewed from the LV perspective highlighting a leaflet cleft/deep indentation (*arrow*) between P2 and P3. **D,** Transillumination imaging with transparency rendering in a patient with MR of mixed etiologies showing the origins of 2 separate MR jets (*arrowheads*), one at A2-P2 (secondary MR component) and another from a perforation of the anterior leaflet near the left trigone (primary MR component). A tricuspid regurgitation (TR) jet is also visualized. A2L, lateral 1/3 of A2; A2M, medial 1/3 of A2; Ao, aorta; LA, left atrium; LV, left ventricle; MPR, multiplanar reconstruction; MV, mitral valve; P2L, lateral 1/3 of P2; P2M, medial 1/3 of P2; TEE, transesophageal echocardiography. (From Fan Y, Chan JSK, Lee AP. Advances in procedural echocardiographic imaging in transcatheter edge-to-edge repair for mitral regurgitation. *Front Cardiovasc Med.* 2022;9:864341, with permission from BMJ Publishing Group Ltd.)

annuloplasty systems aim to reduce the circumference of the mitral annulus to improve coaptation of the leaflets.[88] Transcatheter annuloplasty systems can be categorized as direct or indirect depending on their relation to the mitral annulus.[89] Indirect systems are placed in the coronary sinus given its relation to the posterior mitral annulus to reduce annular dimension, while direct annuloplasty systems are placed directly on the mitral annulus.[90] Transcatheter chordal repair systems are developed for the treatment of primary MR due to flail or prolapsed leaflets.[91-95] Further details of these technologies are beyond the scope of this chapter.

TRANSCATHETER MV REPLACEMENT

Overview

TMVR has emerged as an exciting new frontier in the field of cardiac structural interventions providing an alternative for high-surgical risk patients.[96,97] While transcatheter aortic valve replacement (TAVR) is a well-established treatment option for patients with symptomatic severe calcific aortic stenosis, the experience with TMVR remains at an early stage. There have been important

Anatomic classification associated with stenosis following TEER:
- Carpentier Class IIIa
  - Chronic Rheumatic disease
  - Radiation heart disease resulting in mitral regurgitation
  - Other chronic inflammatory conditions affecting the mitral valve
- Severe mitral annular calcification with mitral stenosis or calcium extension into the leaflets, or restricted leaflet motion
- Severely calcified or fibrotic leaflet(s) (potential for mitral stenosis)
- Prior surgical annuloplasty or ring with potential for stenosis
- Prohibitively small mitral valve area (MVA < 3.5 cm2)

Anatomic classification associated with inadequate reduction in MR:
- Perforation from endocarditis (or other significant loss of leaflet tissue)
- Active endocarditis
- Extreme mitral valve complexity that would preclude a successful mitral valve repair with an E2E device (i.e. severe Barlow's disease, commonly associated with multiple jets; excessive redundancy, calcification, or poor coaptation reserve in the leaflets that inhibits restoration of coaptation with TEER)
- Short or restricted Posterior Mitral Leaflet (<5 mm in the intended grasping location)
- MR is primarily due to clefts

Patient factors associated with inability to perform TEER:
- Intracardiac thrombus that is mobile or may interfere with working in the cardiac chambers
- Imaging limitations that preclude adequate mitral valve visualization to effect an E2E repair
  - Inability to do a TEE
  - Inability to obtain grasping views
- Trans-septal or venous access issues that preclude placement of an E2E device
  - Caval interruption (inferior vena cava filter occluded with thrombus)
  - Large atrial septal occluder device
  - Inability to gain enough height on transseptal for delivery system to work

Clinical Factors associated with futility in performing TEER:
- Patients without meaningful expected survival (12 months) or improvement in quality of life due to non-mitral valve disease
- Patients with less than 3+/4 + mitral regurgitation by quantitative echocardiographic assessment
- Patients with inotropic requirement not thought to be related to mitral valve disease

FIGURE 41.13 Anatomic and patient characteristics associated with unsuitability for mitral transcatheter edge-to-edge repair. (Adapted and edited from Lim DS, Herrmann HC, Grayburn P, et al. Consensus document on non-suitability for transcatheter mitral valve repair by edge-to-edge therapy. *Struct Heart.* 2021;5:227-233. doi:10.1080/24748706.2021.1902595)

challenges in the development of this technology including the complexity of the MV anatomy involving a saddle oval shape, the subvalvular apparatus, the interaction with the left ventricular outflow tract (LVOT) and the aortic valve, as well as the large size of TMVR devices and large catheters for implantation limiting delivery to transapical access in early experience.[98,99] The wide variety of mitral pathology, from stenosis to multiple mechanisms of regurgitation, also adds to the difficulties of valve design.[99] Furthermore, the patients being considered for TMVR are usually at high risk with multiple comorbidities, including frailty, pulmonary hypertension, or severe left ventricular systolic dysfunction, each of which negatively impacts the overall clinical outcome.[100] Despite these technical, anatomic, and clinical limitations, there has been significant progress in the last decade.

The initial TMVR experience started with the use of balloon-expandable aortic THVs in failed mitral bioprostheses with an MViV procedure, failed surgical repairs with annuloplasty rings with MViR, and MV dysfunction in the setting of severe MAC with ViMAC procedures.[97,101,102] In all these procedures, the pre-existing surgical bioprosthesis, annuloplasty ring, or severe MAC serves as a landing zone to anchor the aortic THV in place. Subsequently, dedicated mitral THVs with anchoring mechanisms have been developed for TMVR in noncalcified native MVD.[103] Multiple mitral THV devices are being evaluated. Although transapical access was required in most of the initial experience, several TS technologies are now available. At the time of writing of this chapter, none of the dedicated mitral THV technologies have received FDA approval for use in the United States. Only the Tendyne Mitral Valve System (Abbott Structural Heart, Santa Clara, CA) has received CE mark in January 2020.[104] Therefore, this chapter will focus on technologies with the most robust experience, which are currently in pivotal trials.

Dedicated TMVR Devices

Tendyne MV System

Overview

The Tendyne Mitral Valve System has a self-expanding nitinol double-frame design.[105] The inner stent frame is circular and supports a trileaflet porcine pericardial valve with an effective orifice area of 3.2 cm^2. The outer stent frame has a D-shape to conform to the MV annulus shape. The outer stent has a polyterephthalate cuff for sealing in the annulus. Its anchoring mechanism is an apical tether (**Fig. 41.14**).[103] The valve is delivered via a transapical approach through a 34-French (Fr) sheath. The valve system comes in a standard and low-profile system, which features a smaller valve with a reduced LVOT profile for smaller-sized LVs. The effective orifice area is 3.2 cm^2 for the standard profile prosthesis and 2.2 cm^2 for the low-profile prosthesis.[106]

In the initial feasibility study report that included outcomes of the first 100 patients treated, technical success was 96% with a 30-day mortality of 6% lower than predicted by the Society of Thoracic Surgeons predicted risk of mortality score of 7.8%.[107] Disabling stroke rate at 30 days was 2%, and other adverse event rates were also low. MR at baseline was grade 3 or 4 in 99% of the patients, which was reduced to none or trace in 98.8% at 30 days and 98.4% at 1 year.[108] The valve performance was maintained at 2 years with none or trivial MR in 93/2% of the patients. This was associated with symptom improvement: 66% were in New York Heart Association (NYHA) class III or IV at baseline, whereas 81.6% were in NYHA class I or II at 2 years.[109]

Tendyne was the first dedicated TMVR device to be used in a patient with severe MAC. The initial report of compassionate use experience in the first nine patients with MAC treated with

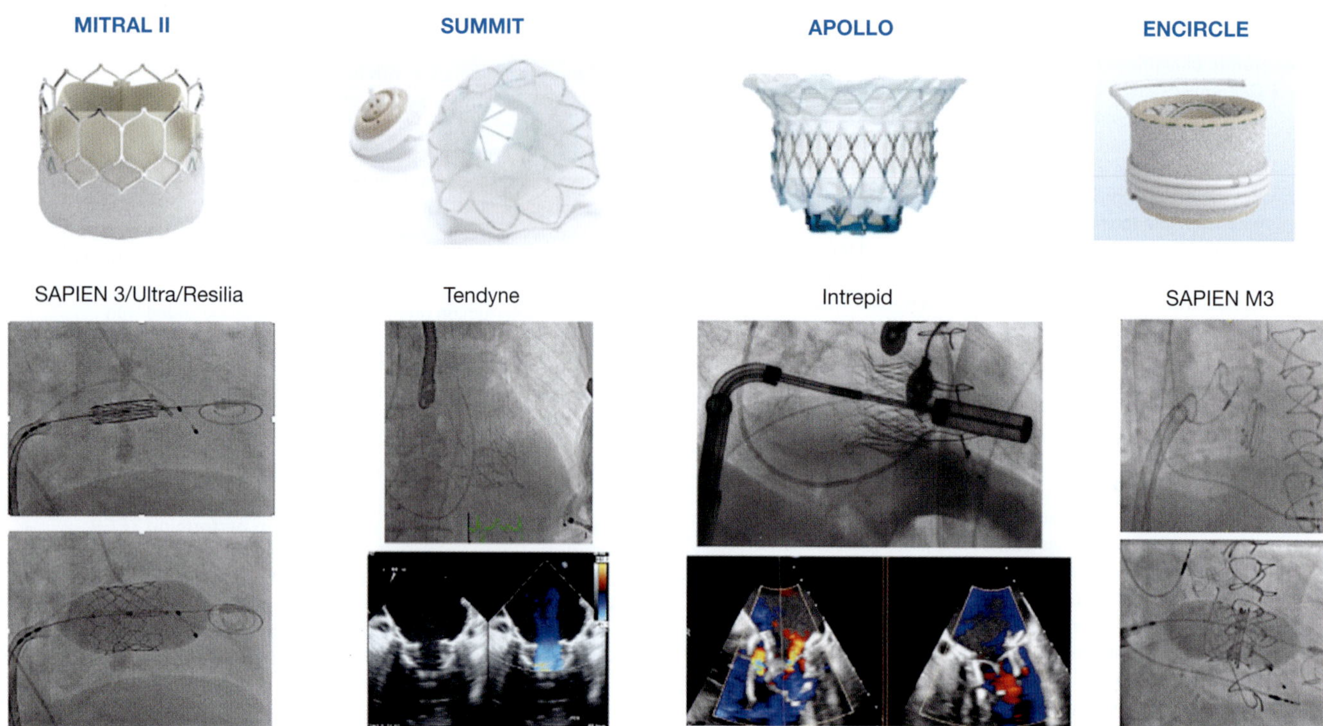

FIGURE 41.14 Transcatheter heart valves being evaluated in transcatheter mitral valve replacement pivotal clinical trials (*Blue font*: Name of Clinical trial. *Black font*: name of transcatheter valve). Images below each transcatheter valve include fluoroscopy images or transesophageal images during valve implantation procedures. (Intrepid procedure image from Zahr F, Song HK, Chadderdon SM, et al. 30-Day outcomes following transfemoral transseptal transcatheter mitral valve replacement: intrepid TMVR early feasibility study results. *JACC Cardiovasc Interv.* 2022;15(1):80-89.)

Tendyne showed no mortality at 30 days, a low procedural complication rate, and complete elimination of MR in all patients.[110] In a subsequent report including an additional 11 patients enrolled in the Tendyne MAC Feasibility Study (NCT03539458), technical success was 95% without intraprocedural deaths. There were 8 deaths at 1 year (40%). Among 12 survivors at 1 year, 100% had none or trivial MR and 92% were in NYHA class I or II.[111]

The SUMMIT (clinical trial to evaluate the Safety and effectiveness of Using the Tendyne Mitral Valve System for the Treatment of Symptomatic MITral Regurgitation, NCT03433274) is the pivotal trial evaluating the Tendyne system. It is the only pivotal trial at the time of writing of this chapter that has a randomized arm comparing Tendyne versus TEER with MitraClip in patients with favorable anatomy for both procedures. For patients who do not have favorable anatomy for TEER, the study has a nonrepairable arm for noncalcified MV and a separate arm for patients with MAC, which completed enrollment in 2023 and has a continued access program for MAC.

Tendyne Valve Implantation Procedure

The TMVR implantation for the Tendyne MV is performed in the operating room under general anesthesia using fluoroscopic and mostly transesophageal echocardiographic guidance. A left thoracotomy is performed to obtain surgical left ventricular access near the apex at the location predetermined by cardiac computed tomography (CT) analysis and confirmed by transesophageal echocardiogram. An 18-gauge needle is introduced in the LV, a 0.035 guidewire is then advanced into the LA, the needle is removed an 8-Fr sheath is placed in the LV. Then, a 7-Fr balloon-tipped catheter is introduced through the sheath and is advanced inflated across the MV into the LA. Then the 0.035 guidewire is introduced through the balloon catheter into the LA, the balloon catheter is pulled back into LV and readvanced in the LA over the guidewire utilizing the "flossing technique" to confirm the guidewire is free and not traversing through chordae. Once proper position of the guidewire is confirmed, the balloon catheter and sheath are removed, and the Tendyne valve delivery system is introduced in the LV. The Tendyne valve is then deployed in the mitral positions using mostly transesophageal guidance (**Fig. 41.14**).

Intrepid Valve

The Medtronic Intrepid THV (Medtronic, Minneapolis, MN) has a self-expandable nitinol outer stent, which provides fixation and sealing, and a circular inner stent, which houses a 27 mm trileaflet bovine pericardium valve with an effective orifice area of 2.4 cm^2 (**Fig. 41.14**). The valve was implanted via transapical access in the early experience.[96] In the initial report that included outcomes of the first 50 patients treated, the valve was successfully implanted in 96% of the patients. About 30-day mortality was 14% in a patient population with the Society of Thoracic Surgeons (STS) score of 6.4%. At 1 year, all-cause mortality was 23.5%. Survivors experienced a reduction of MR with 73.8% having no MR and 79% in NYHA class I or II at the last follow-up (median 173 days).[112] A TS delivery system recently became available. In a recent report describing outcomes of the first 15 patients treated with TS access, the valve was successfully implanted in 14 patients. At 30-day follow-up, 100% had none or trace of MR and 86% were in NYHA I or II class (67% in class III or IV at baseline).[113]

The APOLLO (Transcatheter Mitral Valve Replacement With the Medtronic Intrepid TMVR System in Patients With Severe Symptomatic Mitral Regurgitation, NCT 03242642) pivotal trial has an arm for patients with noncalcified MVs who are not ideal candidates for TEER and has added a registry arm of MAC patients. The Intrepid transcatheter valve implantation procedure using transapical delivery access is similar to the one described in the prior section for Tendyne (**Fig. 41.14**). TS delivery is similar to that described in the subsequent section under special patient populations.

Sapien M3

The Sapien M3 (Edwards Lifesciences, Irvine, CA) is TS balloon-expandable bovine pericardium THV system (**Fig. 41.14**) similar to the Sapien 3 aortic THV but with important differences: the entire stent frame is covered with polyethylene terephthalate cloth to provide sealing, it is a two-piece system that contains a fully retrievable nitinol dock to serve as a landing zone to anchor the THV, and has sleeve guard to decrease PVL rates. The system is currently available in one size (29 mm).[114] The ENCIRCLE (SapiEN M3 system transCatheter mItral valve ReplaCement via transseptaL accEss) pivotal trial (NCT04153292) is currently enrolling. It has 3 arms including anatomy not suitable for TEER (prior surgical repair not excluded), prior failed TEER attempt, and a MAC arm. The Sapien M3 implantation procedure is similar to the TS procedures described in the next section.

TMVR in Special Patient Populations Utilizing Aortic THV

Balloon-expandable aortic THVs have been used to treat patients with failed bioprostheses utilizing an MViV, failing surgical repairs with annuloplasty ring using an MViR procedure, or severe MV dysfunction in the setting of severe MAC using a ViMAC procedure. Although the technical aspects of these procedures have similarities, the patient populations and patient selection are different. We will describe the populations and outcomes data separately followed by a combined procedural overview.

Transcatheter MViV

Mitral bioprosthetic valves are increasingly utilized in the management of patients with MVD.[115] However, bioprosthetic tissue valves have limited durability and are prone to tissue degeneration and disease progression.[116] Reoperation of failed bioprosthetic valves is associated with significant morbidity and mortality, and a significant proportion of patients requiring reoperation are at high surgical risk.[117] TMVR using an aortic THV in an MViV procedure has emerged as alternative to reoperation in high-surgical risk patients.[97] Unlike the aortic position, only stented bioprostheses are implanted in the mitral position. Transapical (TA) and TS are the two procedural access routes for MViV. The TA access enables a more direct implantation and a predictable coaxial deployment. However, studies have demonstrated increased risk of mortality with TA approach compared to TS.[118] This is likely related to the more invasive nature of the TA access with the left thoracotomy as well as the direct myocardial injury. Thus, the TS access is currently the preferred access.

The VIVID registry included 857 patients with a median STS Predicted Risk of Mortality (PROM) score of 9.0% who underwent MViV. TS approach was utilized in 34.5% of the cases, and technical success was achieved in 93.5% with a 30-day mortality rate of 6.5% and 4-year survival estimate of 62.5%.[119] Initial data from the TVT registry included 680 patients with a mean STS score of 10.0% who underwent MViV between 2013 and 2017. TA approach was performed in 41.8%, technical success was achieved in 90.9%, and all-cause mortality at 30 days was 8.1%.[120] Follow-up data from the TVT registry between 2015 and 2019 included 1529 patients with a mean STS PROM score of 8.7% and reported mortality of 5.4% at 30 days and 16.7% at 1 year.[118] TS approach was performed in 86.7% of the patients and was associated with significantly lower 1-year all-cause mortality compared to TA access (TS 15.8% vs TA 21.7%, $P = .03$).[118]

The MITRAL (**M**itral **I**mplantation of **TRA**nscatheter va**L**ves) trial (NCT 02370511) was the first prospective study evaluating TS MViV using aortic THVs.[97] A total of 30 high-surgical risk patients were included with a median STS PROM of 9.4%. Technical success was achieved in 100% of the patients, and 1-year mortality was 3.3%. This was accompanied by improvement in NYHA class and 6-minute walk test at 1 year. At 5-year follow up, all-cause mortality rate was 21.4%, and survivors experienced significant improvement of NYHA class and Kansas City Cardiomyopathy Questionnaire scores with 94.7% of them in NYHA class I or II. Mean mitral gradients remained stable (6.6 ± 2.5 mm Hg), and 100% had none or trace MR at 5 years.[121]

Given the successful results of MViV in high-surgical risk patients, the PARTNER 3 MViV study prospective evaluated the safety of TS MViV in intermediate-risk patients and included 50 patients with a mean STS score of 4.1%. Technical success was achieved in 98.0%. The primary endpoint of all-cause mortality or stroke at 1 year was zero.[122] Patients experienced symptom improvement with 95.7% in NYHA class I or II at 1-year follow-up.

Transcatheter MViR

MR reduction via surgical mitral repair with annuloplasty rings or bands may subsequently degenerate requiring mitral reintervention.[123] Repeat mitral surgery is often associated with higher risk than the index procedure.[124] Accordingly, TMVR in an MViR anatomy has emerged as a therapeutic option in high-surgical risk patients. MViR is a more complex procedure compared to MViV due to varying types of surgical rings, and unlike bioprosthetic valves, not all surgical rings are suitable for an MViR. Surgical rings can be classified as rigid, semi-rigid, or flexible and complete, nearly complete, or incomplete (**Fig. 41.15**).[125] Multiple properties of surgical rings should be considered when assessing their suitability for a THV. This includes the size of the ring, its ability to become circular in shape, and its ability to anchor the THV. Additionally, some surgical rings are not radio-opaque, and MViR in these cases is completely guided by TEE.

There is paucity of data regarding the safety and efficacy of MViR procedures, mostly limited to retrospective registries. The VIVID registry included 222 patients with a median STS PROM of 7.4% who underwent MViR.[119] TS approach was utilized in 46.4% of the patients, and technical success was achieved in 82.0% with a 30-day mortality rate of 8.6% and 4-year survival estimate of 49.7%. In the VIVID registry, survival estimates were significantly lower in patients who underwent MViR compared to those who underwent MViV (MViR 49.7% vs MViV 62.5%, $P = .002$). An early report from the TVT registry included 123 patients with a mean STS PROM of 9.3%. TS approach was performed in 50.4% of the patients, and 30-day mortality rate was 11.5%.[120] The MITRAL trial was the first prospective study to evaluate the safety and feasibility of TS MViR using balloon-expandable aortic THVs.[102] A total of 30 patients were included with a median STS PROM of 7.6%. Technical success was achieved in 66.7% of the patients, and 1-year mortality was 23.3%. Survivors experienced significant improvement in symptoms and quality of life scores, with 84.2% of patients being in NYHA class I or II at 1 year. However, mortality at 5 years was 65.5% similar to the mortality observed in patients in the MAC arm (67.9%) and much higher than the 21.4% mortality observed in MViV patients at 5 years. In addition, only 50% were in NYHA class I or II at 5-year follow-up. Mean mitral gradients

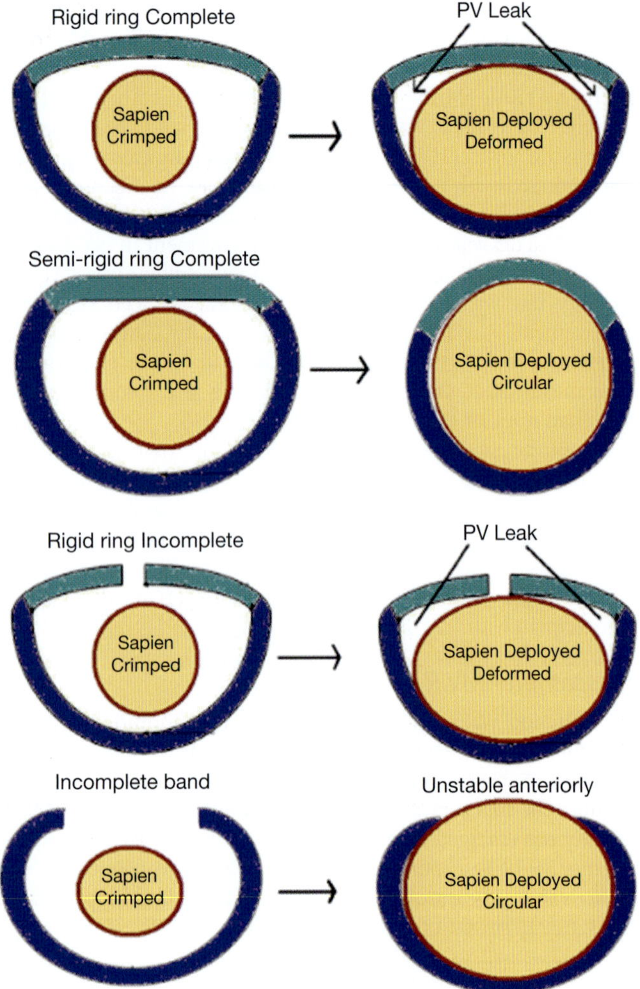

FIGURE 41.15 Different types of surgical rings and their suitability for transcatheter mitral valve replacement. The *yellow circles* represent the SAPIEN transcatheter valves crimped (*Right*) or after deployment (*Left*). PV, paravalvular. (From Little SH, Bapat V, Blanke P, Guerrero M, Rajagopal V, Siegel R. Imaging guidance for transcatheter mitral valve intervention on prosthetic valves, rings, and annular calcification. *JACC Cardiovasc Imaging*. 2021;14(1):22-40. doi:10.1016/j.jcmg.2019.10.027)

remained stable (5.8 ± 0.1 mm Hg), and 66.7% had none or trace MR at 5 years.[121] MViR is a reasonable option for patients with significant symptoms who are not candidates for repeat surgery due to risk. However, further studies are needed to improve patient selection and outcomes.

Transcatheter Mitral ViMAC

MAC is a progressive degenerative process of the MV associated with increased mortality.[126] MAC can extend into the MV resulting in mitral valve dysfunction (MVD) with MS, MR, or both. Patients with MAC and severe MVD are usually very comorbid and are at a high surgical risk.[126] TMVR with a ViMAC procedure using a balloon-expandable aortic THV or dedicated mitral THV device has emerged as a therapeutic option in this challenging patient population.[100] Comprehensive multimodality imaging assessment is crucial in assessing the anatomical extent of MAC and its impact on the MV function.[127] TTE enables qualitative assessment of MAC and the severity of MVD in these patients, which includes visual appearance of the valve, assessing if there is thickening of the leaflets and their mobility as well as assessing its coaptation. Additionally, quantitative assessment of MAC and MVD by TTE includes measuring the MVA, mean diastolic gradient, and indices of regurgitation severity. Furthermore, TEE with 3-dimensional images is excellent in assessing the degree of MR as well as planimetric measurements of valve area.

CT plays a crucial role in preintervention planning, as it enables quantitative anatomical assessment of MAC, including calcium burden, location, and its circumferential extent.[127] A CT-based MAC score has been developed to provide a systematic method to grade MAC severity and predict the risk of THV embolization or migration in patients undergoing ViMAC (**Table 41.5**).[128] A CT-MAC score of ≤6 was associated with a 60% rate of migration or embolization compared with 9.7% of patients with a MAC score of 7 or greater ($P < .001$).[128] Therefore, the use of a Sapien 3 valve for ViMAC in patients with a CT-based MAC score of 6 or less is not recommended. This score is used in current practice in the patient selection of these patients for the various transcatheter procedure options available.

There are limited data available on the safety and efficacy of ViMAC using aortic THVs, mostly from retrospective registries. The MAC Global Registry included 116 patients with extreme surgical risk and a mean STS PROM of 15.3% from 51 centers in 11 countries.[100] Technical success was achieved in 76.7%, and TS approach was utilized in 40.5% of the population. All-cause death at 30 days was 25% at 30 days and 53.7% at 1 year. Additionally, LVOT obstruction with hemodynamic compromise occurred in 11.2% of the population. The MITRAL trial was the first prospective trial that investigated ViMAC using the SAPIEN XT and SAPIEN 3 valves in patients with severe MAC and severe MVD.[101] A total of 31 patients were included with a mean STS PROM of 8.6%. TS access was utilized in 48.4%, and technical success was achieved in 74.2%. LVOT obstruction with hemodynamic compromise occurred in 3 patients, and all-cause mortality was 16.7% at 30 days, 34.5% at 1 year, and 67.9% at 5 years. The high mortality observed in the patients may be related to advanced age and multiple comorbidities that impact long-term outcomes. Nonetheless, survivors experienced sustained improvement in symptoms and quality of life with 83.3% of them in NYHA class I or II at 1 year and 55% at 5 years. Furthermore, THV performance was sustained with stable mean mitral gradients (6.5 ± 2.5 mm Hg) and 83.3% with no or trace MR at 5 years.[121]

TABLE 41.5 A CT-Based MAC Score was Developed to Predict the Risk of Valve Embolization in Patients Undergoing ViMAC

CALCIUM THICKNESS	CALCIUM DISTRIBUTION	TRIGONE INVOLVEMENT	LEAFLET INVOLVEMENT
<5 mm = 1	<180° = 1	None = 0	None = 0
5-9.99 = 2	180°-270° = 2	One = 1	One leaflet = 2
≥10 mm = 3	≥270° = 3	Both = 2	Both leaflets = 2

CT, computed tomography; MAC, mitral annular calcification; ViMAC, valve in mitral annular calcification.

The MITRAL II pivotal trial (NCT 04408430) is a nonrandomized trial investigating the safety and efficacy of SAPIEN 3 and SAPIEN 3 Ultra/RESILA in symptomatic patients with severe MAC and severe MVD. TS approach is the only access used in the trial, and all patients must have a CT MAC score of ≥7 to be included (**Fig. 41.14**). The trial also has a natural history arm for patients who are not candidates for an intervention or not interested in undergoing an intervention. This trial may provide further insights to help define the optimal patient selection strategy and understand the natural history of this condition.

Although THV devices for the MV were initially designed to treat noncalcified MV pathology, several mitral THV devices have been utilized to treat patients with MAC and are being evaluated in pivotal trials as described in the TMVR section of this chapter.

Essentials of TS MViV, MViR, and ViMAC Procedures

Although these procedures are different and are performed in different patient populations, they share several essential steps summarized in this section.[129]

Preprocedural Planning

The use of cardiac CT is essential for planning the important steps of these procedures, including TS access location, mitral annulus sizing, estimating the risk of LVOT obstruction, and determining best fluoroscopy angles during valve deployment or adjuvant procedure such as percutaneous laceration of the anterior leaflet. The risk of LVOT obstruction is assessed by placing a virtual THV using computer software and measuring the remaining LVOT space at the point of closest proximity of the ventricular edge of the THV with the interventricular septum. This is the neo-LVOT (**Fig. 41.16**).

THV Implantation in MV Procedure

TS access is obtained using standard techniques. An inferoposterior location is preferred as it facilitates navigating the anatomy with the Sapien 3 delivery system. Cardiac CT can facilitate predetermine TSP location (**Fig. 41.17**). Once TS access is obtained, intravenous heparin is administered to maintain therapeutic ACT (ideally >300 seconds). Then a 230 cm 0.025″ Toray wire (Toray Industries, Inc, Tokyo, Japan) is introduced in the LA, the TS sheath is removed, and the Edwards e-sheath is introduced in the inferior vena cava over the Toray wire via the right femoral vein. The sheath is oriented in a similar fashion as in the TAVR procedure with the Edwards logo facing up. The sheath is flushed with heparinized saline. A deflectable sheath such as an 8.5-Fr small or medium curve Agilis Steerable Introducer (St. Jude Medical, St. Paul, MN) is introduced in the LA over the Toray wire via the Edwards sheath in the right femoral vein. The Agilis catheter is flexed to point toward the MV under fluoroscopic (**Fig. 41.18A**) and TEE guidance, and the MV is crossed in the deployment fluoroscopy angle using a 6-Fr or 7-Fr pigtail catheter and a J guidewire. The pigtail catheter is advanced to the left ventricular apex, and a 0.035″ extra-small curve Safari2™ guidewire (Boston Scientific, Marlborough, MA) is placed in the left ventricular apex through the pigtail catheter with the wire loop facing down (**Fig. 41.18B**). Once the Safari wire is positioned in the left ventricular apex, the pigtail catheter is removed. A peripheral balloon with 12- or 14-mm diameter 3 to 4 cm long and 110 to 135 cm shaft is introduced over the Agilis

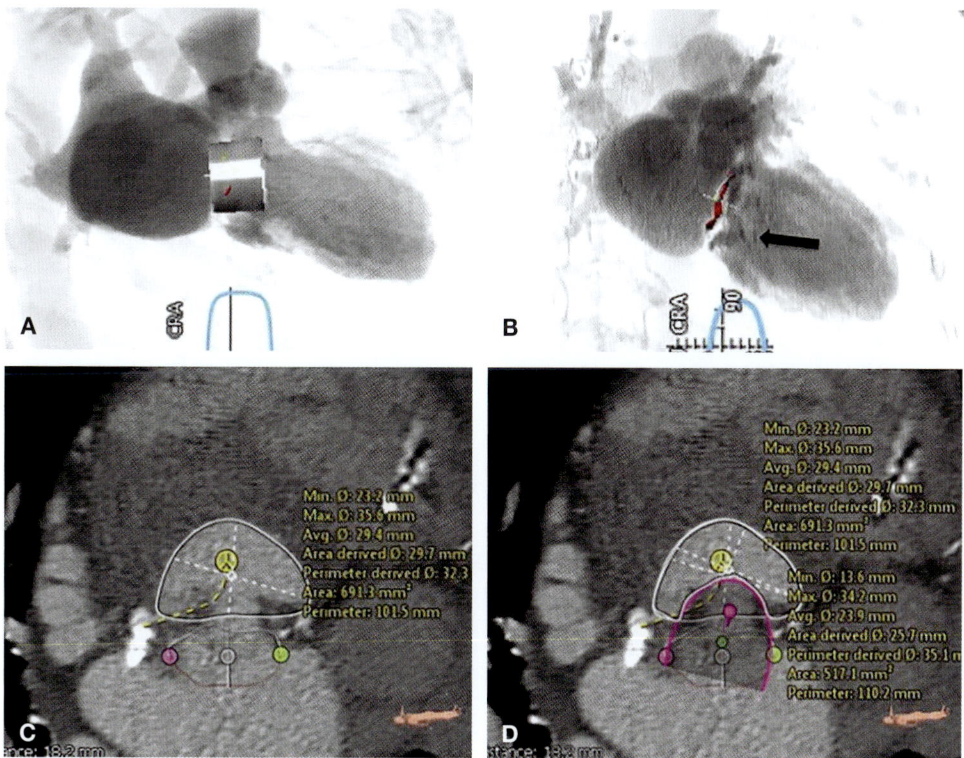

FIGURE 41.16 **A,** Virtual valve placed in the landing zone and visualized in Angio view using 3Mensio Structural Heart Mitral Workflow software version 8.1 (Pie Medical Imaging, Maastricht, The Netherlands). **B,** Calcium deposits when present in the mitral annulus or the left ventricle can be used as fluoroscopic markers of the landing zone (*arrow*) when bioprosthesis is radiolucent. **C,** Measurement of the left ventricular outflow tract area in systole. **D,** Measurement of the Neo-Left ventricular outflow tract area with virtual valve in place in systole. (From Guerrero M, Salinger M, Pursnani A, et al. Transseptal transcatheter mitral valve-in-valve: a step by step guide from pre-procedural planning to post-procedural care. *Catheter Cardiovasc Interv*. 2017;1-12. doi:10.1002/ccd.27128. PMID: 28557344.)

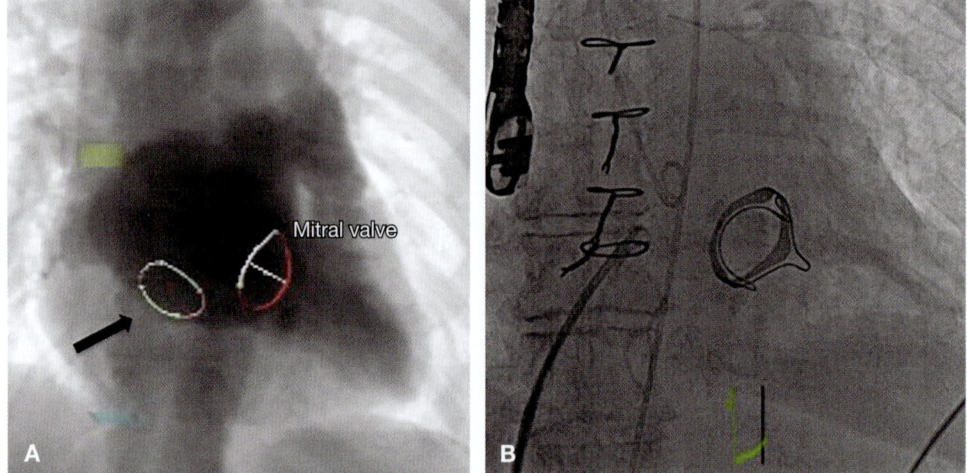

FIGURE 41.17 Cardiac CT analysis using 3Mensio Structural Heart Mitral Workflow software version 8.1 (Pie Medical Imaging, Maastricht, the Netherlands). **A,** The fossa ovalis is marked with a *circle* (*arrow*) and visualized in Angio view. Operators can use this image to predict the position of the trans-septal (TS) needle in fluoroscopy anteroposterior projection during TS puncture. **B,** Fluoroscopy during TS puncture shows the TS needle in the location predicted by CT. CT, computed tomography. *(From Guerrero M, Salinger M, Pursnani A, et al. Transseptal transcatheter mitral valve-in-valve: a step by step guide from pre-procedural planning to post-procedural care. Catheter Cardiovasc Interv.* 2017;1-12. doi:10.1002/ccd.27128. PMID: 28557344.)

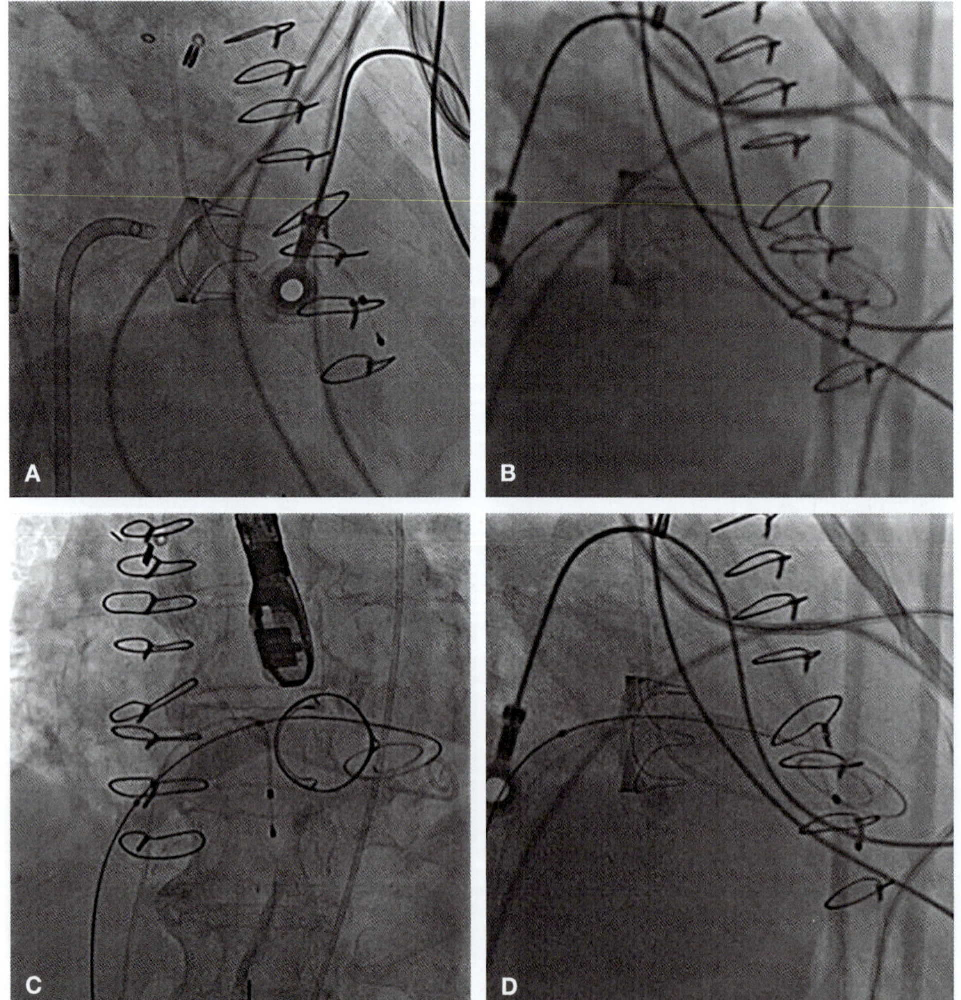

FIGURE 41.18 **A,** Agilis sheath flexed pointing toward the mitral valve. **B,** Safari guidewire placed in the left ventricular apex. **C,** Balloon inflated across the interatrial septum. **D,** Same balloon used for septostomy now inflated across the mitral valve for gentle mitral valvuloplasty in a patient with critical mitral stenosis. (From Guerrero M, Salinger M, Pursnani A, et al. Transseptal transcatheter mitral valve-in-valve: a step by step guide from pre-procedural planning to post-procedural care. *Catheter Cardiovasc Interv.* 2017;1-12. doi:10.1002/ccd.27128. PMID: 28557344.)

sheath to perform atrial septostomy (**Fig. 41.18C**). We use the 12-mm balloon for the 23- and 26-mm SAPIEN 3 valves and the 14 mm for the 29-mm valve if the interatrial septum was instrumented during the initial surgery, as scar may be present. When dealing with thin and intact interatrial septums, a 10- and 12-mm balloon may provide adequate septostomy for the 23- and 26-mm SAPIEN 3 and the 29 mm valve, respectively. After septostomy, the THV is then introduced and deployed under rapid placing (usually 140 bpm) (**Fig. 41.19**).[129]

Strategies to Decrease the Risk of TMVR-Induced LVOT Obstruction

TMVR can cause displacement of the anterior mitral leaflet toward the LVOT resulting in LVOT obstruction, which is associated with very poor outcomes once it occurs.[130] This is the most important complication of TMVR, and the risk of LVOT obstruction is one of the most frequent reasons for exclusion in TMVR clinical trials. Preprocedural assessment of the risk of LVOT obstruction is crucial to determine the eligibility of patients to undergo safe TMVR. This is routinely done with 3-D modeling of virtual prostheses on gated cardiac CT to simulate and measure the neo-LVOT area (**Fig. 41.20**). The neo-LVOT area should be measured during systole when the LV cavity size is the smallest, and a cutoff point of 189 mm^2 or less has been associated with high risk of increased LVOT gradient of 10 mm Hg or greater.[131] This cutoff point has been validated in ViMAC, MViV, and MViR.[131] In the TMVR Global registry, the cutoff of neo-LVOT value associated with LVOT obstruction in patients with MAC was 173 mm^3.[132]

Several strategies have been used to mitigate the risk of LVOT obstruction. Surgical options include a surgical transatrial delivery of a balloon-expandable aortic THV with resection of the anterior leaflet and septal myectomy if needed. However, this is a very invasive procedure, and most patients are not candidates due to high surgical risk. In this chapter, we will focus on percutaneous options including alcohol septal ablation (ASA), electrosurgical laceration of the anterior mitral leaflet, and radiofrequency septal ablation (RFSA).[133-135]

Alcohol Septal Ablation

ASA was initially developed for the treatment of severe symptomatic LVOT obstruction in patients with hypertrophic obstructive cardiomyopathy.[136] The procedure involves percutaneous

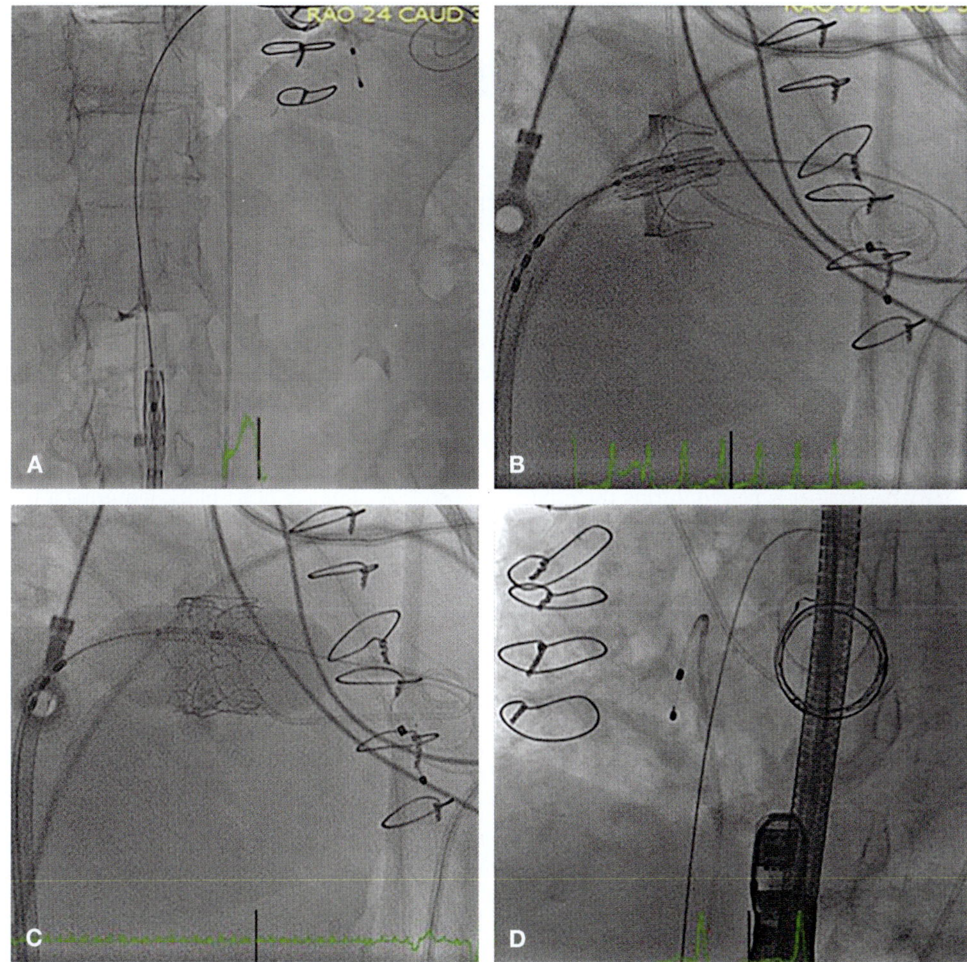

FIGURE 41.19 **A,** SAPIEN 3 valve aligned under fluoroscopy, similar to the alignment done for TAVR procedures. **B,** SAPIEN 3 valve visualized in fluoroscopy deployment angle to position the ventricular edge of the SAPIEN 3 stent frame at the ventricular edge of the pre-existing bioprosthesis. **C,** SAPIEN 3 valve deployed under rapid pacing with additional contrast to flare it in the ventricular side. **D,** LAO caudal view shows adequate expansion and circularity of the SAPIEN 3 valve. LAO, left anterior oblique; TAVR, transcatheter aortic valve replacement. (From Guerrero M, Salinger M, Pursnani A, et al. Transseptal transcatheter mitral valve-in-valve: a step by step guide from pre-procedural planning to post-procedural care. *Catheter Cardiovasc Interv*. 2017;1-12. doi:10.1002/ccd.27128. PMID: 28557344.)

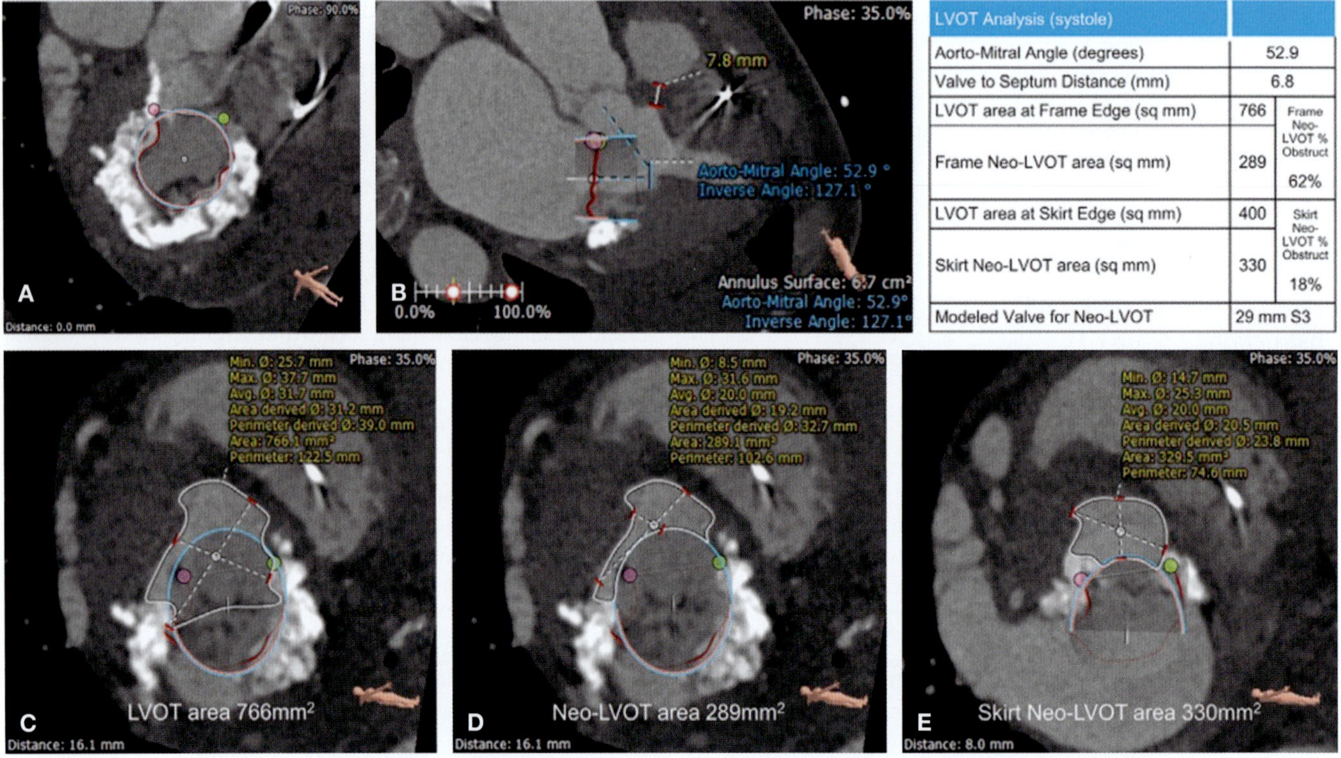

FIGURE 41.20 **A,** Placement of a virtual transcatheter valve on in the mitral annulus and on the intended site of implantation. **B,** Measurement of the ventricular septal thickness and virtual valve frame-to-septum distance. **C,** Measurement of the LVOT area. (**D** and **E**) Measurement of the neo-LVOT area and skirt neo-LVOT areas. (From Eleid MF, Collins JD, Mahoney P, et al. Emerging approaches to management of left ventricular outflow obstruction risk in transcatheter mitral valve replacement. *JACC Cardiovasc Interv.* 2023;16(8):885-895. doi:10.1016/j.jcin.2023.01.357)

cannulation with a 0.014-inch wire and over-the-wire balloon to occlude blood flow to the septal perforator supplying blood to the basal anterior septum. Once the vessel is appropriately localized, microbubble contrast is injected to confirm the opacification of the interventricular septum without involvement of the papillary muscles or other structures. This is followed by the infusion of dehydrated ethanol to achieve septal obliteration. Additionally, a temporary pacemaker is placed during the procedure due to the risk of atrioventricular block. The success of ASA relies on accurate vessel localization and careful confirmation of the target vessel. ASA carries certain risks, including conduction system disease with the development of new right bundle branch block in up to 50% of patients and high-grade AV block in up to 24%.[137] Additionally, the risk of mortality, stroke, pericardial effusion, and major vascular complications is generally low when performed at experienced centers (1%-2%).[137]

This technique was utilized with success-to-treat acute LVOT obstruction after TS ViMAC.[138] During the early experience, one patient who experienced severe LVOT obstruction after ViMAC was treated with salvage ASA. This resulted in initial improvement in LVOT gradient, which reoccurred the following day potentially due to septal edema.[139] This event led to a change in practice favoring pre-emptive alcohol ablation performed 3 to 4 weeks prior to TMVR in those at risk of LVOT obstruction as it is not possible who predict which patients will experience rebound LVOT gradient due to septal edema.

The early experience of pre-emptive ASA was evaluated in a multicenter registry of 30 patients undergoing TMVR.[133] The study demonstrated a median increase of 111.2 mm^2 in the neo-LVOT surface area post ASA, with a 16.7% rate of pacemaker implantation and 6.7% rate of 30-day mortality. A recent single-center study compared outcomes of ASA before TMVR to ASA for HCM.[140] The study found that the total volume of alcohol injected was higher in the HCM group (HCM 1.4 mL vs TMVR 0.8 mL, $P < .001$), and LVOT area significantly increased after ASA in the TMVR patients (HCM 135 mm^2 vs TMVR 233 mm^2, $P < .001$). The incidence of post-ASA complete heart block requiring a permanent pacemaker was numerically higher in the TMVR group (HCM 21% vs TMVR 35%, $P = .195$), and 30-day mortality rate was similar between the groups (HCM 4% vs TMVR 0%).[140] Overall, ASA before TMVR has evolved into a reasonable option to modify the interventricular septum to enlarge the LVOT and help prevent TMVR-induced LVOT obstruction. This strategy has helped more patients be able to safely undergo TMVR, and in some cases, has facilitated enrollment in TMVR trials evaluating dedicated mitral THV devices as well as in the MITRAL II trial evaluating the Sapien 3 valves (**Fig. 41.21**).

Electrosurgical Laceration of the Anterior Mitral Leaflet

Percutaneous laceration of the anterior mitral leaflet to prevent left ventricular outflow tract obstruction (LAMPOON) involves longitudinal splitting of the anterior leaflet to enable the anterior leaflet to splay during the expansion of the transcatheter valve stent frame (**Fig. 41.22**).[135] This deliberate laceration causes the two halves of the anterior leaflet to separate as it is displaced toward the LVOT, thereby minimizing LVOT obstruction. The initial LAMPOON technique was complex and required the use of antegrade and retrograde access to the LV.[141] This has been modified to a slightly

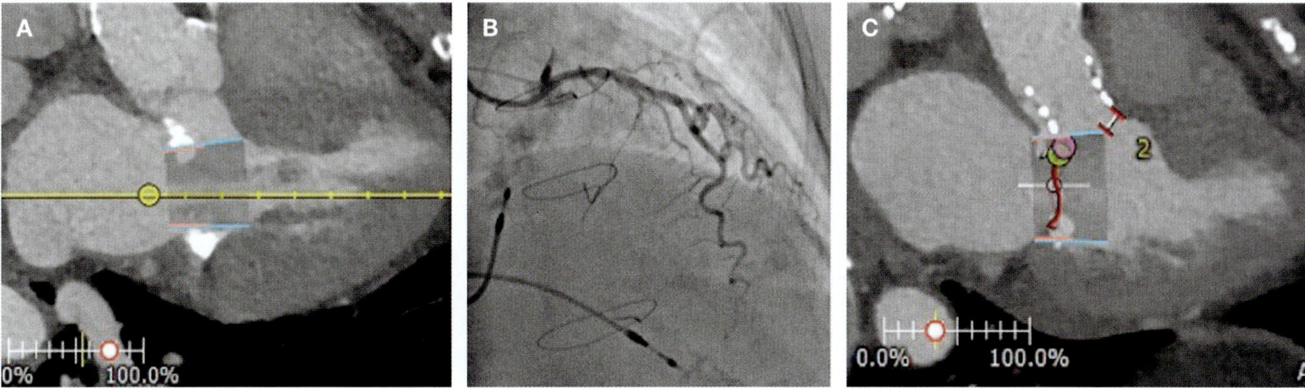

FIGURE 41.21 **A,** A patient with a small neo-LVOT due to a prominent basal septal hypertrophy. **B,** ASA of the first septal perforator is performed using 1 mL of dehydrated alcohol. **C,** The basal septal hypertrophy is decreased 4 weeks after ASA with a resulting increase in the virtual valve-to-septum distance. Additionally, interval placement of transcatheter aortic valve. ASA, alcohol septal ablation; LVOT, left ventricular outflow tract; MAC, mitral annulus calcification. (From Eleid MF, Collins JD, Mahoney P, et al. Emerging approaches to management of left ventricular outflow obstruction risk in transcatheter mitral valve replacement. *JACC Cardiovasc Interv.* 2023;16(8):885-895. doi:10.1016/j.jcin.2023.01.357)

simpler version that requires antegrade entry only. However, it remains complex and requires careful planning as well as experienced operators. The antegrade LAMPOON technique involves transfemoral TS access using two guiding catheters, each equipped with two coronary guiding catheters (usually a 6-F JR4 and 6-F MP). The MP catheter directs an electrified guidewire (Astato wire, Asahi Intecc) through an insulated Piggyback Wire Converter (Teleflex Medical) across the center and base of the anterior mitral leaflet. The JR4 catheter, positioned in the LV, captures the end of the electrified guidewire with a snare. The externalized guidewire forms a loop that is electrified to lacerate the anterior mitral leaflet along its centerline from base to tip. To address the potential

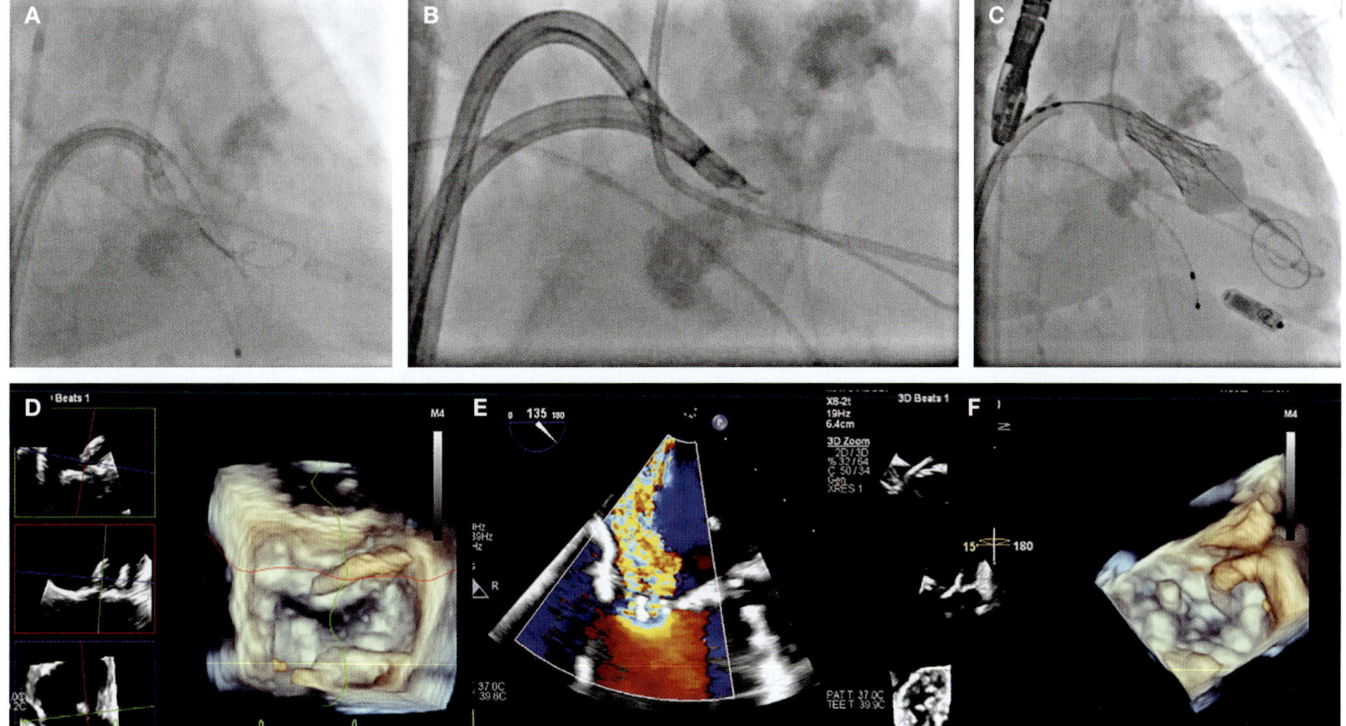

FIGURE 41.22 The simplified trans-septal LAMPOON approach involves anterior leaflet perforation with wire followed by wire snaring **(A)**, anterior leaflet laceration with balloon pump support **(B)** to facilitate balloon-expandable transcatheter mitral valve replacement (TMVR) **(C)**. Transesophageal echocardiography guidance is used to confirm appropriate catheter positioning **(D)**, and following laceration, there is an increase in mitral regurgitation **(E)** and evidence of anterior leaflet splitting on 3-dimensional imaging **(F)**. LAMPOON, left ventricular outflow tract obstruction. (From Eleid MF, Collins JD, Mahoney P, et al. Emerging approaches to management of left ventricular outflow obstruction risk in transcatheter mitral valve replacement. *JACC Cardiovasc Interv.* 2023;16(8):885-895. doi:10.1016/j.jcin.2023.01.357)

development of severe MR, an intra-aortic balloon pump can be utilized for left ventricular unloading.

Clinical experience with the initial LAMPOON technique was reported in 30 patients, 15 with severe MAC and 15 with failed surgical rings.[142] LAMPOON was successfully performed in all patients; however, 10% of patients experienced significant LVOT obstruction. Additionally, the 30-day mortality rate was 7% in the overall cohort (13% in the MAC cohort). Clinical experience with the simplified antegrade LAMPOON was reported in 9 patients with shorter procedure time compared to the initial LAMPOON technique, and none of the patients developed LVOT obstruction.[143] One procedural mortality was secondary to wire-induced ventricular perforation.

Radiofrequency Septal Ablation

RFSA represents another strategy to reduce the septal thickness to mitigate the risk of TMVR-induced LVOT obstruction.[134] The procedure is performed under general anesthesia and using a femoral access. ICE and 3-D electroanatomical mapping are used to facilitate the procedure, and systemic anticoagulation is administrated during the procedure. RFSA can be using TS or retroaortic approaches. Ablation is performed until lesion formation can be detected on ICE and diminutive electrogram signal is noted. Additionally, loss of myocardial capture by high-output pacing is used to confirm lesion formation. An initial case series of 4 patients with severe MAC who underwent RFSA prior to ViMAC, three patients with inadequate neo-LVOT measurements post ASA, and one patient who had unsuitable anatomy for ASA due to blood supply of the septal perforator to an anomalous chord to the papillary muscle.[144] Three patients experienced complete heart block and required pacemaker implantation, while the fourth patient already had a pacemaker. Neo-LVOT area increased, ranging from 30 to 80 mm^2, and all four patients underwent TMVR successfully, with two patients receiving additional anterior mitral leaflet laceration to further enhance the neo-LVOT during the procedure.

SESAME

SESAME (SEptal Scoring Along the Midline Endocardium) has recently been developed to "score" the septum using a retroaortic approach (**Fig. 41.23**).[145] In this technique, the basal septum is accessed using a 6-F HS guiding catheter and a tip-amputated guidewire, followed by the introduction of a microcatheter. A chronic total occlusion guidewire is then exchanged and passed through the targeted path of the basal septum. With the assistance of a second retroaortic guide, the guidewire is snared in the LV, creating a flying V configuration. Electrocautery is subsequently applied while exerting traction on both guiding catheters, resulting in the laceration or scoring of the basal septum. To date, this technique has been reported in a single patient prior to TMVR. The feasibility and effectiveness of SESAME in terms of reducing septal thickness are currently being investigated and require further study.

As described, multiple techniques have been developed to address and minimize the risk of LVOT obstruction in patients undergoing TMVR. Each technique has its advantage in terms of septal reduction or minimizing the displacement of the anterior leaflet. Subsequently, an algorithm has been developed to guide clinicians on how to approach these patients (**Fig. 41.24**).[130] Furthermore, dedicated mitral prostheses have been developed to minimize the risk of LVOT obstruction. The intrepid valve has a low profile that minimizes its protrusion into the LVOT.[96] The Tendyne valve has a tapered shape that limits its protrusion into the LVOT.[110] The SAPIEN M3 uses a dock in the subvalvular apparatus to anchor the THV. The dock pulls the chordae toward the center of the valve, and since the posterior leaflet is shorter, the dock self-centers toward the posterior aspect leaving more space in the LVOT.[114] Similarly, the Innovalve (Innovalve Biomedical) device self-centers toward the posterior aspect, which may help decrease the risk of LVOT obstruction associated with TMVR.[146]

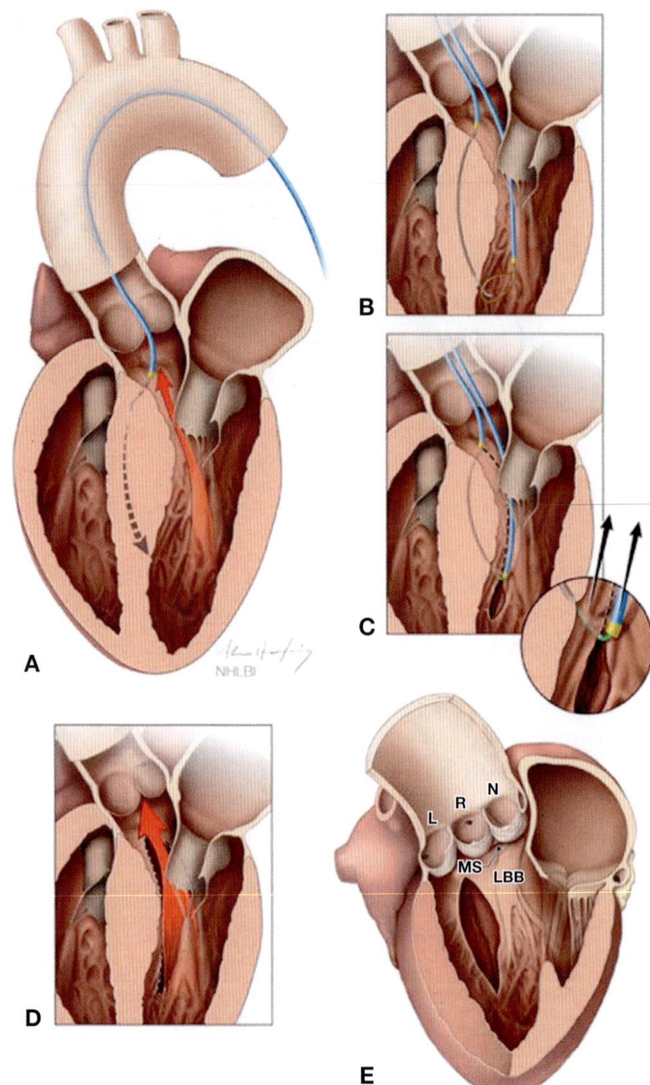

FIGURE 41.23 **A,** Navigation of a stiff guidewire through the interventricular septum. **B,** Re-entry of the guidewire with microcatheter support to the left ventricular cavity into a snare. **C,** Electrification and traction (*black arrows*) are applied to create the myotomy. **D,** Transcatheter SESAME results increased the left ventricular outflow tract and increased blood flow. **(E)** The SESAME laceration avoids the conduction system. L, left cusp; LBB, left bundle branch; MS, membranous septum; N, noncoronary cusp; R, right cusp. (From Khan JM, Bruce CG, Greenbaum AB, et al. Transcatheter myotomy to relieve left ventricular outflow tract obstruction: the septal scoring along the midline endocardium procedure in animals. *Circ Cardiovasc Interv*. 2022;15(6):e011686. doi:10.1161/CIRCINTERVENTIONS.121.011686)

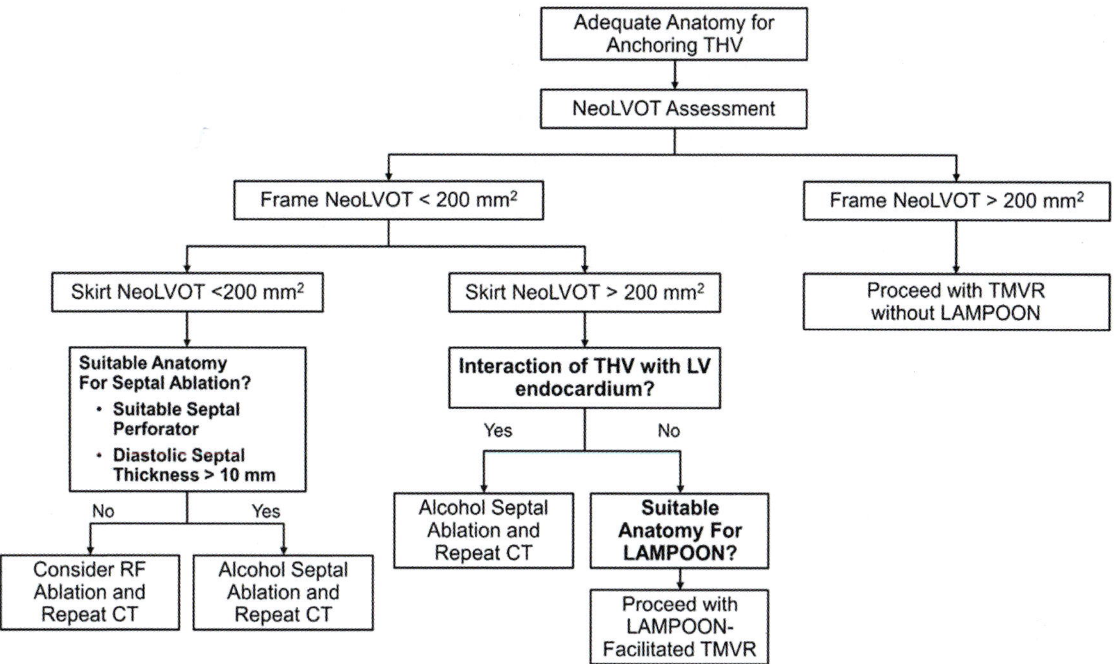

FIGURE 41.24 An algorithm to decrease the risk of TMVR-induced LVOT obstruction after valve-in-MAC. CT, computed tomography, LVOT, left ventricular outflow tract; MAC, mitral annulus calcification, TMVR, transcatheter mitral valve replacement. (From Eleid MF, Collins JD, Mahoney P, et al. Emerging approaches to management of left ventricular outflow obstruction risk in transcatheter mitral valve replacement. *JACC Cardiovasc Interv*. 2023;16(8):885-895. doi:10.1016/j.jcin.2023.01.357)

CONCLUSIONS

Transcatheter MV repair and TMVR are emerging treatment options which aim to address a breadth of mitral pathologies, including RHD, primary or secondary MR, failed surgical bioprostheses or annuloplasty rings, and MAC. Meticulous patient and anatomic review coupled with refined procedural techniques are essential to ensure the continued advancement of this promising field while yielding excellent patient outcomes.

Acknowledgments

The authors thank all the authors involved in the preparation of the prior version of this chapter and acknowledge that some of the prior content (text or figures) was included in this version.

For further review and interactivities, please see the chapter-based multiple choice questions and videos accessible in the complimentary eBook bundled with this text. Access instructions are located in the inside front cover.

References

1. Inoue K, Owaki T, Nakamura T, Kitamura F, Miyamoto N. Clinical application of transvenous mitral commissurotomy by a new balloon catheter. *J Thorac Cardiovasc Surg*. 1984;87(3):394-402.
2. Feldman T, Foster E, Glower DD, et al, EVEREST II Investigators. Percutaneous repair or surgery for mitral regurgitation. *N Engl J Med*. 2011;364(15):1395-1406. doi:10.1056/NEJMoa1009355
3. Stone GW, Lindenfeld J, Abraham WT, et al, COAPT Investigators. Transcatheter mitral-valve repair in patients with heart failure. *N Engl J Med*. 2018;379(24):2307-2318. doi:10.1056/NEJMoa1806640
4. Otto CM, Nishimura RA, Bonow RO, et al. 2020 ACC/AHA guideline for the management of patients with valvular heart disease: a report of the American College of Cardiology/American Heart Association Joint Committee on clinical practice guidelines. *Circulation*. 2021;143(5):e72-e227. doi:10.1161/CIR.0000000000000923
5. Jain S, Mankad SV. Echocardiographic assessment of mitral stenosis: echocardiographic features of rheumatic mitral stenosis. *Cardiol Clin*. 2013;31(2):177-191. doi:10.1016/j.ccl.2013.03.006
6. Iung B, Delgado V, Rosenhek R, et al, EORP VHD II Investigators. Contemporary presentation and management of valvular heart disease: the EURObservational Research Programme Valvular Heart Disease II Survey. *Circulation*. 2019;140(14):1156-1169. doi:10.1161/circulationaha.119.041080
7. Iung B, Vahanian A. Epidemiology of acquired valvular heart disease. *Can J Cardiol*. 2014;30(9):962-970. doi:10.1016/j.cjca.2014.03.022
8. Abramowitz Y, Jilaihawi H, Chakravarty T, Mack MJ, Makkar RR. Mitral annulus calcification. *J Am Coll Cardiol*. 2015;66(17):1934-1941. doi:10.1016/j.jacc.2015.08.872
9. Pibarot P, Herrmann HC, Wu C, et al, Heart Valve Collaboratory. Standardized definitions for bioprosthetic valve dysfunction following aortic or mitral valve replacement: JACC state-of-the-art review. *J Am Coll Cardiol*. 2022;80(5):545-561. doi:10.1016/j.jacc.2022.06.002
10. Giannini C, Mazzola M, Pugliese NR, Petronio AS. Mitral valve stenosis in the current era: a changing landscape. *J Cardiovasc Med*. 2022;23(11):701-709. doi:10.2459/jcm.0000000000001384
11. Vahanian A, Beyersdorf F, Praz F, et al, ESC/EACTS Scientific Document Group. 2021 ESC/EACTS Guidelines for the management of valvular heart disease. *Eur Heart J*. 2022;43(7):561-632. doi:10.1093/eurheartj/ehab395
12. Kim JY, Kim SH, Myong JP, et al. Ten-year trends in the incidence, treatment and outcomes of patients with mitral stenosis in Korea. *Heart*. 2020;106(10):746-750. doi:10.1136/heartjnl-2019-315883
13. Bertrand PB, Mihos CG, Yucel E. Mitral annular calcification and calcific mitral stenosis: therapeutic challenges and considerations. *Curr Treat Options Cardiovasc Med*. 2019;21(4):19. doi:10.1007/s11936-019-0723-6
14. Eleid MF, Nishimura RA, Lennon RJ, Sorajja P. Left ventricular diastolic dysfunction in patients with mitral stenosis undergoing percutaneous mitral balloon valvotomy. *Mayo Clin Proc*. 2013;88(4):337-344. doi:10.1016/j.mayocp.2012.11.018

15. Otto CM, Nishimura RA, Bonow RO, et al. 2020 ACC/AHA guideline for the management of patients with valvular heart disease. Executive summary: a report of the American College of Cardiology/American Heart Association Joint Committee on clinical practice guidelines. *Circulation*. 2021;143(5):e35-e71. doi:10.1161/cir.0000000000000932
16. Bouleti C, Iung B, Laouénan C, et al. Late results of percutaneous mitral commissurotomy up to 20 years: development and validation of a risk score predicting late functional results from a series of 912 patients. *Circulation*. 2012;125(17):2119-2127. doi:10.1161/circulationaha.111.055905
17. Meneguz-Moreno RA, Costa JR Jr, Gomes NL, et al. Very long term follow-up after percutaneous balloon mitral valvuloplasty. *JACC Cardiovasc Interv*. 2018;11(19):1945-1952. doi:10.1016/j.jcin.2018.05.039
18. Watkins DA, Beaton AZ, Carapetis JR, et al. Rheumatic heart disease worldwide: JACC Scientific Expert Panel. *J Am Coll Cardiol*. 2018;72(12):1397-1416. doi:10.1016/j.jacc.2018.06.063
19. Pasca I, Dang P, Tyagi G, Pai RG. Survival in patients with degenerative mitral stenosis: results from a large retrospective cohort study. *J Am Soc Echocardiogr*. 2016;29(5):461-469. doi:10.1016/j.echo.2015.12.012
20. Wilkins GT, Weyman AE, Abascal VM, Block PC, Palacios IF. Percutaneous balloon dilatation of the mitral valve: an analysis of echocardiographic variables related to outcome and the mechanism of dilatation. *Br Heart J*. 1988;60(4):299-308. doi:10.1136/hrt.60.4.299
21. Iung B, Cormier B, Ducimetiere P, et al. Immediate results of percutaneous mitral commissurotomy. A predictive model on a series of 1514 patients. *Circulation*. 1996;94(9):2124-2130. doi:10.1161/01.cir.94.9.2124
22. Sutaria N, Northridge DB, Shaw TR. Significance of commissural calcification on outcome of mitral balloon valvotomy. *Heart*. 2000;84(4):398-402. doi:10.1136/heart.84.4.398
23. Anwar AM, Attia WM, Nosir YF, et al. Validation of a new score for the assessment of mitral stenosis using real-time three-dimensional echocardiography. *J Am Soc Echocardiogr*. 2010;23(1):13-22. doi:10.1016/j.echo.2009.09.022
24. Iung B, Garbarz E, Michaud P, et al. Late results of percutaneous mitral commissurotomy in a series of 1024 patients. Analysis of late clinical deterioration: frequency, anatomic findings, and predictive factors. *Circulation*. 1999;99(25):3272-3278. doi:10.1161/01.cir.99.25.3272
25. Hernandez R, Macaya C, Bañuelos C, et al. Predictors, mechanisms and outcome of severe mitral regurgitation complicating percutaneous mitral valvotomy with the Inoue balloon. *Am J Cardiol*. 1992;70(13):1169-1174. doi:10.1016/0002-9149(92)90050-9
26. Lau KW, Hung JS. A simple balloon-sizing method in Inoue-balloon percutaneous transvenous mitral commissurotomy. *Cathet Cardiovasc Diagn*. 1994;33(2):120-131. discussion 130-121. doi:10.1002/ccd.1810330207
27. Sanati HR, Zahedmehr A, Shakerian F, et al. Percutaneous mitral valvuloplasty using echocardiographic intercommissural diameter as reference for balloon sizing: a randomized controlled trial. *Clin Cardiol*. 2012;35(12):749-754. doi:10.1002/clc.22013
28. Simard T, Thangarasa T, Di Santo P, Labinaz A, Hibbert B. The balloon impasse sign in percutaneous transvenous mitral valvuloplasty. *Oxf Med Case Reports*. 2020;2020(8):omaa062. doi:10.1093/omcr/omaa062
29. Wunderlich NC, Beigel R, Siegel RJ. Management of mitral stenosis using 2D and 3D echo-Doppler imaging. *JACC Cardiovasc Imaging*. 2013;6(11):1191-1205. doi:10.1016/j.jcmg.2013.07.008
30. Elmaghawry LM, El-Dosouky II, Kandil NT, Sayyid-Ahmad AMS. Pulmonary vascular resistance and proper timing of percutaneous balloon mitral valvotomy. *Int J Cardiovasc Imaging*. 2018;34(4):523-529. doi:10.1007/s10554-017-1255-3
31. Wunderlich NC, Dalvi B, Ho SY, Küx H, Siegel RJ. Rheumatic mitral valve stenosis: diagnosis and treatment options. *Curr Cardiol Rep*. 2019;21(3):14. doi:10.1007/s11886-019-1099-7
32. Kulkarni SS, Sakaria AK, Mahajan SK, Shah KB. Lutembacher's syndrome. *J Cardiovasc Dis Res*. 2012;3(2):179-181. doi:10.4103/0975-3583.95381
33. Litwin SE, Borlaug BA, Komtebedde J, Shah SJ. Update on atrial shunt therapy for treatment of heart failure. *Struct Heart*. 2022;6:100090. doi:10.1016/j.shj.2022.100090
34. Hibbert B, Zahr F, Simard T, et al, ALT FLOW Investigators. Left atrial to coronary sinus shunting for treatment of symptomatic heart failure. *JACC Cardiovasc Interv*. 2023;16(11):1369-1380. doi:10.1016/j.jcin.2023.03.012
35. Galusko V, Ionescu A, Edwards A, et al. Management of mitral stenosis: a systematic review of clinical practice guidelines and recommendations. *Eur Heart J Qual Care Clin Outcomes*. 2022;8(6):602-618. doi:10.1093/ehjqcco/qcab083
36. Song JK, Song JM, Kang DH, et al. Restenosis and adverse clinical events after successful percutaneous mitral valvuloplasty: immediate post-procedural mitral valve area as an important prognosticator. *Eur Heart J*. 2009;30(10):1254-1262. doi:10.1093/eurheartj/ehp096
37. Sharma KH, Jain S, Shukla A, et al. Patient profile and results of percutaneous transvenous mitral commissurotomy in mitral restenosis following prior percutaneous transvenous mitral commissurotomy vs surgical commissurotomy. *Indian Heart J*. 2014;66(2):164-168. doi:10.1016/j.ihj.2013.12.007
38. Ralph AP, Noonan S, Wade V, Currie BJ. The 2020 Australian guideline for prevention, diagnosis and management of acute rheumatic fever and rheumatic heart disease. *Med J Aust*. 2021;214(5):220-227. doi:10.5694/mja2.50851
39. Vahanian A, Beyersdorf F, Praz F, et al, ESC/EACTS Scientific Document Group. 2021 ESC/EACTS guidelines for the management of valvular heart disease: developed by the task force for the management of valvular heart disease of the European Society of Cardiology (ESC) and the European Association for Cardio-Thoracic Surgery (EACTS). *Rev Esp Cardiol*. 2022;75(6):524. doi:10.1016/j.rec.2022.05.006
40. Izumi C, Eishi K, Ashihara K, et al, Japanese Circulation Society Joint Working Group. JCS/JSCS/JATS/JSVS 2020 guidelines on the management of valvular heart disease. *Circ J*. 2020;84(11):2037-2119. doi:10.1253/circj.CJ-20-0135
41. Lindley KJ, Bairey Merz CN, Asgar AW, et al, American College of Cardiology Cardiovascular Disease in Women Committee and the Cardio-Obstetrics Work Group. Management of women with congenital or inherited cardiovascular disease from pre-conception through pregnancy and postpartum: JACC focus seminar 2/5. *J Am Coll Cardiol*. 2021;77(14):1778-1798. doi:10.1016/j.jacc.2021.02.026
42. van Hagen IM, Thorne SA, Taha N, et al, ROPAC Investigators and EORP Team. Pregnancy outcomes in women with rheumatic mitral valve disease: results from the registry of pregnancy and cardiac disease. *Circulation*. 2018;137(8):806-816. doi:10.1161/circulationaha.117.032561
43. Siu SC, Colman JM, Sorensen S, et al. Adverse neonatal and cardiac outcomes are more common in pregnant women with cardiac disease. *Circulation*. 2002;105(18):2179-2184. doi:10.1161/01.cir.0000015699.48605.08
44. de Souza JA, Martinez EE Jr, Ambrose JA, et al. Percutaneous balloon mitral valvuloplasty in comparison with open mitral valve commissurotomy for mitral stenosis during pregnancy. *J Am Coll Cardiol*. 2001;37(3):900-903. doi:10.1016/s0735-1097(00)01184-0
45. Nkomo VT, Gardin JM, Skelton TN, Gottdiener JS, Scott CG, Enriquez-Sarano M. Burden of valvular heart diseases: a population-based study. *Lancet*. 2006;368(9540):1005-1011. doi:10.1016/S0140-6736(06)69208-8
46. Zoghbi WA, Levine RA, Flachskampf F, et al. Atrial functional mitral regurgitation: a JACC – cardiovascular imaging expert panel viewpoint. *JACC Cardiovasc Imaging*. 2022;15(11):1870-1882. doi:10.1016/j.jcmg.2022.08.016
47. Carpentier A. Cardiac-valve surgery - the French correction. *J Thorac Cardiovasc Surg*. 1983;86(3):323-337.
48. Feldman T, Kar S, Rinaldi M, et al, EVEREST Investigators. Percutaneous mitral repair with the MitraClip system: safety and midterm durability in the initial EVEREST (Endovascular Valve Edge-to-Edge REpair Study) cohort. *J Am Coll Cardiol*. 2009;54(8):686-694. doi:10.1016/j.jacc.2009.03.077
49. Adminstration USFD. *Approval of MitraClip in Degenerative MR*; 2013. https://www.accessdata.fda.gov/scripts/cdrh/cfdocs/cfpma/pma.cfm?ID=P100009
50. Piriou N, Al Habash O, Donal E, et al. The MITRA-HR study: design and rationale of a randomised study of MitraClip transcatheter mitral valve repair in patients with severe primary mitral regurgitation eligible for high-risk surgery. *EuroIntervention*. 2019;15(4):e329-e335. doi:10.4244/EIJ-D-18-01086
51. McCarthy PM, Whisenant B, Asgar AW, et al. Percutaneous MitraClip device or surgical mitral valve repair in patients with primary mitral

regurgitation who are candidates for surgery: design and rationale of the REPAIR MR trial. *J Am Heart Assoc*. 2023;12(4):e027504. doi:10.1161/JAHA.122.027504

52. ClinicalTrials.Gov. *Percutaneous or Surgical Mitral Valve Repair (PRIMARY)*; 2021. https://classic.clinicaltrials.gov/ct2/show/NCT05051033
53. Lim DS, Kar S, Spargias K, et al. Transcatheter valve repair for patients with mitral regurgitation 30-day results of the CLASP study. *JACC Cardiovasc Interv*. 2019;12(14):1369-1378. doi:10.1016/j.jcin.2019.04.034
54. Webb JG, Hensey M, Szerlip M, et al. 1-Year outcomes for transcatheter repair in patients with mitral regurgitation from the CLASP study. *JACC Cardiovasc Interv*. 2020;13(20):2344-2357. doi:10.1016/j.jcin.2020.06.019
55. Szerlip M, Spargias KS, Makkar R, et al. 2-Year outcomes for transcatheter repair in patients with mitral regurgitation from the CLASP study (vol 14, pg 1538, 2021). *JACC Cardiovasc Interv*. 2022;15:1395. doi: 10.1016/j.jcin.2022.05.024
56. Lim DS, Smith RL, Zahr F, et al, CLASP IID Pivotal Trial Investigators. Early outcomes from the CLASP IID trial roll-in cohort for prohibitive risk patients with degenerative mitral regurgitation. *Catheter Cardiovasc Interv*. 2021;98(4):E637-E646. doi:10.1002/ccd.29749
57. Administration USFaD. *PASCAL Precision Transcatheter Valve Repair System*; 2022. https://www.fda.gov/medical-devices/recently-approved-devices/pascal-precision-transcatheter-valve-repair-system
58. Obadia JF, Messika-Zeitoun D, Leurent G, et al, MITRA-FR Investigators. Percutaneous repair or medical treatment for secondary mitral regurgitation. *N Engl J Med*. 2018;379(24):2297-2306. doi:10.1056/NEJMoa1805374
59. Grayburn PA, Sannino A, Packer M. Proportionate and disproportionate functional mitral regurgitation A new conceptual framework that reconciles the results of the MITRA-FR and COAPT trials. *JACC Cardiovasc Interv*. 2019;12(2):353-362. doi:10.1016/j.jcmg.2018.11.006
60. Pibarot P, Delgado V, Bax JJ. MITRA-FR vs. COAPT: lessons from two trials with diametrically opposed results. *Eur Heart J Cardiovasc Imaging*. 2019;20(6):620-624. doi:10.1093/ehjci/jez073
61. Nishimura RA, Bonow RO. Percutaneous repair of secondary mitral regurgitation - a tale of two trials. *N Engl J Med*. 2018;379(24):2374-2376. doi:10.1056/NEJMe1812279
62. Adminstration USFD. *FDA Approves New Indication for Valve Repair Device to Treat Certain Heart Failure Patients with Mitral Regurgitation*; 2019. https://www.fda.gov/news-events/press-announcements/fda-approves-new-indication-valve-repair-device-treat-certain-heart-failure-patients-mitral
63. Simard T, Reddy YNV, Thaden JJ, et al. Atrial mitral regurgitation: characteristics and outcomes of transcatheter mitral valve edge-to-edge repair. *Catheter Cardiovasc Interv*. 2022;100(1):133-142. doi:10.1002/ccd.30224
64. Doldi P, Stolz L, Orban M, et al. Transcatheter mitral valve repair in patients with atrial functional mitral regurgitation. *JACC Cardiovasc Imaging*. 2022;15(11):1843-1851. doi:10.1016/j.jcmg.2022.05.009
65. Yoon SH, Makar M, Kar S, et al. Outcomes after transcatheter edge-to-edge mitral valve repair according to mitral regurgitation etiology and cardiac remodeling. *JACC Cardiovasc Interv*. 2022;15(17):1711-1722. doi:10.1016/j.jcin.2022.07.004
66. Sodhi N, Asch FM, Ruf T, et al. Clinical outcomes with transcatheter edge-to-edge repair in atrial functional MR from the EXPAND study. *JACC Cardiovasc Interv*. 2022;15(17):1723-1730. doi:10.1016/j.jcin.2022.07.023
67. Tanaka T, Sugiura A, Ozturk C, et al. Transcatheter edge-to-edge repair for atrial secondary mitral regurgitation. *JACC Cardiovasc Interv*. 2022;15(17):1731-1740. doi:10.1016/j.jcin.2022.06.005
68. Popolo Rubbio A, Testa L, Grasso C, et al. Transcatheter edge-to-edge mitral valve repair in atrial functional mitral regurgitation: insights from the multi-center MITRA-TUNE registry. *Int J Cardiol*. 2022;349:39-45. doi:10.1016/j.ijcard.2021.11.027
69. Benito-Gonzalez T, Carrasco-Chinchilla F, Estevez-Loureiro R, et al. Clinical and echocardiographic outcomes of transcatheter mitral valve repair in atrial functional mitral regurgitation. *Int J Cardiol*. 2021;345:29-35. doi:10.1016/j.ijcard.2021.09.056
70. Jung RG, Simard T, Di Santo P, Hibbert B. Transcatheter edge-to-edge repair in patients with mitral regurgitation and cardiogenic shock: a new therapeutic target. *Curr Opin Crit Care*. 2022;28(4):426-433. doi:10.1097/MCC.0000000000000952
71. Thompson CR, Buller CE, Sleeper LA, et al. Cardiogenic shock due to acute severe mitral regurgitation complicating acute myocardial infarction: a report from the SHOCK Trial Registry. SHould we use emergently revascularize Occluded Coronaries in cardiogenic shocK? *J Am Coll Cardiol*. 2000;36(3 suppl A):1104-1109. doi:10.1016/s0735-1097(00)00846-9
72. Jung RG, Simard T, Kovach C, et al. Transcatheter mitral valve repair in cardiogenic shock and mitral regurgitation A patient-level, multicenter analysis. *JACC Cardiovasc Interv*. 2021;14:1-11. doi:10.1016/j.jcin.2020.08.037
73. Simard T, Vemulapalli S, Jung RG, et al. Transcatheter edge-to-edge mitral valve repair in patients with severe mitral regurgitation and cardiogenic shock. *J Am Coll Cardiol*. 2022;80(22):2072-2084. doi:10.1016/j.jacc.2022.09.006
74. Parlow S, Di Santo P, Jung RG, et al. Transcatheter mitral valve repair for inotrope dependent cardiogenic shock - design and rationale of the CAPITAL MINOS trial. *Am Heart J*. 2022;254:81-87. doi:10.1016/j.ahj.2022.08.008
75. St Goar FG, Fann JI, Komtebedde J, et al. Endovascular edge-to-edge mitral valve repair: short-term results in a porcine model. *Circulation*. 2003;108(16):1990-1993. doi:10.1161/01.CIR.0000096052.78331.CA
76. Mackensen GB, Reisman M. Edge-to-Edge repair of the mitral valve with the Mitraclip system: evolution of leaflet grasping technology. *Struct Heart*. 2019;3:341-347. doi:10.1080/24748706.2019.1627015
77. Praz F, Braun D, Unterhuber M, et al. Edge-to-edge mitral valve repair with extended clip arms early experience from a multicenter observational study. *JACC Cardiovasc Interv*. 2019;12(14):1356-1365. doi:10.1016/j.jcin.2019.03.023
78. Kar S, von Bardeleben RS, Rottbauer W, et al. Contemporary outcomes following transcatheter edge-to-edge repair: 1-year results from the EXPAND study. *JACC Cardiovasc Interv*. 2023;16(5):589-602. doi:10.1016/j.jcin.2023.01.010
79. Chakravarty T, Makar M, Patel D, et al. Transcatheter edge-to-edge mitral valve repair with the MitraClip G4 system. *JACC Cardiovasc Interv*. 2020;13(20):2402-2414. doi:10.1016/j.jcin.2020.06.053
80. Praz F, Spargias K, Chrissoheris M, et al. Compassionate use of the PASCAL transcatheter mitral valve repair system for patients with severe mitral regurgitation: a multicentre, prospective, observational, first-in-man study. *Lancet*. 2017;390(10096):773-780. doi:10.1016/S0140-6736(17)31600-8
81. Praz F, Windecker S, Kapadia S. PASCAL: a new addition to the armamentarium of transcatheter repair systems for mitral leaflet approximation. *JACC Cardiovasc Interv*. 2019;12(14):1379-1381. doi:10.1016/j.jcin.2019.05.006
82. Bushari LI, Reeder GS, Eleid MF, et al. Percutaneous transcatheter edge-to-edge MitraClip technique: a practical "Step-by-Step" 3-dimensional transesophageal echocardiography guide. *Mayo Clin Proc*. 2019;94(1):89-102. doi:10.1016/j.mayocp.2018.10.007
83. Fan YT, Chan JSK, Lee APW. Advances in procedural echocardiographic imaging in transcatheter edge-to-edge repair for mitral regurgitation. *Front Cardiovasc Med*. 2022;9:864341. doi:10.3389/fcvm.2022.864341.
84. Lim DS, Herrmann HC, Grayburn P, et al. Consensus document on non-suitability for transcatheter mitral valve repair by edge-to-edge therapy. *Struct Heart*. 2021;5:227-233. doi:10.1080/24748706.2021.1902595
85. Surder D, Pedrazzini G, Gaemperli O, et al. Predictors for efficacy of percutaneous mitral valve repair using the MitraClip system: the results of the MitraSwiss registry. *Heart*. 2013;99(14):1034-1040. doi:10.1136/heartjnl-2012-303105
86. Sugiura A, Kavsur R, Spieker M, et al. Recurrent mitral regurgitation after MitraClip: predictive factors, morphology, and clinical implication. *Circ Cardiovasc Interv*. 2022;15(3):e010895. doi:10.1161/CIRCINTERVENTIONS.121.010895.
87. Alkhouli M, Simard T, El Shaer A, et al. First experience with a novel live 3D ICE catheter to guide transcatheter structural heart interventions. *JACC Cardiovasc Interv*. 2022;15(8):1502-1509. doi:10.1016/j.jcmg.2021.09.015
88. Worthley S, Redwood S, Hildick-Smith D, et al. Transcatheter reshaping of the mitral annulus in patients with functional mitral

regurgitation: one-year outcomes of the MAVERIC trial. *EuroIntervention*. 2021;16(13):1106-1113. doi:10.4244/EIJ-D-20-00484
89. Rogers JH, Boyd WD, Smith TWR, Ebner AA, Grube E, Bolling SF. Transcatheter annuloplasty for mitral regurgitation with an adjustable semi-rigid complete ring: initial experience with the millipede IRIS device. *Struct Heart*. 2018;2:43-50. doi:10.1080/24748706.2017.1385879
90. Witte KK, Lipiecki J, Siminiak T, et al. The REDUCE FMR trial A randomized Sham-controlled study of percutaneous mitral annuloplasty in functional mitral regurgitation. *JACC Heart Fail*. 2019;7(11):945-955. doi:10.1016/j.jchf.2019.06.011
91. Colli A, Manzan E, Zucchetta F, et al. Transapical off-pump mitral valve repair with Neochord implantation: early clinical results. *Int J Cardiol*. 2016;204:23-28. doi:10.1016/j.ijcard.2015.11.131
92. Colli A, Adams D, Fiocco A, et al. Transapical NeoChord mitral valve repair. *Ann Cardiothorac Sur*. 2018;7(6):812-820. doi:10.21037/acs.2018.11.04
93. Wrobel K, Kurnicka K, Zygier M, et al. Transapical off-pump mitral valve repair. First experience with the NeoChord system in Poland (report of two cases). *Kardiol Pol*. 2017;75(1):7-12. doi:10.5603/KP.a2016.0149
94. Seeburger J, Rinaldi M, Nielsen SL, et al. Off-pump transapical implantation of artificial neo-chordae to correct mitral regurgitation: the TACT Trial (Transapical Artificial Chordae Tendinae) proof of concept. *J Am Coll Cardiol*. 2014;63(9):914-919. doi:10.1016/j.jacc.2013.07.090
95. Gammie JS, Wilson P, Bartus K, et al. Transapical beating-heart mitral valve repair with an expanded polytetrafluoroethylene cordal implantation device initial clinical experience. *Circulation*. 2016;134(3):189-197. doi:10.1161/Circulationaha.116.022010
96. Sorajja P, Bapat V. Early experience with the Intrepid system for transcatheter mitral valve replacement. *Ann Cardiothorac Surg*. 2018;7(6):792-798. doi:10.21037/acs.2018.10.03.
97. Guerrero M, Pursnani A, Narang A, et al. Prospective evaluation of transseptal TMVR for failed surgical bioprostheses: MITRAL trial valve-in-valve arm 1-year outcomes. *JACC Cardiovasc Interv*. 2021;14(8):859-872. doi:10.1016/j.jcin.2021.02.027
98. Silverman ME, Hurst JW. The mitral complex. Interaction of the anatomy, physiology, and pathology of the mitral annulus, mitral valve leaflets, chordae tendineae, and papillary muscles. *Am Heart J*. 1968;76(3):399-418. doi:10.1016/0002-8703(68)90237-8
99. Regueiro A, Granada JF, Dagenais F, Rodes-Cabau J. Transcatheter mitral valve replacement insights from early clinical experience and future challenges. *J Am Coll Cardiol*. 2017;69(17):2175-2192. doi:10.1016/j.jacc.2017.02.045
100. Guerrero M, Dvir D, Himbert D, et al. Transcatheter mitral valve replacement in native mitral valve disease with severe mitral annular calcification: results from the first multicenter global registry. *JACC Cardiovasc Interv*. 2016;9(13):1361-1371. doi:10.1016/j.jcin.2016.04.022
101. Guerrero M, Wang DD, Eleid MF, et al. Prospective study of TMVR using balloon-expandable aortic transcatheter valves in MAC: MITRAL trial 1-year outcomes. *JACC Cardiovasc Interv*. 2021;14(8):830-845. doi:10.1016/j.jcin.2021.01.052
102. Guerrero M, Wang DD, Pursnani A, et al. Prospective evaluation of TMVR for failed surgical annuloplasty rings: MITRAL trial valve-in-ring arm 1-year outcomes. *JACC Cardiovasc Interv*. 2021;14(8):846-858. doi:10.1016/j.jcin.2021.01.051
103. Muller DWM, Farivar RS, Jansz P, et al, Tendyne Global Feasibility Trial Investigators. Transcatheter mitral valve replacement for patients with symptomatic mitral regurgitation: a global feasibility trial. *J Am Coll Cardiol*. 2017;69(4):381-391. doi:10.1016/j.jacc.2016.10.068
104. Adminstration USFaD. *Abbott Earns CE Mark for Mitral Regurgitation Therapy*; 2020. https://www.fdanews.com/articles/195689-abbott-earns-ce-mark-for-mitral-regurgitation-therapy#:~:text=Abbott%20Earns%20CE%20Mark%20for%20Mitral%20Regurgitation%20Therapy,%28TMVI%29%20system%2C%20a%20treatment%20for%20significant%20mitral%20regurgitation
105. Lutter G, Lozonschi L, Ebner A, et al. First-in-human off-pump transcatheter mitral valve replacement. *JACC Cardiovasc Interv*. 2014;7(9):1077-1078. doi:10.1016/j.jcin.2014.06.007
106. Niikura H, Gossl M, Sorajja P. Transcatheter mitral valve replacement with Tendyne. *Interv Cardiol Clin*. 2019;8(3):295-300. doi:10.1016/j.iccl.2019.02.003
107. Sorajja P, Moat N, Badhwar V, et al. Initial feasibility study of a new transcatheter mitral prosthesis the first 100 patients. *J Am Coll Cardiol*. 2019;73(11):1250-1260. doi:10.1016/j.jacc.2018.12.066
108. Feasibility Study of the Tendyne Mitral Valve System for Use in Subjects With Mitral Annular Calcification. Last Accessed 10-20-18https://clinicaltrials.gov/ct2/show/NCT03539458.)
109. Muller DWM, Sorajja P, Duncan A, et al. 2-Year outcomes of transcatheter mitral valve replacement in patients with severe symptomatic mitral regurgitation. *J Am Coll Cardiol*. 2021;78(19):1847-1859. doi:10.1016/j.jacc.2021.08.060
110. Sorajja P, Gossl M, Babaliaros V, et al. Novel transcatheter mitral valve prosthesis for patients with severe mitral annular calcification. *J Am Coll Cardiol*. 2019;74(11):1431-1440. doi:10.1016/j.jacc.2019.07.069
111. Gossl M, Thourani V, Babaliaros V, et al. Early outcomes of transcatheter mitral valve replacement with the Tendyne system in severe mitral annular calcification. *EuroIntervention*. 2022;17(18):1523-1531. doi:10.4244/EIJ-D-21-00745
112. Bapat V, Rajagopal V, Meduri C, et al, Intrepid Global Pilot Study Investigators. Early experience with new transcatheter mitral valve replacement. *J Am Coll Cardiol*. 2018;71(1):12-21. doi:10.1016/j.jacc.2017.10.061
113. Zahr F, Song HK, Chadderdon SM, et al. 30-Day outcomes following transfemoral transseptal transcatheter mitral valve replacement: Intrepid TMVR early feasibility study results. *JACC Cardiovasc Interv*. 2022;15(1):80-89. doi:10.1016/j.jcin.2021.10.018
114. Webb JG, Murdoch DJ, Boone RH, et al. Percutaneous transcatheter mitral valve replacement: first-in-human experience with a new transseptal system. *J Am Coll Cardiol*. 2019;73(11):1239-1246. doi:10.1016/j.jacc.2018.12.065
115. Alkhouli M, Alqahtani F, Simard T, Pislaru S, Schaff HV, Nishimura RA. Predictors of use and outcomes of mechanical valve replacement in the United States (2008-2017). *J Am Heart Assoc*. 2021;10(9):e019929. doi:10.1161/jaha.120.019929
116. Goldstone AB, Chiu P, Baiocchi M, et al. Mechanical or biologic prostheses for aortic-valve and mitral-valve replacement. *N Engl J Med*. 2017;377(19):1847-1857. doi:10.1056/NEJMoa1613792
117. Vohra HA, Whistance RN, Roubelakis A, et al. Outcome after redo-mitral valve replacement in adult patients: a 10-year single-centre experience. *Interact Cardiovasc Thorac Surg*. 2012;14(5):575-579. doi:10.1093/icvts/ivs005
118. Whisenant B, Kapadia SR, Eleid MF, et al. One-year outcomes of mitral valve-in-valve using the SAPIEN 3 transcatheter heart valve. *JAMA Cardiol*. 2020;5(11):1245-1252. doi:10.1001/jamacardio.2020.2974
119. Simonato M, Whisenant B, Ribeiro HB, et al. Transcatheter mitral valve replacement after surgical repair or replacement: comprehensive midterm evaluation of valve-in-valve and valve-in-ring implantation from the VIVID registry. *Circulation*. 2021;143(2):104-116. doi:10.1161/CIRCULATIONAHA.120.049088
120. Guerrero M, Vemulapalli S, Xiang Q, et al. Thirty-day outcomes of transcatheter mitral valve replacement for degenerated mitral bioprostheses (valve-in-valve), failed surgical rings (valve-in-ring), and native valve with severe mitral annular calcification (Valve-in-Mitral annular calcification) in the United States: data from the Society of Thoracic Surgeons/American College of Cardiology/Transcatheter Valve Therapy Registry. *Circ Cardiovasc Interv*. 2020;13(3):e008425. doi:10.1161/CIRCINTERVENTIONS.119.008425
121. Guerrero MEM, Eleid MF, Wang DD, et al. 5-Year prospective evaluation of mitral valve-in-valve, valve-in-ring and valve-in-MAC outcomes: mitral trial final results (in press). *JACC Cardiovasc Interv*. 2023.16(18), 2211-2227.
122. Malaisre CS, Guerrero M, Davidson C, Williams M, Sandoli de Brito F, Abizaid A, et al. One-year outcomes of transseptal mitral valve-in-valve in intermediate surgical risk patients. (in press). *Circ Cardiovasc Interv*. 2024.
123. Badhwar V, Rankin JS, He X, et al. The Society of Thoracic Surgeons mitral repair/replacement composite score: a report of the Society of Thoracic Surgeons quality measurement task force. *Ann Thorac Surg*. 2016;101(6):2265-2271. doi:10.1016/j.athoracsur.2015.11.049
124. Mehaffey HJ, Hawkins RB, Schubert S, et al. Contemporary outcomes in reoperative mitral valve surgery. *Heart*. 2018;104(8):652-656. doi:10.1136/heartjnl-2017-312047

125. Okada Y, Shomura T, Yamaura Y, Yoshikawa J. Comparison of the Carpentier and Duran prosthetic rings used in mitral reconstruction. *Ann Thorac Surg*. 1995;59(3):658-663. discussion 662-653. doi:10.1016/0003-4975(94)01008-0
126. Kato N, Guerrero M, Padang R, et al. Prevalence and natural history of mitral annulus calcification and related valve dysfunction. *Mayo Clin Proc*. 2022;97(6):1094-1107. doi:10.1016/j.mayocp.2021.12.015
127. Eleid MF, Foley TA, Said SM, Pislaru SV, Rihal CS. Severe mitral annular calcification: multimodality imaging for therapeutic strategies and interventions. *JACC Cardiovasc Imaging*. 2016;9(11):1318-1337. doi:10.1016/j.jcmg.2016.09.001
128. Guerrero M, Wang DD, Pursnani A, et al. A cardiac computed tomography-based score to categorize mitral annular calcification severity and predict valve embolization. *JACC Cardiovasc Imaging*. 2020;13(9):1945-1957. doi:10.1016/j.jcmg.2020.03.013
129. Guerrero M, Salinger M, Pursnani A, et al. Transseptal transcatheter mitral valve-in-valve: a step by step guide from preprocedural planning to postprocedural care. *Catheter Cardiovasc Interv*. 2018;92(3):E185-E196. doi:10.1002/ccd.27128
130. Eleid MF, Collins JD, Mahoney P, et al. Emerging approaches to management of left ventricular outflow obstruction risk in transcatheter mitral valve replacement. *JACC Cardiovasc Interv*. 2023;16(8):885-895. doi:10.1016/j.jcin.2023.01.357
131. Wang DD, Eng MH, Greenbaum AB, et al. Validating a prediction modeling tool for left ventricular outflow tract (LVOT) obstruction after transcatheter mitral valve replacement (TMVR). *Catheter Cardiovasc Interv*. 2018;92(2):379-387. doi:10.1002/ccd.27447
132. El Sabbagh A, Al-Hijji M, Wang DD, et al. Predictors of left ventricular outflow tract obstruction after transcatheter mitral valve replacement in severe mitral annular calcification: an analysis of the transcatheter mitral valve replacement in mitral annular calcification global registry. *Circ Cardiovasc Interv*. 2021;14(10):e010854. doi:10.1161/CIRCINTERVENTIONS.121.010854
133. Wang DD, Guerrero M, Eng MH, et al. Alcohol septal ablation to prevent left ventricular outflow tract obstruction during transcatheter mitral valve replacement: first-in-man study. *JACC Cardiovasc Interv*. 2019;12(13):1268-1279. doi:10.1016/j.jcin.2019.02.034
134. Guerrero ME, Killu AM, Gonzalez-Quesada C, et al. Pre-emptive radiofrequency septal ablation to decrease the risk of left ventricular outflow tract obstruction after TMVR. *JACC Cardiovasc Interv*. 2020;13(9):1129-1132. doi:10.1016/j.jcin.2020.02.016
135. Khan JM, Rogers T, Schenke WH, et al. Intentional laceration of the anterior mitral valve leaflet to prevent left ventricular outflow tract obstruction during transcatheter mitral valve replacement: pre-clinical findings. *JACC Cardiovasc Interv*. 2016;9(17):1835-1843. doi:10.1016/j.jcin.2016.06.020
136. Sigwart U. Non-surgical myocardial reduction for hypertrophic obstructive cardiomyopathy. *Lancet*. 1995;346(8969):211-214. doi:10.1016/s0140-6736(95)91267-3
137. El-Sabawi B, Nishimura RA, Barsness GW, Cha YM, Geske JB, Eleid MF. Temporal occurrence of arrhythmic complications after alcohol septal ablation. *Circ Cardiovasc Interv*. 2020;13(2):e008540. doi:10.1161/CIRCINTERVENTIONS.119.008540
138. Guerrero M, Wang DD, O'Neill W. Percutaneous alcohol septal ablation to acutely reduce left ventricular outflow tract obstruction induced by transcatheter mitral valve replacement. *Catheter Cardiovasc Interv*. 2016;88(6):E191-E197. doi:10.1002/ccd.26649
139. Guerrero M, Wang DD, Himbert D, et al. Short-term results of alcohol septal ablation as a bail-out strategy to treat severe left ventricular outflow tract obstruction after transcatheter mitral valve replacement in patients with severe mitral annular calcification. *Catheter Cardiovasc Interv*. 2017;90(7):1220-1226. doi:10.1002/ccd.26975
140. Elhadi M, Guerrero M, Collins JD, Rihal CS, Eleid MF. Safety and outcomes of alcohol septal ablation prior to transcatheter mitral valve replacement. *J Soc Cardiovasc Angiograph Interv*. 2022;1. doi:10.1016/j.jscai.2022.100396
141. Babaliaros VC, Greenbaum AB, Khan JM, et al. Intentional percutaneous laceration of the anterior mitral leaflet to prevent outflow obstruction during transcatheter mitral valve replacement: first-in-human experience. *JACC Cardiovasc Interv*. 2017;10(8):798-809. doi:10.1016/j.jcin.2017.01.035
142. Khan JM, Babaliaros VC, Greenbaum AB, et al. Anterior leaflet laceration to prevent ventricular outflow tract obstruction during transcatheter mitral valve replacement. *J Am Coll Cardiol*. 2019;73(20):2521-2534. doi:10.1016/j.jacc.2019.02.076
143. Lisko JC, Greenbaum AB, Khan JM, et al. Antegrade intentional laceration of the anterior mitral leaflet to prevent left ventricular outflow tract obstruction: a simplified technique from bench to bedside. *Circ Cardiovasc Interv*. 2020;13(6):e008903. doi:10.1161/CIRCINTERVENTIONS.119.008903
144. Killu AM, Collins JD, Eleid MF, et al. Preemptive septal radiofrequency ablation to prevent left ventricular outflow tract obstruction with transcatheter mitral valve replacement: a case series. *Circ Cardiovasc Interv*. 2022;15(10):e012228. doi:10.1161/CIRCINTERVENTIONS.122.012228
145. Greenbaum AB, Khan JM, Bruce CG, et al. Transcatheter myotomy to treat hypertrophic cardiomyopathy and enable transcatheter mitral valve replacement: first-in-human report of septal scoring along the midline Endocardium. *Circ Cardiovasc Interv*. 2022;15(6):e012106. doi:10.1161/CIRCINTERVENTIONS.122.012106
146. Mangieri A, Cannata F, Cozzi O, et al. A fully percutaneous transeptal transcatheter mitral valve replacement with a novel device. *JACC Cardiovasc Interv*. 2023;16(16):2050-2052. doi:10.1016/j.jcin.2023.04.040

42 Transcatheter Aortic Valve Replacement

Gregory J. Condos and Christine J. Chung

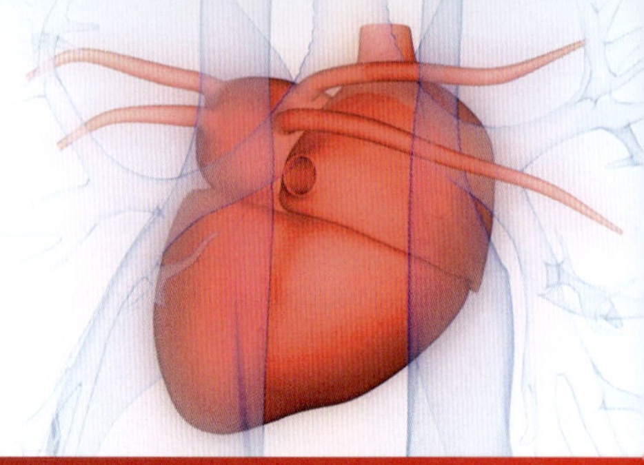

Age-related calcific aortic stenosis (AS) is the most common form of AS. Approximately 3% of patients over the age of 75 years have severe AS. The development of the cardinal symptoms of angina, syncope, or heart failure portends a dismal prognosis,[1] so treatment is recommended at the earliest onset of dyspnea or decline in functional status. Having been the only available intervention for decades, surgical aortic valve replacement (SAVR) remained the standard of care for many years after the advent of transcatheter aortic valve replacement (TAVR), first performed by Dr Alain Cribier in 2002.[2] However, with each iterative clinical trial demonstrating the efficacy and safety of TAVR compared to SAVR in progressively lower risk patient populations, American College of Cardiology (ACC)/American Heart Association (AHA) guidelines currently give a class 1A recommendation for either SAVR or TAVR for patients 65 to 80 years of age and recommend TAVR for those over 80 years. Younger patients with an age less than 65 years retain a class 1A recommendation for SAVR. TAVR volume now far surpasses SAVR volume for the treatment of isolated aortic valve stenosis, accounting for 88% of all such procedures in 2021.[3] Furthermore, the most rapid increase in application of TAVR has been in patients younger than 65 years, such that in 2021, nearly half of this younger cohort received TAVR.

Historically, many patients with severe symptomatic AS were not offered surgery due to advanced age and comorbidities. The widespread availability of TAVR should theoretically increase the proportion of patients receiving treatment. However, the explosive growth of TAVR has occurred concomitantly with significant growth in the aging population with severe symptomatic AS, such that the relative proportion of patients not receiving indicated treatment remains significant.[4] There are also gender, racial, and geographic disparities in access to this intervention. Ongoing efforts are needed to ensure appropriate diagnosis (particularly in low gradient subtypes), referral, and treatment of patients with this lethal but highly treatable disease.

This chapter discusses the pivotal clinical trials and other data supporting the widespread uptake of TAVR, reviews procedural details and potential complications, and addresses the remaining questions about its role alongside SAVR in the management of patients with AS.

CLINICAL DATA

There are two dominant transcatheter valve platforms on the US market – SAPIEN (Edwards Lifesciences, Irvine, CA) and Evolut (which developed from the CoreValve platform) (Medtronic, Minneapolis, MN) – accounting for the vast majority of TAVRs performed today (**Fig. 42.1**). There are many other platforms in various stages of development or more widely used in international markets (**Fig. 42.2**). The current generation SAPIEN 3 Ultra Resilia valve consists of a balloon-expandable (BE) cobalt chromium frame with bovine pericardial leaflets. It has a polyethylene terephthalate outer sealing skirt to reduce paravalvular leak (PVL). The current generation Evolut Pro+ valve has a self-expanding (SE) nitinol frame with porcine pericardial leaflets. It also has an external sealing skirt intended to reduce PVL. The BE SAPIEN valve is deployed in an intra-annular position, whereas the SE Evolut valve has a supra-annular design. The Evolut Pro+ is also recapturable and repositionable. Other notable SE valve platforms include the second-generation Navitor valve (Abbott, St Paul, MN, USA), which recently received Food and Drug Administration (FDA) approval for patients at high or extreme surgical risk, the Trilogy valve (JenaValve Technology, Irvine, CA, USA), which has completed enrollment in its pivotal trial of high-risk patients with aortic regurgitation (AR), and ACURATE neo2 (Boston Scientific, Marlborough, MA, USA), which has an ongoing pivotal trial including patients across all surgical risk levels. Boston Scientific's Lotus valve obtained FDA approval for patients deemed high risk for surgery in 2019 but was discontinued the following year after a voluntary recall of the product for issues with the delivery system. For the remainder of this chapter, the focus will be on the pivotal trials leading to approval of the SAPIEN and CoreValve platforms.

PARTNER TRIALS

In the United States, the landmark PARTNER trial led to FDA approval for TAVR in inoperable patients with severe AS.[5,6] There were two cohorts in this study: A and B. Cohort B consisted of 358 patients with severe symptomatic AS deemed inoperable by two cardiac surgeons, who were then randomized to TAVR or standard medical therapy. In the standard therapy arm, 83.8% of patients underwent balloon aortic valvuloplasty. The primary endpoint was superiority of TAVR in all-cause mortality. At 1 year, there was 50.7% all-cause mortality in those undergoing standard therapy as compared to 30.7% in patients treated with TAVR ($P < .001$). TAVR was associated with a higher rate of major strokes at 30 days (5.0% vs 1.1%, $P = .06$). However, due to the large mortality benefit, the FDA approved the use of the SAPIEN valve for inoperable patients with severe symptomatic AS in November 2011.

PARTNER cohort A examined the role of TAVR in patients with severe symptomatic AS deemed to have high but not prohibitive risk for surgery, with the Society of Thoracic Surgeons (STS) predicted risk of mortality (PROM) of at least 10%.[7] A total of 699 patients were randomized to TAVR, using either transfemoral (TF) or transapical (TA) access depending on the suitability of aortoiliac anatomy or SAVR. Of the 348 patients randomized to TAVR, 244 underwent TF-TAVR. The TA-TAVR patients had higher rates of peripheral vascular disease and prior coronary bypass surgery.

Unlike PARTNER B, the primary endpoint of PARTNER A was noninferiority in all-cause mortality. At 1 year, there were no significant differences in all-cause mortality between TAVR and SAVR, a finding maintained at 3 years. An increased risk of major stroke after TAVR persisted, with a rate of 5.1% in the TAVR group versus

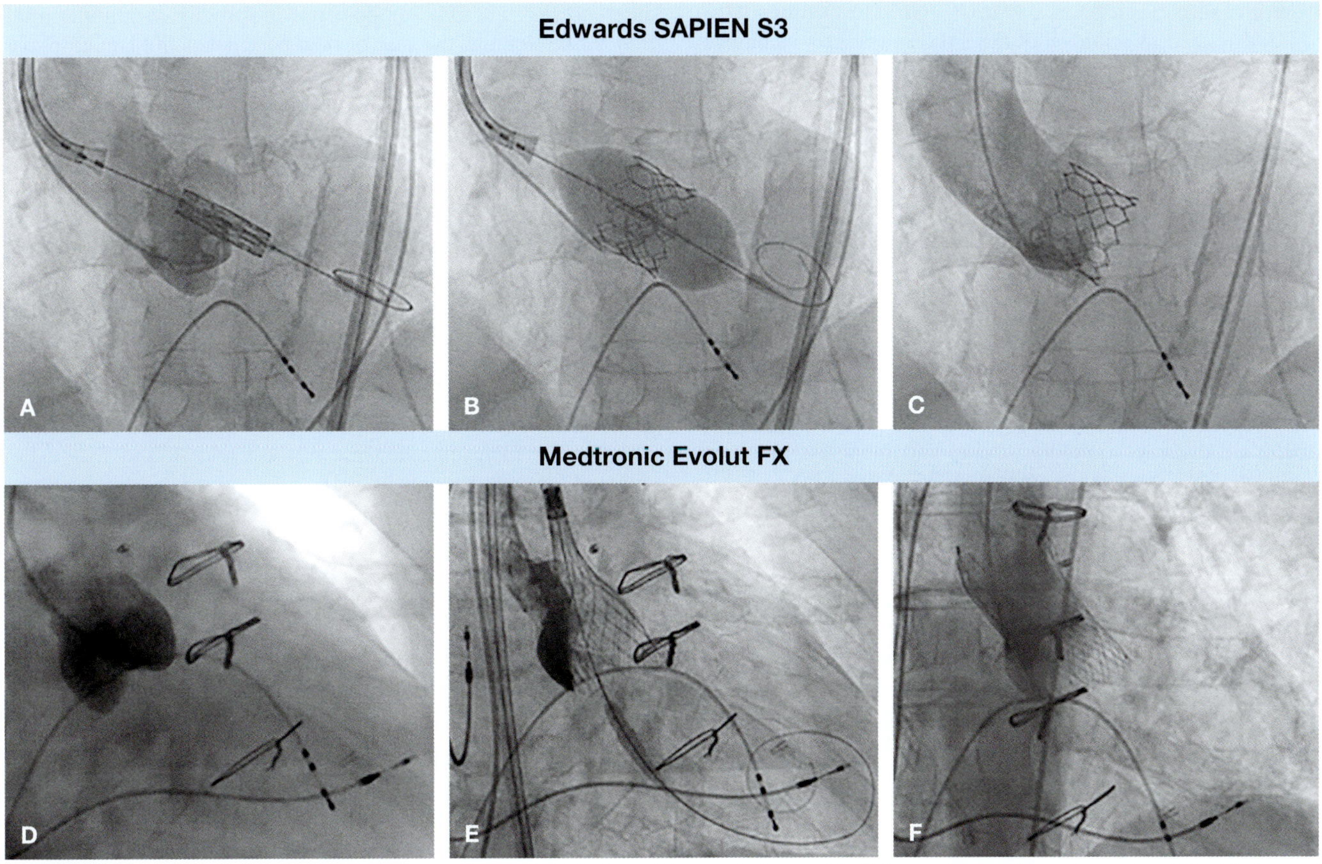

Edwards SAPIEN S3

A B C

Medtronic Evolut FX

D E F

FIGURE 42.1 Valve positioning and deployment for both SAPIEN and Evolut platforms. SAPIEN is positioned in coplanar view **(A)**, with the central marker dot typically located in the middle of the pigtail catheter positioned in the right coronary cusp **(B)**. Final angiography showing appropriate placement approximately 10% to 20% ventricular and no leak **(C)**. Evolut is positioned in the cusp overlap view **(D)** and is retrievable and repositionable up to the point of anchoring in the annulus **(E)**. Final angiography showing appropriate placement at 3 to 4 mm below the noncoronary cusp with no leak **(F)**.

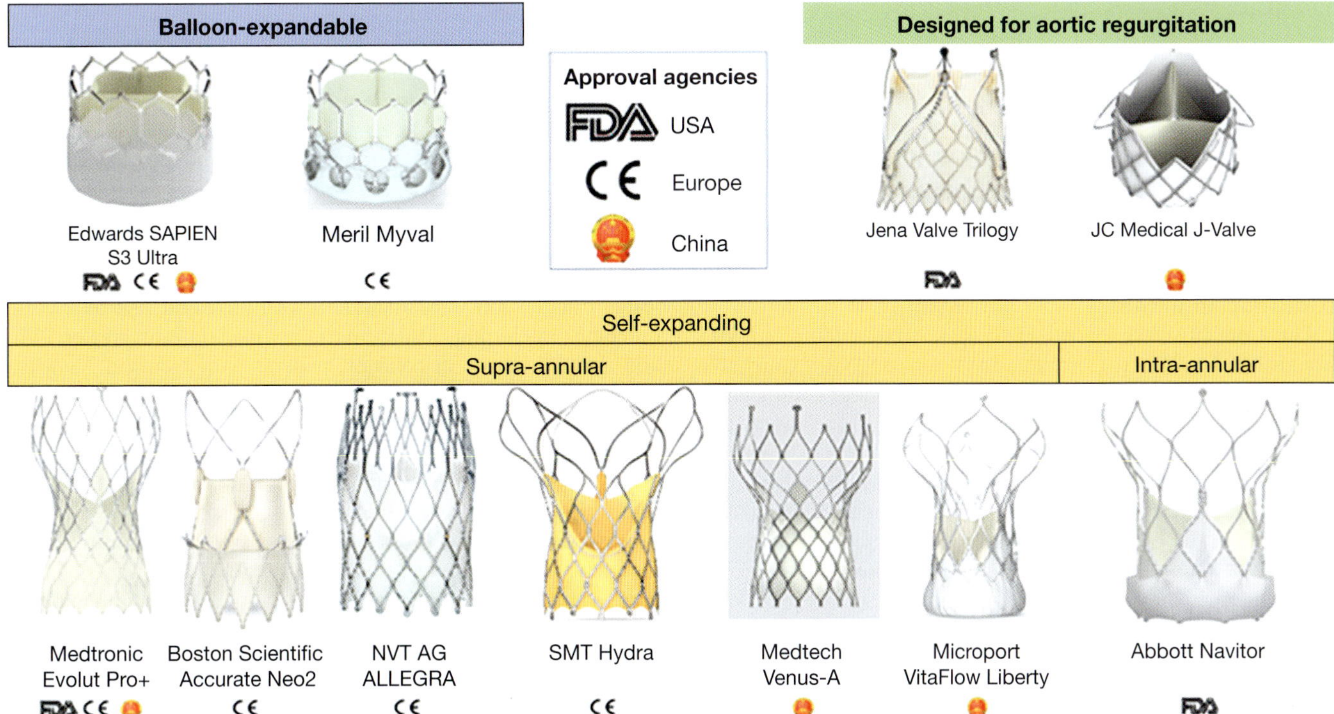

FIGURE 42.2 Overview of commercially available transcatheter aortic valve platforms and which regulatory agencies have approved their use.

2.4% in the surgical group at 1 year (*P* = .07). In October 2012, the FDA extended its approval of the SAPIEN valve to encompass high-risk patients with severe symptomatic AS.

The PARTNER 2A study randomized 2032 intermediate-risk patients (STS PROM 4%-8%) to TAVR with the second-generation SAPIEN XT valve or SAVR.[8] At 2 years, there were no significant differences in the primary endpoint of all-cause mortality or disabling stroke between the groups. Notably, there was no difference in rates of disabling stroke, which was 6.2% in the TAVR group and 6.4% in the SAVR group (*P* = .83).

PARTNER 2 S3i was a prospective registry of intermediate-risk patients undergoing TAVR with the third-generation SAPIEN 3 valve.[5] This cohort of 1032 patients was then compared to the surgical cohort in PARTNER 2A. A propensity-matched analysis showed that SAPIEN 3 TAVR was superior to SAVR for the primary endpoint of all-cause mortality, stroke, and moderate or severe AI (−9.2%, 95% confidence interval [95% CI] −13.0 to −5.4; *P* < .0001). Surgery resulted in superior outcomes compared to those of patients left with moderate or greater AR after TAVR, highlighting the importance of minimizing PVL. In August 2016, on the basis of the results from PARTNER 2A and PARTNER 2 S3i, the FDA approved the use of the SAPIEN XT and SAPIEN 3 valves for intermediate-risk patients with severe symptomatic AS.

Finally, the PARTNER 3 trial randomized 1000 patients at low operative risk, defined as an STS PROM less than 4%, to SAVR or TAVR. Notably, all patients were required to have adequate vascular access to accommodate TF placement of the SAPIEN 3 valve. The composite outcome of all-cause death, stroke, or rehospitalization at 1 year occurred less frequently in the TAVR group (8.5% vs 15.1%, 95% CI for difference, −10.8 to −2.5; *P* < .001 for noninferiority) with a hazard ratio (HR) of 0.54 (95% CI, 0.37-0.79; *P* = .001 for superiority).[6] On the basis of these results, the FDA extended its approval for the SAPIEN valve to encompass patients across the full spectrum of surgical risk.

CoreValve US Pivotal Trials

The approval process for the CoreValve device mirrored that for the SAPIEN valve. However, as the CoreValve entered the market 3 years later than SAPIEN, the CoreValve US Pivotal Extreme Risk Trial did not randomize patients to medical therapy.[9] Instead, it enrolled 489 patients who all underwent attempted TAVR with the CoreValve and met its primary endpoint with a 25.5% rate of death or major stroke at 1 year, which was 40.7% lower (*P* < .0001) than expected based on a performance goal developed in partnership with the FDA. On the basis of these results, in January 2014, the FDA approved the use of CoreValve for extreme-risk patients with severe symptomatic AS.

The CoreValve US Pivotal High Risk Trial randomized 795 patients in 1:1 fashion to CoreValve TAVR versus SAVR.[10] CoreValve TAVR was associated with a lower mortality at 1 year compared to SAVR (14.2% vs 19.1%, *P* = .04 for superiority) and a numerically lower stroke rate (8.8% vs 12.6%, *P* = .1). These benefits were sustained at 3 years. Need for a permanent pacemaker and significant paravalvular regurgitation occurred more frequently with TAVR. In June 2014, the FDA extended its approval of CoreValve for the treatment of high-risk patients with severe symptomatic AS.

The intermediate risk trial, SURTAVI, randomized 1746 patients to SAVR or TAVR with either CoreValve or the second-generation Evolut R.[11] Intermediate risk was defined as an STS PROM between 3% and 15%, and the primary endpoint was death or disabling stroke at 24 months. TAVR was noninferior to SAVR with regard to the primary endpoint (12.6% vs 14.0%, 95% credible interval for difference, −5.2% to 2.3%; posterior probability of noninferiority, *P* > .999). Notably, the rate of new pacemaker implantation was 25.9% in the TAVR group, compared to 6.6% in the SAVR group (95% credible interval for difference, 15.9%-22.7%).

The Evolut Low Risk trial randomized 1403 patients with an STS PROM less than 3% to TAVR, with either Evolut R or the third-generation Evolut Pro, or SAVR.[12] TAVR met the prespecified criteria for noninferiority, with the primary endpoint of all-cause mortality or disabling stroke occurring in 5.3% of patients undergoing TAVR and 6.7% of patients undergoing SAVR at 2 years (*P* < .05 for noninferiority, *P* > .05 for superiority). Rates of major bleeding and new-onset atrial fibrillation were higher in the SAVR group, whereas patients receiving TAVR had higher rates of new pacemaker implantation (17.4% vs 6.1%, *P* < .05) and moderate to severe PVL (3.5% vs 0.5%, *P* < .05). Results were sustained at 3 years. The FDA approved use of the Evolut R and Evolut Pro valves in low-risk patients in 2019.

Special Groups

The pivotal trials for SAPIEN and CoreValve excluded several key groups such as patients with bicuspid valves and severe AR. Patients with low flow, low gradient AS (LGAS) were variably included in the major randomized trials. As a result, there is limited evidence to guide clinical decision making for these subgroups.

Bicuspid Valves

Patients with bicuspid AS were excluded from all pivotal randomized trials, but observational data with early generation TAVR devices demonstrated higher rates of implantation failure, moderate or greater PVL, and pacemaker implantation compared to cases of TAVR in tricuspid AS. Subsequent experiences with later generation devices have been more successful, but several challenges remain. Adding further complexity to their management, these patients tend to present at a younger age and often have concomitant aortopathy that cannot be addressed with a transcatheter approach.

Bicuspid valves display wide variability in anatomy. The Sievers and Schmidtke classification, based on surgical pathology specimens, relies primarily on the number of raphe present and secondarily on the spatial position of fused raphe. However, since the native valve is not excised during TAVR, a more relevant classification scheme in the modern era would anticipate how TAVR devices may interact with various bicuspid morphologies[13] (**Fig. 42.3**). Using computed tomography (CT) analysis of 1034 patients with bicuspid AS, Yoon et al demonstrated that significant raphe and leaflet calcification were associated with increased risk of adverse outcomes, including 30-day mortality, moderate or greater PVL, and annular injury. In contrast, patients with bicuspid AS without calcified raphe and excess leaflet calcification had favorable outcomes.

The annulus tends to be larger in bicuspid valves, sometimes exceeding the treatment range of currently available TAVR prostheses. It is also more often elliptical and asymmetric, which can prove challenging for prosthesis sizing, as well as contribute to the increased occurrence of more than mild PVL. Oversizing may account for the slightly increased risk of pacemaker implantation seen in bicuspid AS patients (9.1% vs 7.5%; *P* = .03) compared to their propensity-matched tricuspid counterparts in the STS/ACC TVT registry.[14,15]

The PARTNER 3 bicuspid registry included low-risk patients ineligible for enrollment in the randomized trial based on the

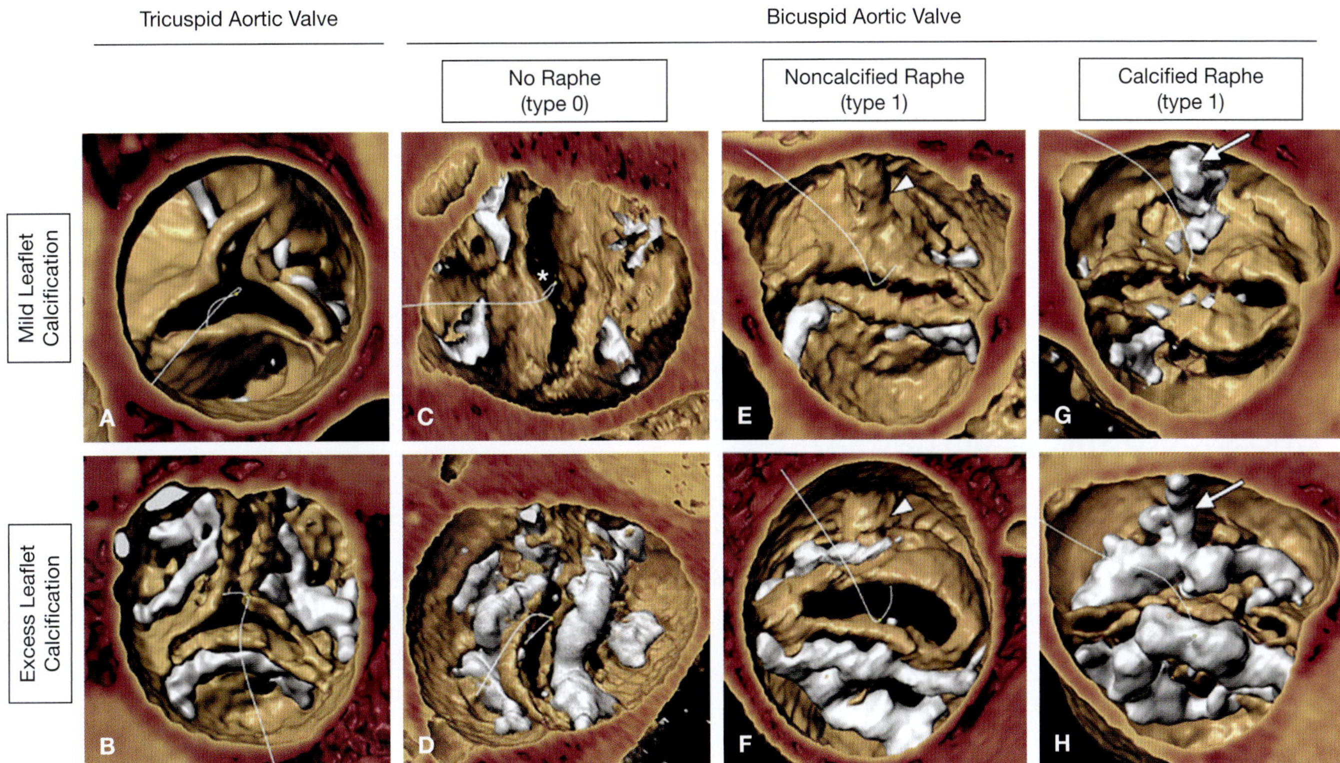

FIGURE 42.3 Various aortic valve morphology on volume-rendered computed tomography for tricuspid **(A and B)** and bicuspid aortic valve stenosis **(C-H)**. The characteristic "fish mouth" opening of the valve (asterisk) is appreciated in bicuspid aortic valve. Bicuspid aortic valve is categorized as no raphe type **(C and D)** and raphe type **(E-H)**. Raphe type is further categorized as noncalcified raphe type **(E and F)** and calcified raphe type **(G and H)**. *Arrowheads* indicate noncalcified raphe, and *arrows* indicate calcified raphe. (*Top*) Aortic valve with mild leaflet calcification; (*bottom*) aortic valves with excess leaflet calcification. (From Yoon SH, Kim WK, Dhoble A, et al. Bicuspid aortic valve morphology and outcomes after transcatheter aortic valve replacement. *J Am Coll Cardiol*. 2020;76(9):1018-1030.)

presence of bicuspid morphology.[16] Patients who met stringent anatomic criteria were included in the single-arm bicuspid valve registry or continued access protocol. There were no differences in key clinical outcomes after TAVR in these highly selected bicuspid patients compared to their propensity-matched counterparts with tricuspid AS. Notably, almost half the screened patients were excluded, predominantly due to significant raphe calcification. These findings suggest that with widespread use of multidetector CT imaging for preprocedural planning and iterative device improvements, carefully selected patients with bicuspid morphology can reasonably be considered for TAVR. Ongoing studies are needed to refine criteria for optimal patient selection. Based on the available data, patients with heavily calcified raphe or leaflets warrant careful consideration of the risk of annular injury, moderate or greater PVL, and pacemaker implant when weighing TAVR against SAVR for the initial treatment in the lifetime management of their valve disease.

Low Flow, Low Gradient AS

LGAS is a well-recognized variant of severe AS with discordant echocardiographic data. Patients have a small calculated valve area (less than 1 cm^2), with a low transvalvular gradient (mean gradient less than 40 mm Hg and peak velocity less than 4.0 m/s) due to decreased stroke volume (less than 35 mL/m^2). It can occur in the setting of depressed left ventricular (LV) systolic function (classical LGAS or ACC/AHA stage D2) or preserved ejection fraction (EF) (paradoxical LGAS or ACC/AHA stage D3). A low flow state is a strong predictor of increased mortality, with about a third of patients dying within 3 years after TAVR in a recent registry.[17] This finding was shown to be independent of LV EF or mean gradient across the aortic valve (above or below 40 mm Hg). However, procedural outcomes and magnitude of symptomatic improvement after TAVR were similar to those in patients with normal stroke volume. Additionally, in a study of nearly 11,000 patients with either a class I or class IIa indication for aortic valve replacement (AVR), the magnitude of mortality benefit for AVR compared to no AVR was consistent between patients with LGAS and classic high gradient AS.[4]

There are conflicting data on the utility of assessing contractile reserve with dobutamine stress echocardiography. While older surgical data support its use for predicting perioperative mortality, contemporary data have shown poor correlation between contractile reserve and outcomes after TAVR.[18] Rather, in cases of diagnostic ambiguity, a CT-derived calcium score greater than 1300 Hounsfield units (HU) in women and 2000 HU in men is highly predictive of mortality and can be used to corroborate severity of AS in the setting of discordant echocardiographic data.[19] Finally, calculation of the dimensionless index (DI), the ratio of the LV outflow tract velocity to the aortic valve velocity, has also been established as a method to confirm severity of AS in the absence of classic hemodynamic patterns. A value ≤0.25 is consistent with severe LGAS.

In summary, while patients with LGAS have poorer overall prognosis compared to those with normal stroke volume, they are expected to experience a comparable magnitude of benefit from AVR.

Aortic Regurgitation

A comprehensive discussion of the off-label use of commercially approved TAVR devices for the treatment of AR is beyond the scope of this chapter. Challenges include lack of adequate calcium for valve anchoring, large annular sizes often exceeding the recommended treatment ranges of commercially approved prostheses, and a higher prevalence of bicuspid morphology. The Trilogy Heart Valve System (JenaValve Technology, Inc, Irvine, CA) is a platform with a novel anchoring mechanism not reliant on the presence of annular calcium that completed enrollment in a pivotal trial of patients at high surgical risk with severe symptomatic AR (**Fig. 42.2**).

WHO SHOULD STILL BE GETTING SAVR?

The considerable data amassed over the past 2 decades have led to a paradigm shift in the approach to the patient with AS, particularly those who are younger and at lower surgical risk. Additionally, patients are increasingly presenting with a preference for TAVR over SAVR at the time of their initial evaluation. While the clinical decision making for an elderly patient is often more straightforward, there are many factors to consider in younger and healthier patients whose life expectancy is likely to extend beyond the lifespan of a single bioprosthetic valve.

SAVR and TAVR have different risk profiles. SAVR is associated with higher risks of postoperative atrial fibrillation and kidney injury, whereas TAVR is associated with higher risks of significant PVL and pacemaker implantation. The key factors framing the discussion in a younger patient include (1) valve durability; (2) feasibility of future valve-in-valve (ViV) procedures; (3) risk of future surgery. The following section will address each of these concerns.

Valve Durability

When TAVR was still a relatively new technology, there was concern that rates of structural valve degeneration (SVD) leading to bioprosthetic valve failure (BVF) may be higher than with surgical bioprosthetic valves. The earliest trials enrolled highly comorbid and sick patients with high mortality rates, limiting the ability to accrue long-term data. The intermediate risk trials (PARTNER 2 and SURTAVI) have reported follow-up at 5 years demonstrating similar mortality rates between SAVR and TAVR. Rehospitalization (33.3% vs 25.2%; HR, 1.28; 95% CI, 1.07-1.53) and repeat valve intervention (3.2% vs 0.8%; HR, 3.28; 95% CI, 1.32-8.13) were more common in patients receiving a BE valve than in those undergoing SAVR in PARTNER 2.[20] Outcomes of SURTAVI were similar at 5 years, with higher reintervention rates in the TAVR cohort (3.5% vs 1.9%; HR, 2.21; 95% CI, 1.10-4.45).[21]

The NOTION trial was the first randomized trial of low-risk patients comparing outcomes of SAVR and TAVR with a first-generation CoreValve prosthesis. At 8 years of follow-up, there was no significant difference in the composite outcome of death, stroke, or myocardial infarction.[22] Importantly, by the time this trial was conducted, the Valve Academic Research Consortium (VARC) had established standardized definitions of the causes of BVF including SVD, thrombosis, endocarditis, PVL, or patient-prosthesis mismatch (PPM).[23] SVD was defined by the presence of one of the following criteria: increase of mean gradient ≥10 mm Hg resulting in a mean gradient ≥20 mm Hg, decrease in aortic valve area (AVA) by ≥0.3 cm^2 or 20%, decrease in DI by ≥0.1 or 20%, or ≥moderate AR. BVF was defined as either severe SVD (increase of mean gradient ≥20 mm Hg resulting in a mean gradient ≥30 mm Hg, decrease in AVA by ≥0.6 cm^2 or 50%, decrease in DI by ≥0.2 or 40%, or severe AR), or SVD resulting in clinical heart failure, valve reintervention, or valve-related death.

In the NOTION trial, investigators found that the TAVR group had higher effective orifice area (EOA) and lower mean gradients at each yearly echocardiogram compared to their counterparts who underwent SAVR. While this correlated with lower rates of SVD (13.7% vs 28.6%, P = .0017), rates of BVF were similar between groups. In contrast, AVALON was a multicenter all-comers registry comparing low-risk patients undergoing elective and isolated SAVR and TAVR.[24] In a propensity score-matched analysis, there was no difference in mortality at 2 years, but SAVR was associated with a 30% reduction in mortality beyond 5 years. One explanation for these findings is selection bias, with healthier, more robust patients being selected for surgery. Additionally, different surgical bioprostheses have widely disparate rates of SVD. Mitroflow (Sorin Group Italia S.r.l., Saluggia, VC, IT) and Trifecta (Abbott Laboratories, Abbott Park, IL, USA) valves were used more frequently in NOTION than in AVALON and have both been associated with earlier SVD. Long-term follow-up from the randomized studies of low-risk patients will be necessary to address the critical question of whether the method of implantation, and consequent implications for valve construction, are key factors impacting their durability.

Indications for Other Procedures

Two common coexisting conditions in patients undergoing evaluation for aortic valve replacement include an ascending aortic aneurysm and significant coronary artery disease (CAD). In the case of a younger lower risk patient with bicuspid AS and concomitant ascending aortic aneurysm, the best approach remains surgery. In the Evolut Low Risk Trial, the presence of moderate comorbid CAD, defined as a SYNTAX score greater than 22, was an exclusion criterion. Similarly, those with severe CAD defined as a SYNTAX score greater than 33 were excluded from the PARTNER 3 trial. A reasonable and practical approach is to determine the optimal method of revascularization independent of the preferred method of treating the AS. A younger patient with concomitant disease in the left main or proximal left anterior descending artery would likely benefit from the durability of a left internal mammary artery graft and should be treated with surgery. Factors impacting need for revascularization and timing of coronary intervention relative to valve replacement will be discussed later in the chapter.

Feasibility of Future ViV Therapy

The options for management of failing bioprosthetic valves are surgical explantation or transcatheter ViV interventions. Early valve failure can occur in the setting of endocarditis or moderate or worse PVL, and patients with these presentations may require an urgent or emergent procedure. Management strategies must consider both the risk profile of the patient and the mechanism of failure. Factors contributing to SVD include smaller prosthesis size and PPM. This section will focus on late BVF with specific attention to risk factors for PPM, strategies to mitigate PPM and coronary obstruction, and the relevant risk of reoperative SAVR compared to ViV TAVR.

Annular Size and Risk of PPM

The concept of PPM is derived from surgical data and is broadly defined as an EOA that is too small in relation to the patient's body size. Obesity, female gender, small annulus size, and ViV status are the primary risk factors for PPM. Variable echocardiographic criteria have been utilized over the years, but in 2021, the VARC-3 Writing Committee defined severe PPM as an indexed EOA (EOAi) ≤0.65 cm^2/m^2. Importantly, this should reflect the hemodynamics of the valve shortly after implant to limit the impact of SVD on calculated valve area. There is disagreement over how to incorporate factors such as obesity, underlying flow state, and the measured or predicted orifice area of specific prostheses.[25] This has led to conflicting data on the impact of PPM on clinical outcomes. However, the preponderance of data suggests that PPM after SAVR or TAVR increases likelihood of SVD, heart failure, and mortality. Therefore, attention must be paid to minimizing risk of PPM, as it not only impacts short- and midterm procedural outcomes but has significant implications for future interventions, particularly in the younger patient who may need a second or even third valve intervention during their lifespan.

Surgical strategies for PPM include aortic root enlargement (ARE), supra-annular implant, use of stentless or sutureless valves, and the Ross procedure. The use of ARE procedures was shown to increase the EOAi and significantly reduce rates of PPM (odds ratio [OR], 0.567, $P = .007$) in a meta-analysis of approximately 40,000 patients undergoing SAVR.[26] In the unadjusted analysis, ARE was associated with a slight increase in perioperative mortality. However, this trend was not seen in mortality analysis of matched populations. As compared to the earlier era preceding FDA approval of the CoreValve for use in ViV procedures in 2015, there was a subsequent increase in the utilization of ARE procedures (3.9% to 6.3%, $P < .001$) and a modest increase in the proportion of implanted valves that were 23 mm or larger (61%-67%, $P = .001$).[27]

It is challenging to compare rates of PPM after SAVR as opposed to TAVR due to significant heterogeneity between the multiple transcatheter platforms and surgical bioprostheses in use. In PARTNER 3, rates of PPM were 4.6% after TAVR and 6.3% after SAVR ($P = .3$) and were associated with worse clinical outcomes in women.[9] Rates of PPM in small- and medium-sized annuli (less than 26 mm) were lower with CoreValve than with SAVR in a subanalysis of the CoreValve US Pivotal High Risk Trial.[28] Rates of PPM and 2-year mortality correlated with annular size in patients undergoing SAVR but not in those undergoing TAVR. There are no guidelines on how best to manage patients at the highest risk of PPM. The ongoing SMART trial is randomizing patients with small annuli to TAVR with either a current generation Evolut or SAPIEN prosthesis and will demonstrate whether there are meaningful differences in SVD and clinical outcomes.

Limitations of ViV TAVR

As increasingly younger patients are being offered TAVR (and bioprosthetic valves in general), there may be increasing numbers of patients who ultimately need two or even three valves over the course of their lives. Each implant introduces constraints on the maximum achievable EOAi, impacting the risk of PPM and potentially limiting valve durability. Another important consideration when assessing the feasibility of ViV TAVR is the risk of coronary obstruction due to sinus sequestration or displacement of the leaflets of the initial bioprosthesis toward the coronary ostium during expansion of the transcatheter valve (see **Fig. 42.7**).

The only way to circumvent all the limitations of ViV TAVR is to perform SAVR with removal of either the initial surgical bioprosthesis or transcatheter valve. Reoperative SAVR is associated with a roughly 2-fold increase in risk compared to native SAVR.[29] When compared to ViV TAVR, a recent meta-analysis showed that re-do SAVR was associated with higher 30-day mortality (OR, 0.52; 95% CI, 0.39-0.68; $P < .001$), but ViV TAVR had higher rates of PPM (OR, 4.63; 95% CI, 3.05-7.03; $P < .001$).[30] There are little long-term data comparing outcomes of re-do SAVR and ViV TAVR, but the risk of PPM will be an important consideration when weighing these options.

The simplest way to decrease risk of PPM is to implant the largest initial prosthesis that can be safely accommodated by the patient's anatomy. Both the CoreValve US Expanded Use Study and PARTNER 2 ViV registry have shown favorable results of ViV TAVR with regard to BVF at 5 years.[31,32] The PARTNER registry excluded patients with labeled valve size <21 mm, while the CoreValve registry included valves with a minimal inner diameter of 17 mm and larger.

In patients with pre-existing PPM conferred by their initial implant, there is an increase in both 30-day and 1-year mortality.[33] Therefore, strategies like balloon valve fracture, high deployment of a BE valve, and use of a supra-annular SE valve have been used to mitigate this risk. However, not all surgical valves are amenable to fracture. The ViV Aortic application, developed by Dr Vinayak Bapat, provides specifications such as internal diameter of numerous surgical bioprostheses, feasibility of fracture, appropriate sizing across transcatheter valve platforms, and suggested deployment techniques for each.

For patients who undergo initial management of their AS with TAVR, then end up having elevated risk for PPM or coronary obstruction with ViV TAVR, there are limited data on outcomes after surgical explantation of transcatheter valves. Jawitz et al described a cohort of 123 patients who underwent SAVR following TAVR between 2011 and 2015.[34] The majority of patients had STS PROM score greater than 8%, recent heart failure, and were categorized as urgent, emergent, or salvage. Mortality within 30 days of surgery was 17% in the overall cohort. The EXPLANT-TAVR registry described another cohort of patients undergoing surgery after TAVR and again showed elevated mortality rates compared to that expected based on STS PROM score.[35] Notably, the mortality rate of TAVR explant was not associated with STS PROM score at the time of index TAVR, suggesting that surgical explantation of a transcatheter valve is an inherently higher risk endeavor due to significant neoepithelialization often resulting in the need for aortic root repair.

Coronary Obstruction

Finally, with subsequent valve in valve procedures, the risk of coronary obstruction rises. Coronary obstruction that occurs in the setting of native TAVR and TAVR-in-SAVR can be treated with snorkel (or chimney) stenting or with a pre-emptive strategy of leaflet laceration (the BASILICA procedure). The effectiveness of BASILICA in TAVR-in-TAVR is limited by the lower rate of commissural alignment during TAVR as compared to SAVR. Sinus sequestration is a unique risk of TAVR-in-TAVR, and a risk stratification scheme based on parameters measured on CT has been proposed.[36] Particularly in cases where adjunct procedures such as BASILICA to mitigate risk of coronary obstruction are necessary, referral to high-volume centers with greater experience should be considered.

SUMMARY

Mapping out a lifetime plan for the management of AS with bioprosthetic valves becomes increasingly complex as the patient's age at initial presentation decreases. As more options for the management of BVF are developed, increasingly younger patients will be offered bioprosthetic over mechanical valves. While the minimally invasive nature of TAVR and associated shorter hospital stay and rapid recovery are naturally appealing to many patients, it does not necessarily confer minimal risk when considered in the context of lifetime management. Further study is needed to delineate which clinical and anatomic features impact risk of future ViV TAVR as compared to surgical reoperation or TAVR explantation.

Preprocedural Evaluation

Paramount to a successful TAVR is a comprehensive preprocedural evaluation of the patient. Patients should be assessed by a multidisciplinary Heart Team, often comprised of clinicians and nurses with expertise in Interventional Cardiology as well as Cardiothoracic Surgery. This initial evaluation should encompass not only the feasibility of the index valve intervention but also implications for future valve interventions. A comprehensive evaluation should include an assessment of symptoms, baseline functional status, severity of the valve disease, presence of CAD and LV dysfunction, presence of medical comorbidities (eg, chronic obstructive pulmonary disease, peripheral arterial disease, or renal insufficiency), and an assessment of the patient's frailty.

The requirement for symptoms prior to consideration of valve intervention has been challenged in recent years. The AVATAR trial demonstrated improved clinical outcomes in asymptomatic patients with severe AS who were randomized to early SAVR as compared to watchful waiting.[37] The EARLY TAVR trial randomizing asymptomatic patients with severe AS to TAVR with a SAPIEN valve or surveillance has completed enrollment.

The diagnosis of severe AS is primarily made via transthoracic echocardiography (TTE). In cases of diagnostic uncertainty with discordant TTE data, a valve calcium score and/or the DI can be used to corroborate severity of AS.

Preprocedural Imaging

Multidetector computed tomography (MDCT) is the preferred imaging modality for the anatomic assessment of the TAVR candidate. In addition to obtaining accurate and reproducible measurements of the iliofemoral anatomy to determine feasibility of TF access, MDCT provides valuable information regarding aortic valve annular dimensions, the presence of ascending aortic calcification (porcelain aorta), and the anatomy of the ascending aorta (**Fig. 42.4**). Measurements of the annular area and perimeter most directly impact sizing of the prosthesis. If the prosthesis is too small, there is increased risk of device embolization and significant PVL. If the prosthesis is too large, there is increased risk of annular rupture, aortic dissection, and coronary obstruction. The aortic annulus accounts for the narrowest part of the aortic root and is defined as a virtual plane connecting three anchor points at the nadir of each coronary cusp.[38] Three-dimensional multiplanar reconstruction of MDCT images enables accurate measurement of the aortic annulus, severity and distribution of annular calcification, height from the annulus to the ostia of the coronary arteries, and dimensions of the sinuses of Valsalva and sinotubular junction (STJ).

Preprocedural evaluation of the vasculature including vessel size, calcification, and tortuosity is another critical aspect to determine suitability for a TF or alternative access. Edwards SAPIEN 3 is available in four sizes (20, 23, 26, and 29 mm). All but the largest valve can be delivered through a 14F sheath (recommended minimum luminal diameter [MLD] 5.5 mm). The 29 mm valve requires a 16F sheath for delivery (recommended MLD 6.0 mm). Evolut Pro is also available in four sizes (23, 26, 29, and 34 mm). Similarly, all but the largest valve can be delivered through a 14F

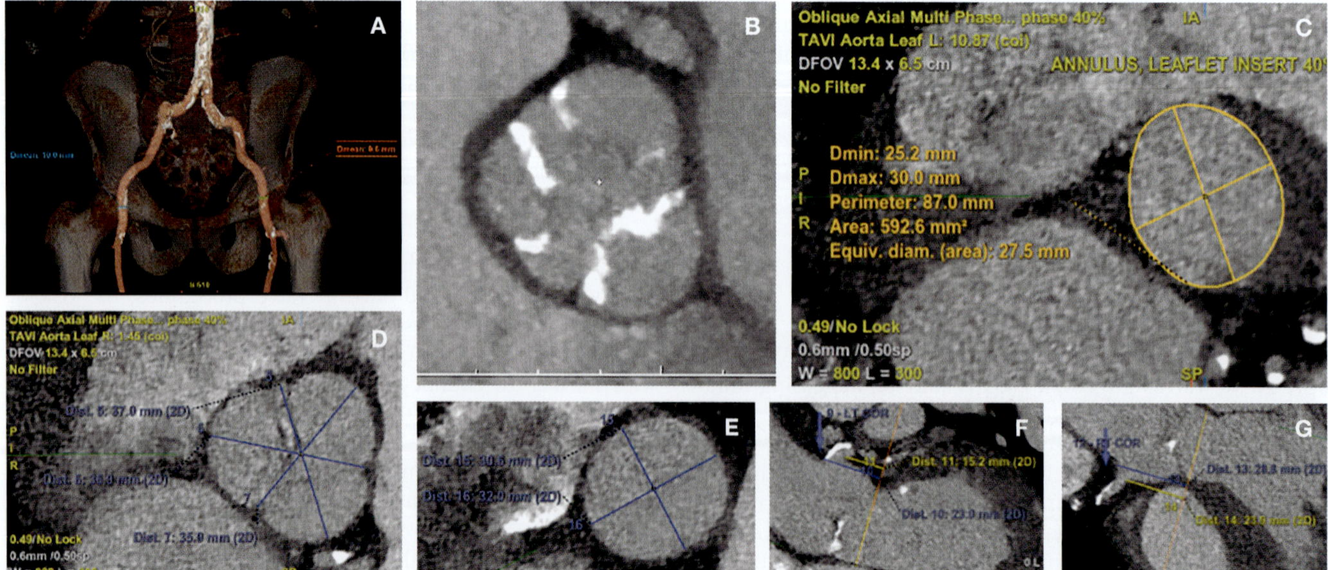

FIGURE 42.4 Typical components of a pre-TAVR CTA including **(A)** iliofemoral angiography with minimum vessel diameter; **(B)** evaluation of aortic valve morphology and the location and severity of commissural and leaflet calcium; **(C)** dimensions at the annulus, **(D)** sinuses of Valsalva, **(E)** sinotubular junction, and **(F and G)** relationship of the coronary ostia to the annular plane. CTA, computed tomographic angiography; TAVR, transcatheter aortic valve replacement.

in-line sheath with a recommended MLD of 5.0 mm. The 34 mm valve is delivered through an 18F in-line sheath with a recommended MLD of 6.0 mm. The iterative reductions in the diameter of the delivery sheaths has drastically reduced vascular complication rates and the need for alternative access, with the rate of TF-TAVR now exceeding 95%.[39] Nevertheless, if a patient does not have adequate iliofemoral anatomy, alternative access sites should be considered. Transaxillary or subclavian access has emerged as the most common alternative approach, followed by transcarotid, transcaval, and direct aortic. Transapical access, previously utilized in approximately a third of cases prior to 2013, has decreased dramatically and now accounts for less than 1% of cases in contemporary practice.

Diagnosis and Management of Concomitant CAD

The optimal method and timing of diagnosis and management of concomitant CAD remains uncertain and is an area of active investigation. Stress tests can be contraindicated (in the case of severe symptomatic AS) and may be less sensitive for ischemia due to increased LV wall tension, so invasive angiography remains the primary method for diagnosis of CAD. However, Chieffo et al showed that computed tomographic angiography (CTA) at the time of MDCT can be safely used as a screening tool for significant CAD with no difference in major adverse cardiovascular and cerebrovascular events at 30 days and 1 year in those who underwent CTA only and those who subsequently had invasive angiography.[40] As data increasingly support the safety of medically managing many, if not most, patients with stable CAD, there has been a gradual shift away from routine revascularization of stable coronary lesions discovered during the evaluation prior to TAVR.

A selective approach to invasive angiography is supported by a recent meta-analysis demonstrating no clinical benefit associated with percutaneous coronary intervention (PCI) prior to TAVR. In fact, patients undergoing PCI had increased risk of bleeding and showed a trend toward higher rates of acute kidney injury.[41] In cases where a patient has angina as the predominant symptom, impaired LV systolic function, or proximal lesions identified on MDCT, selective performance of invasive angiography at the time of TAVR seems a reasonable approach.

Frailty and Futility

When determining the potential benefit of TAVR, it is important to consider the prognosis of other major medical comorbidities. The benefits of TAVR in patients with advanced dementia or frailty are likely to be limited. Current guidelines recommend against TAVR if life expectancy is less than 1 year. There are multiple validated measures of frailty such as the Katz Activities of Daily Living Score that can be easily incorporated into the clinic evaluation.

TRANSCATHETER VALVE DELIVERY, POSITIONING, AND DEPLOYMENT

The following section will focus on the standard TF approach to TAVR (TF-TAVR) as this access route is preferred and feasible in over 90% of cases. In the absence of randomized comparisons, it is not possible to distinguish between the role of patient factors such as increased severity of peripheral vascular disease and procedural factors, but observational studies have consistently reported increased rates of stroke with alternative access.[42] Since most TAVR programs perform small numbers of such cases, consideration should be given to transferring the care of patients requiring alternative access to high-volume centers.

Setting and Personnel

A hybrid operating room/catheterization laboratory that will allow for both fluoroscopy-guided catheter manipulation and emergent conversion to open surgery is necessary for TAVR procedures. It should be large enough to accommodate a team consisting of cardiac anesthesiologists, echocardiographers, perfusionists, cardiac surgeons, and interventional cardiologists. With nearly all procedures being performed percutaneously and rare need for transesophageal echocardiography, most teams have transitioned to a "minimalist" approach to TAVR with avoidance of general anesthesia, pulmonary artery catheterization, and bladder catheterization. Adoption of a "minimalist" approach has been associated with decreased length of stay and hospital costs.

Access Management

Meticulous attention to access technique is required to minimize the risk of vascular complications. Anatomic landmarks such as the location of the groin crease or point of maximal femoral pulsation can be unreliable. Ultrasound-guided access of the femoral vessels using small-bore micropuncture needles is recommended to ensure access in a location without anterior wall calcification, in a compressible location over the femoral head, which will facilitate successful use of vascular closure devices.

Currently, the most common method of TF access site management involves the "preclosure" technique using a Perclose Proglide device (Abbott Vascular Devices, Redwood City, CA, USA). Prior to introduction of the large-bore valve delivery system, either one or two devices are deployed but not locked. In a femoral artery of sufficient caliber, use of a Perclose suture can be combined with an extravascular plug such as an Angio-Seal device (Terumo, Somerset, NJ, USA). Alternatively, the collagen-based MANTA device (Teleflex, Morrisville, NJ, USA) can be used for hemostasis after use of 10 to 20F access sheaths and is deployed after removal of the valve delivery system.

Once percutaneous access is obtained in the common femoral artery, the vessel undergoes serial dilation and the large bore sheath is carefully inserted under fluoroscopic guidance over a stiff supportive wire. Anticoagulation with heparin to attain an activated clotting time of 250 to 300 seconds should be initiated at the time of or immediately following placement of the large bore sheath. Bivalirudin should be avoided as it cannot be reversed in the event of a major bleeding complication.[43] Venous access is obtained in the contralateral groin for placement of a temporary transvenous pacemaker, and a second site of arterial access is obtained to facilitate introduction of a pigtail catheter.

Valve Positioning and Deployment

There are two primary fluoroscopic views currently used to guide positioning and deployment. The coplanar view is perpendicular to the native aortic annular plane such that the right coronary cusp is in the middle. The image detector angulation can be predicted by MDCT, but adjustments at the time of aortography are made using the "follow the right cusp" rule.[44] This is the recommended projection during deployment using the SAPIEN platform. In contrast, the cusp overlap view superimposes the right and left coronary cusps while isolating the noncoronary cusp.

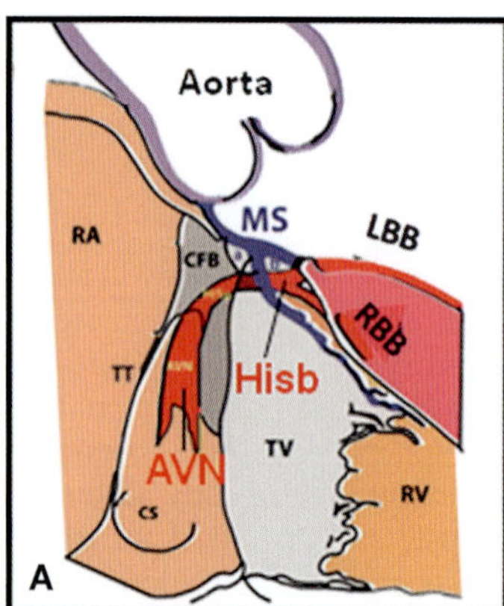

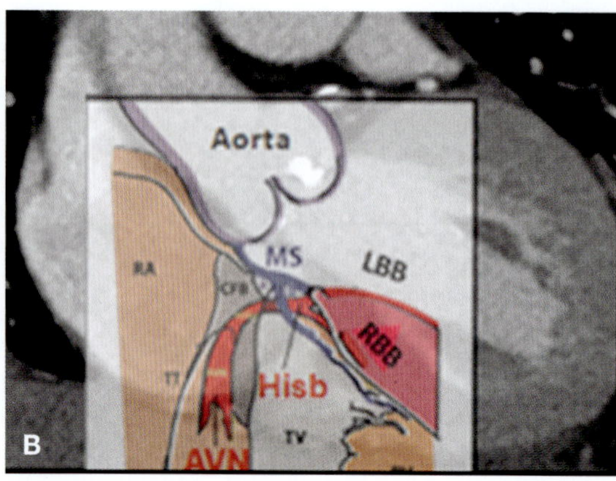

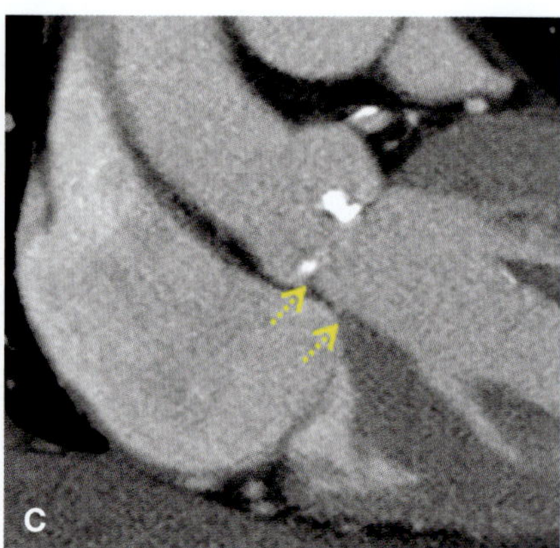

FIGURE 42.5 **A:** Illustration of the conduction system's topographic anatomy. Contrast-enhanced CT coronal view with **(B)** and without **(C)** superimposed illustration of the conduction system. Since the penetrating bundle of His emerges just below the membranous septum at the left ventricular surface, membranous septum (MS) length (*arrows*) serves as an anatomic surrogate of the distance between aortic annulus and the exit point of the bundle of His. AVN, atrioventricular node; CFB, central fibrous body; CS, coronary sinus; CT, computed tomography; His b, penetrating section of the His bundle; LBB, left bundle branch; MS, membranous septum; RA, right atrium; RBB, right bundle branch; RV, right ventricle; TT, tendon of Todazo; TV, tricuspid valve. (From Hamdan A, Guetta V, Klempfner R, et al. Inverse relationship between membranous septal length and the risk of atrioventricular block in patients undergoing transcatheter aortic valve implantation. *JACC Cardiovasc Interv*. 2015;8(9):1218-1228.)

This view elongates the LV outflow tract, thus enabling more accurate assessment of implant depth relative to the membranous septum (**Fig. 42.5**). This has been shown to facilitate higher positioning of the transcatheter valve, resulting in lower rates of conduction disturbances and subsequent need for a pacemaker when using SE valve platforms.[45]

Advancement of the valve delivery system to the native aortic valve is performed under fluoroscopic guidance. An aortogram is performed in either the coplanar or cusp overlap view using a pigtail catheter to assess the depth and coaxiality of the transcatheter valve prior to deployment (**Fig. 42.1A and D**). Once the optimal position is confirmed, steps for valve implantation are initiated (**Fig. 42.1B and E**). For inflation of a BE valve, rapid ventricular pacing at 160 to 200 beats per minute (bpm) is necessary to minimize ventricular ejection and valve embolization into the aorta during balloon inflation. Rapid pacing, albeit at lower rates of 120 to 160 bpm, facilitates stability during deployment of SE valves. In the event of postdilation, regardless of valve type, rapid pacing is mandatory to prevent embolization of the valve during balloon inflation.

Immediately following valve deployment, there may be a period of hypotension requiring administration of inotropes and vasopressors. If blood pressure recovery does not occur quickly in response to resuscitation, a quick yet thorough assessment of valve position, function, presence of either central or paravalvular regurgitation, presence of a pericardial effusion, and ventricular systolic function should be undertaken using a combination of fluoroscopy, angiography, and echo (**Fig. 42.1C and F**). Assessment of valve function immediately after deployment will determine the need for further intervention such as postdilation or placement of a second valve.

TAVR PROCEDURAL RISKS

Stroke

Stroke after TAVR is an infrequent complication and less common after TAVR than SAVR, particularly in low-risk patients. Rates range from 1% to 5% in most contemporary trials and have gradually decreased with iterative improvements in transcatheter delivery systems and valves as well as decline in the age of patients undergoing TAVR. Potential mechanisms for stroke associated with TAVR include embolization of calcific debris from the native aortic valve, atheroma in the aorta, or thrombus from the newly implanted transcatheter valve. Diffusion-weighted magnetic resonance imaging has shown that multiple embolic lesions occur in more than 75% of TAVR patients, but the majority of these are clinically silent with no discernible neurologic deficits or cognitive impairment.[46] Risk factors include high valve calcium score, bicuspid morphology, ViV status, and balloon valvuloplasty.

The Sentinel cerebral protection system (Boston Scientific, Marlborough, MA, USA) is the only device with FDA approval for use during TAVR to reduce the risk of procedural stroke. This approval was granted despite the device not meeting the primary efficacy endpoint in its pivotal trial.[47] More recently, the PROTECTED TAVR trial randomized 3000 patients to TAVR performed with or without a Sentinel device and did not show a statistically significant reduction in stroke within 72 hours or discharge from the hospital. There were numerically fewer disabling strokes (0.5% vs 1.3%). Importantly, the rate of stroke in the entire study population was very low. While the Sentinel device seems safe, its clinical benefit remains unproven, and there has not been widespread adoption of its use.

The antithrombotic strategy used after TAVR has evolved considerably. Use of dual antiplatelet therapy (DAPT) with aspirin and clopidogrel was found to confer increased bleeding risk compared with low-dose aspirin monotherapy without any reduction in ischemic events.[48] Similarly, treatment with rivaroxaban 10 mg daily after TAVR resulted in increased mortality, thromboembolic events, and bleeding compared to an antiplatelet strategy of DAPT for 3 months followed by low-dose aspirin monotherapy.[49] Therefore, low-dose aspirin monotherapy is currently recommended after TAVR in patients without a separate indication for anticoagulation. Patients with atrial fibrillation should take anticoagulation without concomitant antiplatelet therapy as the addition of aspirin does not appear to reduce stroke or major adverse cardiovascular events while increasing the risk of bleeding.[50]

Vascular Complications

Vascular complications include access site events as well as catastrophic aortic dissection and annular rupture. The latter two are rare events but can require emergent surgical repair when severe. Major or life-threatening access site bleeding has occurred at rates around 3% and 2%, respectively, according to the STS/ACC TVT registry.[40] Requisite skills for TAVR operators include the ability to manage vascular complications from the contralateral groin or from the radial artery. Prior knowledge of access vessel diameter and tortuosity is important to quickly tamponade any bleeding with an appropriately sized balloon and deploy a covered stent when conservative measures fail.

Conduction System Abnormalities

The bundle of His is located in the membranous septum of the left ventricular outflow tract inferior to the noncoronary cusp, a location that is susceptible to direct trauma, compression, and ischemia during and after valve deployment (**Fig. 42.5**). Following TAVR, varying degrees of heart block and left bundle branch block can occur. The risk of new pacemaker implantation has steadily declined with improvements in both device technology and implant techniques, but the risk remains higher after TAVR than SAVR. Overall rates remain about 10% in the STS/ACC TVT registry, with higher rates using SE valves than BE valves.[51] While pre-existing right bundle branch block is consistently the strongest predictor of need for a pacemaker, procedural factors such as prosthesis implantation depth and degree of oversizing are modifiable risk factors impacting the risk of a pacemaker after TAVR.

Valvular Insufficiency

Extensive annular and root calcification, underexpansion and undersizing of the prosthesis, as well as improper positioning resulting in the skirt being either too high or too low relative to the native annulus are all risk factors for the development of PVL. Widespread adoption of MDCT evaluation for procedural planning, iterative advances in valve technology (such as modifications to the external skirts), and refinement of implant technique have contributed to significant reductions in the incidence and severity of PVL. Whereas it was previously seen in 10% to 25% of TAVR cases, PVL is now estimated to occur in less than 5% of cases with current generation devices. What has not changed is that when it does occur, moderate or greater PVL portends a worse prognosis, including increased mortality, heart failure hospitalizations, and need for reintervention.[52]

While there is some inconsistency in how best to assess and grade PVL, there is some evidence that even mild PVL may have an effect on clinical outcomes. In the PARTNER A cohort, the presence of mild PVL after TAVR was associated with decreased survival at 2 years.[53] Similarly, survival at 5 years was lower in propensity-matched patients with mild PVL relative to those without PVL (HR, 1.41; 95% CI, 1.04-1.91).[54] Importantly, these studies used a grading scheme comprised of three classes (mid, moderate, and severe), as opposed to another study showing higher mortality only in patients with at least mild-to-moderate (grade 2) PVL on a five-point grading scheme.[55] VARC-3 guidelines recommend shifting to a more granular five-point classification scheme to characterize severity of PVL.

The intraprocedural management of this complication includes balloon dilatation of the valve, either with additional volume in the delivery balloon or with a larger diameter balloon. In severe cases, and depending on the mechanism of PVL, use of a vascular occluder or deployment of a second valve may be required.

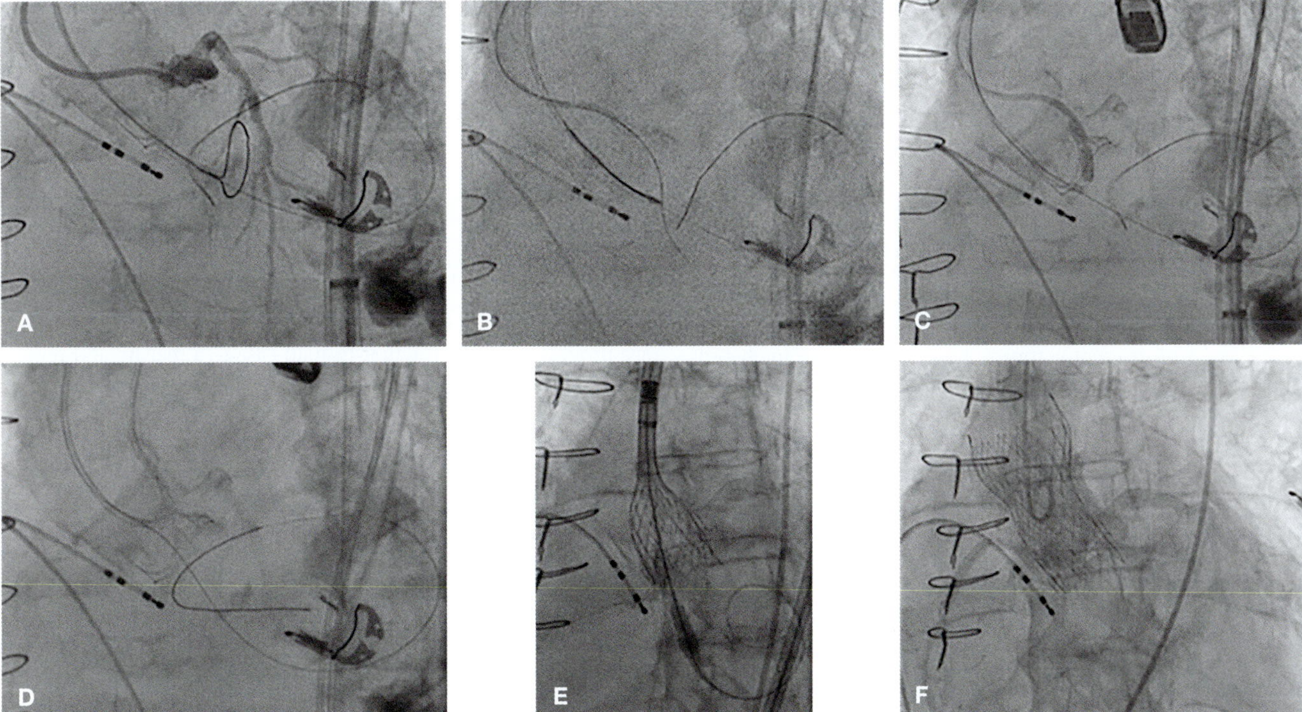

FIGURE 42.6 A case of TAVR-in-SAVR using BASILICA of the left coronary cusp and implantation of 26 mm Evolut Pro valve. Left coronary cusp angiogram demonstrates risk of obstruction from surgical valve leaflet **(A)**. An electrified Astato wire is used to puncture through the left cusp and is snared in the LVOT **(B)**. A coronary balloon is inflated to confirm the wire has traversed the leaflet and facilitate leaflet splaying **(C)**. The externalized Astato is intentionally kinked to create a "V," which is then electrified again and used to lacerate the leaflet **(D)**. The Evolut Pro valve is then positioned **(E)** and deployed **(F)**. LVOT, left ventricular outflow tract; SAVR, surgical aortic valve replacement; TAVR, transcatheter aortic valve replacement. (Courtesy of James McCabe, MD.)

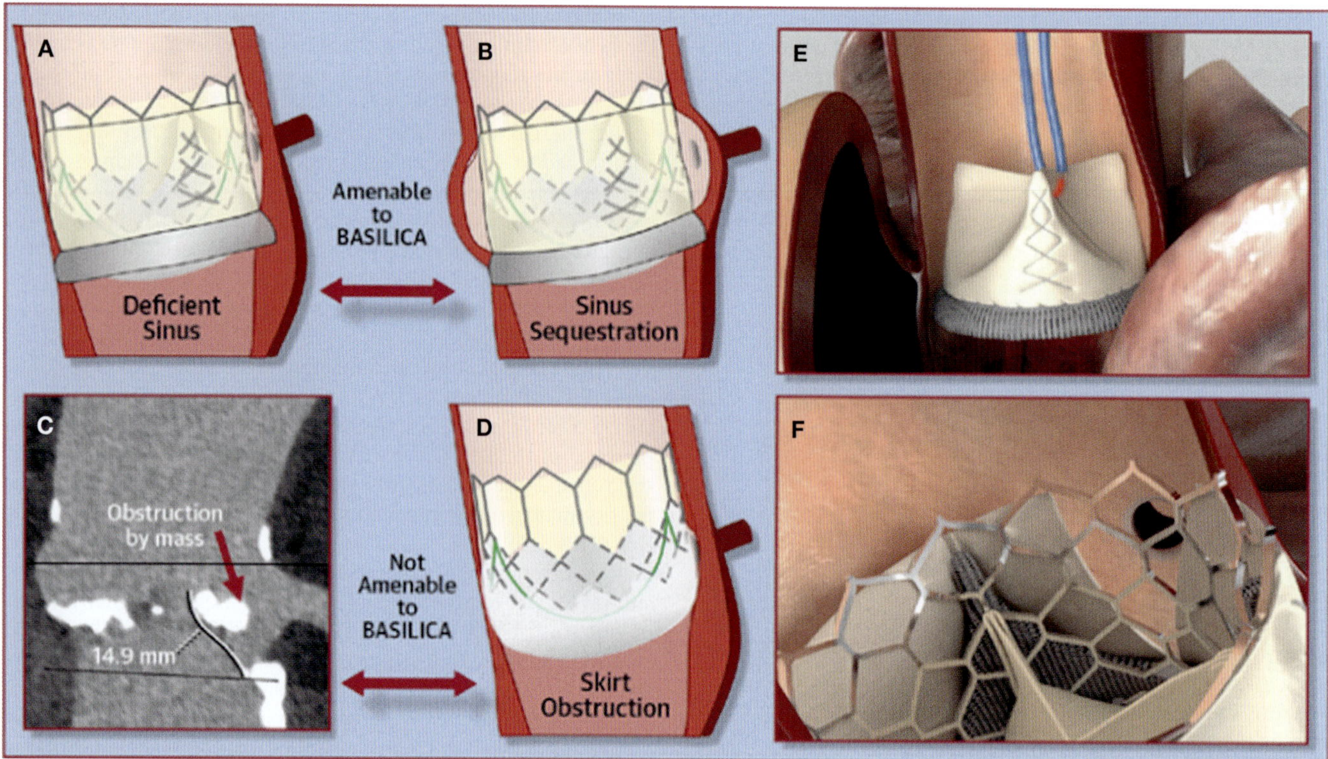

FIGURE 42.7 Mechanisms of transcatheter aortic valve replacement (TAVR)-induced coronary obstruction and mitigation by BASILICA. **A:** In a deficient sinus of Valsalva, the outwardly displaced leaflets directly obstruct the coronary artery ostium. **B:** In a low sinus of Valsalva and narrow sinotubular junction, the outwardly displaced leaflets indirectly obstruct the coronary artery ostium by sequestering the sinus. **C:** A bulky leaflet mass can directly obstruct the coronary ostium. **D:** In a low coronary ostium, the fabric-covered frame or skirt can directly obstruct the coronary artery ostium. **E:** An electrified BASILICA guidewire lacerates the prior aortic valve leaflets. **F:** A TAVR implant splays the lacerated leaflets and ensures inflow to the threatened coronary ostium after BASILICA. (From Lederman RJ, Babaliaros VC, Rogers T, et al. Preventing coronary obstruction during transcatheter aortic valve replacement: from computed tomography to BASILICA. *JACC Cardiovasc Interv.* 2019;12(13):1197-1216.)

Coronary Obstruction

Determining the risk of coronary ostial obstruction is an important aspect of preprocedural planning. The risk of coronary obstruction is higher in ViV procedures, during which either leaflet prolapse across the coronary ostium or sequestration of the sinuses can occur. Key factors impacting risk are the height of the coronary ostia relative to the aortic valve annulus, the dimensions of the sinuses of Valsalva, and the height and diameter of the STJ. Unexpected obstruction of a coronary artery is a potentially catastrophic event with mortality approaching 50%.[56] If an increased risk of obstruction is identified during preprocedural planning, two approaches can be considered: prophylactic wiring of the coronary or the BASILICA (Bioprosthetic or native Aortic Scallop Intentional Laceration to prevent Iatrogenic Coronary Artery obstruction during TAVR) procedure. In the former, a coronary guide and wire are placed into the coronary artery at risk prior to valve deployment. If coronary obstruction occurs, urgent percutaneous coronary revascularization with a stent intentionally protruding into the aorta and "snorkelled" upward toward the top of the valve frame can be performed. Alternatively, BASILICA uses an electrified coronary guidewire to perforate and split the potentially obstructing leaflet, thus enabling flow into the coronary ostium through the open cells of the valve frame (**Figs. 42.6** and **42.7**). The BASILICA trial demonstrated successful leaflet laceration in 95% of attempts with no cases of coronary obstruction.[57] While snorkel stenting is more technically feasible across a broad spectrum of operators, coronary access and risk of in-stent restenosis remain concerns. Particularly in a younger patient, when increased risk of coronary obstruction is identified on MDCT evaluation, SAVR and use of BASILICA in the patient at increased surgical risk should be given preferential consideration.

CONCLUSIONS

TAVR is a truly remarkable success story in interventional cardiology, progressing from the first-in-man case to a mature and reproducible procedure supported by a robust body of clinical outcomes data within a span of 20 years. There has been explosive growth in the number of centers offering TAVR, but significant unmet need persists, with a large proportion of appropriate patients with severe AS remaining untreated. With comparable outcomes to SAVR across a wide range of patient populations, progressively younger patients may be appropriate candidates for TAVR. Given the complexities of planning a lifetime management strategy, the collaborative input of a multidisciplinary Heart Team is necessary to tailor an approach for each individual. MDCT is firmly established as the preferred preprocedural imaging modality to assess feasibility of TF access, size the prosthesis, and predict the risk of postprocedural complications. Two dominant platforms, the SAPIEN and Evolut valves, still account for the vast majority of TAVR performed in the United States, but many others are in various stages of development, seeking to address limitations of existing technology, particularly in the treatment of AR.

The first decade of TAVR witnessed successive improvements in device technology resulting in dramatic expansions of anatomic feasibility, while the subsequent decade gave birth to a robust foundation of clinical data to support its use across a range of patient subgroups. The coming decade appears poised to address critical questions regarding valve durability and lifetime management strategies, perhaps leveraging the increasing capabilities of artificial intelligence and machine learning, such that physicians can 1 day accurately chart a course for each patient starting at the time of the index intervention.

Key Points

- Mortality is high in patients with severe symptomatic AS. Aortic valve replacement is recommended at the earliest onset of symptoms.
- TAVR is now reasonable across the entire spectrum of surgical risk categories and preferred in elderly patients above the age of 80 years.
- A lifetime management strategy accounting for the impact of the index intervention on the feasibility of future interventions must be considered, particularly in young patients expected to live beyond the lifespan of a single bioprosthetic valve. Care must be taken to leave future options that are anatomically feasible and minimize the risks of eventual surgery, PPM, and coronary obstruction.
- Multidetector CT imaging is necessary to assess feasibility of TF access and size the prosthesis as well as the risk of complications.
- Over 90% of patients can be treated using a TF approach. MDCT analysis provides essential information about vessel dimensions, calcification, and tortuosity. If femoral access is not feasible, transaxillary and transcarotid access have emerged as the most commonly used alternative access routes.
- TAVR is associated with higher rates of permanent pacemaker implantation and moderate or greater PVL compared to SAVR, whereas SAVR is associated with higher rates of new-onset atrial fibrillation and acute kidney injury.

References

1. Varadarajan P, Kapoor N, Bansal RC, Pai RG. Clinical profile and natural history of 453 nonsurgically managed patients with severe aortic stenosis. *Ann Thorac Surg*. 2006;82(6):2111-2115.
2. Cribier A, Eltchaninoff H, Bash A, et al. Percutaneous transcatheter implantation of an aortic valve prosthesis for calcific aortic stenosis: first human case description. *Circulation*. 2002;106(24):3006-3008. doi:10.1161/01.cir.0000047200.36165.b8
3. Sharma T, Krishnan AM, Lahoud R, Polomsky M, Dauerman HL. National trends in TAVR and SAVR for patients with severe isolated aortic stenosis. *J Am Coll Cardiol*. 2022;80(21):2054-2056.
4. Li SX, Patel NK, Flannery LD, et al. Trends in utilization of aortic valve replacement for severe aortic stenosis. *J Am Coll Cardiol*. 2022;79(9):864-877.
5. Thourani VH, Kodali S, Makkar RR, et al. Transcatheter aortic valve replacement versus surgical valve replacement in intermediate-risk patients: a propensity score analysis. *Lancet*. 2016;387(10034):2218-2225.
6. Pibarot P, Salaun E, Dahou A, et al. Echocardiographic results of transcatheter versus surgical aortic valve replacement in low-risk patients: the PARTNER 3 trial. *Circulation*. 2020;141(19):1527-1537.
7. Smith CR, Leon MB, Mack MJ, et al. Transcatheter versus surgical aortic valve replacement in high-risk patients. *N Engl J Med*. 2011;364(23):2187-2198.
8. Leon MB, Smith CR, Mack MJ, et al. Transcatheter or surgical aortic-valve replacement in intermediate-risk patients. *N Engl J Med*. 2016;374(17):1609-1620.
9. Popma JJ, Adams DH, Reardon MJ, et al. Transcatheter aortic valve replacement using a self-expanding bioprosthesis in patients with severe aortic stenosis at extreme risk for surgery. *J Am Coll Cardiol*. 2014;63(19):1972-1981.
10. Adams DH, Popma JJ, Reardon MJ, et al. Transcatheter aortic-valve replacement with a self-expanding prosthesis. *N Engl J Med*. 2014;370(19):1790-1798.
11. Reardon MJ, Van Mieghem NM, Popma JJ, et al. Surgical or transcatheter aortic-valve replacement in intermediate-risk patients. *N Engl J Med*. 2017;376(14):1321-1331.
12. Forrest JK, Deeb GM, Yakubov SJ, et al. 4-year outcomes of patients with aortic stenosis in the Evolut low risk trial. *J Am Coll Cardiol*. 2023;82(22):2163-2165.
13. Yoon SH, Kim WK, Dhoble A, et al. Bicuspid aortic valve morphology and outcomes after transcatheter aortic valve replacement. *J Am Coll Cardiol*. 2020;76(9):1018-1030.
14. Yoon SH, Bleiziffer S, De Backer O, et al. Outcomes in transcatheter aortic valve replacement for bicuspid versus tricuspid aortic valve stenosis. *J Am Coll Cardiol*. 2017;69(21):2579-2589.
15. Makkar RR, Yoon SH, Leon MB, et al. Association between transcatheter aortic valve replacement for bicuspid vs tricuspid aortic stenosis and mortality or stroke. *JAMA*. 2019;321(22):2193-2202.
16. Williams M, Jilaihawi H, Makkar R, et al. The PARTNER 3 bicuspid registry for transcatheter aortic valve replacement in low-surgical-risk patients. *JACC Cardiovasc Interv*. 2022;15(5):523-532.
17. Mangner N, Stachel G, Woitek F, et al. Predictors of mortality and symptomatic outcome of patients with low-flow severe aortic stenosis undergoing transcatheter aortic valve replacement. *J Am Heart Assoc*. 2018;7(8):e007977.
18. Ribeiro H, Lerakis S, Gilard M, et al. Transcatheter aortic valve replacement in patients with low-flow, low-gradient aortic stenosis: the TOPAS-TAVI Registry. *J Am Coll Cardiol*. 2018;71(12):1297-1308.
19. Pawade T, Clavel MA, Tribouilloy C, et al. Computed tomography aortic valve calcium scoring in patients with aortic stenosis. *Circ Cardiovasc Imaging*. 2018;11(3):e007146.
20. Makkar RR, Thourani VH, Mack MJ, et al. Five-year outcomes of transcatheter or surgical aortic-valve replacement. *N Engl J Med*. 2020;382(9):799-809.
21. Van Mieghem NM, Deeb GM, Søndergaard L, et al. Self-expanding transcatheter vs surgical aortic valve replacement in intermediate-risk patients: 5-year outcomes of the SURTAVI randomized clinical trial. *JAMA Cardiol*. 2022;7(10):1000-1008.
22. Jørgensen TH, Thyregod HGH, Ihlemann N, et al. Eight-year outcomes for patients with aortic valve stenosis at low surgical risk randomized to transcatheter vs. surgical aortic valve replacement. *Eur Heart J*. 2021;42(30):2912-2919.
23. VARC-3 Writing Committee; Généreux P, Piazza N, et al. Valve Academic Research Consortium 3: updated endpoint definitions for aortic valve clinical research. *Eur Heart J*. 2021;42(19):1825-1857.
24. Kowalówka AR, Kowalewski M, Wańha W, et al. Surgical and transcatheter aortic valve replacement for severe aortic stenosis in low-risk elective patients: analysis of the aortic valve replacement in elective patients from the Aortic Valve Multicenter Registry. *J Thorac Cardiovasc Surg*. 2024;167(5):1714-1723.e4.
25. Herrmann HC, Pibarot P, Wu C, et al. Bioprosthetic aortic valve hemodynamics: definitions, outcomes, and evidence gaps—JACC state-of-the-art review. *J Am Coll Cardiol*. 2022;80(5):527-544.
26. Sá MPBO, Zhigalov K, Cavalcanti LRP, et al. Impact of aortic annulus enlargement on the outcomes of aortic valve replacement: a meta-analysis. *Semin Thorac Cardiovasc Surg*. 2021;33(2):316-325.
27. Hawkins RB, Beller JP, Mehaffey JH, et al. Incremental risk of annular enlargement: a multi-institutional cohort study. *Ann Thorac Surg*. 2019;108(6):1752-1759.
28. Deeb GM, Chetcuti SJ, Yakubov SJ, et al. Impact of annular size on outcomes after surgical or transcatheter aortic valve replacement. *Ann Thorac Surg*. 2018;105(4):1129-1136.

29. Kaneko T, Vassileva CM, Englum B, et al. Contemporary outcomes of repeat aortic valve replacement: a benchmark for transcatheter valve-in-valve procedures. *Ann Thorac Surg*. 2015;100(4):1298-1304.
30. Sá MPBO, Van den Eynde J, Simonato M, et al. Valve-in-valve transcatheter aortic valve replacement versus redo surgical aortic valve replacement: an updated meta-analysis. *JACC Cardiovasc Interv*. 2021;14(2):211-220.
31. Hahn RT, Webb J, Pibarot P, et al. 5-year follow-up from the PARTNER 2 aortic valve-in-valve registry for degenerated aortic surgical bioprostheses. *JACC Cardiovasc Interv*. 2022;15(7):698-708.
32. Bajwa TK, Laham RJ, Khabbaz K, et al. TCT-20 five-year follow-up from the CoreValve expanded use transcatheter aortic valve-in-surgical aortic valve study. *J Am Coll Cardiol*. 2021;78(19_suppl_S):B9-B10.
33. Pibarot P, Simonato M, Barbanti M, et al. Impact of pre-existing prosthesis-patient mismatch on survival following aortic valve-in-valve procedures. *JACC Cardiovasc Interv*. 2018;11(2):133-141.
34. Jawitz OK, Gulack BC, Grau-Sepulveda MV, et al. Reoperation after transcatheter aortic valve replacement: an analysis of the Society of Thoracic Surgeons Database. *JACC Cardiovasc Interv*. 2020;13(13):1515-1525.
35. Bapat VN, Zaid S, Fukuhara S, et al. Surgical explantation after TAVR failure: mid-term outcomes from the EXPLANT-TAVR international registry. *JACC Cardiovasc Interv*. 2021;14(18):1978-1991.
36. Ochiai T, Oakley L, Sekhon N, et al. Risk of coronary obstruction due to sinus sequestration in redo transcatheter aortic valve replacement. *JACC Cardiovasc Interv*. 2020;13(22):2617-2627.
37. Banovic M, Putnik S, Penicka M, et al. Aortic valve replacement versus conservative treatment in asymptomatic severe aortic stenosis: the AVATAR trial. *Circulation*. 2022;145(9):648-658.
38. Kasel AM, Cassese S, Bleiziffer S, et al. Standardized imaging for aortic annular sizing: implications for transcatheter valve selection. *JACC Cardiovasc Imaging*. 2013;6(2):249-262.
39. Carroll JD, Mack MJ, Vemulapalli S, et al. STS-ACC TVT registry of transcatheter aortic valve replacement. *J Am Coll Cardiol*. 2020;76(21):2492-2516.
40. Chieffo A, Giustino G, Spagnolo P, et al. Routine screening of coronary artery disease with computed tomographic coronary angiography in place of invasive coronary angiography in patients undergoing transcatheter aortic valve replacement. *Circ Cardiovasc Interv*. 2015;8(7):e002025.
41. Altibi AM, Ghanem F, Hammad F, et al. Clinical outcomes of revascularization with percutaneous coronary intervention prior to transcatheter aortic valve replacement: a comprehensive meta-analysis. *Curr Probl Cardiol*. 2022;47(11):101339.
42. Chung C, Kaneko T, Tayal R, Dahle TG, McCabe JM. Percutaneous versus surgical transaxillary access for transcatheter aortic valve replacement: a propensity-matched analysis of the US experience. *EuroIntervention*. 2022;17(18):1514-1522.
43. Dangas GD, Lefèvre T, Kupatt C, et al. Bivalirudin versus heparin anticoagulation in transcatheter aortic valve replacement: the randomized BRAVO-3 Trial. *J Am Coll Cardiol*. 2015;66(25):2860-2868.
44. Kasel AM, Cassese S, Leber AW, von Scheidt W, Kastrati A. Fluoroscopy-guided aortic root imaging for TAVR: "follow the right cusp" rule. *JACC Cardiovasc Imaging*. 2013;6(2):274-275.
45. Rawish E, Macherey S, Jurczyk D, et al. Reduction of permanent pacemaker implantation by using the cusp overlap technique in transcatheter aortic valve replacement: a meta-analysis. *Clin Res Cardiol*. 2023;112(5):633-644.
46. Kahlert P, Knipp SC, Schlamann M, et al. Silent and apparent cerebral ischemia after percutaneous transfemoral aortic valve implantation: a diffusion-weighted magnetic resonance imaging study. *Circulation*. 2010;121(7):870-878.
47. Kapadia SR, Kodali S, Makkar R, et al. Protection against cerebral embolism during transcatheter aortic valve replacement. *J Am Coll Cardiol*. 2017;69(4):367-377.
48. Brouwer J, Nijenhuis VJ, Delewi R, et al. Aspirin with or without clopidogrel after transcatheter aortic-valve implantation. *N Engl J Med*. 2020;383(15):1447-1457.
49. Dangas GD, Tijssen JGP, Wöhrle J, et al. A controlled trial of rivaroxaban after transcatheter aortic-valve replacement. *N Engl J Med*. 2020;382(2):120-129.
50. Abdul-Jawad Altisent O, Durand E, Muñoz-García AJ, et al. Warfarin and antiplatelet therapy versus warfarin alone for treating patients with atrial fibrillation undergoing transcatheter aortic valve replacement. *JACC Cardiovasc Interv*. 2016;9(16):1706-1717.
51. Rheude T, Pellegrini C, Allali A, et al. Multicenter comparison of latest-generation balloon-expandable versus self-expanding transcatheter heart valves: ultra versus Evolut. *Int J Cardiol*. 2022;357:115-120.
52. Pibarot P, Hahn RT, Weissman NJ, et al. Association of paravalvular regurgitation with 1-year outcomes after transcatheter aortic valve replacement with the SAPIEN 3 valve. *JAMA Cardiol*. 2017;2(11):1208-1216.
53. Kodali SK, Williams MR, Smith CR, et al. Two-year outcomes after transcatheter or surgical aortic-valve replacement. *N Engl J Med*. 2012;366(18):1686-1695.
54. Yokoyama H, Sugiyama Y, Miyashita H, et al. Impact of mild paravalvular regurgitation on long-term clinical outcomes after transcatheter aortic valve implantation. *Am J Cardiol*. 2023;191:14-22.
55. Okuno T, Tomii D, Heg D, et al. Five-year outcomes of mild paravalvular regurgitation after transcatheter aortic valve implantation. *EuroIntervention*. 2022;18(1):33-42.
56. Ribeiro HB, Rodés-Cabau J, Blanke P, et al. Incidence, predictors, and clinical outcomes of coronary obstruction following transcatheter aortic valve replacement for degenerative bioprosthetic surgical valves: insights from the VIVID registry. *Eur Heart J*. 2018;39(8):687-695.
57. Khan JM, Greenbaum AB, Babaliaros VC, et al. The BASILICA trial: prospective multicenter investigation of intentional leaflet laceration to prevent TAVR coronary obstruction. *JACC Cardiovasc Interv*. 2019;12(13):1240-1252.

Hypertrophic Cardiomyopathy

Atul D. Bali and Srihari S. Naidu

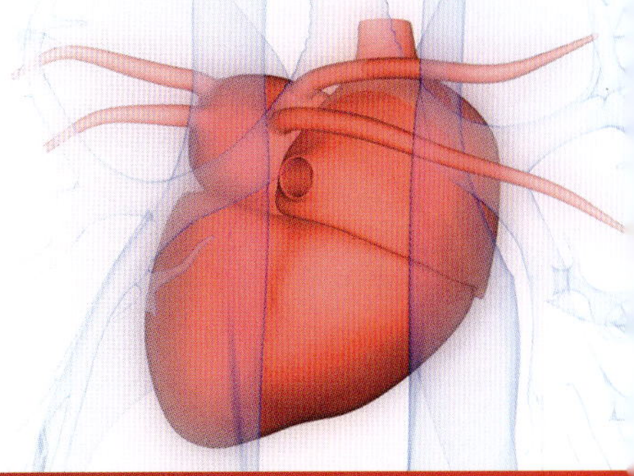

Introduction

Hypertrophic cardiomyopathy (HCM) is a common, inheritable cardiac disorder with an estimated prevalence of 1 in 500 persons in the general population. Clinically, HCM is defined as the presence of severe myocardial hypertrophy in the absence of a known local or systemic etiology.[1] For patients with concomitant conditions that induce hypertrophy such as hypertension or aortic stenosis, the degree of hypertrophy must be out of proportion to the hemodynamic burden imposed by that disease, typically more than 15 mm in maximal wall thickness in any given area, and most commonly asymmetric in its phenotype. Sarcomeric gene mutations are the cause of familial HCM, with 9 established causal mutations, and at least 15 other identified associated mutations that have been identified thus far.[2]

Clinically, the diagnosis of HCM is typically made using cardiac imaging modalities such as two-dimensional transthoracic echocardiography (TTE) or cardiac magnetic resonance imaging (MRI) to detect myocardial hypertrophy with its characteristic thickness and asymmetry. Doppler echocardiography can accurately assess the severity of left ventricular outflow tract (LVOT) gradient; however, concomitant valvular disease or mitral regurgitation can confound the measurements. Invasive evaluation via cardiac catheterization allows for fluoroscopic assessment by way of a left ventriculogram that would demonstrate a small cavity typically with hyperdynamic systolic function (**Fig. 43.1**). Additionally, hemodynamic assessment can reveal the typical gradient, either resting or latent; elevated diastolic pressures; a "spike-and-dome" aortic pressure tracing; postectopic beat drops in stroke volume; and dynamic left ventricular pressure changes in response to loading conditions such as intraprocedural provocative maneuvers (**Fig. 43.2**).

PATHOPHYSIOLOGY

Diastolic dysfunction with elevated ventricular filling pressures is a major pathophysiologic mechanism contributing to the symptomatology of patients with HCM. Abnormalities of diastolic function arise due to poor ventricular relaxation and compliance in the presence of altered loading conditions and sarcomeric dysfunction, chronic microvascular myocardial ischemia with associated fibrosis, ventricular nonuniformity, conduction abnormalities, and severe hypertrophy, which may limit cavity size. The end result of diastolic dysfunction is an increase in left ventricular filling pressures that causes the typical symptoms of dyspnea and angina.

In addition to diastolic dysfunction, the dynamic component of LVOT obstruction is present in 75% of patients with HCM, which often worsens patient symptoms and prognosis.[2] Determining the presence and severity of the LVOT obstruction is essential as this adds granularity to prognosis and provides the basis for targeted therapy. Two mechanisms underlie the development of dynamic LVOT obstruction: (a) septal hypertrophy yielding a narrowed LVOT, which leads to Venturi forces that accelerate during ventricular emptying and push the mitral apparatus anteriorly, and (b) anterior papillary muscle displacement, which subjects the mitral leaflets to intraventricular currents during systole that drag the apparatus anteriorly. Redundancy of the anterior mitral leaflet and/or hypertrophy or abnormalities of the chordal apparatus and papillary muscles may additionally contribute to obstruction. Decreased mitral leaflet coaptation occurs due to systolic anterior motion of the mitral valve, leading to secondary mitral regurgitation, which is also dynamic, characteristically posteriorly and laterally directed, and may be severe in patients with LVOT obstruction.

It is important to note the dynamic nature of LVOT obstruction and secondary mitral regurgitation. LVOT obstruction is exacerbated by increases in inotropy and decreases in either ventricular afterload (eg, vasodilators) or preload (eg, dehydration, diuretic therapy, systemic illness). The severity of LVOT obstruction is highly sensitive to ventricular load and contractility, with changes in the gradient even observed during quiet respiration (**Fig. 43.3**). Importantly, excessive sedation may limit provocation of obstruction and is particularly relevant in the cardiac catheterization laboratory.

MEDICAL THERAPY

Historically, negative inotropic and chronotropic agents, such as β-receptor antagonists, disopyramide, and nondihydropyridine calcium channel blockers (verapamil and diltiazem), are recognized

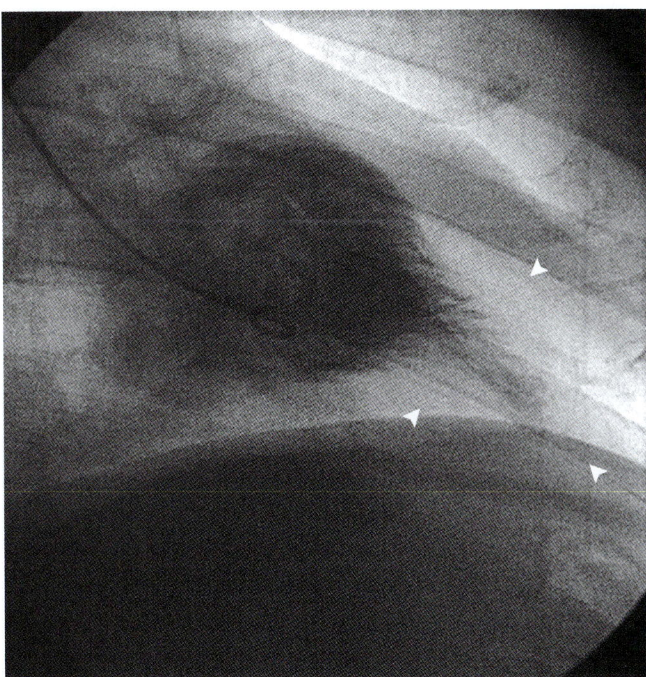

FIGURE 43.1 Left ventriculography of a patient with apical hypertrophic cardiomyopathy. This is an end-diastolic angiographic frame showing severe apical hypertrophy (*arrowheads*).

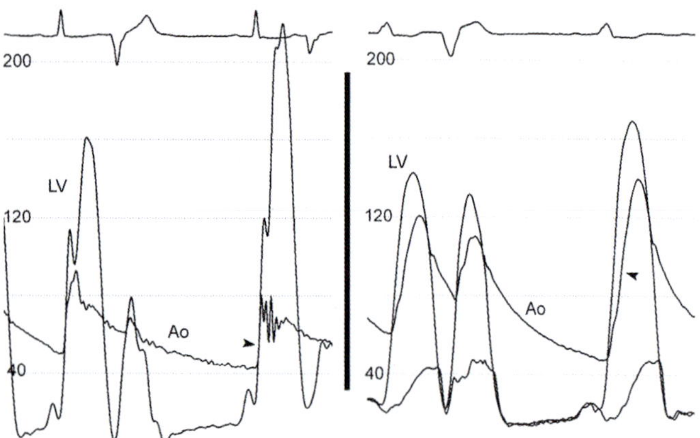

FIGURE 43.2 Dynamic left ventricular outflow tract obstruction during cardiac catheterization in a patient with HCM versus aortic valvular stenosis. **Left:** The patient with HCM has a typical "spike-and-dome" aortic pressure tracing, with dynamic changes in left ventricular pressures in response to changes in loading conditions. In this example, from a postectopic beat, there is an accompanied drop in aortic pulse pressure (*arrowhead*). This is described as the Brockenbrough-Braunwald-Morrow phenomenon. **Right:** In a patient with aortic stenosis, increased contractility on the postectopic beat leads to an increase in stroke volume and an increase in the aortic pulse pressure (*arrowhead*). Ao, ascending aorta; LV, left ventricle.

cornerstones of medical therapy for symptomatic LVOT obstruction. By depressing contractility and reducing chronotropy, these drugs prolong and improve diastolic filling and therefore reduce the degree of LVOT obstruction. Furthermore, these negative inotropic agents can improve myocardial relaxation and reduce the imbalance of myocardial oxygen supply and demand that is present in markedly hypertrophied myocardium, improving angina. It is necessary to note that often large doses of medication or combination therapy with several agents in twice-daily delivery is required to substantially reduce LVOT obstruction and therefore pose the risk of medication side effects (eg, bradycardia, dizziness, hypotension, and

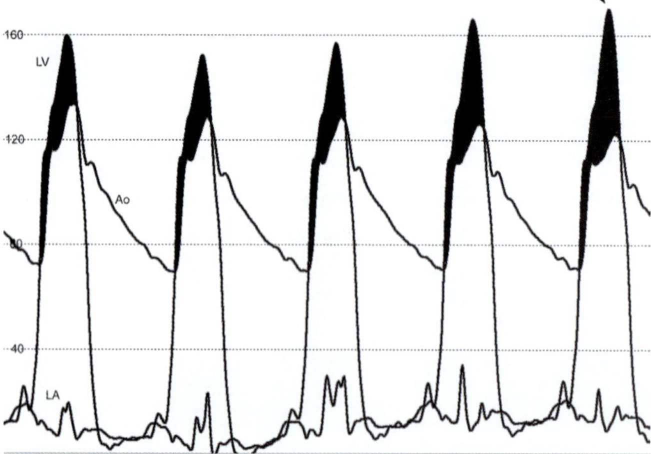

FIGURE 43.3 Dynamic changes in left ventricular outflow tract obstruction related to respiration. The LVOT gradient (*shaded black*) is incredibly sensitive to loading conditions and contractile state, with effects seen even during quiet respiration as demonstrated here. During expiration, an increase in thoracic pressure leads to lower afterload and consequently an increase in the left ventricular outflow tract gradient. Reciprocal changes occur during inspiration. The *arrowhead* indicates peak end expiration. Ao, ascending aorta; LA, left atrium; LV, left ventricle.

atrioventricular [AV] block). Disopyramide should be taken into special consideration as it has been proven to provide symptomatic benefit to patients with obstructive HCM. However, since disopyramide may mechanistically increase AV nodal conduction, potentially leading to fast conduction with the beginning of atrial fibrillation, it should be administered in conjunction with concomitant AV nodal blockers. Lastly, it is necessary to counsel patients on the potential anticholinergic adverse effects of disopyramide, which can be effectively alleviated by pyridostigmine, and the proarrhythmic risks of QT prolongation, which requires early and sustained monitoring.

With the introduction of mavacamten, a cardiospecific allosteric inhibitor of cardiac myosin ATPase that directly targets sarcomere hypercontractility in HCM, a novel therapeutic strategy emerged for obstructive HCM demonstrated in two trials; EXPLORER-HCM and VALOR-HCM. Both studies demonstrated efficacy of mavacamten for patients with obstructive HCM to improve exercise capacity and quality-of-life scores and reduce resting and provocable LVOT gradients, when compared with standard negative inotropic agents. In addition, mavacamten obviated the need for septal reduction therapy in the majority of symptomatic patients slated for invasive treatment.[3,4] Although long-term data are needed, mavacamten and other cardiac myosin inhibitors will be a new and increasing option in the armamentarium of HCM treatment.

Agents that should be avoided are high-dose or potent diuretics that might trigger hypovolemia, peripheral vasodilators, and positive inotropic agents (eg, digoxin, β-receptor agonists), as they will worsen the LVOT obstruction by a combination of mechanisms, namely, hypovolemia and reduced preload, vasodilation and reduced afterload, or increasing contractility and heart rate. Patients should also be counseled on maintenance of adequate hydration to maintain euvolemia. When severe symptoms persist despite optimal drug therapy, definitive septal reduction therapy should be considered in patients with obstructive HCM at recognized centers of excellence.

SURGICAL MYECTOMY

Surgical myectomy, an open-heart procedure where a surgeon widens the LVOT by directly resecting portions of the hypertrophied septal muscle, has been the time-honored standard for septal reduction therapy.[5-7] This surgery has several variations that are related to the type of HCM variant and degree of septal hypertrophy if used to reduce LVOT obstruction and is further modified if there are abnormalities of the mitral valve or associated mitral apparatus. Typically, extended septal myectomies that provide extended resection to papillary bases in the mid ventricle have become the standard of care, with occasional apical myectomies for left ventricular cavity enlargement or in rare cases repair to the mitral valve alone or in combination with myectomy. While early historical studies raised concern about the safety of the procedure, more recent large series have demonstrated very low operative mortality (<1%), with excellent success rates exceeding >90% at experienced centers. Surgical complications are similar to that of most open cardiac surgery, with the addition of certain special considerations of transaortic incisions and septal resection, namely, ventricular septal defects and aortic regurgitation, and possible need for permanent pacemaker (PPM) implantation (<5%). Importantly, long-term studies with greater than 10-year follow-up have demonstrated no limited impairment of survival after surgical myectomy. However, it must be noted that, in a large database series from 2003 through 2011, most septal reduction therapy (SRT) in US institutions were performed in centers with less annual experience than recommended by guidelines and there was an association between low-volume centers with worse in-hospital outcomes including higher mortality, hospital cost, longer length of stay, renal failure, and higher pacemaker implantation rate, strengthening the recommendation for referrals to established, high-volume HCM centers of excellence for such procedures.[8]

ALCOHOL SEPTAL ABLATION

A well-established percutaneous alternative to surgical myectomy was invented in 1994. Now evolved over 25 years, the procedure utilizes standard angioplasty equipment and techniques to induce a localized myocardial infarction by the controlled infusion of ethanol into an appropriate proximal septal artery. This results in akinesis and thinning of the previously hypertrophied septum and relieves LVOT obstruction over the course of approximately 3 to 6 months. In ideal candidates, the procedure can produce a surgery-like result without the associated operative risks.

Patient Selection

As with most percutaneous transcatheter interventions, patient selection is key to success and alcohol septal ablation (ASA) is no exception. A comprehensive evaluation at an HCM center of excellence that has experience with all forms of management including medical and both septal reduction options, surgical or percutaneous, is recommended. Based on the literature and guidelines, a volume threshold of >10 procedures per year has been advocated.

Similar to surgical myectomy, criteria for ASA include the following: (1) drug refractory symptoms (generally New York Heart Association [NYHA] class III/IV) due to HCM; (2) LVOT obstruction with resting gradient >30 mm Hg or >50 mm Hg with provocable maneuvers; (3) septal thickness meeting criteria for HCM (>15 mm); (4) absence of a need for open cardiac surgery such as bypass or valve replacement; (5) informed patient consent; (6) adequate volume and operator and institutional experience. Certain additional characteristics are required for candidacy that are not necessary for surgical myectomy such as appropriate septal artery targets for ethanol delivery and a more basal-predominant area of hypertrophy to target in order to avoid the thinner portions of mid or apical septum. If criteria are met, per the most current HCM guidelines and large series-based data, there is a similar class 1 recommendation for either surgical myectomy or ASA as septal reduction therapy for patients with obstructive HCM with drug-refractory symptoms.

At the foundation of patient selection is an anatomic assessment of the LVOT obstruction, which begins with two-dimensional TTE. The role of a comprehensive TTE is to document the dynamic nature of the LVOT obstruction by establishing both resting and Valsalva-provoked baseline gradients. Additionally, echocardiography evaluates the degree and distribution of hypertrophy and evaluates the mechanism of any associated mitral regurgitation, which is necessary to exclude variants of disease and concomitant intrinsic valvular disease that would impede efficacy of ASA (**Figs. 43.4** and **43.5**).

Given the complex nature of both the disease physiology and treatment both from a medical and procedural standpoint, informed patient consent should be undertaken by a multidisciplinary team with expertise in the care of patients with HCM that involves experienced operators in these procedures. Informed patient consent for ASA requires full understanding of the existing body of data, technical proficiency, systems in place to assure optimal outcomes, durability of the procedure, and possible need for repeat ASA depending on anatomic response to the procedure, elevated risk of pacemaker dependency, and potential complications related to cardiac catheterization, instrumentation of the coronary arteries, and infusion of alcohol.[1]

Although younger age is not a contraindication to the procedure, with several large series demonstrating outcomes comparable with those of surgical myectomy, ASA has traditionally been reserved for the older adult population due to the limited data on long-term survival of the procedure beyond 10 years and occasionally the need for repeated ASA for a durable effect. Additionally, the need for PPM implantation is not insignificant, with some series reporting a rate of up to 8% to 16% PPM placement post ASA.

Hemodynamic Evaluation

Proper performance of septal ablation requires a complete and accurate evaluation of the severity of LVOT obstruction due to HCM. Additionally, a coronary angiogram identifying appropriate septal arteries correlating to areas of culprit hypertrophied myocardium is required. Characteristically, the LVOT obstruction

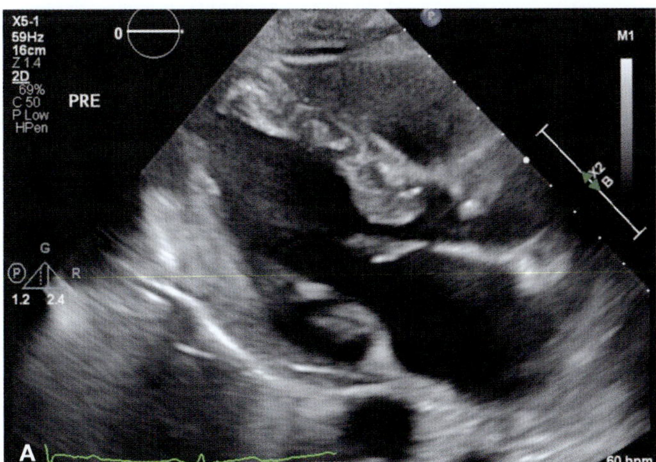

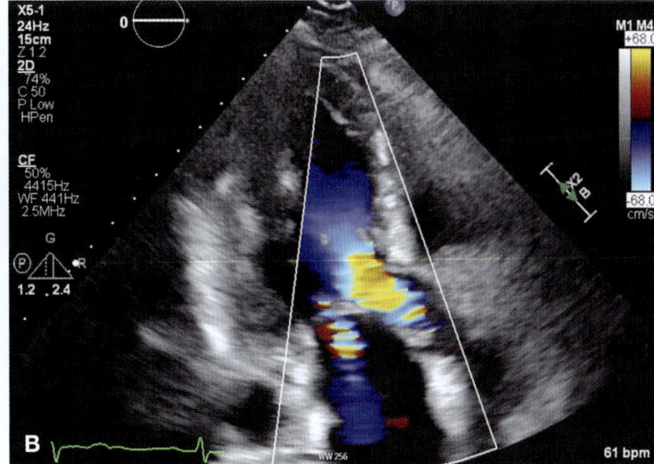

FIGURE 43.4 Patient selection for septal ablation. **A** is a parasternal long-axis view demonstrating focal septal hypertrophy, and **B** is color Doppler showing the typical "Y"-shaped color flow of turbulence through LVOT from the dynamic obstruction and the secondary mitral regurgitation. This patient has appropriate anatomy for consideration of septal ablation.

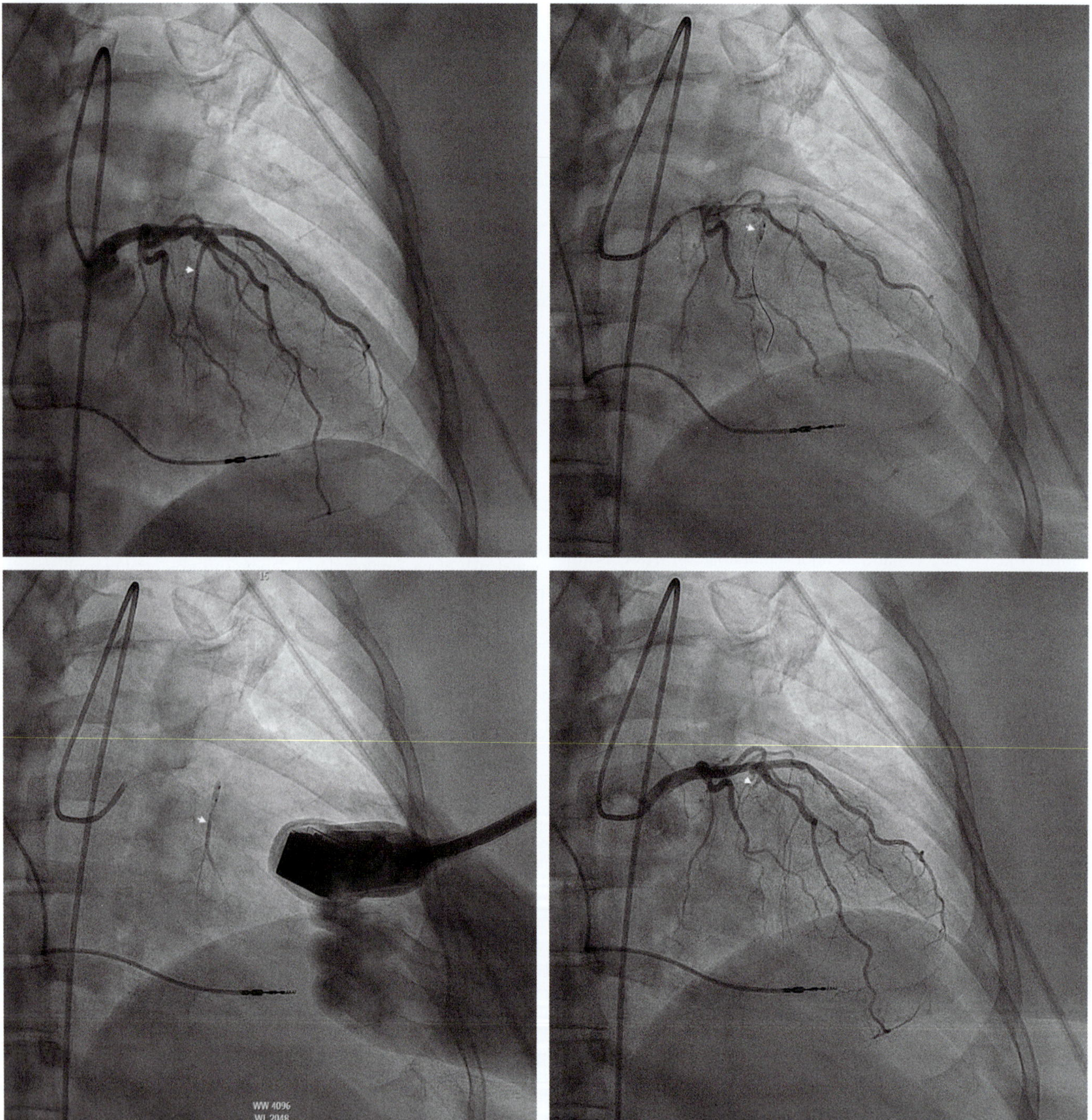

FIGURE 43.6 Percutaneous septal alcohol ablation. **Top left:** Baseline angiogram of the left coronary artery showing the septal perforator artery (*arrow*) to be used for ablation and the externalized actively fixated transvenous pacemaker positioned in the RV apical septum. **Top right:** An over-the-wire balloon is inflated in the perforator artery followed by contrast injection through the balloon for septal angiography (*arrow*). **Bottom left:** Angiographic contrast is injected through the balloon (*arrowhead*) and visualized with simultaneous echocardiography (note the sonographer with probe in hand). **Bottom right:** Following injection of alcohol, the septal artery (*arrow*) is obliterated. LA, left atrium; LV, left ventricle; RV, right ventricle.

of HCM is extremely dynamic and sensitive both to ventricular loading conditions and contractility. The operator should be cognizant of this sensitivity when examining hemodynamic data during the invasive catheterization. Careful attention must be given not only to the initial LVOT gradient observed at rest but also to all dynamic and provocable gradients (eg, variation with respiration, post-PVC accentuation) observed during the procedure, as well as aortic pressure responses to intracavitary gradient manipulation. Furthermore, the operator must take care to assure there is no overlapping fixed gradient of aortic stenosis, which can be present in older patients, and thus must be evaluated carefully with subaortic valve positioning of the catheter.

The invasive evaluation of the dynamic LVOT obstruction in HCM entails simultaneous pressure measurements of both aortic and intracavitary pressures at different LV locations to establish and localize LVOT gradient both at rest and with provocable maneuvers. A 5-F pigtail catheter is placed retrograde across the aortic valve to the LV apex to obtain intraventricular pressure, which is then simultaneously measured with aortic pressure typically obtained by transducing the femoral artery via the 6-F sheath side port. It is notable to mention that ensuring the distal end of the pigtail catheter is not entrapped in aberrant papillary muscles or redundant mitral valve tissue is essential to avoid waveform dampening. In addition, it is imperative to measure the LV pressure at the apex of the ventricle to capture the entirety of provoked gradients. For localization of maximal gradient, the pigtail may be replaced with an end-hole catheter for a slow pullback across the outflow tract. With a meticulous approach, and taking into consideration the possibility of catheter entrapment and peripheral augmentation, this hemodynamic evaluation simplifies the procedure and obviates the need for multiple catheters or the traditional transseptal approach. A hand contrast injection should be performed to ensure that the distal end of the pigtail catheter is adequately positioned in the true LV apex, so as not to miss mid-cavitary gradients, and also to identify aneurysms that may have not been visualized by echocardiography.

Once a resting LVOT gradient is established, provocative maneuvers (namely, PVC stimulation with post-PVC recordings, supervised Valsalva, and respiratory variation) can be performed to determine the degree of dynamic obstruction. In our experience, eliciting a PVC with the right heart catheterization positioned in the right ventricle (RV) apex during the strain phase of the Valsalva maneuver is the most sensitive way to evaluate for and quantify obstruction.

Temporary Pacemaker Placement

The risk of pacemaker dependency from septal ablation varies according to the baseline electrocardiographic (EKG) abnormalities. Septal ablation results in right bundle branch block in approximately 50% to 70% of cases. Thus, for those patients with preexisting left bundle branch block, severe left axis deviation, or a very wide QRS interval, the rate of pacemaker dependency is not insignificant approaching 50%. In patients with a normal EKG, PPM dependency from complete AV block occurs in 10% to 15% based on data from large series.[7-10] Thus, for patients without a PPM, a temporary device is placed at the right ventricular apical septum via the right internal jugular vein prior to septal ablation. We typically use an active fixation RV lead with an externalized generator, so as to allow prolonged ambulation as the patient is evaluated for PPM dependency in the ensuing week. Care must be taken to confirm the RV lead is distal to the septal perforator (ie, more apical), as ablation can change pacing threshold of the lead resulting in loss of capture. There is a noticeable delay in development of conduction abnormalities in patients following alcohol septal ablation, and thus, conventional 5-F or 6-F balloon-tipped temporary pacemakers are less preferable than semipermanent fixed lead attached to an externalized generator as described, which also allows for ambulation and reduced risks of pericardial tamponade. Importantly, it also allows for prolonged monitoring, which may obviate the need for PPM in some patients.

Procedure

Coronary angiography is performed to determine the most appropriate septal artery for the procedure. Both left and right coronary arteries should be evaluated, as basal septal branches occasionally arise from the proximal right coronary artery. With a right anterior oblique angulation of the left coronary artery, straight and caudal views help to examine the angulation of the origin of the proximal septal arteries and area subtended, while cranial projections can assist with the length of the vessel and placement of the balloon. Left anterior oblique projections should be used to demonstrate the course of the artery in the ventricular septum and assure safety of the left anterior descending (LAD) artery during the procedure. It is important to note the septal arteries supplying a hypertrophied basal septum can frequently have branches, which may have to be selectively engaged and ablated for a desired result. In addition, septals can frequently come off the left main, LAD, diagonals, and ramus, and thus, all arteries should be inspected for the optimal septal branch to the target basal septum.

A conventional 6-F guide catheter is used to engage the left main coronary artery with standard procedural anticoagulation to achieve therapeutic activated clotting times (eg, heparin 70-100 U/kg or bivalirudin infusion 1.75 mg/kg/h). A stable guide is necessary as compete opacification is required during angiography for septal artery visualization, and minimal movement of the balloon catheter prior to alcohol infusion. Importantly, since alcohol septal ablation is done without a coronary wire to anchor the balloon, meticulous guide placement and fluoroscopic and echocardiographic monitoring is required throughout the procedure. Both primary and a large secondary bends should be placed on the tip of a standard workhorse long guidewire to facilitate entry into the candidate septal artery. A slightly oversized, short-length, over-the-wire balloon is placed completely into the septal artery using standard catheter techniques. The entire balloon should be advanced into the septal artery to ensure complete occlusion and prevent slippage back into the LAD. Slight oversizing of the balloon allows occlusion of the artery at low pressures, which permits relatively easier injection of material through the wire lumen of the catheter, and decreases the risk of alcohol reflux back into the main vessel. If the operator is having slippage of the balloon into the main vessel despite slight oversizing, a cutting balloon inflated to low pressure can be used to anchor the balloon in the septal artery.[11]

Once the balloon catheter is inflated and the guidewire is removed, angiography of the left coronary artery is performed to demonstrate complete septal occlusion by the balloon. Then contrast is infused into the balloon lumen, with careful attention given to ensure no dye reflux back into the LAD and no dye opening up collaterals to other vessels such as the posterior descending artery or another more distal or proximal septal artery (**Fig. 43.6**). Selective angiography of the septal artery through the balloon catheter also confirms patency of the vessel for ablation and localization by myocardial contrast echocardiography (MCE). MCE is utilized to determine whether the focally enhanced segment of myocardium is appropriate for ablation. Multiple echocardiographic views, namely, standard parasternal long axis and apical two-chamber, three-chamber, and four-chamber views, are used to confirm enhancement of the basal septum without contrast extension to the right ventricle, mid or apical septum, or papillary muscles (**Fig. 43.7**).

Once the targeted myocardium is identified, 1 to 3 mL of ethanol is slowly infused over a 1- to 3-minute period and subsequently followed by a slow flush of 0.3 mL normal saline. The amount of ethanol is usually determined by a combination of septal thickness, septal diameter, and septal length. The patient may experience chest discomfort, and appropriate analgesia should be administered intravenously. During the slow infusion, the echocardiographer should continue to look for ethanol infusion in other areas, indicating spillage or collaterals, and confirm concentration of ethanol in the target septum and should also look at the continuous wave pressure gradient to confirm reduction and transition to an early peaking waveform from a dagger-shaped waveform. Following the flush of normal saline, the balloon catheter should be left inflated for an additional 5 to 10 minutes to ensure adequate washout of the ethanol and reduce the risk of extravasation into the main coronary vessel. Post alcohol infusion, repeat TTE should

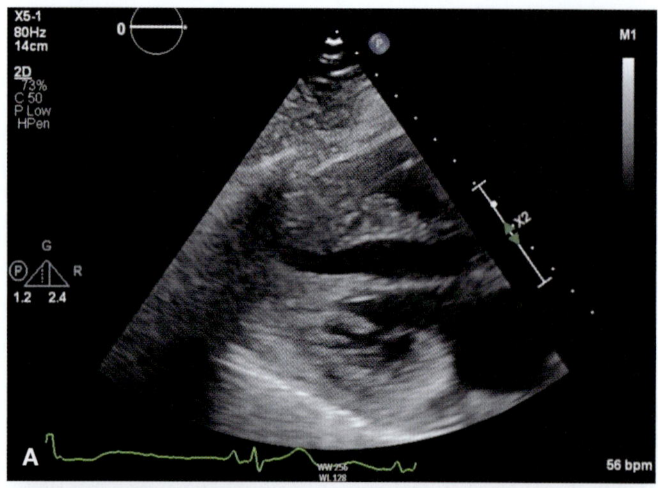

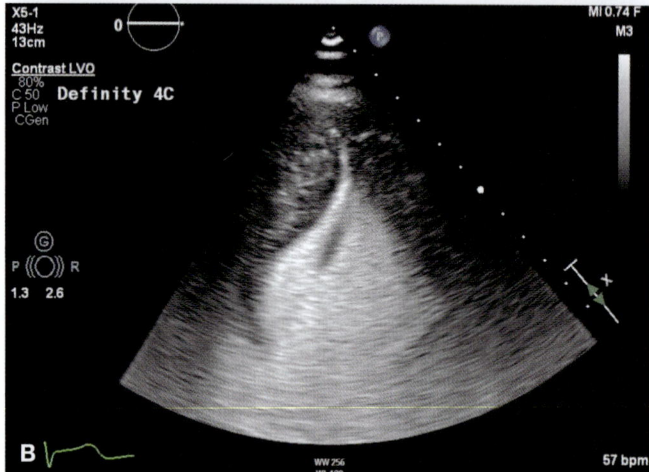

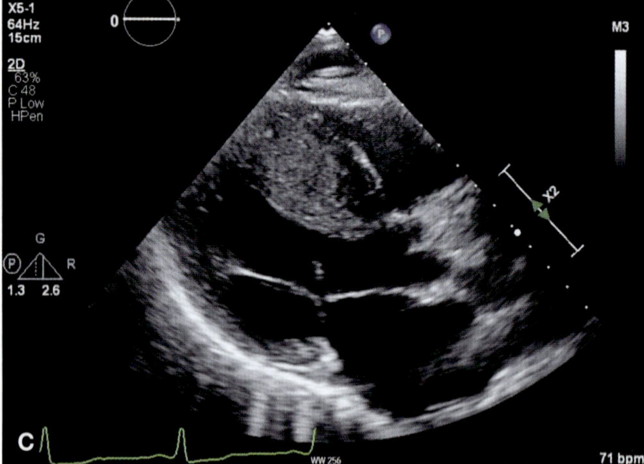

FIGURE 43.5 Patient selection for septal ablation. **Echocardiographic images** demonstrating variants of HCM that are not suitable for ASA. **A** and **B** demonstrate apical HCM with the classic "spade shape" ventricle apparent in **(B)**. **C** demonstrates diffuse massive septal hypertrophy extending beyond basal septum to the mid-cavitary region.

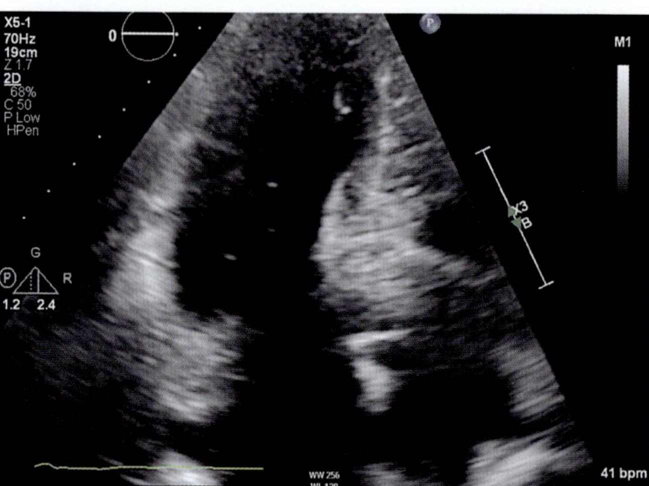

FIGURE 43.7 Myocardial contrast echocardiography. The basal septum is focally opacified after direct contrast injection into the septal artery. This allows for localization of the effect of ethanol effect.

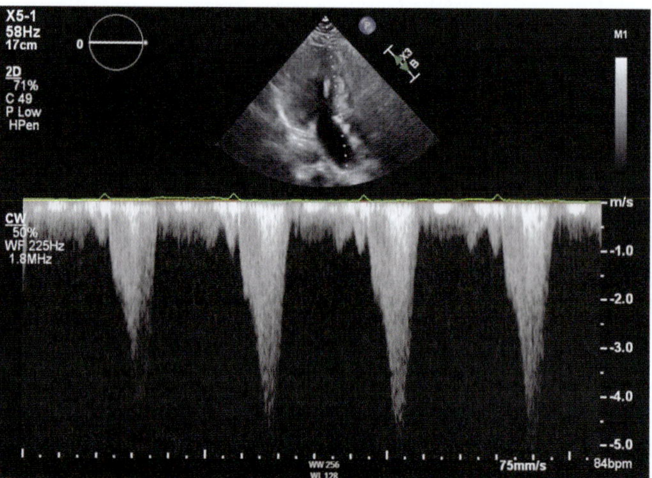

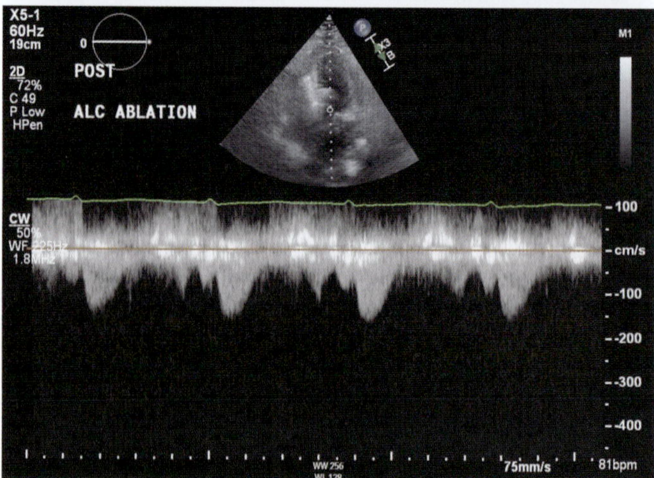

FIGURE 43.8 Hemodynamic effects of septal alcohol ablation evaluated by intraprocedural TTE. **Top:** Baseline LVOT gradient with characteristic late peaking, dagger-shaped gradient of 84 mm Hg. **Bottom:** Postablation LVOT gradient with complete resolution of dynamic obstruction and normalized early-peaking aortic gradient.

be performed to ensure adequate reduction on LVOT gradients, both resting and provoked (**Fig. 43.8**). Final angiography should be performed once the balloon catheter is deflated and removed, to ensure no adverse event in the left coronary artery system and maintained TIMI flow and to confirm the ablation of the septal artery (**Fig. 43.9**).

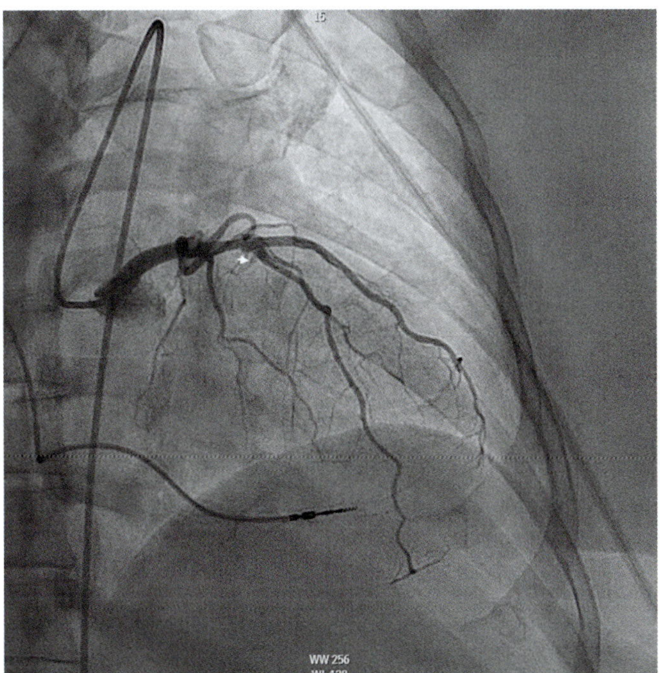

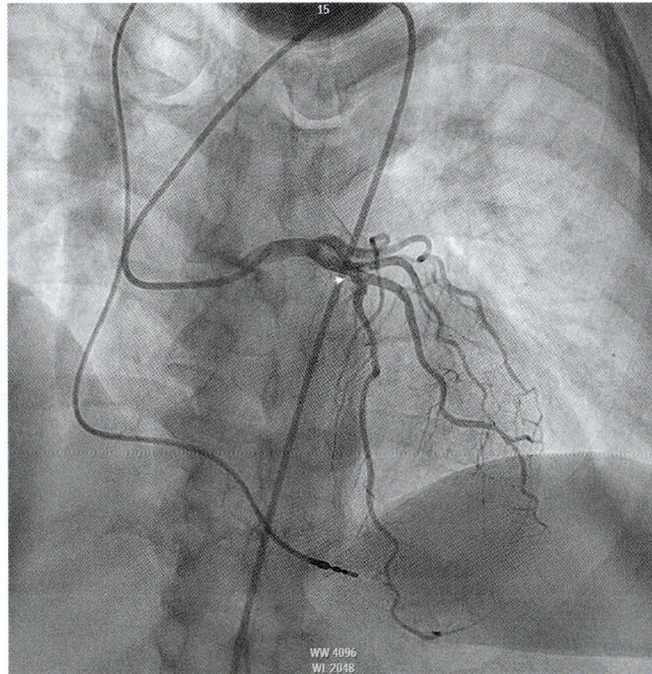

FIGURE 43.9 Final angiography post ablation. The stump of the ablated septal artery is visualized (*arrow*) indicating a successful septal ablation. Furthermore, patency of the LAD is noted without any evidence of injury. **Left:** RAO projection, **Right:** LAO projection.

Acute Procedural Success

Acute procedural success has been previously defined by a >50% reduction in peak LVOT gradient but is more commonly echo guided and based on opacification of the entirety of the offending septum, akinesis in that region, change in the gradient and waveform on echo, and ethanol amount infused, and several series demonstrate the procedural success of an initial ASA for gradient reduction to be as high as 85%.[12,13] Factors that favor procedural success include but are not limited to a predominantly focal basal septal hypertrophy and operator experience.

It is important to note that, due to the myocardial infarction created by the ethanol infusion, focal edema can lead to recrudescence of LVOT gradients in the short-term (1-3 days) post procedural period, so often medical management is continued until the post-ASA TTE is performed at 3 to 6 months after the procedure, which typically demonstrates the completed effects of the ablation (thinning of the septum and widening of the LVOT). Further remodeling and regression of myocardial hypertrophy, with concomitant improvement in diastolic dysfunction, can be seen up to 1 year after the procedure once the LVOT obstruction and intraventricular pressure overload is relieved and has been demonstrated using cardiac MRI.[14]

Temporary or complete AV block is the most common complication after septal ablation, which necessitates PPM placement. Several series report between an 8% and 15% rate of PPM implantation, often with a delayed presentation between the 24- and 96-hour period.[15,16] Heart block can also occur with less frequency after this period, and meticulous evaluation of the EKG can help determine which patients require longer monitoring prior to the decision regarding PPM placement. Risk factors for PPM include female sex, older age, preexisting left bundle branch block, or preexisting first-degree AV block.[9,10] For this reason, patients are observed with semipermanent fixed lead for at least 3 days, with frequent EKG assessment prior to removal. Other possible but rare complications of alcohol septal ablation are ventricular septal defect, tamponade, artery dissection, or myocardial infarction.

Symptom Improvement

ASA leads to a marked improvement in clinical symptomatology measured both subjectively by patient symptom questionnaires and objectively with treadmill exercise time and peak myocardial oxygen consumption. The determining factor of clinical efficacy is related to the reduction of LVOT obstruction, which as mentioned previously, can take up to 3 to 6 months for the full effect and results in continued improvements in diastolic dysfunction and associated mitral regurgitation.[17,18] Clinical improvements have been reported to be sustained in follow-up with effects remaining comparable with that of surgical septal reduction therapy (**Fig. 43.10**).[8,18-24] It is noteworthy that, for younger patients (defined as age <65 years), symptom relief may be greater with surgical myectomy. The reasons for this observation are not clear; however, it might be related to small residual gradients after ASA or higher gradients at baseline in a younger, more active individual. In addition, younger patients are more likely to have massive hypertrophy more amenable to surgical resection.

Survival

Early studies that compared septal ablation with surgical myectomy were limited by short-term follow-up of roughly 4 years. However meta-analyses of medium-term follow-up (~6 years) demonstrate outcomes comparable with those of surgical myectomy with no difference in sudden death or all-cause mortality.[18] In the Mayo Clinic experience (n = 177), survival at 8 years was comparable with that of patients with myectomy and to the expected survival for the US general population.[18] Since the publication of this paper, other series have also shown similar survival curves out to 10 years for both surgical myectomy and alcohol ablation, confirming these

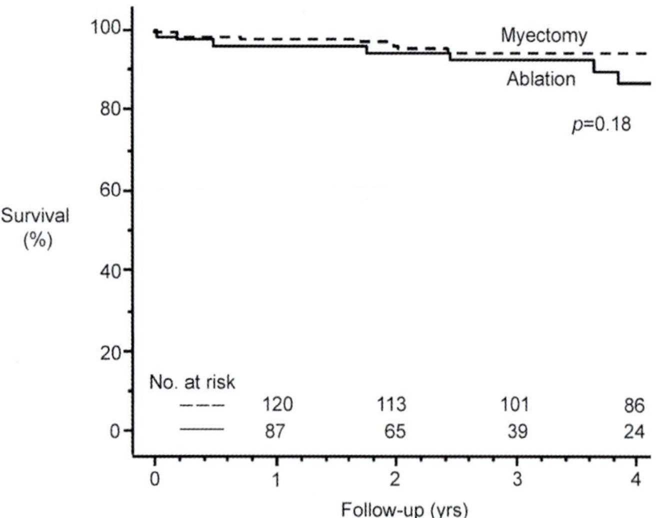

FIGURE 43.10 Comparison of survival after septal ablation with a matched cohort of surgical myectomy patients. The 4-year survival free of all mortality (including defibrillator discharge for lethal arrhythmia) among septal ablation patients was similar to that observed among age- and sex-matched patients who underwent isolated surgical myectomy. (Reprinted from Sorajja P, Valeti U, Nishimura RA, et al. Outcome of alcohol septal ablation for obstructive hypertrophic cardiomyopathy. *Circulation*. 2008;118:131-139, by permission from Lippincott Wilkins.)

benefits, with long-term follow-up of series up to 15 years demonstrating durability of ASA with maintenance of reduced gradients, symptom relief, and comparable outcomes for mortality.[8,21-24] ASA had previously been reserved for the elderly (defined as age >65 years); however, after several large European series demonstrated long-term safety and sustained effect of reduction in LVOT gradients with the average age of patient in their mid-50s, reservations regarding age have lessened.[8,21-26]

Key Points

- The dynamic nature of the LVOT obstruction in HCM is highly dependent on ventricular loading conditions, heart rate, and contractile state. Increases in contractility and decreases in either preload or afterload will lead to worsening of LVOT obstruction and symptoms.
- The dynamic LVOT obstruction is characterized by a "spike-and-dome" pattern in the aortic pressure waveform, with an exaggeration of this contour and subsequent decrease in aortic pulse pressure on the postectopic ventricular beat. Observation of this phenomenon is a key part of the invasive assessment of obstructive HCM (Brockenbrough-Braunwald maneuver).
- Negative inotropic and chronotropic agents are established cornerstones of drug therapy for symptomatic LVOT obstruction. Conversely, peripheral vasodilators, inotropes, and high-dose diuretics should be avoided.
- Mavacamten is a novel cardiomyocyte-specific inhibitor of myosin that has demonstrated in randomized controlled trials to improve NYHA functional status, reduce gradients, and delay or obviate need for SRT.
- Septal reduction therapy is the standard of therapy for symptomatic obstructive HCM refractory to medical therapy, and both surgical myectomy and alcohol septal ablation are class I indications.
- Surgical myectomy and ASA both can be utilized with equal success after a comprehensive evaluation at experienced centers. Both SRT techniques have success rates of >90% with procedural mortality of <1% (at experienced centers).
- Meticulous patient selection is essential to the acute and long-term outcome of alcohol septal ablation.
- The outcomes of alcohol septal ablation are similar to that of surgical myectomy in selected patients and, when performed in experienced centers, with low procedural mortality. The rate of pacemaker dependency after ablation is highly dependent on the baseline conduction abnormalities, age, and gender.

References

1. Gersh BJ, Maron BJ, Bonow RO, et al. 2011 ACCF/AHA guideline for the diagnosis and treatment of hypertrophic cardiomyopathy: a report of the American College of Cardiology Foundation/American Heart Association Task force on Practice guidelines. Developed in collaboration with the American association for Thoracic Surgery, American Society of Echocardiography, American Society of Nuclear Cardiology, Heart Failure Society of America, Heart Rhythm Society, Society for Cardiovascular angiography and interventions, and Society of Thoracic Surgeons. *J Am Coll Cardiol*. 2011;58(25):e212-e260.
2. Marian AJ, Braunwald E. Hypertrophic cardiomyopathy: genetics, pathogenesis, clinical manifestations, diagnosis, and therapy. *Circ Res*. 2017;121(7):749-770.
3. Spertus JA, Fine JT, Elliott P, et al. Mavacamten for treatment of symptomatic obstructive hypertrophic cardiomyopathy (EXPLORER-HCM): health status analysis of a randomised, double-blind, placebo-controlled, phase 3 trial. *Lancet*. 2021;397(10293):2467-2475.
4. Desai M, Owens A, Geske JB, et al. Myosin inhibition in patients with obstructive hypertrophic cardiomyopathy referred for septal reduction therapy. *J Am Coll Cardiol*. 2022;80(2):95-108.
5. Maron MS, Olivotto I, Betocchi S, et al. Effect of left ventricular outflow tract obstruction on clinical outcome in hypertrophic cardiomyopathy. *N Engl J Med*. 2003;348(4):295-303.
6. Ommen SR, Maron BJ, Olivotto I, et al. Long-term effects of surgical septal myectomy on survival in patients with obstructive hypertrophic cardiomyopathy. *J Am Coll Cardiol*. 2005;46(3):470-476.
7. Maron BJ, Dearani JA, Ommen SR, et al. The case for surgery in obstructive hypertrophic cardiomyopathy. *J Am Coll Cardiol*. 2004;44(10):2044-2053.
8. Kim LK, Swaminathan RV, Looser P, et al. Hospital volume outcomes after septal myectomy and alcohol septal ablation for treatment of obstructive hypertrophic cardiomyopathy: US nationwide inpatient database, 2003-2011. *JAMA Cardiol*. 2016;1(3):324-332.
9. Lam M, Kolte D, Kennedy K, et al. Incidence, timing, and predictors of permanent pacemaker placement following alcohol septal ablation for hypertrophic cardiomyopathy. *J Am Coll Cardiol*. 2019;73(9 suppl 1):1175.
10. Veselka J, Liebregts M, Cooper R, et al. Outcomes of patients with hypertrophic obstructive cardiomyopathy and pacemaker implanted after alcohol septal ablation. *JACC Cardiovasc Interv*. 2022;15(19):1910-1917.
11. Polin N, Feldman D, Naidu SS. Alcohol septal ablation for hypertrophic obstructive cardiomyopathy: novel application of the cutting balloon. *J Invasive Cardiol*. 2006;18(9):436-437.
12. Qin JX, Shiota T, Lever HM, et al. Outcome of patients with hypertrophic obstructive cardiomyopathy after percutaneous transluminal septal myocardial ablation and septal myectomy surgery. *J Am Coll Cardiol*. 2001;38(7):1994-2000.
13. Kwon DH, Kapadia SR, Tuzcu EM, et al. Long-term outcomes in high-risk symptomatic patients with hypertrophic cardiomyopathy undergoing alcohol septal ablation. *JACC Cardiovasc Interv*. 2008;1(4):432-438.
14. Van Dockum W, Beek AM, ten Cate FJ, et al. Early onset and progression of left ventricular remodeling after alcohol septal ablation in hypertrophic obstructive cardiomyopathy. *Circulation*. 2005;111(19):2503-2508.

15. Lam MC, Naidu SS, Kolte D, et al. Cardiac implantable electronic device placement following alcohol septal ablation for hypertrophic cardiomyopathy in the United States. *J Cardiovasc Electrophysiol*. 2020;31(10):2712-2719.
16. Kern MJ, Holmes DG, Simpson C, Bitar SR, Rajjoub H. Delayed occurrence of complete heart block without warning after alcohol septal ablation for hypertrophic obstructive cardiomyopathy. *Catheter Cardiovasc Interv*. 2002;56(4):503-507.
17. Nagueh SF, Ommen SR, Lakkis NM, et al. Comparison of ethanol septal reduction therapy with surgical myectomy for the treatment of hypertrophic obstructive cardiomyopathy. *J Am Coll Cardiol*. 2001;38(6):1701-1706.
18. Sorajja P, Ommen SR, Holmes DR Jr, et al. Survival after alcohol septal ablation for obstructive hypertrophic cardiomyopathy. *Circulation*. 2012;126(20):2374-2380.
19. Cuoco FA, Spencer WH III, Fernandes VL, et al. Implantable cardioverter-defibrillator therapy for primary prevention of sudden death after alcohol septal ablation of hypertrophic cardiomyopathy. *J Am Coll Cardiol*. 2008;52(21):1718-1723.
20. Ten Cate FJ, Soliman OII, Michels M, et al. Long-term outcome of alcohol septal ablation in patients with obstructive hypertrophic cardiomyopathy: a word of caution. *Circ Heart Fail*. 2010;3:362-369.
21. Liebregts M, Steggerda RC, Vriesendorp PA, et al. Long-term outcome of alcohol septal ablation for obstructive hypertrophic cardiomyopathy in the young and the elderly. *JACC Cardiovasc Interv*. 2016;9(5):463-469.
22. Nagueh SF, Groves BM, Schwartz L, et al. Alcohol septal ablation for the treatment of hypertrophic obstructive cardiomyopathy. A multicenter North American registry. *J Am Coll Cardiol*. 2011;58(22):2322-2328.
23. Ralph-Edwards A, Woo A, McCrindle BW, et al. Hypertrophic obstructive cardiomyopathy: comparison of outcomes after myectomy or alcohol ablation adjusted by propensity score. *J Thorac Cardiovasc Surg*. 2005;129(2):351-358.
24. Agarwal S, Tuzcu EM, Desai MY, et al. Updated meta-analysis of septal alcohol ablation versus myectomy for hypertrophic cardiomyopathy. *J Am Coll Cardiol*. 2010;55(8):823-834.
25. Liebregts M, Vriesendorp PA, Mahmoodi BK, Schinkel AFL, Michels M, ten Berg JM. A systematic review and meta-analysis of long-term outcomes after septal reduction therapy in patients with hypertrophic cardiomyopathy. *JACC Heart Fail*. 2015;3(11):896-905.
26. Osman M, Kheiri B, Osman K, et al. Alcohol septal ablation vs myectomy for symptomatic hypertrophic obstructive cardiomyopathy: systematic review and meta-analysis. *Clin Cardiol*. 2019;42(1):190-197.

Paravalvular Leaks

John T. Saxon and Adnan K. Chhatriwalla

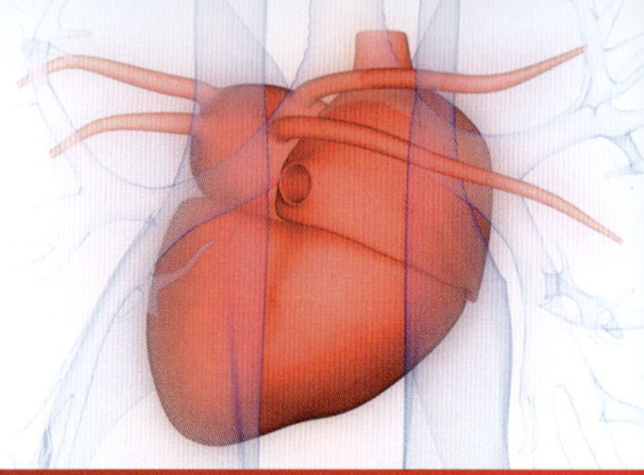

Paravalvular leak (PVL) is a common condition after prosthetic valve replacement wherein a residual gap persists between native tissue and the valve frame, allowing for regurgitant flow. PVL occurs in 5% to 17% of patients with surgical valve replacement and was even more common with early-generation transcatheter valves.[1-5] Although the incidence of PVL has been high following transcatheter aortic valve replacement (TAVR) historically, with improved sizing techniques and newer iterations of transcatheter valves, the incidence of moderate or severe PVL has improved substantially over time.[6-8] Common etiologies for PVL include tissue friability, annular calcification, and infection; an early occurrence of PVL after SAVR typically relates to technical aspects of the surgery. Both bioprosthetic and mechanical valves can be affected, and clinically significant PVL occurs most commonly in the mitral position (~5%), less commonly with aortic prostheses (~3%) and rarely with tricuspid or pulmonary prostheses. The rate of moderate or severe PVL after TAVR with modern transcatheter heart valves is less than 1%.[7,9] The clinical presentation is variable: patients with PVL may be asymptomatic, or they may have symptoms of heart failure, hemolytic anemia, or both. Significant PVL after transcatheter valve replacement has been associated with increased mortality.[10]

Medical therapy for PVL may be helpful to manage symptoms of congestive heart failure (CHF); however, medical therapy alone may not prevent the progression of symptoms or, in the case of hemolytic anemia, the need for repeated blood transfusions. While reoperation has traditionally been the standard of care for management of refractory symptoms, it is associated with increased morbidity and mortality compared with the index surgery and may be unsuccessful due to the underlying annular pathology predisposing to PVL.[11] For these reasons, transcatheter PVL closure has become the preferred approach in many centers. Importantly, catheter-based techniques permit a subsequent surgical attempt in the event of an unsuccessful outcome, if desired. Thus, transcatheter PVL closure is inherently attractive as a less invasive option. Procedural success with transcatheter PVL closure is high[12,13] and has a similar in-hospital survival compared with surgical repair.[14]

In the 2020 American Heart Association/American College of Cardiology guideline for the management of patients with valvular heart disease, transcatheter PVL closure is recommended as reasonable for high-risk surgical patients with severe CHF symptoms or refractory hemolysis and suitable anatomy, when performed at centers with expertise (class IIa recommendation).[15]

CLINICAL EVALUATION AND PATIENT SELECTION

Patients considered for transcatheter PVL closure require a comprehensive, multidisciplinary evaluation with a Heart Team approach, including collaboration between the cardiologist, interventional cardiologist, cardiac surgeon, and imaging specialists. Surgical consultation with objective assessment of operative risk, including use of the Society of Thoracic Surgeons risk calculator, is essential. Although patients' reoperative risk will be increased relative to their initial surgery, this may not be prohibitive in selected patients. All patients with PVL should be evaluated for both hemolytic anemia and endocarditis, even when the index of suspicion is low. Hemolytic anemia is unlikely to resolve unless the PVL is completely closed, which is an important factor in considering management. Active endocarditis is a contraindication to transcatheter PVL closure.

Echocardiography is the primary imaging modality for the evaluation of PVL. PVL is most commonly diagnosed with transthoracic echocardiography (TTE), including color Doppler interrogation; however, in some cases, acoustic shadowing and location of the PVL may render imaging suboptimal. Transesophageal echocardiography (TEE), particularly when paired with three-dimensional echo reconstruction, is essential in characterizing morphology as well as determining the precise location and size of the PVL jet, particularly in the mitral position with the three-dimensional "surgeon's view"[14] (**Fig. 44.1**). As an adjunct to echocardiography, cardiac computed tomography (CT) imaging is quite useful, particularly in determining the size and location of the defect with precision and reconstructing optimal imaging angles for the catheterization laboratory when PVL closure is attempted. In some advanced catheterization laboratories, CT "fusion" imaging may also be used to guide the procedure and enhance the success of transcatheter closure.

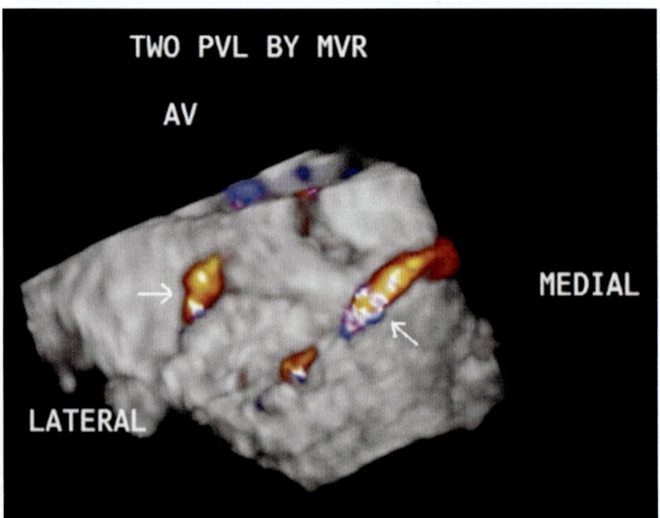

FIGURE 44.1 A three-dimensional transesophageal echocardiography (TEE) image depicting two paravalvular defects around a mechanical mitral prosthesis. This is the so-called surgeons' view, with the aortic valve above (anterior to) the mitral valve, the atrial septum to the right of (medial to) the valve, and the left atrial appendage to the left of (lateral to) the valve. AV, aortic valve; MVR, mitral valve replacement; PVL, paravalvular leak.

Of note, while criteria for echocardiographic quantification of valvular regurgitation are well established, the criteria for quantification of PVL are not as well understood.[16-18] Furthermore, patients with PVL can have symptoms out of proportion to the severity of regurgitation, as assessed by conventional standards. Cardiac magnetic resonance imaging can be beneficial in assessing regurgitant volume, particularly for patients with equivocal echocardiographic findings.[19] For symptomatic patients with inconclusive noninvasive studies, a detailed invasive hemodynamic assessment and aortography or ventriculography may be considered. Even defects that are not quantitatively severe can be hemodynamically significant and may benefit from therapy; thus, direct measurement of intracardiac filling pressures may provide insight. In each case, clinical judgment must be exercised regarding the severity of PVL and the likelihood of associated symptoms, with the decision to pursue treatment individualized for all patients.

Despite the advantages of transcatheter PVL closure, some strict contraindications remain. Patients with active endocarditis, annular dehiscence (a rocking prosthesis), significant valvular regurgitation, or a paravalvular defect comprising >1/3 of the annular circumference should not be treated with transcatheter repair.[20,21]

PROCEDURAL TECHNIQUES

Device Occluders

In the United States, transcatheter PVL closure requires off-label use of vascular occluders. The most commonly used devices are the Amplatzer (Abbott Vascular, Abbott Park, IL) family of vascular plugs (AVP) and duct occluders (ADO). These devices are made of self-expanding nitinol, deliverable through small-caliber catheters, and have retention disks to help reduce the risk of embolization after deployment (**Fig. 44.2**). The AVP-2, AVP-4, and ADO II devices are circular in shape and are available for use in the United States.

The Amplatzer Valvular Plug 3 (AVP-3) is a purpose-built PVL closure device available in Europe and currently under investigational use in the United States (**Fig. 44.2**). The AVP-3 has the advantage of an oval shape, which approximates the shape of most PVL defects, as well as a tighter wire mesh, allowing the device to seal more quickly. The AVP-3 is the most frequently used PVL closure device in Europe, comprising >60% of cases in the largest published series to date.[12]

Other devices include the Amplatzer muscular ventricular septal defect occluder, which requires relatively larger sheaths for delivery, and the Occlutech PLD (Helsingborg, Sweden), which is specifically designed for transcatheter PVL closure but only available in Europe. These devices have a larger delivery profile and larger pores, which may result in suboptimal sealing.[12] Accommodation of occluder devices within delivery catheters with or without wires is not described well in the manufacturers' labeling; however, as transcatheter PVL closure has become more prominent, descriptive tables have been published that may help to facilitate the selection of equipment for the procedure.[22]

Aortic PVL

For patients with aortic PVL, the most common approach for transcatheter closure is retrograde via the femoral artery (**Fig. 44.3**). The echocardiographic imaging modality may be selected based on the location of the defect and the need to minimize acoustic shadowing of the regurgitant jet (TEE for posterior defects; TTE for anterior defects). Intracardiac echocardiography can also be performed from the right atrium, and manipulation of the catheter into the right ventricular outflow tract may provide additional imaging details.

Imaging angles in the catheterization laboratory should be obtained such that no overlap is observed between the defect and the aortic prosthesis, to ensure that the guidewire is being passed into the defect external to the prosthesis. This positioning can be approximated (eg, left anterior oblique cranial for posterior defects; right anterior oblique caudal for anterior defects) or accurately determined from CT imaging. In biplane laboratories, the additional camera can be positioned *en face* to help with external placement of the wire, although this view is not required.

The defect is approached with a coronary guide catheter, and an angled-tip, exchange-length hydrophilic wire is placed through the defect and can be passed antegrade through a bioprosthetic aortic valve in the event that a guidewire rail is desired. A delivery catheter is then advanced over the wire into the left ventricle. Selection of the delivery catheter is dependent on (1) the size and number of device occluders needed, (2) the difficulty encountered in crossing the defect, and (3) the need for an anchor wire. With the delivery catheter in the left ventricle, the device occluder is extruded with retention disks positioned on the ventricular and aortic sides of the defect or, as frequently with AVP-4 plugs, wholly within the defect. Serial occluders can be placed over the anchor wire (if utilized)

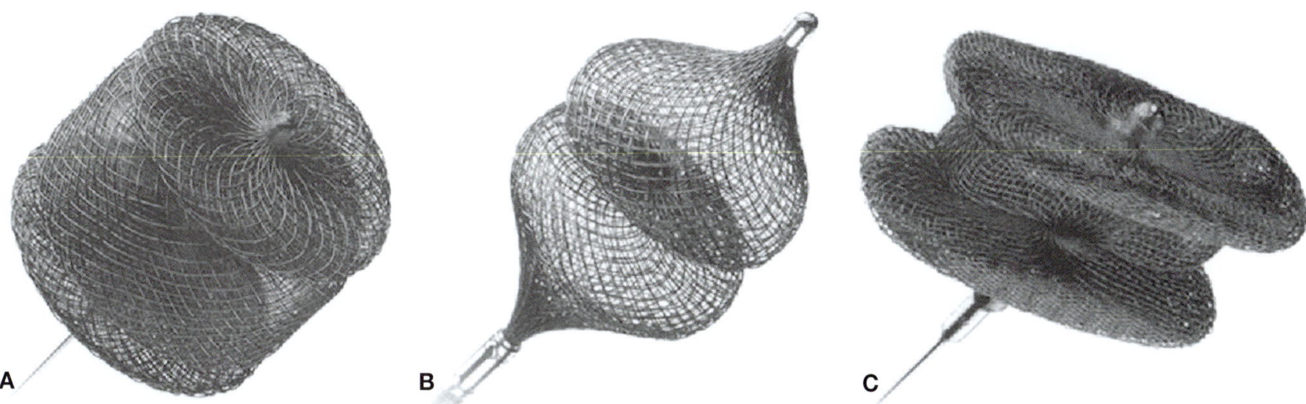

FIGURE 44.2 **A:** Amplatzer Vascular Plug 2 (AVP-2). **B:** Amplatzer Vascular Plug 4 (AVP-4). **C:** Amplatzer Valvular Plug 3 (AVP-3).

or by recrossing the defect adjacent to the deployed device(s). The final assessment must include evaluation for prosthetic leaflet impingement, residual regurgitation, and coronary occlusion. Coronary angiography should be considered in patients requiring large device occluders, and those with small aortic sinuses, low coronary height, or defects located near the coronary ostia, to exclude coronary occlusion. Once the final assessment is satisfactory, the device occluders are released.

Mitral PVL

Transcatheter mitral PVL closure is typically performed with general anesthesia and three-dimensional TEE. Femoral venous access is obtained to permit transseptal puncture, then antegrade cannulation of the defect from the left atrium. Alternatively, direct transapical puncture or a retrograde approach (via the femoral artery) with retrograde cannulation of the defect from the left ventricle also can be successful.[22-24]

For the antegrade approach, standard transseptal technique with guidance from fluoroscopy and echocardiography is used to access the left atrium and approach the defect. A steerable transeptal catheter (eg, Agilis, Abbott Vascular, Minneapolis, MN) is loaded with a telescoped catheter system, eg, a 6-Fr 100-cm multipurpose guide and a 5-Fr 125-cm multipurpose diagnostic catheter (**Fig. 44.4**). A steerable guide with a small-sized curve may be particularly helpful for medial defects. This system is steered toward the defect, which is crossed with a hydrophilic wire. Fluoroscopy should demonstrate positioning of the steerable guide and the guidewires external to the prosthesis ring. The telescoped catheters are placed sequentially into the left ventricle, followed by removal of the diagnostic catheter. A device occluder can be

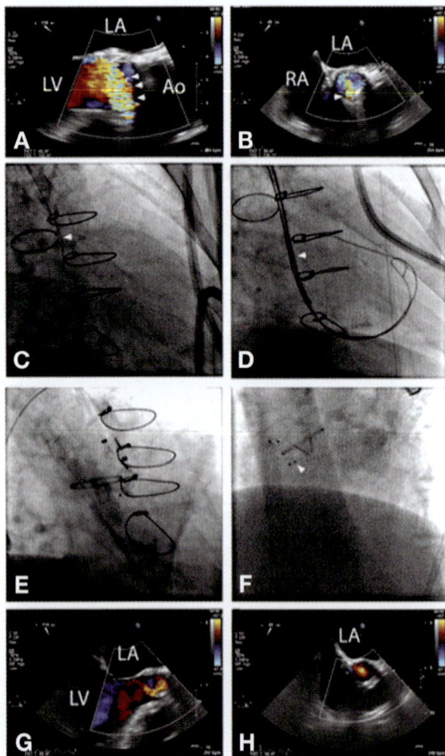

FIGURE 44.3 Transcatheter aortic PVL closure (**A** and **B**) TEE imaging demonstrating PVL (*arrowheads*). **C:** The defect is crossed with a hydrophilic wire (*arrowhead*). **D:** A guide catheter is advanced over the wire to the LV, and the hydrophilic wire is exchanged for two stiff wires. **E:** A delivery catheter is advanced separately over each wire to the LV, and two device occluders are positioned in the defect. **F:** The devices are deployed and released (*arrowhead* marking the ventricular retention disks). **G** and **H:** TEE imaging demonstrates resolution after PVL closure. Ao, ascending aorta; LA, left atrium; LV, left ventricle; PVL, paravalvular leak; RA, right atrium; TEE, transesophageal echocardiography.

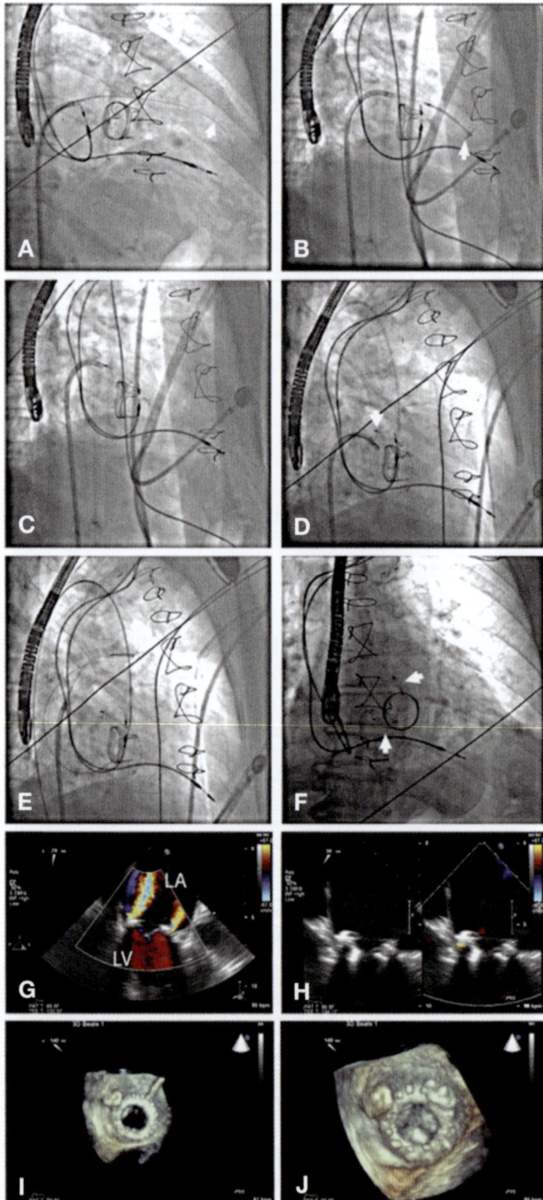

FIGURE 44.4 Transcatheter mitral PVL closure. **A:** A lateral defect is crossed with a hydrophilic wire (*arrow*). **B:** A delivery catheter is advanced over the wire to the LV, and a device occluder is advanced to the LV. The *arrow* indicates the distal retention disk in the LV. **C:** The device is positioned across the defect and further unsheathed. **D:** The device is released with the proximal retention disk positioned on the left atrial side of the defect (*arrow*). **E:** A medial defect is crossed in retrograde fashion with a hydrophilic wire from the LV and snared in the LA to form a guidewire rail. **F:** Two occluder devices are deployed in the medial defect using the guidewire rail. *Arrows* indicate the lateral and medial devices. **G:** TEE imaging demonstrating medial and lateral jets of PVL prior to closure. **H:** TEE imaging demonstrating trivial residual PVL medially and none laterally. **I:** Three-dimensional TEE imaging demonstrating the deployed lateral occluder device and a catheter crossing the medial defect. **J:** Three-dimensional TEE imaging demonstrating device deployment in both the lateral and medial defects. LA, left atrium; LV, left ventricle; PVL, paravalvular leak; TEE, transesophageal echocardiography.

passed through the guide catheter or exchanged over a stiff wire for a larger sheath, depending on the size and number of device occluders needed and the need for an anchor wire. Similar to treatment of aortic defects, the distal retention disk of the occluder is extruded from the guide into the left ventricle, followed by straddling of the defect with the retention disks on both sides. Serial occluders can be placed over the anchor wire (if utilized) or by recrossing the defect adjacent to the deployed device(s). Once leaflet impingement has been excluded on both echocardiography and fluoroscopy, the device occluder is released.

In the retrograde approach from the femoral artery, a coronary catheter is placed into the left ventricle and oriented posteriorly toward the defect. This technique can be used when the transseptal approach is not successful, especially if the defect is located medially. The defect can be crossed with relatively softer wires, such as 0.014-inch or 0.018-inch coronary guidewires, if needed. In the transapical technique, defect cannulation and device placement is similar to the antegrade approach.

PVL After TAVR

PVL occurs more frequently after TAVR than surgical aortic valve replacement (SAVR).[6,10] However, although the incidence of PVL has been historically high after TAVR, with improved annular sizing techniques and newer iterations of transcatheter valves, rates of moderate or severe PVL have been reduced substantially.[6-8] PVL closure after TAVR has thus been less common in case series than treatment of patients with surgical mitral or aortic valves.[12] Closure of TAVR PVL may be challenging, as the native valve leaflets are adjacent to the TAVR valve frame and the etiology of residual PVL is most commonly excess annular calcification, which may encumber catheters advancement through the defect. Furthermore, the TAVR stent frame may be higher profile compared with a surgical valve, resulting in additional complexity wiring the defect as well as obstruction to catheter advancement. Closure of post-TAVR PVL is approached in the same fashion as post-SAVR PVL: retrograde wiring of the defect followed by catheter advancement and deployment of the PVL closure device (**Fig. 44.5**).

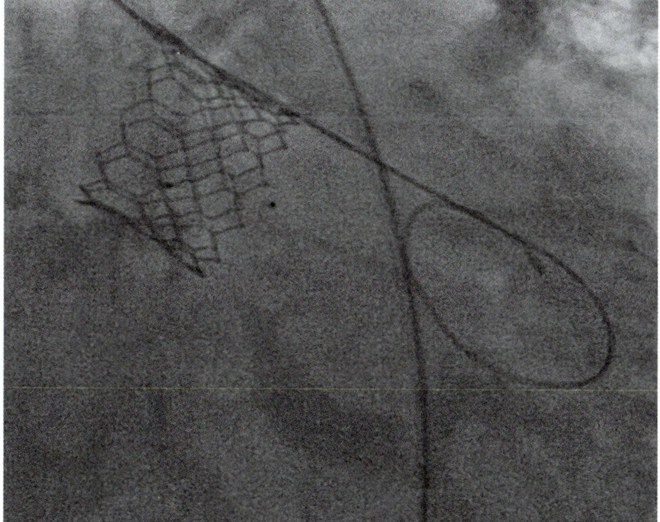

FIGURE 44.5 PVL closure after TAVR. Closure of an aortic PVL after TAVR with a Sapien 3 prosthesis. A stiff guidewire is advanced across the defect with a gentle ventricular curve to prevent injury to the left ventricle. A previously placed Amplatzer Vascular Plug 4 (AVP-4) can be seen in a separate defect.

The AVP series of plugs (AVP-2, AVP-4, Abbot Vascular) are the optimal devices for this purpose. Specifically, the AVP-4 has the advantage of a lower crossing profile and a tighter mesh weave, as well as compatibility with any catheter that can accommodate a 0.035″ wire.

Transcatheter Rails

Advancement of catheters through a paravalvular defect can be challenging, since the defects are often serpiginous and may be calcified. In these instances, transcatheter rails can be utilized for greater support for catheter passage.

Originally described for the treatment of congenital heart lesions, transcatheter rails are created by snaring of a guidewire that has been placed across the paravalvular defect, followed by exteriorization to provide the operator with control of both ends of the wire. For mitral paravalvular defects, a transcatheter rail can be placed left atrial–ventricular–aortic or left atrial–ventricular–apical. For aortic paravalvular defects, the rail can be placed aortic–ventricular–aortic, aortic–ventricular–apical, or left atrial–ventricular–aortic. Once the rail has been created, the operator can advance a guide catheter with support from an assistant who provides tension on both ends of the wire.

Guidewire tension from transcatheter rails can result in injury to the surrounding structures, damage to the prosthetic or native leaflets, as well as myocardial injury, atrioventricular node injury and resultant bradycardia, or disruption of the mitral valve apparatus from chordal entanglement. Therefore, transcatheter heart rails should only be utilized by experienced operators and with careful hemodynamic monitoring and simultaneous echocardiography.

Multiple Device Placement and Anchor Wiring

Paravalvular defects frequently are eccentric and in close proximity to the surgical sewing ring. As a result, successful closure can be challenging with the use of large occluders, because device overhang can result in leaflet impingement of the valve, particularly with mechanical prostheses. An alternative strategy is use of multiple, smaller-device occluders deployed using an anchor wire technique. After the defect is crossed with a hydrophilic guidewire, a larger-bore sheath is placed into the ventricle. The sheath can accommodate multiple, stiff guidewires that can then be used to place the delivery catheters either simultaneously or sequentially over each wire. The anchor wire technique is also useful for maintaining a position across the paravalvular defect in the event that an occluder needs to be exchanged for different or multiple other devices. If anchor wiring is used, large-bore sheaths are required at the arterial or venous access site to accommodate the multiple delivery catheters and wires. The DrySeal sheath (W.L. Gore, Flagstaff, AZ), with its inflatable cuff, is uniquely suited for maintaining hemostasis for this purpose.

CT Guidance

Cardiac CT can identify paravalvular defects and assist with transcatheter PVL closure. Using information from echocardiography, the CT scan is reconstructed using views of the exit point of the regurgitant jet, whose paravalvular continuity can then be examined (**Fig. 44.6**). Imaging with CT can help with sizing of the defect and identifying its course, and can provide information on surrounding calcification. The information gained from CT imaging

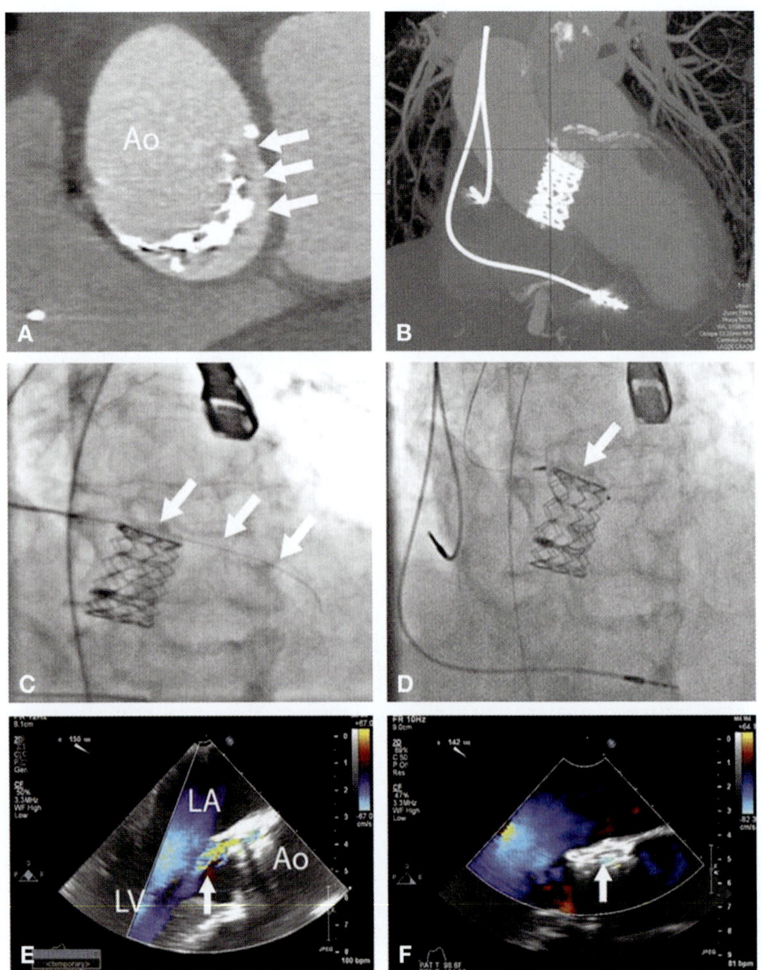

FIGURE 44.6 CT guidance for transcatheter PVL closure. **A:** CT imaging identifies the paravalvular defect (*arrows*). **B:** CT imaging aligns the defect exterior to the prosthesis, providing catheterization laboratory camera angles to facilitate the procedure. **C:** Using the camera angle provided by CT, the defect is easily wired (*arrows*). **D:** A device occluder is deployed in the paravalvular defect (*arrow*). **E:** TEE imaging demonstrating severe paravalvular regurgitation prior to transcatheter PVL closure (*arrow*). **F:** TEE imaging demonstrating mild residual paravalvular regurgitation after transcatheter PVL closure (*arrow*). Ao, aorta; CT, computed tomography; LA, left artery; LV, left ventricle; PVL, paravalvular leak; TEE, transesophageal echocardiography.

may be of particular benefit when there is significant acoustic shadowing on echocardiography.

Fusion CT imaging can also be used to facilitate transcatheter PVL closure. In this technique, CT data are coregistered to cardiac structures (ie, chambers, valves, coronary arteries), enabling overlay onto the fluoroscopy screen. Fusion CT imaging is then used to guide access (transseptal antegrade vs retrograde apical), defect wiring, and device placement.[25]

CLINICAL OUTCOMES

Transcatheter PVL closure was first described over 25 years ago, and interest in this therapy has greatly increased in the last decade.[24] Procedural success in achieving no more than a mild residual leak is approximately 80%, with reduction to moderate or less residual regurgitation in over 90% of cases.[12,13,26] Complications are relatively infrequent. A series of patients[13] reported the following adverse events at 30 days: stroke (2.6%), emergency surgery (0.9%), sudden or unexplained death (1.7%), periprocedural bleeding (5.2%), and device embolization (2.5%). Procedural death is uncommon (~0.5). Coronary artery occlusion is another potential concern in aortic PVL closure and is dependent on the height of the coronary arteries and the location of the defect. New-onset hemolysis requiring transfusion as a consequence of closure has been reported in a minority (1.6%) of patients.[12] Symptomatic improvement following closure is common, with a mean improvement of 1.1 New York Heart Association (NYHA) functional class (baseline 2.7 ± 0.8 vs 1.6 ± 0.8 at follow-up).[12]

The most common reasons for procedural failure are prosthetic leaflet impingement and the inability to cross the defect with a wire or delivery catheter. The rate of leaflet impingement ranges from 5% to 7% and can occur with any prosthesis but is more common in mechanical valves due to the absence of valve struts. The circular shape of some AVP occluders and the close proximity of the defect to the surgical annular ring increase the likelihood of impingement, which can be minimized by using multiple, smaller devices if necessary. Prior to device release, careful assessment using echo, fluoroscopy, and hemodynamics is required to assess leaflet motion and valve gradient. Release of tension on the device after final release can shift the occluder; thus, leaflet impingement should be reassessed after final deployment.

In a long-term evaluation of 126 patients who underwent transcatheter PVL closure, the 3-year survival was 64% (**Fig. 44.7**).[27] Cardiac death occurred in 9.5%, while the incidence of noncardiac death was between 7.1% and 12.7%, indicating the high-risk nature of this patient population. Notably, 72% of survivors were free of severe symptoms or the need for surgical reintervention. Clinical success and relief of symptoms have been shown to be related to the degree of residual regurgitation and are greater for patients with symptoms of CHF than for those with hemolysis (**Fig. 44.7**).[27] Importantly, the NYHA functional class has been demonstrated to improve only in those patients with less than or equal to a mild residual leak. On the other hand, successful treatment of hemolysis ideally requires complete closure of the paravalvular defect. In addition, operator experience with advanced closure techniques (eg, anchor wire, three-dimensional imaging, transcatheter rails) is an important predictor of procedural success (**Fig. 44.8**).[28]

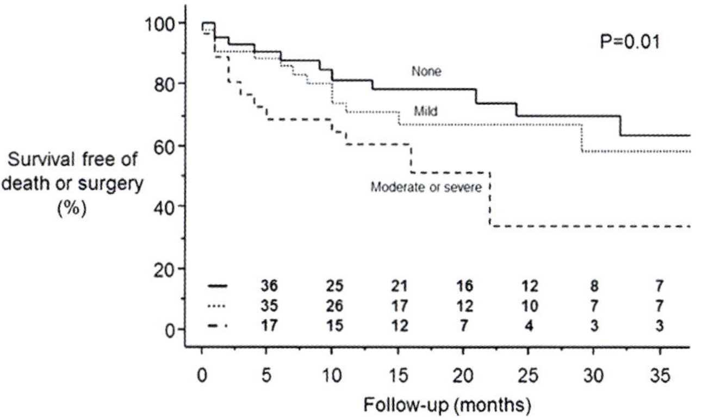

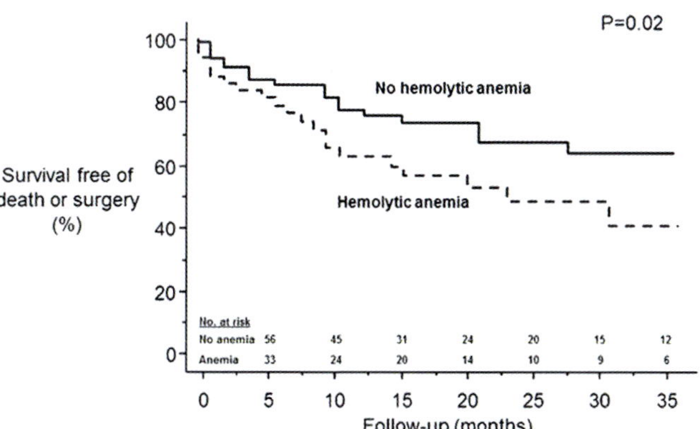

FIGURE 44.7 Survival after transcatheter PVL closure. **Top:** Survival free of death or reoperation according to residual PVL following transcatheter PVL closure. **Bottom:** Survival free of death or reoperation according to the presence or absence of hemolytic anemia. PVL, paravalvular leak. (From Sorajja P, Cabalka AK, Hagler DJ, Rihal CS. Long-term follow-up of percutaneous repair of paravalvular regurgitation. *J Am Coll Cardiol*. 2011;58:2218-2224.)

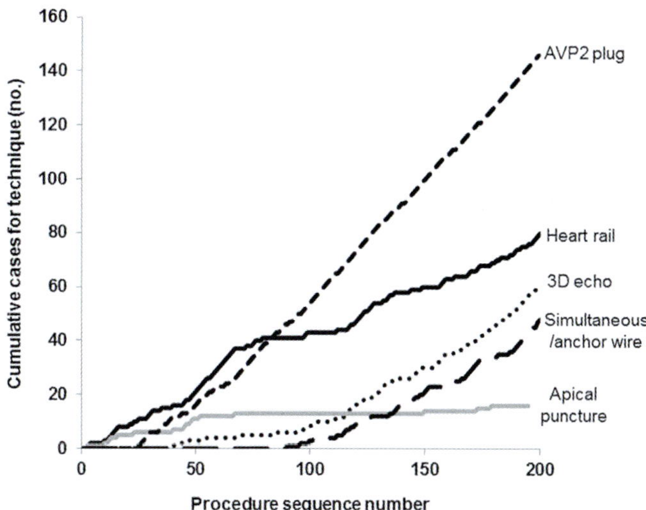

FIGURE 44.8 Adoption of procedural techniques for transcatheter PVL closure at a single center. The graph depicts the cumulative experience with each technique over a series of 200 cases. AVP, Amplatzer Vascular Plug; PVL, paravalvular leak closure. (From Sorajja P, Cabalka AK, Hagler DJ, Rihal CS. The learning curve in percutaneous repair of paravalvular prosthetic regurgitation: an analysis of 200 cases. *JACC Cardiovasc Interv*. 2014;7:521-529.)

Key Points

- PVL after surgical valve replacement is relatively common and may be related to tissue friability, annular calcification, or infection.
- PVL may result in hemolysis, CHF, or both.
- Transcatheter PVL closure is indicated for patients with severe CHF symptoms or refractory hemolysis who are at high risk for reoperation, if their anatomy is suitable.
- Procedural success of transcatheter PVL closure may be as high as 90% through antegrade and retrograde approaches; however, potential complications include bleeding, stroke, valve leaflet impingement, and device embolization.
- Transcatheter PVL closure should be performed at experienced centers using both three-dimensional echocardiographic and fluoroscopic guidance.

References

1. Akins CW, Bitondo JM, Hilgenberg AD, Vlahakes GJ, Madsen JC, MacGillivray TE. Early and late results of the surgical correction of cardiac prosthetic paravalvular leaks. *J Heart Valve Dis*. 2005;14(6):792-800; discussion 9-800.
2. Davila-Roman VG, Waggoner AD, Kennard ED, et al, Artificial Valve Endocarditis Reduction Trial echocardiography study. Prevalence and severity of paravalvular regurgitation in the Artificial Valve Endocarditis Reduction Trial (AVERT) echocardiography study. *J Am Coll Cardiol*. 2004;44(7):1467-1472.
3. Hwang HY, Choi JW, Kim HK, Kim KH, Kim KB, Ahn H. Paravalvular leak after mitral valve replacement: 20-year follow-up. *Ann Thorac Surg*. 2015;100(4):1347-1352.
4. Miller DL, Morris JJ, Schaff HV, Mullany CJ, Nishimura RA, Orszulak TA. Reoperation for aortic valve periprosthetic leakage: identification of patients at risk and results of operation. *J Heart Valve Dis*. 1995;4(2):160-165.

5. Genereux P, Head SJ, Hahn R, et al. Paravalvular leak after transcatheter aortic valve replacement: the new Achilles' heel? A comprehensive review of the literature. *J Am Coll Cardiol*. 2013;61(11):1125-1136.
6. Leon MB, Smith CR, Mack MJ, et al, PARTNER 2 Investigators. Transcatheter or surgical aortic-valve replacement in intermediate-risk patients. *N Engl J Med*. 2016;374(17):1609-1620.
7. Mack MJ, Leon MB, Thourani VH, et al, PARTNER 3 Investigators. Transcatheter aortic-valve replacement with a balloon-expandable valve in low-risk patients. *N Engl J Med*. 2019;380(18):1695-1705.
8. Popma JJ, Deeb GM, Yakubov SJ, et al, Evolut Low Risk Trial Investigators. Transcatheter aortic-valve replacement with a self-expanding valve in low-risk patients. *N Engl J Med*. 2019;380(18):1706-1715.
9. Popma JJ, Reardon MJ. Transcatheter aortic-valve replacement in low-risk patients. Reply. *N Engl J Med*. 2019;381(7):685.
10. Kodali SK, Williams MR, Smith CR, et al, PARTNER Trial Investigators. Two-year outcomes after transcatheter or surgical aortic-valve replacement. *N Engl J Med*. 2012;366(18):1686-1695.
11. Orszulak TA, Schaff HV, Danielson GK, Pluth JR, Puga FJ, Piehler JM. Results of reoperation for periprosthetic leakage. *Ann Thorac Surg*. 1983;35(6):584-589.
12. Calvert PA, Northridge DB, Malik IS, et al. Percutaneous device closure of paravalvular leak: combined experience from the United Kingdom and Ireland. *Circulation*. 2016;134(13):934-944.
13. Sorajja P, Cabalka AK, Hagler DJ, Rihal CS. Percutaneous repair of paravalvular prosthetic regurgitation: acute and 30-day outcomes in 115 patients. *Circ Cardiovasc Interv*. 2011;4(4):314-321.
14. Wells JA, Condado JF, Kamioka N, et al. Outcomes after paravalvular leak closure: transcatheter versus surgical approaches. *JACC Cardiovasc Interv*. 2017;10(5):500-507.
15. Otto CM, Nishimura RA, Bonow RO, et al. 2020 ACC/AHA guideline for the management of patients with valvular heart disease. Executive summary: a report of the American College of Cardiology/American Heart Association Joint Committee on Clinical Practice Guidelines. *Circulation*. 2021;143(5):e35-e71.
16. Kappetein AP, Head SJ, Genereux P, et al. Updated standardized endpoint definitions for transcatheter aortic valve implantation: the Valve Academic Research Consortium-2 consensus document. *J Am Coll Cardiol*. 2012;60(15):1438-1454.
17. Zoghbi WA, Chambers JB, Dumesnil JG, et al, American Society of Echocardiography's Guidelines and Standards Committee, Task Force on Prosthetic Valves, American College of Cardiology Cardiovascular Imaging Committee, Cardiac Imaging Committee of the American Heart Association, European Association of Echocardiography, European Society of Cardiology, Japanese Society of Echocardiography, Canadian Society of Echocardiography, American College of Cardiology Foundation, American Heart Association, European Association of Echocardiography, European Society of Cardiology, Japanese Society of Echocardiography, Canadian Society of Echocardiography. Recommendations for evaluation of prosthetic valves with echocardiography and Doppler ultrasound: a report from the American Society of Echocardiography's Guidelines and Standards Committee and the Task Force on Prosthetic Valves, developed in conjunction with the American College of Cardiology Cardiovascular Imaging Committee, Cardiac Imaging Committee of the American Heart Association, the European Association of Echocardiography, a registered branch of the European Society of Cardiology, the Japanese Society of Echocardiography and the Canadian Society of Echocardiography, endorsed by the American College of Cardiology Foundation, American Heart Association, European Association of Echocardiography, a registered branch of the European Society of Cardiology, the Japanese Society of Echocardiography, and Canadian Society of Echocardiography. *J Am Soc Echocardiogr*. 2009;22(9):975-1084; quiz 82-4.
18. Zoghbi WA, Enriquez-Sarano M, Foster E, et al, American Society of Echocardiography. Recommendations for evaluation of the severity of native valvular regurgitation with two-dimensional and Doppler echocardiography. *J Am Soc Echocardiogr*. 2003;16(7):777-802.
19. Ribeiro HB, Le Ven F, Larose E, et al. Cardiac magnetic resonance versus transthoracic echocardiography for the assessment and quantification of aortic regurgitation in patients undergoing transcatheter aortic valve implantation. *Heart*. 2014;100(24):1924-1932.
20. Eleid MF, Cabalka AK, Malouf JF, Sanon S, Hagler DJ, Rihal CS. Techniques and outcomes for the treatment of paravalvular leak. *Circ Cardiovasc Interv*. 2015;8(8):e001945.
21. Sorajja P. Mitral paravalvular leak closure. *Interv Cardiol Clin*. 2016;5(1):45-54.
22. Gossl M, Rihal CS. Percutaneous treatment of aortic and mitral valve paravalvular regurgitation. *Curr Cardiol Rep*. 2013;15(8):388.
23. Ruiz CE, Hahn RT, Berrebi A, et al, Paravalvular Leak Academic Research Consortium. Clinical trial principles and endpoint definitions for paravalvular leaks in surgical prosthesis: an expert statement. *J Am Coll Cardiol*. 2017;69(16):2067-2087.
24. Hourihan M, Perry SB, Mandell VS, et al. Transcatheter umbrella closure of valvular and paravalvular leaks. *J Am Coll Cardiol*. 1992;20(6):1371-1377.
25. Kliger C, Jelnin V, Sharma S, et al. CT angiography-fluoroscopy fusion imaging for percutaneous transapical access. *JACC Cardiovasc Imaging*. 2014;7(2):169-177.
26. Ruiz CE, Jelnin V, Kronzon I, et al. Clinical outcomes in patients undergoing percutaneous closure of periprosthetic paravalvular leaks. *J Am Coll Cardiol*. 2011;58(21):2210-2217.
27. Sorajja P, Cabalka AK, Hagler DJ, Rihal CS. Long-term follow-up of percutaneous repair of paravalvular prosthetic regurgitation. *J Am Coll Cardiol*. 2011;58(21):2218-2224.
28. Sorajja P, Cabalka AK, Hagler DJ, Rihal CS. The learning curve in percutaneous repair of paravalvular prosthetic regurgitation: an analysis of 200 cases. *JACC Cardiovasc Interv*. 2014;7(5):521-529.

Pericardial Disease Interventions

Jayant Bagai

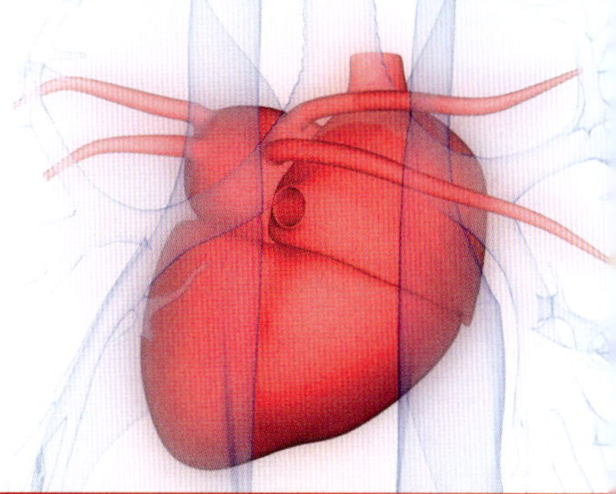

Interventional and invasive cardiologists are frequently required to assess and treat patients with acute and chronic pericardial conditions. The normal pericardial sac, with up to 50 mL of fluid, lies between the tough fibrous parietal pericardium and a thin serous pericardium (the latter is folded upon itself, with one of its two layers adherent to the heart, forming the epicardium, and the other fused with the parietal pericardium). The proximal segments of the great vessels are intrapericardial while most of the left atrium is extrapericardial. Pericardial disease processes, classified into inflammatory, infectious, malignant, metabolic, and traumatic, commonly result in a pathological increase in pericardial fluid and/or thickening. As the pericardial sac is usually a closed space, the end result is a restraining effect on the physiological filling of the heart. This chapter will focus on the diagnosis and management of cardiac tamponade in the cardiac catheterization laboratory.

DIAGNOSIS OF CARDIAC TAMPONADE

Cardiac tamponade develops when the (usually large and circumferential) accumulation of pericardial fluid increases the normally low (−5 to 5 mm Hg) intrapericardial pressure such that it restricts the preload of the right heart. Impaired diastolic filling of the right heart in turn decreases left heart filling with a reduction in cardiac output. It is important to understand that the rapidity of accumulation is as important as the volume of fluid in the sac. Tamponade can result in the rapid accumulation of about 100 to 200 mL of fluid, as seen in traumatic injuries. The most common etiologies in developed countries are idiopathic (presumed viral), malignant, and iatrogenic, related to invasive cardiac procedures. Myocarditis accompanies pericarditis in approximately 15% of cases with elevation of cardiac biomarkers and EKG changes and can therefore be mistaken for acute coronary syndrome. Pericardial infections (bacterial and HIV), bleeding, and neoplastic processes have a high risk of progressing to tamponade, even when initially small.

When the pericardium is stretched beyond its elastic limits, it resists further stretch causing the pressure inside the pericardial sac to rise and be transmitted to the cardiac chambers. The restraining effect of the normal pericardium and its contribution to diastolic interaction between the right and left ventricles (LVs) also increase as the total cardiac volume increases.[1] These physical principles underlie the classic hemodynamic findings in cardiac tamponade, which are summarized in **Table 45.1**. **Fig. 45.1** and **45.2** show right atrial, left ventricular, and aortic tracings in cardiac tamponade.

PERICARDIOCENTESIS

Indications

Pericardiocentesis is typically reserved for relief of actual or threatened cardiac tamponade or a large effusion persistent for >3 months and unresponsive to medical therapy. It is generally not indicated for small- to moderate-sized effusions given its low diagnostic yield, spontaneous resolution in most cases of viral (idiopathic) pericarditis (the most common etiology), and higher procedural risk than with other diagnostic modalities.[2]

Absolute Contraindications

Needle pericardiocentesis is generally contraindicated in patients with ascending aortic dissection or ventricular rupture from trauma or post-myocardial infarction (MI) due to the risk of triggering uncontrollable and recurrent bleeding.[2]

TABLE 45.1 Summary of Hemodynamic Findings in Cardiac Tamponade

FINDING	MECHANISM	COMMENTS
Blunted y descent in RA waveform	Reduced early RV diastolic filling	Concept of fixed total heart volume (blood can only enter when it is also leaving, ie, in systole but not in diastole)
Elevation and approximation of diastolic pressures	RA, RV diastolic, PA diastolic, and wedge pressures are above normal and typically within 5 mm Hg of each other. In patients with pre-existing pulmonary hypertension, PA diastolic and wedge pressures may be disproportionately higher.	Equalization of pressures is closest in inspiration and approximate the intrapericardial pressure. In so-called low-pressure tamponade, smaller effusions can reduce stroke volume due to the low distending pressure of cardiac chambers. This can be seen in patients with decreased intravascular volume, as in dialysis patients or after diuresis
Pulsus paradoxus-reduction in a >10-mm Hg drop in systolic BP during inspiration	Reduced LV filling due to right to left shift of interventricular septum as RV fills during inspiration (increased ventricular interdependence)	Pulsus paradoxus can be noted without tamponade in patients with pulmonary embolism and pulmonary disease (asthma, COPD). It may be absent in severe pulmonary hypertension, aortic insufficiency, atrial septal defect, and chronic LV systolic dysfunction

BP, blood pressure; COPD, chronic obstructive pulmonary disease; LV, left ventricle; PA, pulmonary artery; RA, right artery; RV, right ventricle.

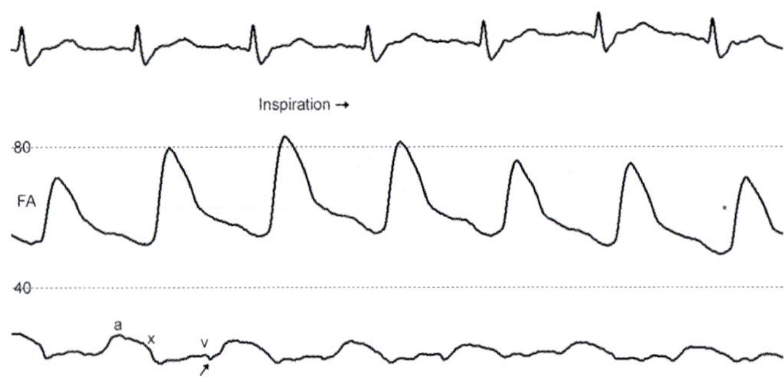

FIGURE 45.1 Invasive hemodynamic findings of cardiac tamponade. On the last beat in the femoral artery (FA) pressure tracing, there is an inspiratory decline in the aortic pulse pressure (*asterisk*), analogous to the bedside finding of pulsus paradoxus. In the right atrial pressure tracing, there is loss of the y descent (*arrow*) that normally follows the V wave.

Preparation for Procedure

Prior to the procedure, coagulopathy should be excluded and corrected, if possible; however, in patients with hemopericardium and tamponade due to excessive oral anticoagulation, pericardial drainage has been safely performed without reversing anticoagulation.[3] This may be because the risk of the procedure is related to inadvertent chamber puncture as opposed to pericardial access itself. In a series of more than 1000 patients, total bleeding or major bleeding complication rates were similar between patients with normal coagulation, International Normalized Ratio (INR) between 1.4 and 1.9 and INR >2, or in the presence of a direct acting oral anticoagulant. No bleeding complications occurred in any of the patients with a platelet count <100,000, including those with a count <50,000.[4]

The proceduralist should personally view the echocardiogram to confirm the presence of sufficient fluid in an accessible location to allow for safe drainage. Small effusions are <10 mm in width, moderate 10 to 20 mm, and large or very large >20 to 25 mm.

Whenever possible, a right heart catheterization should also be performed to assess the effect of pericardial drainage on filling pressures and cardiac output. Persistent elevation of the right atrial pressure with a prominent x and y descent, despite normalization of the pericardial pressure, with persistent equalization of right and left heart filling pressures and a dip and plateau waveform in the right ventricle (RV) signifies the presence of effusive-constrictive pericarditis due to a residual visceral pericardial constraint.[5] In an unstable patient with a clear echocardiographic diagnosis of tamponade, it is reasonable to forgo right-heart catheterization.

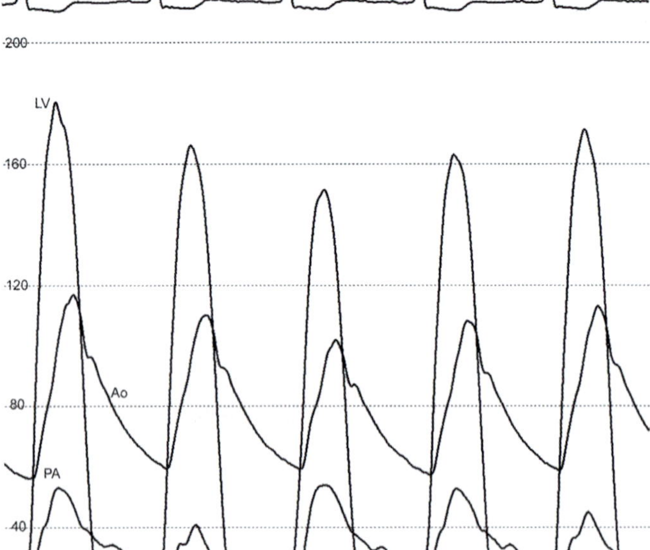

FIGURE 45.2 Change in left ventricular diastolic pressure with cardiac tamponade. This patient underwent retrograde evaluation of her aortic stenosis in the cardiac catheterization laboratory. There is blunting of the left ventricular early diastolic (or minimum) pressure (*arrow*), corresponding to blunting of the y descent that would be seen in the atrial pressure recording. Inspiratory decline in the aortic pulse pressure also is evident on the third beat. Emergent echocardiography confirmed the presence of a pericardial effusion with tamponade physiology. AO, ascending aorta; LV, left ventricle; PA, pulmonary artery.

Technique

The primary objective of the procedure is to successfully access and drain the fluid without causing injury to the cardiac chambers and surrounding structures. The technique for pericardiocentesis has evolved from blind sub-xiphoid puncture with a 11% risk of cardiac chamber perforation to directing the needle under fluoroscopy toward the so-called "epicardial halo" of fluid around the heart[6] and to the contemporary techniques of Echocardiography (ECHO)-assisted or ECHO-guided puncture. The latter technique, pioneered by the Mayo clinic, has been extensively studied and is a safe and predictable procedure which allows for expeditious pericardial drainage in elective and emergency situations.[7] The important principles of this technique are outlined in **Table 45.2**, and the effective use of ECHO to show the optimal site for pericardiocentesis is shown in **Fig. 45.3**.

It is important to note that, in the large Mayo Clinic series, the most common site chosen for both elective and emergency pericardiocentesis, based on the aforementioned principles of ECHO guidance, was not sub-xiphoid (18%-24%) but para-apical (67%).[7,9] In fact, choosing the site based on ECHO guidance is safer and more effective than a routine sub-xiphoid approach.[10]

TABLE 45.2 Summary of Principles of ECHO-Guided Pericardiocentesis

Advantages	Readily available, portable, inexpensive, no radiation exposure, adaptable to bedside, elective and emergency procedures, can assess hemodynamic effects of the effusion, confirm drainage and relief of tamponade physiology, safer and more effective than fluoroscopically guided puncture.
Concept	*Access site is chosen entirely on the basis of* (a) location of largest collection of fluid, (b) proximity to the probe, (c) absence of intervening structures
ECHO-assisted method	Operator estimates optimal needle trajectory based on the angle at which the ultrasound beam intersects the fluid collection, and needle is advanced without continuous ultrasound visualization
ECHO-guided method	Needle entry is visualized in real time with continuous ECHO (a needle mounted on the probe results in high level of safety and efficacy)[8]

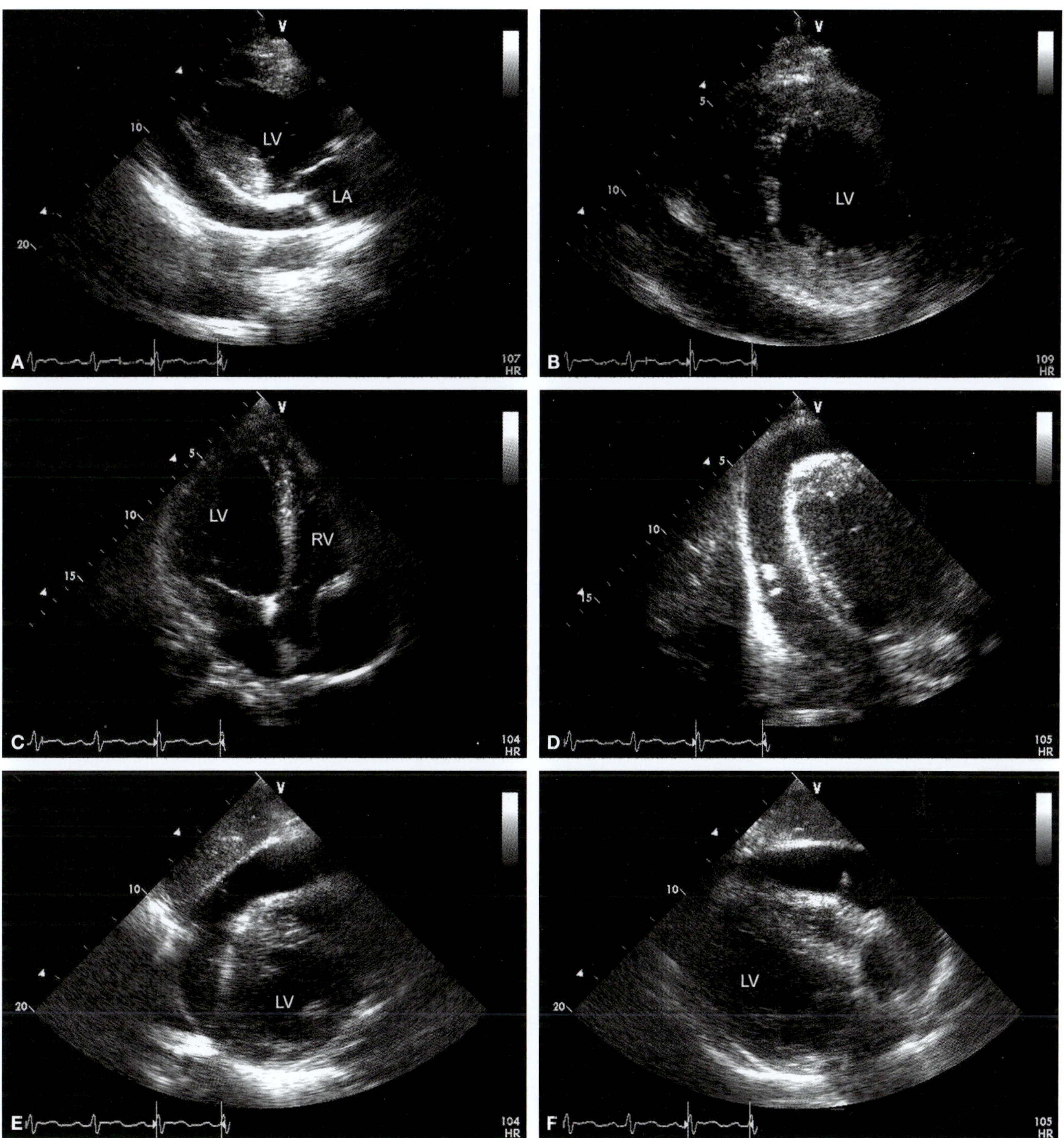

FIGURE 45.3 Echocardiography for site location for pericardiocentesis. Multiple views are required to determine the most appropriate site of pericardiocentesis, with examination of parasternal **(A and B)**, apical **(C and D)**, and sub-coastal **(E and F)** windows. The apical window in panel **D** was chosen for pericardiocentesis. LA, left artery; LV, left ventricle; RA, right artery; RV, right ventricle.

SUB-XIPHOID

The procedure can be performed at bedside or in the cardiac catheterization laboratory. In addition to equipment for monitoring vital signs and resuscitation equipment, it is helpful to have a pressure transducer to confirm the correct location by documenting a right atrial type of pressure, as well as a syringe filled with contrast (provided the patient does not have a contrast allergy). The patient's torso is elevated on a wedge to facilitate pooling of the fluid inferiorly and anteriorly. Even if the chosen location is sub-xiphoid, the chest is prepped broadly to allow for other access sites if the sub-xiphoid is unsuccessful. Using an ECHO probe covered with a sterile sleeve, the depth of the pericardial fluid from the skin is noted along with the angle of the probe. Needle entry is typically just to the left of the xiphoid process, 1 to 2 cm inferior to the costal margin, which allows the needle to clear the costal margin. Needle entry at the apex of the xiphi-sternal angle or further lateral should be avoided. Adequate sedation and analgesia is provided depending on the patient's hemodynamic and clinical status.

After marking the location of the probe, liberal local anesthetic is given in the subcutaneous and deeper tissues. Then, a micropuncture needle attached to a syringe with a mixture of lidocaine and saline via a three-way stopcock is inserted at the marked location and advanced at a 70° angle underneath the rib cage. Alternately, a 16 to 18 G needle in a Teflon sheath can be used. Once the costal margin is cleared, the needle is depressed to a 15°- to 30° angle to the horizontal and advanced along the memorized trajectory of the ECHO probe toward the middle of the left clavicle. Some operators prefer to enter just below the xiphoid process and aim the needle superiorly, but this may increase the risk of right atrial puncture. While advancing the needle, the tip is cleared by injecting lidocaine/saline, and then continuous aspiration is performed till fluid is aspirated. The presence of serous or serosanguineous fluid suggests pericardial entry. If fluid is not aspirated, another pass is made by smoothly withdrawing the needle and then re-advancing slightly more posteriorly and/or medially. Too posterior of an angle increases the risk of peritoneal entry. Advancing the needle during held inspiration may also help as the heart moves lower in the chest. Confirmation that the needle tip is aimed at the so-called epicardial halo, just to the left of the spine, using fluoroscopy helps the operator determine that the needle is aimed at the correct location. In obese/large patients, the pericardial fluid may be located deeper than the 7-cm-long micropuncture needle. In this case, the longer 15-cm 18 G spinal needle, which is included in a pericardiocentesis kit, is used. This needle has a blunt obturator, which is removed after the needle has cleared the costal margin, enabling the needle to be advanced in a similar manner with continuous aspiration. Other variations in technique such as a needle-in-needle technique, marking and tenting the pericardium with contrast, and confirming entry with contrast injection have also been described.[11]

Once fluid is aspirated, one has the choice of either injecting agitated saline/air microbubbles using the second port of the attached stopcock or transducing pressure using a saline-filled tubing. Confirmation of safe entry into the pericardial space is highly recommended before exchanging the needle for a micropuncture sheath or dilator over a wire. ECHO imaging will show stagnant microbubbles in the pericardial space, and contrast will layer sluggishly instead of being washed away. Sometimes the needle enters a hepatic vein or pleural space in which case bubbles are seen in the hepatic vein or not at all. Pericardial pressure will resemble a right atrial tracing, and if needed, it can be compared with a simultaneous right atrial waveform. Once the location is confirmed, a 0.018-in 40-cm-long wire is advanced and noted to loop outside the cardiac borders or coil in the oblique sinus behind the left atrium (**Fig. 45.4**). Two fluoroscopic angles can be used for confirmation if in the catheterization laboratory. Excessive premature ventricular contractions, flailing wire movements, and a wire path of the pulmonary artery should not be noted. Additional local anesthetic is given, if needed, and a generous skin nick is made. The needle is replaced by a 4 French micropuncture sheath. Next, the 0.018-in wire is exchanged for a soft J-tip 80-cm 0.035-in wire. The track is dilated ensuring adequate wire is in place, followed by the placement of either a 6 to 8 French sheath or dilator first, followed by a 65-cm pigtail or straight soft pericardial drain. Alternatives include advancing a 25-cm 6 French radial sheath over a 0.020-in wire or a peel-away 9 French sheath through which a pigtail is advanced, followed by peeling away the sheath. Fluid should be removed slowly to avoid pulmonary edema due to acute diastolic left ventricular failure. After confirming adequate drainage by

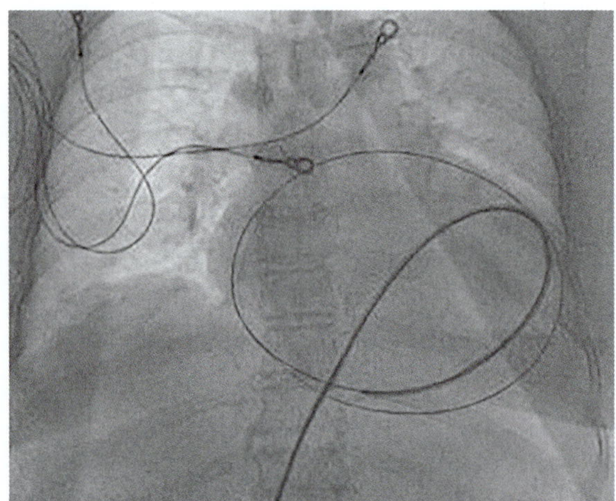

FIGURE 45.4 Wire inserted via sub-xiphoid access looping around the heart suggesting location in the pericardial space.

ECHO, an inspiratory pericardial pressure <0 mm Hg and return of the y descent in the right artery tracing is confirmed. The drain is attached to a closed vacuum accordion-type container and secured in place with a suture.

PARA-APICAL

The needle is advanced in the lower portion of the fifth, sixth, or seventh intercostal space with a trajectory oriented toward the apex of the heart as guided by ECHO, usually 1 cm lateral to the apical impulse. Advancing the needle during held expiration may lower the risk of pneumothorax, which is a concern with this approach. However, since sound does not penetrate air, the use of ECHO guidance ensures the absence of normal intervening lung tissue. There is a higher incidence of LV perforation with this approach.

PARASTERNAL

The needle is advanced perpendicular to the skin in the lower part of the fourth or fifth intercostal space 1 cm from the left or right sternal border as guided by the largest location of fluid on a parasternal long-axis ECHO view of the heart. Care should be taken to avoid being too lateral as the needle can injure the internal mammary artery or vein running down the inner rib cage.

POSTERIOR

Percutaneous ECHO-guided pericardiocentesis for loculated posterior pericardial effusions has been described in cases where compression of the lung by a concomitant large left pleural effusion allows for transmission of the ultrasound beam. More commonly, computed tomography (CT) guidance is used to access such effusions with high efficacy and safety.[12]

Post-pericardiocentesis Management

The pericardial drain is removed when the output is less than 25 to 50 mL in 24 hours. Leaving the drain until daily output is <25 mL (prolonged drainage) is associated with a significant reduction in the need for repeat pericardiocentesis. Absence of prolonged drainage, large effusions, and fluid with positive cytology are independently associated with recurrent effusion.[9] Prolonged drainage is also associated with lower rates of recurrent tamponade and mortality, compared with shorter-duration drainage, in patients with both malignant and nonmalignant effusions.[13] For patients with recurrent malignant pericardial effusions, percutaneous balloon pericardiotomy is a well-described, safe, and effective technique[14] but is infrequently performed when surgical pericardial window is an option.

Complications

ECHO-guided pericardiocentesis is a generally safe procedure with an approximately 1% rate of major complications. The most serious complications are laceration of cardiac chambers and coronary arteries, which can result in uncontrolled bleeding and death, especially in centers where cardiac surgery is not available. The incidence of major complications in the large Mayo Clinic registry of >1100 patients was 1.2%, which included surgery for chamber laceration (0.44%) and pneumothorax (0.44%). Minor complications not requiring specific interventions, such as transient chamber entry, small pneumothorax, arrhythmia, and vasovagal response, occurred in 3.5% of cases.[9] Needle entry, especially into the thick-walled LV, usually seals itself on withdrawal, but inadvertent placement of a sheath into the RV is problematic. In such situations, the sheath should be left in place, and urgent consultation with a cardiac surgeon or structural interventionalist for percutaneous closure of the defect should be sought.[15]

Special Subsets

In case of hemopericardium from coronary or collateral perforation, especially during chronic total occlusion percutaneous coronary intervention (PCI), RV perforation from biopsy or pacemaker insertion, electrophysiological procedures, or during structural interventions like left atrial appendage occlusion, valvuloplasty, or trans-catheter aortic valve replacement, a large pericardial drain or sheath is preferred to rapidly and completely drain the blood in the pericardial space and auto-transfuse the blood via a central vein. Protamine is best reserved after pericardial access and drainage to prevent coagulation of blood in the pericardial sac preventing removal. In the Mayo Clinic series of 92 ECHO-guided pericardiocentesis cases for iatrogenic pericardial tamponade, procedural success rate was 99%, with no mortality related to the procedure and a 3% major complication rate including RV perforation, pneumothorax, and intercostal vessel injury. Sixty-seven percent of cases were performed via an apical approach, and 24% via a subcostal approach. Seventeen percent of cases required an additional cardiac surgery to control ongoing bleeding.[16]

Pericardiocentesis in patients who have undergone prior cardiac surgery is challenging. The pericardium is loosely re-approximated after surgery, and adhesions can result in loculated effusions with compressive effects on the right or left heart causing regional tamponade. Regional tamponade can be difficult to diagnose with a transthoracic ECHO. In cases with a high index of suspicion, right heart catheterization will reveal diastolic equalization of pressures, and a trans-esophageal ECHO or CT can provide a definitive diagnosis. Regional tamponade typically requires surgical evacuation. One subset of regional tamponade, which is difficult to treat and has high mortality, is due to hematoma in the oblique sinus causing left atrial compression due to iatrogenic perforation of the left circumflex coronary artery in the atrioventricular groove such as during chronic total occlusion PCI. This causes refractory shock and requires surgery or CT-guided pericardiocentesis.[17]

Key Points

- The classic hemodynamic findings in cardiac tamponade are blunting or absence of the y descent in the right atrial waveform, associated with elevation and equalization of diastolic pressures in the cardiac chambers and the pericardia space. This is associated with narrowing of the aortic pulse pressure, especially during inspiration (pulsus paradoxus), and reduction in left ventricular stroke volume and cardiac output.
- ECHO-assisted or ECHO-guided pericardiocentesis is the standard of care for management of cardiac tamponade. The use of ECHO guidance allows for increased safety and efficacy.
- Regional tamponade after cardiac surgery or as a complication of PCI can be challenging to manage and requires consultation with the surgery and/or radiology department.

For further review and interactivities, please see the chapter-based multiple choice questions and videos accessible in the complimentary eBook bundled with this text. Access instructions are located in the inside front cover.

References

1. LeWinter MM, *Pericardial diseases*. In: *Braunwald's Heart Disease*. 8th ed. 2008.
2. Adler Y, Charron P, Imazio M, et al. 2015 ESC guidelines for the diagnosis and management of pericardial diseases: the task force for the diagnosis and management of pericardial diseases of the European Society of Cardiology (ESC) endorsed by—The European Association for Cardio-Thoracic Surgery (EACTS). *Eur Heart J*. 2015;36(42):2921-2964.
3. Zhu Y, Zhang C, Xie Y, et al. The safety of pericardiocentesis in patients under antithrombotic therapy: a single-center experience. *Front Cardiovasc Med*. 2022;2022(9):1013979.
4. Ryu AJ, Kane GC, Pislaru SV, et al. Bleeding complications of ultrasound-guided pericardiocentesis in the presence of coagulopathy or thrombocytopenia. *J Am Soc Echocardiogr*. 2020;33(3):399-401.
5. Sagrista-Sauleda J, Angel J, Sanchez A, Permanyer-Miralda G, Soler-Soler J. Effusive-constrictive pericarditis. *N Engl J Med*. 2004;350(5):469-475.
6. Ristić AD, Wagner HJ, Maksimović R, Maisch B. Epicardial halo phenomenon: a guide for pericardiocentesis? *Heart Fail Rev*. 2013;18(3):307-316.
7. Tsang TSM, Freeman WK, Sinak LJ, Seward JB. Echocardiographically-guided pericardiocentesis: evolution and state-of-the-art technique. *Mayo Clin Proc*. 1998;73(7):647-652.
8. Maggiolini S, Gentile G, Farina A, et al. Safety, efficacy, and complications of pericardiocentesis by real-time echo-monitored procedure. *Am J Cardiol*. 2016;117(8):1369-1374.
9. Tsang TS, Enriquez-Sarano M, Freeman WK, et al. Consecutive 1127 therapeutic echocardiographically guided pericardiocenteses: clinical profile, practice patterns, and outcomes spanning 21 years. *Mayo Clin Proc*. 2002;77(5):429-436.
10. Maggiolini S, De Carlini CC, Imazio M. Evolution of the pericardiocentesis technique. *J Cardiovasc Med*. 2018;19(6):267-273.

11. Kumar S, Bazaz R, Barbhaiya CR, et al. "Needle-in-needle" epicardial access: preliminary observations with a modified technique for facilitating epicardial interventional procedures. *Heart Rhythm*. 2015;12(7):1691-1697.
12. Catena E, Addamiano C, Bertoli E, Maggiolini S, Farina A, Achilli F. Pericardiocentesis from back under echographic guidance: an approach for posterior pericardial effusions. *Circulation*. 2011;124(24):e835-e836.
13. Rafique AM, Patel N, Biner S, et al. Frequency of recurrence of pericardial tamponade in patients with extended versus nonextended pericardial catheter drainage. *Am J Cardiol*. 2011;108(12):1820-1825.
14. Viles-Gonzalez J, D'Avilla A, Mauro M. *Pericardial interventions: pericardiocentesis, balloon pericardiotomy and epicardial approach to cardiac procedures*. In: *Grossmman and Baim's Cardiac Catheterization, Angiography and Intervention*. 9th ed. 2021.
15. Saxena A, Karmakar S, Narang R. Successful percutaneous device closure of right ventricular perforation during pericardiocentesis. *JACC Cardiovasc Interv*. 2016;9(22):e221-e222.
16. Tsang TS, Freeman WK, Barnes ME, Reeder GS, Packer DL, Seward JB. Rescue echocardiographically guided pericardiocentesis for cardiac perforation complicating catheter-based procedures. The Mayo Clinic experience. *J Am Coll Cardiol*. 1998;32(5):1345-1350.
17. Wilson WM, Spratt JC, Lombardi WL. Cardiovascular collapse post chronic total occlusion percutaneous coronary intervention due to a compressive left atrial hematoma managed with percutaneous drainage. *Catheter Cardiovasc Interv*. 2015;86(3):407-411.

Interventional Procedures in Adult Congenital Heart Disease

Georges Ephrem

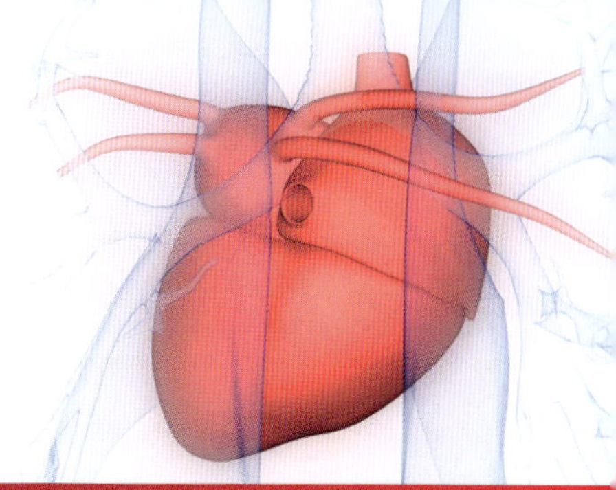

Improved treatment strategies and interventions have increased survival in adult congenital heart disease (ACHD) that up to 90% of children born with cardiac birth defects are expected to live well into adulthood.[1-3] Over the last decade, the field of interventional cardiology has also witnessed a dramatic advancement driven by technologic improvement. Percutaneous therapies are now acceptable alternatives, additions, or treatments of choice when surgical or medical interventions are contemplated in ACHD. Interventional cardiology is a well-established component of any center that provides care to this unique patient population. Guideline recommendations for interventions have been published, including in the context of overall care of ACHD in North America and Europe.[1-6]

In this chapter, we review the most commonly performed percutaneous procedures in adults with congenital heart disease (CHD). The guideline recommendations and level of evidence for these procedures are provided in **Table 46.1**.

TABLE 46.1 Most Commonly Performed Catheter-Based Interventions in Adults With Congenital Heart Diseases: Indications and Guideline Recommendations (Level of Evidence)

INTERVENTION	INDICATION	RECOMMENDATION (LEVEL OF EVIDENCE)
SVSD Closure	Net left-to-right shunt (Qp:Qs ≥ 1.5:1), PA systolic pressure less than 50% systemic and pulmonary vascular resistance less than one-third systemic	I (C)
	Net left-to-right shunt (Qp:Qs ≥ 1.5:1), PA systolic pressure is 50% or more systemic, and/or pulmonary vascular resistance greater than one-third systemic	IIb (C)
VSD Closure	Evidence of LV volume overload and hemodynamically significant shunts (Qp:Qs ≥ 1.5:1), if PA systolic pressure less than 50% systemic and pulmonary vascular resistance less than one-third systemic	I (B)
	Worsening aortic regurgitation (AR) caused by VSD	IIa (C)
	History of IE caused by VSD if not otherwise contraindicated	IIb (C)
	Net left-to-right shunt (Qp:Qs ≥ 1.5:1), PA systolic pressure 50% or more than systemic and/or pulmonary vascular resistance greater than one-third systemic	IIb (C)
PDA Closure	Left atrial or LV enlargement present and attributable to PDA with net left-to-right shunt, PA systolic pressure less than 50% systemic and pulmonary vascular resistance less than one-third systemic	I (C)
	Net left-to-right shunt if PA systolic pressure is 50% or greater systemic, and/or pulmonary vascular resistance greater than one-third systemic	IIb (B)
Balloon Aortic Valvuloplasty	Bicuspid aortic valve stenosis meeting indications for intervention and a noncalcified valve with no more than mild AR	IIb (B)
Balloon Tricuspid Valvuloplasty	Isolated, symptomatic severe tricuspid stenosis without TR	IIb (C)
Balloon Pulmonary Valvuloplasty	Moderate or severe valvular pulmonary stenosis and otherwise unexplained symptoms of HF, cyanosis from interatrial right-to-left communication, and/or exercise intolerance	I (B)
	Asymptomatic adults with severe valvular pulmonary stenosis	IIa (C)
Transcatheter Pulmonary Valve Replacement	Symptomatic patients with moderate or greater PR	I (C)
	Asymptomatic patients with moderate or greater PR with progressive RV dilation and/or RV dysfunction and/or decreased exercise tolerance	IIb (C)
Coarctation of the Aorta	Hypertension and significant native or recurrent coarctation of the aorta	I (B)
	Balloon angioplasty for adults with native and recurrent coarctation of the aorta may be considered if stent placement is not feasible and surgical intervention is not an option	IIb (B)
Pulmonary Artery	Focal branch and/or peripheral pulmonary artery stenosis with >50% diameter narrowing, RVSP >50 mm Hg, and/or symptoms	IIa (B)

(continued)

TABLE 46.1 Most Commonly Performed Catheter-Based Interventions in Adults With Congenital Heart Diseases: Indications and Guideline Recommendations (Level of Evidence) (*Continued*)

INTERVENTION	INDICATION	RECOMMENDATION (LEVEL OF EVIDENCE)
Aortopulmonary Collateral Closure	Unexplained LV or RV dysfunction, fluid retention, chest pain, or cyanosis	IIb (C)
Coronary Artery Fistula Closure	A large fistula, regardless of symptomatology, should be closed via either a transcatheter or surgical route	I (C)
	A small to moderate fistula in the presence of myocardial ischemia, arrhythmia, otherwise unexplained ventricular systolic or diastolic dysfunction or enlargement, or endarteritis should be closed via either a transcatheter or surgical approach	I (C)
Baffle Interventions	In symptomatic patients with baffle stenosis, stenting is recommended when technically feasible	I (C)
	In symptomatic patients with baffle leaks and cyanosis at rest or during exercise, or with strong suspicion of paradoxical emboli, stenting (covered) or device closure is recommended when technically feasible	I (C)
	In patients with baffle leaks and symptoms due to left-to-right shunt, stenting (covered) or device closure is recommended when technically feasible	I (C)
	In asymptomatic patients with baffle leaks with substantial ventricular volume overload due to left-to-right shunt, stenting (covered) or device closure should be considered when technically feasible	IIa (C)
	In patients with a baffle leak who require a PM/ICD, closure of the baffle leak with a covered stent should be considered, when technically feasible, prior to insertion of transvenous leads	IIa (C)
	In asymptomatic patients with baffle stenosis, stenting may be considered when technically feasible	IIb (C)
Fontan Fenestration Closure	In selected patients with significant cyanosis, device closure of a fenestration may be considered but requires careful evaluation before intervention to exclude induction of systemic venous pressure increase or fall in cardiac output	IIb (C)

AR, aortic regurgitation; HF, heart failure; ICD, implantable cardiac defibrillator; IE, infective endocarditis; LV, left ventricle; PA, pulmonary artery; PDA, patent ductus arteriosus; PM, pacemaker; PR, pulmonary regurgitation; Qp, pulmonary flow; Qs, systemic flow; RV, right ventricle; RVSP, right ventricular systolic pressure; SVSD, sinus venosus septal defect; TR, tricuspid regurgitation; VSD, ventricular septal defect.

SHUNT-CENTERED INTERVENTIONS

Correction of Superior Sinus Venosus Septal Defects

Superior sinus venosus septal defect (SSVSD) is a deficiency of the common wall between the superior vena cava (SVC) and right-sided pulmonary veins (PVs) and is associated with an anomalous right upper PV in up to 90% of cases. Patients with SSVSD usually present with symptoms similar to those in patients with atrial septal defect, although they may present earlier because of increased left-to-right shunting from both an atrial-level shunt and >1 anomalous right-sided PVs that drain into the SVC. Treatment is indicated to reverse right-heart enlargement and the following symptoms: dyspnea on exertion, decreased exercise tolerance, or right-heart failure (HF). The standard of care is surgical repair using the Warden procedure or two-patch repair.[1-3] However, over the last several years, transcatheter correction of SSVSD using covered stents has become more established.[6,7] The procedure is technically challenging and is successful only in patients with suitable anatomy. Cardiac CTA (computed tomography angiography) is performed, and virtual or 3-dimensionally printed models are used to help with visualization of SSVSDs, the anomalous PVs, and surrounding structures to assess whether the anatomy is favorable for the placement of a covered stent that will direct SVC blood to the right atrium (RA), allowing for unobstructed anomalous PV flow to then drain into the left atrium through the residual SSVSD. The procedure is usually performed with the patient under general anesthesia given the need for intraprocedural imaging guidance using transesophageal echocardiography. The largest cohort to date demonstrated that the procedure has good short-term outcomes, with no incidence of sinus node dysfunction.[6,7] One of the drawbacks of this procedure is difficulty in using just one stent to adequately cover the SVC superiorly and the SVC-RA junction inferiorly while maintaining stent stability. Forty percent of the patients in the study required covered Cheatham-Platinum stents (B. Braun Inc, Melsungen, Germany) that were longer than 6 cm, which are currently not available commercially in the United States. Fifty-two percent required additional stents to secure the covered stent, and 24% had covered stents that either migrated or embolized during the procedure. Larger studies and more experience with this technique will lead to further iterations and improvements of the procedure; however, a select subset of patients with SSVSDs may benefit from transcatheter correction of the defect as an alternative to surgery.

Ventricular Septal Defects Closure

Ventricular septal defects (VSDs) comprise approximately 20% of all congenital heart lesions and can occur anywhere along the ventricular septum. VSD closure in the adult is usually recommended either when left ventricle (LV) volume overload, unexplained by any alternative mechanism, is present, correlating with Qp:Qs > 1.5:1.0, in the presence of multiple recurrences of otherwise unexplained bacterial endocarditis or when accompanied by progressive aortic regurgitation (AR) as long as the pulmonary artery (PA) pressure or pulmonary vascular resistance is favorable.[1-3]

Percutaneous closure of VSD is an attractive alternative to surgical management in selected patients with isolated uncomplicated defects, increased surgical risk, multiple previous cardiac surgical interventions, or with poorly accessible muscular VSDs. Transcatheter VSD closure is generally performed with intravascular passage through the VSD (if possible using a balloon-tipped catheter to ensure passage via the largest lumen) from the LV side, snaring a guide wire in the PA, formation and externalization of a venous–arterial vascular loop, and subsequent device deployment based on a pathway allowing maximal device arm–septal apposition, without interference from adjacent intracardiac structures. VSD closure can be performed with intravascular passage from the right ventricle (RV), obviating the need for a vascular loop, but entails crossing the defect against the blood flow, which may be complicated depending on the defect location and anatomy.

In the United States, the only currently FDA-approved available device specifically for VSD closure is the AMPLATZER Muscular VSD device (St. Jude Medical, Inc St. Paul, Minnesota, USA). The long-term results are favorable, with procedural success of >90% and complications such as heart block (up to 6%), hemolysis (1%-2%), and embolization (1%-2%) being relatively rare.[8-10] Coils as well as other devices such as the AMPLATZER membranous VSD device, AMPLATZER Septal Occluder, and the AMPLATZER Duct Occluder and Duct Occluder II (St. Jude Medical, Inc St. Paul, Minnesota, USA) are used in an off-label fashion for VSD closure.

Transcatheter closure of acquired VSD secondary to myocardial infarction (MI) is associated with significant morbidity and mortality (up to 50%), similar to surgical closure. This is more due to the underlying critical condition of the patients with HF and cardiogenic shock during acute MI than direct outcome of the percutaneous procedure, which has high rates of success (90%).[11]

Patent Ductus Arteriosus Closure

Patent ductus arteriosus (PDA) is an abnormally persistent arterial connection after birth between the descending aorta and the PA, most commonly to the junction of the main and left PA branches. Similar to VSD, patients with large PDA may develop left-sided volume overload and pulmonary hypertension (PH) at younger ages, leading to diagnosis early in life. It is not uncommon that the diagnosis of PDA is made in adulthood by means of physical examination and the presence of the continuous murmur typical of PDA, or as an incidental finding on echocardiography.[12] Additional problems associated with PDA include infectious endarteritis, aneurysm formation, calcification, and rarely rupture. Large PDA with a significant left-to-right shunt should be closed to reduce occurrence of the sequelae of subaortic ventricular failure or pulmonary arterial hypertension (PAH). There are adult-specific closure issues, such as calcification of ductal tissue, change in orientation of the duct with age, leading to a more horizontal entry into the PA and a higher incidence of PH.

In adults with PDA, percutaneous closure is the preferred mode of therapy given increasing surgical risk with age because of PDA calcification and the potential for intraoperative recurrent laryngeal nerve damage. The current FDA-approved occluder devices (AMPLATZER ductal occluder (ADO), ADO II, and PFM Nit-Occlud (B. Braun Inc, Melsungen, Germany)) are all MRI-safe. The ADO is the most commonly used device typically implanted during an outpatient procedure, with coil embolization reserved for PDA measuring <2 to 3 mm or for residual leaks. Complete closure has been reported in >95% of patients at 3 months without major complications.[13] The postimplantation antiplatelet regimen remains unsubstantiated, and patients continue to receive antibiotic prophylaxis against subacute bacterial endocarditis for 6 months after device implantation.

Ruptured Sinus of Valsalva Aneurysm Closure

The weakness at the junction of the aortic media and annulus fibrosis can lead to formation of a sinus of Valsalva aneurysm (SVA). Aneurysms are asymptomatic in the majority of cases; however, a rupture may cause significant hemodynamic change. The rupture usually occurs into the RA or RV causing a significant left-to-right shunt and HF. Surgical repair remains the treatment of choice; however, transcatheter closure of a ruptured SVA has been successfully performed with success rates of 91%, thus avoiding sternotomy and cardiopulmonary bypass in critically ill patients. The AMPLATZER ductal occluder remains the most commonly used device, with some cases using the muscular VSD occluder.[14] Rare procedure-related AR, as well as severe procedure-related complications, should be considered in the risk assessment.

Shunt Creation

Transcatheter creation of a Potts shunt (from the descending aorta to the left PA) has been described in select patients with severe PH as a way to preserve oxygenated flow to the coronaries and cerebral circulation while allowing right-to-left shunting from the PA to the descending aorta.[15] In select patients, creation or enlargement of a VSD via a transcatheter or hybrid technique may be helpful in improving cardiac output, such as in patients with a double-outlet RV and restrictive VSDs.[16]

VALVE INTERVENTIONS

Mitral Valve Interventions

Balloon Mitral Valvuloplasty

While balloon mitral valvuloplasty (BMV) is frequently performed in the treatment of patients with rheumatic mitral stenosis (MS), there is limited experience with BMV in congenital MS. Surgery is the preferred treatment for adults with congenital MS, in view of their complex anatomy, likely concomitant stenosis of the supra- and/or subvalvular apparatuses, and the potential risk for significant residual mitral regurgitation post dilation.[17]

Aortic Valve Interventions

Balloon Aortic Valvuloplasty

The most common cause for congenital valvular aortic stenosis (AS) is bicuspid aortic valve. In contrast to pulmonary valve stenosis (PS), AS secondary to bicuspid aortic valve disease is a progressive disorder in the adult. The standard approach for balloon aortic valvuloplasty (BAV) in adults is a retrograde transfemoral arterial approach. However, antegrade venous transseptal technique may be an alternative option if needed.[18] Outcomes following BAV vary according to age with repeat intervention more often required in newborns and older patients more likely to develop AR following BAV.[19] The aortic valve leaflets in children are typically pliable and usually easy to dilate. This is in contrast to adult patients with AS in whom the aortic valve becomes thickened and calcified by the fourth decade of life, making them less suitable to effective balloon dilation. The standard approach to BAV results in more than a 50% reduction in gradients in the majority of patients; however, around 15% of the cases develop moderate to severe AR and 10% to 15% have a significant residual gradient that may require repeat BAV.[19,20] Use of an undersized balloon to the annulus diameter (0.9:1.0) and real-time echocardiographic assessment is advised to avoid severe AR. Long-term follow-up data suggest up to 88% survival and just fewer than 50% of the patients requiring aortic valve replacement at 20 years.[21]

In contrast to valvular AS, subvalvular AS does not respond well to balloon dilation. Thus, the appropriate intervention for patients with significant obstruction is surgical resection of the subvalvular membrane. Nevertheless, BAV has been offered as a short-term alternative. Long-term outcomes of patients with discrete subaortic stenosis who underwent balloon dilation suggest a restenosis rate of 15%.[22] Larger annulus diameter and thinner membranes are known to yield better results. Balloon dilation has also been used for congenital supravalvular AS, but this approach has failed to become mainstream therapy.

Tricuspid Valve Interventions

Balloon Tricuspid Valvuloplasty

Tricuspid valve stenosis (TS) is often combined with tricuspid regurgitation (TR) and most frequently of rheumatic origin. Congenital TS is rare, rarely an isolated lesion and rarely intervened on percutaneously. Balloon tricuspid valvuloplasty (BTV) can be considered in patients with severe, symptomatic, native TS without TR.[23] It is less preferable than surgery, because most cases of severe TS have concurrent TR that might worsen after balloon dilation. In addition, there are insufficient data on the long-term outcomes of patients undergoing BTV. While this procedure is most likely to be used in a palliative strategy, it can however be considered as a bridge to percutaneous or surgical valve replacement. Technical considerations for intervention include wire placement (RV or PA) for stability and single or double balloon use. For the latter, assessment with a compliant balloon such as a 34 mm AGA sizing balloon (AGA Medical Corporation, Golden Valley, MN) can yield helpful information regarding the magnitude and the location of the stenosis (annular- and/or leaflet-level) above and beyond what may be available by echocardiographic guidance.[24]

Transcatheter Tricuspid Valve Repair/Replacement

Congenital tricuspid valve lesions are predominantly the result of Ebstein anomaly or tricuspid dysplasia. For these patients, the predominant lesion is TR. In general, tricuspid repair is preferred to replacement; however, the risk of recurrent regurgitation is high and many patients will eventually receive a bioprosthetic tricuspid valve. Operators are mainly adopting the techniques and devices developed for adults without CHD[25] and implementing them as much as possible to those with CHD.[26] For example, transcatheter tricuspid valve (systemic atrioventricular valve) repair with MitraClip (Abbott, USA) has been described in high-surgical-risk patients with congenitally corrected transposition of the great arteries who present with severe TR.[27] In contrast to treatment of the mitral valve, the use of MitraClip on the tricuspid valve aims to clip together two of the three leaflets to create a double orifice tricuspid valve. The choice of leaflets depends on the location of the regurgitant jet and ease of imaging.[28] Over the years, bioprosthetic valves may fail, resulting in stenosis or regurgitation. Multicenter registry data have been compiled and used to evaluate transcatheter tricuspid valve-in-valve and valve-in-ring procedures, and these data have demonstrated high technical success and good clinical outcomes.[29-31] Larger series, and ultimately prospective studies, will determine the safety and efficacy of these techniques and help identify the ideal patients for each approach.

Pulmonary Valve Interventions

Balloon Pulmonary Valvuloplasty

Pulmonary valve stenosis (PS) is almost always congenital in origin and usually results from commissural fusion of thin and pliable leaflets. The majority of the cases are characterized by a narrow central opening with preserved valve motion (ie, dome-type PS). Less frequently, the pulmonary valve is dysplastic, with thickened valve leaflets and a relatively immobile valve. The ACHD guidelines classify the severity of PS by peak velocity and Doppler gradient into mild (peak velocity <3 m/s; peak gradient <36 mm Hg), moderate (peak velocity 3-4 m/s; peak gradient 36-64 mm Hg), and severe (>4 m/s; peak gradient >64 mm Hg, mean gradient>35 mm Hg), respectively.[1]

Balloon pulmonary valvuloplasty (BPV) is the treatment of choice for isolated PS, with high technical success and excellent short- and long-term results. Most patients are free of events in the long term after a single procedure.[6,32,33]

Further reduction in residual gradients may be seen over time because of resolution of residual hypertrophic subvalvular stenosis.[12,32,33] The use of an oversized balloon (1.2-1.25 times the annulus) has been advocated to achieve a successful result, which is defined by a peak valve gradient of <20 mm Hg. More aggressive balloon sizing (>1.4 times the annulus) has been associated with development of moderate to severe pulmonary regurgitation (PR) in 11% of the cases.[34] An undersized balloon (<1.2 times the annulus) is a predictor for restenosis, which is reported in 10% of the patients.[32] Transient severe right ventricular outflow tract (RVOT) obstruction ("suicide" RV) has been reported after BPV, particularly in the pediatric population; however, this may be treated by volume expansion and β-blocker therapy.[32] Surgical intervention is generally recommended in the context of significant obstruction at the supravalvular or subvalvular levels, marked valve dysplasia/annular hypoplasia, or more than moderate PR. The impact of associated aneurysmal dilation of the main pulmonary (and potentially aortic) trunk in patients (and their relatives) with PS remains unclear.

Transcatheter Pulmonary Valve Replacement

Transcatheter pulmonary valve replacement (TPVR) is a less invasive approach than surgical replacement and is available for patients with RVOT dysfunction (stenosis or regurgitation). This includes native RVOTs, dysfunctional pulmonary bioprostheses, and RV to PA conduits.

Two types of valves are commercially available in the United States: The Melody valve (Medtronic, Minneapolis, Minnesota) (18, 20, and 22 mm) and the Edwards Sapien transcatheter heart valve (Edwards Lifesciences, Irvine, California) (23, 26, and 29 mm). Short- and medium-term results of TPVR are available for both platforms, but long-term data (up to 10 years of follow-up) are available for the Melody valve. For the Sapien valve, multicenter registry data show 98% technical success with serious adverse events in 10% of the cases. Valve function at discharge is excellent in most patients with median peak gradient of 5 mm Hg and moderate to severe PR in 2.9% of the patients. During a median follow-up of 12 months, endocarditis was reported in 2.6% and 17 additional patients underwent surgical valve replacement or valve-in-valve TPVR.[35] The data for the Melody valve show a median discharge mean gradient of 17 mm Hg. At 10 years, estimated freedom from mortality was 90%, from reoperation 79%, and from any reintervention 60%. Estimated freedom from TPVR-related endocarditis was 81% at 10 years (95% CI, 69%-89%), with an annualized rate of 2.0% per patient-year.[36]

The implantation technique is similar for the two valves via venous access from the femoral or jugular vein. Because coronary compromise is a life-threatening complication, a balloon test is performed to exclude potential coronary artery compression. This is performed by inflation of a high-pressure balloon equal to the size of the intended diameter of the landing zone for the pulmonary valve in the RVOT conduit, with a simultaneous angiography to visualize coronary arteries. Impairment of coronary blood flow is a contraindication for TPVR. Prestenting of the conduit, usually with a covered stent, is another important measure taken during the procedure to minimize the risk of transcatheter valve fracture or conduit rupture. A valve-in-valve procedure can also be performed in cases of primary device failure.

For regurgitant, native RVOTs that are too large for the Melody or Sapien devices, two platforms based on an "RVOT reducer" concept are now commercially available: The Harmony TPV (Medtronic Inc, Minneapolis MN) and the Alterra Adaptive Prestent coupled with a 29-mm Sapien 3 THV (both Edwards Lifesciences, Irvine, California). The 5-year outcomes from the Harmony native outflow tract early feasibility study demonstrate stable Harmony TPV position and sustained valve function with freedom from moderate-to-severe valve or perivalvular leak or endocarditis.[37] Early feasibility data on the Alterra-S3 platform show 100% device success and no staged procedures necessary. No dysfunction was reported at 6 months follow-up.[38]

GREAT ARTERIES–RELATED INTERVENTIONS

Coarctation of the Aorta

Coarctation of the aorta (CoA) is defined as a narrowing of the aorta usually at the level of the ductus arteriosus. The presence of cystic medial necrosis in the aortic wall adjacent to the coarctation site predisposes the patients to aortic wall rupture and aneurysm formation with percutaneous or surgical interventions. When left untreated, CoA is associated with a mean survival rate of 35 years, with 75% mortality at 46 years of age.[1-3] This is due to uncontrolled systemic hypertension, accelerated coronary artery disease, stroke, aortic dissection, and HF.

Studies suggest that balloon angioplasty and surgical correction are equally effective in reducing the peak systolic pressure gradient early after intervention; however, the surgical approach is associated with higher immediate procedural complications and longer hospital stays, whereas balloon angioplasty is associated with a higher incidence of recoarctation (up to 25%) and aneurysm (7%) formation at follow-up.[39,40] Therefore, stent placement with the advantage of sustained hemodynamic benefit is now considered the treatment of choice for older children and adults with native coarctation. Balloon angioplasty for adults with native and recurrent CoA may be considered if stent placement is not feasible and surgical intervention is not an option.

Long-term (up to 5 years) outcomes of the CoA stent (COAST and COAST II) trials demonstrate the efficacy and safety of stent placement with a notable decrease in the use of antihypertensive medication, from 53% at immediate, to 42% at early, and 29% at late follow-up. The cumulative incidence of stent fractures was 0% immediately, 2.9% at early, and 24.4% at late follow-up. Independent predictors for stent fractures at late follow-up were age <18 years, male sex, minimum stent diameter ≥12 mm, and use of bare metal stent. The cumulative incidence of reintervention was 1.6% at immediate, 5.1% at early, and 21.3% at late follow-up. Independent predictors for reinterventions at late follow-up were age <18 years, postimplantation systolic arm-leg blood pressure gradient ≥10 mm Hg, minimum stent diameter at implantation <12 mm, and initial coarctation minimum diameter <6 mm. The cumulative incidence of aortic aneurysms was 6.3% at late follow-up.[41]

When an intervention is considered, detailed imaging of the coarctation site using cardiac computed tomography (CT) or cardiac magnetic resonance imaging (CMR) is recommended. If the CoA site is long and tubular or if there is concomitant diffuse arch hypoplasia, a surgical approach is usually favored because of concerns about perfusion and injury to spinal arteries. Long-term complications after interventions might include systemic hypertension or premature coronary artery disease despite adequate relief of the obstruction. Re-CoA occurs in 10% to 20% of patients. Possible additional long-term complications include true and/or pseudo aneurysm formation at the site of the intervention. Regular follow-up with CT or CMR (possibly every 5 years) should be considered for these patients.

Pulmonary Artery

PA stenosis (PAS) in patients with CHD may occur anywhere in the pulmonary vascular tree. Isolation of a PA due to ductal constriction is congenital. PAS is typically associated with other congenital defects or syndromes, such as tetralogy of Fallot, VSD, or genetic conditions such as Williams, Alagille, Noonan, rubella, and Ehlers-Danlos syndromes. Additionally, PAS may result as sequelae of surgical interventions (including systemic-pulmonary shunts, homograft or conduit implantation, PA banding, pulmonary arterioplasty, or after arterial switch operation) or may be a residue of acquired diseases (including chronic thromboembolic disease).[42]

In persons with abnormal pulmonary resistance, isolated branch obstruction can result in PH, increased subpulmonary ventricular afterload, PR, or a sufficient perfusion-ventilation imbalance that may lead to symptoms.

Quantitative radiographic assessment of lung perfusion and ventilation should be part of the diagnostic algorithm and should be used as a tool to evaluate the results of dilation procedures in such patients. Surgical access and correction of PAS may be cumbersome and limited. Consequently, percutaneous therapy is the preferred treatment method to restore pulmonary blood flow and balance and to decrease resistance for patients with PAS. PA procedures such as balloon angioplasty and/or stenting (PA rehabilitation) may account for up to 20% of all catheter-based interventions in this population.[43]

Data from multicenter registries (NCDR and Congenital Cardiac Catheterization Project on Outcomes) suggest major adverse events in up to 10% of patients.[43,44] While vascular/cardiac tear is the most common adverse event, balloon rupture (5%) and stent embolization/malposition (6%) have also been reported.[44] Technological advances allowed for improved success rates (up to 90%) with balloons of lower profile, high and ultrahigh burst pressure, cutting balloons, scoring balloons, and drug-eluting balloons. Success rates for PA stenting surpass those of angioplasty alone, reaching 75% to 100% anatomic resolution in addition to reducing the pressure gradient and RV pressure and improving the disparity of pulmonary blood flow. Restenosis post-angioplasty has been reported in 15% to 35% and may be unpredictable. Following stenting, long-term results report a low incidence of in-stent restenosis (<5%), apart from that which occurs because of somatic growth. Reinterventions on PAS are frequent during follow-up (22% by 16 months of follow-up) and more common in peripheral lesions. The presence of significant PR predisposes to stent embolization. Certain lesions remain problematic for stent therapy, such as proximal main PA stenosis close to the pulmonary valve and bifurcation stenoses. Both pulmonary angioplasty and PA stenting can be performed in the hybrid environment, via a surgical access site or under direct visualization in open procedures with concomitant cardiothoracic surgery. Recanalization of an occluded vessel can be performed from a transcatheter approach, using radiofrequency (RF) perforation or coronary chronic total occlusion wires, followed by angioplasty and stenting.[45] Whether congenital or acquired, PA aneurysms are rare and, if associated with elevated PA pressure, may require embolization or covered stent therapy.[46] PA aneurysms are unlikely to rupture in the absence of PH.

Aortopulmonary Arterial Collaterals

Aortopulmonary (AP) collaterals may be observed in patients with congenital malformations associated with decreased pulmonary flow, including pulmonary atresia, as well as variations of single-ventricle physiology, or after a Glenn shunt or Fontan palliation. These collaterals can arise from any systemic artery and connect directly to the PAs at the lung hilum or at the periphery.[6] Resulting left-to-right systemic arterial to pulmonary arterial shunting may cause pulmonary vascular disease, elevation of systemic ventricular filling pressure, systemic ventricular volume loading, and ultimate failure. Residual surgically created systemic to pulmonary arterial shunts share the same pathophysiologic sequelae. In addition to the aforementioned factors, AP collateral embolization is indicated before the final stage of surgical subpulmonary ventricle to PA connection because the left-to-right shunt directly into the PAs complicates cardiopulmonary bypass, and the dual supply to the vascular branches leads to overcirculation and development of PAH. Embolization is typically performed in those collaterals that share significant flow from the main or additional unifocal PAs to avoid lung infarction. Embolization is typically performed with coils oversized to 30% to 50% larger than that of the target artery; however, use of AMPLATZER vascular plugs (St. Jude Medical, Inc. St. Paul, Minnesota, USA), microspheres, and copolymers of ethylene vinyl alcohol has also been reported with similar success.[47]

Coronary Artery Fistulae

Coronary fistulae can originate from all major epicardial coronary arteries (55% from right coronary artery), and drainage usually occurs to the RV (40%), RA (25%), coronary sinus, or PA. These collaterals can become markedly enlarged and can lead to significant left-to-right shunting with right-sided volume overload and effective coronary arterial steal leading to ischemia. Surgical correction is associated with low mortality and morbidity; nevertheless, percutaneous catheter techniques have become the method of choice. Embolization has been reported predominantly with coils (Gianturco coils; interlocking detachable coils); however, other devices such as AMPLATZER duct occluders and AMPLATZER vascular plugs have been used successfully as well.[48,49] Risks include MI (15%) and the migration of coils or discs to extracoronary vascular structures or within the coronary artery branches. Long-term follow-up suggests that patients with distal type, large fistulae, and older age at presentation may be at highest risk for coronary thrombosis.[48,49]

VENOUS-RELATED INTERVENTIONS

Systemic Veins

Venous stenosis is rarely congenital in nature. Lesions in the iliac venous system are typically due to thrombus secondary to deep vein thrombosis or to prior surgical interventions, and lesions in the SVC are due to either malignant intrathoracic lesions, indwelling central venous catheters, pacemaker leads, or enlarged nodes due to granulomatous disease. Stents in the venous system are associated with few complications at the time of insertion and have excellent long-term patency.[50]

Pulmonary Veins

Congenital PV stenosis is rare (0.4% of CHD) and frequently associated with other defects.[51] PV stenosis acquired after RF ablation procedures has been treated almost exclusively by transcatheter techniques. Balloon angioplasty of the involved vessels usually leads to a reasonably good initial result. Restenosis, however, occurs in >50% of patients within 1 year. Stent implantation has been associated with a better medium-term prognosis.[51] Use of other added technologies such as intravascular ultrasound to achieve adequate stent apposition to the PV walls, as well as limit vessel overdilation, has been described as an effort to minimize future in-stent stenosis and need for reintervention.[52]

ATRIAL SWITCH-RELATED INTERVENTIONS

Baffle Obstruction

Systemic baffle obstruction is observed in up to 25% of patients undergoing atrial switch (Mustard or Senning) procedures. Obstruction of atrial baffles might be challenging to detect using echocardiography, and CMR or CT imaging is helpful to define the anatomy. Balloon angioplasty occasionally results in long-term relief and can be preferred in situations such as the presence of functional device leads; however, stent deployment has been highly successful in relieving obstruction, with low complication rates and superior results, especially when performed in the superior portion of the systemic venous baffle after atrial switch operations.[6,12] This may require the performance of a combined procedure whereby a device lead is extracted followed by stenting of the superior systemic baffle and then lead replacement in the same setting in order to avoid "jailing" and damaging the initial lead. Depending on the anatomic complexity, the operator may consider dual venous access with wire externalization to create a "rail" for additional support and stability. Pulmonary venous obstruction is a potential complication of systemic venous stenting. Careful review of preprocedure imaging, three-dimensionally printed models, and intraprocedural pulmonary angiography are advised to pre-empt and rule out potential PV obstruction.

In addition to compression due to stenting of a systemic venous baffle limb, pulmonary venous baffle obstructions can occur de novo. Surgery or a hybrid procedure is usually required, because the pulmonary venous compartment is not easily amenable to percutaneous intervention. However, transseptal transcatheter intervention is an available option to relieve obstruction.[53] Such intervention can be facilitated by the use of intraprocedural echocardiography guidance for transseptal access and steerable sheath and/or catheter for optimal navigation.

Baffle Leak

Up to 25% of patients undergoing Mustard or Senning operations will demonstrate late baffle leaks, likely as the result of suture dehiscence. Although many of these shunts are hemodynamically unapparent and do not require therapy, closure is indicated for large defects, resulting in significant intracardiac shunting. Percutaneous closure has been reported with the closure devices, covered stents, or a combination of both.[54]

SINGLE VENTRICLE-RELATED INTERVENTIONS

Fenestration

Following Fontan operations, patients may have spontaneous or surgically created residual fenestrations that may lead to a right-to-left shunt and consequent systemic oxygen desaturation, systemic emboli, and exercise incapacity. These fenestrations can be closed with the use of the AMPLATZER or Gore CardioForm septal occluder devices (W. L. Gore & Associates, Inc, Newark, DE, USA). Patients typically receive long-term anticoagulation and prophylaxis against subacute bacterial endocarditis. Recent studies have suggested that closure of fenestrations may contribute to late tachyarrhythmias in this patient population.[55]

Fontan Circuit

Conduit stenosis can be observed after Glenn or Fontan operations. Patients with obstructions in the Fontan pathway can have significant symptoms because they lack a subpulmonary ventricle. Any obstruction in this circuit, even with only a low (1-3 mm Hg) gradient, may be hemodynamically significant. Thus, interventions such as balloon angioplasty or stenting of the Fontan circuit, the branch PAs, or residual aortic obstructions such as CoA are often performed with few adverse events.[56]

Collaterals

Collaterals from the systemic to the PVs (veno-venous collaterals) can occur in patients with single ventricle physiology, especially after Glenn or Fontan operations, in part because of chronically elevated systemic venous pressures. Pulmonary arteriovenous fistulae may also present late after Glenn anastomosis, as well as in patients with chronic liver failure or with hereditary hemorrhagic telangiectasia (Osler-Weber-Rendu syndrome). In both instances, there is a right-to-left shunt, with various degrees of cyanosis. Both types of abnormal connections can be treated successfully with coil embolization or AMPLATZER vascular plugs; however, this is rarely indicated.[57] In addition, the recurrence of collaterals is not uncommon unless the underlying physiology driving their development is modified significantly.

Lymphatic System

Percutaneous lymphatic embolization is a novel and specialized technique to identify pathways of lymphatic decompression and occlude these abnormal channels to treat protein-losing enteropathy and plastic bronchitis.[58] Only a few centers are specialized in these interventions because they require magnetic resonance lymphangiograms[59]; however, these procedures can be very effective.

CONCLUSION

Interventions in patients with ACHD present unique challenges to caregivers. As these patients grow older and develop more sequelae of their residual defects, more patients will need transcatheter interventions in the context of physiologic occurrences, risks, and complications encountered less frequently in typical pediatric or adult transcatheter interventions. It is important that these patients are treated in centers of excellence equipped with appropriately trained and experienced operators. Multidisciplinary team evaluation, including clinical ACHD, interventional cardiology, anesthesia, surgery, and advanced cardiac imaging, is critical for preprocedural planning. Building the unique expertise required to care for adults with CHD requires focused training, continuous research and quality improvement, and lifelong learning supported by a nationwide and international community of experts.

Key Points

- Percutaneous closure of VSD is an attractive alternative to surgical management in selected patients with isolated uncomplicated defects, increased surgical risk, multiple previous cardiac surgical interventions, or with poorly accessible muscular VSDs.
- In adults with PDA, the ADO is the most commonly used device with MRI-compatible coil embolization reserved for PDA measuring <2 to 3 mm or for residual leaks.
- In contrast to valvular AS, subvalvular AS does not respond well to balloon dilation.
- BPV is the treatment of choice for isolated PS. The use of oversized balloon (1.2-1.25 times the annulus) has been advocated to achieve a successful result, which is defined by a peak valve gradient of <20 mm Hg.
- TPVR is a less invasive alternative to surgical replacement for stenosis and/or regurgitation and is now available for patients with regurgitant large native RVOTs through the RVOT reducer platforms.
- Stent placement is the treatment of choice for older children and adults with native CoA. Covered stents may reduce the risk of aneurysms.
- Quantitative radiographic assessment of lung perfusion and ventilation should be part of the diagnostic algorithm and should be used as a tool to evaluate the results of dilation procedures in patients with PAS.
- PA stenting provides an effective relief for PAS in adults with congenital heart disease; however, multiple and bilateral stents may be required.

For further review and interactivities, please see the chapter-based multiple choice questions and videos accessible in the complimentary eBook bundled with this text. Access instructions are located in the inside front cover.

References

1. Stout KK, Daniels CJ, Aboulhosn JA, et al. 2018 AHA/ACC guideline for the management of adults with congenital heart disease: a report of the American College of Cardiology/American Heart Association Task Force on clinical practice guidelines. *Circulation*. 2019;139(14):e698-e800.
2. Baumgartner H, De Backer J, Babu-Narayan SV, et al. 2020 ESC Guidelines for the management of adult congenital heart disease. *Eur Heart J*. 2021;42(6):563-645.
3. Warnes CA, Williams RG, Bashore TM, et al. ACC/AHA 2008 guidelines for the management of adults with congenital heart disease: a report of the American College of Cardiology/American Heart Association Task Force on Practice Guidelines (writing committee to develop guidelines on the management of adults with congenital heart disease). *Circulation*. 2008;118(23):e714-e833.
4. Nishimura RA, Otto CM, Bonow RO, et al. 2014 AHA/ACC guideline for the management of patients with valvular heart disease: a report of the American College of cardiology/American Heart Association task force on practice guidelines. *J Thorac Cardiovasc Surg*. 2014;148(1):e1-e132.
5. Marelli AJ, Beauchesne L, Colman J, et al. Canadian Cardiovascular Society 2022 guidelines for cardiovascular interventions in adults with congenital heart disease. *Can J Cardiol*. 2022;38(7):862-896.
6. Tan W, Schmidt ACS, Horlick E, Aboulhosn J. Transcatheter interventions in patients with adult congenital heart disease. *J Soc Cardiovasc Angiogr Interv*. 2022;1(6):100438.
7. Hansen JH, Duong P, Jivanji SGM, et al. Transcatheter correction of superior sinus venosus atrial septal defects as an alternative to surgical treatment. *J Am Coll Cardiol*. 2020;75(11):1266-1278.
8. Dua JS, Carminati M, Lucente M, et al. Transcatheter closure of postsurgical residual ventricular septal defects: early and mid-term results. *Catheter Cardiovasc Interv*. 2010;75(2):246-255.
9. Chessa M, Butera G, Negura D, et al. Transcatheter closure of congenital ventricular septal defects in adult: mid-term results and complications. *Int J Cardiol*. 2009;133(1):70-73.
10. Carminati M, Butera G, Chessa M, et al. Transcatheter closure of congenital ventricular septal defects: results of the European Registry. *Eur Heart J*. 2007;28(19):2361-2368.
11. Schlotter F, de Waha S, Eitel I, Desch S, Fuernau G, Thiele H. Interventional post-myocardial infarction ventricular septal defect closure: a systematic review of current evidence. *EuroIntervention*. 2016;12(1):94-102.
12. Inglessis I, Landzberg MJ. Interventional catheterization in adult congenital heart disease. *Circulation*. 2007;115(12):1622-1633.
13. Wilson WM, Shah A, Osten MD, et al. Clinical outcomes after percutaneous patent ductus arteriosus closure in adults. *Can J Cardiol*. 2020;36(6):837-843.
14. Zhong L, Tong SF, Zhang Q, et al. Clinical efficacy and safety of transcatheter closure of ruptured sinus of valsalva aneurysm. *Cathet Cardiovasc Interv*. 2014;84(7):1184-1189.
15. Esch JJ, Shah PB, Cockrill BA, et al. Transcatheter Potts shunt creation in patients with severe pulmonary arterial hypertension: initial clinical experience. *J Heart Lung Transplant*. 2013;32(4):381-387.
16. Lin CH, Huddleston C, Balzer DT. Transcatheter ventricular septal defect (VSD) creation for restrictive VSD in double-outlet right ventricle. *Pediatr Cardiol*. 2013;34(3):743-747.
17. McElhinney DB, Sherwood MC, Keane JF, del Nido PJ, Almond CSD, Lock JE. Current management of severe congenital mitral stenosis: outcomes of transcatheter and surgical therapy in 108 infants and children. *Circulation*. 2005;112(5):707-714.
18. Cubeddu RJ, Jneid H, Don CW, et al. Retrograde versus antegrade percutaneous aortic balloon valvuloplasty: immediate, short- and long-term outcome at 2 years. *Cathet Cardiovasc Interv*. 2009;74:225-231.
19. Brown DW, Dipilato AE, Chong EC, Lock JE, McElhinney DB. Aortic valve reinterventions after balloon aortic valvuloplasty for congenital aortic stenosis intermediate and late follow-up. *J Am Coll Cardiol*. 2010;56(21):1740-1749.
20. Boe BA, Zampi JD, Kennedy KF, et al. Acute success of balloon aortic valvuloplasty in the current era: a national cardiovascular data registry study. *JACC Cardiovasc Interv*. 2017;10(17):1717-1726.
21. Maskatia SA, Ing FF, Justino H, et al. Twenty-five year experience with balloon aortic valvuloplasty for congenital aortic stenosis. *Am J Cardiol*. 2011;108(7):1024-1028.
22. de Lezo JS, Romero M, Segura J, et al. Long-term outcome of patients with isolated thin discrete subaortic stenosis treated by balloon dilation: a 25-year study. *Circulation*. 2011;124(13):1461-1468.
23. Nishimura RA, Otto CM, Bonow RO, et al. 2014 AHA/ACC guideline for the management of patients with valvular heart disease: a report of the American College of cardiology/American Heart Association task force on practice guidelines. *J Am Coll Cardiol*. 2014;63(22):e57-e185.
24. Ephrem G, Gorocica-Romero R, Day J, Flores-Umanzor E, Abrahamyan L, Horlick E. Balloon valvuloplasty for annular- and leaflet-level tricuspid stenosis: report of cases and literature review. *J Invasive Cardiol*. 2024;36(1).
25. Praz F, Muraru D, Kreidel F, et al. Transcatheter treatment for tricuspid valve disease. *EuroIntervention*. 2021;17(10):791-808.
26. Barry OM, Bouhout I, Kodali SK, et al. Interventions for congenital atrioventricular valve dysfunction: JACC focus seminar. *J Am Coll Cardiol*. 2022;79(22):2259-2269.
27. Picard F, Tadros VX, Asgar AW. From tricuspid to double orifice morphology: percutaneous tricuspid regurgitation repair with the MitraClip device in congenitally corrected-transposition of great arteries. *Catheter Cardiovasc Interv*. 2017;90(3):432-436.
28. van Melle JP, Schurer R, Willemsen M, Hoendermis ES, van den Heuvel AFM. Percutaneous tricuspid valve repair using MitraClip® for the treatment of severe tricuspid valve regurgitation in a patient with congenitally corrected transposition of the great arteries. *Neth Heart J*. 2016;24(11):696-697.
29. Taggart NW, Cabalka AK, Eicken A, et al. Outcomes of transcatheter tricuspid valve-in-valve implantation in patients with Ebstein anomaly. *Am J Cardiol*. 2018;121(2):262-268.
30. McElhinney DB, Cabalka AK, Aboulhosn JA, et al. Transcatheter tricuspid valve-in-valve implantation for the treatment of dysfunctional surgical bioprosthetic valves: an International, Multicenter Registry study. *Circulation*. 2016;133(16):1582-1593.
31. McElhinney DB, Aboulhosn JA, Dvir D, et al. Mid-term valve-related outcomes after transcatheter tricuspid valve-in-valve or valve-in-ring replacement. *J Am Coll Cardiol*. 2019;73(2):148-157.
32. Rao PS. Percutaneous balloon pulmonary valvuloplasty: state of the art. *Cathet Cardiovasc Interv*. 2007;69(5):747-763.
33. Fawzy ME, Hassan W, Fadel BM, et al. Long-term results (up to 17 years) of pulmonary balloon valvuloplasty in adults and its effects on concomitant severe infundibular stenosis and tricuspid regurgitation. *Am Heart J*. 2007;153(3):433-438.
34. Harrild DM, Powell AJ, Tran TX, et al. Long-term pulmonary regurgitation following balloon valvuloplasty for pulmonary stenosis risk factors and relationship to exercise capacity and ventricular volume and function. *J Am Coll Cardiol*. 2010;55(10):1041-1047.
35. Shahanavaz S, Zahn EM, Levi DS, et al. Transcatheter pulmonary valve replacement with the Sapien prosthesis. *J Am Coll Cardiol*. 2020;76(24):2847-2858.
36. Jones TK, McElhinney DB, Vincent JA, et al. Long-term outcomes after Melody transcatheter pulmonary valve replacement in the US investigational device exemption trial. *Circ Cardiovasc Interv*. 2022;15(1):e010852.
37. Gillespie MJ, Bergersen L, Benson LN, Weng S, Cheatham JP. 5-Year outcomes from the Harmony native outflow tract early feasibility study. *JACC Cardiovasc Interv*. 2021;14(7):816-817.
38. Shahanavaz S, Balzer D, Babaliaros V, et al. Alterra adaptive prestent and SAPIEN 3 THV for congenital pulmonic valve dysfunction: an early feasibility study. *JACC Cardiovasc Interv*. 2020;13(21):2510-2524.
39. Rodes-Cabau J, Miró J, Dancea A, et al. Comparison of surgical and transcatheter treatment for native coarctation of the aorta in patients > or = 1 year old. The Quebec Native Coarctation of the Aorta study. *Am Heart J*. 2007;154(1):186-192.
40. Fawzy ME, Fathala A, Osman A, et al. Twenty-two years of follow-up results of balloon angioplasty for discreet native coarctation of the aorta in adolescents and adults. *Am Heart J*. 2008;156(5):910-917.
41. Holzer RJ, Gauvreau K, McEnaney K, Watanabe H, Ringel R. Long-term outcomes of the coarctation of the aorta stent trials. *Circ Cardiovasc Interv*. 2021;14(6):e010308.

42. Goldstein BH, Kreutzer J. Transcatheter intervention for congenital defects involving the great vessels: JACC review topic of the week. *J Am Coll Cardiol*. 2021;77(1):80-96.
43. Lewis MJ, Kennedy KF, Ginns J, et al. Procedural success and adverse events in pulmonary artery stenting: insights from the NCDR. *J Am Coll Cardiol*. 2016;67(11):1327-1335.
44. Holzer RJ, Gauvreau K, Kreutzer J, et al. Balloon angioplasty and stenting of branch pulmonary arteries: adverse events and procedural characteristics—results of a multi-institutional registry. *Circ Cardiovasc Interv*. 2011;4(3):287-296.
45. Qureshi AM, Hill JA, Prieto LR, et al. Transcatheter recanalization of totally occluded proximal pulmonary arteries and major systemic veins in patients with congenital heart disease. *Am J Cardiol*. 2013;111(3):412-417.
46. Gupta M, Agrawal A, Iakovou A, Cohen S, Shah R, Talwar A. Pulmonary artery aneurysm: a review. *Pulm Circ*. 2020;10(1):2045894020908780.
47. Alex A, Ayyappan A, Valakkada J, Kramadhari H, Sasikumar D, Menon S. Major aortopulmonary collateral arteries. *Radiol Cardiothorac Imaging*. 2022;4(1):e210157.
48. Gowda ST, Latson LA, Kutty S, Prieto LR. Intermediate to long-term outcome following congenital coronary artery fistulae closure with focus on thrombus formation. *Am J Cardiol*. 2011;107(2):302-308.
49. Valente AM, Lock JE, Gauvreau K, et al. Predictors of long-term adverse outcomes in patients with congenital coronary artery fistulae. *Circ Cardiovasc Interv*. 2010;3(2):134-139.
50. Lee MM, Hines GL. Stents in the management of stenotic and occlusive lesions in the venous system. *Cardiol Rev*. 2022;30(6):314-317.
51. Latson LA, Prieto LR. Congenital and acquired pulmonary vein stenosis. *Circulation*. 2007;115(1):103-108.
52. Kops SA, Strah D, Lee KS, Seckeler MD. Intravascular ultrasound for pulmonary vein stenosis interventions in congenital heart disease. *J Invasive Cardiol*. 2021;33(4):E259-E262.
53. Poterucha JT, Taggart NW, Johnson JN, et al. Intravascular and hybrid intraoperative stent placement for baffle obstruction in transposition of the great arteries after atrial switch. *Catheter Cardiovasc Interv*. 2017;89(2):306-314.
54. Bradley EA, Cai A, Cheatham SL, et al. Mustard baffle obstruction and leak - how successful are percutaneous interventions in adults? *Prog Pediatr Cardiol*. 2015;39(2 pt B):157-163.
55. Ono M, Boethig D, Goerler H, Lange M, Westhoff-Bleck M, Breymann T. Clinical outcome of patients 20 years after Fontan operation—effect of fenestration on late morbidity. *Eur J Cardio Thorac Surg*. 2006;30(6):923-929.
56. Mets JM, Bergersen L, Mayer JE Jr, Marshall AC, McElhinney DB. Outcomes of stent implantation for obstruction of intracardiac lateral tunnel Fontan pathways. *Circ Cardiovasc Interv*. 2013;6(1):92-100.
57. Wiegand G, Sieverding L, Bocksch W, Hofbeck M. Transcatheter closure of abnormal vessels and arteriovenous fistulas with the Amplatzer vascular plug 4 in patients with congenital heart disease. *Pediatr Cardiol*. 2013;34(7):1668-1673.
58. Dori Y, Keller MS, Rome JJ, et al. Percutaneous lymphatic embolization of abnormal pulmonary lymphatic flow as treatment of plastic bronchitis in patients with congenital heart disease. *Circulation*. 2016;133(12):1160-1170.
59. Biko DM, Smith CL, Otero HJ, et al. Intrahepatic dynamic contrast MR lymphangiography: initial experience with a new technique for the assessment of liver lymphatics. *Eur Radiol*. 2019;29(10):5190-5196.

Introduction to Statistics in Clinical Research for Interventional Cardiology

Neel M. Butala and Stephen W. Waldo

As clinical cardiologists, including those in interventional specialties, it is essential to understand the quantitative issues in clinical research to make informed decisions about patient care. This chapter provides an introduction to statistics in clinical research, covering the basic concepts of study design, analytical techniques, and the critical role of clinical research in shaping medical practice. Whether or not clinicians are involved in clinical investigation, a familiarity with these foundational principles is crucial to choosing therapies and technologies that benefit patients and avoiding those that may be harmful or ineffective. Although study results are subjected to peer review before publication in leading medical journals, individual clinicians need to understand quantitative methods to evaluate potentially conflicting sources of evidence to make informed decisions about patient care.

Thus, this chapter aims to equip interventional cardiologists with the foundational knowledge necessary to effectively integrate evidence-based medicine into their practice and ensure the best and most reliable care for their patients.

CARDIOVASCULAR EVIDENCE AND GUIDELINES

Evidence-based medicine is defined as combining quantitative evidence with expert medical judgment to ensure that medical care is provided with reproducibly high quality.[1] In cardiology, the American College of Cardiology (ACC) and the American Heart Association (AHA) have issued a series of clinical practice guidelines that provide evidence-based practice recommendations, often in collaboration with the Society for Cardiovascular Angiography and Intervention (SCAI). These guidelines span a wide range of topics relevant to interventional cardiologists, including acute coronary syndromes, percutaneous coronary intervention (PCI), coronary artery bypass grafting (CABG), and valvular heart disease.[2,3]

All ACC/AHA guidelines follow a similar format of grading evidence and issuing recommendations (**Table 47.1**). Understanding how to read and interpret ACC/AHA guidelines is crucial for contemporary clinical practice. Recommendations in guidelines are assigned a class (I, II, or III). Class I recommendations are useful and effective interventions, and Class III recommendations are for interventions that are not useful or effective. Familiarity with Class I and III recommendations is particularly important for those taking the board examinations. Class II recommendations indicate situations where the evidence is more controversial and are further broken down into IIa recommendations, in which the weight of the evidence overall leans toward benefit, and IIb recommendations, in which the weight of the evidence leans against benefit.

All recommendations are accompanied by a grade of evidence (A, B, or C), with Grade A indicating the highest level of evidence derived from many trials or a single large, randomized clinical trial. Grade B denotes evidence derived from smaller randomized trials or nonrandomized observational studies, while Grade C denotes expert consensus, which carries the lowest weight of evidence.

TABLE 47.1 Levels of Evidence for Clinical Practice Recommendations

MEASURE	DESCRIPTION
Class of Recommendation	
I	Intervention is useful and effective
IIa	Evidence conflicts/opinions differ but lean toward efficacy
IIb	Evidence conflicts/opinions differ but lean against efficacy
III	Intervention is not useful/effective and may be harmful
Level of Evidence	
A	Data from many randomized clinical trials
B	Data from single randomized trial or nonrandomized studies
C	Expert consensus

Adapted from Gibbons RJ, Smith S, Antman E, et al. American College of Cardiology/American Heart Association clinical practice guidelines: part I—where do they come from? *Circulation*. 2003;107:2979-2986, with permission.

INTERPRETING STUDY RESULTS

Although guidelines are updated regularly, new clinical evidence is constantly being generated that can directly impact patient care. Therefore, it is crucial for clinicians to be able to interpret individual studies to ensure appropriate care for their patients. Most clinical research study results begin with a summary of baseline characteristics of the study sample, typically split up by treatment arm (often **Table 47.1** of a research manuscript), followed by differences in outcomes between treatment groups.

Baseline Characteristics

Characteristics can be summarized differently based on the type of data they contain. Data can be categorical or continuous.

Categorical variables are further split into nominal and ordinal variables. Nominal variables are made up of discrete categories without a particular order (eg, ethnicity). Binary variables are a subset of nominal variables that only contain two categories. The presence or absence of cardiovascular risk factors are frequently reported in clinical research as binary variables (yes/no). Ordinal data are categorical but have an inherent order, such as number of diseased coronary vessels (one, two, or three). Categorical variables are typically summarized in cardiovascular clinical research by the number and percentage of each sample that fall into each category.

Continuous variables are those in which the differences between numbers have meaning, such as age or height. In dealing with continuous variables, it is important to consider the shape of the distribution. Continuous variables can have a normal (bell shaped) distribution, can be skewed, or can have a bimodal distribution with multiple peaks. Statistical analysis must take special considerations into account in cases of data that are not normally distributed. Continuous variables should be summarized by a measure of the center of their distribution and the spread of the distribution. The center can be described by the mean, which is the average value in the distribution, or the median, which is the middle value of the distribution. Means are more affected by skewed distributions and outliers than medians. The spread or variability of the data around the center can be described by the standard deviation (square root of the variance), range (maximum value – minimum value), or the percentile (eg, interquartile range or the 25th-75th range).

Differences Between Treatment Groups

Differences in variables between two groups can be evaluated further with statistical tests. For example, when data are normally distributed, one can use a chi-square test or Fisher's exact test for categorical variables or a Student's *t* test for continuous variables.

Differences between treatment groups are often presented as rates, odds ratios, and/or risk ratios (also called relative risk). Odds ratios and risk ratios are often confused. A risk ratio compares the probability of an outcome occurring in two groups, while an odds ratio compares the odds of an outcome occurring in two groups. The odds of an event happening is the ratio of the number of times an event occurs to the number of times it does not occur. **Table 47.2** provides examples for calculating each of these and the key differences. Odds ratios are frequently reported in clinical literature because they are a direct output of logistic regression, which is frequently used to evaluate the association of an exposure of interest with a binary outcome of interest (eg, mortality, MI, or a composite endpoint).

TABLE 47.2 Examples of Calculating Odds Ratios and Risk Ratios in the ASCEND-HF Trial

One of the two primary endpoints—death from any cause or hospitalization for heart failure to 30 days—was compared in patients receiving intravenous nesiritide vs placebo. In the nesiritide group, 321 out of 3496 patients experienced an event. In the placebo group, 345 out of 3511 experienced an event.

Odds ratios

Odds in the nesiritide group: 321/3175 = 0.101

Odds in the placebo group: 345/3166 = 0.109

Odds ratio: 0.101/0.109 = 0.929

Risk ratios

Risk in the nesiritide group: 321/3496 = 9.2%

Risk in the placebo group: 345/3511 = 9.8%

Risk ratio: 9.2/9.8 = 0.934

Data from O'Connor CM, Starling RC, Hernandez AF, et al. Effect of nesiritide in patients with acute decompensated heart failure. *N Engl J Med.* 2011;365:32-43.

Results are also frequently presented using survival analysis, which is a statistical method that accounts for the time it takes for an event of interest to occur, such as death, disease progression, or relapse. In clinical research, survival analysis is commonly used to analyze the time-to-event outcomes in clinical trials, cohort studies, and other types of observational studies. Event rates may be plotted using Kaplan-Meier curves or cumulative incidence functions. Differences between treatment groups may be quantified by using a hazard ratio, which is a measure of the relative risk of an event occurring in one group compared to another group over time. In observational studies, a Cox proportional hazards model can be used to adjust other variables, similar to multivariate regression as described previously.

The "number needed to treat" (NNT) is a clinically significant value that is frequently cited in medical literature. It represents the number of patients who must receive a particular treatment to prevent one adverse event. This is calculated by dividing one by the absolute risk reduction. For example, if the absolute risk difference between two therapies is 2%, the NNT is 1 divided by 0.02, which is 50 patients. The NNT gives a good representation of the clinical significance of a statistically significant treatment effect. However, it is important to note that this is the expected average treatment effect across the entire population, and it may not capture the effect of a therapy of specific patient subgroups, which may be more or less likely to benefit.

Statistical Measures

The *P*-value is frequently reported in clinical literature to quantify the statistical significance of a difference between two or more groups. A *P*-value is the probability of obtaining the results one has observed by random chance alone.[4] A *P*-value of ≤.05 suggests that in less than 5 out of 100 similar experiments, a difference equal to or greater than the amount observed in the experiment would be expected if the treatment had no effect on the outcome being measured. When designing a clinical study, especially a randomized clinical trial, it is important for investigators to specify the hypothesis being tested, the statistical test to be employed on this hypothesis (to reject the null hypothesis, which means that there is no difference between treatment groups), and the critical (or nominal) value for declaring significance (the Type I error rate).

The critical value for declaring significance in most clinical research is commonly set at 0.05, although for certain types of studies, a different nominal significance level, such as 0.025 or 0.001, may be more appropriate. It is important to follow the prestated declaration when stating a nominal level of significance. For instance, if the nominal level of significance is 0.05, a final study *P*-value of 0.053 cannot be considered statistically significant, while a *P*-value of 0.048 under the same conditions would allow for the declaration of a statistically significant difference between the treatment groups. To properly interpret clinical trial results, it is necessary to carefully review the study methods and understand the prospectively set Type I error for the clinical experiment.

Performing multiple statistical tests within one study to obtain a desired *P*-value is especially problematic and violates this conservative approach. If one performs 20 *post-hoc* secondary comparisons of a completely null treatment effect, it is likely that one will be statistically significant at a *P*-value threshold of ≤0.05 based on chance alone. This is why findings of many *post-hoc* subgroup analyses in clinical trials are considered exploratory in nature and not definitive in identifying a treatment effect.

A confidence interval (CI) provides complementary information to a *P*-value. A 95% CI indicates that if the same study were

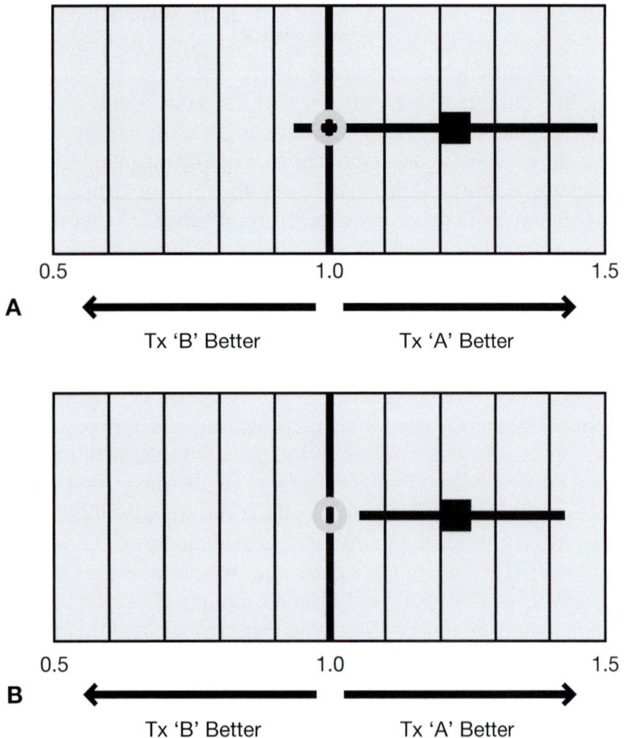

FIGURE 47.1 Interpreting the ratio plots. If the confidence interval crosses the value of no difference (1.0 for a ratio), as in **(A)**, then the *P*-value is >.05. If it does not, as in **(B)**, the *P*-value is <.05, and the comparison is statistically significant, which, in this case, shows that Treatment A is better.

performed an infinite number of times, 95% of the effect estimates would fall within the interval's bounds. A ratio of two event rates that are the same gives a value of 1. Thus, a CI that overlaps with 1 signifies that there is no statistically significant difference between the treatment groups, while an interval that does not include one indicates statistical significance. When the *P*-value and the CI are derived using the same test statistic, they will yield the same interpretation for statistical significance. Ratio plots, which depict the point estimate and the associated 95% CI, are frequently used to present data. **Figure 47.1** illustrates study outcomes using ratio plots that display superiority and uncertainty results.

INCORPORATING CARDIOVASCULAR EVIDENCE INTO PRACTICE

In addition to understanding whether a study's results are statistically significant, it is important to understand whether the effect size of a study is clinically significant and meaningful to patients. One must also consider whether the study sample was too homogenous and whether its results are broadly generalizable. More specifically, it is important for a clinician to determine whether patients included in a clinical study represent the patient sitting in front of them. Is there an important subgroup that better represents one's patient, and are the results different from that group? Or would the patient have been included in the study at all?

Ultimately, incorporating evidence from guidelines or individual studies into clinical decision-making for a particular patient requires skill, judgment, a familiarity with key statistical methods in clinical research, and an understanding of different study designs.

TYPES OF STUDY DESIGNS

There are two major types of study designs: observational studies and experimental studies. An experimental study design relies on the introduction of an intervention into a population, and the effect of the intervention on the study subjects is subsequently observed. Observational studies attempt to determine the effect of an intervention via more indirect means, often through simulating an experimental study through methodological or statistical approaches.

OBSERVATIONAL STUDIES

Observational studies make inferences about the effect of an intervention by attempting to identify conditions in which equipoise exists between two treatment options and then studying outcomes of those who received a treatment and those who did not receive a treatment. Because treatment is not randomly assigned in the real world, investigators attempt to create conditions in which it could be assigned by chance. This can be done by matching patients with similar baseline characteristics or controlling for characteristics known to affect treatment choice in a statistical model.

The two major types of observational study designs to investigate the effects of an intervention are case-control and cohort studies.

Case-Control

Case-control studies start with identifying whether an outcome of interest was present or absent for each individual in a retrospective dataset. Individuals that have that outcome of interest are deemed "cases." Additional individuals that are matched on common characteristics as cases but do not have the outcome of interest are included as "controls." Next, an investigator looks at the history of cases and controls to detect possible causes or risk factors that were not controlled for in the matching process. Finally, the investigator attempts to determine whether an exposure of interest can explain the difference between cases and controls that might explain the outcome of interest. For instance, a case-control study may be useful in examining whether a medication is related to the development of a disease. An investigator may match an array of demographics and risk factors related to the development of that disease between cases and controls and then examine whether those who developed a disease were more likely to receive a medication of interest. **Figure 47.2** and **Table 47.3** illustrate examples of case-control studies.

The main advantage of a case-control study design is the ability to detect diseases or conditions that are rare or may develop over a long period of time since an investigator begins with a set of cases that have the condition. Case-control studies can also be conducted very rapidly since data are typically already collected and available for analysis. The major disadvantage of the case-control study design is that the data used for the study may be subject to a fair degree of bias or error since they are typically collected for other reasons. For instance, key factors associated with both the treatment and the outcome may not have been collected. Therefore, it may not be possible to test whether differences in factors other than the treatment of interest are responsible for any of the outcomes. Factors that are associated with both the exposure and outcome are often termed "confounders," meaning that they may "confound" the observed relationship between the exposure

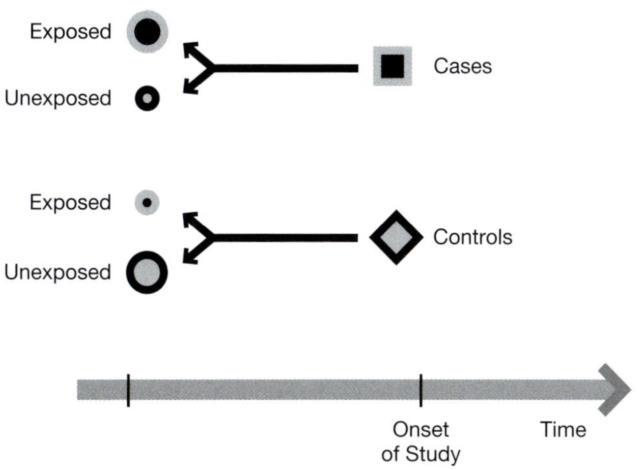

FIGURE 47.2 Example of a case–control study design.

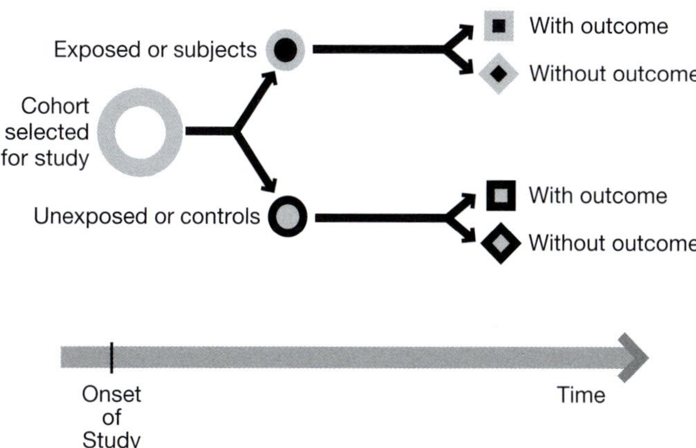

FIGURE 47.3 Example of a cohort study design.

and outcome, making it more challenging to interpret the results. In addition, patient care may have changed since data were collected, making the results no longer applicable. Finally, it is critical to choose an appropriately matched control group, but this can be challenging.

Cohort Studies

Cohort studies first identify whether an exposure of interest was present or absent for each individual in a group of subjects. This group of subjects is then followed up over a period of time to determine whether an outcome of interest occurs. Risk factors or other possible causes of the outcome of interest are either controlled for in a statistical model or matched for to ensure similarity between exposed and nonexposed groups. A cohort study can be prospective, meaning that data are collected after the study is initiated, or retrospective, meaning that data were already collected and analysis is being conducted *post hoc*. Nevertheless, in both prospective and retrospective cohort studies, patients are still followed up in time after an exposure to understand whether an outcome occurs subsequently. **Figure 47.3** and **Table 47.4** provide examples of cohort studies.

The main advantage of a cohort study design is the ability to study the impact of an exposure of interest over time. The Framingham Heart Study, which has provided critical knowledge regarding the associations between cardiac risk factors and cardiac outcome, is an example of a cohort study. One of the major disadvantages of a cohort study is difficulty proving causation, as no intervention is introduced into the population. Another disadvantage specific to a prospective cohort study is the amount of time necessary for completion and the amount of resources needed to ensure follow-up. A retrospective cohort study can be conducted using pre-existing data collected for another purpose, but it may then suffer from the same issues with regards to data bias or unmeasured confounders as described with case-control studies. Finally, a cohort design may be challenging to study a rare disease because the large sample size needed to include enough outcomes may be prohibitive.

Statistical Methods in Observational Studies

Observational studies rely on identifying a situation in which there is equipoise between two treatment choices to draw valid inferences. The most common statistical methods used to accomplish this are multivariate regression and matching or weighting. **Figure 47.4** illustrates the difference between these two methods.

MULTIVARIATE REGRESSION

A regression model is a statistical method used to examine the relationship between a dependent variable and one or more independent variables. In clinical research, the dependent variable is the outcome of interest, and the primary independent variable is the exposure of interest. Additional variables thought to be associated with both the outcome and the exposure that could potentially

TABLE 47.3 Example of a Case–Control Study: Is There an Association Between the Use of Aspirin and the Development of Reye's Syndrome?

We have 30 patients with Reye's syndrome, of whom 28 used Aspirin. There were 60 patients drawn from a large population of patients with minor viral illnesses, but not Reye's syndrome. Of these, 35 used aspirin.

Odds of exposure in cases: 28/2 = 14

Odds of exposure in controls: 35/25 = 1.4

Odds ratio: 14/1.4 = 10

Interpretation: Odds of being on aspirin is 10 times greater with Reye's syndrome than without.

TABLE 47.4 Example of a Cohort Study Design

The association of smoking with coronary heart disease (CHD) is investigated by selecting a group of 3000 smokers (exposed) and a group of 5000 nonsmokers (unexposed) who, in both groups, are free of heart disease at the beginning of the study. Both groups are followed up for the development of CHD, and the incidence in the groups is compared. Suppose CHD develops in 84 smokers and 87 nonsmokers.

Risk of CHD in smokers: 84/3000 = 2.8%

Risk of CHD in nonsmokers: 87/5000 = 1.74%

Risk ratio: 2.8/1.74 = 1.61

Interpretation: The risk of CHD is 61% times greater in patients who smoke than in those who do not.

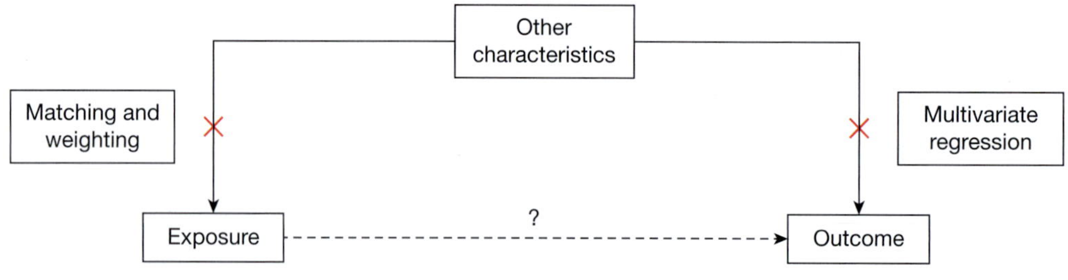

The goal of statistical methods in observational studies is to reduce the effect of characteristics known to influence both the exposure and outcome in estimating the treatment effect. Matching and weighting addresses the influence of these variables by making exposed groups similar. Multivariate regression addresses the influence of these variables by controlling for their presence in evaluating the outcome.

FIGURE 47.4 Statistical methods in observational studies. The goal of statistical methods in observational studies is to reduce the effect of characteristics known to influence both the exposure and outcome in estimating the treatment effect. Matching and weighting addresses the influence of these variables by making exposed groups similar. Multivariate regression addresses the influence of these variables by controlling for their presence in evaluating the outcome.

confound the estimation of the relationship between the exposure and outcome are included in the model as additional independent variables to "control for" their presence. For example, in examining the relationship between the choice of PCI or CABG for coronary revascularization and mortality, older age is thought to be a factor influencing the decision to choose PCI over CABG and is associated with higher mortality. One can include age in the regression model to account for this. The model would then report the average association of PCI relative to CABG with mortality in the sample studied, adjusted for age.

The most common types of regression in clinical research are linear regression and logistic regression. In linear regression, the relationship between an exposure and outcome is modeled as a line, and the results are reported as the change in the outcome associated with one unit change in the exposure. In logistic regression, the outcome of interest in binary (such as mortality) and the results are typically reported as odds ratios, particularly if the exposure is also binary (such as PCI or CABG).

A key limitation of multivariate regression models is the inability to account for unobserved confounders, which are variables that are associated with both the exposure and the outcome but are not captured in the dataset. One such example of an unmeasured confounder in interventional cardiology research is frailty, which can often be challenging to capture and quantify reliably. Another limitation of regression models is that they typically make assumptions about the nature of the relationship between an exposure and an outcome, and the true nature of this relationship is often unknown. For instance, a regression model will not perform well if one assumes a linear relationship between an exposure and an outcome, but in reality, the relationship is U-shaped.

MATCHING OR WEIGHTING

Matching or weighting can be used to make exposed and unexposed individuals look similar based on observed characteristics prior to making inferences in observational data. With matching, investigators compare differences in the outcome of interest between exposed and unexposed individuals that are identical on other observed characteristics. However, it is often hard to find exact matches between exposed and unexposed groups, particularly when many characteristics are included. With weighting, investigators use a statistical model to create a propensity score, which reflects a subject's probability of receiving an exposure based on observed characteristics of interest. This propensity score can then be used to assign weights to exposed and unexposed individuals to make them look similar. In clinical research, the most common method of weighting is inverse probability of treatment weighting, which applies a weight to each individual that makes the exposed and unexposed as a whole look balanced on the propensity score.

The major limitation of matching and weighting is similar to multivariate regression in its inability to account for unknown or unobserved confounders.

EXPERIMENTAL STUDIES

Experimental studies make inferences about the effect of an intervention by introducing an intervention into a group of subjects. Experimental studies can be controlled or uncontrolled. In uncontrolled experiments, investigators make observations about the outcomes of a group exposed to an intervention, often in comparison to a historical reference standard. Uncontrolled experiments in interventional cardiology include many studies of investigational devices, such as Disrupt CAD III, which investigated coronary intravascular lithotripsy for calcified coronary disease.[5] While uncontrolled experiments can be easier to conduct and facilitate introduction of novel technologies into practice, there is a risk that they may not capture the full safety and efficacy of an intervention, particularly if comparisons are made to historical reference standards that may not represent modern practice.

In controlled experiments, investigators compare outcomes of those exposed to the intervention with a prospective group of similar individuals who are not exposed to the intervention. This overcomes many of the issues that uncontrolled experiments face with respect to historical reference standards. However, there is a risk that patients who are exposed to a treatment are fundamentally different from those that are not exposed to a treatment. Such experiments can face the same issues with accounting for confounding that observational studies may face, and similar statistical techniques may be needed to establish equipoise between treatment options.

A subset of controlled experiments is randomized controlled trials, in which treatment is assigned to subjects enrolled in the trial at random. Randomized controlled trials use randomization to establish equipoise. They provide the strongest evidence for reaching a conclusion of causation and represent the gold standard for evidence-based medicine. Because treatments are randomly allocated, risk factors should occur equally between the exposed and unexposed groups, thus leaving only the intervention to be different.

The next several sections will review key concepts relevant to interpreting randomized controlled trials focusing on study endpoints, sample size, trial design, and analytic strategy.

Study Endpoints

The goal of a clinical study is to assess the effect of an intervention on an outcome of interest, or a study endpoint. Endpoints can be classified into hard endpoints and soft endpoints. Hard endpoints are those that are well-defined, measurable, and objective, such as death, myocardial infarction (MI), revascularization, or rehospitalization. Soft endpoints are those that may be more challenging to define or measure, such as quality of life, symptom scales, and clinical impression. Hard clinical endpoints typically allow an investigator to make more definitive statements about the value of a treatment, although soft endpoints are also important for patients.

Most cardiovascular trials use standardized endpoints to enable comparison across different studies.[6,7] Notably, definitions of these endpoints are frequently updated, so careful consideration should be taken in comparing older and newer studies. The sensitivity of trial results to subtleties in endpoint definitions was made apparent in the Evaluation of XIENCE versus Coronary Artery Bypass Surgery for Effectiveness of Left Main Revascularization (EXCEL) trial, which compared PCI and CABG for left main disease.[8] The rate of periprocedural MI defined according to the pre-specified study protocol favored PCI, but CABG had the advantage when periprocedural MI was defined according to the Universal Definition of MI.

COMPOSITE ENDPOINTS

Because some cardiovascular outcomes can be rare, cardiovascular trials frequently combine endpoints into one composite endpoint to increase the number of anticipated outcome events and decrease the potential sample size necessary to detect a difference between groups. Common examples of composite endpoints in interventional cardiology trials include a combination of death or MI; death, MI, or revascularization; death or heart failure hospitalization; or death or disabling stroke.

Typically, one measures the occurrence of any one of the components of the composite endpoint versus none of the events. In such cases, it is important for the clinician interpreting the study to ensure that endpoints of different severity do not cancel each other out and obscure any potential treatment effect. For instance, if one treatment leads to greater occurrence of death, but the other leads to substantially more MI, performance on a composite endpoint of death or MI may not be reflective of the subtleties in the relative efficacy of treatments. Any study reporting a composite endpoint should also report individual rates of component events by treatment groups to aid the clinician in understanding the key drivers of differences observed in the composite endpoint.

Composite endpoints can also be evaluated via other methods, such as a win ratio.[9] To calculate a win ratio, patients in treatment and control groups are first formed into matched pairs based on their risk profiles. For each pair, each patient is labeled as a "winner" or "loser" depending on who had the most severe endpoint (typically death), first. If that is unknown, then they are labeled as a "winner" or "loser" based on who had the next most severe endpoint first. The win ratio is calculated as the total number of winners divided by the total number of losers.

TRIAL SAMPLE SIZE

Determination of a sample size of a trial is a fundamental part of its design. Clinicians need to understand how a sample size is determined in order to understand whether an appropriate sample size was chosen to support the validity of a study's findings. Calculation of sample size depends on many factors, such as the endpoint to be analyzed, the estimated value of the endpoint in the control arm, the estimated improvement in the treatment arm, the amount of variation in the endpoint measured, the statistical method used to analyze the endpoint, and the prespecified rates of Type I and Type II errors. In general, a larger sample size is needed if the estimated incidence of the endpoint in the control arm is low, the estimated improvement in the treatment arm is low, and the amount of variation in the endpoint measured is high.

It is important for all clinicians to understand the differences between Type I and Type II errors (**Table 47.5**). Type I error (α) occurs when one observes an effect, but in fact, no effect exists. The Type I error rate in a trial is determined by a prespecified critical value of a statistical test for declaring statistical significance in rejecting a null hypothesis that there is no difference between treatment groups. In most clinical research, this critical value is set at 0.05. Type II error (β) occurs when one observes no treatment effect, but in fact a treatment effect does exist. Power is equivalent to 1 minus Type II error ($1 - \beta$). Randomized trials should have a large-enough sample size to have enough power to detect a clinically important treatment effect to be valid.

TRIAL DESIGN

Interventional cardiology trials are typically classified into three types: superiority, noninferiority, and equivalence. A superiority trial aims to establish a statistically significant and clinically meaningful improvement or harm from using an experimental treatment compared to the standard of care. In contrast, an equivalence trial determines if the difference in outcome between the experimental treatment and standard of care falls within a clinically defined minimally important difference (MID) boundary. This boundary represents the largest acceptable difference between the two groups while still being considered clinically comparable. A noninferiority trial evaluates the experimental treatment assuming that it is not worse than the standard of care by a clinically meaningful amount. Although noninferiority studies still use the MID to determine the boundary of noninferiority, they do not look for small improvements over the standard therapy. **Figure 47.5** graphically

TABLE 47.5 Sample Size Estimation: Type I and II Errors

TEST RESULTS			
		NO TREATMENT EFFECT	TREATMENT HAS AN EFFECT
Truth	No treatment effect	—	Type 1 error (α)
	Treatment has an effect	Type II error (β)	Power ($1 - \beta$)

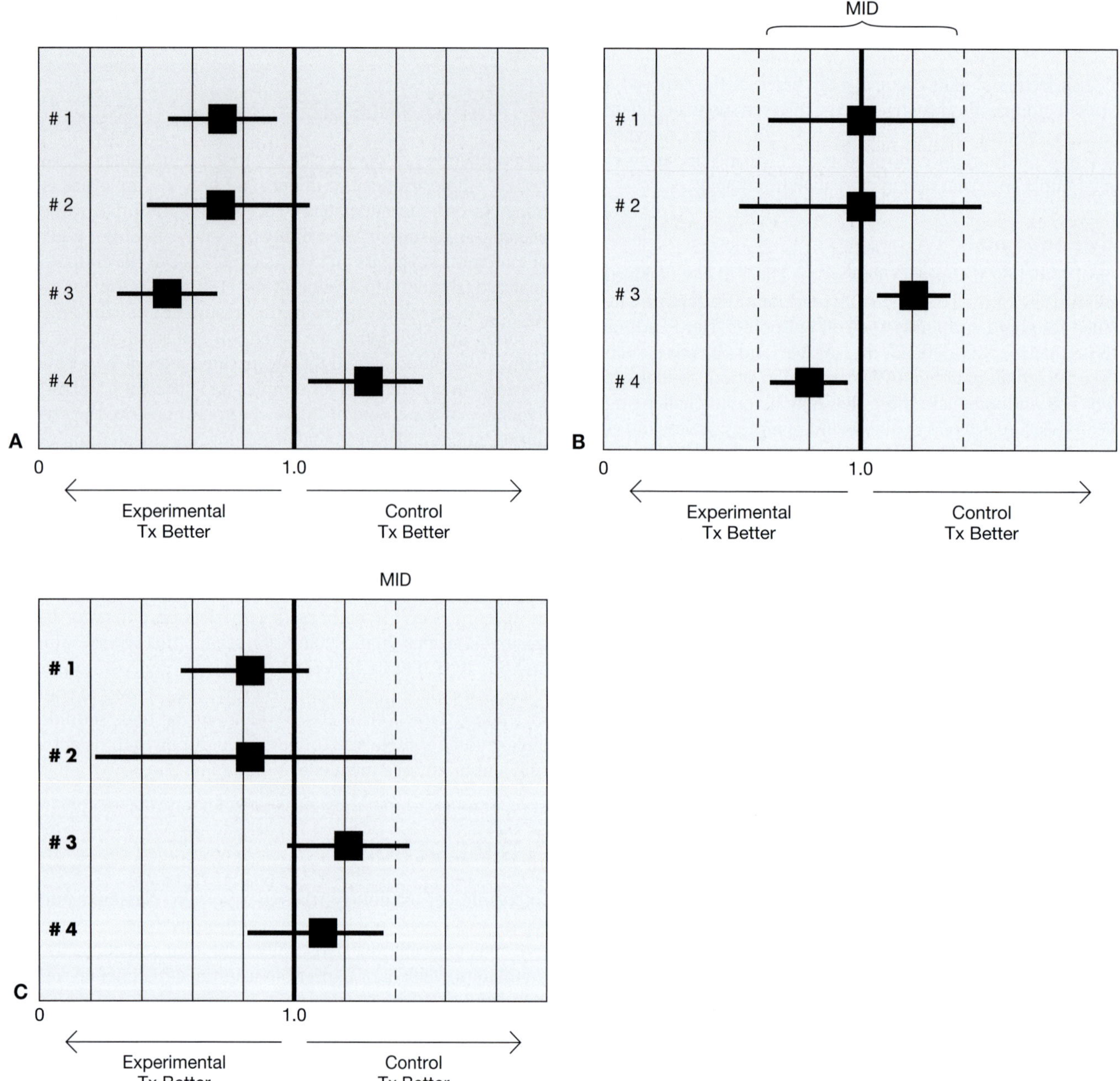

FIGURE 47.5 Sample results of superiority, equivalence, and noninferiority studies. In **(A)**, Studies #1 and #3 show that the experimental therapy is statistically significantly *superior* to the control therapy, while in Study #4, the control therapy is statistically better. Study #2 does not show statistical significance at all because the confidence interval crosses the line of no difference. In **(B)**, Study #1 shows that the experimental therapy is clinically and statistically *equivalent* to the control therapy because the confidence interval crosses the line of no difference and falls within the minimally important difference (MID). In Study #2, the experimental therapy cannot be considered either statistically equivalent or different because the confidence interval crosses both the line of no difference and the MID. Studies #3 and #4 show statistical equivalence as well; had these results come from a superiority trial, the experimental therapy would be considered clinically equivalent but statistically inferior (#3) or superior (#4). In **(C)**, Studies #1 and #4 show that the experimental treatment is *noninferior* to the control therapy because the confidence interval does not cross the MID. The confidence interval of Study #2 is too wide to draw a conclusion. Study #3 crosses the MID, indicating that the experimental treatment is inferior to the control. MID, minimally important difference.

demonstrates the results of a variety of studies and the potential results in superiority, equivalence, and noninferiority study designs.

Two recent examples from the interventional cardiology literature help demonstrate the concept of noninferiority. The Placement of Aortic Transcatheter Valves (PARTNER) 3 Trial was designed to test the noninferiority of transcatheter aortic valve replacement (TAVR) compared to surgical aortic valve replacement (SAVR).[10] The trial had a prespecified upper boundary of less than 6% of the risk difference in rates of a composite endpoint of death or disabling stroke for TAVR compared to SAVR. If the requirement for noninferiority was met, testing for the superiority of TAVR to SAVR with regards to the primary endpoint was to be performed. The rate of the primary endpoint was 6.6% lower with TAVR than that with SAVR, with a 95% CI of −10.8% to −2.5%, which was well below the noninferiority boundary of 6%, so noninferiority was met. Therefore, superiority testing was performed, and TAVR was found to be superior to SAVR (0.54; 95% CI 0.37-0.79;

P = .001 for superiority). The Fractional Flow Reserve (FFR) versus Angiography for Multivessel Evaluation (FAME) three trial was designed as a noninferiority trial testing whether FFR-guided PCI was noninferior to CABG in patients with three-vessel coronary artery disease.[11] This trial had a prespecified upper boundary of less than 1.65 of the hazard ratio for the primary composite endpoint of death, MI, stroke, or repeat revascularization. The hazard ratio for the primary endpoint was 1.5 with a 95% CI of 1.1 to 2.2, which exceeded 1.65. Thus, FAME-3 found that FFR-guided PCI was not found to be noninferior to CABG with respect to the primary endpoint at 1 year. Notably, FAME-3 was not designed or powered to test for superiority, so these results do not imply that CABG is superior to FFR-guided PCI for patients with multivessel disease.

Equivalence and noninferiority trials are becoming more common in evaluating new therapies, particularly in the realm of interventional cardiology when multiple active therapies are available. These types of trial designs have the most value when an experimental therapy is felt unlikely to be better than an established therapy but could offer other incremental benefits, such as improved safety, ease of use, or lower cost.

The key challenge in noninferiority and equivalence methodologies is in setting the MID boundary, as there is no firmly accepted definition for this. Hence, it is crucial for clinicians to carefully consider the construction of the boundary when interpreting medical literature. A large MID could raise questions about the validity of a noninferiority or equivalence claim, whereas an overly narrow boundary provides minimal advantage over a traditional superiority design. The MID can be established subjectively based on clinical judgment or mathematically based on the expected treatment effect of the standard treatment over placebo. In the latter case, the MID boundary is derived such that it will not be crossed if the experimental treatment can maintain at least 50% of the treatment effect over placebo.

TRIAL ANALYTIC STRATEGY

In a randomized controlled trial, enrolled patients are randomly assigned to a treatment, but they may not always receive that treatment. This may be due to a variety of issues such as changes in patient preference after randomization or crossover from one treatment to another during the follow-up period. There are several analytic strategies to deal with such issues.

Intention-to-treat (ITT) analysis is the notion that any patient who signs an informed consent and is assigned a randomized treatment remains in that treatment arm for the purposes of analysis, even if that patient drops out before any treatment was received or if that patient receives a different treatment from that which was allocated.

In the purest form, ITT analysis preserves the equipoise that is generated through randomization. Thus, most randomized controlled trials report ITT analysis results. However, ITT analysis may not generalize to settings where adherence to a treatment does not reflect adherence in the study. In addition, an ITT analysis estimates the effect of being assigned to a treatment, and if there is significant crossover between treatment arms, the estimated treatment effect in a trial will be biased downward toward no effect. This can make an ITT analysis challenging to interpret in the case of a noninferiority trial because nonadherence to assigned treatment paradoxically improves the chances of declaring a noninferior result. For example, if none of the patients in a randomized trial were given the assigned novel therapy to be tested, it would be an extreme case where the two groups would show no discernible difference, thereby meeting the noninferiority criteria.

Other forms of analyzing trial results estimate the effect of receiving a treatment. In a "per-protocol" analysis, one only analyzes data from participants who follow the prespecified protocol and excludes participants once there is a deviation from the protocol. In an "as-treated" analysis, one assigns participants to treatment groups based on which treatment they actually received, regardless of what they were assigned in the protocol. Both per-protocol and as-treated analyses are subject to systematic bias in treatment assignment. Randomization and ITT analysis ensure balance between baseline characteristics of different treatment groups through randomization. In contrast, treatment groups in a per protocol or as-treated analysis may differ on important baseline characteristics that can also influence the outcome of interest.

The Catheter Ablation vs Antiarrhythmic Drug Therapy for Atrial Fibrillation (CABANA) trial comparing catheter ablation to medical therapy for atrial fibrillation illustrates the importance of analytic approach in randomized controlled trials, as there was significant crossover between treatment groups.[12] In addition to an ITT analysis, a per protocol analysis was undertaken in which medical therapy patients were excluded once they underwent a catheter ablation. In addition, an as-treated analysis was undertaken in which patients were counted as being in the medical therapy group until they received an ablation and then counted in the ablation group afterward. The ITT analysis showed no significant difference between treatment strategies (HR 0.86, 95% CI 0.65-1.15) with respect to the primary composite outcome of death, disabling stroke, serious bleeding, or cardiac arrest. The per protocol analysis showed a possible effect in favor of catheter ablation, but this was not statistically significant (HR 0.75, 95% CI 0.54-1.01). However, in the as-treated analysis, the benefit of undergoing catheter ablation was statistically significant (HR 0.67, 95% CI 0.50-0.89). Taken together, these results suggest a possible benefit of catheter ablation for the primary endpoint among those who underwent the procedure, although this could be confounded by patients with more comorbidities not undergoing subsequent ablation in the medical therapy arm.

CONCLUSION

Clinicians must be acquainted with common quantitative issues to accurately interpret and incorporate the medical literature to advance patient care. Evidence-based medicine involves providing conscientious clinical care based on the most reliable data available for a particular topic. Interventional cardiologists who are preparing for their board exams should possess a grasp of fundamental statistical concepts, as well as how the widely used ACC/AHA Practice Guidelines are developed and utilized.

Key Points

- Incorporating evidence from guidelines or individual studies into clinical decision-making for a particular patient requires skill, judgment, and a familiarity with key statistical methods in clinical research
- Identifying different types of study designs is critical to understanding statistics and interpreting study results
  - Case-control studies compare exposures among patients who did versus did not experience an outcome of interest

- Cohort studies compare outcomes among patients who did versus did not experience an exposure of interest
- Experimental studies determine the treatment effect of a therapy by introducing an intervention and utilizing randomization to establish equipoise between treatment options, while observational studies use statistical methods to approximate equipoise between treatment options that have already been selected.

- Composite endpoints are often used in clinical trials to increase the number of anticipated outcome events, and therefore decrease the potential sample size.
- Calculation of sample size depends on many factors, such as the endpoint to be analyzed, the estimated value of the endpoint in the control arm, the estimated improvement in the treatment arm, the amount of variation in the endpoint measured, the statistical method used to analyze the endpoint, and the prespecified rates of Type I and Type II errors.
- Superiority trials aim to show that a new treatment is better than an existing treatment, noninferiority trials aim to show that a new treatment is not significantly worse than an existing treatment, and equivalence trials aim to show that a new treatment is as effective as an existing treatment.
- Intention-to-treat analysis includes all randomized participants in their original group, as-treated analysis only includes participants who received the full treatment as planned, and per-protocol analysis only includes participants who strictly adhered to the study protocol.
- Differences between treatment groups are evaluated with statistical tests and often presented as rates, odds ratios, risk ratios, hazard ratios, or number needed to treat.

Disclosures

The views expressed in this article are those of the authors and do not necessarily reflect the position or policy of the Department of Veterans Affairs, the U.S. Government, or National Institutes of Health. Dr. Butala is supported by grants from the Boettcher Foundation and the American Heart Association and reports consulting fees from Shockwave Medical and Boston Scientific and consulting fees and ownership interest in HiLabs and Catch Bio, outside the current work. Dr Waldo has received investigator-initiated research support to the Denver Research Institute from Abiomed, Cardiovascular Systems Incorporated, and Janssen Pharmaceuticals, as well as grants from the National Institutes of Health and VA Health Services Research.

References

1. Sackett DL, Rosenberg WM, Gray JA, Haynes RB, Richardson WS. Evidence based medicine: what it is and what it isn't. *BMJ*. 1996;312(7023):71-72. doi:10.1136/bmj.312.7023.71
2. Writing Committee Members; Lawton JS, Tamis-Holland JE, Bangalore S, et al. 2021 ACC/AHA/SCAI guideline for coronary artery revascularization: executive summary—a report of the American College of Cardiology/American Heart Association Joint Committee on clinical practice guidelines. *J Am Coll Cardiol*. 2022;79(2):197-215. doi:10.1016/j.jacc.2021.09.005
3. Writing Committee Members; Otto CM, Nishimura RA, Bonow RO, et al. 2020 ACC/AHA guideline for the management of patients with valvular heart disease: executive summary—a report of the American College of Cardiology/American Heart Association Joint Committee on clinical practice guidelines. *J Am Coll Cardiol*. 2021;77(4):450-500. doi:10.1016/j.jacc.2020.11.035
4. Moyé LA. P-value interpretation and alpha allocation in clinical trials. *Ann Epidemiol*. 1998;8(6):351-357. doi:10.1016/s1047-2797(98)00003-9
5. Hill JM, Kereiakes DJ, Shlofmitz RA, et al. Intravascular lithotripsy for treatment of severely calcified coronary artery disease. *J Am Coll Cardiol*. 2020;76(22):2635-2646. doi:10.1016/j.jacc.2020.09.603
6. Hicks KA, Mahaffey KW, Mehran R, et al. 2017 cardiovascular and stroke endpoint definitions for clinical trials. *Circulation*. 2018;137(9):961-972. doi:10.1161/circulationaha.117.033502
7. Généreux P, Généreux P, Piazza N, et al. Valve Academic Research Consortium 3: updated endpoint definitions for aortic valve clinical research. *Eur Heart J*. 2021;42(19):1825-1857. doi:10.1093/eurheartj/ehaa799
8. Stone GW, Kappetein AP, Sabik JF, et al. Five-year outcomes after PCI or CABG for left main coronary disease. *N Engl J Med*. 2019;381(19):1820-1830.
9. Pocock SJ, Ariti CA, Collier TJ, Wang D. The win ratio: a new approach to the analysis of composite endpoints in clinical trials based on clinical priorities. *Eur Heart J*. 2012;33(2):176-182. doi:10.1093/eurheartj/ehr352
10. Mack MJ, Leon MB, Thourani VH, et al. Transcatheter aortic-valve replacement with a balloon-expandable valve in low-risk patients. *N Engl J Med*. 2019;380(18):1695-1705. doi:10.1056/NEJMoa1814052
11. Fearon WF, Zimmermann FM, De Bruyne B, et al. Fractional flow reserve–guided PCI as compared with coronary bypass surgery. *N Engl J Med*. 2022;386(2):128-137. doi:10.1056/NEJMoa2112299
12. Packer DL, Mark DB, Robb RA, et al. Effect of catheter ablation vs antiarrhythmic drug therapy on mortality, stroke, bleeding, and cardiac arrest among patients with atrial fibrillation: the CABANA randomized clinical trial. *JAMA*. 2019;321(13):1261-1274. doi:10.1001/jama.2019.0693

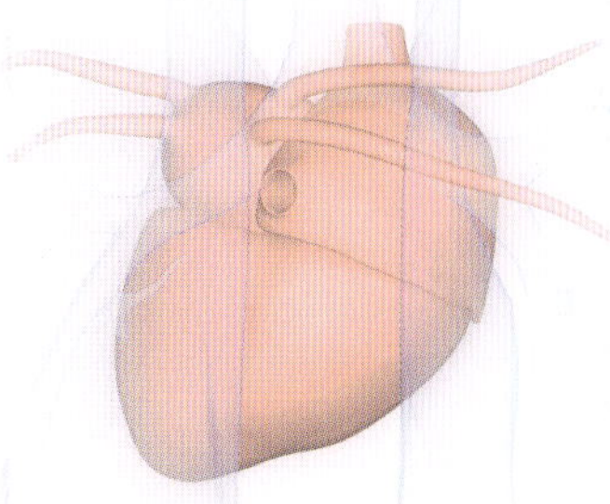

INDEX

Note: Page numbers followed by *f* indicate figures and *t* indicate tables.

A

B

D

E

F

G

H

I

J

K

L

M

N

O

P

Q

R

S

T

U

V

QUADM0824